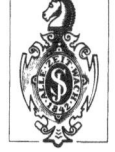

K. Nabeya · T. Hanaoka · H. Nogami (Eds.)

Recent Advances in Diseases of the Esophagus

Selected Papers in 5th World Congress of the
International Society for Diseases of the Esophagus
Kyoto, Japan, 1992

With 446 Figures

Springer-Verlag
Tokyo Berlin Heidelberg
New York London Paris
Hong Kong Barcelona
Budapest

Professor KIN-ICHI NABEYA, M.D.
Professor TATEO HANAOKA, M.D.
HIROSHI NOGAMI, M.D.
Second Department of Surgery, Kyorin University School of Medicine,
6-20-2, Shinkawa, Mitaka, Tokyo, 181 Japan

ISBN-13:978-4-431-68248-6   e-ISBN-13:978-4-431-68246-2
DOI: 10.1007/978-4-431-68246-2

Printed on acid-free paper

Preface

The Fifth World Congress of the International Society for Diseases of the Esophagus was held in the historic city of Kyoto, Japan, from August 5 through 8, 1992. Approximately 40 countries throughout the world participated and roughly 500 presentations were made. Excellent authors were selected and they were requested to send in their manuscripts for publication of this book. It is our ardent hope that this book will prove to be beneficial to the doctor interested in the esophagus and that it will provide the reader with first-hand information from leading scientists and clinicians in this field.

The incidence of esophageal diseases vary greatly from country to country and in recent years, worldwide interest in these diseases has resulted in various international studies. The International Society for Diseases of the Esophagus was inaugurated by Professor Komei Nakayama in 1979 and since that time it has actively contributed to the exchange of information regarding these diseases and has made endeavors in bringing about advancement in the struggle against diseases of the esophagus in every way possible.

It is my firm belief, that discussions and presentations made at congresses such as these, make great contributions in the progress of medicine, and communications between young promising researchers and the older experienced generation is truly significant. The "March in Medicine" must go on and it is my fervent wish that seeds sowed at this congress will flourish and that this book comprised of presentations made at the Fifth World Congress may serve as a tool to cultivate those seeds.

Lastly, but not leastly, I would like to express my heartfelt appreciation to all the people involved in making this publication possible, especially to those who generously gave of their time and cooperation in editing this book: Dr. Tateo Hanaoka, Dr. Hiroshi Nogami, and the doctors of the Second Department of Surgery of Kyorin University School of Medicine.

KIN-ICHI NABEYA
Congress President
The Fifth World Congress of
the International Society
for Diseases of the Esophagus

V

Foreword

Every three years the world's top esophagologists convene at different locations all over the world under the leadership of the International Society for Diseases of the Esophagus. The ISDE world congress has meanwhile come to occupy a solid position as an international scientific forum.

Most recently, the congress was held in Kyoto, Japan, thus returning to its country of birth: In 1980, the first session of the ISDE world congress was convened in Tokyo. The decision to meet in Japan for a second time may be seen as a gesture of reverence on the part of the Society to a country whose achievements in esophagology research have been of great merit.

The international community of scientists involved in esophagology research came to Kyoto to present its newest investigational results and to discuss them with the experts in this field. The quintessence of their findings is presented in this book, which could perhaps be described as documenting the "Olympics of esophagology". For all those interested in keeping up with the "state of the art" of current esophagology research, this book will therefore be the definitive source of information.

The ISDE and its president would like to extend their thanks to Professor Nabeya, whose outstanding hospitality made this congress unforgettable. This book will be a tribute to the congress and to him.

J. RÜDIGER SIEWERT
President of the ISDE 1989–1992

Foreword

In August, 1992 the fifth triennial Congress of the International Society for Diseases of the Esophagus was held in Kyoto. In the twelve years since the first Congress took place in Tokyo in 1980, ISDE, founded by Professor Komei Nakayma, has become a robust and healthy international organization. At the time of the Kyoto Congress there were approximately 650 official participants representing 45 different countries. The Congresses held previously in Tokyo, Rome, Munich, and Chicago were scheduled every three years to provide sufficient time for major advances and accomplishments to be made in the interim, thus enabling each Congress to offer many new and original presentations. This was the theme at the 1992 Congress under the leadership of Congress President Professor Kin-ichi Nabeya and ISDE President Professor Rüdiger Siewert. Professor Nabeya's Scientific Committee was able to select a superb program from more than 500 abstracts submitted from countries around the world. A series of first-rate paper and poster presentations filled the days in Kyoto, and the social programs scheduled for the evenings were equally memorable.

As has been the case following previous ISDE Congresses, the outstanding presentations were compiled and edited for presentation in book form. This volume offers the highlights of what is new and exciting in the management of esophageal disease in 1992. The triennial ISDE volumes have become the standard reference works for students of esophageal disease and define the "state of the art" in the interim between Congresses. This volume admirably serves this important purpose.

While ISDE has always encouraged participation from various specialties that have a strong interest in esophageal disorders, the major portions of the Congresses have usually reflected surgical approaches. At the 1992 Congress it was decided to make a concerted effort to broaden the membership and scope of the organization in order to develop a more balanced program among gastro-enterologists, oncologists, radiologists, and pathologists as well as thoracic and general surgeons. This book will be of interest to all of these specialists, and the next Congress scheduled for Milan in September 1995 promises to have an even larger representation of original work presented from a variety of disciplines that are contributing to advances in knowledge concerning the esophagus.

DAVID B. SKINNER
President of the ISDE

Table of Contents

Esophageal Varices

Esophageal Perforation

Other Diseases and Strictures

Esophageal Cancer

Epidemiology and Biology

Diagnosis and Cancer Staging

Resection for Esophageal Cancer

Esophageal Cancer: Surgical Treatment

Multimodality Treatment for Esophageal Cancer

List of Contributors

Abe, S.   249, 359, 947
Abo, S.   448, 891
Adachi, Y.   316, 473
Adams, I.P.   224
Addario Chieco, P.   236
Aikou, T.   657, 709, 795, 905
Akaishi, T.   780, 841
Akamine, S.   771
Akazawa, S.   1029
Akiyama, H.   600, 697, 884
Albertucci, M.   392
Alloisio, M.   871
Altorjay, Á.   307, 351, 644
Altorki, N.K.   657, 709
Ando, N.   417, 766
Andrews Jr. C.W.   760
Aoki, H.   249
Aoki, K.   173
Aoki, T.   249, 359
Aoyama, N.   978
Arai, T,   173
Arens, S.   1050
Argente-Navarro, P.   139
Asakura, S.   580
Asakura, T.   580
Asami, M.   580
Asolati, M.   726
Attwood, S.E.A.   156
Ayabe, H.   771, 786
Ayres-de-Campos, D.   281
Baba, H.   354
Baba, K.   473
Baba, M.   657, 709, 795
Bardini, R.   630, 726
Barlow, A.P.   156
Barreca, M.   236

Bartels, H.   623
Basile, R.   240, 676
Becker, H.   685, 1007
Bedini, V.   871
Bercedo, M.J.   663
Bettineschi, F.   207
Bhatnagar, N.K.   84
Bidoli, P.   871
Bollschweiler, E.   546, 651, 703
Bonavina, L.   207
Borzellino, G.   532
Brazzale, A.   412
Bremner, C.G.   108, 230
Bremner, R.M.   34, 169
Bumm, R.   651, 755
Busch, R.   714
Byrne, P.J.   134
Calle, S.A.   39
Calvo-Bermúdez, M.A.   139
Cantu, G.   871
Cardoso, V.   281
Carrette, M.   2
Casciani, C.U.   1003
Castoro, C.   630
Catania, G.   78
Cecconello, I.   91, 606
Cejalvo-Lapeña, D.   139
Chanvitan, A.   381
Chen, C.   673
Chen, C.-L.   731
Chen, C.-Y.   731
Chikuba, K.   441
Chongsuvivatwong, V.   381
Coosemans, W.   162, 404
Cordiano, C.   532, 823
Costantini, M.   34

Crookes, P.F.   34
Csanádi, J.   150
Darnton, S.J.   224
Daschner, C.   746
De Boeck, K.   2
De Giacomo, T.   240
De Leyn, P.   162
De Manzoni, G.   532, 823
De Toledo Viana, A.   343
Decker, D.   302
Decker, P.   14, 302
DeMeester, T.R.   27, 34, 169, 197
Deschamps, C.   115
Desmet, V.   336
Devilieger, H.   2
Dhar, D.K.   507
Dillemans, B.   162
Dittadi, R.   412
Dittler, H.J.   877
Doki, Y.   514
Domene, C.E.   102
Duffy, J.P.   224
Duranceau, A.   115
Ebener, C.   1007
Eeckels, R.   2
Eggermont, E.   2
Eguchi, R.   462, 568, 916, 959, 1039
Ellis Jr., F.H.   760
Enbom, H.   65, 72
Endo, M.   540
Endo, T.   916, 1039
Endo, Y.   922
Endoh, Y.   1056
Falkowski, S.   927
Felix, V.   91

Congenital Disease

Pulmonary Status During Childhood After Corrected Congenital Esophageal Atresia

D. Van Gysel[1], K. De Boeck[1], T. Lerut[2], T. Willems[1], M. Carrette[1], H. Devlieger[1], E. Eggermont[1], and R. Eeckels[1]

Introduction

The pulmonary consequences during childhood of corrected congenital esophageal atresia and its treatment have not been extensively studied. In the literature, there are only a few reports with small numbers of patients [1–3]. We, therefore, made a study of a larger group of patients treated at our institution.

Patients and Methods

From 1977 to 1984, 72 children underwent repair of congenital tracheo-esophageal atresia at the University Hospital of Leuven. Sixty-one (85%) were discharged alive. Three children died after discharge: one died accidentally, one from bacterial meningitis and one after a history of recurrent pneumonias caused by aspiration through the reopened tracheoesophageal fistula (TEF). Forty-nine patients had regular follow-up visits. All but one set of parents agreed to enter the study and one retarded patient was excluded due to inability to perform some of the tests. Thus, 47 children (81% of the surviving patients) were studied, 19 girls and 28 boys. Information on both the events and management in the neonatal period and at follow-up had been collected prospectively. The data included: presence of polyhydramnios, postmenstrual age (PMA), birth weight, associated congenital malformations, respiratory signs and symptoms during the neonatal period and at follow-up, the presence of a TEF, the age at diagnosis, diagnosis before or after starting oral feedings, the use of contrast medium to ascertain the diagnosis, age at the time of the first intervention, therapeutic aspiration before intervention, the type of correction (end-to-

Departments of [1] Pediatrics and [2] Thoracic Surgery, Leuven University Hospital, Herestraat 49, 3000 Leuven, Belgium

end anastomosis alone, end-to-end anastomosis after preliminary elongation, or colonic interposition), intra- and postoperative respiratory complications (pneumonia, pneumothorax, and/or atelectasis), number of esophageal dilatations, respiratory problems during childhood, the presence of gastroesophageal reflux (documented by upper gastrointestinal tract radiography and/or gastroesophageal scintigraphy), and presence of the characteristic barking cough. Age at the time of the study ranged from 6–13 years. Each patient and one or both of the parents were interviewed using a detailed questionnaire. All the patients were examined by the same physician.

Static lung volumes and three maximal expiratory flow volume curves were measured on a Morgan dry-sealed spirometer. The curve with the highest sum of vital capacity (VC) and forced expiratory volume in 1 s (FEV1) was examined. All values were compared to the expected values for sex and height according to Zapletal [4]. In order to allow comparison between patients of different age and sex, measurements were reported as percentages of predicted values. The following were considered to be indicative of restrictive lung disease: a TLC below the mean minus 2 SD, together with a high or normal ratio of FEV1/VC. The following were considered to be indicative of obstructive airway disease: a normal or elevated total lung capacity (TLC) and FEV1/VC or forced expiratory flow between 25% and 75% of VC (FEF25-75) below the mean minus 2 SD or residual volume (RV)/TLC higher than the mean plus 2 SD. The following were considered to be indicative of mixed restrictive/obstructive lung disease: a TLC below the mean minus 2 SD, together with FEV1/VC and/or FEF25-75 below the mean minus 2 SD or RV/TLC higher than the mean plus 2 SD.

For variables with a normal distribution, statistical analysis was done using the Student t-test. When the distribution was not normal, the Mann-Whitney U-test was used. The Chi-squared test and stepwise linear regression were used as appropriate. P values of <0.05 were considered statistically significant. The Z score was used to compare our study group with a normal population according to Zapletal [4].

Results

Mean (range) age, height and weight at follow-up study were, respectively, 9.7 years (6.4–14.1), 135 cm (110–167) and 29 kg (16.5–49.9).

Twenty-seven patients (57%) had recurrent episodes of croup in early childhood, but these subsided by the age of 5–6 years; 6 (13%) had more than one episode of pneumonia; 17 children (36%) had no more respiratory problems than children of their age without esophageal atresia. Thirty-six (77%) had a history of barking cough until 7 years of age.

The results of the lung function tests for the whole group are depicted in Fig. 1. The values for TLC, VC, FEV1, FEV1/VC, and FEF25-75 significantly differed from those in a normal population according to Zapletal [4] when analyzed using the Z score ($P < 0.000001$).

Twenty-three patients (49%) had restrictive lung disease; 8 patients (17%) had obstructive airway disease; 5 patients (11%) had combined restrictive and obstructive lung function changes and 11 patients (23%) had normal lung function.

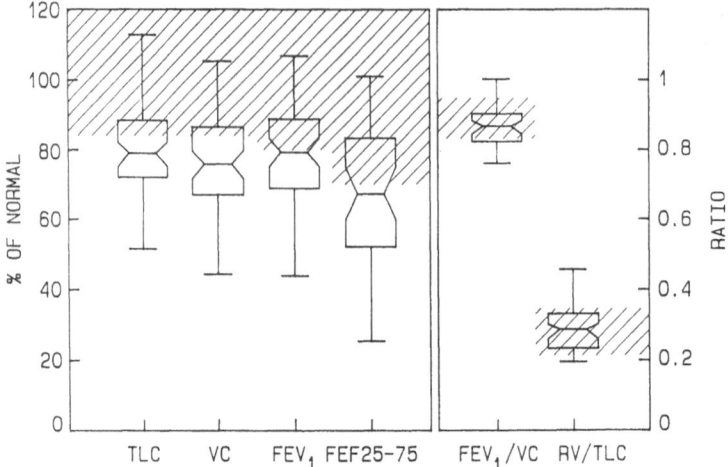

Fig. 1. The results for TLC, VC, FEV1, and FEF25-75, expressed as a percentage of normal values for height, sex, and age according to Zapletal [4]. FEV1/VC and RV/TLC are plotted as the actual ratios. Each variable is represented by a notched boxplot. The box is limited by the 25th and the 75th percentiles; the lines extending from the box indicate the 10th and the 90th percentiles. The notch indicates the 95% confidence interval around the median. The hatched area represents the 95% confidence limits for the normal population according to Zapletal [4]. *FEF25-75*, forced expiratory flow between 25% and 75% of the vital capacity; *FEV1*, forced expiratory volume in 1 s; *RV*, residual volume; *TLC*, total lung capacity; *VC*, vital capacity

Both static and dynamic lung function variables were compared to the recorded data from the neonatal period and previous follow-up. Factors associated with significant differences in pulmonary function are shown in Table 1.

Patients born before 37 weeks of gestation had lower TLC ($P < 0.0005$), FEV1 ($P < 0.005$), and VC ($P < 0.005$) than those born at or after 37 weeks. TLC, FEV1 and VC were lower ($P < 0.05$) in the group of patients with a birth weight below the tenth percentile as compared to heavier babies. Patients in whom contrast studies had been used to establish the diagnosis, had significantly lower TLC ($P < 0.05$) and higher FEV1/VC ($P < 0.005$) and FEF25-75 ($P < 0.05$). In the group with colonic interposition, TLC, FEV1 and VC were significantly lower ($P < 0.005$) than in the group with end-to-end anastomosis. Postoperative respiratory problems were associated with lower FEV1/VC and FEF25-75 ($P < 0.05$). No significant differences were found for the other variables mentioned above.

Discussion

In this study, 47 (81%) of the long-term survivors of corrected congenital esophageal atresia were examined. This contrasts with previous papers on this topic, which report results in a minority of patients: Milligan et al. [2] examined 24 (15%) of 159 patients, Couriel et al. [3] examined 20 (17%) of 118 patients and Biller et al. [5] examined 12 (24%) of 50 patients.

Table 1. Medians of pulmonary function variables for specific risk factors, current weight, and drug use

	TLC	VC	FEV1	FEF25-75	FEV1/VC	RV/TLC
PMA						
<37 w ($n = 10$)	72	69	70	62	87	30
⩾37 w ($n = 37$)	86	82	82	67	87	28
	***	**	**			
Birth weight						
⩽P[a]10 ($n = 10$)	75	69	71	62	84	29
>P10 ($n = 37$)	82	77	80	65	86	29
	*	*	*			
Use of contrast						
+ ($n = 32$)	76	74	78	68	88	29
− ($n = 13$)	84	79	79	60	82	29
	*			*	**	
Type of surgery						
Colon ($n = 7$)	68	65	67	59	88	29
End-to-end	83	80	80	65	86	29
alone ($n = 34$)	**	**	**			
Postop. compl.						
+ ($n = 27$)	82	74	77	60	84	28
− ($n = 20$)	79	75	79	71	88	29
				*	*	
Current weight						
⩽P10 ($n = 11$)	73	64	66	59	86	31
>P10 ($n = 36$)	82	79	80	68	87	27
	*	*	**			
Drug use						
+ ($n = 10$)	85	78	76	56	83	31
− ($n = 37$)	76	75	79	67	88	28
				*		*

TLC, VC, FEV1, and FEF25-75 are expressed as a percentage of normal; the values of FEV1/VC and RV/TLC are the absolute values. *FEF25-75*, forced expiratory flow between 25% and 75% of the vital capacity; *FEV1*, forced expiratory volume in 1 s; *RV*, residual volume; *TLC*, total lung capacity; *VC*, vital capacity; *PMA*, postmenstrual age; *W*, weeks. Comparison of groups was done using Mann-Whitney U-test. [a] tenth percentile.
* $P < 0.05$; ** $P < 0.005$; *** $P < 0.0005$

Most patients with esophageal atresia have abnormal pulmonary function. Both restrictive and obstructive changes were observed. The etiology of the impaired pulmonary function is still unclear, but several factors may play a role:

1. Thoracotomy adversely affects pulmonary lung function (reduction of TLC and VC) [6] by reducing the expansion of the thorax.
2. Prandial and interprandial aspiration: the former is related to anastomotic stricture [7], the latter to an insufficient gastroesophageal sphincter [8]. Both are exacerbated by abnormal esophageal peristalsis, resulting from changes in the myenteric plexus in the distal portion of the esophagus [9, 10].

3. Impaired mucociliary clearance as a result of tracheomalacia [2], tracheal squamous metaplasia [11, 12] and other factors (i.e. congenital abnormality of the intrinsic tracheal nervous plexuses [13]).

Certain neonatal variables are significantly associated with a more restrictive and/or obstructive lung function pattern. The lower the PMA and/or birth weight, the more restrictive the lung function pattern is. This could be because the smaller the child at the time of the insult to the chest wall, the more important is the effect on chest wall movements later on.

A restrictive lung function pattern was more common in the group of children in whom diagnostic contrast studies had been used at birth. Aspiration of this material might cause chemical pneumonitis and lead to some degree of pulmonary fibrosis.

Several factors are responsible for the more restrictive pulmonary function in the group of children with colonic interposition: They have undergone a bilateral thoracotomy, whereas the other patients have undergone one or two thoracotomies on the right side.

The large volume of the intrathoracic colon segment might impair lung growth, resembling the sequence of events in congenital diaphragmatic hernia. Also, repeated episodes of aspiration might occur more frequently following colonic interposition.

In addition, postoperative respiratory problems worsened pulmonary outcome and were associated with obstructive lung changes.

From the variables obtained during follow-up, only present weight and current drug use correlated with outcome. We found a more restrictive pattern in the patients with a lower weight for height and a more obstructive lung function pattern in the group of patients requiring current drug use. These differences are more likely a consequence rather than a cause of impaired pulmonary function. As a group, our patients have both a low weight and small lungs in proportion to their height. Although present weight was clearly a function of birth weight, it is possible that pulmonary function adversely affects growth in this population.

However, in spite of 75% of patients having abnormal pulmonary function, only 25% of the patients are currently symptomatic. Being asymptomatic in the presence of abnormal pulmonary function is encountered in other diseases, the most common example being asthma. It is likely that patients adapt to their chronic respiratory handicap. In addition, spirometry is a sensitive tool and detects abnormalities before overt complaints of limited exercise tolerance occur.

In conclusion, when studied at the age of 6–13 years, the majority of our patients operated on for esophageal atresia do have impaired pulmonary function. About half have signs of moderately restrictive lung disease, another quarter have obstructive or combined restrictive plus obstructive lung disease, and only one quarter of the patients have normal pulmonary function tests. Use of contrast studies to establish the diagnosis of esophageal atresia clearly emerges as a preventable risk factor of impaired pulmonary function in later life. Despite a high incidence of abnormal pulmonary function, the majority of patients report no problems and lead a normal, active life.

References

1. Dudley NE, Phelan PD (1976) Respiratory complications in long-term survivors of oesophageal atresia. Arch Dis Child 51:279–82
2. Milligan DWA, Levison H (1979) Lung function in children following repair of tracheoesophageal fistula. J Pediatr 95:24–7
3. Couriel JM, Hibbert M, Olinsky A, Phelan PD (1982) Long-term pulmonary consequences of oesophageal atresia with tracheo-oesophageal fistula. Acta Pediatr Scand 71:973–8
4. Zapletal A (1987) Lung function in children and adolescents: Methods, reference values. Karger (Basel, München, Paris, London, New York, New Delhi, Singapore, Tokyo, Sydney) pp 114–140
5. Biller JA, Allen JL, Schuster SR, Treves ST, Winter HS (1987) Long-term evaluation of esophageal and pulmonary function in patients with repaired esophageal atresia and tracheoesophageal fistula. Dig Dis Sci 32:985–90
6. Beasley SW (1991) Influence of anatomy and physiology on the man-agement of esophageal atresia. Prog Pediatr Surg 27:53–61
7. Desjardin JG, Stephens CA, Moes CAF (1964) Results of surgical treatment of congenital tracheoesophageal fistula, with a note on cine-fluorographic findings. Ann Surg 160:141–5
8. Parker AF, Christie DL, Cahill JL (1979) Incidence and significance of gastroesophageal reflux following repair of esophageal atresia and the tracheoesophageal fistula and the need for anti-reflux procedures. J Pediatr Surgery 14:5–8
9. Nakazato Y, Landing BH, Wells TR (1986) Abnormal Auerbach plexus in the esophagus and stomach of patients with esophageal atresia and tracheoesophageal fistula. J Pediatr Surg 21:831–7
10. Romeo G, Zuccarello B, Proietto F, Romeo C (1987) Disorders of the esophageal motor activity in atresia of the esophagus. J Pediatr Surg 22:120–4
11. Vailoo MP, Emery JL (1979) The trachea in children with tracheoesophageal fistula. Histopathology 3:329–38
12. Emery JL, Haddadin AJ (1971) Squamous epithelium in respiratory tract of children with tracheoesophageal fistula. Arch Dis Child 46:236–42
13. Nakazato Y, Wells TR, Landing BH (1986) Abnormal tracheal innervation in patients with esophageal atresia and tracheoesophageal fistula: study of the intrinsic tracheal nerve plexuses by a microdissection technique. J Pediatr Surg 21:838–44

Investigations of Reoperated Cases of Congenital Disorders of the Esophagus in Children: Reports of Two Cases

Hiroo Takehara[1], Nobuhiko Komi[1], Akira Okada[1], Masaharu Nishi[1], and Kazuhiro Kameoka[2]

Summary. Two pediatric cases of esophageal atresia, with or without a tracheoesophageal fistula (TEF), required secondary surgical intervention to the esophagus because of unexpected or unusual morbidities. Case 1 is an 8-year-old girl who required a reoperation for late recurrence of TEF 8 years after initial surgery at 1 day of age. Case 2 is a male newborn who was operated on at 3 days of age for left diaphragmatic hernia. He also underwent a second surgery 12 days later for lower esophageal atresia associated with a diverticulum-like abscess cavity, in which an abnormal air bubble was misinterpreted as being in the fundus of the herniated stomach. Patient 1 has had an uneventful course since surgery, but patient 2 died at 161 days of age due to severe aspiration pnuemonia caused by gastroesophageal reflux.

Introduction

Although the literature contains several large series of patients with esophageal atresia and tracheoesophageal fistula (TEF) [1, 2], the question of secondary operative procedures to the esophagus after repair of esophageal atresia has not been addressed. In this paper, we report two cases of esophageal atresia (with or without TEF) that required secondary surgical intervention to the esophagus, with specific reference to late recurrent TEF as a rare complication and lower esophageal atresia caused by an unusual etiology.

---

[1] First Department of Surgery, School of Medicine, University of Tokushima, 3-18-15, Kuramoto-cho, Tokushima, 770 Japan
[2] Division of Pediatric Surgery, Ehime Prefectural Central Hospital, 83 Kasuga-cho, Matsuyama, 790 Japan

Case Reports

Thirty-eight patients with congenital esophageal disorders were treated at our institution and an associated hospital between 1972 and 1991. Surgical interventions were carried out in 36 cases: 29 had esophageal atresia with or without a TEF, 5 had tracheal remnants, and 2 had fibromuscular hypertrophy. The survival rate in the 29 surgical cases with esophageal atresia was 62.1%, while all other surgical patients survived. Of the 36 patients, 2 underwent reoperation for unexpected or unusual morbidities.

Case 1

An 8-year-old girl presented with a 3-month history of coughing with eating and repeated episodes of upper respiratory infection and pneumonia. At the age of 1 day, she had undergone a primary esophagoesophagostomy for esophageal atresia with TEF. The surgery was easily performed by a one-layer, end-to-end anastomosis using interrupted sutures without any tension. Esophageal bouginage was performed twice at 39 days and 48 days after the surgery for the anastomotic stenosis. The clinical course had been uneventful after the esophageal bouginage until the most recent 3 months. An esophagram showed part of the trachea via a TEF (Fig. 1). She, therefore, underwent a second operation for closure of the

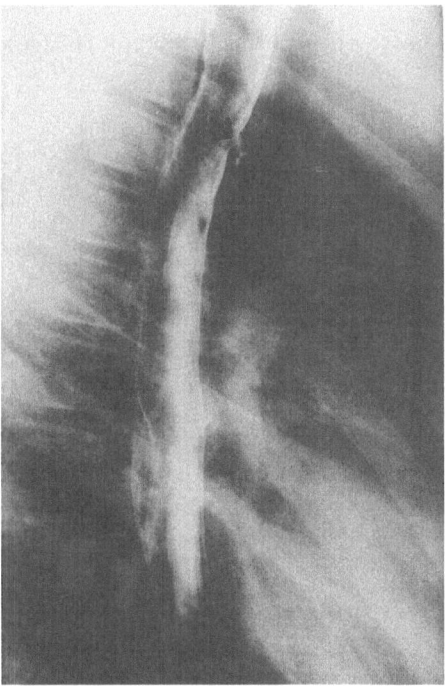

Fig. 1. Esophagram at 8 years after initial operation reveals a recurrent fistula between the esophagus and the trachea (*arrow*)

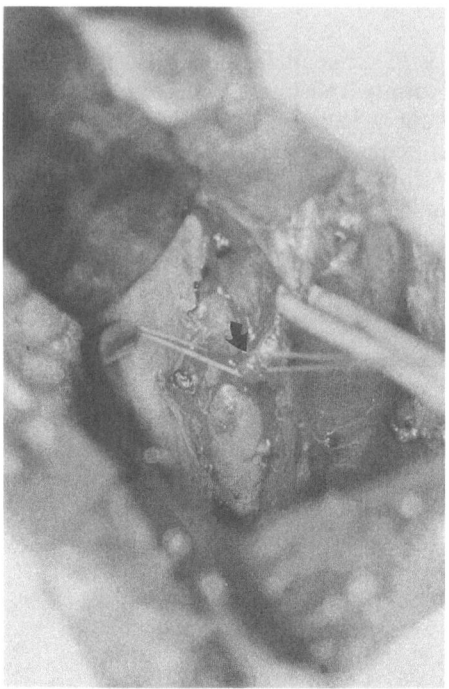

Fig. 2. Photograph during second operation. The recurrent TEF (diameter of 3 mm and length of 10 mm) is indicated by two stitches (*arrows*)

recurrent TEF (diameter of 3 mm and length of 10 mm) by a right transpleural approach (Fig. 2). The postoperative course has been uneventful since the second operation.

Case 2

A male newborn (weighing 3,078 g) was born by vaginal delivery at 36 weeks and 4 days of gestation. The mother's pregnancy was complicated by maternal hydramnios. After birth, the infant suffered excessive choking and coughing and produced abundant frothy saliva. A plain chest-abdominal roentgenogram showed a rightward shift of the central shadow, haziness in the left lower chest, an abnormal air bubble resembling a gastric bubble in the left lower mediastinum, and a gasless abdomen (Fig. 3a). An esophagram revealed that the esophagus was seen terminating in a blind end, and a nasogastric tube could not be passed into the stomach. The gas seen on the left side of the chest was thought to be the gastric bubble of a herniated stomach. A barium enema showed that the transverse colon was in the left chest, and a diagnosis of a left diaphragmatic hernia was made (Fig. 4). The patient (at the age of 3 days) had surgery to return the liver, stomach, and transverse colon to the abdominal cavity from the left thoracic cavity and to repair the defect in the left hemidiaphragm. The lower esophageal obstruction, however, was not relieved by repositioning of the stomach

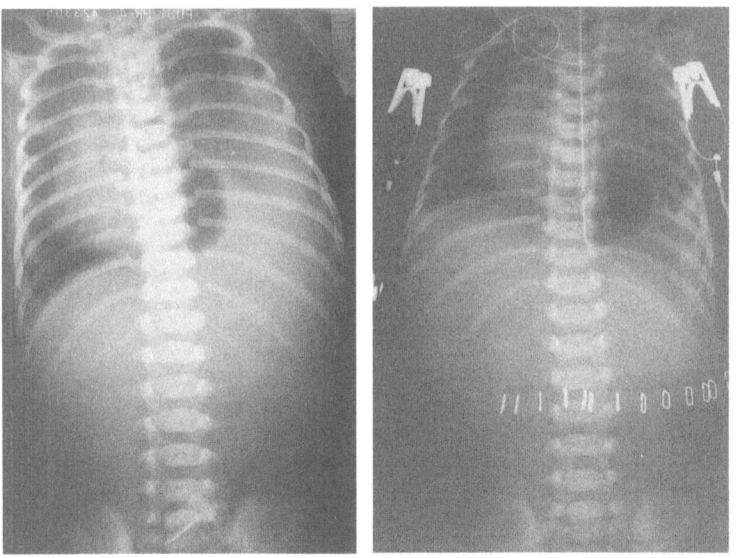

a   b

Fig. 3a,b. Chest-abdominal roentgenogram at 1 day of age shows **a** a rightward shift of the central shadow, haziness in the left lower chest, and an abnormal air bubble resembling a gastric bubble in the left lower mediastinum. **b** In spite of repositioning of the stomach in the abdominal cavity, the abnormal air bubble, which resembled the gastric fundus, is still observed on a postoperative roentgenogram

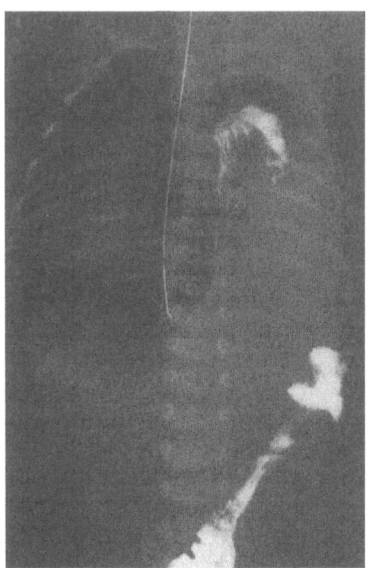

Fig. 4. A barium enema shows the transverse colon was in the left chest

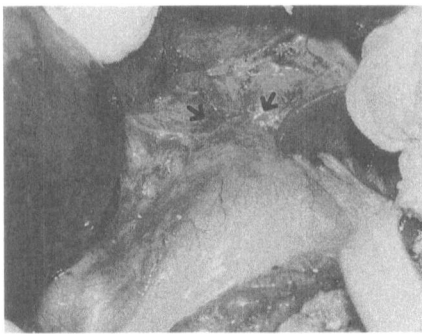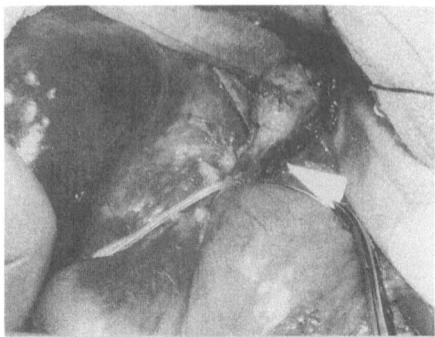

a   b

Fig. 5a,b. Intraoperative photograph of the second surgery 12 days after the initial operation. **a** The esophagocardiac junction is found to be embedded in fibrotic scar tissue (*arrows*) which extended from the diaphragm to the cardia at the esophageal hiatus. **b** The lower esophagus and esophagocardiac junction are exposed after dissection of the fibrotic scar tissue. The *black arrows* show a diverticulum-like abscess cavity, and the *white arrow* shows the atretic portion of the lower esophagus in which there is no lumen to the stomach

in the abdominal cavity, and the abnormal air bubble (which resembled the gastric fundus) was still observed in the left lower mediastinum on a postoperative roentgenogram (Fig. 3b). Twelve days after the first operation, a second procedure was performed. At surgery, the esophagocardiac junction was found to be embedded in fibrotic scar tissue, which extended from the diaphragm to the cardia at the esophageal hiatus (Fig. 5a). Partial resection of the lower esophagus, including an atretic segment contiguous with a diverticulum-like abscess cavity, and esophagogastrostomy were performed (Fig. 5b). Histologic examination of the wall of the resected diverticulum-like cyst did not reveal any epithelia or smooth muscle. The wall consisted of granulation tissue with infiltration of inflammatory cells, suggesting an abscess. Unfortunately, the patient died at 161 days of age due to sepsis and aspiration pneumonia caused by gastroesophageal reflux while awaiting further reconstructive surgery.

Discussion

The survival rate of infants with congenital esophageal atresia with or without TEF has steadily improved during the past 3 decades as a result of earlier recognition, improved anesthetic management, and better surgical technique. Recurrent TEF is a troublesome and not an uncommon complication of surgery for esophageal atresia. Estimation of the incidence of TEF is difficult. Figures from 0% [3] up to 40% [4] have been reported, but the actual figure seems to be between 5% and 15% [5]. The various factors responsible for recurrent TEF are esophageal leakage, direct apposition of the tracheal and esophageal suture lines, erosion of the suture line, and mechanical trauma during esophageal dilatation [6]. More than 50% of recurrent fistula are diagnosed within 2 months after the initial repair. However, a very rare case diagnosed as a recurrent TEF 9 years after the initial operation (like case 1) was reported [7]. The mechanism of late recurrence of TEF is unclear. Most observers agree that the symptoms are probably directly related to the size of the fistula. The smaller the fistula, the less material gets through from the esophagus to the trachea and vice versa [3]. The recurrent fistula may be subtle in its presentation or even totally asymptomatic. This accounts for some fistula not being discovered for years, if at all [8, 9].

Esophageal atresia is usually located in the mid-esophagus and is associated with a TEF. Membranous atresia of the lower esophagus, not associated with a fistula, has also been reported [10]. Similar lesions have been found elsewhere in the alimentary tract. The diaphragm usually involves only mucosa. However, there was no mucosa in the atretic portion of the esophagus in case 2. The embryogenesis of the atresia in this case, therefore, appears to be different than the usual etiology of membranous atresia. We hypothesize that local necrosis, due to the interruption of blood flow, was caused by prolonged kinking of the esophagocardiac junction following herniation of the stomach into the left thoracic cavity. Necrosis of the lower esophagus progressed to perforation, and leakage of the esophageal contents produced an abscess which resembled a diverticulum of the distal esophagus. Initially, we misinterpreted the air bubble in the abscess cavity as in the fundus of the herniated stomach. To reduce the likelihood of making this error, we recommend insertion of a nasogastric tube into the stomach after repositioning of the herniated organs during surgery.

References

1. Louhimo I, Lindahl H (1983) Oesophageal atresia: Primary results of 500 consecutively treated patients. J Pediatr Surg 18:217–229
2. Holder TM, Cloud DT, Lewis JE Jr, Pilling GP (1964) Esophageal atresia and tracheoesophageal fistula: A survey of its members by the surgical section of the American Academy of Pediatrics. Pediatrics 34:542–549
3. Daum R (1971) Postoperative complications following operation for oesophageal atresia and tracheo-oesophageal fistula. In: Rickham PP, Hecker WC, Prevot J (eds) Progress in pediatric surgery. University Park Press, Baltimore, pp 209–237
4. Ein SH, Theman TE (1973) A comparison of the results of primary repair of esophageal atresia with tracheoesophageal fistula using end-to-side and end-to-end anastomosis. J Pediatr Surg 8:641–645
5. Cudmore RE (1978) Oesophageal atresia and tracheo-oesophageal fistula. In: Rickham PP, Lister J, Irving IM (eds) Neonatal surgery. Butterworth, London, pp 200–201
6. Randolph JC (1986) Esophageal atresia and congenital stenosis. In: Welch KJ, Randolph JC, Ravitch MM, O'Neill JA Jr, Rowe MI (eds) Pediatric surgery. Chicago, Year Book Medical, pp 682–697
7. Ein SH, Stringer DA, Stephens CA, Shandling B, Simpson J (1983) Recurrent tracheoesophageal fistula: 17-year review. J Pediatr Surg 18:436–441
8. Slim MS, Tabry IF (1974) Left extrapleural approach for the repair of recurrent tracheoesophageal fistula. J Thorac Cardiovasc Surg 68:654–657
9. Kiser JC, Peterson TA, Johnson FE (1972) Chronic recurrent tracheo-esophageal fistula. Chest 62:222–224
10. Schwartz SI (1962) Congenital membranous obstruction of esophagus. Arch Surg 85:480–482

Problems Associated with Congenital Esophageal Atresia and Their Treatment

Pan Decker, J. Jakschik, C.H. Siebert, and A. Hirner[1]

Introduction

Congenital esophageal atresia is seen in 1 out of 3000 living births today. The cause of this malformation is a disturbance of the separation of the esophagus, trachea, and lung during their embryonic development. The resulting abnormalities have many different forms but can classified into five major groups as described by Gross-Vogt [1] (Fig. 1). During pregnancy, a hydramnion can frequently be noted, and the postpartum clinical consequences can include choking or coughing. Already during the first hours, the regurgitated gastric juices can pass into the lungs and cause chemical pneumonia and atelectasis. Therefore, an early diagnosis and proper treatment are of vital importance.

Patients and Methods

From February 1, 1989, to January 31, 1992, seven newborns with esophageal atresia (Fig. 2) were treated in our hospital. Three infants presented with type C, two with type B, one with type A, and one with a type E esophageal atresia. In each instance, the atresia was treated in a single procedure, and all of the infants have survived. In a single case, a type E or H fistula, a second operation was necessary due to a recurrence of the fistula. In one patient with a long-gap atresia, a primary gastric transposition was carried out (Fig. 3).

The postoperative examinations did not reveal a single case of esophageal stenosis. One child developed a reflux esophagitis, while the early surgical intervention could not prevent the development of a pneumonia in two patients. All the children survived and were discharged from hospital care.

---

[1] Department of Surgery, University of Bonn, Sigmund-Freud-Str. 25, D-5300 Bonn 1, Germany

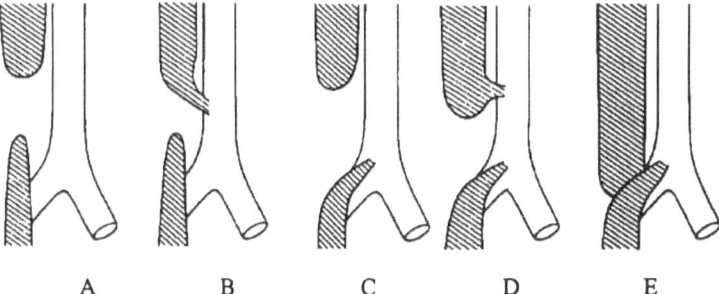

Fig. 1. Gross-Vogt [1] classification of congenital esophageal atresia. Five major categories of esophageal atresia and tracheoesophageal fistula. *A*, Atresia without fistula; *B*, atresia with proximal tracheoesophageal fistula; *C*, atresia with distal fistula; *D*, atresia with fistula between both proximal and distal ends of esophagus and trachea; *E*, tracheoesophageal fistula with esophageal atresia (H-type fistula)

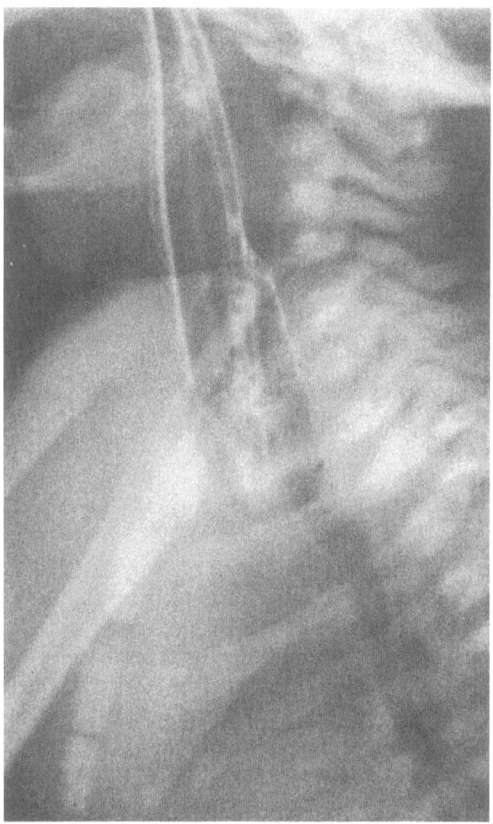

Fig. 2. Esophageal atresia

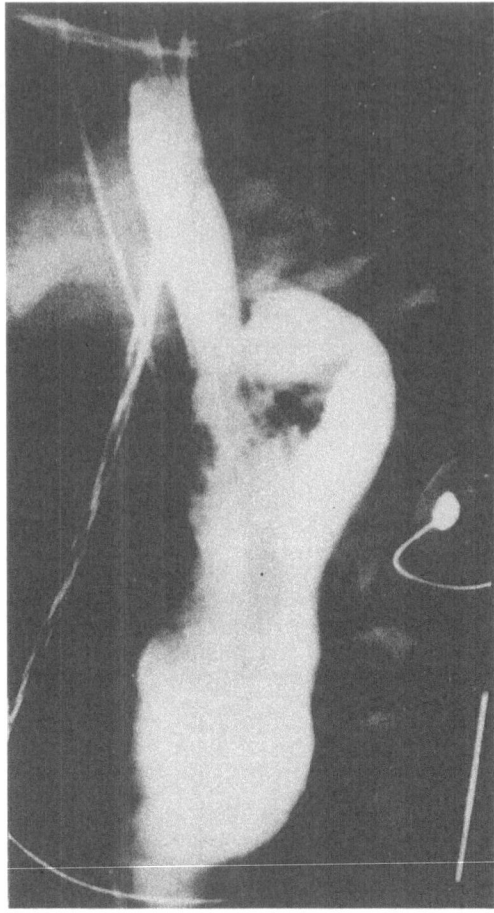

Fig. 3. Patient with gastric transposition

Discussion

The infants prognosis depends not only on the early diagnosis and on the associated anomalies but also on the surgical procedure. It is always desirable to reconstruct the gastric passage in a single operation if the patient's condition permits. In most instances, the small distance between both the proximal and distal esophageal ends allows for a direct end-to-end anastomosis and transsection of the fistula. To avoid development of a stenosis, it is important to use a meticulous single row suture technique as well as using a limited exposure of the esophageal ends so as not to damage the vascular supply.

In those patients in whom a primary suture is not possible, the choice of operative techniques becomes essential. Generally, one has to differentiate primary repairs and staged, possibly as a combination of conservative and operative treatment modalities and procedures. A primary repair is generally preferred in our hospital if the patient can tolerate a single procedure. A staged procedure is only carried out in children with severe pulmonary alterations, a birth weight under 1800 g, or associated anomalies. During the first procedure, an extrapleural transsection of the fistula and a gastrostomy are performed. At a later date, a reconstruction of the passage is carried out in form of a gastric transposition.

The various combinations of conservative and surgical treatment, as described by Rehbein and Schweder [2], Kato et al. [3], Hendren and Hale [4], and Howard and Myers [5], all entail numerous narcosis and a long hospital stay. Until the final reconstruction of the gastric passage, normal intake of food is not possible. It would seem plausible that this negatively influences the psychological development of the infant. Also, a high rate of esophageal stenosis requiring renewed surgical intervention are encountered with these treatment regimens [6, 7]. A final resolution of the dispute in regard to which reconstructive procedure has the best long term results has not been found at this point in time. In 1984, Spitz et al. [7] first described the gastric transposition in the treatment of long-gap atresias. The successful use of a colon interposition and reverse gastric tube reconstruction have also been reported.

We believe the primary gastric transposition without a gastrotomy to be the procedure of choice because it offers the following advantages:

- No danger of compromising the gastric vascular supply.
- No long suture rows, as seen in the reverse gastric tube.
- Transposition into the anatomic, physiologic esophageal bed.
- In the case of a staged repair, scar tissue may make a retrosternal transposition necessary.
- A relatively short period of restricted food intake permits early enteral nutrition.

The surgical treatment should adhere to the following rules:

- Immediate surgical treatment to avoid pulmonary problems.
- A single operative procedure when the patient can tolerate it.
- Limited exposure of the ends of the esophagus.
- Primary suture with single row.
- In the case of long-gap atresia not amenable to primary suture, we presently prefer the use of gastric transposition as an esophageal replacement.

Table 1. Comparison of our results and those found in the literature

	n	Fisula recurr.	Stenosis	Reflux	Pneumonia	Mortality
Krichenja and Almashi (1991) [8]	29	9%	4%	39%	13%	33%
Holschneider et al. (1991) [9]	94	4%	4%	16%	20%	13%
Spitz et al. (1988) [7]	148	21%	18%	—	—	14%
Own results	7	1/7	0/7	1/7	2/7	0/7

With the help of the described treatment regimen, we were able to achieve favorable results, especially in regard to postoperative complications. This is shown by the comparison of our rates to those found in other publications (Table 1). Thanks to the improvements in early diagnostics, the diagnosis of esophageal atresia should no longer be a matter of chance. Only the early surgical treatment and the cooperation of pediatric surgeons, pediatricians, and anesthesiologists can avoid pulmonary complications and lead to a normal development of the infants.

References

1. Gross RE (1953) The surgery of infancy and childhood. W.B. Saunders, Philadelphia
2. Rehbein F, Schweder UG (1972) Neue Wege in der Rekonstruktion der kindlichen Speiseröhre. Dtsch Med Wschr 97:757–770
3. Kato T, Hollyman G, Höpner F, Ohashi E, Hecker W Ch (1980) Ein neues Instrument zur Fadenlegüng ohne Thorakotomie in ausgewöhlten Fällen von Ösophagoatresie. Z Kinderchir 29:20–23
4. Hendren W, Hale, JR (1976) Esophageal atresia treated by electromagnetic bougienage and subsequent repair. Ped Surg 11:713–722
5. Howard R, Myers NA (1965) Esophageal atresia: A technique for elongating the upper pouch. Surg 58:725–727
6. Sauer H, Kurz R (1986) Experiences in the treatment of esophageal atresia with Rehbein's olive technique. In: Wurnig P (ed) Long-gap esophageal atresia—prenatal diagnosis of congenital malformations. Springer, Berlin Heidelberg New York, pp 93–102
7. Spitz U, Hagberg S. Rubenson A, Werkmäster, K (1988) Management of esophageal atresia: Review of 16 years' experience. J Ped Surg 23:805–809
8. Krichenja DU, Almashi GG (1991) Spätergebnissse nach Behandlung der Ösophagusatresie durch End-zu-End-Anastomose. In: Hasse W (ed) Funktionsgerechte Chirurgie der Ösophagusatresie. Gustav-Fischer, Stuttgart, pp 209–212
9. Holschneider AM, Slany E, Holzki J, Gharib M (1991) Postoperative Kom-plikationen nach Primäranastomose einer Ösophagusatresie—eine prospektive Studie. In: Hasse W (ed) Funktionsgerechte Chirurgie der Ösophagusatresie. Gustav-Fischer Stuttgart, pp 62–70

Gastroesophageal Reflux

Esophageal Motility in Gastroesophageal Reflux Disease

S.M. FREYS, K.H. FUCHS, J. HEIMBUCHER, and A. THIEDE[1]

Introduction

The correlation between gastroesophageal reflux disease (GERD) and motility disorders of the esophagus is still a matter of discussion (Table 1). Bumm [1] reports on a chronologic relation between motility events and reflux episodes in the esophagus in healthy volunteers. He found that GER episodes mainly influence frequency and type rather than amplitude and duration of contractions. Other investigators demonstrate that an increasing degree of esophagitis leads to a decrease in contraction amplitude and to an increase in pathologic contractions [2], as well as to an accumulation of defective primary peristalsis or hypertensive peristalsis in the distal esophagus [3]. A clear trend as to the correlation of the two pathophysiologic findings, esophagitis and esophageal motility disorder, cannot be derived from these reports. Two other studies investigating esophageal motility before and after healing of esophagitis by omeprazol come to exactly opposite conclusions: on the one hand an improvement in peristaltic force and clearance could be demonstrated, leading to the conclusion that motility disorders are caused by an inflammatory dysfunction of the plexus myentericus [4]. On the other hand, a significant difference could not be demonstrated comparing contraction amplitudes before and after healing of esophagitis, leading to the conclusion that motility disorders are a primary phenomenon and not the result of mucosal damage [5].

In the present prospective study, we investigated the correlation of esophagitis and esophageal motility disorder within the realm of GERD. The aim of this study was to determine whether esophageal motility disorders are the cause or the consequence of esophagitis.

---

[1] Department of Surgery, University of Würzburg, Josef-Schneider-Str. 2, 8700 Würzburg, Germany

Table 1. Current publications on the correlation of esophagitis and motility disorder

Esophagitis → Motility disorder

- Jehle and Blum—1990 [11]
- Kahrilas, Dodds, Hogan, Kern, Arndorfer, Reece—1986 [3]
- Olsen and Schlegel—1965 [10]
- Rühl and Erckenbrecht—1990 [9]
- Walker, Maiorana, Chakkaphak, Ferguson, Skinner, Little—1990 [2]
- Williams, Thompson, O'Hanrahan, Bancewicz—1990 [4]

Motility disorder → Esophagitis

- Hotz—1990 [8]
- Jehle and Blum—1990 [11]
- Rühl and Erckenbrecht—1990 [9]
- Singh, Adamopoulos, Taylor, Colin-Jones—1990 [5]

Materials and Methods

The study population was comprised of 10 healthy control volunteers and 58 patients. In all individuals, the following investigations were performed:

1. History and physical examination
2. Endoscopy of the upper GI tract
3. Stationary pull-through perfusion manometry of the esophagus, performing five voluntary wet swallows
4. Ambulatory 24-h pH-monitoring of the esophagus (Digitrapper/Synectics)

Evaluation was performed on three occasions in each of the 68 individuals: (1) at endoscopy according to the Savary-Miller classification of esophagitis, (2) at esophageal manometry according to the criteria for esophageal motility disorders by Eypasch [6] (Table 2), and (3) at pH-monitoring according to the criteria for pathologic acid exposition according to DeMeester [7] (Table 3). After evaluation of these investigations, the individuals were divided into seven groups according to the presence or absence of the following criteria: Esophagitis, positive reflux score, dysphagia, and peptic stenosis (Table 4).

Once an individual had been assigned a group according to the above criteria, the following parameters were investigated:

1. Progression of contractions
2. Duration of contractions
3. Amplitude of contractions
4. Amount of pathologic contractions

The median values of these parameters were compared with the Wilcoxon-rank test for unpaired parameters (parameter 1–3) and the Fischer-exact test (parameter 4).

Results

Looking at the progression and duration of contractions (Figs. 1 and 2, respectively), we did not find any significant differences when comparing all seven

Table 2. Stationary esophageal manometry: Criteria for pathologic esophageal peristalsis [6]

Pathologic single contraction	Pathologic sequence of contractions
Amplitude >180 mmHg	Simultaneous (=progression >20 cm/s)
Amplitude <20 mmHg	Non—progressive (=amplitude <10 mmHg)
Duration >7 s	Repetitive (>30% of cases)
Multi-peaked	
Repetitive	

Table 3. Ambulatory 24-h pH-monitoring of the esophagus: Criteria for pathologic acid exposure [7]

Percentage time	<pH 4 (total, upright, supine)
Max. duration	<pH 4
No. reflux episodes	<pH 4
No. reflux episodes	<pH 4 >5 min

Table 4. Study population

Group	
1	10 Healthy volunteers
2	10 Patients with "healthy esophagus"
3	10 Patients with positive reflux score without esophagitis/dysphagia
4	10 Patients with GERD (esophagitis I or II) without dysphagia
5	10 Patients with GERD (esophagitis III or IV) without dysphagia
6	10 Patients with GERD (peptic stenosis) with dysphagia
7	8 Patients with GERD (without peptic stenosis) with dysphagia

GERD, gastroesophageal reflux disease

groups. The course of the amplitude of contractions in the individual groups is suggestive of a certain trend: with increasing degrees of esophagitis, we find a decrease in the amplitude of contractions (Fig. 3). Comparing the individual groups, we found a significant difference between group 1 and groups 6 and 7 ($P < 0.02$), between group 2 and groups 5–7 ($P < 0.05$), and between group 3 and group 6 ($P < 0.005$).

Evaluation of the amount of pathologic contractions in the individual groups underscores this trend (Fig. 4): The highest amount of pathologic contractions is found in the two groups with dysphagia (groups 6 and 7), reaching a level of significance in comparison with all other five groups.

Discussion

In accordance with the investigations by Walker [2] our results demonstrate that the amplitude of contractions in the esophagus decreases with increasing degrees of esophagitis. However, the findings by Bumm [1] in healthy volunteers do not support our results. Walker explained the increase in amplitude in patients

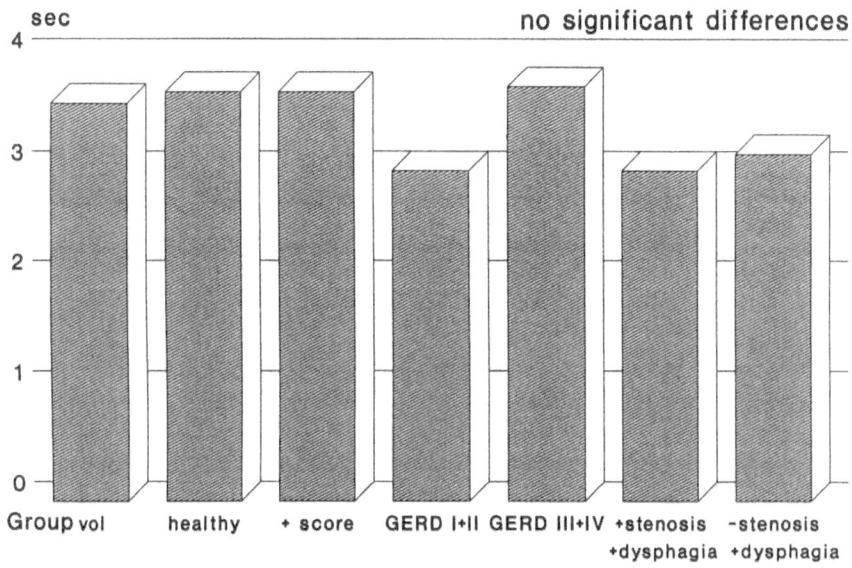

Fig. 1. Progression of contractions. (Explanation of groups: see Table 4)

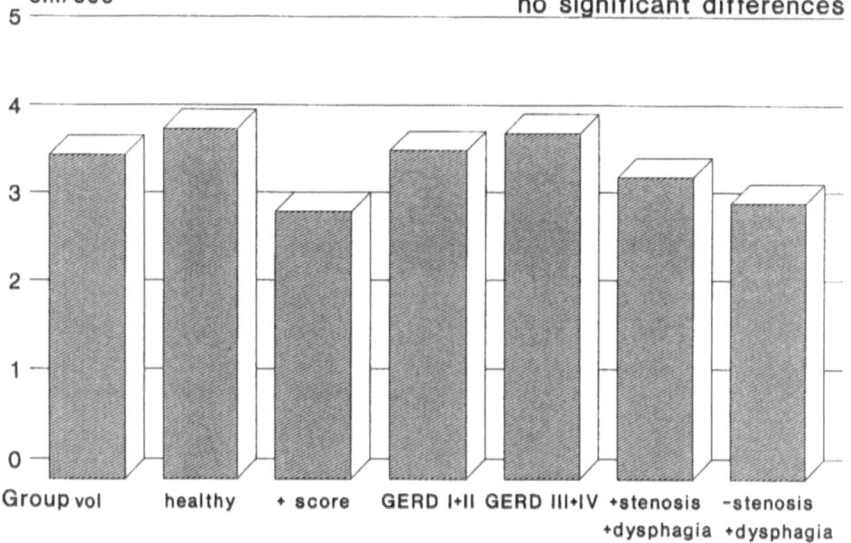

Fig. 2. Duration of contractions

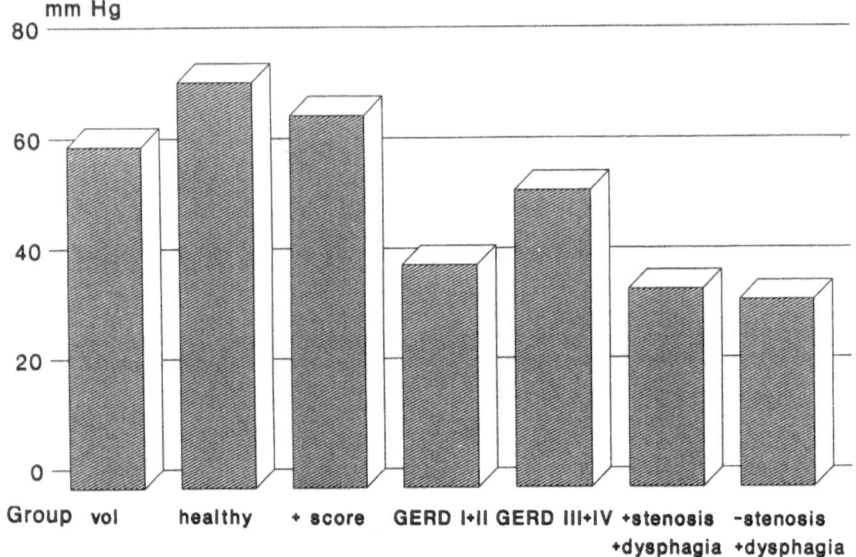

Fig. 3. Amplitude of contractions

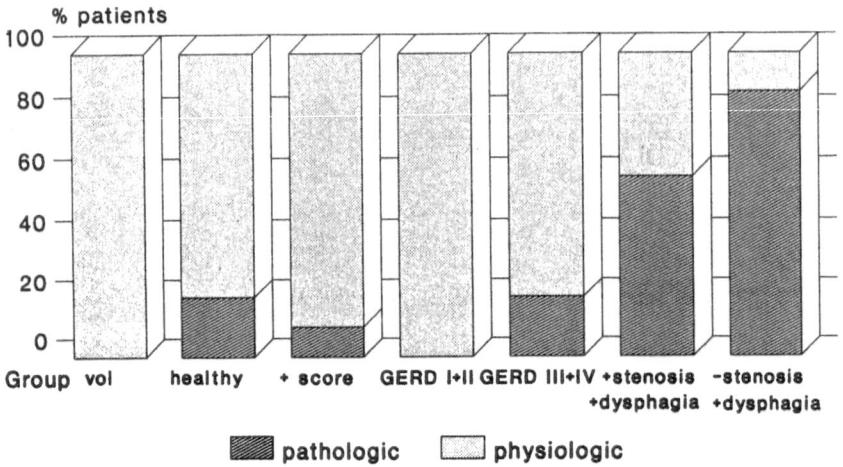

Fig. 4. Percentage of patients with pathologic contractions

with mild degrees of esophagitis as a compensatory mechanism of esophageal musculature that is only slightly injured. In accordance with similar investigations [1–4], we found an increasing amount of pathologic contractions with increasing degrees of mucosal damage. In a further differentiation, we found that there was no linear correlation between the degree of esophagitis and the amount of pathologic contractions. Group 7 comprises patients with GERD and dysphagia. The endoscopic findings in these patients are equivalent to the findings in the patients of group 4 showing mild to moderate degrees of esophagitis; however, we found the highest amount of pathologic contractions in the dysphagia patients in group 7, while there was no motility disorder found in group 4.

Thus, the pathologic contractions in group 7 (88%) cannot be explained by the amount of esophageal mucosal damage as can be done in group 5, comprising patients with GERD and showing severe degrees of esophagitis; the rate of pathologic contractions in group 5 was only 20%. Even the patients in group 6 who presented with stenosis as a complication of a longstanding mucosal damage, only presented pathologic contractions at a rate of 60%. It appears that the pathologic contractions found in group 7 represent primary motility defects wtih a secondary development of esophagitis. The applied methods of investigations, however, are not able to qualitatively separate those primary motility disorders from secondary motility disorders.

In summary, our results suggest two principally opposite pathophysiologic mechanisms within the field of GERD: On the one hand, increasing mucosal damage leads to secondary changes of the esophageal motility pattern, which in turn forms the basis for a progressive inflammatory reaction. On the other hand, primary motility disorders can provoke inflammatory reactions by way of a reduction in the clearance and a prolonged exposure of the esophageal mucosa to acid refluxate.

We conclude from these results that esophageal motility disorders may be the cause of as well as the result of, esophagitis.

The conservative therapeutic approach is similar in both cases: promotion and support of motility by procinetics (Cisapride) and reduction of the acid exposure by H_2-antagonists. In cases of an intended surgical intervention, primary motility disorders may lead to persisting emptying problems of the esophagus.

References

1. Bumm R, Feussner H, Emde C, Hölscher A, Siewert JR (1990) Interaction of gastroesophageal reflux and esophageal motility in healthy men undergoing combined 24-hour Mano/pH-metry. In: Little AG, Ferguson MK, Skinner DB (eds) Diseases of the esophagus, vol. 2. Benign diseases. Futura, Mount Kisco, pp 101–112
2. Walker SJ, Maiorana AM, Chakkaphak A, Ferguson MK, Skinner DB, Little AG (1990) Gastroesophageal reflux and esophageal body function: Correlation with severity of mucosal changes. In: Little AG, Ferguson MK, Skinner DB (eds) Diseases of the esophagus, vol. 2. Benign diseases. Futura, Mount Kisco, pp 113–120
3. Kahrilas PJ, Dodds WJ, Hogan WJ, Kern M, Arndorfer RC, Reece A (1986) Esophageal peristaltic dysfunction in peptic esophagitis. Gastroenterology 91:897–904
4. Williams D, Thompson DG, Marples M, Mani V, Bate M, O'Hanrahan T, Bancewicz J (1990) Improvement in esophageal function after healing of esophagitis. Gut. 31:A1165

5. Singh P, Adamopoulos A, Taylor RH, Colin-Jones DG (1990) Healing of esophagitis does not improve esophageal function. Gut. 31:A1165
6. Eypasch EP, Stein HJ, DeMeester TR, Johansson KE, Barlow AP, Schneider GT (1990) A new technique to define and clarify esophageal motor disorders. Am J Surg 159:144–152
7. DeMeester TR, Johnson LF, Guy JJ, Toscano MS, Hall AN, Skinner DB (1976) Patterns of gastroesophageal reflux in health, and disease. Ann Surg 184:459–470
8. Hotz J (1990) Pathophysiologie der oesophagealen Motilität. Z Gastroenterolog 28 [Suppl 1]:52–55
9. Rühl A, Erckenbrecht JF (1990) Therapeutische Ansätze bei gastroösophagealer Reflux-krankheit: Z Gastroenterol 28 [Suppl 1]:60–66
10. Olsen AM, Schlegel JF (1965) Motility disturbances caused by esophagitis: J Thoracic Surg. 50:607–612
11. Jehle EC, Blum AL (1990) Ambulante Langzeit-pH-Manometrie beim gastrooesophagealen Reflux (GOR): Diagnostikum der Wahl und Basis einer differenzierten Therapie. Z Gastroenterol 28 [Suppl 1]:56–59

Symptoms and Functional Foregut Abnormalities in Patients with Complications of Gastroesophageal Reflux Disease

SEBASTIAN HOEFT, HUBERT J. STEIN, and TOM R. DEMEESTER[1]

Summary. The factors predisposing to the development of Barrett's esophagus in patients with gastroesophageal reflux disease are unclear. Assessing symptoms, esophageal acid and alkaline exposure (pH <2, <3, <4, and >7), lower esophageal sphincter resistance, esophageal clearance function, the gastric secretory state, gastric emptying, and duodenogastric reflux, we compared 15 patients with Barrett's esophagus to 24 patients with esophagitis, and 22 normal subjects. Compared to patients with esophagitis, patients with Barrett's esophagus had less heartburn and regurgitation, but an increased frequency and duration of reflux episodes, and increased percentage of time at pH <2, <3, <4 and pH >7 on ambulatory 24-hour esophageal pH monitoring. This was associated with decreased lower esophageal sphincter resistance, a decreased contraction amplitude in the distal esophagus, an increased frequency of nonperistaltic contractions and contractions <30 mmHg on 24-h ambulatory esophageal motility monitoring, increased basal and stimulated gastric acid secretion, and a higher prevalence of excessive duodenogastric reflux. These data show that despite having less symptoms, patients with Barrett's esophagus have a markedly increased esophageal acid and alkaline exposure compared to patients with esophagitis. This appears to be due to persistent reflux of concentrated gastric acid and duodenal contents across a mechanically defective lower esophageal sphincter, in combination with inefficient esophageal clearance function.

Introduction

Gastroesophageal reflux disease is a common foregut disorder. It is complicated by columnar cell metaplasia in the distal esophagus, the so-called Barrett's

---

[1] Department of Surgery, University of Southern California, 1510 San Pablo Street, Los Angeles, CA 90033-4612, USA

esophagus, in approximately 10%–15% of patients in whom increased esophageal exposure to gastric juice is documented by 24-hour esophageal pH monitoring [1, 2]. The factors predisposing to the development of columnar lined epithelium with its known premalignant potential are unclear. Loss of lower esophageal sphincter resistance, compromised esophageal clearance, and the composition of the refluxate, i.e. gastric acid, pepsin, pancreatic enzymes, and bile acids, may individually or in combination contribute to columnar metaplasia in patients with gastroesophageal reflux disease. Detailed functional studies to assess the relative importance of these factors in a single patient population are, however, not available. We therefore compared symptoms, esophageal acid (pH < 2, pH < 3, pH < 4) and alkaline (pH > 7) exposure, lower esophageal sphincter characteristics, esophageal clearance function, the secretory and motor function of the gastric reservoir, and duodenogastric reflux in patients with Barrett's esophagus to normal volunteers and patients with esophagitis.

Patients and Methods

The study population consisted of 22 normal asymptomatic volunteers (mean age 34.2 years, male/female ratio 13/9) and 39 patients with increased esophageal acid exposure documented by ambulatory 24-h esophageal pH monitoring. Fifteen of the patients (mean age 49.7 years, male/female ratio 10/5) had a Barrett's esophagus diagnosed by the endoscopic observation of a segment of the lower esophagus, at least 3 cm in length, lined by columnar epithelium in continuity with the gastric mucosa. In all 15 patients the presence of columnar epithelium was confirmed by histology. The remaining 24 patients (mean age 45.3 years, male/female ratio 13/11) had esophagitis characterized by mucosal erythema in 12 patients, linear erosions and friability in 7 patients, or coalescent erosions, the so-called cobblestone mucosa, in 5 patients.

Esophageal acid (pH < 2, pH < 3, pH < 4) and alkaline (pH > 7) exposure was measured in all subjects with ambulatory 24-h esophageal pH monitoring. The function of the lower esophageal sphincter was evaluated with standard manometry. The clearance function of the esophageal body was studied with standard and ambulatory 24-h esophageal manometry of the esophageal body. Gastric acid secretion was quantitated in all patients with standard gastric acid analysis. Gastric emptying of a radiolabeled oatmeal was evaluated scintigraphically. Duodenogastric reflux was assessed with cholescintigraphy and gastric pH monitoring. All functional studies were performed as described in detail elsewhere [3, 4]. The severity of heartburn, regurgitation, and dysphagia were scored 0 (symptom not present), 1 (mild), 2 (moderate), or 3 (severe).

Symptoms, esophageal acid and alkaline exposure, manometric parameters of the lower esophageal sphincter and esophageal body, basal and maximum gastric acid secretion, and the gastric half-emptying time were compared between groups using standard tests for nonparametric data sets. The prevalence of a mechanically defective sphincter and excessive duodenogastric reflux was compared between the groups using the Fisher exact test. A P-value below 0.05 was considered significant. All data are expressed as mean ± standard error of the mean (SEM).

Table 1. Symptoms and results of foregut function tests in normal volunteers, patients with esophagitis, and patients with Barrett's Esophagus

	Volunteers	Esophagitis	Barrett's
Heartburn score	0 ± 0	2.3 ± 0.2[1]	1.4 ± 0.3[1,2]
Regurgitation score	0 ± 0	2.1 ± 0.3[1]	1.6 ± 0.2[1,2]
Dysphagia score	0 ± 0	1.1 ± 0.3[1]	1.9 ± 0.4[1,2]
LES resting pressure (mmHg)	12.1 ± 2.1	8.2 ± 1.7[1]	4.3 ± 0.7[1,2]
LES overall length (cm)	3.4 ± 0.5	2.5 ± 0.3[1]	1.7 ± 0.3[1,2]
LES abdominal length (cm)	2.2 ± 0.3	1.7 ± 0.3[1]	0.8 ± 0.2[1,2]
Isolated contractions (%)	3.2 ± 1.2	5.1 ± 1.9	18.8 ± 6.6[1,2]
Contractions <30 mmHg (%)	15.4 ± 3.5	18.9 ± 4.2	32.4 ± 5.9[1,2]
Basal acid output (mMol/h)	—	2.7 ± 0.4	6.3 ± 1.3[2]
Maximum acid output (mMol/h)	—	13.2 ± 3.1	23.4 ± 5.2[2]
DGR on cholescintigraphy	2/22	9/24	7/15
DGR on gastric pH monitoring	0/22	6/24	6/15[2]
Gastric emptying ($t_\frac{1}{2}$ mins)	57.4 ± 4.9	71.1 ± 7.5[1]	75.2 ± 7.7[1]

Means ± SEM,
[1] $P < 0.01$ vs normal volunteers
[2] $P < 0.01$ vs patients with esophagitis
LES, lower esophageal sphincter; DGR, duodenogastric reflux

Results

Compared to patients with esophagitis, patients with Barrett's esophagus complained of less heartburn and regurgitation, but a higher degree of dysphagia (Table 1). On pH monitoring, esophageal acid exposure at all measured thresholds, i.e., pH < 2, pH < 3, and pH < 4, was markedly higher in patients with columnar epithelium than in patients with esophagitis (Fig. 1). This was due to an increased number of reflux episodes and reflux episodes lasting longer than 5 min (Fig. 2). Patients with Barrett's esophagus also had an increased esophageal alkaline exposure, i.e., % time pH > 7, as compared to normal volunteers or patients with esophagitis (Fig. 1).

As shown in Table 1, resting pressure, overall length, and abdominal length of the lower esophageal sphincter were markedly decreased in patients with Barrett's esophagus as compared to patients with esophagitis or normal volunteers. The lower esophageal sphincter was mechanically defective, i.e., resting pressure below 6 mmHg or overall length below 2 cm or abdominal length below 1 cm [3], in 1/25 volunteers (4%), 11/24 patients with esophagitis (46%), and 14/15 patients with Barrett's esophagus (93%).

On standard manometry of the esophageal body, the mean amplitude of contractions in the distal three segments of the esophagus, i.e., 11, 16, and 21 cm below the upper esophageal sphincter, was significantly reduced in patients with Barrett's esophagus as compared to normal volunteers or patients with esophagitis (Fig. 3). This was confirmed by 24-h esophageal motility monitoring which showed a significantly increased frequency of isolated, i.e., nonpropulsive, contractions, and low amplitude (<30 mmHg) contractions in patients with Barrett's esophagus (Table 1).

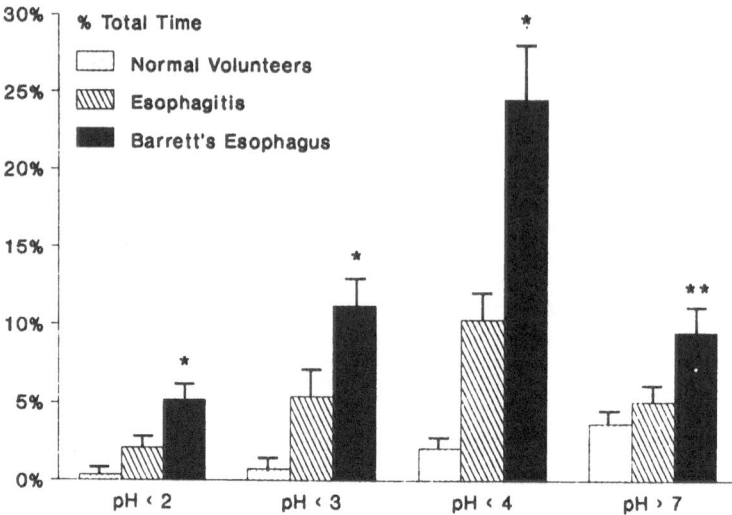

Fig. 1. Mean esophageal acid and alkaline exposure on ambulatory 24-h esophageal pH monitoring in normal volunteers, patients with esophagitis, and patients with Barrett's esophagus. * $P < 0.01$ vs esophagitis and normal volunteers, ** $P < 0.05$ vs esophagitis and normal volunteers

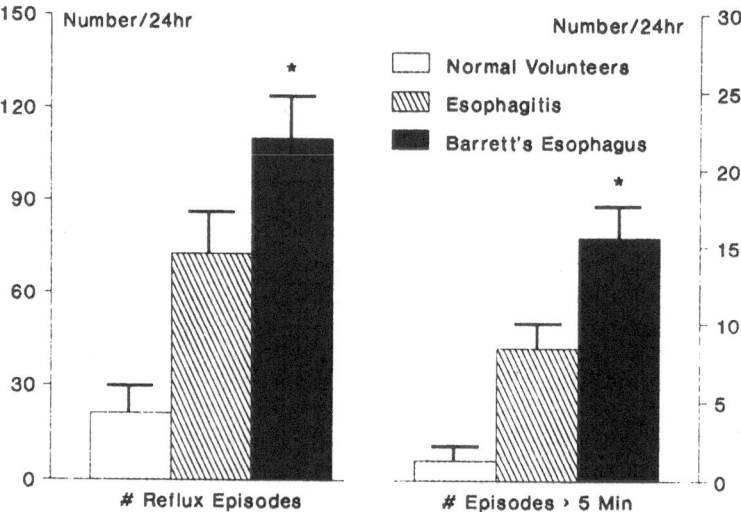

Fig. 2. Frequency of reflux episodes and reflux episodes lasting longer than 5 min (pH < 4) on ambulatory 24-h esophageal pH monitoring in normal volunteers, patients with esophagitis, and patients with Barrett's esophagus. * $P < 0.01$ vs esophagitis and normal volunteers

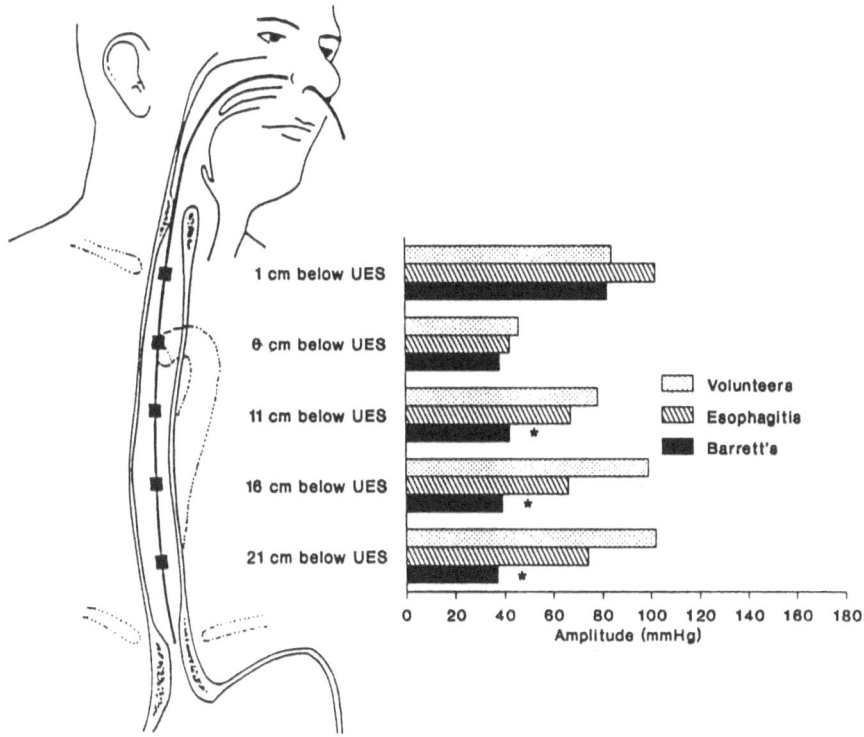

Fig. 3. Mean of amplitude of esophageal contractions following 10 wet swallows measured 1, 6, 11, 16, and 21 cm below the upper esophageal sphincter (*UES*) in normal volunteers, patients with esophagitis, and patients with Barrett's esophagus. * $P < 0.01$ vs esophagitis and normal volunteers

Gastric acid analysis showed a higher basal and stimulated gastric acid secretion in patients with Barrett's esophagus compared to those with esophagitis (Table 1). This was associated with an increased prevalence of excessive duodenogastric reflux on cholescintigraphy and gastric pH monitoring (Table 1). Gastric emptying was delayed in patients with esophagitis and Barrett's esophagus, but there was no difference in gastric emptying between reflux patients with or without columnar epithelium (Table 1).

Discussion

Columnar lined esophagus, i.e., Barrett's esophagus, is today commonly regarded as an acquired condition resulting from replacement of the normal squamous esophageal epithelium by columnar epithelium [1, 2, 5, 6]. The present study indicates that Barrett's esophagus is associated with end-stage reflux disease characterized by a markedly increased esophageal exposure to acidity and alkalinity, the loss of lower esophageal sphincter resistance and clearance function of the esophageal body, increased gastric acid secretion, and excessive duodeno-gastric reflux.

Esophageal pH monitoring showed that the pattern of esophageal exposure to gastric juice is different in patients with Barrett's esophagus as compared to patients with esophagitis. The increased frequency and duration of reflux episodes, with a longer esophageal exposure time to a higher degree of acidity in Barrett's esophagus, appears to be due to a loss of lower esophageal sphincter resistance and effective esophageal clearance, in combination with increased gastric acid secretion. These observations are in concert with those of previous studies and may represent a predisposing condition for the development of columnar cell metaplasia in patients with gastroesophageal reflux disease [7, 8, 9].

An important observation was that the mean amplitude of contractions in the distal esophagus is decreased in patients with Barrett's esophagus. On ambulatory 24-h esophageal motility and pH monitoring, this was paralleled by a markedly increased frequency of isolated contractions, contractions with an amplitude below 30 mmHg, and an increased frequency of reflux episodes lasting longer than 5 min indicating a compromised clearance function of the esophageal body. This is supported by the observation that nonpropulsive contractions or con-tractions of low amplitude, even if they are peristaltic, may not propel swallowed food or clear the esophagus of refluxed gastric contents [10]. In addition to prolonging the clearance of refluxed gastric contents, the observed loss of esophageal contractility may also be responsible for the higher degree of dys-phagia observed in patients with Barrett's esophagus.

In contrast to patients with esophagitis, patients with Barrett's esophagus also had an increased exposure time to pH > 7 on esophageal pH monitoring. If there is assiduous attention to the technical details of the esophageal pH monitoring, the presence of an increased esophageal exposure to pH > 7 reflects reflux gastric juice containing bile or other duodenal contents [11]. This is confirmed by the high prevalence of excessive duodenogastric reflux in patients with Barrett's esophagus observed in the present and previous studies [12, 13].

Regardless of the underlying physiologic abnormality leading to columnar cell metaplasia in patients with gastroesophageal reflux disease, current medical therapy is aimed at suppressing its acid component. In patients with a defective lower esophageal sphincter and excessive duodenogastric reflux, this approach allows the duodenal components of the refluxate to continue to cause tissue destruction. This may explain why medical therapy fails to reduce the prevalence of Barrett's esophagus and allows upward progression of the columnar epithelium [14]. In contrast, reconstruction of an effective barrier at the gastroesophageal junction by a surgical antireflux procedure can effectively abolish reflux of any gastric content, halt the progression of columnar epithelium, and provide more effective protection against malignant degeneration of the columnar epithelium than medical management [15, 16]. When performing an antireflux procedure consideration must be given to the reduced length and the compromised con-tractility of the esophageal body. In this situation a Collis gastroplasty with a Belsey antireflux repair is most suitable to avoid postoperative dysphagia and breakdown of the repair [4].

References

1. Sarr MG, Hamilton FR, Marone GC, Cameron JL (1985) Barrett's esophagus: Its prevalence and association with symptoms of gastroesophageal reflux. Am J Surg 149:187–193
2. Winters C, Spurling TJ, Chobanian SJ, et al (1987) Barrett's esophagus: A prevalent, occult complication of gastroesophageal reflux disease. Gastroenterology 92:118–124
3. DeMeester TR, Stein HJ, Fuchs KH (1991) Diagnostic studies in the evaluation of the esophagus: Physiologic diagnostic studies. In: Shackelford RT, Zuidema GD (eds) Surgery of the alimentary tract, vol 1, 3rd edn. WB Saunders, Philadelphia, pp 94–126
4. Stein HJ, DeMeester TR, Hinder RA (1992) Outpatient physiological testing and surgical management of foregut motor disorders. Curr Probl Surg 29:415–555
5. Naef AP, Savary M, Ozello L (1975) Columnar lined lower esophagus: An acquired lesion with malignant predisposition. Report on 140 cases of Barrett's esophagus with 12 adenocarcinomas. J Thorac Cardiovasc Surg 70:826–834
6. Iascone C, DeMeester TR, Little AG, Skinner DB (1983) Barrett's esophagus: Functional assessment, proposed pathogenesis and surgical therapy. Arch Surg 118:543–549
7. Gillen P, Keeling P, Byrne PJ, Hennessy TPJ (1987) Barrett's oesophagus: pH profile. Br J Surg 74:774–776
8. Mulholland MW, Reid, Levine DS, Rubin CE (1989) Elevated gastric acid secretion in patients with Barrett's metaplastic epithelium. Dig Dis Sci 34:1329–1335
9. Stein HJ, DeMeester TR, Naspetti R, Jamieson J, Naspetti R, Perry R (1991) The three dimensional lower esophageal sphincter pressure profile in gastroesophageal reflux disease. Ann Surg 214:374–384
10. Kahrilas PJ, Dodds WJ, Hogan WJ (1988) Effect of peristaltic dysfunction on esophageal volume clearance. Gastroenterology 94:73–80
11. Stein HJ, Feussner H, Barthlen W, DeMeester TR, Siewert JR (1992) Alkalischer gastroösophagealer Reflux—Quantifizierung und klinische Relevanz. Langenbecks Arch Chir For Suppl 87–91
12. Attwood SEA, DeMeester TR, Bremner CB, Barlow AP, Hinder RA (1989) Alkaline gastroesophageal reflux: Implications in the development of complications in Barrett's columnar-lined lower esophagus. Surgery 106:764–770
13. Waring JP, Legrand J, Chibichian A, Sanowski RA (1990) Duodenogastric reflux in patients with Barrett's esophagus. Dig Dis Sci 35:759–762
14. Bremner CG (1989) Barrett's oesophagus. Br J Surg 76:995–996
15. DeMeester TR, Attwood SEA, Smyrk TC, Therkildsen DH, Hinder RA (1990) Surgical therapy in Barrett's esophagus. Ann Surg 212:528–542
16. McCallum RW, Polepalle S, Davenport K, Boyd S (1991) Role of antireflux surgery against dysplasia in Barrett's esophagus. Gastroenterology 100:(A)121

The Value of a Scoring System in Gastroesophageal Reflux Disease: Does It Predict the Response to Surgical Treatment?

P.F. Crookes, R.M. Bremner, M. Costantini, S.F. Hoeft, J.A. Hagen,
J.H. Peters, and T.R. DeMeester[1]

Introduction

Gastroesophageal reflux disease (GERD) is the commonest disease of the upper gastrointestinal tract. Despite its high prevalence in Western society, there is little agreement on the indications for, and outcome of, antireflux surgery. One factor contributing to this controversy is the difficulty in comparing results from different institutions, because of the lack of an agreed method of assessing the spectrum of severity of GERD from a given institution.

The ISDE Subcommittee for Classification of Gastroesophageal Reflux Disease recently proposed a simple classification for GERD in which a score is given for three separate components of the disease process. The aim of this study was to assess the value of this scoring system in predicting the outcome of surgery in GERD.

Patients and Methods

The AFP score is calculated by giving a score for each of three separate components of the disease, namely **A**natomical (presence of hiatal herniation), **F**unctional (esophageal acid exposure), and **P**athologic (presence of mucosal injury). The derivation of these scores is described in Table 1, and scores for each component are summed to produce the AFP score.

One hundred and thirty-five patients undergoing primary antireflux surgery were studied. The indications for surgery were for control of symptoms or complications of GERD, or for repair of paraesophageal hernia. All patients had barium esophagogram, upper GI endoscopy, esophageal manometry and

[1] University of Southern California, School of Medicine Department of Surgery 1510 San Pablo Street, Suite 514 Los Angeles, CA 90033-4612, USA

Table 1. Derivation of AFP score

A = Anatomy	0	No hernia
	1	Small or intermittent hernia
	2	Constant hernia >3 cm on endoscopy
	3	Mixed or paraesophageal hernia
F = Function	0	Time pH <4 0%–4%
	1	Time pH <4 4%–8%
	2	Time pH <4 8%–12%
	3	Time pH <4 >12%
P = Pathology	0	No mucosal changes
	1	Isolated erosive mucosal lesions
	2	Confluent erosive mucosal lesions
	3	Stricture, ulcer, or shortening

Table 2. Antireflux surgery performed in 135 patients

Procedure	No. of patients
Nissen fundoplication	119
(Abdominal)	89
(Thoracic)	30
Belsey	8
Collis-Belsey	2
Esophageal replacement	4
Hill	1
Angelchik	1

24-h pH monitoring. Stationary esophageal motility was performed using an eight-lumen catheter perfused via a pneumohydraulic low compliance pump, and 24-h esophageal pH was measured using a glass pH electrode positioned 5 cm above the manometrically determined upper border of the lower esophageal sphincter, as previously described [1]. The AFP score was calculated for each patient based on these investigations.

The operations performed in the 135 patients are listed in Table 2. Outcome after surgery was assessed symptomatically on a standard questionnaire at clinic visits or by telephone interview. Follow-up ranged from 6–96 months (median 50 months). Patient satisfaction with surgery was graded from 1 (no symptoms at all) to 4 (persistent or recurrent symptoms or troublesome side effects not controlled by medication) similar to Visick grading. Patients with grade 1 or 2 symptoms were classified as having a good result, and grade 3 or 4 symptoms were classified as a poor result. In addition to symptomatic follow-up, a subgroup of 26 patients volunteered to have follow-up endoscopy, manometry, and pH testing, allowing the calculation of the AFP score postoperatively.

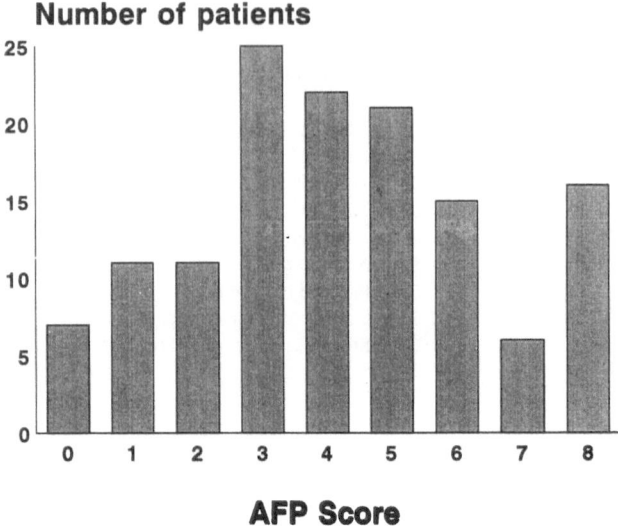

Fig. 1. The spectrum of severity as assessed by the AFP score in 135 patients

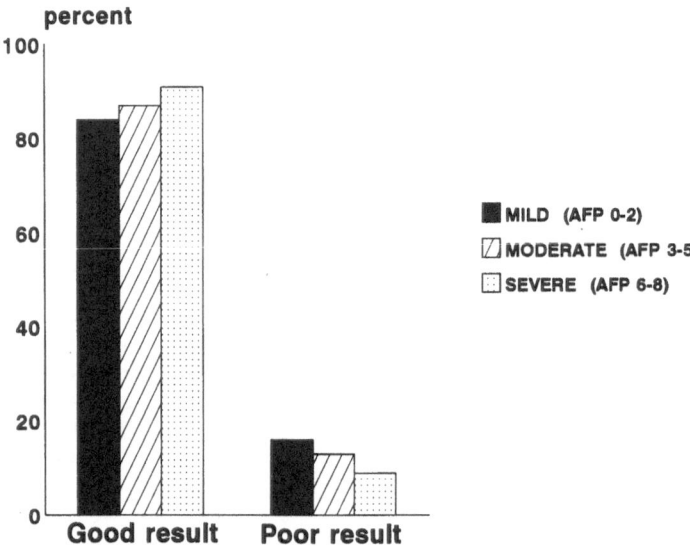

Fig. 2. The symptomatic outcome of antireflux surgery in patients with disease classified as mild, moderate, or severe using the AFP score

Results

Figure 1 shows the spectrum of disease as shown by the AFP score in the 135 patients. Patients were classified as having mild (AFP score 0–2), moderate (score 3–5), or severe (score 6–8) disease. Figure 2 shows that symptomatic

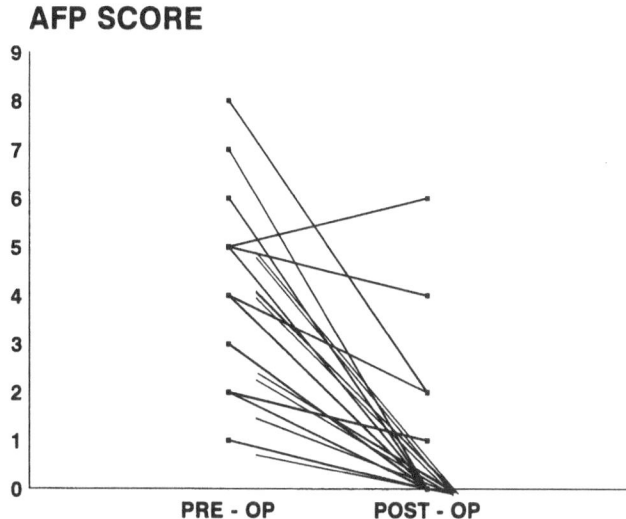

Fig. 3. Individual pre- and postoperative AFP scores in 26 patients studied postoperatively

Table 3. Reason for patient dissatisfaction in mild versus severe disease

Mild Disease (AFP 0–2)	5
Persistent cough	4
Recurrent reflux	1
Severe Disease (AFP 3–8)	13
Recurrent reflux	4
Gastritis	6
Persistent dysphagia	1
Scleroderma	1
Post-thoracotomy pain	1

outcome after surgery was not related to the preoperative severity of disease as assessed by AFP score, in that a similar percentage of poor results was seen in each category. In the 26 patients with postoperative studies allowing the calculation of a postoperative AFP score, the AFP score was reduced from a mean of 4.8 preoperatively to 0.5 postoperatively. However, the five patients with postoperative AFP scores of 1 or greater were not those with high preoperative scores (Fig. 3).

The reasons for poor results after surgery were analyzed (Table 3). In patients with mild disease, the commonest reason was persistence of respiratory symptoms. In those with moderate or severe disease (AFP score 3–8), epigastric pain and nausea suggestive of gastritis was the commonest reason for patient dissatisfaction. Four patients developed recurrent reflux in this group.

Discussion

The need for an agreed measure of severity in GERD is widely accepted. Using the proposed scoring system, this study has shown that in our surgical practice, all degrees of severity of GERD are referred for surgery. The data also show that preoperative severity of GERD as assessed by the AFP score does not predict the symptomatic outcome of antireflux surgery. One reason for this may be because the associated respiratory and gastric symptoms are not assessed by this scoring system. The subgroup with paraesophageal hiatal hernias all had uniformly good results after surgery, and the AFP score was not relevant to decision making in that condition.

Other workers have described the use of the AFP score to give an objective assessment of the effect of antireflux surgery [2]. Although our results are in agreement with Feussner et al. [2], limited conclusions can be drawn from the postoperative AFP score, since the patients in whom the AFP score is obtained represent a selected subgroup. Comparison of pre- and postoperative AFP scores may be useful in giving the surgeon an objective means of assessing if the goal of the operation has been attained, and may encourage him to modify the technique in the light of the results.

References

1. Zaninotto G, DeMeester TR, Schwizer W, et al (1988) The lower esophageal sphincter in health and disease. Am J Surg 155:104–111
2. Feussner H, Petri A, Walker S, et al (1991) The modified AFP score: An attempt to make the results of anti-reflux surgery comparable. Br J Surg 78:942–6

Patients With Gastroesophageal Reflux: Differences in Esophageal pH-Monitoring Between Patients Undergoing Surgery (Nissen) and Patients Undergoing Medical Treatment

S.R. Gómez, G.E. Moreno, P.I. Gonzalez, G.J. Seoane, S.A. Calle, S.J. Palomo, M. Marcello, L.A. Lopez, and M. Musella[1]

Introduction

The pathologic gastroesophageal reflux (PGER) can be treated medically or surgically [1–6]. To date, there is not an accepted criterion to divide the patients in each category of treatment. Neither the symptoms, manometry, image studies (baritate or isotopic) nor endoscopy lesions alone have achieved this purpose. The introduction of the ambulatory esophageal pH monitoring for 24 h has permited us a more reliable method for the diagnosis of PGER [7–9].

In the present study, we tried to identify differences in esophageal pH monitoring between patients medically and surgically treated. If differences were present, we could establish the more appropriate treatment for each patient based on an objective criterion.

Material and Methods

We prospectively analyzed 51 patients with PGER (typical symptomatology, endoscopy, imaging studies—baritate and isotopic—manometry and pH esophageal monitoring compatible with PGER) treated medically or surgically, based on the efficacy of medical treatment or esophageal complications. We established two groups Group A consisted of 20 patients who were surgically treated by means of Nissen fundoplication due to (a) failure of correct medical treatment to control symptoms ($n = 13$), (b) hemorrhage secondary to esophagitis and/or gastritis of the hiatal hernia ($n = 5$), and (c) esophageal stricture resistant to dilatations ($n = 2$). Group B consisted of 31 patients with successful medical

[1]Servicio de Cirugia General y AP. Digestivo C. University Hospital "12 de Octubre", Carretera de Andalucia Km. 5, 400, 28041, Madrid, Spain

Table 1. Characteristics of groups

	Group A	Group B	P
Mean age (years)	46.1 ± 3.7	47.6 ± 2.9	ns
Sex M/F	11/9	14/17	ns
Symptoms (%)			
Heartburn	90	93.5	ns
Pain	65	54.8	ns
Regurgitation	55	41.9	ns
Dysphagia	20	25.8	ns
Time with PGER	7.5 ± 1.3	4.5 ± 0.7	0.05
Number of symptoms	3 ± 0.2	3 ± 0.2	ns
Endoscopy (%)			
Esophagitis 0–I	50	74.2	ns
Esophagitis II–IV	50	25.8	ns
Manometry			
LESP (mmHg)	11.3 ± 1.4	14.7 ± 1.2	ns
LESL (cm)	2.7 ± 0.2	3.1 ± 0.1	ns
Simult. waves (%)	7.8 ± 5.5	14.1 ± 4	ns
Amplitude (mmHg)	62.5 ± 8.6	64.8 ± 9	ns
W duration (s)	5.5 ± 0.2	5.3 ± 0.3	ns

W, waves; *LESP*, lower esophageal sphincter pressure; *LESL*, lower esophageal sphincter length; *ns*, not significant; *PGER*, pathologic gastroesophageal reflux

treatment against PGER. Patients' characteristics (mean age, sex, symptomatology, and time with PGER) are shown in Table 1.

We performed endoscopy, manometry, imaging studies (baritate and isotopic) and esophageal pH monitoring for 24 h in both group A and group B.

Surgical Technique

We performed an esophageal fundoplication of 360 degrees through an abdominal approach in group A patients. The length of the fundoplication with gastric fundus was from 3 to 4 cm and moreover, we closed the diaphragmatic crura with 3–4 stitches [6].

Medical Treatment

We administered metoclopramide and H_2-blockers which were taken in conjunction with the appropriate diet regimen and postural habits. Intermittent ingestion of antacids was used against transitory heartburn.

Ambulatory pH Monitoring

We used a portable pH meter (Proxima light). The glass probes were positioned by means of instantaneous esophagogastric pH measures with the pH meter. A posterior-anterior (P-A) and lateral chest x-ray permitted us to check the correct

Table 2. Characteristics of esophageal pH monitoring

	Group A (n = 20)	Group B (n = 31)	P
Total reflux time (min)	404.9 ± 80	387 ± 63	ns
Upright	159.4 ± 43.8	187 ± 33	
Supine	245.4 ± 47.2	200 ± 40	
No. of episodes >5 min	11.3 ± 1.6	6.5 ± 1.2	ns
Upright	4.5 ± 1.2	5.6 ± 1.1	
Supine	6.7 ± 1.2	5.6 ± 1.1	
Duration longest episode	106.1 ± 30	72.1 ± 14.6	ns
Upright	67.6 ± 31	40.2 ± 9	
Supine	60 ± 12	62.4 ± 15	
Number of episodes	119 ± 16.3	156 ± 18.7	ns
Upright	80.6 ± 16.6	107 ± 13.3	
Supine	38.4 ± 6.5	48 ± 9.2	
Clearance (min)	4.1 ± 0.8	3.5 ± 0.9	ns
Upright	1.9 ± 0.6	3.8 ± 2	ns
Supine	13.3 ± 5.2	6.2 ± 1.7	0.05
Median esophageal pH	4.6 ± 0.2	4.2 ± 0.3	ns
DeMeester test value	163.9 ± 31	162 ± 26.4	ns

position of the probes (the end of the esophageal probe was 5 cm over the cardia). The pH readings were stored and processed by the Proxima computer program.

Statistical Analysis

The Student's t-test was used for statistical evaluation of the data. The values were expresed as the mean ± SE.

Results

The time with PGER was longer in group A (Table 1). We did not find any statistically significant differences between the two groups in endoscopy lesions or manometric values (Table 1). Table 2 shows the esophageal pH monitoring characteristics for each group. Only the esophageal clearance in the supine position was worse in the surgical group ($P < 0.05$).

Discussion

To date, in spite of the sophistication of the diagnostic techniques for PGER, the appearance of severe esophageal complications or the failure of the medical treatment to adequately control symptomatology result in the need for surgery in patients with PGER. Esophageal pH monitoring is a very sensitive technique for the diagnosis of PGER, but in our experience it does not establish (quantitatively) clinically useful differences between the patients with medical treatment and operated patients. Therefore, ambulatory esophageal pH monitoring is not a useful for establishing better therapeutic options for patients with PGER. Perhaps, the time of day or the body position in which the PGER predominantly is present could be important for the therapeutic indication. Fuchs et al. [7] think that the PGER in the supine position is more dangerous and they operates on patients with this type of esophageal reflux. Therefore, in our experience, although the operated patients (group A) had a worse clearance in the supine position (generally at night), they did not have more esophageal lesions or quantitatively more total reflux (Table 2). We think that the best approach for a more correct treatment of patients with PGER is a global qualitative and quantitative evaluation of the esophageal pH monitoring over 24 h which can be used to augment other diagnostic techniques.

References

1. Johnson F, DeMeester T (1981) Evaluation of elevation of the bed, bethanechol and antiacid foam tablets on gastroesophageal reflux. Dig Dis Sci 26:673–680
2. Hill LD (1967) An effective operation for hiatal hernia: An 8-year appraisal. Ann Surg 166:681–683
3. Jamielson GG (1987) Anti-reflux operations: How do they work? Br J Surg 74:155–156
4. Lieberman DA (1897) Medical therapy for chronic reflux esophagitis. Arch Intern Med 147:1717–1720
5. Lieberman DA, Keefe EB (1986) Treatment of severe reflux esophagitis with cimetidine and metoclopramide. Ann Intern Med 104:21–26
6. Nissen R, Rosseti M (1965) Surgery of hiatal and other diaphragmatic hernias. J Int Coll Surg 43:663–668
7. Fuchs K, DeMeester TR, Albertucci M (1987) Specificity and sensitivity of objective diagnosis of gastroesophageal reflux disease. Surg 102:575–580
8. DeMeester TR, Johnson LF, Guy JJ, Toscano M, Hall A, Skinner D (1976) Patterns of gastroesophageal reflux in health and disease. Ann Surg 184:459–470
9. DeMeester TR, Ching-I W, Wernly J, et al. (1980) Technique, indications, and clinical use of 24-hour esophageal pH monitoring. J Thorac Cardiovasc Surg 79:656–670

Indication and Technique of Laparoscopic Antireflux Operations

K.-H. Fuchs, S.M. Freys, J. Heimbucher, and A. Thiede[1]

Introduction

The basic pathophysiologic abnormality of gastroesophageal reflux disease is an excessive exposure of the esophagus to gastric juice, resulting in damage to the esophageal mucosa [1]. Prior to any therapy, a precise diagnosis as to the cause of this abnormal exposure is necessary. Therefore, nowadays antireflux surgery should not be planned without a diagnostic workup, including detection of the functional defect [2]. There are three main causes of gastroesophageal reflux disease known which can occur isolated or in combination. These causes are a mechanically defective distal esophageal sphincter, inefficient esophageal clearance of refluxed gastric juice, and abnormalities of the stomach or gastroduodenal segment such as increased gastric pressure, excessive gastric dilatation, delayed gastric emptying, and/or increased gastric acid secretion [1, 3].

Diagnostic Considerations

Mechanical failure of the antireflux barrier is diagnosed by measuring inadequate mechanical characteristics of the lower esophageal sphincter by manometry. This criterion was defined as having any one or a combination of the following: an average lower esophageal sphincter pressure of less than 6 mmHg, an average lower esophageal sphincter length exposed to the positive pressure environment of the abdomen of 1 cm or less, and average lower esophageal sphincter overall resting length of 2 cm or less [4, 5]. The most common cause of a mechanically incompetent cardia is inadequate lower esophageal sphincter pressure, but the

[1] Chirurgische Universitätsklinik Würzburg, Josef-Schneider-Str. 2, 8700 Würzburg, Germany

efficiency of a normal lower esophageal sphincter pressure can be nullified by an inadequate abdominal length or an abnormally short overall resting length.

Increased esophageal exposure to gastric juice can also be caused by a failure of the propulsive pump-like function of the body of the esophagus resulting in inefficient esophageal clearance of refluxed gastric juice [6, 7]. This can be due to damage to the esophageal wall by noxes such as excessive reflux, a myogenic abnormality, a motility disorder, or reduction in salivary flow.

An increased esophageal exposure to gastric juice, secondary to a gastric disorder, has not been recognized as a cause of the disease for a long time. Clinical studies have indicated that nearly 30% of patients with gastroesophageal reflux have a disturbance of upper gastrointestinal motility that is manifested by delayed gastric emptying [8]. This results in gastric retention and an increased probability of reflux through a normal sphincter. Gastric distention can result in shortening of the length of a normal sphincter, like the shortening of the neck of a balloon on inflation. With excessive distention, the sphincter is shortened, resulting in low resistance to prevent reflux. There is evidence that increased gastric acid secretion can lead to increased esophageal acid exposure [9, 10]. This is most likely due to augmentation of physiologic reflux by increased gastric volume and the high acidity of that volume.

Indications for Operation

Antireflux surgery is symptom-driven and the indication for surgery is the presence of uncontrolled symptoms of heartburn or regurgitation. Since surgery is a mechanical therapeutic approach to gastroesophageal reflux disease, patients with a mechanically incompetent cardia will benefit the most from surgery. Consequently, an antireflux procedure should be considered only for those patients who have: (1) uncontrolled symptoms of increased acid esophageal exposure to gastric juice; i.e., heartburn, regurgitation, chest pain, chronic cough, wheezing, or dysphagia; (2) a documented increase in esophageal exposure to gastric juice by 24-hour esophageal pH monitoring; and (3) a documented mechanical defect of the lower esophageal sphincter [4].

However, these clear statements are not fully accepted by gastroenterologists. At present, potent medication is available to reduce gastric acid secretion, which allows for successful reduction of reflux symptoms as well as pathologic acid exposure of the esophageal mucosa, as long as the medication is taken by the patient. But long-term treatment with these drugs over years can cause side effects and patients' compliance can be a problem. Many gastroenterologists do not discuss any more with their patients the possibility of surgical treatment. However, with the advance of minimally invasive surgery, surgeons have the opportunity to gain new confidence from their gastroenterologic colleagues and the patients.

With a high prevalence of gastroesophageal reflux disease in western populations, the optimal therapy of this disease is very important. Most of the reflux patients, especially patients with border line sphincter incompetence of the lower esophageal sphincter will be treated with a high rate of success by conservative antisecretory therapy with H2-blockers, antiacids, or Omeprazol, a proton-pump inhibitor. In these patients, the existing esophagitis is usually minor and will be reduced quickly, and the patients will be symptom-free within a few weeks. However, in a lot of patients compliance can be a problem. In young patients, the willingness for long-term medical treatment—in many cases lifelong—still leads to request for surgery in order to gain a permanent solution of this disease. On the other hand, it must be emphasized that a large group of patients with a defective antireflux mechanism continue treatment over a long period of time with unsuccessful medical therapy resulting in the development of complications, such as ulcers, bleeding, and strictures.

Therefore, there is a need for definitive surgical therapy of the functional defect. The procedure must be safe with minimal morbitity for the patient. It is obvious that the new laparoscopic techniques should be applied in these operations. Looking at the design of a 180° hemifundoplication, it is evident that this kind of operation can be done laparoscopically with very limited risk in a reasonable time.

Prior to a surgical antireflux repair, two important factors must be considered [11]. First, the patient should be queried for complaints of epigastric pain, nausea, vomiting, and loss of appetite. These symptoms can be due to bile reflux gastritis which occurs independently or in association with gastroesophageal reflux. The problem is usually seen in patients who have had previous upper GI surgery, although this is not always the case. The correction of only the incompetent cardia in such patients will result in a disgruntled individual who continues to complain of nausea and epigastric pain made worse by eating. Gastric function tests such 24-hour gastric pH monitoring, and gastric emptying scintigraphy will reveal the underlying gastric causes of reflux disease. Second, the propulsive force of the body of the esophagus should be measured. There should be sufficient power to propel a bolus of food through the newly constructed valve. This is done by stationary and 24-hour ambulatory esophageal manometry or a radioisotope esophageal transit time study [12]. Failure to recognize inadequate esophageal contractility can lead to postoperative dysphagia.

Available Antireflux Procedures

Currently, the Nissen fundoplication, the Belsey Mark IV operation, the Toupet posterior hemifundoplication, the Watson anterior fundoplication, the Hill posterior gastropexy, and the Angelchik prosthesis are the most widely published antireflux repairs [13–19].

Aware of the complications and troublesome side effects of the full wrap of the Nissen fundoplication, authors have looked for better alternatives [14, 16, 17, 20]. The hemifundoplication of Watson and that of Toupet involve a 180° wrap with less obstructing effect on the distal espophagus, causing less gas-bloat and persistent dysphagia. Critics comment that there is a higher risk of reflux recurrency due to the limited sphincter augmentation and a possible higher risk of wrap breakdown.

The primary goal of all antireflux operations is the mechanical augmentation of the high pressure zone in the distal oesophagus to improve the resistance of the lower esophogeal sphincter. However, extensive augmentation bears side effects. Simple gastropexy or fundopexy have not been successful in open surgery to sufficiently correct pathologic gastroesophageal reflux. On the basis of the pathophysiologic background of gastroesophageal reflux disease, it is known that partial and especially 360° fundoplication techniques are able to control pathologic gastroesophageal reflux completely since their effect of augmentation of the distal esophageal high pressure zone is greatest. Troublesome symptoms due to mechanical problems of the total 360° fundoplication, such as the gas-bloat phenomenon or persistent dysphagia postoperatively, have been reported and have been a major reason why most gastroenterologists object to this kind of operation [14, 20, 21]. However, in the past year, surgeons have with increas-ing understanding of the pathophysiology tried to limit the size of the fundoplica-tion and to successfully reduce postoperative persistent dysphagia [14].

Laparoscopic Techniques

Without question, the 360° Nissen fundoplication is the most popular antireflux operation among the surgeons. However, the original version has been modified with a great variety. We think the full 360° Nissen fundoplication is indicated in patients with a clear incompetence of the lower esophageal sphincter, with severe symptoms, and/or severe reflux esophagitis refractory to conserva-tive medical treatment. We performed the laparoscopic Nissen procedure in the same way as we do the open 360° wrap in laparotomy according to the DeMeester-Nissen sandwich technique. In patients with concomitant esophageal pump failure, we prefer a hemifundoplication. In addition, as an alternative for long-term treatment of gastric acid reduction, such as H2-blocker or Omeprazol therapy especially in patients with border line incompetence of the lower esoph-ageal sphincter, we prefer the usefulness of a 180° partial fundoplication or hemifundoplication.

The technique involves the usual tools for laparoscopic operations. The pro-cedure can be facilitated by a number of special instruments, such as curved dissection forceps to work behind the esophagus and special grasping forceps for the stomach, but it also can be done with the regular instruments. It has to be emphasized, that a laparoscopic Babcock clamp is optimal to hold the distal esophagus and stomach in order to optimally dissect the target area. Via a supraumbilical incision after insufflation of a proper pneumoperitoneum a 10 mm trocar is entered into the abdominal cavity and a 30° 10 mm optic is inserted. Additional 10 mm trocars preferably with automatic valves, are brought into the right and left subcostal area. Via the trocar in the right upper quadrant, the left liver lobe is held back to allow dissection of the hiatus. The left lateral trocar is used to pull the stomach and especially the gastroesophageal junction caudally in order to expose that area. Then via the other two trocars with scissors and grasping forceps, the gastroesophageal junction and especially a present hiatal hernia is dissected. The preparation starts left from the angle of HIS cranially to the right. Care is taken not to harm the branches of the vagal nerve. The dissection of the lower esophageal sphincter and the hiatal crura is taken over to the right. These structures must clearly be identified. The proximal fundus is also mobilized towards the spleen but without extensive dissection of the small gastric vessels all the way along the spleen. It must be possible that the fundic flap can be pulled with ease across the lower esophageal sphincter towards the right crus of the hiatus. If that cannot be done with ease, mobiliza-

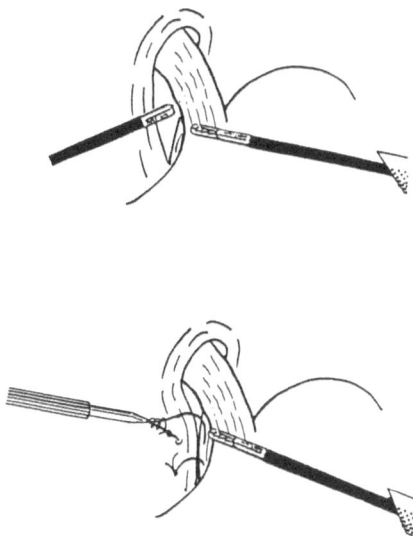

Fig. 1. Approximation of hiatal crura and posterior hiatoplasty with two endosutures

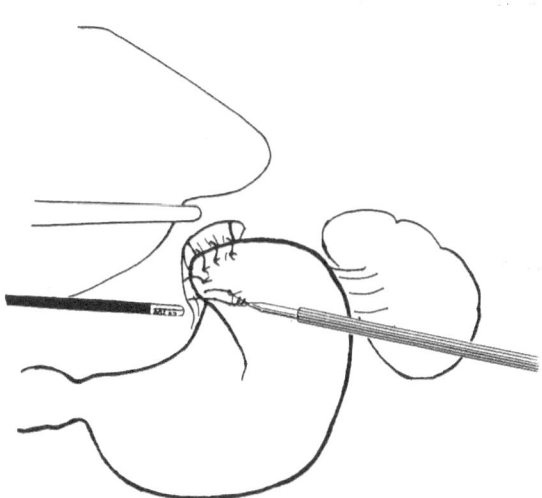

Fig. 2. Anterior hemifundoplication (180°) with fixation of the fundic flap at the lower esophageal sphincter and the right crus

tion of the fundus must be expanded, but usually this is not necessary. Now the posterior area of the esophagus is dissected by pulling the gastroesophageal junction up with a Babcock placed through the middle trocar using the left lateral trocar for dissection of the hiatal crura. In most cases, a posterior hiatal approximation and suture is performed using two u-stitches in extracorporal technique (Fig. 1). Then the fundic flap is fixed with two or three non-resorbable endosutures at the middle portion of the lower esophageal sphincter. The right lateral part of the flap is fixed on the right crura with another two to three sutures. Again these sutures are closed with extracorporal tying. Now the antireflux 180° anterior hemifundoplication is finished (Fig. 2).

In case of a defective lower esophageal sphincter, the mobilization of the fundus is carried out further down dissecting the short gastric vessels between clips. When the fundus is completely mobilized, a floppy wrap is possible. If necessary also a posterior crural closure of the hiatus is performed. Then the posterior portion of the fundus is brought around the posterior wall of the esophagus with a Babcock clamp and taken over at the right crus with another Babcock (Fig. 3). Now the 360° fundoplication is finished by typing one u-stitch

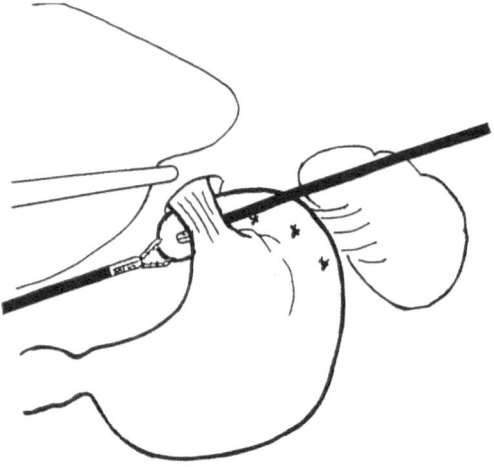

Fig. 3. Preparation of the gastroesophageal junction for a 360° Nissen fundoplication

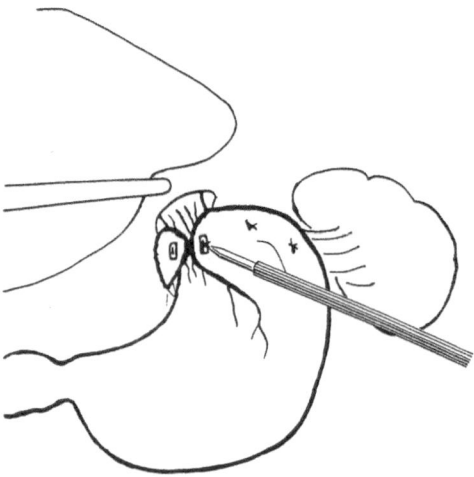

Fig. 4. Wrap of a DeMeester-Nissen fundoplication (360°) in the sandwich technique

with non resorbable 0 suture in the sandwich technique (Fig. 4). This involves also the anterior right lateral wall of the lower oesphageal sphincter. In order to place the wrap as loose as possible, a 45 french NG tube is placed into the cardia during the suturing procedure.

Discussion

Early functional results show an improvement of the lower esophageal sphincter pressure with less effect on sphincter length. The symptomatic improvement of the patients has been shown in comparison to patients after laparotomy. The recovery time of the patients in the first postoperative days after the laparoscopic procedure has been shortened, as is the case with other laparoscopic operations as well [22]. Patients can be discharged quicker. However, one has to wait to objectively decide whether the laparoscopic techniques, especially the 180° hemifundoplication, has better long-term results than long-term medication treatment. Until then, laparoscopic antireflux procedures should be performed in centers under study control in order to gather as much data as possible.

A wide-spread application of laparoscopic techniques in antireflux surgery, especially without objective assessment of the functional defects of patients without clear indications can cause bad postoperative results for the patients. The consequences of this can be distastrous, since it generates a negative criticism of laparoscopic techniques. Such criticism, however, can only be prevented if these operations are performed after extensive training, with the right indications, and with minimally invasive techniques.

References

1. DeMeester TR (1985) Gastroesophageal reflux disease. In: Moody FG, Carey LC, Jones RS, et al (eds) Surgical treatment of digestive disease. Year Book Medical, Chicago, pp 132–158
2. Fuchs KH, DeMeester TR, Albertucci M (1987) Specificity and sensitivity of objective diagnosis of gastroesophageal reflux disease. Surgery (102) pp 4:575–580
3. DeMeester TR, Fuchs KH (1988) Comparison of operations for uncomplicated reflux disease. In: Jamieson GG (ed) Surgery of the Oesophagus. Churchill Livingstone, pp 299–308
4. Bonavina L, Evander A, DeMeester TR, Walther W, Cheng SC, Palazzo L, Concannon JL (1986) Length of the distal esophageal sphincter and competency of the cardia. Am J Surg 151:25–34
5. Zaninotto G, DeMeester RR, Schwizer W, Johansson KE, Cheng SC (1988) The lower esophageal sphincter in health and disease. Am J Surg 155:104–111
6. Joelsson BE, DeMeester RR, Skinner DB, et al (1982) The role of the esophageal body in the antireflux mechanism. Surg 92:417–424
7. Kahrilas PJ, Dodds WJ, Hogan WG, et al (1986) Esophageal peristalic dysfunction in peptic esophagitis. Gastroenterology 91:897
8. Schwizer W, Hinder RA, DeMeester TR (1989) Does delayed gastric emptying contribute to gastroesophageal reflux disease? Am J Surg 157:74–81
9. Boesby S (1977) Relationship between gastroesophageal acid reflux, basal gastroesophageal sphincter pressure and gastric acid secretion. Scand J Gastroenterol 12:547–551
10. Barlow AP, DeMeester TR, Boll CS, Eypasch EP (1989) The significance of the gastric secretory state in gastroesophageal reflux disease. Arch Surg 124:937–940

11. Fuchs K-H (1991) Die chirurgische Therapie der gastroösophagealen Refluxkrankheit. In: Fuchs K-H, Hamelmann H (eds) Gastrointestinale Funktionsdiagnostik in der Chirurgie. Blackwell, Berlin, pp 86–98

12. Stein HJ, DeMeester TR, Naspetti R, Jamieson J, Perry RE (1991) Three-dimensional imaging of the lower esophageal sphincter in gastroesophageal reflux disease. Ann Surg, pp 374–384

13. Nissen R (1961) Gastropexy and fundoplication in surgical treatment of hiatal hernia. Am J Dig Dis 6:954–961

14. DeMeester TR, Bonavina L, Albertucci M (1986) Nissen fundoplication for gastro-esophageal reflux disease. Evaluation of primary repair in 100 consecutive patients. Ann Surg 204:19

15. Skinner DB, Belsey RHR (1967) Surgical management of esophageal reflux with hiatus hernia: Long-term results with 1030 cases. J Thorac Cardiovasc Surg 53:33–54

16. Toupet A (1963) Technique d'oesophago-gastroplastie avec phrénogastropexie appliquée dans la cure radicale des hernies hiatales et comme complément de l'opération d'Heller dans les cardiospasmes. Mem Acad Chir 89:394

17. Watson A, Jenkinson LR, Ball CS, Barlow AP, Norris TL (1991) A more physiological alternative to total fundoplication for the surgical correction of resistant gastro-oesophageal reflux. Br J Surg 78:1088–1094

18. Hill LD (1978) Intraoperative measurement of lower esophageal sphincter pressure. J Thorac Cardiovasc Surg 75:378–382

19. Angelchik JP, Cohen R (1979) A new surgical procedure for the treatment of gastro-esophageal reflux and hiatal hernia. Surg Gynecol Obstet 148:246–248

20. Fuchs K-H, Freys SM, Thiede A (1992) Laparoskopische Antirefluxoperation an der Cardia. In: Fuchs K-H, Hamelmann H, Manegold BC (eds) Chirurgische Endoskopie im Abdomen. Blackwell, Berlin, pp 415–420

21. Richter JE, Castell DO (1982) Gastroesophageal reflux: Pathogenesis, diagnosis and therapy. Ann Intern Med 97:93–103

22. Fuchs K-H, Freys SM, Heimbucher J, Thiede A (1992) Laparoskopische Cholecystektomie—Lohnt sich die laparoskopische Technik in "schwierigen" Fällen? Chirurg 63:296–304

The Reproducibility of Ambulatory Intra-Esophageal pH Monitoring

S.J. WALKER, S. HOLT, C.J. SANDERSON, and C.J. STODDARD[1]

Introduction

Prolonged intra-esophageal pH monitoring is regarded as the "gold standard" test for the diagnosis of abnormal gastro-esophageal reflux, with a reported sensitivity of 88% and specificity of 98% [1]. Its use has also been advocated in patients with atypical chest pain [2], lung disease [3], and to evaluate medical and surgical treatment [4]. Although a routine investigation in many centers, the reproducibility of current ambulatory techniques has received little attention. The aim of this research project was to undertake a series of investigations in patients with suspected gastro-esophageal reflux disease and asymptomatic controls, in order to:

1. Determine the reproducibility of ambulatory intra-esophageal pH monitoring under standardized conditions (Study I).
2. Discover whether activity influences the results of pH monitoring (Study II).
3. Assess day-to-day variation in pH results during 5 days of continuous monitoring (Study III).

Methods

Patients and Controls

Two separate groups of 35 consecutive patients with regular symptoms, suggestive of gastro-esophageal reflux (predominantly heartburn and/or regurgitation [5]), and 5 asymptomatic control subjects, were entered into Study I (Patients: 23 males; mean age 45 years, range 22–69. Controls:

[1] University Department of Surgery, Royal Liverpool Hospital, PO Box 147, Liverpool L69 3BX, UK

4 males; mean age 31 years, range 19–56) and Study II (Patients: 20 males; mean age 44 years, range 21–70. Controls: 3 males; mean age 33 years, range 21–42). Five patients (four males; mean age 45 years, range 34–64) with abnormal acid reflux, confirmed by pH monitoring, and five asymptomatic control subjects (four males; mean age 31 years, range 19–54) were entered in Study III. The entry and exclusion criteria were similar to those used by other researchers [6, 7].

Study I

Standardized esophageal pH monitoring was performed on day 1 (Period I) and again between 5 and 28 days later (mean 12 days) (Period II). Monitoring was performed over 22 h on an outpatient basis. Drugs known to affect gastro-esophageal function were withheld for 24 h both prior to and during monitoring. Patients and controls were instructed to abstain from smoking, alcohol, and food or drink with a pH less than 5.0 during both recording periods. All subjects were instructed to maintain a similar daily routine during Periods I and II, and to keep a timed record of diet, activity, and periods when supine.

Study II

Esophageal pH monitoring was performed on day 1 (Period I) and between 5 and 32 days later (mean 8 days) (Period II). Test conditions were the same as for Study I with one exception: during Period II, patients and controls were instructed to "double" their level of physical exertion.

Study III

Changes in intra-esophageal pH was monitored over five consecutive 24-h periods. Restrictions on medication, smoking, alcohol, and an "acid" diet were imposed, as for Study I. All subjects were instructed to continue their normal daily routine. At the end of each recording period, the pH electrode was removed, cleaned, and the equipment recalibrated. Subjects were allowed a rest period (5–480 min) before the electrode was re-inserted and the next recording cycle commenced.

pH Monitoring

Details of the pH equipment (Ormed, Welwyn Garden City, UK; Microelectrode MI 506, Londonderry, New Hampshire, USA) and technique of ambulatory monitoring used in this study are described elsewhere [8]. Normal values had previously been obtained from a group of 20 asymptomatic control subjects using the method of Johnson and DeMeester [Normal: total reflux % time (Tot%) $<7\%$, upright (Upr%) $<9\%$, supine (Sup%) $<10\%$, total number of reflux episodes (TRef) <30, number over 5 min (Ref >5) <5, time for longest episode (Tmax) <50 min) [9, 10]. These six reflux parameters were examined at the standard pH <4.0 level.

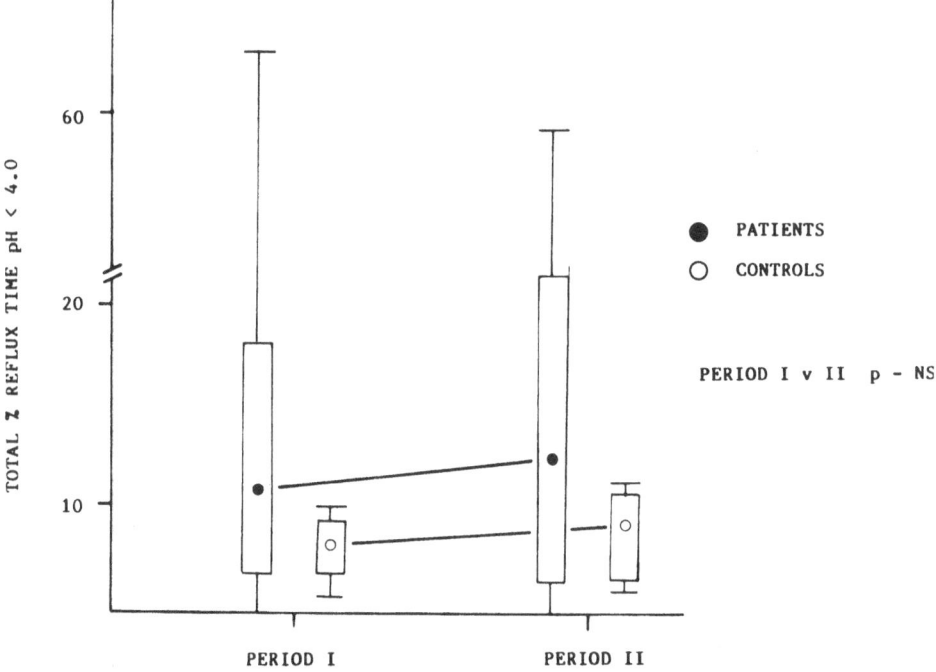

Fig. 1. The reproducibility of standardized intra-esophageal pH monitoring: Comparison of total percentage reflux time (median, IQR, group range; pH < 4.0) between Periods I and II in patients ($n = 35$) and controls ($n = 5$). Respective correlation coefficients (degrees of concordance) $r = 0.56$ (32%) and $r = 0.07$ (0.4%). *IQR*, Interquartile range

Statistical Analysis

Median values were compared by the Wilcoxon signed rank test and the Mann-Whitney U-test. In Studies I and II, reproducibility was analyzed by linear regression analysis. Results were expressed as the square of the correlation coefficient converted to a percentage [7]. In Study III, results were examined using analysis of variance and calculation of the "F-ratio" for equality of two variances.

Results

Prolonged pH monitoring was well tolerated without serious complication. Patients had more acid reflux than control ($P < 0.05$), in spite of 9 of 35 patients (26%) from Study I and 8 of 35 patients (23%) from Study II having normal values for all six parameters examined during both recording periods. A degree of overlap was encountered in the results of patients and controls in all three studies.

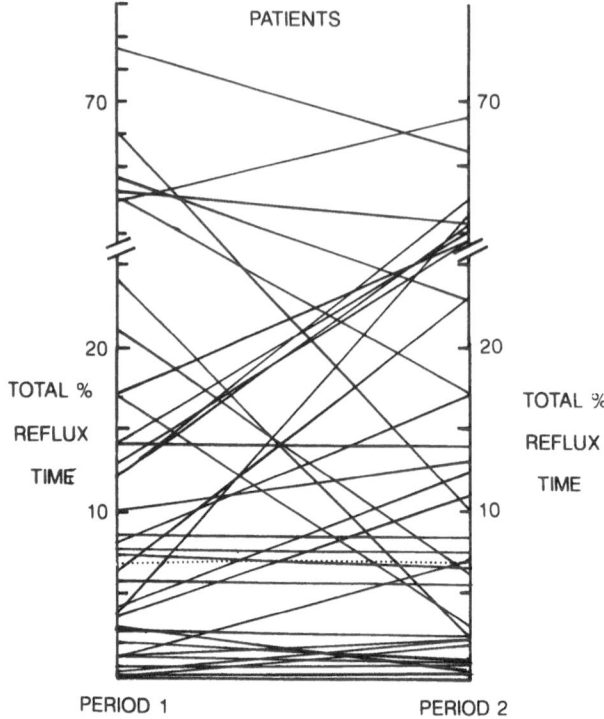

Fig. 2. The reproducibility of standardized intra-esophageal pH monitoring in patients ($n = 35$): Comparison of individual results for total percentage reflux time (pH < 4.0) between Periods I and II (some lines overlap)

Study I

There were no significant differences ($P > 0.05$) between the corresponding median values obtained during Periods I and II for patients or controls (Fig. 1). Correlation coefficients (and degrees of concordance) varied in the patient group between $r = 0.7$ (50%) for TRef to $r = 0.08$ (0%) for Tmax [Tot% $r = 0.56$ (32%), Upr% $r = 0.57$ (32%), Sup% $r = 0.5$ (25%), Ref >5 $r = 0.69$ (47%)]. Among control subjects, correlation coefficients (and degrees of concordance) varied between $r = 0.97$ (94%) for Sup% to $r = 0.07$ (0%) for Tot% [Upr% $r = 0.19$ (3%), TRef $r = 0.43$ (18%), Ref >5 $r = 0.43$ (18%), Tmax $r = 0.6$ (36%)].

Important changes in results were occasionally seen (Fig. 2). Five patients (14%) acquired a different status on repeat pH testing based on the results of the parameter Tot% (normal Period I to abnormal Period II: $n = 3$; abnormal Period I to normal Period II: $n = 2$). They were classified as abnormal refluxers. One control subject was found to have excessive supine acid reflux during both recording period, another demonstrated abnormal upright reflux during Period II. The patterns of reflux were examined in 26 patients with abnormal results. Fourteen patients (54%) changed their predominant reflux status between

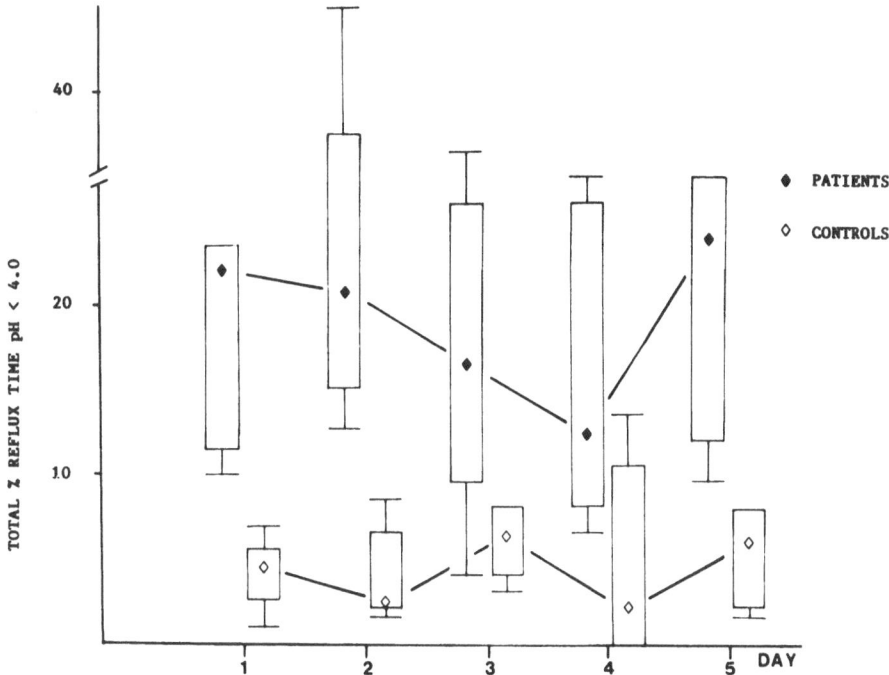

Fig. 3. Day-to-day variation in the rsults of pH monitoring over 5 days of recording in patients ($n = 5$) and controls ($n = 5$): Total percentage reflux time pH < 4.0 (median value, IQR, group range)

Periods I and II: upright to supine ($n = 2$), upright to mixed ($n = 3$), supine to upright ($n = 4$), mixed to upright ($n = 3$), and mixed to supine ($n = 2$).

Study II

The "events" diary confirmed that all subjects had increased their level of activity during Period II. Symptoms occurred more often as indicated by the increased use of the marker button. With the exception of Sup% ($P = 0.07$), corresponding median values in the patient group were significantly higher ($P < 0.05$) during Period II than Period I. Median values among control subjects were higher during Period II, but this difference did not reach statistical significance.

In patients, the correlation coefficient (and degree of concordance) varied between 0.53 (28%) for TRef to 0.04 (0%) for Tmax [Tot% 0.24 (6%), Upr% 0.44 (19%), Sup% 0.11 (1%), Ref >5 0.43 (19%)]. In controls, the correlation coefficient (and degree of concordance) varied between 0.84 (71%) for Ref >5, to 0.05 (0%) for Sup% [Tot% 0.48 (23%), Upr% 0.44 (19%), TRef 0.51 (26%), Tmax 0.26 (7%)]. Though in the majority of subjects acid reflux increased with activity, ten patients (29%) and one control (20%) were found to have a lower result for Tot% time during Period II.

Study III

The mean length of analyzable recording was 21 h 41 min. Examination of corresponding median values failed to demonstrate a significant difference between the results of pH monitoring on different days in either patients or controls ($P > 0.05$) (Fig. 3). Fluctuation in individual results did occur and such variation was greater in the patient than in the control group (P values between <0.001 and <0.054).

Discussion

This investigation confirms that symptoms are an unreliable guide to the presence of acid reflux [11] and that pH monitoring may be used to separate refluxers from non-refluxers [12]. Unfortunately, problems of reproducibility, individual variability, and overlap of pH values in patients and controls mean that a degree of caution is needed when interpreting the results of this investigation.

The reproducibility of standardized ambulatory intra-esophageal pH monitoring proved only to be moderately good. This outcome contrasts with the more positive findings of Johnsson and Joelsson [7]. The latter examined pH values during two consecutive 24-h periods in 20 patients and found, for example, that the correlation coefficient (degree of concordance) for the parameter Tot% was 0.87 (77%) compared to 0.56 (32%) in the present study. We suggest, therefore, because our patient population was larger and the recording periods were separated by at least 5 days, the results of Study I give a truer picture of the reproducibility of this test.

The results of Study II point to the need for standardization of activity when performing serial intra-esophageal pH recordings. A deliberate increase in activity in the patient group led to a significant increase ($P < 0.05$) in the median value of five out of the six reflux parameters under investigation. Interestingly, supine percentage reflux time only just failed to reach statistical significance, suggesting that the effects of a busy day on the level of esophageal acidity may continue into the night. Similar non-significant trends were seen among our small group of control subjects.

Markedly different results were occasionally obtained by repeat pH monitoring. In all three studies, such differences were so great in a minority of individuals to change their status from non-refluxer to refluxer, or vice versa, while others altered their predominant reflux type. The latter finding challenges the assertion of DeMeester et al. [13] that it is important to separate patients into their predominant reflux type (i.e., upright, supine, or mixed) both in terms of pathophysiology and subsequent treatment. How median values and individual pH results can vary from day to day is well illustrated by the findings of Study III. Such changes in the patient group were often dramatic, while among control subjects pH values were generally contained within a relatively narrow range. It is concluded that widely fluctuating pH results are a feature of patients with gastro-esophageal reflux disease.

A further problem apparent from this investigation is what constitutes "normal" esophageal pH. Our previously obtained control range, though supported by other researchers [14, 15] is wider than that reported by Johnson and DeMeester [10]. It is therefore conceiveable that some of the subjects included in this investigation may have been misclassified. Examination of Fig. 1 and 3 shows that, because of the overlap in the results of patients and controls, the assumption of a narrower control range may still have led to a minority of subjects being misclassified. Therefore, the results of pH monitoring are not clear-cut, rather a spectrum of values exists between what is "normal" and "abnormal". Care is required when interpreting results in the "grey" area between the two.

References

1. Richter JE, Castell DO (1981) Gastroesophageal reflux. Pathogenesis, diagnosis and therapy. Ann Int Med 97:93–103
2. Bennett JR (1983) Chest pain: Heart or gullet? BMJ 286:1231–1232
3. Pellegrini CA, DeMeester TR, Johnson LF, Skinner DB (1979) Gastroesophageal reflux and pulmonary aspiration. Incidence, functional abnormality, and results of surgical therapy. Surgery 86:110–119
4. Walker SJ, Holt S, Sanderson CJ, Stoddard CJ (1989) Why is anti-reflux surgery superior to medical treatment for refractory gastro-oesophageal reflux? Br J Surg 75:639
5. Ishmail-Beigi F, Horton PF, Pope CE (1970) Histological consequences of gastroesophageal reflux in man. Gastroenterology 58:163–174
6. Fink SM, McCallum RW (1984) The role of prolonged esophageal pH monitoring in the diagnosis of gastroesophageal reflux. JAMA 252:1160–1164
7. Johnsson F, Joelsson B (1988) Reproducibility of ambulatory oesophageal pH monitoring. Gut 29:886–889
8. Walker SJ, Holt S, Sanderson CJ, Stoddard CJ (1992) Comparison of Nissen total and Lind partial transabdominal fundoplication in the treatment of gastro-oesophageal reflux. Br J Surg 79:410–414
9. Walker SJ (1990) Ambulatory intra-oesophageal pH monitoring and its role in the medical and surgical management of refractory gastro-oesophageal reflux. MD Thesis, University of Birmingham
10. Johnson LF, DeMeester TR (1974) Twenty-four hour pH monitoring in the distal esophagus. Am J Gastroenterol 62:325–332
11. DeMeester TR (1984) Pathophysiology of gastro-oesophageal reflux. In: Watson A, Celestin LR (eds) Disorders of the oesophagus. Advances and controversies. Pitman, London, pp 73–93
12. Branicki FJ, Evans DF, Ogilvie AL, Atkinson M, Hardcastle JD (1982) Ambulatory monitoring of oesophageal pH in reflux oesophagitis using a portable radiotelemetry system. Gut 23:992–998
13. DeMeester TR, Wernly JA, Little AG, Bermudez G, Skinner DB (1980) Technique, indications, and clinical use of 24-hour esophageal pH monitoring. J Thorac Cardiovasc Surg 79:656–670
14. Schlesinger PK, Donahue PE, Schmid B, Layden TJ (1985) Limitations of 24-hour intraesophageal pH monitoring in the hospital setting. Gastroenterology 89:797–804
15. Schindlbeck NE, Heinrich C, Konig A, Dendorfer A, Pace F, Muller-Lissner S (1987) Optimal thresholds, sensitivity and specificity of long-term pH-metry for the detection of gastroesophageal reflux disease. Gastroenterology 93:85–90

pH-Monitoring Patterns of Gastroesophageal Reflux: Differences Between Populations

J.B. Seoane, E. Moreno, S. Merigliano, C. Jimenez, I. Gonzalez-Pinto, P. Rico, F. Palma, and V. Maffettone[1]

Introduction

Esophageal pH measurement was initialy proposed by Tuttle in 1958 [1]. The further evolution of his concept was the basis of the standard acid reflux test (SART), the acid clearance tests, and recently ambulatory 24-hour esophageal pH monitoring. Using the latter method, the amount of acid refluxed to the esophagus can be quantified and related to the time of day when it occurs [2, 3]. Ambulatory 24-hour pH meters (Holter), mimics as closely as possible the normal circadian variation in gastric pH, although having one or two micro-electrodes in the esophagus and/or the stomach can alter the physiologic status of the esophagus, lower esophageal sphincter (LES), or the stomach. The fact that individual pH values can vary physiologically throughout the day, as well as from day to day, or it can be influenced by enviromental factors such as elevation above sea level.

Some of the multiple cofactors that play a role in the pathogenesis of gastro-esophageal reflux (GER) include increased reflux (infectious, chemical, estasic, anatomical malposition, etc.), which can alter the esophageal muscular layer itself or peristalsis; the quality and quantity of the refluxed material; and sphinc-teric dysfunction (alteration of LES—authentic valve mostly unidirectional located between the esophageal and gastric chambers). Thereafter, we must consider GER as a phenomenon encompassing wide physiological limits, which only when it exceeds the mucosal resistance in addition to a mucosal pathological disease (esophagitis), must be considered abnormal. Twenty-four hour pH monitoring has allowed quantification of the cause of the esophagitis, although it

[1] Servicio de Cirugia General, Aparato Digestivo y Trasplante de Organos Abdominales, University Hospital "12 de Octubre", Universidad Complutense de Madrid, Carretera of Andalucia Km 5,5. 28045 Madrid, Spain

is not sufficient itself to establish surgical indications in the absence of esophagitis [4, 5].

Manometric studies of LES have established its paramount importance in the control of GER [6], and even though it is accepted that LES hypotony is a cause of reflux, there are patients with a hypotonic sphincter without esophagitis and patients with esophagitis (with or without symptoms) whose LES show pressures within normal ranges. The sphincter pressures calculated with manometry by means of a rapid passage of the probe through the high pressure zone (HPZ) vary according to the procedure and the equipement, with values between 10 and 25 mmHg. We consider normal values to be 20.57 ± 6.22 mmHg. Comparing·the values obtained from GER patients with the mean, an important overlap of populations is observed. Other parameters such as the total length of LES and particularly its abdominal segment (short portion) seem to have a decisive influence in a subgroup of patients with a normal mean pressure who nevertheless have reflux. The presence of the so-called inappropriate episodes of LES relaxation (Dodds and Dent) in patients with normal mean pressures could partially justify these abnormalities in the records. Nowadays, the need for manometry before 24-hour pH monitoring with the aim of localization of LES and positioning of the pH microelectrode is debatable [7, 8].

Certain kinds of food or drugs can alter the esophageal motor activity and LES tone. Gastric emptying with its cofactors (type of food, volume, gastric secretion, duodenal reflux, etc.) determine the severity of reflux in terms of quantity and quality of refluxed material to the esophagus.

Twenty-four-hour pH monitoring measures esophageal and/or gastric pH values, but does not differentiate qualitatively the nature of the content in which the measurement is done. The technique itself is conditioned by factors derived of the positioning of the microelectrodes, their type and the material of which they are made, and the measuring equipment and its algoritm for transforming mV into pH [9–15]. Accepting that such factors are correctly controlled by the investigator, the concepts of normality can be defined and thereafter universally applied to any kind of population, not forgetting that gastric secretion is a dynamic factor, which follows cycles clearly related to the presence of food during the day of the test and can oscillate between wide ranges of normality in consecutive days [16–21]. To try to demonstrate this dynamic behaviour with differentiated responses according to the populations under analysis, we designed a study comparing two different populations analyzed with the same procedure. Others have performed similar studies with the aim of finding the normality criteria through one or more predictive variables of GER [22–24].

Material and Methods

Two samples of asymptomatic volunteers from different countries, Madrid (Spain) and Padova (Italy) were compared. The M group (Madrid) included 23 volunteers and the P group (Padova) 16.

The following inclusion criteria were established: age between 14 and 65 years, diet and social habits usual in their enviroment (including the presence of smokers), absence of personal or familial antecedents of GER, hiatal hernia, abnormal esophageal motor activity, peptic ulcer, or bile duct disease. Informed consent was obtained after the nature of the study was explained, and they were asked to follow a normal regimen of life during the test. Both groups were studied with the same methodology and equipement, using a portable measuring system (Holter) based in microprocessors and solid memory (RAM C MOS), enough to record at the same time gastric and/or esophageal pH values every 6 s over a 24-hour period. An informatic system allows the results to be expressed as graphics. The Holter itself can communicate through an RS 232 C output to any MS-DOS compatible system, which by means of the appropriate software can display the results as tables or graphics. In both groups Ingold type crystal electrodes were used with internal reference incorporated in one of them.

The esophageal probe was positioned 5 cm above the LES and the gastric probe 5 cm below. A positioning control was always made by x-ray examination. We considered esophageal reflux to be any prolonged drop in esophageal pH below 4. The results of the study were associated to 97 variables, which underwent a computerized statistical analysis by means of a data base developed by professors of the Department of Biostatistics of the Universidad Autonoma de Madrid (software Sigma).

A p value less than 0.05 was considered statistically significant using the Student's t-test (two-tailed comparison) , multiple correlation and/or regression coefficients, or analysis of variance for one or more factors (Scheffé technique). From the total of 97 variables studied, we will refer specifically to the more universally accepted, as well as to the values obtained with the DeMeester and Kaye Scores, which are included in Tables 1, 2, 3, and 4 (exclusively referred to group M).

Table 1. Basic statistics total population

Variable	Mean	SD	Size	SE	Min	Max
N. episodes	72.4	59.76	23	12.46	13	286
N. EPI. >5 min	2.73	4.12	23	0.86	0	18
Longest EPI.	20	22.44	23	4.68	1	82
T. reflux time	5.8	6.79	23	1.41	0.4	31.2
U. reflux time	5.78	5.95	23	1.24	0.6	27.4
S. reflux time	5.86	9.13	23	1.9	0	36.5
Score DM	32	39.9	23	8.32	0	168
Score Kaye	110.04	126	23	26.28	5	451

EPI, episode; *T*, total; *U*, upright; *S*, supine; *DM*, De Meester

Table 2. Basic statistics men

Variable	Mean	SD	Size	SE	Min	Max
N. episodes	91.63	73.27	11	22.09	21	286
N. EPI. >5 min	2.81	2.99	11	0.90	0	9
Longest EPI.	22.81	18.44	11	5.56	3	50
T. reflux time	6.30	4.40	11	1.32	1.3	15.9
U. reflux time	6.28	4.21	11	1.27	2.2	16.9
S. reflux time	6.51	6.27	11	1.89	0	16
Score DM	36.27	28.71	11	8.65	2	88
Score Kaye	113	114.95	11	34.66	7	353

Table 3. Basic statistics women

Variable	Mean	SD	Size	SE	Min	Max
N. episodes	54.83	39.44	12	11.38	13	150
N. EPI. >5 min	2.66	5.08	12	1.46	0	18
Longest EPI.	17.41	26.13	12	7.54	1	82
T. reflux time	5.33	8.62	12	2.48	0.4	31.2
U. reflux time	5.33	7.37	12	2.12	0.6	27.4
S. reflux time	5.26	11.41	12	3.29	0	36.5
Score DM	28.08	48.99	12	14.14	0	168
Score Kaye	107.33	140.56	12	40.57	5	451

Table 4. Basic statistics comparison by sexes

Variable	Men		Women		P
	Mean	SD	Mean	SD	
N. episodes	91.63	73.27	54.83	39.44	NS
N. EPI. >5 min	2.81	2.99	2.66	5.08	NS
Longest EPI.	22.81	18.44	17.41	26.13	NS
T. reflux time	6.30	4.40	5.33	8.62	NS
U. reflux time	6.28	4.21	5.33	7.37	NS
S. reflux time	6.51	6.271	5.26	11.41	NS
Score DM	36.27	28.71	28.08	48.99	NS
Score Kaye	113	14.95	107.33	140.56	NS

Table 5. Comparison of populations (Madrid-Padova)

	Total series Madrid	Total series Padova	Statistical significance
N Tot EPI	72.4 ± 59.8	25.6 ± 24.1	$P < 0.01$
N EPI >5 m T	2.7 ± 4.1	1.6 ± 3.3	NS
Longest T m	20.0 ± 22.4	7.4 ± 7.8	$P < 0.05$
% Time T	5.8 ± 6.7	2.6 ± 3.7	NS
% Time U	5.8 ± 5.9	2.2 ± 1.9	$P < 0.05$
% Time S	5.8 ± 9.1	2.9 ± 6.7	NS
Score DM	32 ± 39.9	14.3 ± 24.2	CS*
Score Kaye	110 ± 126	87 ± 93	NS

*CS, $P < 0.1$

Results

When both groups were compared (M and P), differences were seen in the number of total episodes, the total length of the longest episode, and the percentage of reflux time in the upright position. There are two cumulative variables close to statistical significance: the total percentage of reflux time and the total, DeMeester Score (Tables 5 and 6). The multiple correlation coefficient

Table 6. Comparison of populations. Madrid-Padova

	Madrid-Padova men & women	Madrid-Padova men	Madrid-Padova women
N. Tot EPI	$P < 0.01$	$P < 0.05$	NS
N. EPI >5 m T	NS	NS	NS
Longest T m	$P < 0.05$	$P < 0.05$	NS
% Time T	CS*	CS*	NS
% Time U	$P < 0.05$	$P < 0.05$	NS
% Time S	NS	NS	NS
Score DM	CS*	CS*	NS
Score Kaye	NS	NS	NS

* CS, $P < 0.1$

Table 7. Analysis of variance by population and sex

Variable	Anova 1 (pop.)	Anova 2 (pop. and sex)
N. EPI	$P < 0.01$	$P < 0.01$
N. EPI >5 m	NS	NS
Lg Max EPI	$P < 0.05$	NS
% T Total	CS. $P < 0.1$	NS
% T Bipe	$P < 0.05$	$P < 0.01$
% T Sup	NS	NS
DeMeester	NS	NS
Kaye	NS	NS

in both populations scores studied together and separately, shows a significant correlation between all of them, as well as between both where $r = 0.75$ or 0.83 depending on the population studied. When the variance is analyzed for one factor (origin of the population) or two factors (population and sex), the significant values are again the number of total episodes, the total length of the longest episode, and the percentage of reflux time in the upright position, and the total percentage of reflux time is nearly significant. If both the sex and origin of the population are analyzed, the same factors are significant, except for the length of the longest episode [which, even though it is longer in Spanish men compared to women (Table 4), is not statistically significant] (Table 7).

Discussion

From the statistical analysis, it is possible to deduce that there are significant differences between both populations under study in the number of total episodes, the total length of the longest episode, and the percentages of the reflux time in the upright position, and also that both populations behave in different ways.

When the meaning of the studied variables are analyzed, it can be observed that the total percentage of reflux time is a cumulative vriable, which is to say that it is influenced by all the others, and subsequently it could be deduced that this one should be actually the predictive value to be used as the universal parameter for comparison.

Twenty-four-hour pH monitoring is basically a quantitative test, and the results can be altered by individual factors such as age, ethnic origin (population), social habits (alcohol, tobacco, etc.), as well as the physical activity of the individual (exercise, posture, etc.). To the individual factors, it is necessary to add other external ones related to the methodology such as the type and characteristics of the probe, calibration, and esophageal positioning. We must also take into account possible recording errors derived from the nature of the esophageal content (mucus, food, etc.), which alter its meaning; or even errors derived from the Holter itself (hardware) or from differences in the algorithms (software), which elaborate the final results.

These factors together with our own results lead us to think that even though 24-hour pH monitoring is the best of the possible tests to study GER, it is influenced by factors of variability which make it necessary for each research group to study their populations of reference and, if possible, using the same methodology to compare them with control populations that minimize these variables.

References

1. Tuttle S, Grossmann MJ (1958) Detection of gastroesophageal reflux by simultaneous measurement of intraluminal pressure and pH. Proc Soc Exp Biol Med 98:225–229
2. De Caestecker JS, Heading RC (1990) Esophageal pH monitoring. Gastroenterol Clin North Am 19(3):645–669
3. Zaninotto G, Merigliano S, Baessato M, Costantini M, Nosadini A, Sorrentino P, Pianalto S, Ancona E (1984) Gastro-oesophageal reflux in Italian healthy volunteers and patients: Relationship between gastro-oesophageal reflux, endoscopic oesophagitis and symptoms. Dig Surg 1:211–216
4. Masclee AA, De Best AC, De Graaf R, Cluysenaer OJ, Jansen JB (1990) Ambulatory 24-hour pH-metry in the diagnosis of gastroesophageal reflux disease. Determination of criteria and relation to endoscopy. Scand J Gastroenterol 25(3):225–230
5. Mattox HE 3d, Richter JE (1990) Prolonged ambulatory esophageal pH monitoring in the evaluation of gastroesophageal reflux disease. Am J Med 89(3):345–356
6. Zaninotto G, Demeester TR, Schwizer W, Johansson KE, Cheng SC (1988) The lower esophageal sphincter in health and disease. Am J Surg 155:104–111
7. Klauser AG, Schindlbeck NE, Muller-Lissner SA (1990) Esophageal 24-h pH monitoring: is prior manometry necessary for correct positioning of the electrode? Am J Gastroenterol 85(11):1463–1467
8. Kraus BB, Wu WC, Castell DO (1990) Comparison of lower esophageal sphincter manometrics and gastroesophageal reflux measured by 24 hour pH recording. Am J Gastroenterol 85:692–696
9. Andersen J, Naesdal J, Strom M (1988) Identical 24-hour gastric pH profiles when using intragastric antimony or glass electrodes or aspirated gastric juice. Scand J Gastroenterol 23:375–379
10. Emde C (1990) Electrochemical aspects of pH electrodes. Dig Dis 8:18–22
11. Emde C (1990) Graphical display and statistical evaluation of data gained by long-term ambulatory intragastric pH monitoring. Dig Dis 8:82–86
12. Jonard P, Fiasse R, Tome G, Dive C (1990) pH-metrie ambulatoire de l'oesophage: revue critique de la methodologie (appareillage, reproductibilite, normes), interet clinique et experience personnelle. Acta-Gastroenterol-Belg 53(5–6):554–558

13. Kuit JA, Schepel SJ, Bijleveld CM, Kleibeuker JH (1991) Evaluation of a new catheter for esophageal pH monitoring. Hepatogastroenterology 38(1):78–80

14. Londong W, Angerer M, Bosch R, Koelzow H (1990) Standardization of electrode positioning and composition of meals for long-term intragastric pH-metry in man. Dig Dis [Suppl 8] 1:46–53

15. Mela GS, Savarino V, Moretti M, Sumberaz A, Bonifacino G, Zentilin P, Caputo E, Villa G, Celle G (1990) Antimony and glass pH electrodes can be used interchangeably in 24-hour studies of gastric acidity. Dig Dis Sci 35:1473–1481

16. Dreizzen E, Escourrou P, Odievre M, Guilleminault C, Gaultier C (1990) Esophageal reflux in symptomatic and asymptomatic infants: postprandial and circadian variations. J Pediatr Gastroenterol Nutr 10:316–321

17. Mattioli S, Felice V, Pilotti V, Bacchi ML, Di Simone MP, Pastina M, Gozzetti G (1991) Definizione di normalita di un tracciato pH-metrico. Minerva chir 46 [Suppl 7]:93–101

18. Mela GS, Savarino V (1990) Doubt on pH-metry as an absolute gold standard for measuring acid gastroesophageal reflux. Dig Dis Sci 35:282–283

19. Savarini V, Mela GS, Zentilin P, Cutela P (1991) pH-metria esofagea: fattori influenzanti la definizione di normalita. Minerva chir 46 [Suppl 7]:103–109

20. Vandenplas Y, Goyvaerts H, Helven R (1990) esophageal pH monitoring data depend on recorrding equipment and probes? J Pediatr Gastroenterol Nutr 10(3):322–326

21. Vandenplas Y, Helven R, Goyvaerts H, Sacre L (1990) Reproducibility of continuous 24 hour oesophageal pH monitoring in infants and children. Gut 31:374–377

22. Colson DJ, Campbell CA, Wright VA, Watson BW (1990) Predictive value of oesophageal pH variables in children with gastro-oesophagealp reflux. Gut 31:370–373

23. Hampton FJ, Macfadyen UM, Simpson H (1990) Reproducibility of 24 hour oesophageal pH studies in infants. Arch Dis Childhood 65:1249–1254

24. Hampton FJ, Macfadyen UM, Mayberry JF (1992) Variations in results of simultaneous ambulatory esophageal pH monitoring. Dig Dis Sci 37(4):506–512

Examination of the Hiatal Defence Mechanism with Manometry Including an Abdominal Pressure Test. A Comparative Study with 24-Hour pH Monitoring and Esophagoscopy

BJÖRN SANDMARK, HÅKAN ENBOM, and STIG SANDMARK[1]

Introduction

A normally efficient clamping mechanism between the stomach and the esophagus prevents backflow of gastric contents into the esophagus. There is a widespread conception that the lower esophageal sphincter (LES) constitutes the most important protection against reflux, irrespective of whether the location of the sphincter is in the hiatal channel or, as in the case of a sliding hernia, in the thoracic cavity [1–2]. However, there is also conflicting evidence, and some authors have stressed the importance of the hiatal mechanism in preventing reflux [3–9]. On contraction of the diaphragm, the muscles around the hiatus also contract, thereby pinching the esophagogastric tract which passes through the hiatus. One can also consider the hiatus simply as a gap. When there is an increased pressure difference across the diaphragm, the stomach wall and/or other viscera are forced towards and into the hiatal channel. Herniation may occur, and thereby the hiatal channel can be plugged, thus constricting the lumen of the esophagogastric tract.

On recording intraluminal pressures in the esophagus and the stomach, two important factors may be identified: the pressure inversion point (PIP) and LES. PIP can be identified by different pressure waves due to respiratory movements. On inspiration, the diaphragm descends and the pressure within the abdomen increases, with positive pressure swings on intraluminal recordings and negative pressure swings within the thoracic cavity. At the level of the effective diaphragmatic hiatus, a pressure inversion point is recorded. LES can be identified as a high pressure zone in the distal esophagus with a characteristic pressure response during deglutition.

[1] Department of Otorhinolaryngology, Örebro Medical Center Hospital, S-701 85 Örebro, Sweden

By using an abdominal pressure test, the barrier function at the level of hiatus and LES can be investigated [5–6]. If, on abdominal compression, a segment of increased pressure is demonstrated 2 cm or more above PIP, there is strong reason to suspect an incompetent hiatal mechanism and/or gastroesophageal reflux.

The aim of the study was to show the existence of a hiatal mechanism and to compare the clinical relevance of manometry with an abdominal pressure test with findings by endoscopy and 24-hour pH monitoring.

Methods

A catheter assembly with six tubes with lateral openings was used. It was composed of six polythene tubes (Portex), each with an inner diameter of 0.86 mm, an outer diameter of 1.27 mm, and a length of 130 cm. The openings were situated 1, 5, 6, 7, 11, and 24 cm from the distal tip and radially oriented 120 degrees from each other. The tubes were connected to 5 pressure transducers (746 Siemens-Elema, Solna, Sweden) and these were connected to a pressure amplifier (863 Siemens-Elema). Two tubes with the openings 7 and 11 cm from the distal tip were put through a 3-way stopcock connected to the same transducer. The tubes were constantly perfused with distilled water via a low compliance, pneumohydraulic capillary infusion pump at a rate of 0.7 ml/min in each tube. All pressures were recorded on a direct-writing automatic 8-channel ink-writer (Mingocard 7, Siemens-Elema) with a paper speed of 2.5 mm/s. For calibration, standard hydrostatic pressures were introduced in the system. On the occlusion of each recorded orifice, the recorded pressure rise rate exceeded 150 mm Hg/sec (20 kPa/sec).

To establish a constant increased intra-abdominal pressure as part of the examination, a large rubber bladder (23 cm × 50 cm) surrounded by firm cloth was fixed over the patients abdomen. The bladder was connected to an electric blowing fan which at constant speed maintained a constant pressure in the bladder.

The recording catheter was introduced through the nose into the esophagus and the stomach. The tranducers were positioned at the level of the mid-axillary line. All recordings were made with the patients in the supine position. Immediately prior to the examination, the patients were given 200 ml of water. The patients were told to relax, to breath calmly, and refrain from swallowing.

The four distal orifices of the catheter were then positioned in the stomach, well below the PIP and the pressure at end expiration was recorded as reference pressure. A station pull-through technique with 1-cm steps was used. At each step, intraluminal pressures were recorded, and the levels of PIP and LES were estimated. For LES pressure, we used the openings situated 5, 6 and 7 cm from the distal tip and calculated the avarage of the pressure readings. By abdominal compression, the pressure within the bladder was increased 60 mmHg for 10–20 s and any pressure increase above PIP and LES, as well as changing respiratory pressure swings, were recorded.

24-Hour pH Monitoring

Portable pH recording equipment designed by Synetics was used. It consists of an antimony pH electrode, a silver-silver chloride cutaneous reference electrod, and a solid-state memory unit. After calibration with buffer solutions (pH 7.0 and 1.0) the pH electrode was introduced through the nose and placed 5 cm above the LES. The reference electrode was placed on the chest. The patients were told to avoid acid liquids and not to use long-acting anti-reflux medications before the investigation. The patients were also told to record erect and supine periods. The data were analysed with standard computer program (Esophagogram, Synectics; IBM PC).

The 24-hour pH-metric limits used were chosen in accordance with the findings of DeMeester et al. [10]. Endoscopy was performed with flexible endoscopes (Olympus). Degree of esophagitis was classified in accordance with Savary-Miller [11]. For statistical analysis of cross tabulations, we used two different Chi-squared tests: Pearsson (Pe) and Mantel–Haenszel test for linear association (M-H).

Subjects

Patients examined in our esophageal laboratory between 1988 and 1990 were reviewed. All patients in whom manometry, 24-hour pH monitoring, and endoscopy were performed participated in this study (143 patients, 87 men and 56 women, aged 19–76 years, median 54.6 years).

Results

Manometry

When the pressure in the rubber bladder was increased to 60 mmHg, the intra-abdominal pressure was increased by approx. 15–20 mmHg. Abdominal compression also increased the pressure in a segment above the PIP. The pressure at end expiration in this segment was about the same as within the abdomen, and positive or negative pressure swings could be recorded at inspiration. The pressure increment occured within 20 s and could be demonstrated repeatedly.

According to the length of the segment with increased pressure and behaviour of respiratory pressure swings during abdominal compression, the data can be divided into five groups:

(A) No pressure increase recordable 2 cm or more above the PIP;

(B1) Increased pressure at the end of expiration at least 2 cm above the PIP and negative pressure swings at inspiration still recordable but with no pressure increase above LES;

(B2) Increased pressure at the end of expiration at least 2 cm above the PIP, with positive pressure swings at inspiration in this segment but no pressure increase above LES;

(C1) Increased pressure at the end of expiration above the LES with negative pressure swings at inspiration; and

Table 1. Results of manometry with abdominal compression

Manometric groups	Number of patients	Increased pressure ≥ 2 cm above PIP	Increased pressure above LES
A	36	no	no
B1	36	yes	no
B2	8	yes	no
C1	18	yes	yes
C2	45	yes	yes

PIP, pressure inversion point; *LES*, lower esophageal sphincter

Table 2. Resting pressure in the lower esophageal sphincter and distribution of esophagitis in the different manometric groups

Manometric groups	LES pressure (mmHg)		Percent of cases with esophagitis
	Mean	Range	
A	9.8	4–20	31%
B1	8.6	2–18	44%
B2	13.3	7–17	63%
C1	9.2	3–17	72%
C2	6.3	0–13	71%
Total	8.5	0–20	54%

Table 3. Distribution of esophagitis in the different manometric groups

Manometric groups	Grade of esophagitis					Total
	0	I	II	III	IV	
A	25	8	3	0	0	36
B1	20	7	6	0	3	36
B2	3	2	2	0	1	8
C1	5	7	3	1	2	18
C2	13	8	14	7	3	45

(C2) Increased pressure at the end of expiration with positive pressure swings above the LES.

Tables 1 and 2 show the results. Thirty six patients were placed in group A. Thirty six patients in group B1 and 18 patients in group C1 showed negative pressure swings in the segment with increased pressure. Eight patients in group B2 and 45 patients in group C2 showed positive pressure swings above the level of the PIP (before abdominal compression), thus the level of PIP changed considerably when abdominal compression was applied.

Esophagoscopy showed esophagitis in 54% of the patients (Table 3).

PH monitoring showed pathologic reflux time in 70% of the patients (total time) and in 62% of the patients (supine period) (Table 4).

Table 4. Outcome of 24-hour pH monitoring in relation to manometric groups

Manometric groups	24-hour pH monitoring					
	Reflux time total			Reflux time supine		
	<4.2%	4.2%–10%	>10%	<1.2%	1.2%–10%	>10%
A	18	12	6	26	6	4
B1	11	11	14	12	13	11
B2	3	3	2	3	3	2
C1	5	4	9	5	8	5
C2	6	19	20	9	20	16

Table 5. Outcome of 24-hour pH monitoring in relation to endoscopy

Grade of esophagitis	24-hour pH monitoring					
	Reflux time total			Reflux time supine		
	<4.2%	4.2%–10%	>10%	<1.2%	1.2%–10%	>10%
0	30	18	18	35	19	12
I	8	16	8	14	15	3
II	3	13	12	5	12	11
III	0	0	8	0	0	8
IV	2	2	5	1	4	4

Table 3 compares findings on manometry and esophagoscopy. The frequency of esophagitis was 31% in group A, 48% in group B1 + B2 and 71% in group C1 + C2. Only 11 patients in group A had esophagitis and none of them had grade III–IV. In group C, nearly 50% had severe esophagitis, grade II or more.

Table 4 compares findings on manometry and the total reflux time by 24-hour pH monitoring: 50% in group A, 68% in groups B1 + B2 and 83% in group C1 + C2 had values above the limit for the test. Patients with the longest time for acid exposure were included in group C, and nearly 50% in this group had a pH reflux time of over 10%.

Comparing findings on manometry and reflux time in the supine position we found that 28% in group A, 66% in group B1 + B2 and 78% in group C1 + C2 had values above 1.2%.

Table 5 compares findings on esophagoscopy and pH monitoring. Patients with esophagitis had longer time for acid exposure.

Chi square tests between the two variables in Tables 3–5 showed that there is good evidence of a relationship in all of them. The following P-values were calculated. In manometry, we used three groups: A, B1 + B2 and C1 + C2. Manometry and endoscopy Pe = 0.0014, M-H < 0.00001. Manometry and 24-hour pH monitoring: Total period Pe = 0.0078, M-H = 0.0003, and supine period Pe = 0.00006, M-H = 0.00003. Endoscopy and 24-hour pH monitoring: total period Pe = 0.00008, M-H = 0.00003, and supine period Pe = 0.0001, M-H < 0.00001.

Discussion

The function of the antireflux barrier is not fully understood. Normally, LES is situated within the hiatal channel. In the case of sliding herniation, hiatus and LES are situated at different levels and the barrier function at each level can be tested separately. In this study, recorded resting pressures in the LES showed considerable overlap between the manometric groups.

If no pressure increase is recorded 2 cm or more above the PIP, then the LES and/or the hiatal mechanism is competent. In patients with a competent hiatal mechanism, a more pronounced pressure increase was often recorded at the hiatal level than the corresponding pressure increment within the abdomen. This can be explained as an effect of plugging the mucosa within the hiatal channel.

If there is increased pressure at the end of expiration at least 2 cm above the PIP, this indicates an incompetent hiatal mechanism of varying degree. If negative pressure swings at inspiration are still recorded, then there is a partial barrier at the hiatus level. If positive pressure swings at inspiration are recorded in this segment, then there is no barrier at the hiatus level.

If no pressure increase is demonstrated above LES, then there is a competent sphincter. If the manometric test indicates that both the hiatal mechanism and the sphincter is incompetent, it is probable that the patient has an advanced stage of gastroesophageal reflux disease.

Results of the inter-group comparisons showed the same trends. In patients who showed manometric evidence of hiatal incompetence, it was more likely that at least one of the other tests indicated that there was gastroesophageal reflux disease. In conclusion, this study demonstrated that the hiatal mechanism is an important part of the anti-reflux barrier. The competence of the hiatal mechanism and the sphincter can be tested separately in patients with hiatal herniation by an abdominal pressure test. The test is clinically useful as a complement to endoscopy and 24-hour pH monitoring in the selection of patients for surgical treatment and intensive medical treatment.

References

1. Castell DO (1992) The esophagus. Little, Brown, Boston
2. Cohen S, Harris LD (1971) Does hiatus hernia affect competence of the gastroesophageal sphincter? N Engl J Med 284:1053–1056
3. Edwards DAW (1982) The anti-reflux mechanism, its disorders and their consequences. In: Connel AM (ed) Clinics in gastroenterology, vol 11. WB Saunders, London, pp 479–496
4. Sandmark S (1963) Hiatal incompetence. Acta Radiol [Suppl] (Stock) 919:1–46
5. Sandmark S (1963) Intraluminal pressures and pH in hiatus hernia and gastroesophageal reflux. Acta Otolaryngol 56:683–698
6. Lindell D, Sandmark S (1979) Hiatal incompetence and gastro-oesophageal reflux. Acta Radiol 20:626–636
7. Mittal RK, Rochester DF, McCallum RW (1988) Electrical and mechanical activity in the human lower esophageal sphincter during diaphragmatic contraction. J Clin Invest 81:1182–1189
8. Mittal RK, Rochester DF, McCallum RW (1989) Sphincteric action of the diaphragm during a relaxed lower esophageal sphincter in humans. Am J Physiol 256:G139–G144

9. Mittal RK, Fisher M, McCallum RW, Rochester DF, Dent J, SLUSS J (1990) Human lower esophageal sphincter pressure response to increased intra-abdominal pressure. Am J Physiol 258:G624–G630

10. DeMeester TR, Wang CI, Werkly JA, Pellegrini CA, Little AG, Klementschitsch P, Bermudez G, Johnson LF, Skinner DB (1980) Technique, indications and clinical use of 24-hour esophageal pH monitoring. J Thorac Cardiovasc Surg 79:656–670

11. Savary M, Miller G (1978) The esophagus. Gassmann, Solothurn

Gastroesophageal Reflux Due to Hiatal Incompetence—Influence of the Viscosity of the Gastric Content

STIG SANDMARK, BJÖRN SANDMARK, and HÅKAN ENBOM[1]

Introduction

The lower esophageal sphincter provides important protection against gastro-esophageal reflux [1]. Some authors have also stressed the importance of the hiatal mechanism in preventing reflux [2–6]. On contraction of the diaphragm, the muscles around the hiatus also contract and thereby pinch the esophago-gastric tract. When the pressure difference across the diaphragm increases, the stomach wall and/or other viscera are forced towards and into the hiatal channel. In this way, the folds of the mucous membrane can be compressed so that the gastric contents cannot pass into a herniated part of the stomach or into the esophagus, making the hiatus competent. If the hiatal channel is wider, the gastric contents can pass the folds which means that the hiatus is incompetent. If the sphincter is also forced, reflux will occur. Earlier investigations have shown that substances with a high viscosity increase hiatal competence and decrease reflux. This observation provided the background for the invention of Gaviscon [3, 7]. The aim of the present study was to investigate the effect of varying the viscosity of gastric content on intraluminal pressures in patients with hiatal incompetence and incompetent sphincter.

Methods

Manometric measurements were made with a catheter assembly with 6 open-tipped tubes, and a station pull-through technique was used. The examination technique has been described in detail in another chapter (B. Sandmark et al., this volume). To provoke the anti-reflux mechanism, a square rubber balloon

---
[1] Department of Otorhinolaryngology, Örebro Medical Center Hospital, S-701 85 Örebro Sweden

with an encircling bandage was fixed over the patients abdomen. The pressure in the balloon was increased to 60 mm Hg.

The patients were first given 200 ml of water to drink after which the intraluminal pressures were recorded both without and with abdominal compression. Then the patients were given a highly viscous preparation of 4 g of Gaviscon powder containing alginate in 100 ml of water. Afterwards, 100 ml 0.1 mmol HCl was instilled into the stomach. After resting for 10 min, patients were reexamined in the same position with abdominal compression for at least 20 s.

Subjects

Eighty consecutive patients (56 men and 24 women, aged 22–70 years, mean 56 years) in whom the "common cavity phenomenon" had been demonstrated within 10 s by abdominal compression, were selected for the study. Of these patients, 72 were also examined by endoscopy with flexible endoscope. Esophagitis was graded according to Savary and Miller [8].

Results

Abdominal compression increased the end expiratory pressure within the abdomen and also in a segment above the pressure inversion point (PIP). A previous investigation showed that increased pressure at least 2 cm above PIP indicated an incompetent hiatal mechanism and/or gastroesophageal reflux. If a pressure increase was demonstrated above the sphincter, then reflux had occured. The following abdominal five compression patterns of pressure changes are demonstrable above the PIP: (A) No pressure increase recordable 2 cm or more above the PIP (Fig. 1); (B1) Increased pressure at the end of expiration at least 2 cm above the PIP and negative pressure swings at inspiration still recordable but with no pressure increase above the lower esophageal sphincter (LES) (Fig. 2); (B2) Increased pressure at the end of expiration at least 2 cm above the PIP with positive pressure swings at inspiration in this segment but no pressure increase above the LES (Fig. 3); (C1) Increased pressure at the end of expiration above the LES with negative pressure swings at inspiration (Fig. 4); and (C2) Increased pressure at the end of expiration with positive pressure swings above the LES (Fig. 5).

Tables 1 and 2 show the results. With watery stomach contents, all patients showed gastroesophageal reflux and positive pressure swings within 10 s by abdominal compression. After the intake of the preparation which contained alginate, improved hiatal competence and a reduced tendency to gastroesophageal reflux by abdominal compression for 20 s were found in more than half of the patients (n = 46). In 35 of these patients, gastroesophageal reflux was inhibited when the viscosity of the gastric contents was increased. The interval of time when increase in pressure was noted above the PIP was extended after the intake of the alginate preparation.

In 33 patients, no positive pressure swings could be demonstrated further. On esophagoscopy, 50 patients (69%) had varying degrees of esophagitis. In the group showing no improvment, the majority of esophagitis (80%) was found by

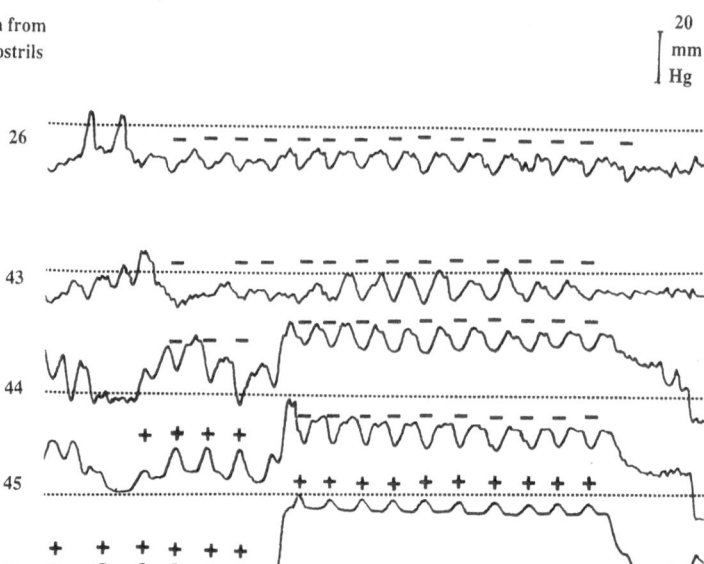

Fig. 1. Recordings of intraluminal pressures. During abdominal compression (*A* to *B*) no pressure increase is recordable 2 cm above PIP between levels 44 and 45. Reference pressure levels are represented by *broken lines*. +, positive pressure swings on inspiration; −, negative pressure swings; *PIP*, pressure inversion point

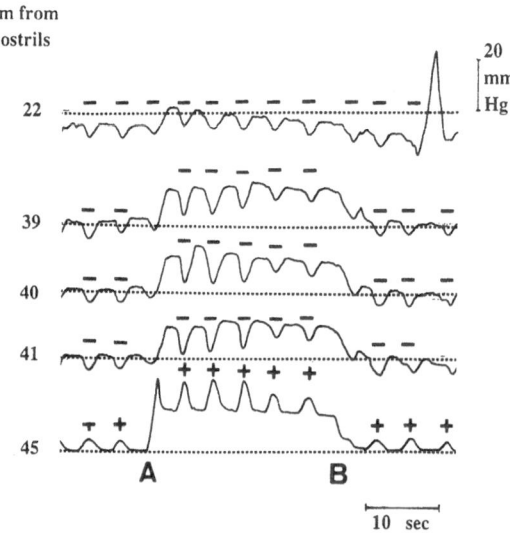

Fig. 2. Recordings of intraluminal pressures. During abdominal compression (*A* to *B*) increased pressure at the end of expiration is recordable at least 2 cm above PIP and with negative pressure swings at inspiration but no pressure increase above LES. Reference pressure levels are represented by *broken lines*. +, positive pressure swings on inspiration; −, negative pressure swings; *LES*, lower esophageal sphincter

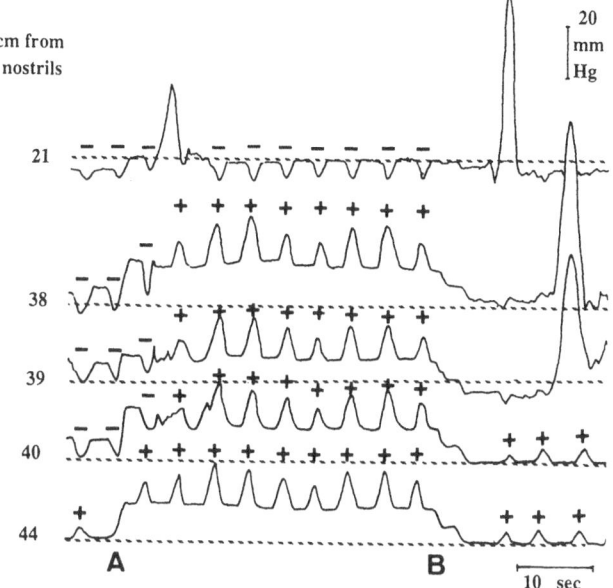

Fig. 3. Recordings of intraluminal pressures. During abdominal compression (*A* to *B*) increased pressure at the end of expiration is recordable at least 2 cm above PIP and with positive pressure swings at inspiration but no pressure increase above LES. Reference pressure levels are represented by *broken lines*. +, positive pressure swings on inspiration; −, negative pressure swings

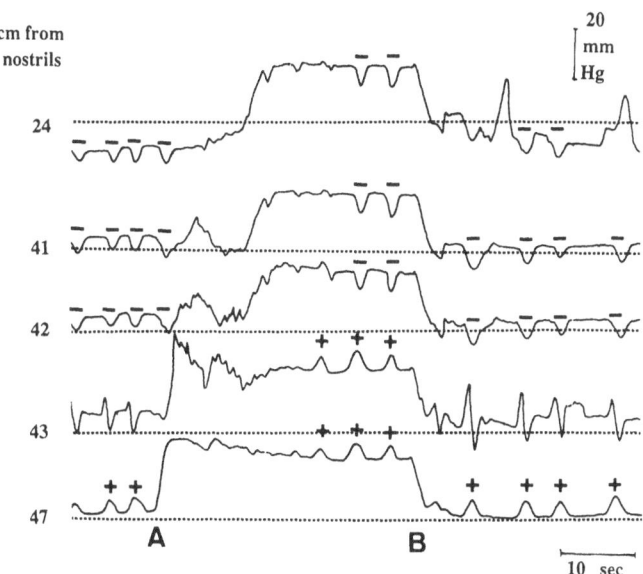

Fig. 4. Recordings of intraluminal pressures. During abdominal compression (*A* to *B*) increased pressure at the end of expiration is recordable after 10 s above LES and with negative pressure swings at inspiration. Reference pressure levels are represented by *broken lines*. +, positive pressure swings on inspiration; −, negative pressure swings

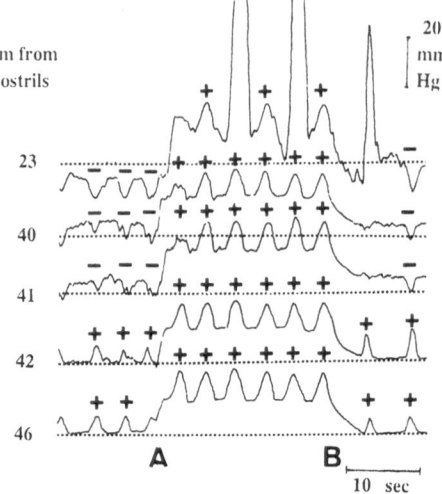

Fig. 5. Recordings of intraluminal pressures. During abdominal compression (*A* to *B*) increased pressure at the end of expiration is recordable above LES and with positive pressure swings at inspiration. Reference pressure levels are represented by *broken lines*. +, positive pressure swings on inspiration; −, negative pressure swings

Table 1. Results of viscosity test

Manometric groups	Hiatal incompetence and/or reflux	
	Before alginate	After alginate
A		4
B1		18
B2		13
C1		11
C2	80	34

Table 2. Distribution of esophagitis in the different manometric groups

Manometric groups	Grade of esophagitis					No endoscopy
	0	I	II	III	IV	
A	1	2	1	0	0	0
B1	8	3	2	0	3	2
B2	4	3	3	0	0	3
C1	3	2	3	0	1	2
C2	6	9	9	5	4	1
Total	22	19	18	5	8	8

endoscopy. Patients who had no demonstrable reflux after the intake of alginate had a lower incidence of esophagitis compared with those who had remaining tendency to reflux.

Discussion

The hiatal mechanism provides important protection against increased gastro-esophageal reflux, and this study demonstrates that the protection capacity can be improved by increasing the viscosity of the gastric contents. The viscosity test is an interesting method for distinguishing patients with a relatively good functioning hiatal mechanism from those with a completely incompetent hiatal defence and in whom severe reflux disease is likely. Patients showing instanta-neous reflux at repeated abdominal compression are a group at high risk for complications such as esophagitis or stricture. The latter group are thus can-didates for anti-reflux surgery or lifetime medical treatment.

In patients with advanced gastroesophageal reflux disease, the effect of increased viscosity of the gastric contents can clearly be demonstrated. The test has also been used in the examination of other patients and we have found the measurements to be of prognostic value and useful as a guide to therapy.

References

1. Castell DO (1992) The esophagus. Little, Brown, Boston
2. Edwards DAW (1982) The Anti-reflux Mechanism, its Disorders and their Consequences. In: Clinics in gastroenterology, vol 11, 3rd edn. London, WB Saunders, pp 479–496
3. Sandmark S (1963) Hiatal incompetencc. Acta Radiol [Suppl] (Stockh) 919:1–46
4. Mittal RK, Fisher M, McCallum RW, Rochester DF, Dent J, Sluss J (1990) Human lower esophageal sphincter pressure response to increased intra-abdominal pressure. Am J Physiol 258:G624–G630
5. Lindell D, Sandmark S (1979) Hiatal incompetence and gastro-oesophageal reflux. Acta Radiol 20:626–636
6. Sandmark S (1963) Intraluminal pressures and pH in hiatus hernia and gastroesophageal reflux. Acta Otolaryngol 56:683–698
7. Sandmark S, Zenk L (1964) Treatment with Gaviscon in hiatus hernia. Lakartidningen 61:1940–1943
8. Savary M, Miller G (1978) The esophagus. Gassmann, Solothurn

Correlation Between Preoperative and Postoperative Manometry After Nissen-Rossetti Fundoplication

Marcello Migliore, Gaetano Catania, and Gaetano Romeo[1]

Introduction

There are several factors to be considered in the pathogenesis of gastroesophageal reflux (GER) as recognized by Skinner in 1985 [1]. The three most common surgical procedures are Nissen-Rossetti fundoplication [2], the Belsey Mark IV repair [3], and the Hill procedure [4]. The principle of the first two operations is to reinforce the lower esophageal sphincter (LES) with a cuff of gastric fundus wrapped around the intra-abdominal distal esophageal segment, and the principal of the last is a posterior gastropexy [5].

The clinical result of these operations is the resolution of gastroesophageal reflux symptoms such as heartburn, regurgitation, cough, belching, and dysphagia. However, the physiological mechanisms responsible for the development and disappearance of postoperative dysphagia are still unknown.

We undertook a prospective study to assess the changes in motility of the middle and lower esophagus and changes in pressure in the LES following the Nissen-Rossetti fundoplication for gastroesophageal reflux and correlation with postoperative symptoms.

Method

Between January 1988 and December 1991, 273 patients presented with GER to our unit. Failure to respond to conservative medical treatment including dietary, postural advice, and drugs (omeprazole, cisapride) after a period of 6 months was seen in 27 patients (9.9%), which constitutes our surgical group.

[1] Department of Surgery, University of Catania, Patologia Chirurgica II, C/O Ospedale Vittorio Emanuele, Via Plebiscito 624-95124, Catania, Italy

There were 9 male and 18 female patients, with a mean age of 50 (range 28–79 years). None had any previous esophageal or gastric surgery.

Thus, 27 patients entered our study protocol which consisted of:

(a) questionnaire: heartburn, regurgitation, dysphagia, cough, and belching.
(b) preoperative studies including a barium swallow, endoscopy, manometry, and esophagogastric pH-metry.
(c) postoperative manometric studies performed at 10 days and 12 months; 24-h pH-metry was performed when necessary. The questionnaire was repeated at the time of the manometric studies.

Manometry was performed using a standard motility catheter consisting of six water-filled polyvinyl tubes bonded together with lateral openings spaced 5 cm apart. The proximal ends of the polyvinyl tubes are connected to pressure transducer and in turn to a polygraph (Synectics Medical, Inc., Sweden) connected to a computer system (IBM compatible). A constant infusion of distilled water was delivered by a (Arndorfer) (Medical Specialties, Greenfield, WI, USA) pneumohydraulic system with an infusion rate of 0.6 ml/min. The slow pull-through technique was used to study the LES pressure and the sphincter relaxation (complete when sphincter pressure drops to intragastric baseline). The inferior two-thirds of the body of the esophagus (smooth muscle) were evaluated with ten dry and ten wet swallows every 30 s (recording sites 5 and 10 cm above LES). Simultaneus, repetitive, high (>150 mmHg) and low amplitude (<20 mmHg) contractions were studied.

Esophagogastric pH-metry was carried out using two glass electrode (Ingold Eletro Wilmington, MAI) and a portable solid state monitor (Digitrapper; Synectsis Medical) that sampled and stored pH at 7-s intervals.

All the manometric studies were performed and evaluated by the same investigator, and two authors were always on the operating team. One investigator performed 92.5% of the operations. Informed consent was obtained from all patients.

Fourteen patients met our criteria and thus are the subject of this study. There were two late deaths (one myocardial infarction at 6 months and one cardiomyopathy at 8 months), two patients refused, and nine patients are awaiting manometry at 1 year.

In our laboratory, we are currently forming the control group. Statistical analysis was performed using the Student's t-test for paired data. Regression line was used to obtain a relationship between preoperative and postoperative data. A probability value less than 0.05 was considered significant. All the values were expressed as the mean ± SD.

Clinical Results

There was recurrence of heartburn in two out of eight patients at 1 year, of which one had positive gastroesophgeal reflux as evidenced by pH-metry. Dysphagia was present in two patients preoperatively, in five patients at 10 days, and in one patient at 1 year postoperatively. Preoperative symptoms of regurgitation (n = 4), cough (n = 3), and belching (n = 4) were not present at 1 year postoperatively.

Manometric Results

LES

The preoperative resting LES pressure mean was 6.3 ± 2 mmHg (range 2–14 mmHg). Ten days postoperatively, the mean LES pressure was 24.4 ± 5 mmHg which was significantly higher than preoperative results ($P < 0.005$); 1 year postoperatively the mean was 20.2 ± 3 mmHg with no statistical significance as compared with the early postoperative results ($P < 0.1$). The mean decrease of LES pressure was 4.2 mmHg (range from 0–15 mmHg). The regression line of LES pressure after 10 days and after 12 months is shown in Fig. 1.

LES Relaxation

Eight out 14 (57%) patients had incomplete relaxation at 10 days, and 3 out 14 (21%) had incomplete relaxation at 1 year postoperatively.

Body Motility

The mean wave amplitude was 41 ± 17 mmHg preoperatively, 40 ± 13 mmHg at 10 days ($P < 0.01$) and 72 ± 29 mmHg ($P < 0.025$) at 12 months postoperatively. Peristalsis was normal in 4 patients preoperatively and in 12 patients 1 year postoperatively. One patient with total esophageal body incordination had normal peristalsis in both postoperative manometric studies.

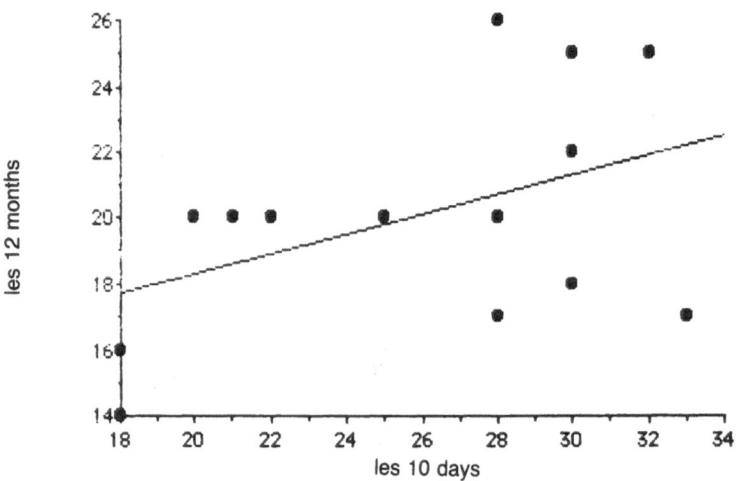

Fig. 1. Regression line of LES pressure after 10 days and after 12 months

Five out of eight patients with preoperative repetitive waves had normal peristalsis 10 days postoperatively, and only two had repetitive contractions 12 months later. Three patients with preoperative low amplitude waves had similar manometric characteristics early and late postoperatively. High amplitude waves were present in one patient preoperatively and in six (43%) 1 year postoperatively. Two patients had simultaneous waves preoperatively that were not detected at 10 days or 1 year postoperatively.

Discussion

Manometric changes in the motility of the esophagus after antireflux surgery have not been clearly demonstrated. Although postoperative motility studies [6, 7] have been performed these are retrospective with variable patterns. Prospective postoperative studies performed [8, 9] have not monitored the LES early after Nissen-Rossetti fundoplication.

The most important clinical outcome is the onset and disappearance of dysphagia [7, 8, 10, 11]. Our study shows that dysphagia is transient and tends to disappear after surgery, associated with a decrease of LES pressure, improvement of LES relaxation, and increase in the amplitude of contractions in the oesophageal body.

The mean LES pressure decreases from 10 days to 1 year with no statistical significance ($P < 0.1$); the regression line (Fig. 1) shows that the higher the early postoperative LES pressure, the greater the decrease in LES pressure at 1 year, which stabilizes at 16–18 mmHg.

The LES relaxation is abnormal in 57% (8/14) of patients in the early postoperative manometric studies, which could be secondary to surgical manipulation. Three patients had abnormal LES relaxation late postoperatively and are the same patients with low amplitude contractions. Therefore, we believe that hypotonic peristaltic contractions do not improve after surgery and that the amplitude of the esophageal contractions may play a role in the LES relaxation.

In our experience, the motility of the body shows some interesting changes. Motility disorders manifested as esophageal body incoordination (repetitive, spontaneous, or simultaneous contractions) are not a contraindication for surgery, as the majority of these problems will disappear after surgery [10]. These observations are confirmed in our experience. Of interest was one patient who had total esophageal body incoordination preoperatively and normal peristaltic contractions postoperative.

The mean contraction amplitude shows a slight drop early after surgery and increases significantly 12 months postoperatively ($P < 0.001$). Our findings are in contrast to those of DeMeester et al. [6], who showed a decrease in the amplitude after surgery (measured between 6 months and 9 years postoperatively). However, our results agree with those of Grande et al. [8] who reported an increase in amplitude 14 months versus 6 months after surgery.

The question that arises is obvious: Why did we find an increase in esophageal amplitude contractions? We believe that this is related to improved motility of the body of the esophagus with regards to both peristaltic and amplitude waves which could be due to the absence of acid reflux. We also believe that this phenomena is not related to a tight wrap, otherwise dysphagia would persist postoperatively.

Conclusion

Our Experience Indicates that:

1. The mean LES pressure decreases from 10 days to 1 year with no statistical significance.
2. LES relaxation and esophageal body function improve from 10 days to 1 year postoperatively.
3. Hypotonic esophageal contractions are associated with incomplete LES relaxation at 1 year postoperatively.
4. Esophageal peristalsis abnormalities, as total body incordination or repetitive contractions, return toward normal after Nissen-Rossetti fundoplication.
5. No correlation has been found between increase in the amplitude of contractions postoperatively and clinical dysphagia.
6. Postoperative dysphagia tends to disappear as a result of a concomitant decrease in LES pressure, improvement of LES relaxation, and increase in the amplitude of contractions.

Acknowledgment. We gratefully acknowledge Mr. Wallid Dihimis, who helped us in writing the manuscript.

References

1. Skinner DB (1985) Pathophysiology of gastroesophageal reflux. Ann Surg 202:546–556
2. Nissen R (1956) Einfache operation zur beeinflussung der reflux oesophagitis. Schweiz Med Wochenschz 86:590–592
3. Skinner DB, Belsey R (1967) Surgical management of esophageal reflux and hiatus hernia. J Thorac Cardiovasc Surg 53:33
4. Low DE, Anderson RP, Ilves R, Ricciardelli E, Hill LD (1989) Fifteen to 20 year result after the Hill antireflux operation. J Thorac Cardiovasc Surg 98:444–450
5. DeMeester T, Hill LD, Skinner DB (1988) Indications for and technique of hiatal hernia repair. Symposium Contemp Surg 33:83–104
6. DeMeester T, Bonavina L, Albertucci M (1986) Nissen fundoplication for gastroesophageal reflux disease: evaluation of primary repair in 100 consecutive patients. Ann Surg 204: 9–20
7. Breumelhof R, Feelinger HW, Vlablom V, Jansen A, Smout AJPM (1991) Dysphagia after Nissen Fundoplication. Dysphagia 6:6–10
8. Grande L, Lacima G, Ros E, Puiol A, Garcia Caldecasa JC, Fuster J, Visa J, Pera C (1991) Dysphagia and esophageal motor dysfunction in gastroesophageal reflux are corrected by fundoplication. J Clin Gastroenterol 13(1):11–16
9. Cooper JD, Gill SS, Nelems JM, Pearson FG (1977) Intraoperative and postoperative esophageal manometric findings with Collis gastroplasty and Belsey hiatal hernia repair for gastroesophageal reflux. J Thorac cardiovasc Surg 74(5):744–751

10. DeMeester T, Johnson LF, Kent AH (1974) Evaluation for current operation for the prevention of gastroesophageal reflux. Ann Surg 180:511–525
11. Kaul BK, DeMeester TR, Oka M, Ball CS, Stein HJ, Kim CB, Cheng S (1990) The cause of dysphagia in uncomplicated sliding hiatal hernia and its relief by hiatal herniorrhaphy. Ann Surg 211:406–410

A Continuous 10-Year Assessment of the Results of Surgery for Shortened Esophagus

K. Jeyasingham, N.K. Bhatnagar, G. Peppas, and H.R. Payne[1]

Introduction

The problem of shortened esophagus complicating gastro-esophageal reflux and hiatal herniation was first tackled by Collis [1] by creating a vertical gastroplasty. The purpose of the gastroplasty was to create an acute angle of entry of the esophagus into the stomach. In doing so, he also achieved a lengthening of the esophagus. Pearson, in dealing with peptic stricture complicating gastro-esophageal reflux associated with shortening, combined the procedures of a Collis gastroplasty with a Belsey type partial fundoplication [2]. The short- and long-term results of such a procedure however, revealed that the anti-reflux maneuver was not successfully accomplished by a partial fundoplication. As a result, Henderson modified the procedure by incorporating a total fundoplication of the Nissen type to the Collis gastroplasty [3].

Both Orringer [4] and Henderson [5] have described the short- and long-term results of the Collis-Nissen procedure, which are far superior to those achieved by the Pearson operation. The poor results of the Pearson operation are in fact attributable to the distortion of the neofundus by the taking up of some of the stomach in the creation of a neo-esophagus. We have described a V-Y modification to the gastroplasty which renders the neofundus globular and therefore more akin to a normal fundus, enabling a truly Belsey type partial fundoplication to be achieved [6]. The aim of this paper is to present the short- and long-term continuous assessment of patients undergoing V-Y gastroplasty and partial fundoplication.

---

[1] Department of Thoracic Surgery, Frenchay Hospital, Bristol, BS16 1LE, UK

Materials and Methods

In the 10- year period from March 1981—March 1991, 58 patients underwent a
V-Y gastroplasty and partial fundoplication in our department. There were 28
men (48.2%) and 30 women. The average age was 64.7 years (range 23–84
years). Six patients had associated pharyngeal pouch, two had esophageal webs
and one patient suffered from scleroderma. Two patients had severe chronic
obstructive airways disease. In 15 patients (25.8%), one or more anti-reflux
procedures had been performed previously. Twenty-two patients (37.9%)
presented with dysphagia preoperatively. All of these patients had a dilatable
stricture. On preoperative radiology with contrast screening a sliding hiatal
hernia was found in 47 (81%) patients, and gastro-esophageal reflux was demonstrated in only 32 (51.8%) patients. Preoperative ambulatory pH metry
was carried out successfully on 25 patients, using an antimony electrode
connected to a digitrapper (Syncetics) and analyzed on an Apple II E computer
using Syncetics pH software. Esophageal manometry was carried out using a
triple solid state terminal tipped Gaeltec transducer probe, with transducers
offset 120° and situated 5 cm apart, connected by an amplification system to
a Bryans U-V recorder set at a speed of 5 mm/s. The station pull-through
technique was applied for both wet and dry swallows. The technique of V-Y
gastroplasty and partial fundoplication was as described previously [6] and is
depicted in Fig. 1. The indication for V-Y gastroplasty and partial fundoplication was the presence of a shortened esophagus assessed either prior to
operation or at operation, whether or not associated with a dilatable stricture.
All patients were continuously assessed postoperatively at regular intervals,
clinically, radiologically, with pH metry, manometry, and endoscopy. Postoperative pH metry was successfully completed in 46 patients but the results
were meaningfully interpreted only in 31 patients. Errors of interpretation were
caused in those patients in whom the pH and manometry probes were mal-
positioned due to breathing or coughing movements, and also brought into close
proximity of the neo-esophagus, where the ambient pH was acidic [7].

Results

The operation carried an early mortality (hospital and 30 day) of 5.2%. One
patient died of pulmonary embolism complicating peritonitis as a result of
leakage of the suture line. A second patient died as a result of acute myocardial
ischemia, and a third patient died from a cerebral infarct. There were three late
deaths (5.2%), all due to natural causes, unrelated to V-Y gastroplasty and
partial fundoplication. One patient emigrated and was lost to follow-up. Two
other asymptomatic patients refused invasive postoperative investigations and
were excluded from the study. One patient developed an adenocarcinoma in
the neo-esophagus 3.5 years after V-Y gastroplasty partial fundoplication and is
now alive 2.5 years after esophago-gastric resection and reconstruction. Thus, 48
patients were available for follow-up from 6 months to 10.5 years (mean 4.8
years). Overall clinical status was assessed on Visick scale. Thirty-three patients
were in Visick class I, 12 in class II, 2 patients in class IIIu, and 1 patient in class
IIIs. There were none in class IV. The co-relation between reflux demonstrated

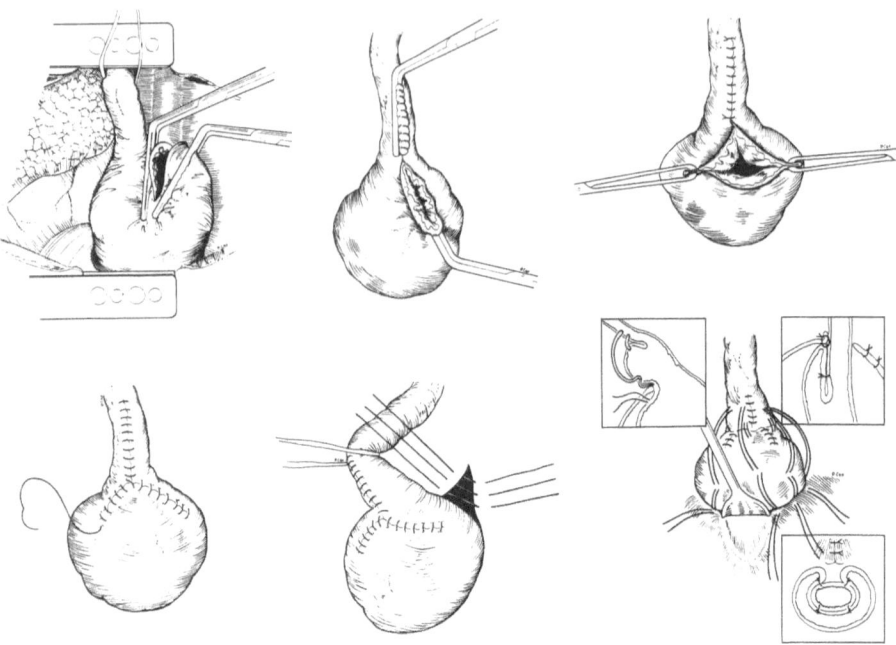

Fig. 1. The technique of V-Y gastroplasty and partial fundoplication is shown in stages from *left to right top to bottom*. The final stages of the fundoplication are as performed in a partial fundoplication of 240 in the Mark IV Belsey fashion but using more sutures in the inversion wrap as there is sufficient neofundus available for this purpose

on radiology, with clinical evidence of reflux, was present in three patients only. In the long-term, 36 patients have remained entirely asymptomatic from the time of surgery. One patient developed dysphagia for the first time within weeks of the operation and required one dilatation only. Only two others who presented preoperatively with a stricture continue to have dysphagia, while five continue to manifest dysphagia, although stricture has been adequately dilated. Two of these patients who subsequently were shown to have disordered motor activity persisted with their dysphagia despite control of reflux and adequate dilatation of stricture.

Of the 31 patients who successfully underwent postoperative esophageal manometry, 24 showed a normal motility pattern. Seven patients showed abnormalities in their motility and Table 1 shows the nature of the abnormality in co-relation to the symptoms and the treatment required. In patients in whom both pre- and postoperative manometry was successfully completed, it was possible to compare the results to assess the effects of surgery. In ten patients, the lower esophageal high pressure zone showed an elevation of the tone by a mean of 4.8 mmHg. In four patients, the tone remained unchanged, while in three other patients there was a decrease of the tone by a mean of 2.75 mmHg (Fig. 2). The changes in lower esophageal high pressure zone did not co-relate with the Visick grading of symptomatology. In 31 patients whose ambulatory pH

Table 1. Postoperative esophageal manometry 7 in abnormal patients out of a total of 31 patients; 24 patients were normal

Patient	Manometry	Symptoms and treatment
EP	Poor peristalsis Non-relaxation of HPZ	None No dilatation required for past 12 months
US	DMA Non-relaxation of HPZ	Dysphagia reflux, required dilatation
LT	DMA Poor peristalsis	Dysphagia Dilated × 9 Now asymptomatic
AC	Poor peristalsis HPZ—non-relaxation	Dysphagia Dilated × 5
LB	HPZ—non-relaxation	Asymptomatic
EF	DMA	Dysphagia Dilatations required
EL	Poor peristalsis HPZ—low tone, non-relaxation	Asymptomatic

DMA, disordered motor activity; *HPZ*, high pressure zone
Each of the abnormal patients showed a variety of motility disturbances and these findings are correlated with the symptoms and the need for dilatation

metry was successfully interpreted, 18 have no demonstrable reflux. Eleven patients show minimal reflux but not reaching significant levels on the DeMeester score [8].

One patient shows significant acid reflux and one other shows significant alkaline reflux, both of whom have their symptoms controlled on a medical regimen. Endoscopically, three patients who showed grade III–IV esophagitis preoperatively have all required medical treatment postoperatively and have shown complete healing since. However, each required one, four, and five dilatations respectively, despite total healing of the esophagitis. Of the entire series of 16 patients who presented with preoperative dysphagia, associated with stricture in all patients, only two currently require dilatations 7–8 years after surgery. Radiologically, there was no incidence of recurrence of herniation. Pylorospasm and gastro-esophageal reflux was seen in three asymptomatic patients.

Discussion

Acquired shortening of the esophagus is one of the sequelae of severe gastro-esophageal reflux, transmural esophagitis ultimately leading to longitudinal and circumferential shortening. Esophageal lengthening by Collis gastroplasty allows the creation of a neo-esophagus which can then be brought down intra-abdominally enabling a fundoplication procedure without tension. The tube of

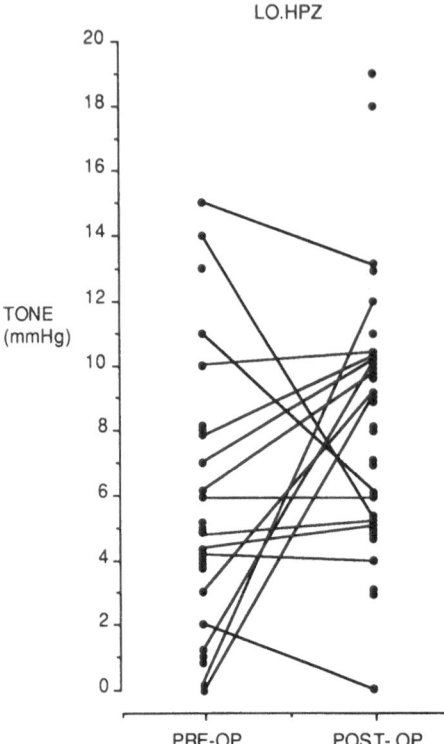

Fig. 2. Shows the pre- and postoperative values of the lower esophageal high pressure zone (*LOHPZ*). The mean length of the pressure zone measured 3.8 cm with a range of 2–4 cm. The mean value for the tones was 11.5 mmHg in the postoperative assessment. There were some patients who had preoperative values but did not successfully complete the postoperative study. Similarly, there were some who underwent the postoperative study successfully but did not complete the preoperative studies adequately

stomach thus created provides a healthy tissue free of peri-esophagitis in which sutures can be placed safely without the risk of breakdown. Henderson [3] has reported a recurrent reflux rate of 44.6% after a Collis-Belsey procedure and Orringer [4] found a 19% incidence of failure to control symptoms of reflux and a 30% incidence of moderate to serious reflux on pH testing after a Collis-Belsey repair. It is clear that following a Collis gastroplasty, the sausage shape of the neofundus lacks lateral mobility and thus, is not suitable for a Belsey type fundic wrap. With the V-Y modification that we have described, this feature is overcome and an ample, broad neofundus is available for a partial fundoplication of the Belsey mark IV type. The effectiveness of any anti-reflux operation is best judged on the basis of long-term subjective and objective clinical results.

In this report, a total of 58 patients were operated upon and the long-term follow-up of 10.5 years is now available with a mean 4.8 years. Routine postoperative esophageal function testing was utilized and overall clinical status was assessed on the Visick scoring system. On pH metry, one patient showed acid reflux and another alkaline reflux. Both patients have remained asymptomatic on medical therapy. However, a physiological degree of reflux was seen in 11 patients who remain entirely asymptomatic. This is in contrast to the standard Collis-Belsey operation, where 30% showed abnormal reflux after a mean follow-up of 13 months [9], while only 9% of patients following the Collis-Nissen operation continue to have objective pH evidence of abnormal reflux [10]. Any operation designed to augment the lower esophageal high pressure zone has a potential for producing postoperative dysphagia. The Collis-Nissen operation has the added potential for gas bloat syndrome. Following the latter operation, a significant degree of postoperative dysphagia requiring regular dilatations, has been reported in 12% of patients, while a further 10% require occasional dilatations [10]. With the Collis-Belsey operation, an incidence of 11% dysphagia requiring regular dilatations were reported by Pearson et al. [11].

A previous history of anti-reflux operation has been recognised as a significant risk factor for an unsatisfactory result from any additional anti-reflux procedure. An overally unsatisfactory result has been reported in nearly 49% of the patients undergoing a Collis-Nissen operation [10]. However, in our series of V-Y gastroplasty, in the series of 15 patients who required this operation for recurrent reflux problems, the incidence of unsatisfactory results has been reduced to 13%. Disordered motor activity of the esophagus continue to pose a problem. Scleroderma is clearly a risk factor for poor results after an anti-reflux operation. However, our single patient with scleroderma remains symptom-free despite having required dilatations in the early years after surgery. Pearson [12] also has reported excellent results with the Collis-Belsey procedure in this group of patients.

The operative treatment of gastro-esophageal reflux, with or without a dilatable stricture and with or without a previous anti-reflux operation, remains a challenge. However, a V-Y gastroplasty and partial fundoplication offers excellent long-term results: 77% of our patients in the series of 58 remain symptom free. Allowing for those not available for full assessment, this figure rises to 94% (45 out of 48 patients). None of the patients has required a re-operation for gastroesophageal reflux or recurrent hiatal herniation following a V-Y gastroplasty.

References

1. Collis JL (1961) Gastroplasty. Thorax 16:197–206
2. Pearson FG, Tanger B, Henderson RD (1971) Gastroplasty and Belsey—Hiatal Hernia repair. J Thor Cardiovasc Surg 61:50–63
3. Henderson RD (1977) Reflux control following gastroplasty. Ann Thorac Surg 24:206–214
4. Orringer MB (1985) The combined Collis gastroplasty—Nissen fundoplication for gastro-esophageal reflux. In: De Meester TR, Skinner DB (eds) Esophageal disorders. Raven, New York, pp. 203–208
5. Henderson RD (1986) Surgical management of the failed gastroplasty. J Thorac Cardiovasc Surg 91:45–52
6. Reilly KM, Jeyasingham K (1984) A modified Pearson gastroplasty. Thorax 39:67–69
7. Choiniere L, Payne HR, Jeyasingham K (1986) Pre- and postoperative prolonged pH and manometric studies in patients undergoing V-Y gastroplasty with partial fundoplication. In: Siewert JT, Holscher AH (eds) Diseases of the esophagus. Springer, Berlin Heidelberg New York, pp 1193–1197
8. Demeester TR (1985) Limitations of twenty-four hour pH monitoring of the esophagus. In: Demeester TR, Skinner DB (eds) Esophageal disorders. Raven, New York, pp 109–117
9. Orringer MB, Sloan H (1977) Complications and failing of the combined Collis-Belsey operation. J Thorac Cardiovasc Surg 74:726–735
10. Stirling MC, Orringer MB (1989) Continued assessment of the combined Collis-Nissen operation. Ann Thorac Surg 47:224–230

11. Pearson FG, Cooper JD, Nelems JM (1978) Gastroplasty and fundoplication in the man-
    agement of complex reflux problems. J Thorac Cardiovasc Surg 76:665–672
12. Pearson FG (1985) Collis-Belsey procedure for peptic strictures five to fifteen years follow-
    up. In: Demeester TR, Skinner DB (eds) Esophageal disorders. Raven, New York,
    pp 257–259

Reflux Esophagitis and Development of Ectopic Columnar Epithelium in the Esophageal Stump After Gastric Transposition: A Prospective Study

I. Cecconello, J. Mariano Da Rocha, B. Zilberstein, V. Felix, and H.W. Pinotti[1]

Summary. Fifty-eight consecutive cases submitted to esophagectomy and gastric transposition because of advanced achalasia were followed prospectively. All patients underwent endoscopy and acid secretion studies both pre- and post-operatively (6 and 48 months after resection). Esophagitis was observed in 7 cases after 6 months (15.9%) and 24 cases at the second evaluation (41.3%). Of these, 12 complained of heartburn (50%). In 4 of the 58 cases (7%), ectopic columnar epithelium ranging in length from 1.5 to 3.0 cm was observed in the esophageal stump. An ulcer was present in one case and intestinal metaplasia was diagnosed in another. All subjects were treated clinically with continuous antacid therapy, mandatory in 8 cases. Regurgitation and bile in the transposed stomach were noted frequently (50%) in cases with and without esophagitis. Regarding preoperative status, basal and stimulated acid output decreased in the first p.o. evaluation but increased over the long term, and higher mean levels were observed in the group with esophagitis. In conclusion, reflux esophagitis was found to occur even after high anastomoses positioned above the aortic arch. Furthermore, as the period of observation increases, the incidence and intensity of reflux esophagitis rise due to greater exposure of the stump to reflux, regurgitation, and the constant presence of bile and progressively higher acid output in the transposed stomach. Endoscopic follow-up is mandatory because of the possibility of developing ectopic columnar epithelial lining. Lastly, employment of the stomach after esophagectomy is not contraindicated by esophagitis.

[1] Digestive Surgery Division, São Paulo University Medical School, Av. Arnolfo Azevedo, 201 01236-030, São Paulo, Brazil

91

Introduction

Esophagectomy with esophagogastroplasty and cervical anastomosis is presently the procedure of choice in the management of Chagas' megaesophagus. This is explained in part by the advances which have made possible a one-stage operation with low morbidity and mortality and good postoperative clinical results [1–8].

However, careful follow-up has revealed some mild complications that so long as they are diagnosed and adequately treated do not markedly influence the clinical progress of these patients. The scope of this paper is to describe a new complication, that is, the development of ectopic columnar epithelium (ECE) (Barrett's esophagus) in the cervical esophageal stump (CES). This finding has already been reported on this Service [9].

The development of ECE had never been described at this site and under these conditions. This situation seems to be intimately related to reflux esophagitis.

Both qualitative and quantitative reflux esophagitis was also assessed in this study. With this objective, pre- and postoperative gastric acid secretion and the condition of the esophageal mucosa using endoscopic examinations were studied. It was possible that changes that characterize ECE, might occur in the CES in the cases of chronic esophagitis of long-standing duration. This hypothesis was confirmed with the endoscopic diagnosis and histologic proof of the existence of ECE in the remaining cervical esophagus.

Material and Methods

Between January 1976 to December 1991, a prospective study of 58 patients with Chagas' megaesophagus submitted to transmediastinal subtotal esophagectomy (Pinotti's technique) with transposition of the stomach to the cervical region. The mean length of the cervical esophageal stump was 5 cm.

Pre- and postoperative endoscopic examinations of the esophagus, stomach and duodenum as well as acid secretion of the stomach were carried out on all patients. The postoperative study was undertaken 6 to 48 months after esophageal resection.

Results

The surgery and postoperative course of all these subjects was uneventful. The specific goal of this report was to study gastroesophageal reflux and its effect on the esophageal stump. Therefore, the studies in these patients included gastric acid secretion, endoscopy and biospies of the esophageal mucosa during the times mentioned.

The results are demonstrated in Tables 1–5.

Table 1. Endoscopic results (58 cases)

Endoscopy	Preop	6 months	3–16 years (mean = 4 years)
Normal esophagus (superior 1/3)	58	51	34
Esophagitis (superior 1/3)	—	7 (15.9%)	24 (41.3%)

Table 2. Results of the study of gastric acid secretion

Acid secretion	Basal (mEq/l)	MAO (mEq/l)
Preop	1.2 + 0.6	19.7 + 7.3
6 months postop	0.9 + 1.3	8.0 + 7.5
48 months postop	1.6 + 0.8	18.2 + 10.3

MAO, maximal acid output

Table 3. Type of endoscopic reflux esophagitis after gastric transposition (24 cases)[a]

Type of esophagitis	6 months	3–16 years (mean = 4 years)
Hyperemic	4	9
Erosive	3	11
Columnar epithelium	—	4 (16.6%/6.8%)
Total	7	24

[a] Continuous medical treatment in 8 cases (33.3%/13.8%)

Table 4. Types of ectopic columnar epithelium in the esophageal stump after gastric transposition (4 cases)

Case	1	2	3	4
6 months	normal	esophagitis	normal	normal
Time interval	esophagitis	esophagitis	esophagitis	esophagitis
Time of diagnosis	columnar epithelium 3 years	columnar epithelium 18 months	columnar epithelium 6 years	columnar epithelium 7 years

Table 5. Length of ectopic columnar epithelium in the esophageal stump after gastric transposition

Case	1	2	3	4
Length	3 cm	3 cm	1.5 cm + Esophageal ulceration	3 cm
Type of epithelium	Intestinal + fundic	Fundic	Pyloric + fundic	Pyloric

Discussion

Reflux esophagitis in the esophageal stump after subtotal esophagectomy and esophagogastroplasty with cervical anastomosis has been reported by several authors: Mariano da Rocha [6] in a prospective study, reported a rate of 20%; Cecconello et al. [7], 14.5%; and Pinotti et al. [5], 25%.

It is well-known that bile salts injure both the gastric and the esophageal mucosa and their harmful effects are strengthened by the action of gastric secretion. The latter mechanism seems to be responsible for esophagitis in the CES, similarly to what occurs in patients with reflux esophagitis and Barrett's esophagus with the organ in the normal position. However, some authors [8, 10], deny the presence of reflux esophagitis after esophagogastroplasty with cervical anastomosis. A possible explanation for this might be that these investigators studied subjects with esophageal cancer whose gastric acid secretion is usually low and who were followed-up for time intervals varying from 6 to 12 months. In our opinion, the presence of reflux esophagitis after gastroplasty is unquestionable both in patients followed over the mid- as well as the long-term.

The development of ECE in the CES after subtotal esophagectomy with transposition of the stomach and esophagogastric anastomosis had never been described either at this site or under these conditions. This factor seems to be closely related to the gastroesophageal reflux (bile and gastric secretions), culminating in a new challenge in the follow-up of these patients.

The increase in the incidence of esophagitis in the esophageal stump over time, together with the progressive rise in gastric acid secretion and the continuing biliary reflux has been the subject of study by our group. The latter are always on the alert to possible complications that might occur at this level with time.

In 1990, we were able to confirm and report four cases with development of ECE in the CES.

All 58 patients in the present prospective study underwent endoscopy and gastric acid secretion studies pre- and postoperatively (6 and 84 months after resection). Esophagitis was noted in 7 patients (15.9%) after 6 months and in 24 patients (41.3%) at the time of the second assessment (Tables 1 and 2). Twelve subjects (50%) reported heartburn and in 4 of them (7%) the development of finger-like ECE was observed in the CES (Tables 3 and 4), varying from 1.5 to 3.0 cm above the esophagogastric anastomosis. An ulcer was present in one case and in another, intestinal metaplasia associated with fundic type epithelium was diagnosed (Table 5). A pyloric type of epithelium was also confirmed (Fig. 1).

The preoperative levels of basal and stimulated acid secretion decreased at the first postoperative assessment, but increased over the long-term, with higher mean values noted in the group with esophagitis (Table 2). The observed tendency of marked increase in the intensity of reflux esophagitis (Table 3), accompanying the significant rise in gastric acid secretion (Table 2) had already been reported by Cecconello et al. [7].

In addition, on endoscopic examination persistent gastroesophageal regurgitation (79%) and biliary reflux (70%) were noted in the cases of esophagitis. However, gastroesophageal reflux (41%) and biliary reflux (64%) were also present in the cases without esophagitis.

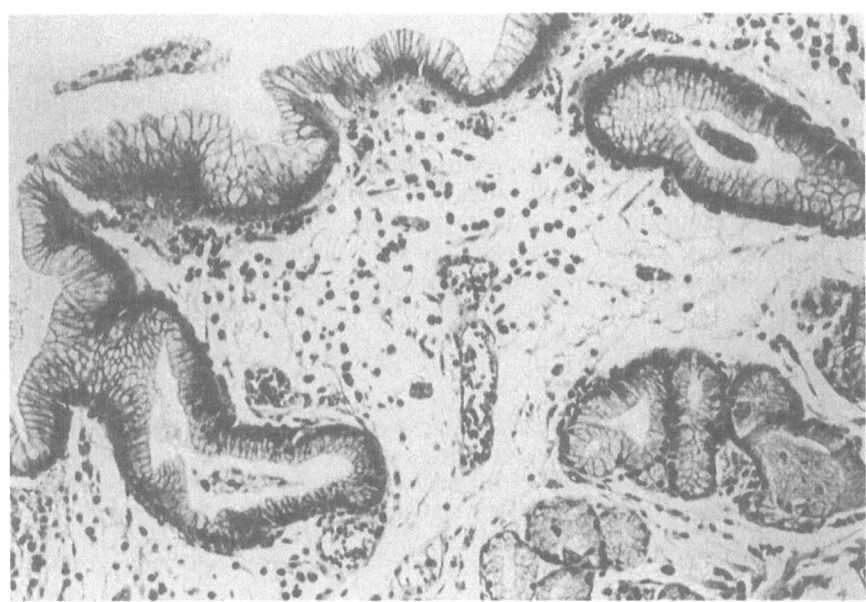

Fig. 1. Ectopic columnar epithelium (pyloric type) obtained from the cervical esophageal stump at the site of Barrett's epithelium. (H&E, ×85)

The mean length of the esophageal stump was 5 cm. The diagnosis of ECE in the CES was established from 18 to 84 months after esophagogastroplasty. The importance of a follow-up of at least 18 months for the analysis of metaplasic epithelium is stressed because the earliest case in which this condition was diagnosed was at 18 months p.o. (Table 4). In subjects without esophagitis, the pale rose color of the esophageal stump on endoscopy is in marked contrast with the reddish-rose (salmon) color of those cases developing ECE. It is emphasized that this diagnosis was always preceded by esophagitis of the stump, lasting for at least a year before the appearance of ECE. It is noteworthy to underscore that with time, in spite of the increase in symptoms of heartburn and the cases of esophagitis, at the time of diagnosis of ECE of the CES, no marked change in the clinical picture was noted in any patient. This factor is significant because it demonstrates the necessity of yearly endoscopy in these patients, even when they are asymptomatic. All cases of esophagitis of the stump were managed clinically, with antacid therapy maintained in 8 cases.

The complications previously diagnosed and treated in our follow-up (reflux esophagitis, alkaline reflux esophagitis, diarrhea and dumping) are of low incidence and clinically controllable.

Nevertheless, it is necessary to emphasize that the mention of rare complications resulting from esophagogastroplasty, in no way discredit the merits of this procedure which in addition to solving the serious problem of dysphagia and effecting a gain in weight and nutritional status, returns the patient promptly to society and the work force. The low mortality and ease of the procedure should also be stressed.

Conclusion

Our study showed that reflux esophagitis can occur even after high anastomoses positioned above the aortic arch. Furthermore, as the period of observation increases, the incidence and intensity of reflux esophagitis rise due to greater exposure of the stump to reflux, regurgitation, and the constant presence of bile and progressively higher acid output in the transposed stomach. Endoscopic follow-up is mandatory because of the possibility of developing ectopic columnar epithelial lining. Lastly, we were able to show that employment of the stomach after esophagectomy is not contraindicated by esophagitis.

References

1. Ferreira-Santos R (1963) Surgical treatment of aperistalsis of the esophagus (in Portuguese). Ribeirão Preto, Thesis, São Paulo University Medical School
2. Ferreira EAB (1975) Subtotal esophagectomy and posterior transmediastinal esophagogastroplasty without thoracotomy in the treatment of megaesophagus (in Portuguese). Thesis, São Paulo University Medical School
3. Pinotti HW (1977) Transmediastinal subtotal esophagectomy without thoracotomy (in Portuguese). AMB Rev Assoc Med Bras 23:395
4. Pinotti HW, Zilberstein B, Pollara WM, Raia AA (1981) Esophagectomy without thoracotomy. Surg Gynecol Obstet 152:344–346
5. Pinotti HW, Cecconello I, Mariano da Rocha J, Zilberstein B (1991) Resection for achalasia of the esophagus. Hepatogastroenterology 38:470–473
6. Mariano-da-Rocha J (1986) Surgical treatment of the advanced megaesophagus by subtotal esophagectomy associated with gastroplasty: Clinical evaluation and study of the gastric acid secretion and levels of serum pepsinogen and gastrin (in Portuguese). Thesis, São Paulo University Medical School
7. Cecconello I, Mariano da Rocha JR, Pollara WM, Zilberstein B, Pinotti HW (1988) Long-term evaluation of gastroplasty in achalasia. In: Siewert JR, Holscher AH (eds) Diseases of the esophagus. Springer, Berlin Heidelberg New York, pp 975–979
8. Holscher AH, Voit H, Buttermann G, Siewert JR (1988) Function of the intrathoracic stomach as esophageal replacement. World J Surg 12:835
9. Mariano da Rocha JR, Cecconello I, Sallum RAA, Sakai P, Zilberstein B, Pinotti HW (1991) Barrett esophagus in the esophageal stump, after subtotal esophagectomy with cervical esophagogastroplasty (in Portuguese). ABCD Arq Bras Cir Dig 6 [Suppl 2]:20
10. Okada N, Nishimura O, Sakurai T, Tsuchihashi S, Juhri M (1986) Gastric functions in patients with intrathoracic stomach after esophageal surgery. Ann Surg 204:144

Gastroesophageal Reflux After Gastric Surgery

Mamoru Hiraishi, Toshiro Konishi, Kiyoshi Mori, Ken-ichi Mafune, Takeshi Miyama, Tooru Hirata, Haruhiro Nishina, and Yasuo Idezuki[1]

Summary. Esophageal and gastric pH monitoring and endoscopic examination of the esophagus were performed in patients after gastric surgery. The duration time and frequency of gastroesophageal reflux were studied using an ambulatory 24-h pH monitoring system. The subjects consisted of 43 patients with distal gastrectomy, 3 patients with proximal gastrectomy, 19 patients with total gastrectomy, 9 patients with reflux esophagitis without previous gastric surgery, and 53 preoperative patients. Esophageal and gastric pH were measured 5 cm above and 5 cm or 10 cm below the esophagogastric junction (EGJ). The duration, ratio and frequency of acid (pH < 4.0) and alkaline (pH > 7.4) reflux, acid and alkaline clearance time, and mean and median pH were measured. From the pattern of the esophageal pH curve, patients were divided into four groups: normal, acid reflux, alkaline reflux, and mixed type. In patients who received distal gastrectomy, acid reflux time (pH < 4) was longer than in preoperative patients. The most common reflux patterns were acid reflux and alkaline reflux. There were some tendencies to reflux when in the supine position, and before and after meals. Endoscopic findings of the esophagus were almost normal, but after iodine staining, slightly unstained patchy areas were recognized in patients in these two groups. After total gastrectomy, alkaline reflux time (pH > 7.4) and alkaline clearance time were longer than in preoperative patients. There were a few patients who showed small changes in esophageal pH in spite of esophagitis; the esophagitis in these patients was considered to be due to pancreatic enzymes.

[1] Second Department of Surgery, University of Tokyo, 7-3-1 Hongo, Bunkyo-ku, Tokyo, 113 Japan

Table 1. Subjects

Preoperative patients		53
Distal gastrectomy		43
Billroth I	37	
Billroth II	6	
Total gastrectomy		19
Roux-Y	18	
Interposition	1	
Reflux esophagitis		9

Table 2. Analysis system and components

Recorder	Digitrapper MKII or Medilog 1010
Electrode	antimony or glass electrode (MI 506)
Location	5 cm above EGJ, 5 cm or 10 cm below EGJ
Computer	NEC 9801
Analysis	Gastrosoft
Variables	
Acid	< pH 4.0
Alkaline	> pH 7.4
Duration (time %)	
Reflux number	
Frequency	
Clearance time	
Mean pH, median pH	

EGJ: Esophago-Gastric-Junction

Introduction

Gastroesophageal reflux or reflux esophagitis is one of the post-gastrectomy syndromes. In patients with reflux esophagitis who have not undergone gastric surgery, the most common cause is acid reflux. On the other hand, after total gastrectomy, esophagitis is considered to be caused by alkaline reflux such as bile and pancreatic juice. After distal gastrectomy, the refluxate is considered to be acidic or alkaline, or a mixture of the two. The acid production of the remnant stomach is very poor in many patients after subtotal gastrectomy for gastric carcinoma, but there are some patients who have the ability to produce gastric acid. In these patients, acid reflux is sometimes observed in the lower esophagus. It is important to know the contents of the refluxate because the therapy is quite different in cases of acid or alkaline reflux.

We performed ambulatory 24-h pH monitoring of the esophagus and stomach after gastric surgery. By measuring the gastric pH and esophageal pH simultaneously, we can easily know what is the refluxate. The aim of this study was to clarify the status of gastroesophageal reflux after gastric surgery.

Materials and Methods

Ambulatory 24-h pH monitoring was performed in 65 patients after gastric surgery, 53 preoperative patients, and 9 patients with reflux esophagitis. Details of patient numbers are shown in Table 1. These numbers include both symp-

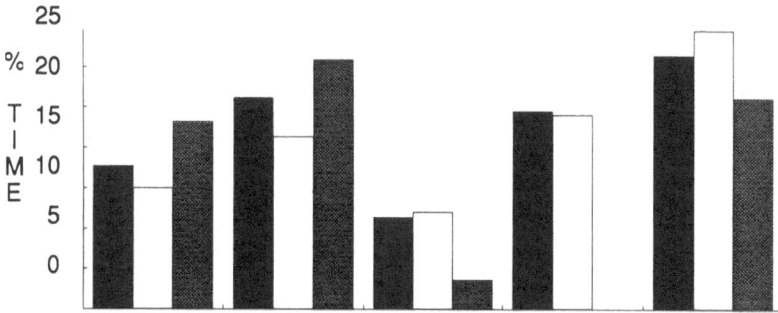

Fig. 1. Acid reflux time (pH < 4.0). *Solid columns*, whole day; *open columns*, upright; *stippled columns*, supine; *DIST*, distal; *GAST*, gastrectomy; *PROX*, proximal; *REFL.ESOPH*, reflux esophagitis

tomatic and asymptomatic patients. All the patients were in-patients at our hospital and received ordinary hospital food. We used digitrapper MK II (Synectic Medical) or Medilog 1010 (Oxford Medical) as pH monitoring systems. The monitoring systems, electrodes, and variables analyzed are shown in Table 2. The pH catheter was located 5 cm above, and 5 cm or 10 cm below the esophago gastric junction. The location of the catheter was determined by x-ray examination with barium swallowing. The duration, clearance time, ratio and frequency of acid reflux (pH < 4.0) and alkaline reflux (pH > 7.4) were measured, and mean and median pH were calculated in the supine and upright positions.

Results

From the pattern of the esophageal pH curve, patients were divided into four groups: normal, acid reflux, alkaline reflux, and mixed type. In patients after distal gastrectomy, the mean percentage duration of acid reflux (pH < 4) was $5.7 \pm 1.7\%$ in one 24-h-period (whole day), which was much greater than that of preoperative patients ($3.2 \pm 0.4\%$). Figure 1 shows the acid reflux time below pH 4.0. The time is shown as a percentage in a 24-h-period, in the upright and supine positions. The most common reflux patterns were acid and alkaline reflux. There were some tendencies to reflux in the supine position, before and after meals (pH < 4.0; supine, $4.7 \pm 1.8\%$, upright, $6.2 \pm 2.7\%$). The acid clearance time was also prolonged. Figure 2 shows the acid clearance time below pH 4.0 (the mean duration time of each acid reflux in the esophagus). The acid clearance time was prolonged in the supine position, except in patients who underwent total gastrectomy; in these patients acid was present only with food and acid reflux was observed mostly in upright position in the daytime. Endoscopic findings in the esophagus were almost normal, but after iodine staining, slightly stained patchy areas were recognized in patients with acid and alkaline reflux.

After total gastrectomy, alkaline reflux time (pH > 7.4) was $7.9 \pm 3.1\%$, being greater than that of preoperative patients ($4.6 \pm 1.4\%$); it was prolonged in the supine position. Figure 3 shows the alkaline reflux time which was

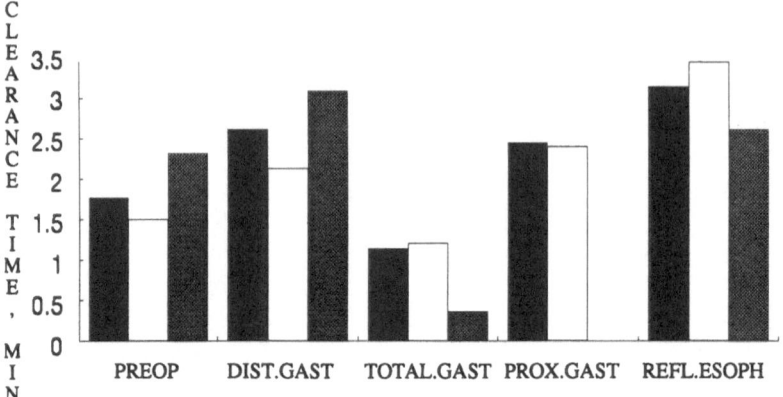

Fig. 2. Acid clearance time (pH < 4.0)

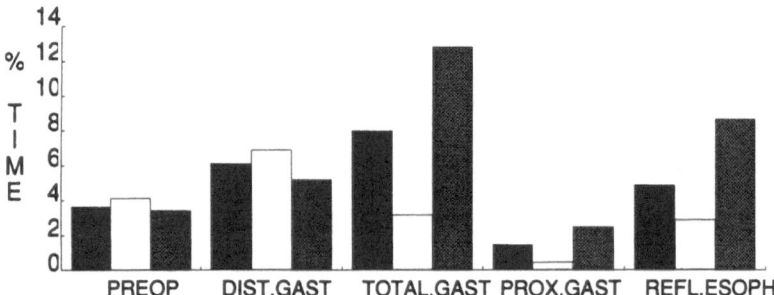

Fig. 3. Alkaline reflux time (pH > 7.4)

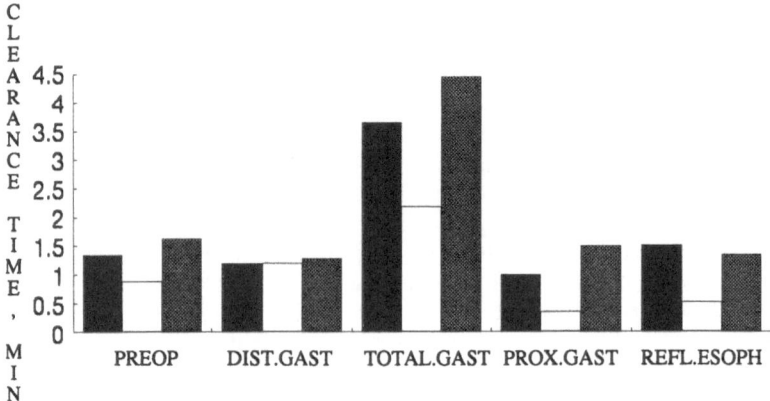

Fig. 4. Alkaline clearance time (pH > 7.4). The alkaline clearance time was much prolonged in patients after total gastrectomy, especially in the supine position

prolonged in patients after total gastrectomy and distal gastrectomy. The alkaline clearance time was greatly prolonged in patients after total gastrectomy, especially in the supine position. Figure 4 shows the alkaline clearance time. There were a few patients who showed small changes in esophageal pH in spite of esophagitis; esophagitis in these patients was considered to be due to pancreatic enzymes. After distal gastrectomy, the mean esophageal pH was 5.8 and the median esophageal pH was 5.9. The mean gastric pH was 5.4 and median gastric pH was 5.6. After distal gastrectomy, five patients showed reflux esophagitis endoscopically. One patient was considered to have acid reflux, and four were considered to have either alkaline reflux or mixed type esophagitis.

Discussion

Esophageal pH monitoring has been performed previously in gastroesophageal reflux and reflux esophagitis patients [1, 2]. In many reports, refluxate was acidic, and medical treatment using H_2 blockers and antacids, or surgical treatment, was performed. On the other hand, there are relatively fewer reports of alkaline reflux [3, 4]. Stoker and Williams reported alkaline reflux esophagitis after gastrectomy, the esophagitis being considered to be due to bile salts and pancreatic enzymes; the mixture of acids and these substances led to toxic synergism [5]. Gotley et al. performed continuous aspiration of refluxate in the lower esophagus in patients after gastrectomy. They observed conjugated bile acids and trypsin in patients in the supine position [6]. In our study, gastroesophageal reflux was studied after various types of gastric surgery. After distal gastrectomy, alkaline, acidic, or mixed type reflux was identified. After total gastrectomy, alkaline reflux occurred predominantly in the supine position. For the treatment of alkaline and mixed type reflux, oral administration of camostat mesilate was effective. We set the alkaline pH above pH 7.4. That is the physiologically normal serum pH. The alkaline reflux time did not always correspond with the degree of esophagitis, but it was considered to be a good indicator of alkaline reflux.

References

1. Johnson LF, DeMeester TR (1974) Twenty-four-hour pH monitoring of the distal esophagus: A quantitative measure of gastroesophageal reflux. Am J Gastroenterol 62:325–332
2. DeMeester TR, Johnson LF, Joseph GJ, Toscano MS, Hall AW, Skinner DB (1976) Patterns of gastroesophageal reflux in health and disease. Ann Surg 184:459–470
3. Cortesini C, Marcuzzo G, Pucciani F (1985) Relationship between mixed acid-alkaline gastroesophageal reflux and esophagitis. It J Surg Sci 15i:9–15
4. Penagini R, Yuen H, Misiewict JJ, Bianchi PA (1988) Alkaline intraesophageal pH and gastrooesophageal reflux in patients with peptic oesophagitis. Scand J Gastroenterol 23: 675–678
5. Stoker DL, Williams JG (1991) Alkaline reflux esophagitis. Gut 32:1090–1092
6. Gotley DC, Ball DE, Owen RW, Williamson RCN, Cooper MJ (1992) Evaluation and surgical correction of esophagitis after partial gastrectomy. Surg 111:29–36

Surgical Treatment

Video-Assisted Laparoscopic Surgery in Achalasia

HENRIOUE WALTER PINOTTI, ARY NASI, CARLOS EDUARDO DOMENE, MARCO AURELIO SANTO, and HILTON TELLES LIBANORI[1]

Introduction

The management of achalasia should depend on the degree of esophageal involvement assessed individually in order to indicate precisely the therapeutic measures for each case. Staging based on morphological and functional variables is used to distinguish the different degrees of esophageal involvement more accurately. Radiologic and manometric studies are used for assessment as follows:

Incipient

Undilated esophagus, with some stasis of contrast and/or radiologic evidence suggestive of motor changes and some manometric confirmation of megaesophagus.

Intermediate

Esophageal dilatation less than 7 cm, x-ray of the esophagus shows it is still in its normal position and manometric studies indicate esophageal aperistalsis, swallowing patterns with amplitude of over 10 cm of water.

Advanced

Esophageal dilatation over 7 cm and/or a "sigmoid" appearance of the esophagus on x-ray. Manometric studies reveal esophageal aperistalsis, swallowing patterns with amplitudes of less than 10 cm of water.

[1] Department of Gastroenterology, [1] Hospital das Clinicas of the University of São Paulo Medical School, Av. Dr. Eneas de Carvalho Aguiar. 255—9o. andar São Paulo, Brazil Cep: 05403

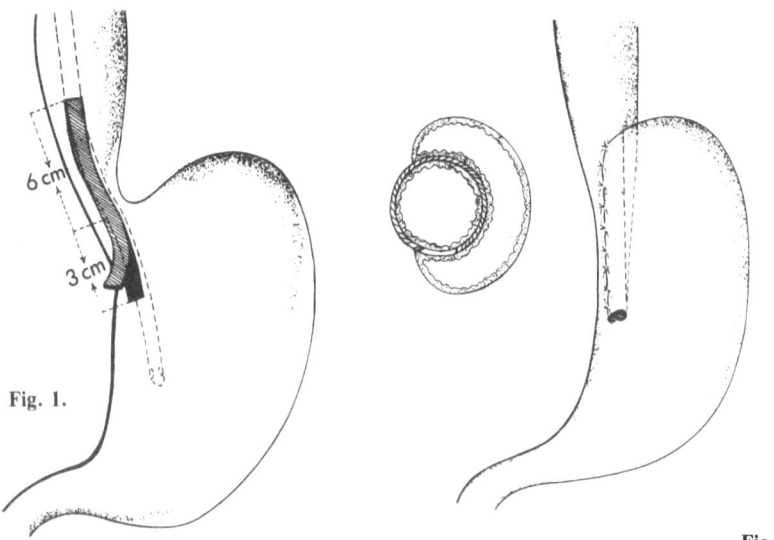

Fig. 1.

Fig. 2.

Fig. 1. Cardiomyectomy

Fig. 2. Partial valvuloplasty. In the cross section of the valvuloplasty region, notice that the esophagus is partially wrapped by the gastric fundus using three suture lines: A posterior one, another in the left margin of the myectomy, and the third in the right margin

Our guidelines for management of achalasia are based on the above staging. Therefore, for subjects with the non-advanced type of the disorder (incipient and intermediate), we recommend a 9-cm-long cardiomyectomy, 6 cm in the distal esophagus and 3 cm in the stomach (Fig. 1), together with Pinotti's anti-reflux valvuloplasty [1] (Fig. 2).

Although satisfactory results were achieved [2] in over 1000 patients with achalasia, managed during the last 15 years by the open procedure, we feel motivated to open new horizons with the modern technique of video assisted laparoscopic surgery (VALS).

After technical training and our past experience utilizing VALS for cholecystectomies since November 1990, we felt secure enough in April 1991, to perform the first VALS cardiomyotomy for management of megaesophagus.

The current series with the procedure, technical details and initial results will be presented.

Material

From April 1991 to September 1992, 11 patients with non-advanced achalasia, 6 males and 5 females with ages ranging from 29 to 67 underwent VALS. The preoperative work-up included a clinical interview, x-rays of the esophagus, stomach and duodenum, manometric study of the esophagus, esophagogastroduodenoscopy, and abdominal ultrasound. One patient also suffered from chronic gallbladder stones.

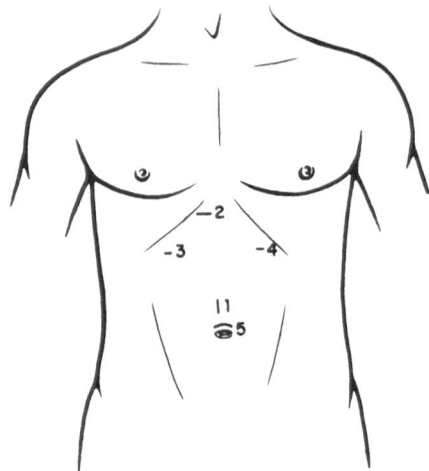

Fig. 3. Location of the ports for the abdominal approach

Operative Technique

After induction of general anesthesia, the surgeon takes a position between the patient's legs. On the left the assistant handles the video camera; the first assistant and scrub nurse are to the patient's right.

Five trocar incisions provide access to the peritoneal cavity, as shown in Fig. 3, according to the following sequence: Pneumo-peritoneum is accomplished via a Veres needle inserted in the first port. An automatic device is used to insufflate the necessary volume of CO_2 to maintain the intra-abdominal pressure at 14 mmHg.

After insertion of the first 11-cm trocar for introduction of the laparoscope, the peritoneal cavity is explored and the other trocars guided through the ports. The 11-mm trocar is introduced into the second port for the liver retractor. This retractor was designed on our service. It consists of a hinged metal shaft covered by a soft rubber protector to avoid hepatic injury.

The liver is deviated by the first assistant, exposing the region of the eso-phagogastric junction. At this point, the third and fourth ports, 11 and 5 mm, respectively, are made for the dissecting forceps. The surgeon holds these forceps one in each hand. After dissection of the esophagogastric junction and isolation of the distal esophagus, a supraumbilical incision is made to introduce and position the esophageal retractor. The latter also designed and made on the Service is useful when pulling the esophagus caudally, exposing the distal eso-phagus. This permits slight rotation of the organ to simplify execution of the valvuloplasty.

After positioning the esophageal retractor and applying traction in a caudal direction and counterclockwise rotation, the valvuloplasty is accomplished. The gastric fundus is sutured with a continuous suture to the posterior region of the distal esophagus for about 6 cm (Fig. 4). At the end of this stage, the esophageal rotation is released slightly in order to facilitate the next suture line (Fig. 5).

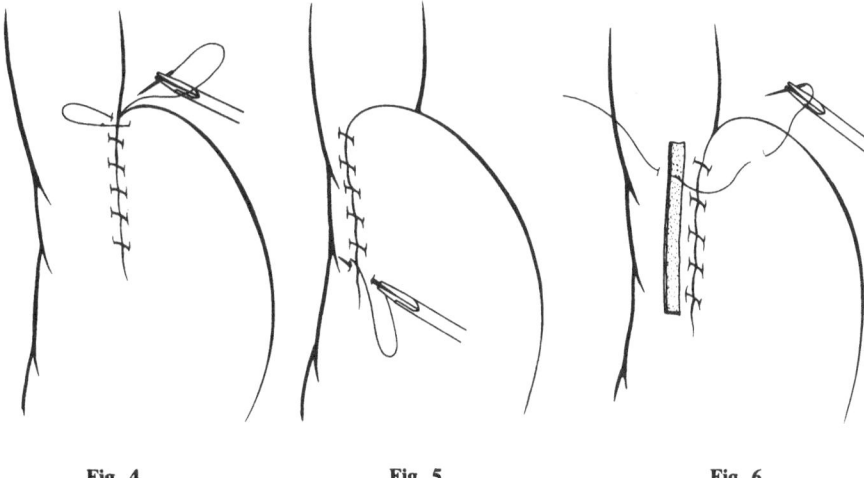

Fig. 4.   **Fig. 5.**   **Fig. 6.**

Fig. 4. The first suture line of the gastric fundus to the posterior region of the esophagus
Fig. 5. Second suture line of the gastric fundus to the esophagus
Fig. 6. Third suture line of the gastric fundus to the right margin of the myectomy, covering it completely

After concluding the two suture lines of the valvuloplasty, one in the posterior and the other in the left lateral region of the esophagus, the cardiomyotomy is begun. The adventitia and muscle layers of the distal 6 cm of the esophagus and serosa and muscle layers of 3 cm of the proximal stomach are cut, resulting in a 9-cm-long myotomy. Fragments of the cut layers are resected so that not only a cardiomyotomy but a cardiomyectomy is also accomplished.

The resected strip is sent for histopathologic study. After checking the integrity of the exposed mucosa, the counterclockwise traction on the esophageal retractor is completely released and the third and last suture line is taken on the gastric fundus, now on the right margin of the cardiomyectomy (Fig. 6).

In the last seven patients, the surgeries were performed as described. A cardiomyectomy without associated valvuloplasty was accomplished on the first three patients of our series.

Results

The procedure was feasible in all the patients, and it was unnecessary to convert to the open technique. Intra-operative complications included: two cases of perforation of the esophageal mucosa and two cases of subcutaneous cervical emphysema. It should be mentioned that these problems occurred in the first four cases of the series. After refinement in technique with proper utilization of the esophageal and liver retractors, and the execution of the first two suture lines of the valvuloplasty prior to the cardiomyectomy, these complications no longer occurred.

Perforation of the mucosa was closed with a continuous mucomucosal suture and protected by wrapping the suture line with the gastric fundus during the valvuloplasty and drainage with a Penrose drain. The problem of subcutaneous emphysema was resolved by reducing the intra-peritoneal pressure. The region of the emphysema was carefully observed by the anesthetist, it eventually stabilized during the operation and regressed completely postoperatively.

The postoperative complication of a small esohageal fistula was noted in one of the cases of esophageal perforation. It was suspected because of the characteristic drainage and confirmed by x-ray using iodated contrast. The fissure closed spontaneously after 7 days of fasting and parenteral feeding with satisfactory recovery on the patient's part. This was the only postoperative complication observed.

Ten of the 11 patients were ready to be discharged 48 h postoperatively but they remained hospitalized longer for a better clinical evaluation and to carry out the initial studies of the functional assessment.

Immediate functional results were assessed by a clinical interview, barium roentgenograph, and manometric study. The initial interview and x-ray studies were accomplished during the early days of oral feeding and the manometry 7–10 days postoperatively.

Improvement of dysphagia and patient satisfaction with the results was noted in all cases at the first clinical interview. Regarding the x-ray evaluation, the contrast passed more easily to the stomach in all patients.

Esophageal manometry was feasible in seven patients preoperatively and eight postoperatively. At this time, a reduction in pressure levels of the lower esophageal sphincter (LES) was observed. The mean LES pressure was reduced from 50 cm of water preoperatively to 23 cm postoperatively.

The patients are still being followed clinically to assess the results over the long term. Presently, with follow-up time ranging from 1 to 15 months, dysphagia has improved in almost 90% of cases.

Five patients (45.4%) still have some degree of residual dysphagia for solid foods in spite of their improvement compared to the preoperative dysphagia. Five subjects (45.4%) no longer complain of dysphagia, and dysphagia improved temporarily in one (9%), but 10 months postoperatively his symptoms returned with the same intensity as before the operation.

One patient, currently followed-up for 13 months, who underwent cardiomyectomy only, has complained of symptoms suggestive of gastroesophageal reflux. However, they are easily controlled clinically by sleeping on a bed with elevation of the head, dietetic orientation, and periodic utilization of H_2-blocking agents.

Discussion

The appearance of VALS and the rapid design and development of equipment facilitating its use, has made possible the extension of its applications, employing it for more complex procedures, where wider dissections, sutures, resections, and even anastomoses are necessary.

Due to the rapid progress of VALS and the experience acquired in the management of achalasia, we felt this approach could be used to carry out the conservative operation utilized for the "non-advanced" type of the disorder, similarly to the open procedure, dispensing with the classical incision and its inherent morbidity.

This limited experience suggests that this is a valuable technique with a low rate of inter-operative and postoperative complications, certifying to the safety of the procedure. This factor added to the satisfactory results achieved over the short and medium term attest to the value of the modality. However, we realize that a longer period of clinical observation is required for better judgement of the results of the operation.

In looking over our series, we note that with growing experience of the team, development of techniques and equipment for suturing and proper retraction of the liver and esophagogastric junction, the operative time is being considerably reduced and is becoming gradually similar to the "open procedure" (conventional surgery).

We also believe that the functional results can be just as good. This new technical option is an extremely valuable adjunct providing safety and effectiveness, comparable to the standard technique, with the additional advantages of shortened recovery time, better cosmetic results, speedier return to normal activities, reduced postoperative pain, and elimination of complications inherent to conventional laparotomy.

References

1. Pinotti HW, Gama-Rodrigues JJ, Ellenbogen G, Raia A (1974) Nova técnica no tratamento cirúrgico do megaesôfago. Esofagocardiomiotomia associada a esofagofundogastropexia. *Rev Goiana de Med* 20:1
2. Ellenbogen G (1979) Megaesôfago não avançado. Tratamento pela cardiomiectomia associada a esofagofundogastropexia. Avaliação clínica, morfológica e funcional dos seus resultados. Thesis, Faculdade de Medicina da Universidade de São Paulo

Re-Operation for Failed Antireflux Operations

C.G. Bremner and R. Mason[1]

Introduction

In the best series published, antireflux surgery will give an excellent to good result in about 90% of cases [1], and these results are sustained for up to 10 years. There are series reported, however, where the results have not been long-lasting, and reflux returns. Recurrent reflux is not the only cause of unsatisfactory results. Side effects of the operations such as dysphagia, bloating, diarrhea and persistent pain are also described [2].

In the last 17 years, the senior author (C.G.B.) has operated on 51 patients who have had failed antireflux surgery. Five of these patients were failures after operation by the author and the rest had been operated on by other surgeons. These patients underwent a full investigation to illustrate the cause of the failed initial operation, and were reoperated to correct the defect. An analysis of the investigations, surgery performed, and results is reported.

Patients and Methods

Of the 51 patients, 30 were female and 21 male, with a mean age of 51.5 years (35–82). Forty-four patients had undergone a single previous operation, 5 had undergone two previous operations and 2 patients had undergone three and four operations, respectively. Eighteen patients had re-operations by a thoracic approach and 33 had an abdominal approach via the previous operation scar. Following the second operation, four patients were lost to follow-up. The mean follow-up period in the 47 remaining patients was 3.16 years (1 month to 17 years). All patients had a barium swallow radiographic examination to define

[1] Department of Surgery, University of the Witwatersrand Medical School, 7 York Road, Park Town, 2193 Johannesburg, South Africa

Table 1. Previous procedures that failed

Known			
Nissen	27	2 Operations	×6
Hill	1	3 Operations	×1
Belsey	1	4 Operations	×1
Es-gastric	1		
Unknown		Vagotomy	×4
Abdominal	14		
Thoracic	7		

anatomy, and endoscopy. Motility was measured in 29 patients, and in a further 6 patients the motility tube could not be passed. Reflux was assessed by either radiology (free reflux) the standard acid reflux test (SART), or pH monitoring. Gastric emptying studies using technetium-labelled chicken liver and labelled liquid, and an extended hepato-biliary HIDA (hydroxy-imino-diacetic acid) scan to detect duodenogastric reflux was also carried out. Patients were assessed according to a modified Visick grading. Grade I patients had excellent results and were free of reflux symptoms and required no further treatment. Grade II patients had non-reflux symptoms related to mild epigastric discomfort, chest discomfort, and did not require medication. Grade III patients had symptoms requiring medication for heart-burn, epigastric pain, diarrhea, or fullness. Grade IV had poor results and were considered to be failures because they were not improved by the operation and required medication or repeat surgery. The procedures which had been done prior to recurrent symptoms are listed in Table 1.

Results of Investigations Prior to Re-Operation

Symptoms

The main symptoms in this group of patients were heartburn ($n = 34$) heartburn and dysphagia ($n = 12$), dysphagia alone ($n = 5$). Other symptoms were bilious vomiting and nausea ($n = 2$), epigastric pain ($n = 3$), and vomiting ($n = 2$).

Radiological Examination

Radiology demonstrated a recurrence of the hernia ($n = 31$), a slipped Nissen fundoplication ($n = 3$), paraesophageal hernia ($n = 2$), tight Nissen ($n = 2$), and stricture ($n = 3$) (Figs. 1 and 2).

Manometry

The lower esophageal sphincter pressures (LESP) are listed in Table 2, and the causes for high LESP are detailed in Fig. 3. The body of the esophagus was hypomotile in four patients, incoordinate in one, and spastic in five.

HIDA Scan for Duodenogastric Reflux

There was positive reflux in three patients.

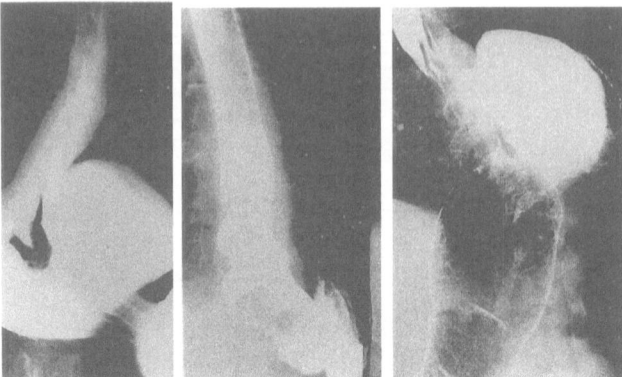

Fig. 1. Radiographs of three patients with failed antireflux surgery. The hernia has recurred in each case, and there is no sign of a fundoplication

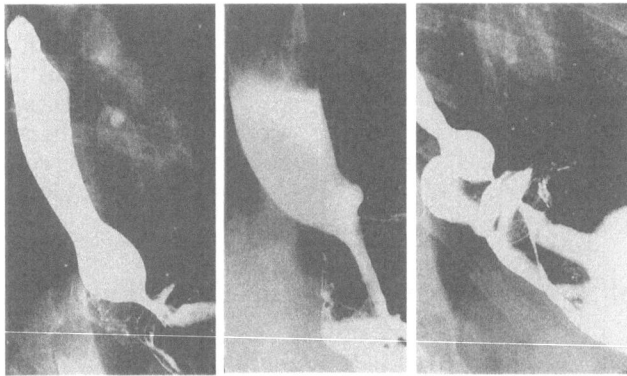

Fig. 2. Radiographs of 3 patients with failed results despite intact Nissen fundoplication. Nissen too tight with stasis (*left*). Nissen too long with retention (*middle*). Paraesophageal hernia causing dysphagia (*right*)

Table 2. Manometric results of the lower esophageal sphincter

	n		
Defective	25	LESP <6 mm	20
		LESL <2 cm	1
		IAL <1 cm	4
Normal	5	(3 Reflux; 2 Dysphagia)	
High	8	Dysphagia	

LESP, lower esophageal sphincter pressure; LESL, lower esophageal sphincter

Table 3. Reasons for Failure of Primary Antireflux Operation

	n
Recurrence of hernia and reflux	32
Recurrent reflux	4
Bilious vomiting	2
Slipped Nissen	3
Paraesophageal hernia	2
Nissen too long or tight	5
Unresolved stricture	2
"Secondary" achalasia	1

Fig. 3. The diagnosis in eight patients who had a high lower esophageal sphincter pressure. *Incarc*, incarcerated hernia; *DGR*, duodenogastric reflux

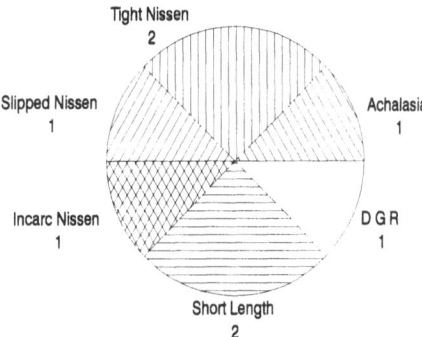

Manometry - high LESP

Table 4. Re-operation procedures performed in 51 patients

Operation (n)		
Nissen (38)	Revision	31
	+V+ drain	4
	+Duod switch	1
	+Collis	1
	+Thal	1
Belsey (3)		
Reduction only (2)		
Resection (4)		
Roux + Duod. stapling (1)		
Angelchik (1)		
Gastrogastrostomy (1)		
Esophagoplasty (1)		

Assessment of the Cause of Failed Results

The overall assessment of the cause of failure in this group of patients is summarized in Table 3.

Re-Operation Procedures

The revision procedures performed are listed in Table 4.

Results of Re-Operation

There was no mortality. One patient had a gastric leak from gastric damage resulting from a takedown of a previous Nissen fundoplication. The results of the operations are summarized in Table 5. Excellent to good results were

Table 5. Results of Re-operation

Visick I Excellent 57% ($n = 27$)	Visick II Good 11% ($n = 5$)	Visick III Fair 21% ($n = 10$)	Visick IV Poor 11% ($n = 5$)
Late DU—1 Late Cencer—1	Dysphagia ($n = 2$) Epigastric discomfort 　($n = 3$)	Thoracic pain 　($n = 2$) Bile Reflux 　($n = 3$) GER ($n = 2$) Anastomotic 　stricture ($n = 1$) Nutcracker 　($n = 1$) Inadequate LES Relaxation ($n =$ 　1)	Dumping ($n = 1$) Dysphagia ($n = 1$) Bile Reflux ($n = 2$) GER ($n = 1$)

DU, duodenal ulcer; *GER*, gastroesophaged reflux; *LES*, lower esophageal sphincter

Table 6. Unsatisfactory Results in 15 patients

Cause	(n)	Treatment	Results	Visick
GER	(3)	Medical	Fair	3
Bile gastritis	(5)	Medical (2)	Fair	3
		Roux (2)	Mid stasis (1)	2
		Switch (1)	Mid stasis (1)	2
Dumping + 　gastritis	(1)	Roux Reversed 　segment	Good	1
Stricture	(1)	Resection	Fair	2
Nutcracker	(1)	Medical	"	2
Thoracotomy 　pain	(2)	Medical	"	2
Poor LES relax	(1)	Pneumatic	"	2
Anast stricture	(1)	Dilate	"	2

Table 7. Details of five failed patients

Type of operation		Treatment	Results
1. Resection	(anastomotic 　stricture)	Dilated	Good
2. Nissen	(D-G reflux)	Roux	Good
3. Nissen	(D-G reflux)	Prokinetics	
4. Gastro- 　gastrostomy	(reflux)	H_2-receptor 　block	Fair
5. Colon interpos.	(gastric stasis)	Prokinetics	Fair

D-G, Duodenogastric

documented in 68% of the patients. Unsatisfactory results (Visick III and IV grades) are listed in Table 6. Only three of these patients had recurrence of gastroesophageal reflux. Following treatment, results were fair in six of the patients. All four patients in the group who had two previous operations had an excellent or good result, and the patients who had three and four operations had satisfactory results. Details of the five failed cases are given in Table 7.

Discussion

Failure of the initial procedure was clearly technical in most cases. Failure to control reflux was obvious in 36 cases in which reflux was present. Failure to close the hiatus adequately resulted in recurrent hernia in 32 cases. The Nissen fundoplication was too long or too tight in five cases. The failures not obviously related to technical problems were duodenogastric reflux ($n = 2$) and achalasia ($n = 1$). There is no evidence to suggest that antireflux surgery causes duodeno-gastric reflux, and in the experimental animal a Nissen fundoplication did not cause pyloric dysfunction [3]. It is suggested that duodenogastric reflux was present prior to the first procedure and this raises the question as to whether HIDA scans should be routinely performed or not before antireflux surgery. It is the policy of this unit to investigate all patients with a battery of tests. Manometry was most helpful in making the diagnosis of an incompetent lower esophageal sphincter, nutcracker esophagus ($n = 1$), and achalasia ($n = 1$). Gastric emptying studies revealed marked stasis in only one patient (retention of 80% after 1 h) and a pyloroplasty was added to the procedure. HIDA scans showed severe duodenogastric reflux in two patients and bile diverting procedures were performed. The initial overall satisfactory result of 68% increased to 78% following re-operation on the five failed patients. It was our preference to perform a revision Nissen fundoplication re-operation in 31 patients, and a revision associated with either a gastric drainage procedure ($n = 1$), bile diversion ($n = 1$), lengthening ($n = 1$) or Thal patch ($n = 1$). Ellis and Crozier [4] reported a 92% satisfactory outcome in their series of 24 re-operation fundoplication patients. However, after takedown of the fundus there may be a tissue shortage making refundoplication technically impossible. Either a Belsy (if transthoracic) or Hill procedure are good alternative procedures.

In one patient, it was technically impossible to undo the Nissen fundoplication which had welded to the gastric wall, and a gastrogastrostomy was performed. This was predictably unsuccessful and the patient now requires a colon replacement. The esophagoplasty was performed for a strictured lower esophagus due to suture misplacement by the referring surgeon.

Unsatisfactory results after reoperation were due to recurrent reflux in four cases only. Patient dissatisfaction in these cases was due to a variety of problems related to other sequelae of surgery such as chest pain, duodenogastric reflux, dumping, and unexplained spasticity of the esophagus. One of the five patients with poor results required reoperation for duodenogastric reflux, and following treatment (Table 7) results improved to grades of Visick II ($n = 2$) and III ($n = 3$).

Conclusions

Most cases of failed antireflux procedures are the result of technical problems. Failure to close the hiatus adequately may result in recurrent hernia. Nissen fundoplications are also prone to disrupt, and the use of Teflon pledgets would seem to be a wise precaution against this mishap [1]. Achalasia following a Nissen fundoplication has been described previously [5]. In our particular case, preoperative manometry had been performed and achalasia was not diagnosed. It is probable that the patient was in the period of minimal achalasia, a condition difficult to diagnose which sometimes simulates reflux. The problem of duodenogastric reflux following antireflux surgery is not a new one, and it is the authors' opinion that duodenogastric reflux was present before the procedure. Generally, the results suggest two important aspects. Preoperative evaluation should be complete, and should include radiological studies, endoscopy, motility, gastric emptying, and HIDA scan studies. The complete pathophysiological problem should be carefully analyzed before any procedure and, in particular, before reoperation. Secondly, meticulous care should be given to technique. Failure to close the hiatus adequately begs for recurrence of the hernia. It is probable that this step is less important in the posterior gastropexy procedure of Hill.

References

1. DeMeester TR, Bonavina L, Albertucci M (1986) Nissen fundoplication for gastroesophageal reflux disease: Evaluation of primary repair in 100 consecutive patients. Ann Surg 204:2–9
2. Leonardi HK, Ellis FH Jr (1983) Complications of the Nissen fundoplication. Surg Clin North Amer 63:1155–65
3. Bremner CG (1978) Pyloric competence and gastric emptying after the Nissen fundoplication operation. S Afr J Surg 16:202(A)
4. Ellis FJ Jr., Crozier R (1984) Reflux control by fundoplication: A clinical and manometric assessment of the Nissen operation. Ann Thorac Surg 38:387–92
5. Smart HL, Mayberry JF, Atkinson M (1986) Achalasia following gastro-oesophageal reflux. J R Soc Med 79:71–3

Gastroesophageal Reflux Control in Operated Scleroderma Patients

A. Duranceau, P. Topart, C. Deschamps, and R. Taillefer[1]

Summary. Over a 14-year period, 12 patients with documented scleroderma had an antireflux operation: eight short total fundoplication, two Collis-Nissen, one Collis-Belsey, and one Roux-en-Y. They were assessed before and after their operation with a follow-up range of 14–169 months (mean, 71 months) (Table 1). The functional abnormalities of scleroderma remained unchanged following antireflux surgery. Despite a decrease in total acid exposure, 6/12 patients still show significant episodes of acid pH in their esophagus, causing symptoms in 5. The esophageal mucosa reverted to normal in two patients. Ten of 12 still show extensive columnar lined mucosa. Despite a total fundoplication in 10/12 patients, significant acid exposure persists in 50% of operated scleroderma patients.

Introduction

Scleroderma eventually results in an inability to achieve normal food transit at the level of the esophagus, stomach, and lower gut. Gastroesophageal reflux (GER) represents a challenging problem in sclerodermic patients. Control of this reflux, although purely palliative in this condition, remains essential in order to prevent progression of simple esophagitis toward more severe lesions such as peptic stricture and Barrett's esophagus. [1–4] The operation is usually proposed to protect the esophagus from reflux damage and to limit the extent of existing mucosal abnormalities. Several techniques are offered, usually a partial fundoplication, often in conjunction with a lengthening procedure [2, 5]. The aim of the present study is to assess the functional results in patients presenting with reflux complications of scleroderma following their operative treatment.

[1] Department of Surgery, Université de Montréal, Division of Thoracic Surgery, Hôtel-Dieu de Montréal, 3840 St Urbain Ave., Montreal, Québec, H2W 1T8 Canada

Subjects and Methods

Twelve sclerodermic patients (9 women and 3 men) aged 37–60 (mean 48.5) were operated on between 1977 and 1990. They all underwent extensive functional esophageal evaluation before and after their operation: Clinical assessment, endoscopy, esophagogram, emptying scintiscan, manometry, and 24-h pH recording were obtained preoperatively. The same investigation was obtained at 18 and 36 months for 12 and 10 patients, respectively. Four patients had further control studies 60 months after their antireflux surgery.

Operation

Ten of the 12 patients underwent an antireflux operation performed through the left chest. For eight of these patients, the operation was a modified Nissen fundoplication with a short 2-cm wrap over a large (56 French) mercury bougie. A Collis-Nissen was the operation of choice for two patients and a Collis-Belsey operation was performed in one patient. The last patient underwent, through laparatomy, a truncal vagotomy with an antrectomy and a Roux-en-Y diversion.

Manometry

Recordings are made using a four-lumen catheter (R4 A 5-5-5, MUI Scientific Mississauga, Ont.) with four lateral openings spaced 5 cm apart and radially oriented at 90 degrees. Each lumen is water perfused at a rate of 0.7 ml/min by means of a low compliance pneumohydraulic Arndorfer-Mui Pump (Model PIP-3, Mui Scientific Mississauga, Ont.) rated at 15 PSI. The four lumen are connected to external quartz transducers (Hewlett Packard 1290 AOPT-002). Pressures are recorded on a four-channel physiograph (Hewlett Packard 7754A) through Hewlett Packard 8805D preamplifiers.

Each scleroderma patient served as their own control in a preoperative and postoperative situation. They were assessed manometrically with all having one or two preoperative recordings. Postoperatively, one to four manometric assessment were obtained.

Radiology

Radiographic studies used conventional barium esophagograms under fluoroscopic control. Four to six picture frames per second were obtained using this method and all patients had pre- and postoperative radiologic assessment.

Scintigraphy

Esophageal emptying scintiscans were obtained using a bolus of 1.0 Ci of 99 m Technitium (Tc) sulfur colloid diluted in 10 ml of water. Data was acquired during a 3-min period. The clearance of radioactivity was studied in each of three esophageal segments (proximal, middle, and distal). The total remaining activity at 2 min was computed in both supine and upright positions. Eight patients were assessed preoperatively, and there was a total of 18 postoperative esophageal emptying scans in nine patients.

24-H pH Recording

Twenty-four-h pH recordings were obtained from an ambulatory software reflux monitor (RMS, Sandhill—Littleton, Colorado, USA) using an antimony probe. The data were analyzed and displayed through an IBM computer interface. Three patients had a preoperative recording when it became available. All 12 patients had control 24-h pH recordings after the operation.

Statistical Analysis

Student's t-test for unpaired values was used to compare preoperative and postoperative quantitative information. Differences were considered significant at the level of $P < 0.05$.

Results

Clinical

The follow-up ranged from 17 to 169 months (mean 71.7 months). Before the operation, regurgitations and heartburn were reported by all 12 patients, and 11/12 had obstructive symptoms at their initial presentation. Following the operation and after the most recent symptom assessment, only two patients are totally asymptomatic from their esophagus. One patient remained asymptomatic for 10 years, but regurgitation and heartburn have since reappeared. Five of the 12 patients still complain of a substernal burning pain. Three describe regurgitation episodes while two have only the burning sensation. One patient describes regurgitation only, without the heartburn. Only one patient has reported frank dysphagia. However, eight patients are aware of slow esophageal emptying, and are otherwise asymptomatic. Two patients presented with postoperative cmplications: One with a wound infection and the other atelectasis and pericardial effusion. There was no postoperative death.

Endoscopy

Preoperative and postoperative findings at endoscopy are summarized as follows: 7 out 12 patients had a circumferential columnar lined esophagus observed during their initial assessment. Four additional patients who were interpreted as having extensive ulcerative esophagitis showed by their evolution that they probably had in fact a circumferential columnar lined mucosa with a stricture. All 12 patients underwent a total of 36 endoscopic reassessments over a follow-up period of 72 months. At present, only two patients show a normal esophageal mucosa: The first had minimal esophagitis with no lower esophageal sphincter (LES) function and the second had persistent reflux with active ulcers and stricture following a first antireflux operation. The remaining 10 patients show persistent columnar lined mucosa which has decreased however from a length of 7.5 cm above the esophagogastric junction to 4.2 cm after the antireflux operation.

Radiology

Preoperative radiologic findings suggested a hiatal hernia in 7 of 12 patients. None of these patients showed a hernia at operation. In nine patients, free reflux episodes were noted. Following the operation, three patients still revealed radiological reflux episodes. The maximal transverse diameter remained stable after the antireflux operation (4.1 cm before, 4.0 cm after). In the one patient who had vagotomy, antrectomy, and a Roux-en-Y diversion, a large pseudodiverticulum formed above the diaphragm despite the absence of any type of fundoplication at the gastroesophageal junction. Esophageal stricture was observed in 4/12 patients before the operation. Following repair, 11/12 patients show the imprint of their operation of the GE junction. And while atony and stasis could be observed in eight patients before surgery, it was present on the radiological assessment of all patients following their operation.

Manometric Evaluation

Pre- and postoperative manometric recordings were obtained in all patients. Details of the motility studies are shown in Table 1.

Only 1 out of 12 recordings revealed normal preoperative propulsion with acceptable contraction pressures in the esophageal body. Nine patients showed a total absence of peristalsis with very hypotonic contractions in both the proximal

Table 1. Patient characteristics and motility studies

Clinical symptoms		Preoperative	Postoperative	P value
Reflux		12/12	5/12	$P < 0.01$
Obstructive		11/12	9/12	N.S.
Radiology				
Atony		8/12	12/12	N.S.
Transverse diameter		4.1 ± 1.6	4.0 ± 1	N.S.
Mucosal Damage grade IV		7	10	
III		4	0	
II		4	0	
I		1	0	
0		0	2	
Motility				
Proximal Resting	(mmHg)	6.3 ± 2.1	11.3 ± 7.2	$P < 0.01$
Peak contraction	(mmHg)	25.7 ± 15.8	28.1 ± 18.1	N.S.
Primary peristalsis	(%)	18.5	11	
Distal Resting	(mmHg)	6.0 ± 2.6	9.9 ± 6.9	$P < 0.02$
Peak contraction	(mmHg)	13.8 ± 7.9	16.8 ± 9.9	N.S.
Primary peristalsis	(%)	16.8	8.4	
LES LES Resting		9.0 ± 4.7	13.8 ± 6.4	$P < 0.02$
Gastric resting		6.4 ± 3.1	8.9 ± 4.7	$P < 0.05$
Gradient		3.4 ± 3.2	4.8 ± 3.9	N.S.
24-h pH Studies				
% Time exposure to acid		21	8.4	
Esophageal Emptying Scintiscan				
% Retention at 2 min		24	38	$P < 0.05$

UES, upper esophageal sphincter; *LES*, lower esophageal sphincter and distal esophagus. This hypomotility was coupled with a hypotensive LES in 11 of the 12 patients. Following the operation, contraction abnormalities remained unchanged and resting intraesophageal pressures increased. LES gradient values were slightly increased from 3.4 ± 3.2 mmHg on the preoperative recording to 4.8 ± 3.9 mmHg after the operation. This difference was not statistically significant.

Twenty-Four-H pH Studies

Five patients underwent a 24-h pH recording before their operation. All 12 patients had one to three 24-h pH studies following their operation. There was a decrease in acid exposure in the esophagus from 21% before to 8.4% after the operation. Even in those in whom reflux persisted, it was reduced by the operation. Despite the use of a total fundoplication in eight patients, acid exposure persisted in the esophagus for 50% of these patients.

Esophageal Scintiscans

The emptying capacity of the esophagus is decreased following antireflux operations. Eight patients were assessed preoperatively and nine patients had from one to four postoperative evaluations. Radionuclide stasis at 2 min showed preoperatively a retention of 21% of the radionuclide. After antireflux surgery, this retention increased to 38%.

Discussion

The esophageal complications of scleroderma are a difficult challenge both for the physician and the surgeon. The motor disturbances seen in this condition are highly variable. They may range from normal peristalsis and LES function to altered contractions, wave amplitude, and LES values, to total paralysis of the esophageal body and absent LES. Only one of our patients showed normal propulsion for a majority of her esophageal body contractions. She still had weaker peak contraction pressures in both the distal and proximal esophagus and no LES zone could be recorded. All other patients showed loss of peristalsis and powerless contractions averaging 17 mmHg in the distal half of the esophagus. The LES gradient was virtually nonexistent, averaging 3.4 mmHg for the whole group.

When esophagus and LES have been structurally damaged, it is difficult to obtain significant functional improvement by medication alone. Progression of reflux lesions is thus virtually certain. Seven of our 12 patients showed a circumferential columnar lined mucosa in their distal esophagus and 3 more were interpreted as extensive ulcerative esophagitis which persisted as columnar epithelium after their operation. These lesions are witnesses to the long-term exposure of the esophageal mucosa to the damaging effect of the free flowing refluxate.

Good postoperative results are more difficult to obtain in scleroderma patients, especially if strictures [6–8] or columnar epithelium replacement [9] have occurred. One report shows the long-term results of surgical treatment in scleroderma patients. Orringer et al. [5, 10] reports their experience with 37 patients with scleroderma who have undergone either a Collis-Belsey fundoplication or a Collis-Nissen operation. Good to excellent symptomatic improvement had been observed in 89% of all patients. Reflux control was considered inadequate in 11% of their group. When documented by pH studies, excellent reflux control was present in 68% of the group. Moderate to severe reflux was observed in 32% of the patients. When looking at manometric changes brought by the operation, Orringer found that LES pressures were increased from 4.6 to 8.6 mmHg by the Collis-Belsey gastroplasty and from 2.5 to 12 mmHg by the Collis-Nissen operation. The Collis-Belsey gastroplasty still allowed gastroesophageal reflux in 41% of the patients while the Collis-Nissen permitted reflux episodes to occur in 25% of operated patients. Henderson [6] found persistent reflux in 6 of 11 patients who were offered partial fundoplication gastroplasty. A 0.5–1 cm total gastroplasty fundoplication was considered to be adequate control of reflux in six patients while avoiding dysphagia. No pH studies were carried in his report. Orringer [5, 10] reports persistent reflux in 26%–54% of operated scleroderma patients. This is consistent with our observation that 6 of 12 patients still show esophageal exposure to acid as documented by 24-h pH studies.

Altered defense mechanisms in the atonic esophagus and progression over time of the systemic condition might be involved in explaining the poor acid reflux control [11] Mansour [12] reported recurrence of reflux disease complications 4 years after the initial reflux operation. In our group, three patients who were initially improved from 67 to 108 months after their operation now show evidence of either persistent or recurrent symptomatic reflux disease. The effectiveness of a total fundoplication may well be altered by the underlying disease. Four of the five patients assessed pre and postoperatively by 24-hour pH studies still show diminished although persistent exposure to acid. The fifth patient shows the same acid level exposure as before the operation. The exact mechanism by which total fundoplication loses its antireflux properties still needs to be clarified. However, it may be that a simple reduction in frequency and duration of reflux episodes allows some healing in the damaged esophagus. This is certainly a possibility since neither resting and contracting pressures or peristalsis in the esophageal body are altered by the operation. The LES tone is virtually unchanged by the short total wrap. Thus, a simple mechanical effect of the fundoplication may reduce the reflux episodes enough to allow at least some healing and protection to take place. Reduction of mucosal damage in three patients despite persistent exposure to acid seems to support that hypothesis. Since 10 of 12 patients showed documented Barrett's mucosa, the functional status of that mucosa in regard to acid production also needs to be clarified: This point is raised in regard to diminished level of damage in two of the patients despite the presence of acid in the esophageal body during 24-hour pH recording. Persisten esophageal exposure to acid may be due to either acid secretion in the esophageal body by an abnormal columnar mucosa or results from active gastroesophageal reflux.

Radiologic and scintigraphic evaluation of the sclerodermic esophagus affords an objective visualization and quantitation of its emptying capacity both preoperatively and postoperatively. After a total fundoplication, even if made shorter and over a large bougie, the esophagus shows significant retention at 2 min. A combination of atony and functional obstruction at the LES level are logical explanations for this retention. Such a situation may also explain the occurence of esophageal moniliasis, requiring active antifungal medication in two of our patients.

The persistence and/or recurrence of reflux in scleroderma patients must be assessed with the perspective of mucosal damage evolution. Treatment must be weighed between the severity of esophagitis and its complications against functional obstruction created by any type of fundoplication at the distal esophageal level. On a long-term basis, reduced or stable damage should be treated conservatively. Total gastroplasty fundoplication of the cut or uncut variety needs to be assessed in the management of this condition especially in the perspective of persistent and/or recurrent reflux damage. Resection of the esophagus should be limited to extreme complication especially with the notion that none of the available organs for reconstruction are more functional, due to the underlying systemic condition. Complete Roux-en-Y diversion after antrectomy and vagotomy may afford valuable protection, although at the expense of the stomach which is then lost as a replacement organ.

The ideal treatment for esophageal complications of reflux esophagitis in scleroderma patients still remains to be found. An antireflux repair which will afford sufficient antireflux control without significant functional obstruction is needed to help these patients.

References

1. Brain RHF (1973) Surgical management of hiatal herniae and oesophageal strictures in systemic sclerosis. Thorax 28:515–520
2. Gimmon Z, Katz S, Eyal Z (1982) Surgical aspects of multifocal involvement of the gastrointestinal tract in progressive systemic sclerosis. Int Surg 67:471–473
3. McLaughlin JS, Roig R, Woodruff MFA (1971) Surgical treatment of strictures of the esophagus in patients with scleroderma. J Thorac Cardiovasc Surg 61:641–645
4. Poirier TJ, Rankin GB (1972) Gastrointestinal manifestations of progressive systemic scleroderma based on a review of 364 cases. Am J Gastroent 58:30–44
5. Orringer MB, Dabich L, Zarafonetis CJD, Sloan C (1976) Gastroesophageal reflux in esophageal scleroderma: Diagnosis and implications. Ann Thorac Surg 22:122–129
6. Henderson RD, Pearson FG (1973) Surgical management of esophageal scleroderma. J Thorac Cardiovasc Surg 66:686–692
7. Netscher DT, Richardson D (1984) Complications requiring operative intervention in scleroderma. Surg Gynecol Obstet 158:507–512
8. Payne WS (1970) Surgical treatment of reflux esophagitis and stricture associated with permanent incompetence of the cardia. Mayo Clin Proc 45:553–562
9. Cameron AV, Payne WS (1978) Barrett's esophagus occuring as a complication of scleroderma. Mayo Clin Proc 53:612–615
10. Orringer MB., Orringer JS., Dabich L., Zarafonetis C.: Combined Collis gastroplasty fundoplication operations for scleroderma reflux esophagitis. Surgery, 1981; 90: 624–630.
11. Garrett JM, Winkelmann RK, Code CF (1971) Esophageal deterioration in scleroderma. Mayo Clin Proc 46:92–96
12. Mansour KA, Malone CE (1988) Surgery for scleroderma of the esophagus: 12 years experience. Ann Thorac Surg 46:513–514

Barret's Esophagus

Barrett's Esophagus—Open and Answered Questions 1993*

J.R. SIEWERT and H.J. STEIN[1]

Introduction

In 1950, Norman Barrett first reported on an area of tubular esophagus lined with gastric mucosa associated with peptic stenosis and transition ulcers [1]. Barrett, however, needed the help of the functional studies performed by Allison and Johnstone to realize that this area of intestine indeed was the distal esophagus [2, 3]. At about the same time, columnar epithelial lining of the distal esophagus was also observed in Paris by Lortat-Jacob and termed "endobrachyoesophagus", i.e. an esophagus, which is too short from the interior or mucosal aspect [4].

Today, columnar cell lining of the distal esophagus or Barrett's esophagus is an accepted entity which is defined by circumferential columnar epithelial lining of the distal esophagus which measures more than 3 cm in length and is in continuity with the gastric mucosa [5]. With this definition, it is easy to differentiate Barrett's esophagus from the congenital "inlet patches", i.e. isolated areas of gastric mucosa which are usually located in the proximal esophagus [6].

Epidemiology and Pathophysiology

The typical patient with Barrett's esophagus is older than 50 years, male, white, and has a long history of reflux symptoms [7, 8]. This description demonstrates that Barrett's esophagus today is primarily a problem of the Western

* Special Lecture, 5th World Congress of the International Society for Diseases of the Esophagus, Kyoto, August 5–8, 1992

[1] Department of Surgery, Technische Universität München, Klinikum rechts der Isar, Ismaningersstr 22, W-8000 München 80, Germany

hemisphere. With the changing lifestyle of the Japanese, Barrett's esophagus may, however, soon also become a problem of the Eastern hemisphere.

It is commonly accepted that in the vast majority of patients, Barrett's esophagus is caused by longlasting gastroesophageal reflux. Physiologic studies show that the underlying functional abnormalities in patients with Barrett's esophagus are more severe as compared to patients with primary reflux disease but no columnar epithelium. On manometry, there is a marked reduction or complete absence of a resting pressure in the lower esophageal sphincter in over 90% of patients with Barrett's esophagus. The clearance function of the esophageal body is disturbed in about 80% of patients with the condition and about half of the patients have hypersecretion of gastric acid. Excessive duodenogastric reflux can also frequently be documented in patients with Barrett's esophagus and ulcers or strictures [9].

Large series show that a Barrett's esophagus can be observed in 1%–5% of patients undergoing upper gastrointestinal endoscopy [8]. This prevalence increases to 10%–20% if only patients with symptoms of gastroesophageal reflux disease are analyzed [8, 10, 11]. On autopsy studies, a Barrett's esophagus can be found in about 400/100 000 patients [12]. The real incidence of the condition is, however, not clear but estimated to be similar to the incidence of Crohn's disease or lung cancer. The apparent increase in the incidence of Barrett's esophagus described during recent years matches the increasing number of endoscopies performed [12]. This suggests that, the true incidence of Barrett's esophagus remains stable.

Pathogenesis and Complications of Barrett's Esophagus

On the basis of the available data, Barrett's esophagus is without any question an aquired condition. It should not be considered a complication of reflux disease itself but rather a special form of healing of reflux induced defects in the normal squamous esophageal epithelium. A Barrett's esophagus, however, predisposes to some potentially severe complications in the further course of the underlying reflux disease. The complications of Barrett's esophagus and their prevalence are shown in Fig. 1. The development of strictures usually is the result of scars arising from transition ulcers, i.e. ulcers at the squamocolumnar epithelial border. Peptic ulcers may also develop within an area of Barrett's esophagus and are termed Barrett's ulcer. The most severe and, from the surgical point of view, interesting complication of Barrett's esophagus is the development of an adenocarcinoma in the columnar cell-lined esophagus [13]. In retrospective analyses, the prevalence of adenocarcinomas arising in Barrett's esophagus is between 12% and 15%. Of some 1400 patients with Barrett's esophagus described in the recent literature, 38 devolped an adenocarcinoma during prospective follow-up, accounting for an incidence of 1 carcinoma in 158 patient years. Compared to the normal population, this correlates to a 56-fold increase in the risk for developing esophageal adenocarcinoma in patients with Barrett's esophagus [14]. Of interest is, that the incidence and prevalence of adenocarcinomas in the distal esophagus and at the gastroesophageal junction

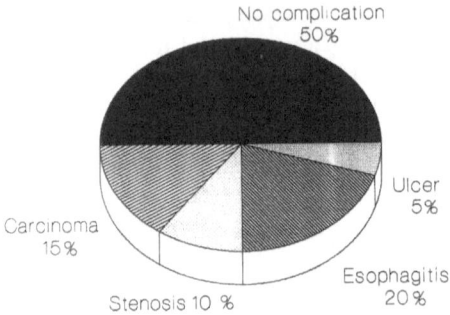

Fig. 1. Prevalence of complications in patients presenting with Barrett's esophagus

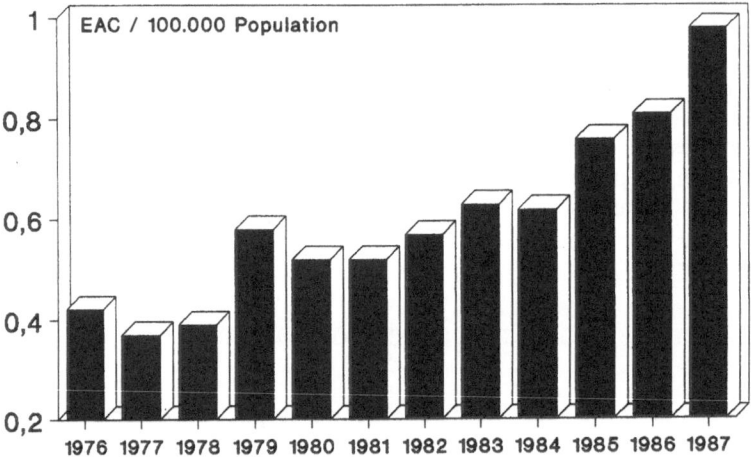

Fig. 2. Incidence of esophageal adenocarcinoma (*EAC*) in nine cancer registries of the United States. (Based on data from [15])

has shown an epidemic increase over the past two decades (Fig. 2) [15]. The reasons for this observation are not known.

These data indicate that Barrett's esophagus is a possible dangerous phenomenon. Agressive antireflux treatment of all patients with Barrett's esophagus has therefore been suggested by some investigators. This approach would, however, result in overtreatment of at least 50% of the patients who will never develop a complication (Fig. 2). There is no question, however, that patients with manifest complications should receive treatment of the underlying reflux disease. In our opinion, aggressive treatment should be initiated as soon as patients with Barrett's esophagus develop esophagitis above the columnar epithelial border.

Management of Gastroesophageal Reflux in Patients with Barrett's Esophagus

With the development of H2-blockers and proton pump inhibitors, medical treatment of gastroesophageal reflux has become very successful. These powerful drugs should be the initial line of medical treatment in a patient with Barrett's esophagus. Life style modifications, antacids, and prokinetic agents usually are not effective in these patients. As medical treatment of gastroesophageal reflux has improved, there have also been advances in antireflux surgery. Surgical antireflux procedures are now standardized and well evaluated. The modern antireflux procedure of choice is a 360 degree fundoplication with a short and floppy cuff which provides complete suppression of reflux with minimal side effects [16]. Mobilization of the gastric fundus is an essential part of this procedure.

The last years have shown that a fundoplication can also be performed laparoscopically [17]. This minimizes the trauma of access to the gastroesophageal junction, decreases postoperative pain, shortens hospital and recovery time, and may reduce pulmonary and thromboembolic complications. Consequently, the indications for an antireflux procedure may broaden in the future [18]. At the moment, however, we recommend a surgical antireflux procedure only in patients who have persistent or recurrent symptoms and/or complications of reflux despite aggressive medical management.

Recent studies, indicate that antireflux surgery is superior to aggressive medical management in the treatment of esophagitis, ulcers, and stenoses in patients with Barrett's esophagus [19, 20]. Whether an antireflux procedure can induce regression of Barrett's epithelium and prevent malignant degeneration remains, however, unclear. In the literature, regression of Barrett's esophagus has been described in about 7% of the patients and similar results were achieved with both medical and surgical therapy. In many instances, the described regression was only partial and the quality of the documentation and measurements of the extent of the columnar epithelium was poor. Progression to invasive cancer has also been reported in individual patients while on medical therapy or after antireflux surgery. In most of these patients, the effectiveness of antireflux therapy was not proven [21]. Consequently, the issue of regression of Barrett's esophagus and protection against malignant degeneration with medical or surgical management remains open.

Dysplasia in Barrett's Esophagus

Progressively severe grades of dysplasia in the columnar mucosa have been postulated as precursors for the development of an invasive adenocarcinoma in patients with Barrett's esophagus. Hameeteman et al. reported on five such patients with no dysplasia in their columnar epithelium on initial evaluation who developed low-grade dysplasia, then high-grade dysplasia, and eventually an invasive carcinoma during prospective follow-up confirming the dysplasia—carcinoma sequence [22].

There are, however, several pitfalls and open questions with dysplasia as an indicator for malignant degeneration. First, areas of dysplasia usually have a

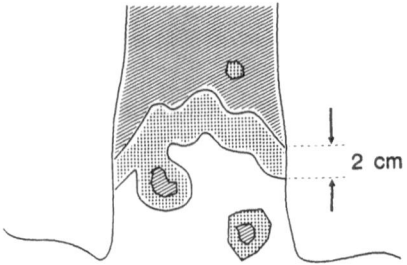

Fig. 3. High-risk area for the development of adenocarcinoma in patients with Barrett's esophagus (*dotted area*). *Cross hatched area* shows squamous epithelium, *blank area* columnar epithelium. (Modified from [24] with permission)

patchy distribution, can not be differentiated from normal columnar mucosa on endoscopy, and may consequently be missed when biopsies are taken. Second, pathologists frequently do not agree on the presence and severity of the dysplasia [23]. Third, low grade dysplasia may only reflect inflammation. Finally, it remains open whether dysplasia is reversible after successful antireflux therapy. In general, high grade dysplasia seen on more than one occasion and confirmed by two independent pathologists must, however, be considered a dangerous situation and deserves close surveillance or even prophylactic esophagectomy.

In our opinion, there are several good arguments for close surveillance rather than prophylactic esophageal resection in patients with high-grade dysplasia. First, it is not clear how frequently and after what time period dysplasia develops into an invasive cancer. Second, close endoscopic follow-up will allow detection of an invasive cancer at an early stage. Finally, esophagectomy is associated with considerable risks which may not be justified in a prophylactic procedure. Close endoscopic follow-up of patients with high-grade dysplasia is also supported by the report of Nishimaki et al. who observed that invasive cancers in patients with Barrett's esophagus appear to develop only in specialized columnar epithelium within 2 cm of the squamocolumnar epithelial junction (Fig. 3) [24]. This high-risk area should be observed carefully by endoscopy and extensive biopsy during follow-up.

On the other hand, there are several good arguments for esophageal resection in patients with high-grade dysplasia. First, an invasive cancer can be detected in the removed specimen in up to 50% of the patients who had resection because of areas with high-grade dysplasia [25]. Second, all tumors apparently develop within areas of high-grade dysplasia [26]. Finally, an invasive carcinoma can be cured only when resected at an early stage [27]. An algorithm for the management of patients with dysplasia in Barrett's esophagus is shown in Fig. 4 [28].

Due to the shortcomings of dysplasia as a marker for malignant degeneration, several other parameters have been investigated in the past years to identify patients at risk [29]. Of these parameters, assessment of mutations in the tumor suppressor gene coding for the protein p53 currently appear most promising [30]. Prospective studies are, however, necessary to confirm this finding.

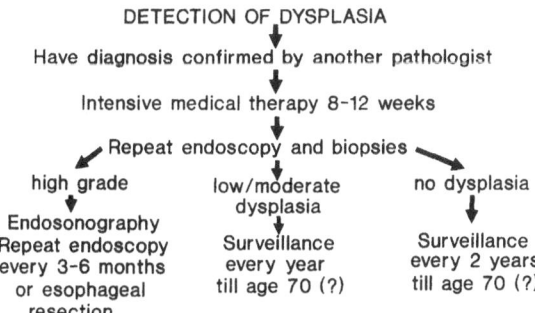

Fig. 4. Management of patients with dysplasia in Barrett's esophagus. (Modified from [28] with permission)

Surgical Approach to Barrett's Carcinoma

The definition of a carcinoma arising in Barrett's esophagus, i.e. a Barrett's carcinoma, is controversial. In our opinion, the very strict and academically correct definition of Barrett's carcinoma proposed by Moghissi is not practical for daily clinical use (Table 1) [31]. We and most other investigators prefer the more pratical definition of Barrett's carcinoma shown in Table 1 [27].

As for all other tumors of the gastrointestinal tract, the aim of any surgical approach to Barrett's carcinoma must be the removal of all macroscopic and microscopic tumor, i.e. an R0-resection according to the UICC 1987 classification. The importance of complete tumor resection is illustrated by the superior survival curves of patients with an R0-resection as compared to those who had an R1- or R2-resection, i.e. an incomplete resection [27].

For the selection of the correct surgical procedure, it is necessary to accurately determine the location of the tumor and its lymphatic drainage. As shown in Fig. 5, over 80% of early and advanced Barrett's carcinomas are located in the lower third of the esophagus. Only in very rare situations we have seen a Barrett's carcinoma located in the middle third of the esophagus. Of the patients with lymph node metastases, 84.2% had positive nodes around the celiac axis and 63.2% in the lower third of the mediastinum. More proximal lymph node metastases were found in only 19% of these patients. Usually, these were patients with very advanced tumor stages.

These observations led us to the following choice of procedures in patients with Barrett's carcinoma: In patients with a distal tumor, a transmediastinal esophagectomy is adequate. In this situation, we perform a regional lymph node

Table 1. Definitions of Barrett's carcinoma

Strict: Adenocarcinoma in the esophagus whose mucosa is covered by columnar epithelium for 3 cm or more above the site of insertion of the phrenoesophageal membrane. (After [31])
Practical: Adenocarcinoma with the center of tumor in the area of the tubular esophagus as long as Barrett's epithelium has been proven by endoscopy or histopathologic examination of the removed specimen

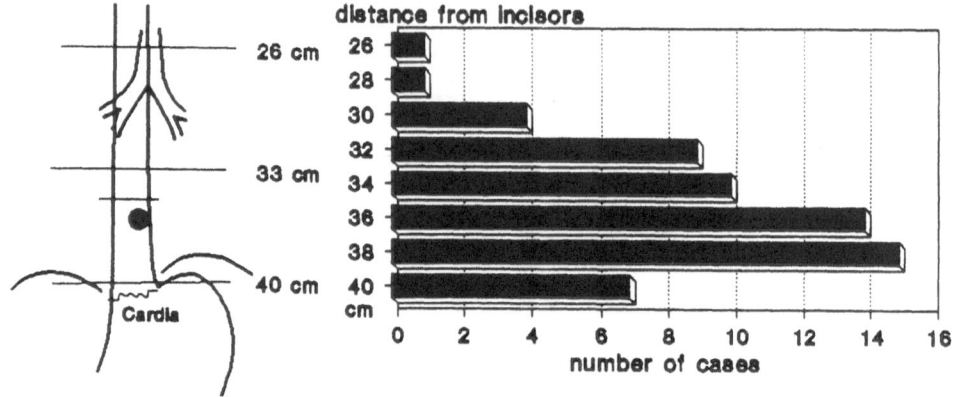

Fig. 5. Distribution of the tumor center in patients with Barrett's carcinoma

Table 2. Postoperative residual tumor stages in 106 patients with Barrett's carcinoma

	Total N	R0-Resection	R1/2-Resection
pT1	21	21 (100%)	0
pT2	17	15 (88.2%)	2 (11.8%)
pT3	40	32 (80.0%)	8 (20.0%)
pT4	28	16 (57.1%)	12 (42.9%)
pT1–4	106	84 (79.3%)	22 (20.7%)

R0, Complete macroscopic and microscopic tumor resection [32]
R1/2, Residual microscopic (R1) or macroscopic (R2) tumor [32]

dissection of the lower posterior mediastinum and around the celiac axis. If the tumor is located in the middle third of the mediastinum, we perform a transthoracic enbloc esophagectomy together with a 2-field lymphadenectomy [27]. With this approach, a R0-resection can be achieved in more than 80% of patients with tumor stages T1, T2, and T3. In 12 of 28 patients with a T4 tumor a complete macroscopic and microscopic tumor resection was not possible (Table 2). Since the presence of a T4 tumor can be demonstrated preoperatively by endoscopic ultrasound, we have started a trial with preoperative chemotherapy (EAP) followed by surgical resection in the patients with T4 tumors.

Results of Surgical Treatment of Barrett's Carcinoma

Over a period of 10 years, 457 patients with esophageal cancer had a resection at our institution. Histopathologic evaluation showed an adenocarcinoma in

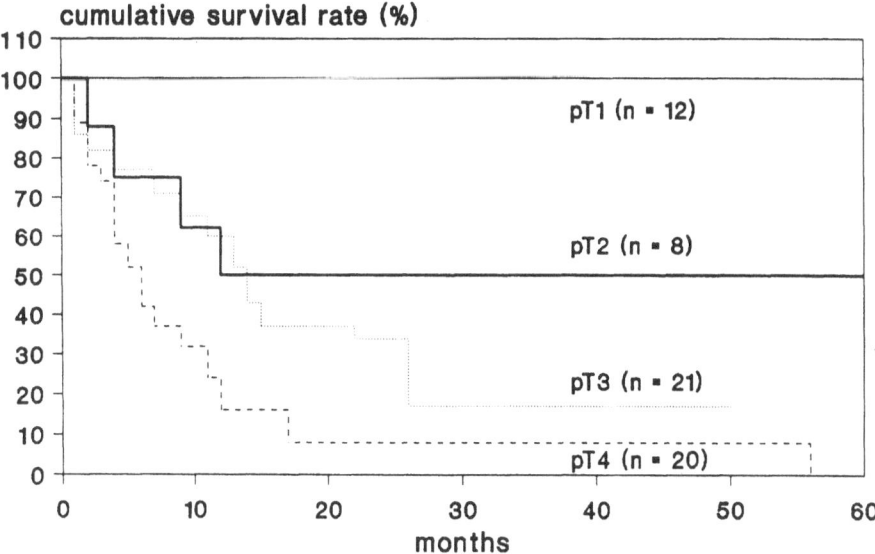

Fig. 6. Survival curve in patients with resected Barrett's carcinoma shown according to the T stages. (Modified from [27] with permission)

129/457 (28%) of the patients. According to the practical criteria shown in Table 1, the tumor was diagnosed as a Barrett's carcinoma in 106 of these patients.

Compared to the patients with squamous cell carcinoma, the patients with Barrett's carcinoma were more frequently male and on average 10 years older. The comparison of tumor stages between squamous and Barrett's carcinoma showed a higher rate of T1 tumors in the Barrett's group. On the other hand, lymph node metastases were more frequent in patients with Barrett's carcinoma.

The overall mortality after surgical resection of Barrett's carcinoma was 5.4%. Mortality was only 2.6% in patients with early Barrett's cancer, while the mortality markedly increased in patients with advanced tumors. The most frequent postoperative complications were pulmonary and a leakage of the cervical esophagogastrostomy which were observed in 25% and 17% of the patients, respectively.

The survival rates according to the T stages in patients with Barrett's carcinoma are shown in Fig. 6. Patients with T-1 tumors arising in Barrett's esophagus can be considered cured after resection. This is in contrast to patients with a T-1 squamous cell carcinoma of the esophagus. With all other T stages, survival is very similar between Barrett's carcinoma and squamous cell esophageal carcinoma. These data compare favourably to those reported in the literature.

Open and Answered Questions

In summary, today there is no question that in patients with Barrett's esophagus:

- The condition is acquired.
- Severe reflux disease is present.
- The antireflux mechanism is severly compromised.
- The risk for malignant degeneration is markedly increased.
- High-grade dysplasia is an ominous sign.
- Early tumors can be cured by surgical resection.

On the other hand, there remain several open questions:

- The predisposing factors for Barrett's esophagus and its complications are controversial.
- The factors leading to malignant degeneration are unknown.
- Regression of Barrett's esophagus is unproven.
- There is no good marker to identify patients at risk for malignant degeneration.

References

1. Barrett NR (1950) Chronic peptic ulcer of the esophagus and esophagitis. Br J Surg 38:175–182
2. Allison PR, Johnstone AS (1953) The esophagus lined with gastric mucous membrane. Thorax 8:87–101
3. Barrett NR (1957) The lower esophagus lined by columnar epithelium. Surgery 41:881–894
4. Lortat-Jacob JL (1957) L'endobrachy-ösophage. Ann Chir 11:1247–1252
5. Skinner DB, Walter BC, Riddel RH, Schmidt H, Iascone C, DeMeester TR (1983) Barrett's esophagus: Comparison of benign and malignant cases. Ann Surg 198:554–566
6. Borhan-Manesh F, Farnum JB (1991) Incidence of heterotopic gastric mucosa in the upper oesophagus. Gut 32:968–972
7. Cameron AJ, Lomboy CT (1992) Barrett's esophagus: Age, prevalence, and extent of columnar epithelium. Gastroenterology 103, 1241–1245
8. Gruppo Operativo Per Le Studio Delle Precancerosi Dell'Esophago (GOSPE) (1991) Barrett's esophagus: Epidemiological and clinical results of a multicentric survey. Int J Cancer 48:364–368
9. Stein HJ, Hoeft S, DeMeester TR (1992) Reflux and motility pattern in Barrett's esophagus. Dis Esoph 5, 21–28
10. Sarr MG, Hamilton FR, Marone GC, Cameron JL (1985) Barrett's esophagus: Its prevalence and association with symptoms of gastroesophageal reflux. Am J Surg 149:187–193
11. Winters C, Spurling TJ, Chobanian SJ, et al (1987) Barrett's esophagus: A prevalent, occult complication of gastroesophageal reflux disease. Gastroenterology 92:118–124
12. Cameron AJ, Zinsmeister AR, Ballard DJ, Carney AJ (1990) Prevalence of columnar lined (Barrett's) esophagus: Comparison of population-based clinical and autopsy findings. Gastroenterology 99:918–922
13. Siewert JR, Weiser HF, Lepsien G, Peiper HJ (1979) Endobrachyösophagus und Adenocarcinom der Speiseröhre. Chirurg 50:675–680
14. Stein HJ, Siewert JR (1993) Endobrachyösophagus: Pathogenese, Epidemiologie, Funktionsstörungen und maligne Degeneration. Dtsch Med Wschr 18:511–519
15. Yang PC, Davis S (SEER-Report) (1988) Incidence of cancer of the esophagus in the U.S. by histologic type. Cancer 61:612–617

16. Siewert JR, Feussner H, Walker SJ (1992) Fundoplication: How to do it? Periesophageal wrapping as therapeutic principle in gastroesophageal reflux prevention. World J Surg 16:326–334

17. Dellemagne B, Weerts JM, Jehaes C, Markiewicz S, Lombard R (1991) Laparoscopic Nissen fundoplication: Preliminary report. Surg Laparosc Endosc 1:138–143

18. Stein HJ, Feussner H, Siewert JR (1992) Minimally invasive antireflux procedures. World J Surg 16, 347–348

19. Spechler SJ, and the Dept. of Veterans Affairs Gastroesophageal Reflux Study Group (1992) Comparison of medical and surgical therapy for complicated gastroesophageal reflux disease in veterans. N Engl J Med 326:786–792

20. Attwood SEA, Barlow AP, Norris TL, Watson A (1992) Barrett's oesophagus: Effect of antireflux surgery on symptom control and development of complications. Br J Surg 79, 1050–1053

21. Skinner DB (1990) Controversies about Barrett's esophagus. Ann Thor Surg 49:523–524

22. Hameeteman W, Tytgat GNJ, Houthoff HJ, van den Tweel JG (1989) Barrett's esophagus: Development of dysplasia and adenocarcinoma. Gastroenterology 96:1249–1256

23. Reid BJ, Haggit RC, Rubin CE, et al (1988) Observer variation in the diagnosis of dysplasia in Barrett's esophagus. Hum Pathol 19, 166–178

24. Nishimaki T, Hölscher AH, Schuler M, Bollschweiler E, Becker K, Siewert JR (1991) Histopathologic characteristics of early adenocarcinoma in Barrett's esophagus. Cancer 68:1731–1736

25. Pera M, Trastek VF, Carpenter HA, Allen MS, Deschamps C, Pairolero PC (1992) Barrett's esophagus with high-grade dysplasia: An indication for esophagectomy? Ann Thor Surg 54, 199–204

26. Hamilton SR, Smith RRL (1987) The relationship between columnar epithelial dysplasia and invasive adenocarcinoma arising in Barrett's esophagus. Am J Clin Pathol 87, 301–312

27. Siewert JR, Hölscher AH, Bollschweiler E (1992) Surgical therapy of cancer in Barrett's esophagus. Dis Esop 5:57–62

28. Tytgat GNJ, Hameeteman W (1992) The neoplastic potential of columnar-lined (Barrett's) esophagus. World J Surg 16, 308–312

29. Schneider PM, Casson AG, Roth JA (1992) Detection of malignant potential in Barrett's epithelium. Dis Esoph 5, 45–50

30. Casson AG, Mukopadhay T, Clearry KC, Ro JY, Levine B, Roth JA (1991) p53 Gene mutations in Barrett's epithelium and esophageal cancer. Cancer Res 52, 4495–4499

31. Moghissi K (1992) Definition of adenocarcinoma arising in columnar epithelial lined oesophagus (Barrett's adenocarcinoma) Dis Esoph 5, 37–44

32. Hermanek P, Sobin LM, Union Internationale Contre le Cancer (1987) TNM classification of malignant tumors, 4th eds. Springer-Verlag Berlin Heidelberg

Regression of Columnar Metaplasia of the Lower Esophagus in a Canine Model

H. Li, T.N. Walsh, G. O'Dowd, P.G. Gillen, P.J. Byrne, and T.P.J. Hennessy[1]

Introduction

It is generally accepted that Barrett's esophagus is acquired due to longstanding gastroesophageal reflux which destroys the squamous epithelium, replacing it with acid resistant gastric-type epithelium [1–3]. Regression of this epithelium should reduce the risk of cancer and other complications. The evidence that regression can occur is conflicting and no large series has demonstrated it convincingly. This study compared regeneration in the presence of stimulated acid reflux with healing in the presence of acid control.

Methods

Study Protocol

Twelve adult mongrel dogs of mixed sex weighing between 14 and 20 kg acted as their own controls. All had a strip of esophageal mucosa excised from the lower end of the esophagus. A Wendel cardioplasty was created and acid secretion was promoted with daily pentagastrin injections. At 3 months, the mucosa which had regenerated in this milieu was resected. Six of these animals then had reflux controlled by repair of the hiatus hernia and reconstruction of cardia, and acid secretion was suppressed by administration of omeprazole (Astra Pharmaceuticals, UK). They were then followed up for an additional 3 months after which they were sacrificed and the esophagogastric specimens examined histologically.

[1] University Department of Surgery, St James's Hospital, Dublin 8, Ireland

Reflux-Inducing Procedure

Through a left thoracotomy, the esophagus was mobilized, the vagus nerve protected, the cardia opened through a vertical incision and a mucosal strip measuring 1 × 3 cm was removed from the lower esophagus, above a 1-cm barrier of normal squamous mucosa, which was left between it and the squamo-columnar junction. The esophagogastric incision was closed transversely and a fixed hiatus hernia was established by securing the cardioplasty and fundus of the stomach above the diaphragm with interrupted nylon sutures. From the 5th postoperative day, subcutaneous injections of pentagastrin (ICI Pharmaceuticals, UK) 100 μg were administered daily.

Excision of Regeneration Mucosa

Three months later, surviving animals underwent re-operation when the transverse incision was reopened. The squamous barrier was intact in all cases. The re-epithelialized area was then completely re-excised, leaving a further 1 × 3 cm defect surrounded by a squamous barrier and once again the cardia was reconstructed, this time by closing the esophagotomy longitudinally and the diaphragmatic hernia was also repaired. Pentagastrin was discontinued and omeprazole (20 mg) was given daily to suppress gastric acid secretion. Three months later, these animals were sacrificed and the esophagogastrectomy specimens removed en bloc.

Intra-Esophageal pH Monitoring

Intra-esophageal pH monitoring was performed for a 2-h period in awake, unanesthetized animals preoperatively, at 6 weeks following the reflux-inducing procedure, and again at 6 weeks following anti-reflux surgery. Recordings were made using a Digitrapper (Synectics, UK) and analysed using the Gastrosoft (Synectics, UK) analysis program.

Endoscopy

Upper gastrointestinal endoscopy was performed in all animals preoperatively and in ten at 10 weeks postoperatively.

Specimen Processing

Multiple longitudinal sections, 2–3 mm in width, were taken from the resected specimen of the normal esophagus, from the regenerated mucosa at 3 months, and from the posterior wall of the specimen of esophagus and stomach removed en bloc, to include normal esophagus, regenerating mucosa, the gastroesophageal junction, and the upper stomach. Sections were stained using hematoxylin and eosin.

Statistical Analysis

The pH data is represented as mean ± SEM. The significance of differences was determined by means of the Wilcoxon rank sum test.

Results

Intra-Esophageal pH Monitoring

No acid reflux occurred in control animals; the mean (SEM) percentage time when esophageal pH < 4 was 2.9% (1.0). Following the reflux-inducing procedure, the mean percentage time at pH < 4 increased significantly to 55.9% (5.6) (P < 0.001). Following reconstruction of the cardia and omeprazole therapy, the percentage time at pH < 4 fell significantly, to 0.7% (0.45) (P < 0.001), a value similar to controls.

Endoscopy

Endoscopy was normal in all control animals. Following the reflux-inducing procedure, the hiatus hernia was confirmed at endoscopy and varying degrees of esophagitis were noted in the lower esophagus which was graded using the classification of Savary and Miller [4]. Five animals had grade I, three had grade II, and two had grade IV esophagitis. The squamous barrier between the squamo-columnar junction and healing mucosal defect was frequently noted to be inflamed but remained intact in all cases.

Complications

Of the 12 dogs entered in the study, 6 had an uncomplicated course, 2 animals were sacrificed at 1 and 5 weeks post-operatively due to severe stricture and extensive gastric herniation, respectively, and 4 had non-fatal complications including mild stricture in 2 which responded to dilatation and diaphragmatic hernia in 2 which was successfully repaired.

Histology

Histological examination of the mucosal strips taken from control animals revealed normal squamous epithelium in all cases. Some esophageal glands and gland ducts remained after stripping the superficial mucosa. Biopsy specimens from the lower esophagus demonstrated reflux change with mucosal inflammation and ulceration. Foci of non-specialized gastric-type glandular mucosa with villiform surface and tall foveolar epithelial cells, consistent with Barrett's mucosa, were also identified on biopsy of the regenerated epithelium at 10 weeks following initiation. Intestinal type metaplasia with goblet cells was not seen.

Following 3 months of stimulated gastroesophageal reflux, columnar metaplasia was seen in seven of ten dogs. There was no evidence of regenerating squamous "islands". The regenerating columnar epithelium was villiform in pattern. The columnar epithelium was continuous with the columnar lined ducts of the deep esophageal glands. There was no continuity demonstrated macroscopically or microscopically between the columnar mucosa of the esophageal defect and the gastric mucosa. In three dogs, re-epithelialisation occurred by squamous epithelium alone.

Following 3 months of reflux control, the re-epithelialisation was by columnar epithelium, consistent with Barrett's mucosa in all six cases. On this occasion, however, interspersed with the metaplastic columnar epithelium were small foci of squamous epithelium. Islands ranged in number from two to six per strip and measured from 0.12 mm to 0.86 mm in length. The squamous islands appear to be directly continuous with the adjacent columnar epithelium with focal overlap and two epithelial types at the interface. Examination of multiple histological levels of these regenerating squamous "islands" and their surrounds suggested a direct continuity with the squamous-lined superficial portion of the esophageal gland ducts. The squamous barrier was again identified surrounding the columnar mucosa and was intact in all instances.

Discussion

It has previously been shown that repair of a mucosal defect in the lower esophagus heals by squamous epithelium in the presence of free reflux [5]. When acid production is stimulated by histamine or pentagastrin, however, Bremner et al. [6] and Gillen et al. [7] both found that regeneration was by columnar epithelium. In the current study, where esophageal pH-metry confirmed that the esophageal pH was less than 4 for a significant period, re-epithelialisation was by columnar mucosa in seven of ten dogs. When reflux was controlled, however, the mucosal defect was repaired in each case by columnar epithelium with islands of squamous mucosa scattered throughout.

The cell of origin of the columnar epithelium in Barrett's esophagus is much debated. Bremner et al. [6] suggested that the epithelium resulted from proximal migration of columnar cells from the cardia. Gillen et al. [7] demonstrated that columnar epithelium could develop in a mucosal defect above a squamous barrier. They presented evidence that the columnar mucosa is intrinsic to the esophagus itself and offered further evidence suggesting that it developed from the ducts of the esophageal glands. The current study adds further weight to this suggestion, as the mucosal defect was completely surrounded by squamous epithelium which remained intact for the 12 weeks of observation. On histological examination, the deep esophageal glands, lined in their proximal two-thirds by cuboidal or columnar epithelial cells, are in direct continuity with the columnar mucosa repairing the defect.

The origin of the squamous islands has also been unclear. The ducts of the esophageal glands are lined in their distal third by squamous epithelium, and it is postulated that the squamous islands seen in this study arise from proliferation of these cells. As the turnover of columnar cells is approximately five times faster than that of squamous cells [8], columnar epithelial growth will predominate. It is also suggested that for squamous regeneration to occur, remnants of the squamous lined ducts must be present and reflux must be controlled to prevent damage by bile or acid to this vulnerable epithelium. If, therefore, reflux causes severe damage to the esophageal mucosa, denuding it down to a level which destroys the superficial squamous portion of the gland ducts, regeneration will be by columnar epithelium only. If the mucosal damage is less severe, leaving portions of the squamous-lined ducts intact, regeneration will include squamous islands.

References

1. Borrie J, Goldwater L (1976) Columnar cell-lined esophagus: Assessment of etiology and treatment. A 22-year experience. J Thorac Cardiovasc Surg 71:825–834
2. Iascone C, DeMeester TR, Little AG, Skinner DB (1983) Barrett's esophagus: functional assessment, proposed pathogenesis, and surgical therapy. Arch Surg 118:543–549
3. Bremner CG (1989) Barrett's esophagus. Br J Surg 76:995–996
4. Savary M, Miller G (1978) The esophagus. Handbook and atlas of endoscopy. Gassman, Saluthurn, pp 119–205
5. Hennessy TPJ, Edlich RF, Buchin RJ, Tsung MS, Prevost M, Wangensteen OH (1968) Influence of gastroesophageal incompetence on regeneration of esophageal mucosa. Arch Surg 97:105–107
6. Bremner CG, Lynch VP, Ellis FH Jr (1970) Barrett's esophagus: Congenital or acquired? An experimental study of esophageal mucosal regeneration in the dog. Surgery 68:209–216
7. Gillen P, Keeling P, Byrne PJ, West AB, Hennessy TPJ (1988) Experimental columnar metaplasia in the canine esophagus. Br J Surg 75:113–115
8. Creamer B, Shorter RG, Bamforth J (1961) The turnover and shedding of epithelial cells. Part I. The turnover in the gastrointestinal tract. Gut 2:110–118

Endobrachyesophagus Without Mucosectomy: An Experimental Model in Dogs

BENJAMIN NARBONA-ARNAU, PILAR ARGENTE-NAVARRO,
JOSE MIGUEL LLORIS-CARSÍ, MIGUEL ANGEL CALVO-BERMÚDEZ,
and DOLORES CEJALVO-LAPEÑA[1]

Introduction

Barrett's esophagus is regarded us a precancerous disease, with a neoplastic degenerative tendency some 40 times that of the normal mucosa [1]. The condition lacks efficient medical treatment and antireflux surgery is insufficient and controversial. In turn, prophylaxis, involving endoscopic control and biopsies to afford curative exeresis or preventive resection, is both problematic and unsatisfactory, since endoscopy-biopsy is uncertain and expensive, while esophagectomy involves excessive morbidity and mortality.

This situation could be remedied if it were possible to demonstrate that acquired Barrett's esophagus is the result of distal mucoesophageal reflux lesions, particularly when summing both refluxes—gastric and duodenal—since the former alone does not seem capable of producing the metaplastic-neoplastic cellular and architectural alterations of endobrachyesophagus. The underlying etiopathogenic factors would involve duodenogastric reflux plus an incontinent lower esophageal sphincter (LES), duodeno-gastroesophageal reflux being the outcome.

Nevertheless, this cause and effect relationship has not yet been established with certainty [2]. It is difficult to obtain reliable data from clinical studies that must not only be longitudinal and prospective but also cover a long period of time and involve a great many patients and data—thus requiring multicenter efforts [3] that tend to accumulate subjective variables affecting the significance of the results obtained.

Experimental research could overome these problems, although not without a certain risk in extrapolating the results to humans. Generally [4–8], Barrett's esophagus is induced by exposing denuded esophageal areas (occasionally

[1] Centro de Investigación Hospital General Universitario Tres Cruces s/n, 46014-Valencia, Spain

140   B. Narbona-Arnau et al.

even with an intermediate squamous mucosal zone between the gastroesophageal junction and the mucosectomy) to gastroesophageal reflux [9]. This
process does not imply "creeping substitution" from the cardio-fundus mucosa,
but rather metaplasia of superficial cells of the esophageal glands (which possess
greater potential than the deeper lying cells) [9]. When reflux is cancelled by
fundoplicature (H. Li et al., see this volume), regeneration of the denuded
mucosal area is mixed and includes squamous areas.

The major inconvenience posed by such models is that in associating mucosectomy with acid reflux, they present an artificial etiopathogenic basis far
removed from that presumed in human clinical practice.

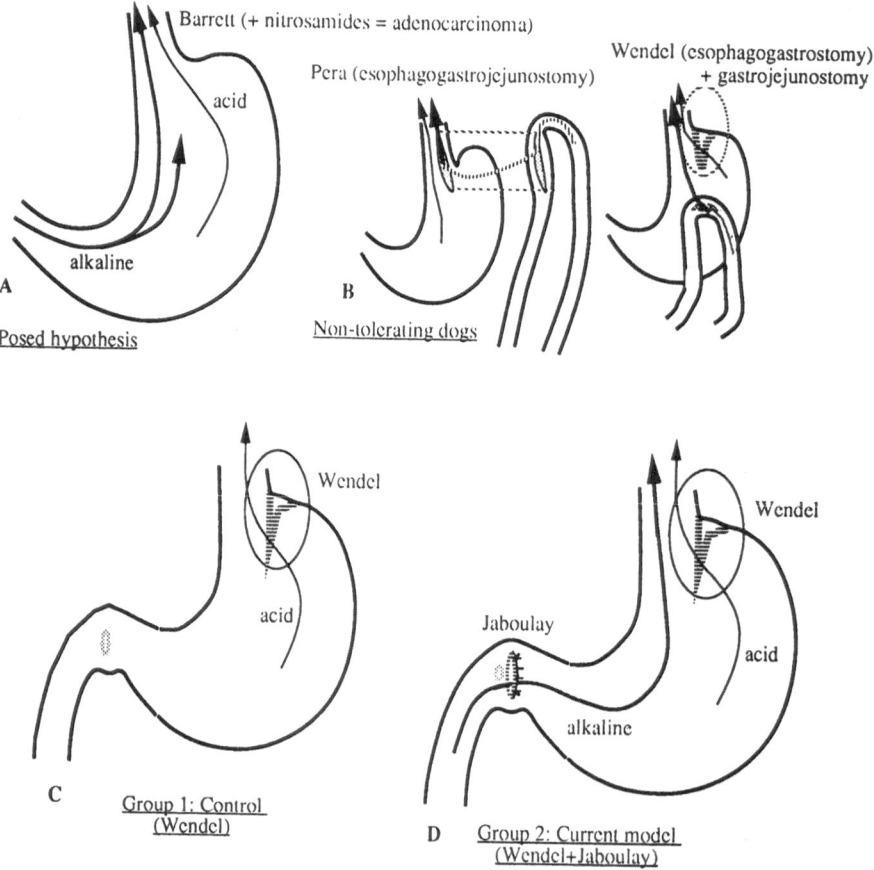

Fig. 1A–D. Experimental protocols. **A** Posed hypothesis: dual reflux (acid and alkaline) effect
on the esophageal mucosa. **B** Preliminary experiments: esophagogastrojejunostomy, not
tolerated by the dogs, and Wendel vertical esophagogastropeasty plus gastrojejunostomy—which
was likewise not tolerated. **C** Current model: Group 1 (control), limited to Wendel surgery. **D**
Current model: Group 2, where a prepyloric antroduodenostomy or Jaboulay operation is
performed in addition to the Wendel, to obtain dual reflux. This protocol was adequately
tolerated

Pera et al. [10], and more recently Attwood et al. [11], have found that the association of nitrosamides with reflux or esophageal exposure to biliopancreatic secretions causes adenocarcinoma in rats. Moreover, in 1 out of 14 cases, bile exerted a cancerigenic effect in the absence of nitrosamides [11]. These studies indicate that duodenoesophageal reflux causes cylindrical metaplasia in these animals while converting the habitual nitrosamide-induced esophageal epidermoid neoplastic response to adenocarcinoma.

If this etiopathogenic route towards the adenocarcinomatous transformation of Barrett's esophagus is confirmed, then undoubtedly suppression of the causes of the meta/dysplastic/cancerous alteration of the esophageal mucosa and prevention of mixed acid-alkaline exposure (in particular out of the duodenum) would be more efficient and economical that controlling Barrett's esophagus and/or surgical removing this segment of the digestive tract at an early curative or prophylactic stage.

Inspired by the studies by Pera et al. [12], we have investigated a canine model in which the contents of the two immediately distal digestive tract segments—the stomach and duodenum—combine to act upon the esophagus (Fig. 1a).

Material and Methods

Beagle dogs of either sex (15–20 kg) were examined to exclude possible esophageal pathology and gastroesophageal reflux.

The preoperative examination included fibroendoscopic biopsy, manometry (automatic catheter extraction and paper inscription at the same semi-show rate of 1 cm/5 s) and 24-h pH-metry (Synectics, monocrystal pH electrode, Model 91-0205, Ref. 4001) (Microdigitrapper, Synmed).

These preoperative explorations showed the absence of esophagitis, LES location, alkaline esophagus and the habitual absence of basal gastric acid secretion.

The dogs were operated on after overnight fasting according to habitual asepsia-anesthetic protocol. Preanesthesia was performed using atropine (0.05 ml/kg) and diethyl phenothiazine (0.05 ml/kg). Anesthesia consisted of thiobarbital (20–22 mg/kg), atracuronium bezylate (0.3 mg/kg) and N_2O—O_2 (2:1 v/v) (Engström respirator). Postanesthesia was carried out with prostigmine-atropine.

Antibiotherapy consisted of cephalozine 0.1 g preoperatively and then every 6 h for 24 h.

Preliminary Experiments

The jejunoesophagogastrostomy that appears to cause cylindrical metaplasia and adenocarcinoma in rats (H. Li et al., see this volume) [11] was attempted in four Beagles. The procedure was not tolerated however, due to intractable vomiting (Fig. 1b).

The same happened on summing stapled vertical gastroesophagoplasty (Wendel operation with the GIA stapler) and gastrojejunostomy in another four dogs.

The latter had to be undone, leaving only the Wendel operation. Along with a further 6 animals, this constituted the control group (Group 1).

Current Models

Group 1 (controls) was subjected to surgery to secure gastroesophageal incontinence. A vertical Wendel esophagogastrostomy (4–5 cm) was performed. A 1-cm anterior gastrotomy allowed introduction of the two GIA stapler arms—one in the esophagus and the other in the fundus (Fig. 1c). Group 1 consisted of ten dogs (four originating from the Wendel-gastrojejunostomy group in which persistent severe vomiting forced us to undo the gastrojejunostomy, plus the additional 6 animals) that were limited to the Wendel procedure.

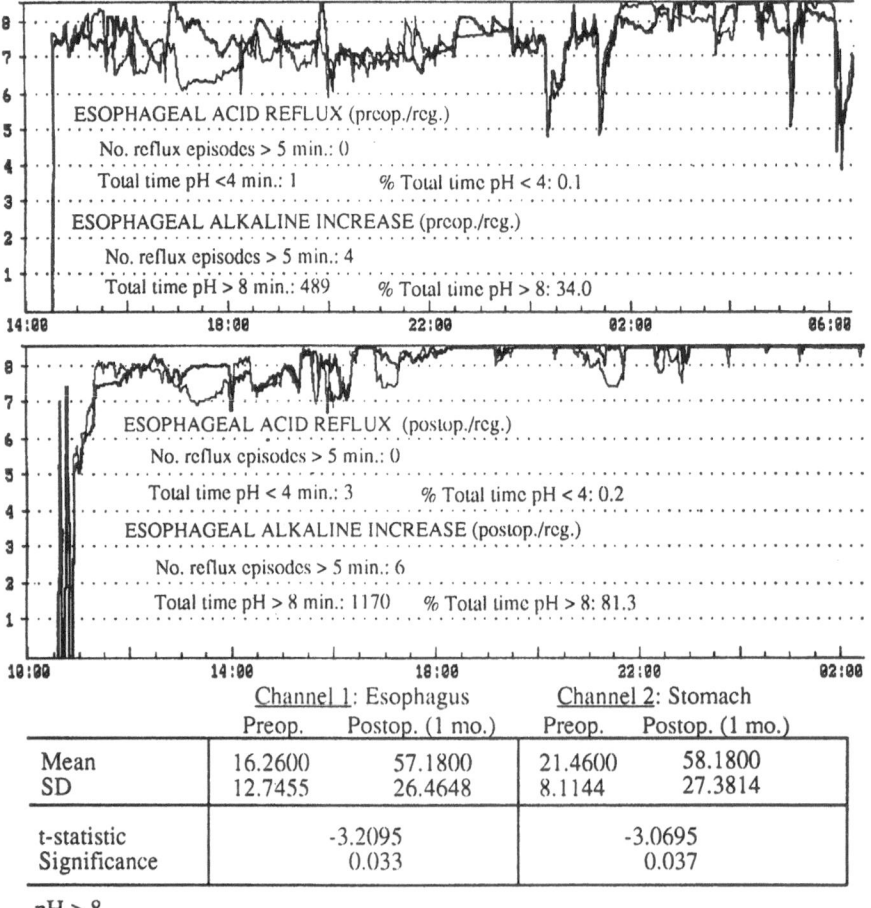

| | Channel 1: Esophagus | | Channel 2: Stomach | |
	Preop.	Postop. (1 mo.)	Preop.	Postop. (1 mo.)
Mean	16.2600	57.1800	21.4600	58.1800
SD	12.7455	26.4648	8.1144	27.3814
t-statistic	-3.2095		-3.0695	
Significance	0.033		0.037	

pH > 8

Fig. 2. Pre- and postoperative (1 month) pH-metric recording. The time difference with pH readings above 8 was significant

Group 2 was in turn subjected to double incontinence (gastroesophageal and duodenogastric) through a middle laparotomy. The same vertical esophago-gastroplasty plus a Jaboulay-type prepyloric gastroduodenostomy, some 2 cm long and about 1.3 cm in diameter, was performed (Fig. 1d).

The postoperative examination in both groups consisted of 24-hour pH-metry, manometry and endoscopy-biopsy in the 1st, 6th and 12th months. Endoscopy-biopsy and pH-metry was performed in the 2nd, 4th and 9th months.

Results

Two dogs died of anesthetic complications and bowel loop necrosis.

As to the postoperative explorations, manometry clearly revealed, in both groups, the almost total disappearance of the LES.

In Group 2, pH-metry revealed a significant increase in alkaline reflux with respect to the preoperative levels. During 24-hour pH-metry, the recordings were for most of the time at $pH > 8$, this result being statistically significant (Fig. 2). No significant changes were seen in Group 1.

Endoscopy-biopsy in the control group showed either no or minimal esophagitis. Conversely, Group 2 ("double refluxers") revealed Stage II–IV esophagitis after only 4 weeks, with rivulets of possible metaplasia after 10–12 weeks. After the 2nd month, we noted gastric-type glands among the esophageal glands, with occasional cylindrical metaplastic foci. In this sense, however, quite a few biopsies were too superficial to allow confirmation of these changes.

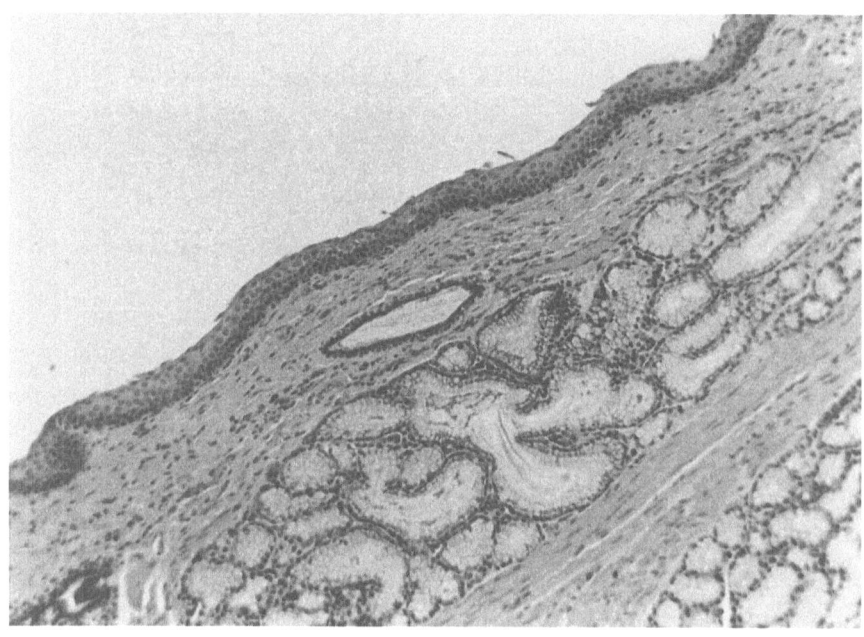

Fig. 3. Group 1 autopsy specimen. The microscopic appearance is normal

Three dogs (one in Group 1, and two in Group 2) were autopsied after between 16 and 25 weeks. The first animal developed bowel occlusion and died in spite of reoperation. The other two animals had been developing severe nutritional problems.

The stomach was opened along the greater curvature, together with the esophagus. These organs were macroscopically examined and 2 mm by 7 mm esophageal strips were subjected at 3, 6, 9 and 12 h to microscopic scrutiny over every 2 cm measured from the gastroesophageal junction.

In Group 1 (only Wendel surgery) both the macro- and microscopical examinations were negative (absent or minimal esophagitis) (Fig. 3). In the two Group 2 autopsied dogs ("double refluxers"; Wendel plus Jaboulay procedures)

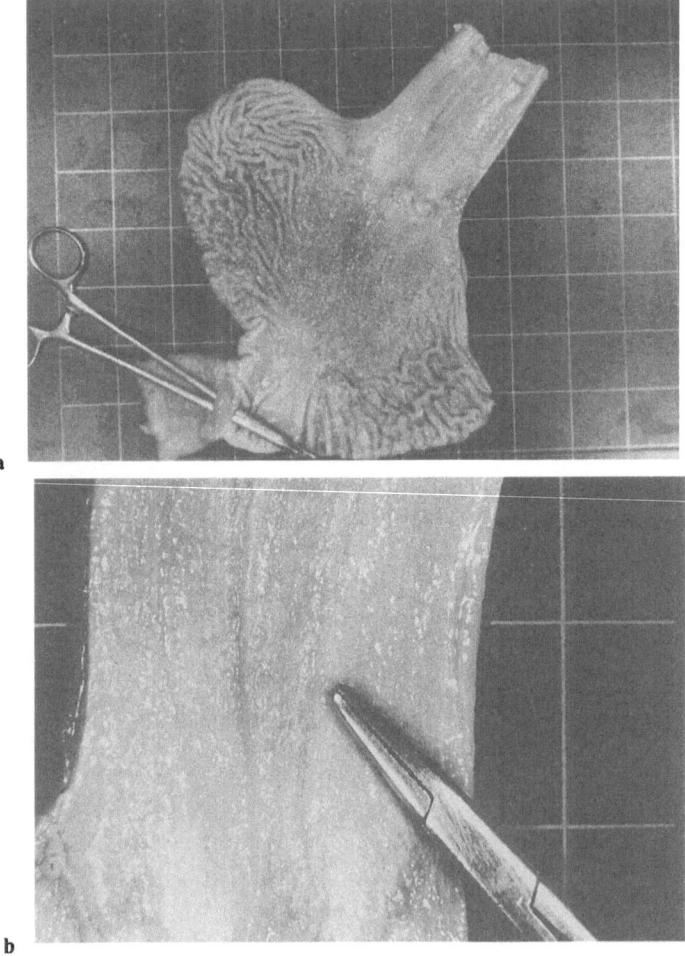

Fig. 4a,b. Group 2 autopsy specimen. **a** Esophagus and stomach opened along the greater curvature and through the Jaboulay region. The forceps are passed through the intact pylorus. **b** Macroscopic appearance, with rivulets and dark red areas

there were rivulets and areas of different coloring in the midst of intense esophagitis (Fig. 4). Multiple samples were obtained above 2 cm from the gastroesophageal junction (Fig. 5a). Thus, gastric glands were seen interspersed among the esophageal glands, and even goblet cells were seen in one case. Also, peptic ulceration was seen (Fig. 5b) over an esophageal glandular background. There were evident, extensive areas of cylindrical metaplasia (Fig. 5c,d) interspaced among squamous epithelium. Finally, thick papillas and a highly dense inflammatory infiltrate were noted. No mucin assays were performed.

Discussion

The treatment best suited to Barret's esophagus-preneoplastic pathology remains controversial. Medication to reduce acidity cannot cure the endobrachyesophagus, and antireflux surgery cannot eliminate the possibility of degenerative changes (9.4% of adenocarcinomas over Barrett's esophagus in the series reported by Streitz et al. [13] were operated on). Controversy continues to center on whether to perform prophylactic resection or carry out continued endoscopic control.

The latter is both expensive and uncertain, and its efficacy remains to be established [14]. The detection of severe dysplasia remains the "gold standard" but is endoscopically indistinguishable [14]; although its most likely location is close to the epdermoid-cylindrical mucosal limit [15], "blind" biopsy taking would have to be multiplied and systemized, without even then being able to obviate the possibility of false-negative results. The cost of detecting each adenocarcinoma is about US\$62 000 [16]. Even if endoscopic control were limited to those patients eligible for esophageal resection, the financial costs would be very considerable.

The second alternative, prophylactic esophagectomy, is mentioned because severe dysplasia—in spite of its diagnostic subjectivity [15]—must unequivocally be regarded [17] as a neoplastic alteration or even as *carcinoma in situ*. Consequently, while some surgeons opt for radical prophylaxis [13, 15] (T. Lerut et al., see this volume; J.M. Mendes-Almeida et al., see this volume), particularly in the case of endobrachyesophagus with a high risk of neoplastic degeneration, in patients without surgical problems, others are contrary to this approach because of the excessive risk posed by such preventive measures [1]. Moreover, the possibility of an adenocarcinoma developing somewhere in the remaining esophagus persists in 6.2% of patients [13]. In any case, redical prophylaxis may undoubtedly cause unnecessary operative deaths.

For as long as no easily determined unambiguous marker is encountered or the risks associated with esophagectomy can be minimized, this controversy will persist.

As pointed out initially, it is clear that if the etiopathogenic mechanism involved in Barrett's esophagus were clarified, showing that biliopancreatic secretion is responsible for the metaplasia/dysplasia/neoplasia observed, and means were available to free the esophagus of contact with these duodenal contents, then the current controversy between an uncertain endoscopic control and prophylactic morbidity and mortality would be put to rest.

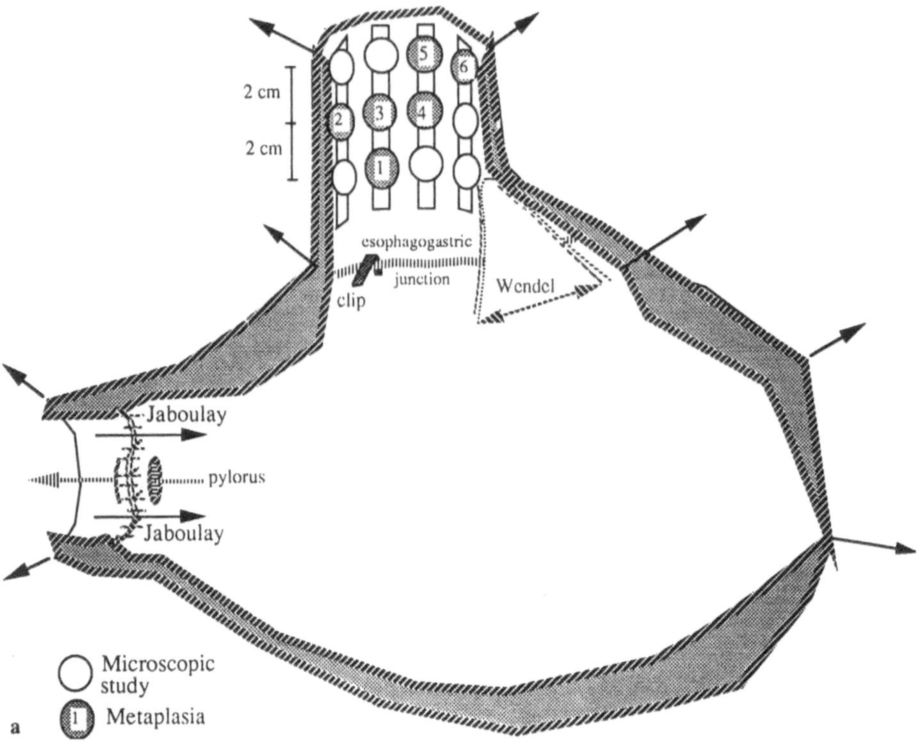

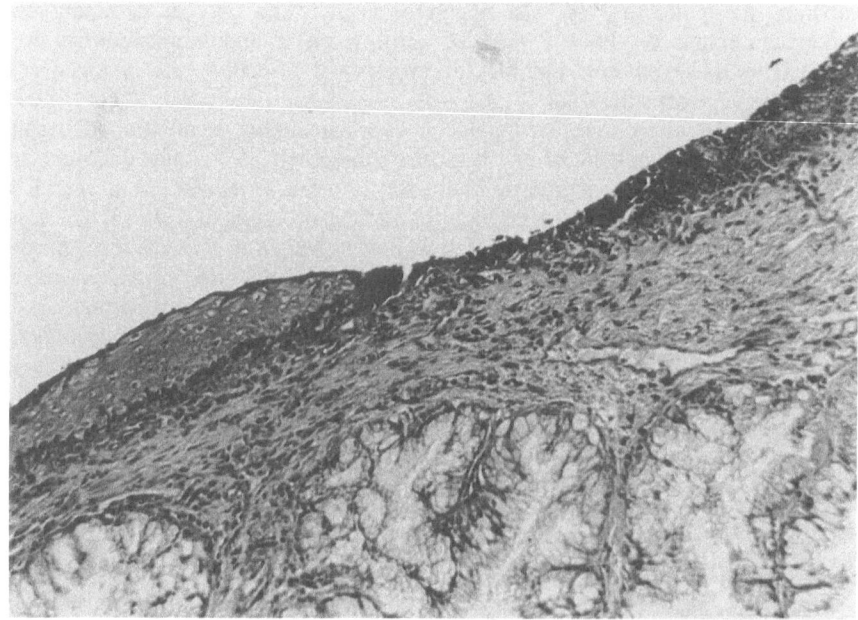

Fig. 5. a Esophageal sampling points for microscope study. The cylindrical metaplasia-positive areas are numbered. Micrographs of **b** peptic ulcer, **c,d** cylindrical epithelium out of glands and at this surface

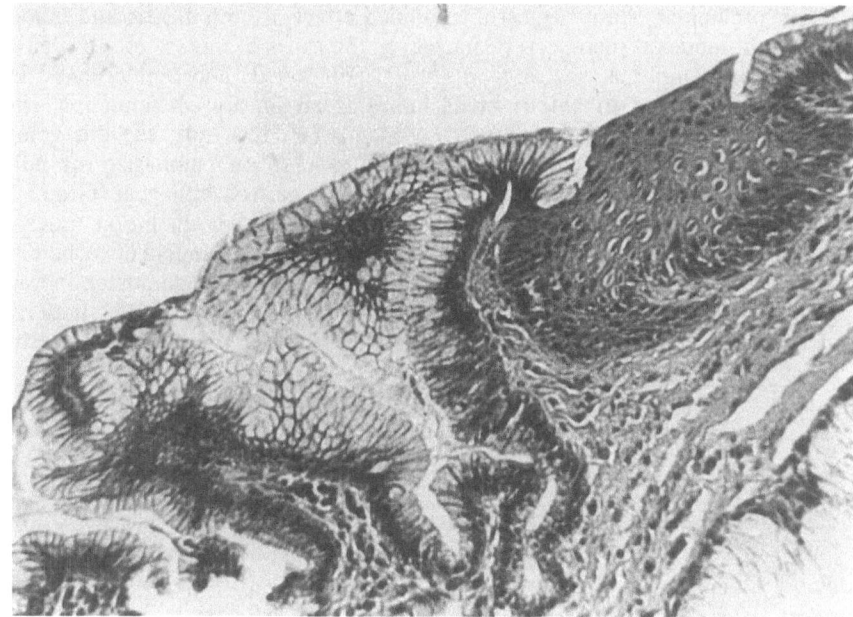

c

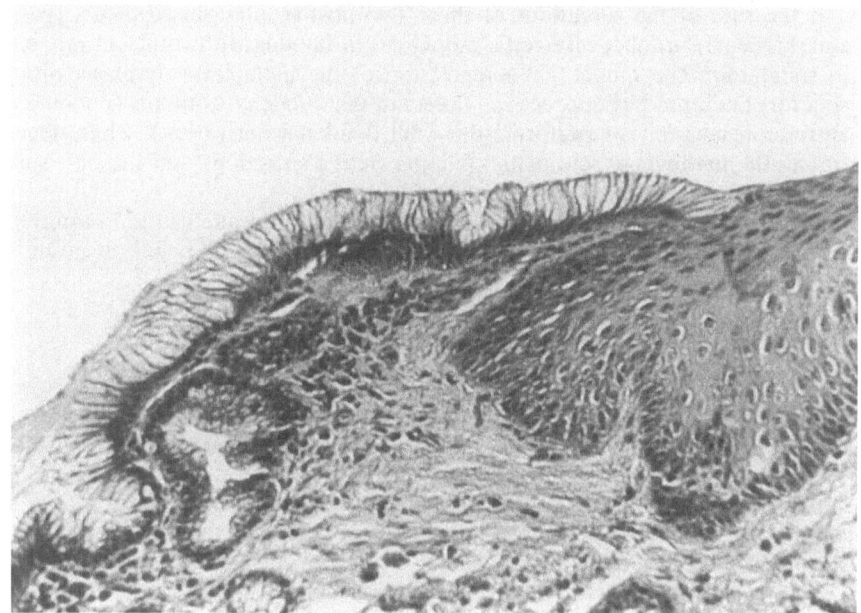

d

Fig. 5. *Continued*

Our preliminary data suggest a combined effect of both gastric and biliopancreatic or duodenal secretions (Group 2) as the cause of intense esophagitis with cylindrical metaplasia, gastric-type glands, goblet cells and peptic ulcer. Their distribution among squamous areas indicates an in situ phenomenon arising from the cubic cells of the esophageal glands (H. Li et al., see this volume) rather than a "creeping substitution". In this sense we emphasize the null or minimal esophagitis observed when reflux is only gastroesophageal (Group 1).

When a more extensive series is studied, with longer evolution times and additional study parameters including electron microscopy, mucin histochemistry, and flow cytometry, etc., the existence of Barrett's esophagus or endobrachyesophagus may be confirmed in this experimental canine model. The underlying mechanisms may then be investigated, and possible therapeutic approaches tested.

If these studies using a model to reproduce mixed reflux finally supports the Barrett's esophagus-adenocarcinoma etiopathogenic hypothesis of duodenogastric reflux with LES insufficiency and medium-low acid gastroesophageal reflux, then the best suited therapeutic approach would be to prevent the possibility of esophageal exposure to the duodenal contents. The latter at this level would thus be prevented from causing lesions equivalent to those observed in the stomach in the presence of a competent LES, i.e., atrophic gastritis, gastric ulcer, intetinal metaplasia, dyspepsia, and cancer (A. Yasui et al., see this volume).

If the sum of the secretions of these two post-esophageal segments (gastric and duodenal) produces Barrett's esophagus in the dog with sufficient reliability to standardize the model, then regression of the metaplasia dysplasia process could be attempted by suppressing access of the duodenal contents (undoing the antroduodenostomy or performing a total duodenal derivation), while demontrating the pathogenic role of the biliopancreatic secretions and the best suited therapeutic approach.

These aspects should of course be regarded with the due caution required in extrapolating results from experimental studies to the human clinical setting.

Conclusion

These initial double reflux (duodenal and gastric) experiments in dogs suggest the existence of effects of the esophageal mucosa compatible with Barrett's esophagus or endobrachyesophagus (cylindrical cells, metaplastic foci, goblet cells, severe esophagitis, and peptic ulcer).

If these obervations are confirmed and moreover undergo regression after the interrupting arrival of the second (duodenal) reflux, then the best suited therapeutic approach could be clarified.

We consider that this mixed acid and bile-alkaline model—once adequately standardized—may be used to perform therapeutic trials in endobrachyesophagus.

References

1. Tygat GNS (1992) Incidence of cancer in esophageal columnar metaplasia (Barrett's esophagus). Dis Esoph 5:29–35

2. Skinner DB (1990) Controversies about Barrett's esophagus. Ann Thorac Surg 49:523–524
3. Giuli R, De Vathaire F (1988) OESO collaborative studies. Launching of a international study on esophagitis: Barrett's esophagus and esophageal dysphasia. Dis Esoph 1:139–146
4. Hennessy TPJ, Edlich RF, Buchin RJ, et al (1968) Influence of gastroesophageal incompetence on regeneration of oesophageal mucosa. Arch Surg 95:105–107
5. Bremner CG, Lynch VP, Ellis FM (1970) Barrett's esophagus: congenital or acquired? An experimental study of esophageal mucosal regeneration in dog. Surgery 68:209–216
6. Bremner CG (1982) Benign strictures of the esophagus. Curr Prob Surg 19:460–449
7. Martin CJ, Funk NA, Ewing ME, et al (1992) Reversal of experimental Barrett's esophagus by endoscopic laser ablation and reduction of acid reflux. Fifth World Congress ISDE, 5–8 August 1992, Kyoto. Abstracts SP 151 p 188
8. Pollara WM, Zilberstein B, Cercoconello I, Filho UL, Pinotti HW (1985) Regeneration of eophageal epithelium in the presence of gastroesophageal reflux. In: DeMeester TR, Skinner DB (eds) Esophageal disorders: Pathophysiology and therapy, Raven, New York
9. Guillen P, West AB, Keeling P, Hennessy TPJ (1988) Barrett's oesophagus: A pathophysiological study. In: Siewert JR, Hölschner AH (eds) Diseases of the esophagus. Springer, Berlin Heidelberg New York, pp 540–541
10. Pera M, Cardesa A, Bombi JA, Ernst H, Pera C, Mohr U (1989) Influence of esophagojejunostomy on the induction of adenocarcinoma of the distal esophagus in Sprague-Dawley rats by subcutaneous injection of 2,6-dimethylnitrosomorpholine. Cancer Res 49:6803–6808
11. Attwood SFA, Smyrk ThC, DeMeester TR, et al (1992) Duodenoesophageal reflux and the development of esophageal adenocarcinoma in rats. Surgery 111:503–510
12. Pera M, Cardesa A, Bombi JA, Ernst H, Pera C, Mohr U (1989) Experimental adenocarcinoma of the distal esophagus after exposure to 2,6-dimethylnitrosomorpholine under the influence of reflux esophagitis. Fourth World Congress ISDE, 6–8 Sept. 1989, Chicago. Abstracts p 100
13. Streitz JM, Ellis FH, Gibb SP, et al. (1991) Adenocarcinoma in Barrett's esophagus: a clinical pathologic study of 65 cases. Ann Surg 313:122–125
14. Schneider PM, Casson AG, Roth JA (1992) Dectection of malignant potential in Barrett's epithelium. Dis Esoph 5:45–50
15. Siewert JR, Hölscher AH, Bollschweller E (1992) Surgical therapy of cancer in Barrett's esophagus. Dis Esoph 5:57–62
16. Achkar E, Carey WC (1988) The cost of surveillance for adenocarcinoma complicating Barrett's esophagus. Am J Gastroenterol 81:580–584
17. Appelman HD, Kallsh RJ, Chancy PE, Orringer MB (1985) Distinguishing features of adenocarcinoma in Barrett's esophagus and in the gastric cardia. In: Spechler SJ, Goyal RK (eds) Barrett's Esophagus. Pathophysiology, diagnosis and management. Elsevier, New York

Adenocarcinoma Arising in Barrett's Esophagus After Esophageal Resection and Jejunal Interposition

Örs Péter Horváth[1], Jolán Csanádi[2], and Vilmos Szendrényi[2]

Introduction

There are a lot of open questions about the pathogenesis of Barrett's esophagus. Some of them are listed below:

1. Is the presence of gastroesophageal reflux necessary to elicit development of a columnar-lined esophagus?
2. Is Barrett's esophagus merely due to an excessive alkaline exposure or are there some specific factors, such as certain components of bile or pancreatic enzymes, also necessary for the formation of a columnarlined esophagus?
3. Where does the metaplastic epithelium arise from? (The new adenomatosus lining develops either from submucosal glands of the esophageeal mucosa or from adjacent tissues.)
4. Does columnar epithelium regress after a successful antireflux repair?

We tried to answer these questions having diagnosed esophageal adenocarcinoma in two patients who had been operated upon for peptic stricture when an esophageal resection with jejunal interposition had been performed 17 and 18 years earlier.

Material, Methods, and Results

Between 1965 and 1980, 72 esophageal resections and jejunal interpositions were performed for undilatable peptic and mixed-type stricture at the Surgical Clinic of the Medical University of Szeged. A left thoracolaparotomy approach was chosen in all cases.

[1] Department of Surgery, Medical University of Pécs, Ifjúság u. 13. 7643. Pécs, Hungary
[2] Department of Surgery and Pathology, Albert Szent-Györgyi Medical University of Szeged, Pécsi út 4. 6720. Szeged, Hungary

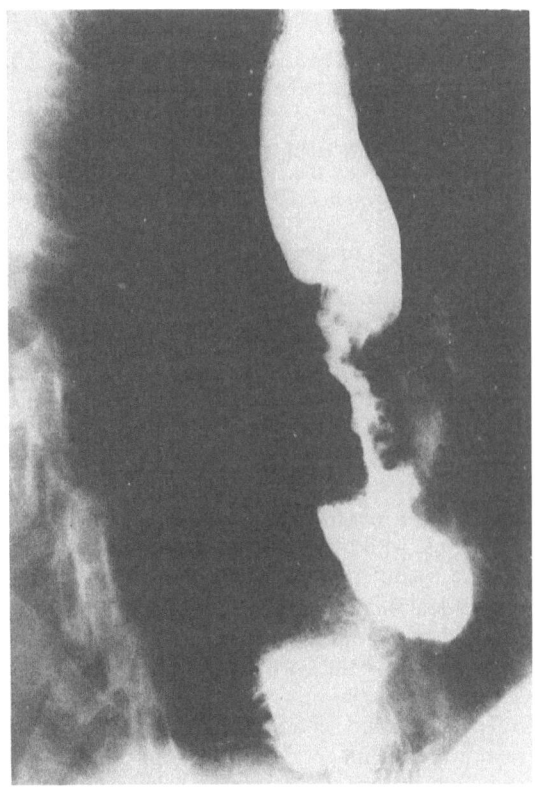

Fig. 1. Adenocarcinoma in the esophagus 17 years after esophagus resection and jejunum interposition

The first patient suffering from severe dysphagia caused by an adenocarcinoma of the remainder esophagus above the esophago-jejunal anastomosis, was admitted in 1989 (Fig. 1). Earlier, in 1971 an esophageal resection was performed for the treatment of a peptic stricture. At that time, the patient was 41 years old. The histologic examination revealed a cardia-type Barrett esophagus in the resected specimen. We performed an esophagectomy without thoracotomy with additional colonic replacement 18 years later. This time histology showed an intestinal-type Barrett esophagus with severe dysplasia in addition to adenocarcinoma.

The second patient with adenocarcinoma following esophageal resection and jejunal interposition was admitted in 1991 with progressive dysphagia. The 57-year-old man was operated on for peptic stricture in 1974. Then histology showed an intestinal-type metaplasia with ulceration and fibrosis.

At the second admission (in 1991), biopsies showed adenocarcinoma and an intestinal type columnar-lined epithelium in the adjacent tissue. He refused esophagectomy.

We started a follow-up study on 12 patients with high cancer risk who underwent esophageal resection and jejunal interposition 12–20 years previously. Esophageal resection was indicated in seven cases with peptic stricture and in five cases with mixed-type stricture. There were eight men and four women. The mean age was 67 years.

Table 1. Data of the two control patients with Barrett's esophagus

Variable	Patient 1	Patient 2
Date of birth	1921	1923
Sex	Male	Male
Date of esophagus resection	1975	1976
Indication for resection	Peptic stricture	Mixed stricture
Histology (after resection)	No Barrett's	Intestinal-type Barrett's
Histology (biopsy prior to resection)	Intestinal-type Barrett's	Intestinal-type Barrett's

During the follow-up study, we performed endoscopy and took four biopsies from four quadrants of the esophagus 2 cm proximal to the esophago-jejunal anastomosis. In ten cases, histology revealed normal squamous epithelium or mild non-specific changes. In two cases, a columnar-lined epithelium was found. The data of these patients are shown in Table 1.

Patients with columnar-lined esophagus were further investigated by means of barium roentgenography and 24-h pH monitoring.

The length of interposed jejunal segments was estimated in the course of contrast radiography and was found to be 50 cm on average.

As found by the 24-h pH monitoring, pH values fluctuated between 6.2 and 7.4 in both cases.

The histologic sections of the resected esophagus were reevaluated and new sections were made. In one of the control patients—in whom the esophageal resection had been performed earlier due to peptic stricture—we did not find Barrett's epithelium in the resected specimen.

In the original sections of the second control patient, an intestinal type Barrett was to be seen. Of special interest was the finding in this patient at the follow-up study whereby epithelium regenerated in areas where Barrett's epithelium was previously found. Remnants of columnar epithelium could be found under the squamous layer (Fig. 2).

Discussion

It is widely accepted that jejunal interposition following esophageal resection prevents gastro-esophageal reflux if the jejunal segment is longer than 40–60 cm [1]. In both control patients, the length of interposed jejunal segments was about 50 cm, therefore acidic reflux could not be detected by pH monitoring. In cases of adenocarcinoma, we did not perform pH monitoring because the highly obstructive tumor would have made results unappreciable.

Esophageal resection had been performed earlier in three patients (two with adenocarcinoma and one in the control group) for the treatment of peptic stricture. In cases of Barrett's esophagus, the stricture usually develops at the squamo-columnar border [2] and therefore the whole columnar segment is removed with resection of the strictured part. In one patient, esophageal resection was made for a mixed-type stricture; and, under such circumstances, the

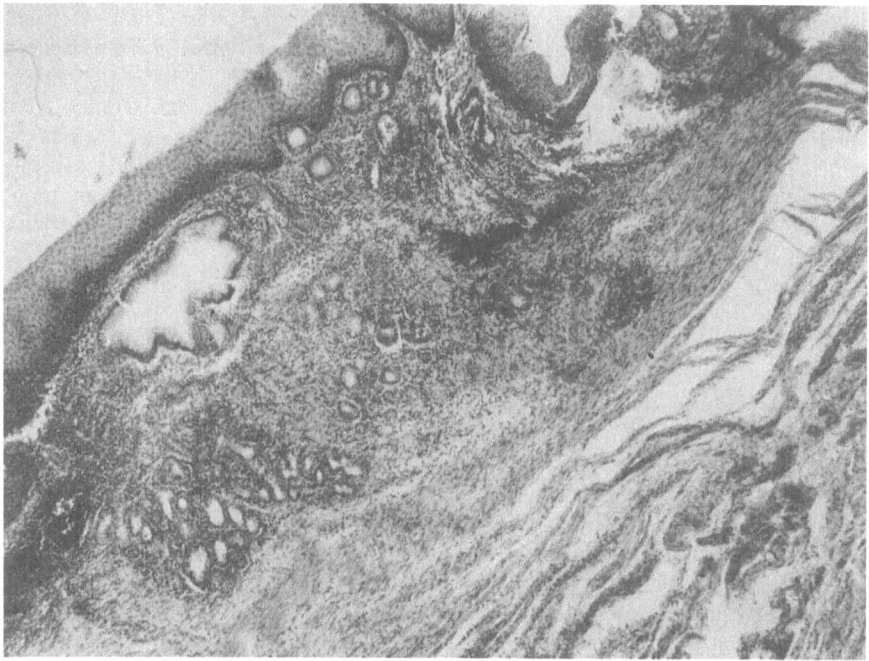

Fig. 2. Endoscopic biopsy taken 16 years after esophagus resection from a region previously lined with intestinal type metaplasia. Squamous epithelium is overlying the residual Barrett's epithelium (H & E, ×300)

stricture and the squamo-columnar border did not always coincide. Consequently, residual Barrett's epithelium could remain in the esophagus after resection.

Based on our follow-up data, a columnar epithelium newly developed in three patients after esophageal resection and jejunal interposition. Accordingly, acid reflux seems to be not necessary in the development of Barrett's esophagus.

Some authors believe that alkaline or mixed reflux can play an important role in the pathogenesis of Barrett's esophagus [3, 4]. Bremner [2] states that the components of the refluxate are more important than pH.

After esophago-jejuno-gastrectomy, bile or pancreatic juice can not reach the esophageal mucosa, so the role of alkaline pH in itself becomes negligible.

Meyer et al. [5] described a patient in whom Barrett's esophagus had developed after total gastrectomy. Hamilton et al. [6] reported that an adenocarcinoma had developed 8 years after esophageal resection and colonic replacement. These two cases and our own findings support the theory that the new adenomatous lining may develop either from submucosal glands, by metaplasia of the squamous epithelium, or from the adjacent jejunum or colon.

If reflux cannot be implicated as a causative factor lending support to the acquired theory of columnar-lined esophagus, a congenital origin with or without reflux must be considered.

The type of epithelium found in cases with adenocarcinoma was an intestinal type Barrett-lining. Skinner et al. [7] reported similar findings and suggested that a specialized type of intestinal metaplasia is the type most likely to undergo malignant transformation.

Whether or not antireflux operations protect the columnar segment from malignant changes is still controversial [8]. There are reports on adenocarcinomas that have developed after antireflux surgery [9, 10]. The jejunal interposition is one of the most reliable antireflux procedures, nevertheless, adenocarcinomas have developed in our two cases 17 and 18 years after resection of the stricture together with jejunal replacement.

There is also some debate as to whether the columnar segment regresses after antireflux surgery [11, 12]. Brand et al. [13] reported on regression of the epithelium after surgery, but this has not been a uniform finding. We observed squamous epithelium regeneration after surgery in areas where Barrett's epithelium had previously been found in one patient. This phenomenon was first described by Skinner et al. [7]. Whether the glandular epithelium will persist deep to the squamous layer, will gradually atrophy and disappear completely or even persist and become malignant, is unknown.

There is still much to learn about Barrett's esophagus. It is very likely that there are great individual differences regarding predisposition to development of metaplastic epithelium in the esophagus. According to our data, Barrett's esophagus may develop again in a new environment after esophageal resection. Therefore, endoscopic surveillance is indicated even after esophageal resection and jejunal interposition presuming the operation has been performed for Barrett's esophagus.

Since the columnar epithelium can develop again after its removal, it is advisable to consider this fact by the indication of preventive surgery to be performed (e.g., resection, antireflux op.) in cases with Barrett's esophagus.

References

1. Polk HC, Richardson JD (1981) Non-functional esophagogastric junction: Treatment of jejunal interposition. In: Stipa S, Belsey RH, Moraldi H (eds) Medical and surgical problems of the esophagus. Academic, New York, pp 188–194
2. Bremner CG (1987) Barrett's esophagus. In: DeMeester TR, Matthews HR (eds) International trends in general thoracic surgery. Benign esophageal disease. Mosby, St Louis, pp 227–239
3. Attwood SE, DeMeester TR, Bremner CG, Barlow AP, Hinder RA (1989) Alkaline gastroesophageal reflux: Implications in the development of complications in Barrett's columnar-lined lower esophagus. Surgery 106:764–770
4. Gillen P, Keeling P, Byrne PJ, Healy M, O Moore RR, Henessy TPJ (1988) Implication of duodenogastric reflux in the pathogenesis of Barrett's esophagus. Br J Surg 75:540–543
5. Meyer W, Vollmar F, Bar W (1979) Barrett's esophagus following total gastrectomy. A contribution to its pathogenesis. Endoscopy 12:121–126
6. Hamilton SR, Hutcheon DF, Ravich WJ, Cameron J, Paulson M (1984) Adenocarcinoma in Barrett's esophagus after elimination of gastroesophageal reflux. Gastroenterology 86: 356–360
7. Skinner DB, Walther BC, Riddell RH, Schmidt H, Iascone C, DeMeester TR (1983) Barrett's esophagus. Comparison of benign and malignant cases. Ann Surg 198:554–566

8. DeMeester TR, Attwood SEA, Smyrk TC, Therkildsen DH, Hinder RA (1990) Surgical therapy in Barrett's esophagus. Ann Surg 212:526–540

9. Skinner DB (1990) Controversies about Barrett's esophagus. Ann Thor Surg 49:523–524

10. Szendrényi V, Oláh T, Csanádi J, Horváth ÖP (1992) Barrett's esophagus. Orv Hetil 133:2079–2084

11. Mangla JC (1980) Barrett's epithelium: regression or no regression? N Engl J Med 303: 529–530

12. Naef AP, Savary M, Ozello L, Pearson FG (1975) Columnar-lined lower esophagus. Surgery 70:826–834

13. Brand DL, Ylvisaker JT, Gelfand M, Pope CE (1980) Regression of columnar esophageal (Barrett's) epithelium after anti-reflux surgery. N Engl J Med 302:844–848

Therapy in Barrett's Esophagus: Medical Treatment Versus Antireflux Surgery

S.E.A. Attwood, A.P. Barlow, T.L. Norris, and A. Watson[1]

Introduction

Barrett's columnar lined esophagus (CLO) has a marked propensity to develop serious complications [1]. In more than 50% of patients there is an associated stricture or ulceration, and tendency to hemorrhage, perforation, or malignant degeneration [2, 3]. Gastroesophageal reflux disease is almost invariably present in patients who have Barrett's CLO but the reason why only a portion of the patients with reflux develop an abnormal glandular lining in the esophagus, and why some of these are more prone to complications, is not known.

Patients with Barrett's CLO frequently have a severe degree of gastroesophageal reflux and this, associated with the high frequency of complications, presents a therapeutic challenge [4]. The management of Barrett's CLO remains controversial, ranging from no treatment in the absence of symptoms to pharmacological acid suppression and antireflux surgery, but the relative merits of each form of treatment are unknown. The aim of this study was to compare the efficacy of pharmacological acid suppression and antireflux surgery on symptom control and the incidence of complications in Barrett's CLO.

Patients and Methods

Forty-five patients with Barrett's CLO were treated at the Royal Lancaster Infirmary over a 9-year period. Patients with an esophageal carcinoma at first presentation were not included in the study. The initial symptoms were recorded using a standard questionnaire. Table 1 shows the grading used for symptom severity. Flexible endoscopy was performed to document the length of colum-

[1] Department of Surgery, Royal Lancaster Infirmary, Ashten Road, Lancaster, UK
[2] Department of Surgery, Wallace Freeborn Professional Block, Royal North Shore Hospital, Sydney NSW 2065, Australia

Table 1. Symptom grading for the assessment of heartburn, dysphagia, and epigastric pain

Score	1	2	3	4
Heartburn	Monthly	Weekly	Daily	—
Dysphagia	Occasional	Solids only	Semi-solid	Liquid
Epigastric pain	Monthly	Weekly	Daily	—

Table 2. Age, sex, extent and length of follow up in patients treated for Barrett's esophagus

	Medical $n = 26$	Surgical $n = 19$
Median (range) age, years	70 (40–91)	62 (26–74)
Male : Female	12:14	11:8
Median (range) length of Barrett's mucosa in cm	5.0 (3–10)	6.0 (3–11)
Median (range) duration of follow-up in years	3.0 (1–9)	3.0 (1.5–9)

narization above the gastroesophageal junction and to identify the presence of a stricture or other complication. Strictures were dilated before commencing therapy, using Celestin dilators passed over a guide wire. Full dilatation to 56Fr gauge was achieved in all patients. Patients underwent esophageal manometry and 24–h ambulatory esophageal and gastric pH monitoring as described previously [5, 6]. Each patient was treated for a period of 3–6 months with high-dose H2 antagonist therapy (ranitidine, 600 mg daily), and Gaviscon (10 mls four times daily) in addition to standard general measures. Symptoms were assessed after the initial trial of medical therapy. Patients with residual reflux symptoms, or dysphagia due to a persistent or recurrent stricture, were offered antireflux surgery. Twenty-one of the 45 patients had an initial good response to medical treatment at three months and continued to take high-dose ranitidine. Five of the remaining 24 were considered ineligible on the basis of age and general condition. Nineteen patients underwent antireflux surgery, which comprised restoration of the lower esophageal sphincter to the abdominal cavity, accentuation of the flap valve mechanism of the cardia, and partial anterior fundoplication as previously described [7, 8]. Endoscopic surveillance was performed annually. Symptoms of heartburn, dysphagia, and epigastric pain were recorded and graded using the standard questionnaire at each endoscopic visit. The number of recurrent strictures was recorded as the number of patients who required redilatation during the course of the study. In addition, the number of dilatations required for each patient was also recorded. The age and sex ratio of the two groups is shown in Table 2. The extent of the lower esophagus covered by circumferential glandular epithelium is also shown and was similar in each group. The length of follow-up was a median of 3 years with a similar range of 1–9 years in each group.

Table 3. The manometric assessment of the esophageal body and lower esophageal sphincter

	Medical n = 16		Surgical n = 13
Defective lower sphincter	10	NS	11
Weak esophageal peristalsis	9	NS	5

NS, no significant difference, *P* > 0.05 Fishers exact test

Table 4. pH profile in Barrett's esophagus before medical or surgical therapy

	Medical n = 16	Surgical n = 13
% time pH < 4		
Median (range)	14.4 (1–49)	14.5 (2.6–68)
Score[a] pH < 4		
Median (range)	40.6 (2.1–139)	43 (8–182)
% time pH > 7		
Median (range)	7.5 (0–58.9)*	15.7 (0–47)

[a] DeMeester composite score [6]
* *P* < 0.05 Wilcoxon rank sum

Statistical Analysis

Patients' symptoms were assessed annually and the median score for each post-treatment symptom in each patient was recorded to compare the pre- and post-treatment symptoms in the two groups using the Wilcoxon Signed Rank test. Inter-group comparisons of symptoms were made using the Wilcoxon Rank Sum test. The proportion of patients with persistent or absent symptoms and the incidence of complications were compared using the Fisher's exact test. *P* values were considered significant at the 5% level.

Results

Pretreatment manometry and esophageal pH monitoring showed that patients treated medically or surgically had similar severe degrees of gastroesophageal reflux disease. (Tables 3 and 4). There was no significant difference in the pretreatment acid pH profile of the medically and surgically treated groups, but there was a greater exposure to pH > 7 in the surgically treated group prior to surgery.

Pretreatment symptoms were similar in both groups, with heartburn and dysphagia being the most troublesome (Table 5), and these improved more after surgery than after medical therapy. Symptoms of heartburn (grade 2 or higher) and or dysphagia (grade 1 or higher) persisted or recurred in 23 (88%) patients on medical treatment and in four (21%) after antireflux surgery (*P* value <0.01, Fisher's exact test, Table 6). Complications developed in ten (38%) after medical

Table 5. Mean symptom scores before and after medical and surgical therapy for Barrett's esophagus

Symptom	Medical		Surgical	
	Pre median (range)	Post median (range)	Pre median (range)	Post median (range)
Heartburn	2 (2–3)	2.0 (0–3)	3 (2–3)	*0 (0–2)
Regurgitation	1 (0–2)	0.0 (0–2)	1 (0–3)	0 (0–0)
Dysphagia	2 (0–4)	1.0 (0–4)	2 (0–4)	*0 (0–2)
Epigastric pain	1 (0–3)	0.0 (0–3)	1 (0–3)	0 (0–3)

* $P < 0.05$ Wilcoxon signed rank test

Table 6. Symptoms and complications after medical or surgical therapy for Barrett's esophagus

	Medical $n = 26$		Surgical $n = 19$
Symptom resolved	3		15
Symptom persisted	23	*	4
Stricture resolved	2		4
Stricture recurred	6		2
New stricture developed	3		0

* difference between Medical and Surgical significant at $P < 0.01$, Fisher's exact test

therapy, and included stricture in nine patients and a carcinoma in one. After antireflux surgery, three patients (16%) developed a complication: stricture in two and carcinoma in one ($P < 0.05$). The mean extent of the Barrett's mucosa was unchanged in each group although after surgery it regressed completely in two patients. Nine strictures required dilatation in the medically treated group compared to two after surgery.

Discussion

While there is general agreement concerning the need for surveillance of patients with Barrett's CLO [9, 10], it is surprising that no clear guidelines exist regarding the treatment of these patients or indeed whether they should be treated at all in the absence of significant symptoms [11]. Where treatment is recommended, both pharmacological acid suppression and antireflux surgery have been espoused [9, 12, 13]. Although not randomized, this study was performed prospectively as part of ongoing surveillance, and reflects our current clinical management of Barrett's CLO. The long-term symptomatic response in patients treated medically was poor and the rate of stricture redevelopment was high, in contrast to the good symptomatic response and the low rate of stricture recurrence after surgery. No new strictures occurred after antireflux surgery. Our results of medical therapy are comparable with those of Atkinson and Robertson [13] who compared stricture recurrence in patients with and without Barrett's esophagus.

This study indicates failure of medical therapy in over half of the patients treated and is consistent with the large multi-centre study of medical and surgical therapy of gastroesophageal reflux disease reported by Spechler [14]. Since medication was aimed at acid suppression, the implication is that either the degree of acid suppression was insufficient or the presence of non-acid injurious agents in the refluxed material continued unabated and indeed may have been enhanced by the neutralising effect of acid. We believe that duodenogastric reflux may play a role in the development of complications in Barrett's CLO [15]. Successful antireflux surgery creates a mechanical barrier to refluxed material regardless of composition, and the greater efficacy of antireflux surgery over pharmacological acid suppression supports the hypothesis that components of the refluxate other than acid/pepsin may play a role in the development of complications. Maximal acid suppression with Omeprazole is still associated with a significant failure rate in healing esophagitis within the first 8 weeks [16–18], a rate which approaches 50% in the most severe grades of esophagitis, and so the results of our study are likely to apply to any form of medical therapy aimed purely at acid suppression.

Our study has not shown any overall reduction in the length of Barrett's epithelium with either therapy, but similar to previous reports [19] there were two cases (10.5%) of complete regression of the Barrett's epithelium after surgery. There was no difference in the rate of malignant degeneration as one patient from each group subsequently developed cancer. The occurrence of malignant degeneration in both groups encourages vigilance in the follow-up of patients with Barrett's esophagus, regardless of treatment modality. The reason for malignant degeneration in Barrett's esophagus is not understood but it has been proposed that this may be consequent on continued gastroesophageal reflux [6, 20]. Animal studies indicate a co-carcinogenic effect of duodenal juice but not of gastric juice in the esophagus of the rat [20]. Whether duodenal juices play a role in the development of carcinoma in the human esophagus is not known.

The results of this prospective, nonrandomized study strongly suggest that antireflux surgery is more effective than pharmacological acid suppression in symptom control and the prevention of complications in patients with Barrett's CLO.

Acknowledgment. The data in this chapter has been published in the British Journal of Surgery (1992) 79:1024–1028.

References

1. Barrett NR (1950) Chronic peptic ulcer of the oesophagus and "oesophagitis". Br J Surg 38:175–182
2. Bremner CG (1987) Barrett's esophagus. In: DeMeester TR, Matthews HR (eds) International treads in general thoracic surgery, vol 3: Benign esophageal diseases. CV Mosby, St Louis, pp 227–238
3. Naef AP, Savary M, Ozello L (1975) Columnar lined lower esophagus: an acquired lesion with malignant predisposition. Report on 140 cases of Barrett's esophagus with 12 carcinomas. J Thorac Cardiovasc Surg 70:826–834

4. DeMeester TR, Attwood SEA, Smyrk TC, Therkildsen DH, Hinder RA (1990) Surgical therapy in Barrett's esophagus. Ann Surg 212:528–542
5. Jenkinson L, Norris TL, Watson A (1986) Dietary guidelines for ambulatory pH recording. Gut 27:594–595
6. DeMeester TR (1987) Definition, detection and pathophysiology of gastro-oesophageal reflux disease. In: DeMeester TR, Matthews HR (eds) International trends in general thoracic surgery, vol 3: Benign esophageal disease. CV Mosby, St. Louis, pp 99–127
7. Watson A (1984) A clinical and pathophysiological study of a simple effective operation for the correction of gastro-oesophageal reflux. Br J Surg 71:991–993
8. Watson A, Jenkinson LR, Ball CS, Barlow AP, Norris TL (1991) A more physiological alternative to total fundoplication for the surgical correction of resistant gastro-oesophageal reflux. Br J Surg 78:1088–1094
9. Bremner CG (1989) Barrett's Oesophagus. Br J Surg 76:995–996
10. Robertson CS, Mayberry JF, Nicholson DA, James PD, Atkinson M (1988) Value of endoscopic surveillance in the detection of neoplastic change in Barrett's oesophagus. Br J Surg 75:760–763
11. Scarpignato C, Franze A (1990) Columnar-lined (Barrett's) esophagus. Curr Opin Gastroenterol 6:580–585
12. Sampliner RE, Garewal HS, Fennerty MB, Aickin M (1990) Lack of impact of therapy on extent of Barrett's esophagus in 67 patients. Dig Dis Sci 35:93–96
13. Atkinson M, Robertson CS (1988) Benign oesophageal stricture in Barrett's columnar epithelialised oesophagus and its responsiveness to conservative management. Gut 29: 1721–1724
14. Spechler SJ (1992) Comparison of medical and surgical therapy for complicated gastroesophageal reflux disease in veterans. The Department of Veterans' Affairs gastroesophageal reflux disease study group. N Engl J Med 326:786–792
15. Attwood SEA, DeMeester TR, Bremner CG, Barlow AP, Hinder RA (1989) Alkaline gastroesophageal reflux: implications in the development of complications in Barrett's columnar-lined lower esophagus. Surgery 106:764–770
16. Hetzel DJ, Dent J, Reed WD, Narielvala FM, Mackinnon M, McCarthy JH, Mitchell B, Beveridge BR, Laurence BH, Gibson GG, Grant AK, Shearman DJC, Whitehead R, Buckle PJ (1988) Healing and relapse of severe peptic esophagitis after treatment with omeprazole. Gastroenterology 95:903–912
17. Bate CM, Keeling PWN, O'Morain CA, Wilkinson SP, Foster DN, Mountford RA, Temperley JM, Harvey RF, Thompson DG, Davis M, Forgacs IC, Bassett KS, Richardson PDI (1990) Comparison of omeprazole and cimetidine in reflux oesophagitis: symptomatic, endoscopic and histological evaluations. Gut 31:968–970
18. Hameeteman W, Tytgat GN (1986) Healing of chronic Barrett ulcers with omeprazole. Am J Gastroenterol 81:764–766
19. Brand DL, Ylvisaker JT, Gelfand M, Pope CE (1980) Regression of columnar esophageal (Barrett's) epithelium after anti-reflux surgery. N Engl J Med 102:844–848
20. Attwood SEA, Smyrk TC, DeMeester TR, Mirvish SS, Stein HJ, Hinder RA (1992) Duodenoesophageal reflux and the development of esophageal adenocarcinoma. Surgery 111:503–510

Surgical Treatment of Barrett's Carcinoma: Correlation Between Morphologic Findings and Prognosis

T. Lerut, W. Coosemans, B. Dillemans, D. Van Raemdonck,
P. De Leyn, J.M. Marnette[1], and K. Geboes[2]

Introduction

Barrett's esophagus or columnar epithelium-lined lower esophagus is a disorder in which the normal squamous cell epithelium is replaced by a metaplastic columnar mucosa. It is estimated that it occurs in about 10% of the patients suffering from gastroesophageal reflux. The importance of Barrett's esophagus is related to the high frequency of its association with degeneration into adenocarcinoma with a prevalence varying from 10% to 45% [1, 2]. The true risk is estimated at 30–40 times higher than within the general population [3]. As the diagnosis is frequently made in an advanced stage, the prognosis of a Barrett adenocarcinoma is reported to be poor [4]. Early diagnosis of such adenocarcinomas certainly could improve significantly the prognosis, and this opens the debate concerning surveillance programs in patients with Barrett's metaplasia. We have been analyzing our experience with Barrett's adenocarcinomas focusing on the results of surgical treatment and trying to establish a correlation between histomorophological findings of Barrett's metaplasia and risk of degeneration.

Clinical Results

From 1975 until 1991, 331 adenocarcinomas of the esophagus and gastroesophageal junction have been treated. Amongst them, 66 (20%) were Barrett's adenocarcinomas and the mean age was 62.8 years. Thirty-two patients (48.5%) had a history positive for reflux, 33 (58%) for alcohol, and 34 (51.5%) for tabacco. The mean length of the metaplastic zone was 7.37 cm for the whole

[1] Departments of General Thoracic Surgery and [2] Histopathology, University Hospitals, K.U.
U.Z. Gasthuisberg, Herestraat 49, 3000 Leuven, Belgium

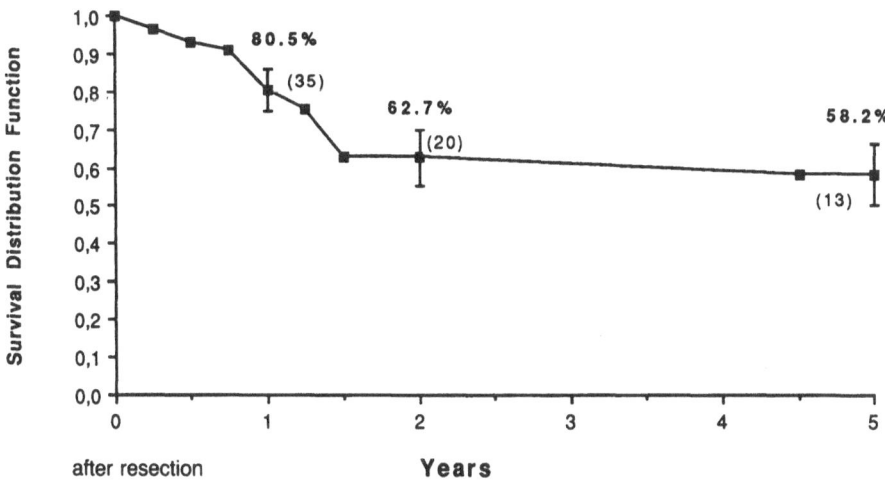

Fig. 1. Overall 5-year survival. *Solid box* represents all stadia ($n = 63$)

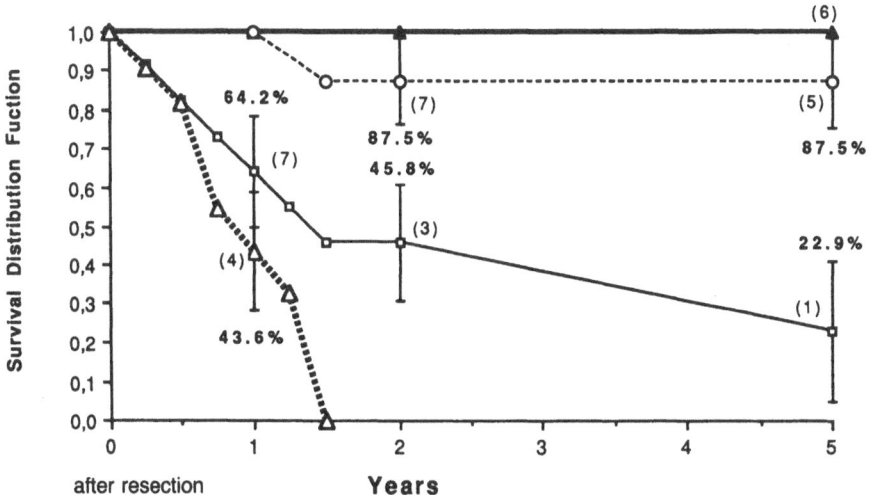

Fig. 2. Five-year survival according to TNM staging. *Solid triangle*, stage I ($n = 24$); *open circle*, stage II ($n = 13$); *open box*, stage III ($n = 14$); *open triangle*, stage IV ($n = 12$)

group. Operability was 98.5% (65/66) while resectability was 95.5% (63/66). Postoperative and hospital mortality was zero.

The pathologic staging was as follows: stage I, 38.3%; stage II, 20.6%; stage III, 22.2%; and stage IV, 19%.

The overall survival was 80.5% at 1 year, 62.7% at 2 years, and 58.2% at 5 years (Fig. 1). According to the pTNM staging, the 5-year survivals rates were: 100% for stage I, 87.5% for stage II, 22.2% for stage III, and no survival in stage IV (Fig. 2). Five year survival in lymph node-negative patients was 85.3%,

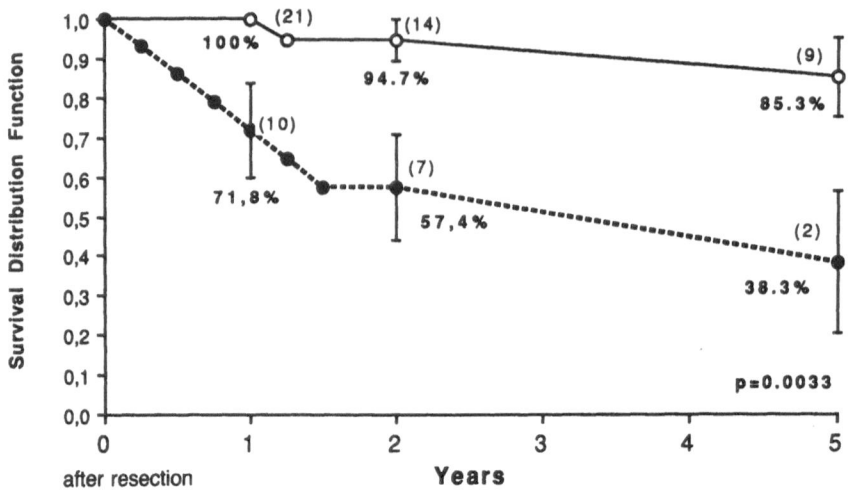

Fig. 3. Five-year survival according to lymph node status. *Open circle*, TXN0M0 ($n = 34$); *closed circle*, TXN1M0 ($n = 17$)

Table 1. Relationship between medical history and lymph node status

51.5%	Under medical screening before diagnosis of cancer	73.5%	LN	—
48.5%	Diagnosis of cancer at first medical contact	22%	LN	—

LN, lymph node

significantly better than lymph node positives patients (38.8%, $P = 0.0033$) (Fig. 3).

Thirty-four patients (51.5%) were under medical screening for a related or unrelated upper G.I. condition before diagnosis. Out of them, only nine (26.5%) patients had positive lymph nodes. Thirty-two had their diagnosis established at the occasion of their first medical contact. Here, the number of positive lymph nodes was as high as 78% (Table 1).

Morphological Findings

As a substantial number of patients were under medical screening before diagnosis of cancer, 19 patients were documented has having a biopsy-proven history of Barrett's metaplasia before carcinoma occurred. The mean time between diagnosis of metaplasia and degeneration was 3.8 years (89% > 1 year). Length of metaplasia remained unchanged in all patients. Barrett's ulcer was present from the beginning in 14 patients, and at the time of resection 12 patients had an ulcer (Table 2). Only three patients had never had an ulcer. The tumor was located in the ulcer zone in nine patients. Intestinal metaplasia was present in 18 patients either as a mosaic pattern together with junctional and fundic metaplasia or as a rather well-defined zonation separating the three different types of

Table 2. Morphologic findings in barrett's carcinoma. Macroscopic characteristics at the time of resection $n = 18$

		Tumor
Ulcer	9 ⎫ 12	9/12
Ulcer + elevated lesion	3 ⎭	
Elevated lesion	2	2/2
Irregular mucosa	4	4/4

Table 3. Morphologic findings in barrett's carcinoma. Histologic characteristics and type of metaplasia $n = 18$

Surface epithelium		
Mosaic:	9	
Zonation:	9	
	Intestinal	2
	Intestinal-junctional	6
	Intestinal-indeterminate	1
Glandular epithelium		
Mosaic:	6	
Zonation:	12	
	Intestinal	5
	Intestinal-junctional	5
	Intestinal-junctional-fundic	1
	Intestinal-indeterminate	1
Tumor always in zone of intestinal metaplasia		

Table 4. Morphologic findings in barrett's carcinoma. Histologic characteristics, and incidence of dysplasia and its relation to type of metaplasia $n = 18$

Dysplasia: 16		
Severe	5 ⎫	14 Patients
Low-grade + severe	9 ⎭	
Low-grade	2	
No dysplasia	2	
Dysplasia—type metaplasia		
Intestinal	11	
Mosaic	3	
Indeterminate	2	

metaplasia (Table 3). The adenocarcinoma in all 18 patients was located in an intestinal metaplastic tissue (5 mosaic, 13 zonation).

Ulcers were found in intestinal metaplastic tissue in 11 patients. Dysplasia was present in the resection specimens of 16 patients. Severe dysplasia, which today has to be considered as carcinoma in situ showing unequivocal neoplastic characteristics, was seen in 14 patients (Table 4).

Only in one patient was an evolution form low grade to carcinoma in situ noticed. In another patient, the diagnosis of carcinoma in situ was made but he refused surgery for 5 years. At the time of operation, his condition remained unchanged.

As 17 of 19 patients in the group with documented history of Barrett's metaplasia were under very close endoscopic monitoring, early diagnosis was possible in 14 (82%), the other three, however, all had stage III carcinoma at the time of operation.

Discussion

The debate whether there is an increased risk of developing adenocarcinoma in Barrett's metaplasia remains open: As in many other reports, our study confirms a high prevalence rate of 20%. This prevalence may even be higher as advanced carcinomas in the distal esophagus or gastroesophageal junction, or in carcinoma arising in zones of metaplasia of less than 3 cm in length, progress to carcinoma of the gastric cardia or a non-Barrett adenocarcinoma of the distal esophagus in which the columnar lined segment has been overgrown by the tumor.

The discussion about the true incidence of adenocarcinoma in Barrett's esophagus is even more difficult as indeed many patients with Barrett's metaplasia, as much as 50% in our series, are asymptomatic for reflux and are non-smokers and non-drinkers. This means that there are probably many people having Barrett's metaplasia who will never be diagnosed as they never come to see a doctor and therefore never will be candidates for surveillance programs.

The fact that as much as half of our patients with Barrett's adenocarcinoma were non-smokers and non-drinkers is perhaps partially explaining the high operability rate (98.5%) and why there was no hospital mortality in this series together, of course, with the fact that over the years enormous progress has been made in controlling peri- and postoperative mortality and morbidity. These data are of paramount importance in determining whether or not to perform esophagectomy in cases of carcinoma in situ.

In this series, 51.5% of the patients were under medical screening before the diagnosis of carcinoma was made. In those patients, 73% had no lymph node invasion and overall as much as 58.9% of the patients were in the early stages (I and II) which is much higher than for other esophageal carcinomas where usually no more than one-third of the patients will have a early stage. This, of course, explains the high 58.2% 5-year survival rate proving that Barrett's adenocarcinoma has no worse prognosis than esophageal carcinoma, provided a early diagnosis can be made [5, 6]. As expected, the most important survival related prognostic factor is lymph node involvement with 38.8% 5-year survival for lymph node positive versus 85.3% for lymph node negative patients. Therefore, early detection is of paramount importance as this will result in clearly better chances for cure.

The group of 19 patients in which there was a biopsy-proven history of Barrett's metaplasia offers a unique opportunity to evaluate retrospectively which morphologic characteristics are of importance in determining the risk of degeneration and therefore perhaps allowing earlier diagnosis.

From the macroscopic point of view, it seems that a more extensive length (mean 7.37 cm) is a more predisposing factor and all but three patients had an ulcer within the zone of metaplasia either preoperatively or at the time of resection. Tumor was found in the majority of the ulcers but not exclusively, and the ulcers were located in almost every patient (11/12 patients) in a zone of intestinal metaplasia.

From the microscopic point of view, intestinal metaplasia is invariably present in all patients. It's presentation can be as a zonation pattern or as a mosaic pattern and these patterns are noticed in both the surface epithelium and glandular epithelium as well. Tumor, however, was mainly found in the zonation pattern (13 patients) rather than in the mosaic pattern (5 patients) but always tumor was found in zones of intestinal metaplasia.

Thus, it seems that patients with extensive Barrett's metaplasia presenting themselves with an ulcer in a zone of intestinal metaplasia are to be considered as a high risk group for degeneration, and here the debate is open as to the treatment of choice when there is no evidence of malignancy or dysplasia on the biopsy specimens: medical treatment, antireflux procedure, or even resection.

Dysplasia was seen in 16 patients again mostly located in a zone of intestinal metaplasia (14 patients). Out of those 16 patients, 14 had high grade dysplasia (carcinoma in situ) showing unequivocal neoplastic characteristics. Only in one patient was an evolution from low grade dysplasia to carcinoma in situ noticed.

The significance of high grade dysplasia still remains controversial as its natural history is not well known. As in other reports and also in our experience, there were patients who did not show any change of high-grade dysplasia over a period as long as 5 year [2]. For this reason, some authors advocate a conservative attitude with close surveillance using endoscopy and biopsy. Stating that the risks of such an approach are less than the risk of postresection surgical mortality [7].

However, there are reports of some series in which patients with only high grade dysplasia on the preoperative biopsies were diagnosed histologically as having microinvasion or invasive carcinoma in up to 50% [2] consequently exposing those patients to the risk of metastasis.

Certainly, today close echoendoscopic and endoscopic surveillance will enable early diagnosis of degeneration. This was also the case in our group of 17 patients who were under very close endoscopic monitoring, allowing early diagnosis in 82%. However, in the remaining three patients, the final staging showed are advanced stage III carcinomas.

Therefore we believe that patients with high grade dysplasia in Barrett's metaplasia should undergo esophageal resection and reconstruction whenever possible for the following reasons: (1) the risk of degeneration in high grade dysplasia is distinctly higher than in the general population, (2) close endoscopic and echoendoscopic monitoring even in the hands of the most experienced groups still does not guarantee successful early diagnosis in all patients, and (3) esophageal resection can be done safely with a zero mortality in our series.

References

1. Hameeteman W, Tytgat GNJ, Houthoff HJ, van den Tweel JG (1988) Barrett's esophagus: Development of dysplasia and adenocarcinoma. Gastroenterology 96:1249–1256
2. Reid BJ, Weinstein WM, Lewin KJ, Haggitt RC, Van Deventer G, Den Besten L, Rubin CE (1988) Endoscopic biopsy can detect high-grade dysplasia or early adenocarcinoma

in Barrett's esophagus without grossly recognizable neoplastic lesion. Gastroenterology 94:81–90

3. Spechler SJ, Goyal RK (1986) Barrett's esophagus. New Engl J Med 315:361–371
4. Sanfey H, Hamilton SR, Smith RRL, Cameron JL (1985) Carcinoma arising in Barrett's esophagus. Surg Gynecol Obstet 161:570–574
5. Lerut T, De Leyn P, Coosemans W, Van Raemdonck D, Scheys I, Lesaffre E (1992) Surgical strategies in esophageal carcinoma with emphasis on radical lymphadenectomy. Ann Surg 216:583–590
6. de Meester TR, Attwood SA, Smyrk TC, Therkildsen DH, Hinder RA (1990) Surgical therapy in Barrett's esophagus. Ann Surg 212:528–542
7. De Baecque C, Potet F, Molas G, Flejou JF, Barbier P, Martignon C (1990) Superficial adenocarcinoma of the oesophagus arising in Barrett's mucosa with dyplasia: A clinico-pathological study of 12 patients. Histopathology 16:213–220

An Alkaline Stomach Is Common to Barrett's Esophagus and Gastric Carcinoma

Akihiro Yasui[1], Sebastian F. Hoeft[2], Hubert J. Stein[2],
Tom R. DeMeester[2], Ross M. Bremner[2], and Yuji Nimura[1]

Introduction

The interdigestive pH environment of the stomach fluctuates from 1 to 2. A rise in pH to above 3 occurs either from decreased acid secretion, as in achlorhydria, or iatrogenic acid reduction (anti-secretory drugs: H_2-blockers, proton pump inhibitors), neutralization of acid from swallowed food, or reflux of alkaline pancreatic and biliary secretions from the duodenum.

Reflux of duodenal juice has been implicated in the pathogenesis of gastric cancer and in the development of complications of Barrett's esophagus, i.e., stricture, giant ulcer, and dysplasia [1].

In the present study, we investigated the pattern of alkalinity in stomach and esophagus as measured by 24-h pH-monitoring, in patients with early gastric carcinoma and patients with complications of Barrett's esophagus.

Subjects and Methods

Forty-two patients with Barrett's esophagus confirmed by histologic documentation of at least 3-cm columnar epithelium above the gastroesophageal junction were studied. These patients were divided on the basis of whether complications, i.e., stricture, ulceration, or dysplasia were present. Of the 42 patients complications were present in 24: stricture ($n = 15$), ulcer ($n = 3$), and dysplasia ($n = 13$). Eighteen patients were free of complications.

Seventeen patients with early gastric carcinoma confined to the submucosal layer were studied. None were achlorhydric.

[1] First Department of Surgery, Nagoya University School of Medicine, 65 Tsurumai-cho, Showa-ku, Nagoya, Aichi, 466 Japan
[2] University of Southern California, School of Medicine, Department of Surgery, 1510 San Pablo Street, Suite 514, Los Angeles, CA 90033-4612, USA

A control group consisted of 60 normal volunteers, who were asymptomatic and had a normal barium swallow to exclude the presence of unrecognized esophageal disease.

All patients underwent esophageal manometry using a water-perfused system and a stationary pull-through technique. The lower esophageal sphincter was defined as defective when the resting pressure was below 7 mmHg, the overall length was less than 2.0 cm, or when the abdominal length was less than 1.0 cm. Twenty-four-h esophageal pH monitoring was performed with a glass electrode (Ingold Electronics) placed 5 cm above the manometrically determined lower esophageal sphincter. Analysis of the data was performed with commercially available software (EsopHogram, Gastrosoft, Irving, Tex.).

Simultaneous 24-h gastric pH monitoring was performed with a glass electrode positioned 5 cm below the lower border of the lower esophageal sphincter. The data were stored on Synectics (Stockholm, Sweden) digitrappers. Analysis of the tracings was performed with Gastrosoft software (Irving, Tex.) according to a previously published method [1]. Briefly, the gastric pH recording was analyzed according to the time the pH spent at a specific pH interval and the number of times the pH moved from a lower into a higher pH interval. A discriminant analysis of the data which emphasized a repetitive rise rather than a continuous rise in gastric pH (as in achlorhydria) separated normal subjects from patients with clinical symptoms and signs of duodenogastric reflux [1].

Statistical analysis of the difference between groups was performed using a commercially available software package, SAS 6.04 (SAS Institute, Cary, N.C.).

Results

A defective lower esophageal sphincter was not seen in normal subjects or patients with superficial gastric cancer, whereas 76% of patients with Barrett's esophagus without complications and 92% of those with complications had a mechanically defective sphincter. Results from the gastric pH-recording are

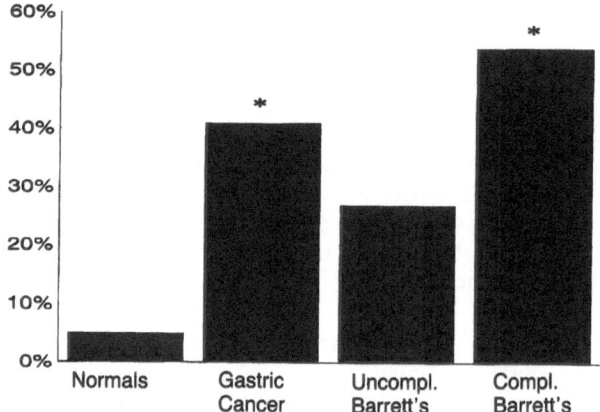

Fig. 1. Prevalence of positive duodenogastric reflux (*DGR*) score. *$P < 0.05$ normals and uncomplicated Barrett's vs gastric cancer and complicated Barrett's

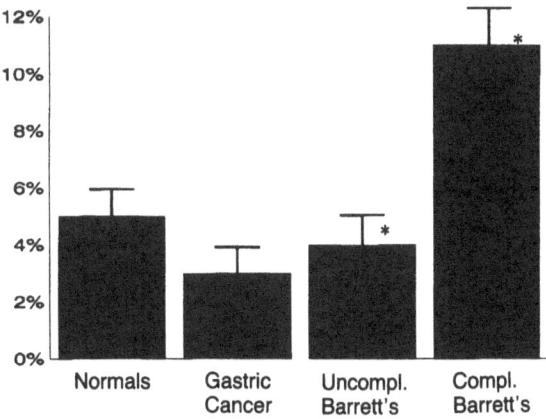

Fig. 2. Mean exposure time to pH > 7 (as percentage of total time). *$P < 0.05$ uncomplicated Barrett's vs complicated Barrett's (mean ± SEM)

summarized in Fig. 1. The prevalence of pathologic duodenogastric reflux was significantly higher in patients with early gastric carcinoma ($P < 0.001$) than in normal volunteers. Patients with Barrett's esophagus who had complications, i.e., stricture, ulcer, or dysplasia, showed a higher prevalence of pathologic duodenogastric reflux than Barrett's patients without complication ($P < 0.05$).

Results from the esophageal pH-recording are summarized in Fig. 2. There was a marked increase in alkaline esophageal exposure in patients with complications of Barrett's esophagus compared to those with uncomplicated Barrett's, gastric cancer, and normals ($P < 0.05$). Exposure to a pH < 4 was highest in the complicated Barrett's group (29% ± 6%, mean ± SEM).

Discussion

Reflux of alkaline duodenal contents has been implicated in the development of gastric intestinalization and Barrett's esophagus [2, 3]. The damaging component appears to be not only the elevated alkaline pH, but also the composition of the refluxed juice. Bile acids have been shown experimentally to stimulate cell proliferation in ileal and colonic mucosa, and have been considered as possible endogenous cocarcinogens [4, 5]. The observed effect of duodenogastric reflux on antral mucosa with foveolar hyperplasia supports these observations [6]. Animal studies with experimental duodenoesophageal reflux show that, besides the bilious content, the enzymatic component of pancreatic secretions plays an important role, possibly together with bacterial overgrowth caused by reduced acidity and thus increased bacterial degradation of procarcinogens from the food.

The alkaline pH of duodenal juice, although not in itself potentially damaging to the mucosa, is a suitable tool for detecting duodenogastric reflux [7]. When using a discriminate analysis program previously evaluated in our institution [1], normal volunteers could be distinguished from patients with pathologic duodenogastric reflux. The basis of the differential analysis emphasizes repetitive alkalinization episodes of reflux rather than a continuous rise in pH as an indicator of duodenogastric reflux. In a clinical study this analysis was superior to radionuclide scanning (DISIDA) [8].

Assessment of alkaline reflux into the lower esophagus can be problematic for several reasons. First of all, the median pH in the esophagus is close to neutral, which makes it difficult to assess the significance of pH rises in the alkaline range. This requires the use of glass electrodes, which are more stable especially in the alkaline range than antimony probes. The latter show a drift to higher pH and consequently do not provide a reliable pH tracing in the alkaline range. Second, swallowed saliva can influence the pH in the lower esophagus, and the passage of duodenal juice through the acid environment of the stomach can acidify the refluxate to pH values in the mid- to low-acid range. Consequently, the exposure time of the lower esophagus to a pH > 7 could be the tip of the iceberg, and the actual exposure to duodenal contents might be much larger. Our data from the gastric pH-recording in gastric cancer patients suggest that a similar exposure to duodenal juice might be involved. In these patients, the presence of a mechanically normal lower esophageal sphincter prevents the duodenal juice from reaching the esophagus. Partial gastrectomy, which increases the chance of enterogastric reflux, has been considered as a risk factor for gastric cancer [9]. Bechi et al. demonstrated cell kinetic abnormalities in patients with duodenogastric reflux that have been shown to be oncogenic [6].

Our results suggest that alkaline exposure in the stomach and esophagus might promote the development of dysplastic mucosa and malignant transformation.

References

1. Fuchs KH, DeMeester TR, Hinder RA, Stein HJ, Barlow AP, Gupta N (1991) Computerized identification of pathologic reflux using 24-h gastric pH monitoring. Ann Surg 213:13–20
2. Attwood SEA, DeMeester TR, Bremner CG, Barlow AP, Hinder RA (1991) Alkaline gastroesophageal reflux: Implications in the development of complications in Barrett's esophagus. Surgery 106:563–566
3. Williamson RCN, Bauer FLR, Ross JS, et al (1978) Contributions of bile and pancreatic juice to cell proliferation in ileal mucosa. Surgery 83:570–576
4. Deschner EE (1988) Cell proliferation and colonic neoplasia. Scand J Gastroenterol 23 [Suppl 151]:94–97
5. Williamson RCN, Rainey JB (1984) The relationship between intestinal hyperplasia and carcinogenesis. Scand J Gastroenterol 19 [Suppl 104]:57–76
6. Bechi P, Balzi M, Becciolini A, Amorosi A, Scubla E, et al (1991) Gastric cell proliferation and bile reflux after partial gastrectomy. Am J Gastroent 86(10):1424–1432
7. Pellegrini CA, DeMeester TR, Wernly JA, Johnson LF, Skinner DB (1978) Alkaline gastroesophageal reflux. Am J Surg 135:177–184
8. Stein HJ, Hinder RA, DeMeester TR, Lloyd BA, Fuchs KH, Attwood SEA, Gupta NC (1990) Clinical use of 24-h gastric pH monitoring vs o-diisopropyl iminodiacetic acid (DISIDA) scanning in the diagnosis of pathologic duodenogastric reflux. Arch Surg 125:966–971
9. Domellof L, Janunger KG (1977) The risk for gastric carcinoma after partial gastrectomy. Am J Surg 134:581–584

A Histopathological Study of Barrett's Esophagus with Special Reference to the Specialized Columnar Epithelium

SHIN-ICHI NAKAMURA[1]*, ISAMU KINO[2], TOMIO ARAI[2], and KATUNORI AOKI[3]

Introduction

Barrett's esophagus is defined as a lesion in which the squamous epithelium of the lower esophagus is replaced extensively by columnar epithelium [1–3]. Three different kinds of columnar mucosa are observed in Barrett's esophagus: Atrophic gastric fundic mucosa, junctional mucosa similar to the gastric cardia, and an intestinal type bearing "specialized columnar epithelium" (SCE) [4, 5].

We studied the characteristics of the columnar epithelium of Barrett's esophagus, and compared them with that of intestinal metaplasia of the stomach. Our findings indicate that the columnar epithelium of Barrett's esophagus closely resembles that of intestinal metaplasia of the stomach morphologically, histochemically, and immunohistochemically. Tall columnar mucous epithelium, regarded as SCE in Barrett's esophagus, is also found in gastric intestinal metaplasia.

Based upon these and other data [6] we feel that the term "specialized columnar epithelium" is vague, unhelpful, and misleading.

Subjects and Methods

Two patients, a 60-year-old male and a 69-year-old female had undergone the resection of the esophagus because of adenocarcinoma of the lower esophagus at Hamamatsu University Hospital.

[1] Department of Pathology, Hamamatsu University Hospital, [2] First Department of Pathology, Hamamatsu University School of Medicine and [3] Emergency Department, Hamamatsu University Hospital, 3600 Handa-cho, Hamamatsu, 431-31 Japan
* Current address: Department of Pathology, St Mark's Hospital, City Road, London EC1V 2PS, UK

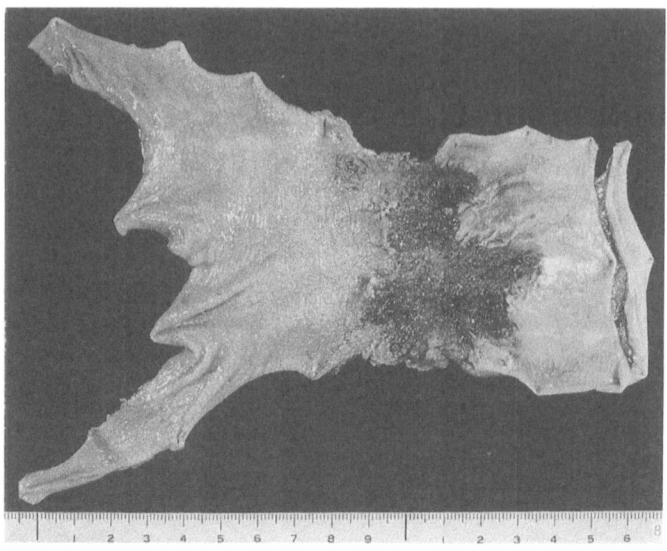

Fig. 1. Macroscopic finding of resected esophagus (case 2)

Histologic sections of several cases of surgically resected stomach for gastric cancer at the same hospital, were used for the comparison of gastric intestinal metaplasia and the epithelium of Barrett's esophagus.

Histopathology: Resected surgical specimens were routinely examined using paraffin-embedded, hematoxylin and eosin (H&E) stained sections to make the pathological diagnosis. Mucosa surrounding the adenocarcinoma was examined and classified according to the histological features as follows: stratified squamous, cardiac, fundic, and intestinal with SCE.

Several representative sections were examined for epithelial mucin content, using the high iron-diamine and alcian blue (pH 2.5) (HID-alcian blue) to identify and distinguish sulpho- and sialo-acid mucins [7]. Specific gastric antral type (labile type III) mucin was identified using the paradoxical concanavalin A method [8]. Argyrophil endocrine cells were identified using the Grimelius stain. Carcinoembryonic antigen (CEA) was identified immunohistochemically using a polyclonal antiserum (DAKO Japan, Kyoto).

Results

Case study: The gross specimens of both patients revealed multiple elevated lesions in the lower esophagus: case 1 measuring $35 \times 45\,\mathrm{mm}$ and case 2 $40 \times 55\,\mathrm{mm}$. Well differentiated adenocarcinoma infiltrated the submucosa of the esophagus associated with adjacent metaplastic columnar epithelium (case 1). In case 2, mucinous adenocarcinoma invaded the muscularis propria with lymph node metastasis; and the three types of metaplastic mucosa, predominantly the intestinal type, covered the lower esophagus surrounding the adenocarcinoma (Fig. 1).

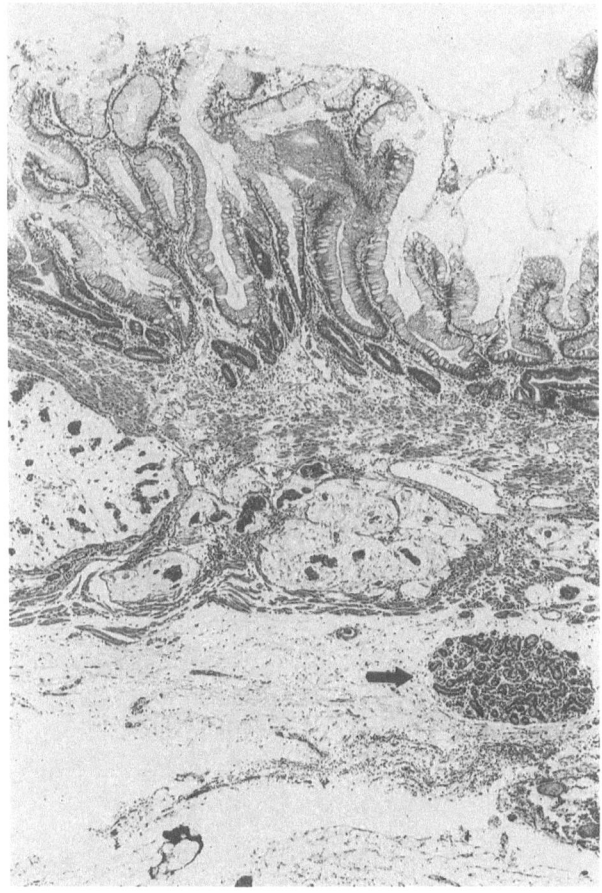

Fig. 2. Barrett's esophagus lined by columnar epithelium with villous structure. Mucinous carcinoma invading the muscularis mucosae. An island of esophageal gland in the submucosa (*arrow*). (H&E, ×10)

Histopathology: Characteristic of these cases of Barrett's esophagus was the tall columnar epithelium with a villous architecture (Fig. 2). This epithelium was composed of three cell types: absorptive cells, interspersed goblet cells, and tall columnar mucous cells (Fig. 3). In intestinal metaplasia of the stomach, the same three types of cells were usually observed. Mucin staining with HID-alcian blue revealed that both the tall columnar mucous cells and goblet cells in Barrett's epithelium contained both sialomucin and sulphomucin (Fig. 4). Pyloric type glands found in Barrett's esophagus showed mucin staining positively with paradoxical concanavalin A. Argyrophil endocrine cells were present at the lower part of the glands of both Barrett's mucosa and gastric intestinal metaplasia. CEA expression was identified at the apical surface of the columnar cells of both epithelia. A summary of the comparison of Barrett's epithelium and gastric intestinal metaplasia is shown in Table 1.

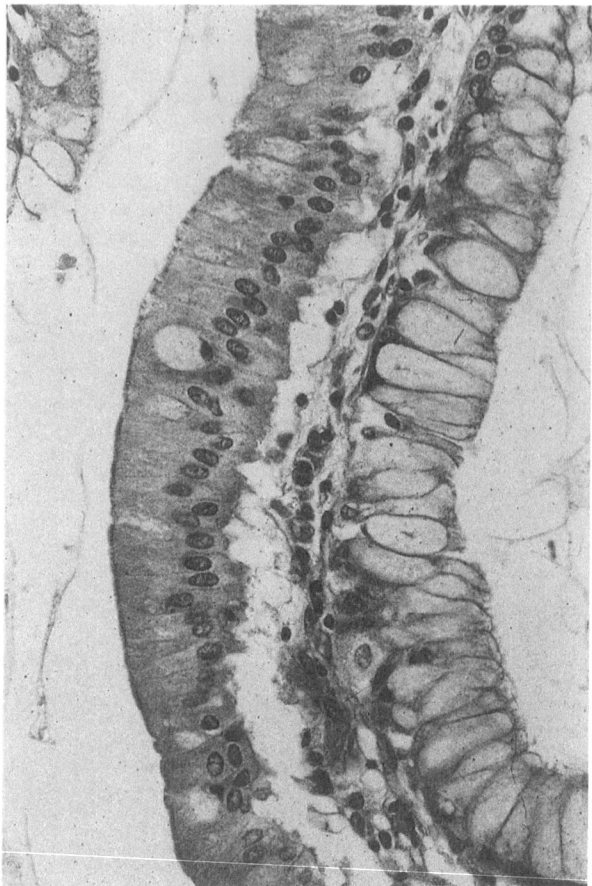

Fig. 3. Three types of cells in the columnar epithelium. Absorptive cells with apical brush border and interspersed goblet cells on the left side of the lamina propria. On the right, tall columnar mucous cells, SCE, with abundant clear cytoplasm and basally located nucleus. (H&E, ×100)

Discussion

Trier first described the columnar cells which had microvilli and cytoplasmic secretory granules among the goblet and absorptive cells in Barrett's esophagus; and considered them distinct from normal fundic, cardiac, or intestinal epithelia, morphologically and physiologically. He named it the principal cell [4]. Berenson et al. [9] supported Trier's findings and the epithelium containing the principal cell was regarded as SCE. Levine et al. [10] found that SCE showed the features of a transitional form between mucous and absorptive cells. Ultrastructural studies have also revealed that similar transitional forms between absorptive and foveolar cell types among the epithelium of gastric intestinal metaplasia [11, 12].

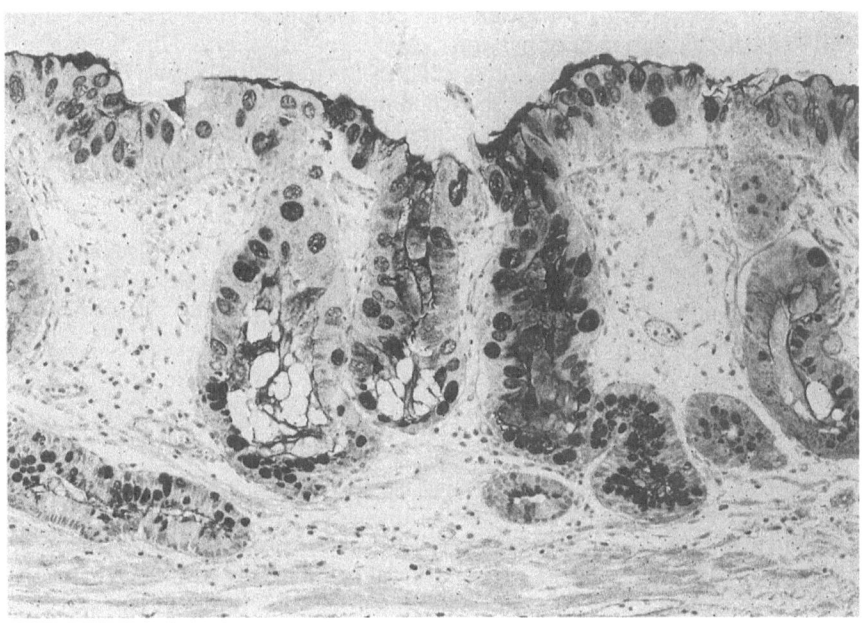

Fig. 4. Both sulphomucin and sialomucin detected in the Barrett's epithelium. (HID-alcian blue stain, ×33)

Table 1. Comparison of Barrett's epithelium with intestinal metaplasia of the stomach

Histopathology	Barrett's epithelium	Intestinal metaplasia
Goblet cell	+	+
Absorptive cell	+	+
SCE	+	+
Paneth cell	−	+
Type III mucin[a]	+	+
Sialomucin	+	+
Sulphomucin	+	+
Argyrophil granules	+	+
CEA	+	+

[a] Type III mucin was stained by paradoxical concanavalin A method. *SCE*, specialized columnar epithelium. *CEA*, carcinoembryonic antigen

Our findings indicate that this columnar epithelium closely resembles the incomplete type of intestinal metaplasia of the stomach morphologically, histochemically, and immunohistochemically [13], and that SCE was also one of the components of gastric intestinal metaplasia.

It is obvious that Barrett's mucosa arises in morbid processes and that the columnar epithelium differs from normal. SCE might be considered to be specialized or distinct morphologically and physiologically compared with normal epithelia of the gastrointestinal tract, but is not specialized in the sense of terminal differentiation. It is not specific to Barrett's esophagus, but indistinguishable cells are seen in gastric intestinal metaplasia.

The term "specialized columnar epithelium" is not helpful and it may be better to avoid its use to prevent misunderstanding and confusion in the study of pathogenesis of Barrett's esophagus.

Acknowledgments. We are grateful to Dr. Ian W. Thompson, Department of Pathology, St Mark's Hospital, for instructive suggestions. We also thank Mr. Takaharu Kamo and Hisayoshi Igarashi for histologic technical assistance and Mr. Tuneji Noguchi for photography.

References

1. Barrett NR (1950) Chronic peptic ulcer of the oesophagus and "oesophagitis'. Br J Surg 38:175–182
2. Barrett NR (1957) The lower esophagus lined by columnar epithelium. Surgery 41:881–894
3. Burgess JN, Payne WS, Andersen HA, Weiland LH, Carlson HC (1971) Barrett's esophagus. The columnar-epithelial-lined lower esophagus. Mayo Clin Proc 46:728–734
4. Trier JS (1970) Morphology of the epithelium of the distal esophagus in patients with midesophageal peptic strictures. Gastroenterology 58:444–461
5. Paull A, Trier JS, Dalton D, Camp RC, Loeb P, Goyal RK (1976) The histologic spectrum of Barrett's esophagus. N Engl J Med 295:476–480
6. Mangla JC (1981) Barrett's esophagus: An old entity rediscovered. J Clin Gastroenterol 3:347–356
7. Filipe MI, Bogomoletz W, Dawson P, Fabiani B, Potet F (1983) Intestinal metaplasia subtypes in the assessment of gastric cancer risk. A multicentric prospective study. Gut 24:A974–A975
8. Katsuyama T, Spicer SS (1978) Histochemical differentiation of complex carbohydrates with variants of the concanavalin A-horse radish peroxidase method. J Histochem Cytochem 26:233–250
9. Berenson MM, Herbst JJ, Freston JW (1974) Enzyme and ultrastructural characteristics of esophageal columnar epithelium. Dig Dis Sci 19:895–907
10. Levine DS, Rubin CE, Reid BJ, Haggitt RC (1989) Specialized metaplastic columnar epithelium in Barrett's esophagus. A comparative transmission electron microscopic study. Lab Invest 60:418–432
11. Ming SC, Goldman H, Freiman DG (1967) Intestinal metaplasia and histogenesis of carcinoma in human stomach. Light and electron microscopic study. Cancer 20:1418–1429
12. Iida F, Murata F, Nagata T (1978) Histochemical studies of mucosubstances in metaplastic epithelium of the stomach, with special reference to the development of intestinal metaplasia. Histochemistry 56:229–237
13. Matsukura N, Suzuki K, Kawachi T, Aoyagi M, Sugimura T, Kitaoka H, Numajiri H, Shirota A, Itabashi M, Hirota T (1980) Distribution of marker enzymes and mucin in intestinal metaplasia in human stomach and relation of complete and incomplete types of intestinal metaplasia to minute gastric carcinomas. JNCI 65:231–240

Motility Disorders (Achalasia)

Clinical Approach to Achalasia of the Esophagus from the Viewpoint of Gastrointestinal Hormone

Akira Tangoku, Takuo Murakami, Hiroto Hayashi, Hiroyuki Uchisako, Masahiro Nishikawa, Hiroaki Ozasa, Hiroshi Kusanagi, Masashi Tsurumi, and Takashi Suzuki[1]

Summary. Twenty-seven patients with achalasia of the esophagus were treated at the Department of Surgery II, Yamaguchi University Hospital.

Lower esophageal sphincter pressure (LESP) was measured and the response to exogenous gastrointestinal hormones were examined in patients with achalasia and in controls. Gastrin increased the LESP and secretin decreased the LESP in both achalasia patients and in controls. Achalasia patients showed hypersensitivity to gastrin induced LESP and hypersensitivity to secretin reduced LESP compared to controls. Twenty-four of 27 patients underwent the modified Jekler-Lhotka's operation which consist myectomy and antireflux fundoplication. Gastroscintigraphy showed delayed retention of food in the esophagus before surgery and smooth emptying into the stomach after surgery. Long-term efficacy of this procedure was 91.7%. Specimens from myectomized LES were examined to study the pathophysiology of achalasia. The amount of vasoactive intestinal polypeptide (VIP) in the specimen was measured by radioimmunoassay and the specimen was also examined immunohistochemically. The specimens from achalasia patients have less radioimmunoreactive VIP, fewer VIP cells, and fibers were observed in Auerbach's plexus in the LES. Decreased VIP in the LES may cause incomplete relaxation of achalasia esophagus.

Introduction

Esophageal achalasia is a disorder of the lower esophageal sphincter (LES). A lot of studies have been done to elucidate the mechanism of this disease, but the etiology of esophageal achalasia is still unclear. The diagnosis for this disease is usually made based on radiologic features, endoscopy, and manometry; how-

[1] Department of Surgery II, Yamaguchi University School of Medicine, 1144 Kogushi, Ube, Yamaguchi, 755 Japan

ever, correct diagnosis is sometimes hard. Drug therapy, dilation, and surgical procedures are performed for this disease, however, the best treatment is still controversial. In this paper, we present our own diagnostic method with gastrointestinal hormones and surgical treatment. Further, we will discuss our specific study with myectomized specimens to study pathophysiology of achalasia of the esophagus.

Patients and Methods

Between 1971 and 1992, 27 patients with achalasia of the esophagus were treated at the Department of Surgery II, Yamaguchi University Hospital. Preoperative manometric study was made in recent cases according to the following method.

Measurement of Intraluminal Pressure of the Esophagus

Lower esophageal sphincter pressure (LESP) was measured by manometry. The side-opened three-lumen polyvinyl tube (Argile Ltd.), 1.3 mm in diameter, with each lumen opening 5 cm apart at 120° to each other, was connected to the transducer by a three-way stopcock. Each stopcock was connected to a short polyvinyl tube, in which 30 ml/h of distilled water was constantly infused. Intraluminal pressure was recorded by a multichannel polygraph (RM-6000, Nihon Koden, Japan), which was connected to the transducer.

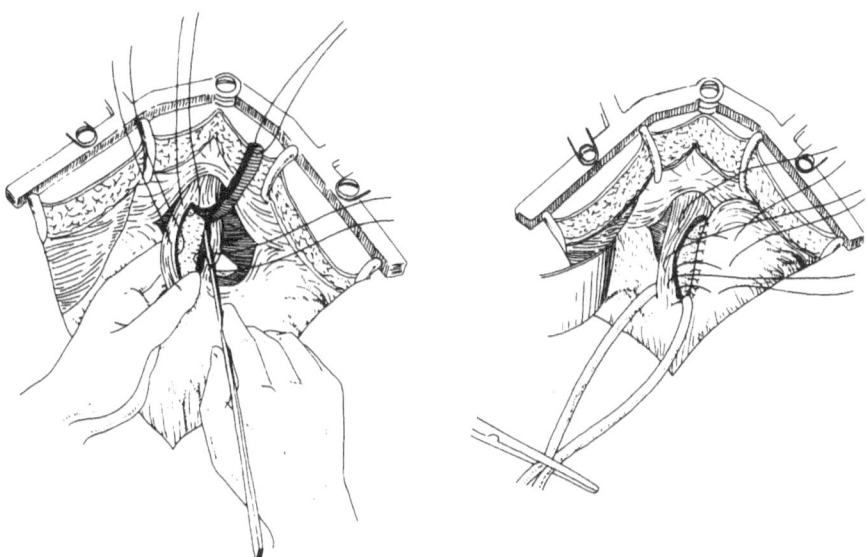

Fig. 1. Modified Jekler-Lhotka's method. Through a laparotomy, wide (1–1.5 cm) and long (6–8 cm) myectomy in the lower esophagus and the bulging esophageal mucosa is covered by anterior wall of the gastric fundus

Table 1. Summary of patient data

Case no.	Age	Sex	Period	Type	Grade	Operation (myectomy length)	Result
1.	15	F	1 year 2 months	Sp	II	J-L (6 cm)	Good
2.	76	M	10 years	Sp	II	J-L (10 cm)	Good
3.	29	M	20 years	S	III	J-L (6 cm) relapsed after 14 months	Poor
4.	15	M	1 year 7 months	Sp	II	J-L (7.5 cm)	Good
5.	38	F	2 years	F	II	J-L (8.2 cm)	Good
6.	63	M	2 years	Sp	II	J-L (10 cm) post gastrectomy	Unknown
7.	52	M	20 years	S	III	J-L (5.2 cm)	Good
8.	22	F	1 year	Sp	II	J-L (7 cm)	Good
9.	18	F	3 years	Sp	II	J-L (8.6 cm)	Good
10.	26	M	1 year	Sp	II	J-L (8.2 cm)	Good
11.	42	M	2 years	Sp	II	J-L (6.8 cm) + part. gastrectomy	Good
12.	12	F	6 years	Sp	II	J-L (6.8 cm)	Good
13.	53	F	10 years	F	II	J-L (6.6 cm)	Good
14.	34	M	1 year	Sp	II	J-L (11.2 cm)	Good
15.	34	M	4 years	Sp	II	J-L (9.6 cm)	Good
16.	16	M	2 years	Sp	III	J-L (7 cm)	Good
17.	51	M	3 years	Sp	II	J-L (6 cm) + part. gastrectomy	Good
18.	33	F	2 years	Sp	II	J-L (6 cm)	Good
19.	16	M	2 years	Sp	II	J-L (7 cm)	Good
20.	16	F	2 years	F	III	J-L (8.7 cm)	Good
21.	71	F	6 years	Sp	III	J-L (7 cm)	Good
22.	55	F	2 years	Sp	III	J-L (7 cm)	Good
23.	50	F	10 years	Sp	II	J-L (7.5 cm)	Good
24.	42	F	2 years	Sp	II	J-L (7 cm)	Good

S, Sigmoid type; *Sp*, spindle type; *F*, flask type; *J-L*, Jekler-Lhotka procedure

Resting LESP was measured by the withdrawal method. After 5 µg/kg tetragastrin (Teikoku Zouki, Japan) injection, peak-response pressure was measured in 13 patients with achalasia of the esophagus and compared to the LESP changes in 4 control patients. In 4 healthy volunteers and 7 clinical patients with achalasia, 3 IU/kg of secretin was injected intravenously, and LESP changes were measured.

Surgery

Twenty four of 27 patients underwent a modified Jekler-Lhotka's operation. There were 12 men and 12 women, aged from 12 to 76 years (mean 36.7) (Table 1). Figure 1 shows the modified Jekler-Lhotka's operation in which wide (1–1.5 cm) and long (6–8 cm) myectomy are carried out in the lower esophagus and the bulging esophageal mucosa is covered by the anterior wall of the gastric fundus through a laparotomy. The average length of myectomy was 7.5 cm. During the procedure, intraoperative manometry was made to determine the adequate pressure of the myectomy and the fundoplication (Fig. 2). In two

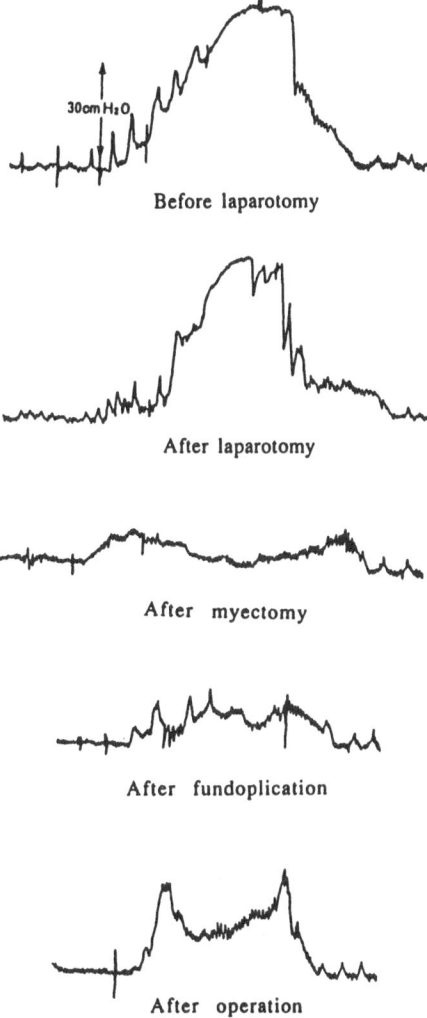

Fig. 2. Intraoperative manometry. Intraoperative manometry was carried out to decide the adequate pressure of the myectomy and the fundoplication

cases, distal partial gastrectomy was added for gastric ulcer (Table 1). Long-term efficacy of our operation was followed up by telephone and letter interview.

Gastroscintigraphy

After a 12-hour fast, the patients were positioned semireclined in front of a large field of view gamma camera (Digital gamma camera GCAA/W2, Toshiba, Japan) fitted with a diverging collimator (Toshiba medium energy general purpose collimator model ROC-930A) on line to a scintigraphic data analyzer (Toshiba medical image processor model GMS-550J). Each patient was given 60 g of

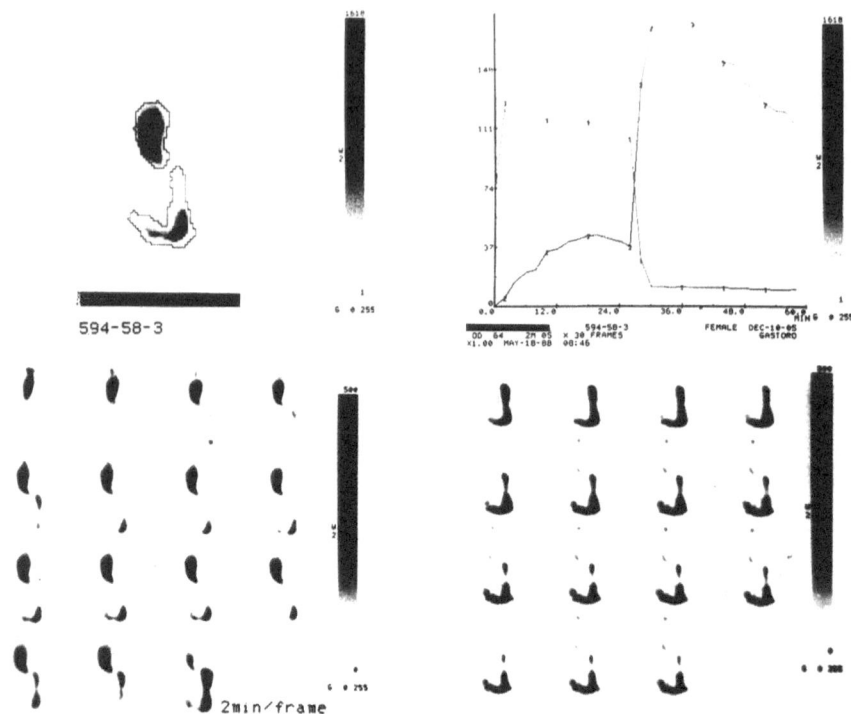

Fig. 3. Gastroscintigraphy (1). Patients were given the radiolabeled meal and the time-activity curve was calculated for the esophagus and stomach

semiliquid meal containing 10 g of Clinimeal (Eisai Co., Tokyo, Japan) labeled with ^{99m}Tc or ^{111}In-diethylene triaminepentaacetic acid (DTPA). This agent was imaged using the two windows on the gamma camera every minute for 60 min and all data was stored in a computer. The time-activity curve was calculated in the area of the esophagus and the stomach (Fig. 3). Radiological estimation was made by this scintigraphy before and after surgery.

Radioimmunoassay and Immunohistochemical Study

Specimens were excised from the LES in patients with achalasia and patients with esophageal varices. Radioimmunoassay and immunohistochemical studies were performed with anti-vasoactive intestinal polypeptide (VIP) antibody.

Results

Manometric Study

The resting levels of LESP in achalasia patients were significantly greater than those in control patients ($P < 0.05$). Achalasia patients showed a significant increase (40.7 ± 3.6%) in the LESP to tetragastrin injection when compared

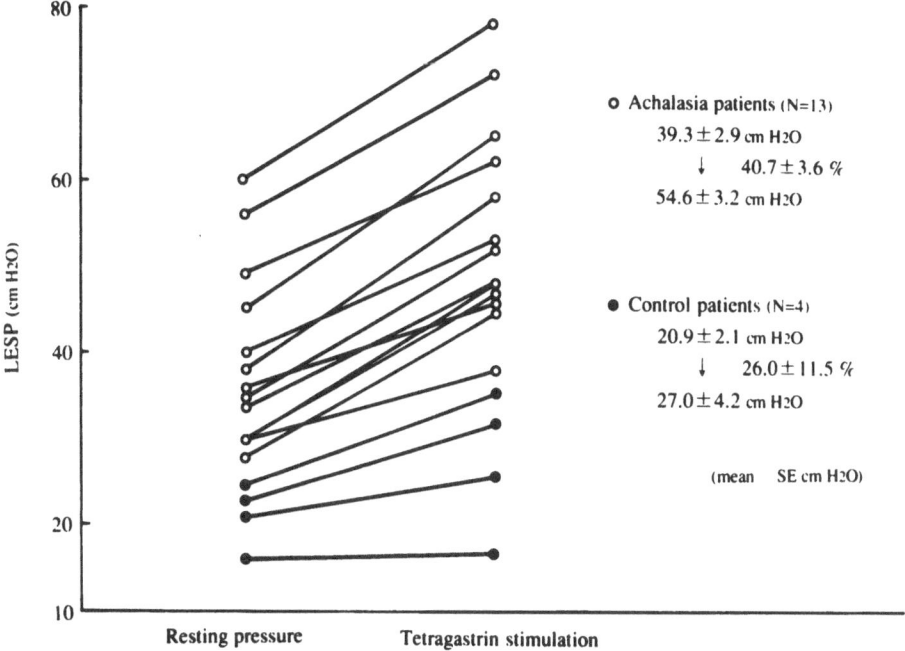

Fig. 4. Lower esophageal sphincter pressure (*LESP*) changes to exogenous gastrin injection. Tetragastrin (5 μg/kg) injection increased the LESP both in achalasia patients and controls. The increase rate was greater ($P < 0.05$) in achalasia patients compared to the controls

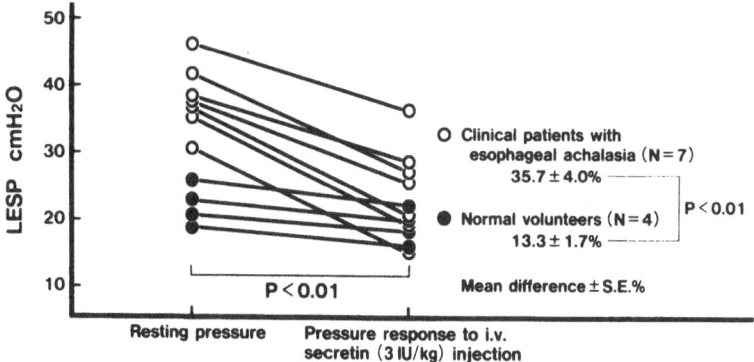

Fig. 5. LESP changes to exogenous secretin injection. The resting pressure was greater in achalasia patients. Both in normal volunteers and achalasia patients, secretin (3 IU/kg) reduced the LESP ($P < 0.01$). The reduction rate was greater ($P < 0.01$) in achalasia patients compared to normal controls

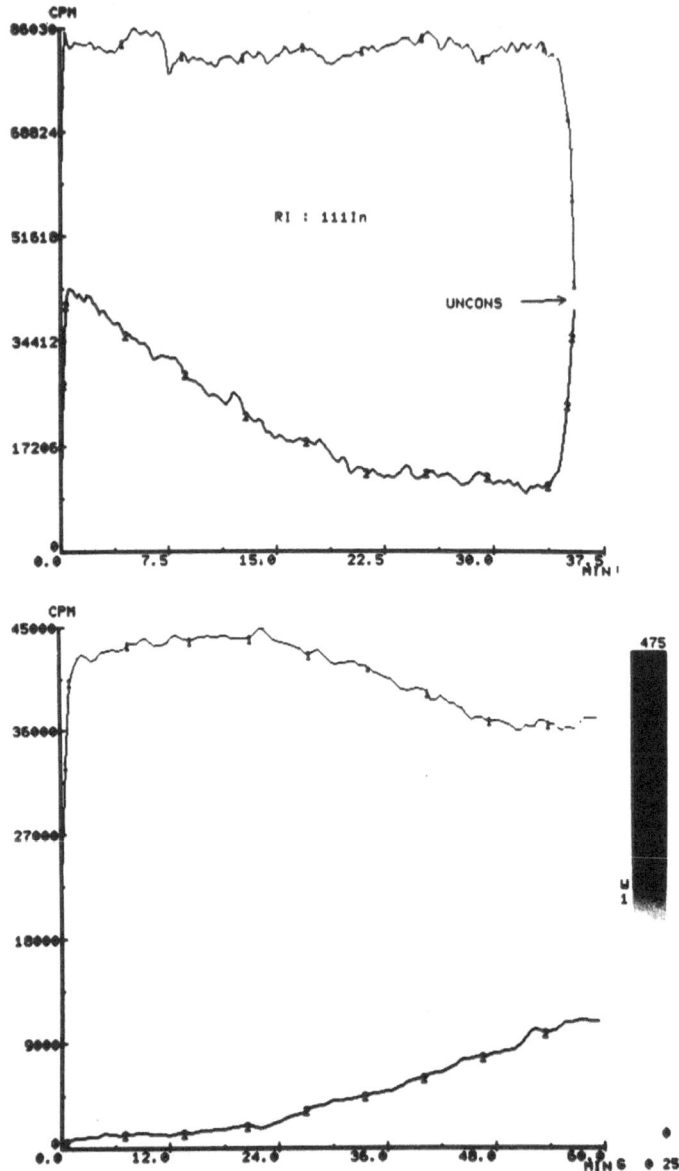

Fig. 6. Gastroscintigraphy (2). Radiolabeled meal was retained in the esophagus and the emptying was very slow in patients with achalasia of the esophagus

with the controls (26.0 ± 11.5%) ($P < 0.05$) (Fig. 4). In both patients with achalasia and controls, LESP was reduced remarkably by an injection of 3 IU/kg of secretin ($P < 0.01$). The percentage of LESP reduction was significantly greater in achalasia patients (35.7 ± 4.0%) as compared to normal volunteers (13.3 ± 1.7%) ($P < 0.01$) (Fig. 5).

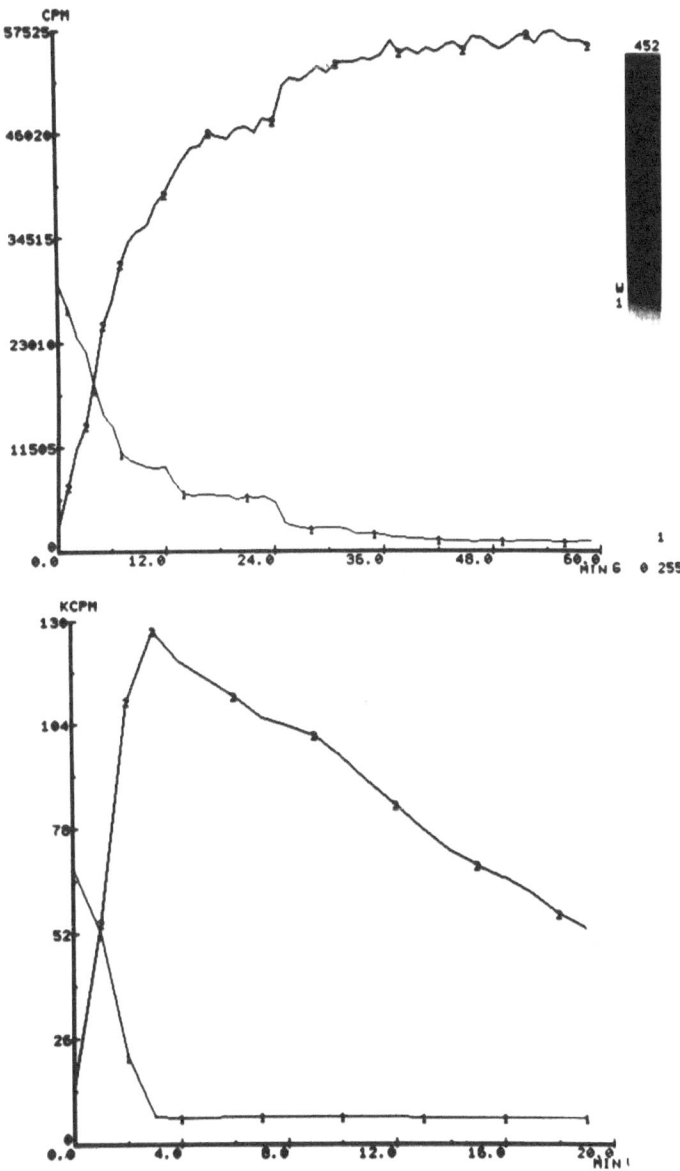

Fig. 7. Gastroscintigraphy (3). After surgery, the meal passed smoothly into the stomach

Surgery

In one case with sigmoid type achalasia, dysphagia relapsed 14 months after surgery, and lower esohagectomy and proximal gastrectomy was done. Overall efficacy of our operation was 91.7% according to follow-up data.

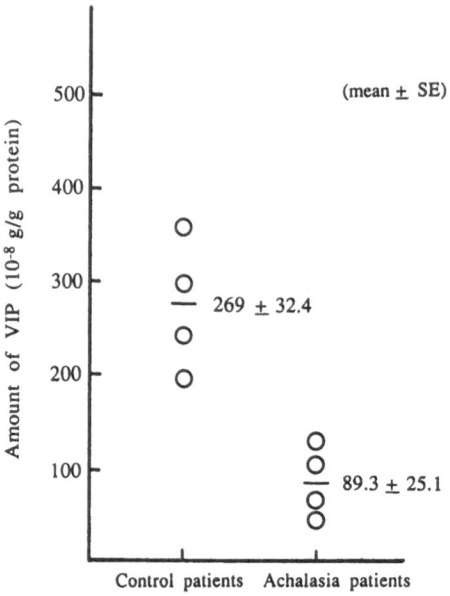

Fig. 8. Concentration of vasoactive intestinal polypeptide (*VIP*) by radioimmunoassay. Amount of VIP was smaller ($P < 0.05$) in the specimens from achalasia patients compared to control patients

Gastroscintigraphy

Before surgery, the radiolabeled meal was left in the esophagus over 30 min. One of our patients showed retention for 60 min (Fig. 6). Food went into the stomach smoothly after surgery (Fig. 7).

Radioimmunoassay and Immunohistochemical Study

Radioimmunoassay showed VIP immunoreactivity was smaller in the specimens from achalasia patients ($P < 0.05$) (Fig. 8).

VIP-immunoreactive nerve cells and fibers were observed in the myenteric plexus of the control patients. In achalasia patients, VIP nerves were rarely noted (Fig. 9).

Discussion

Esophageal achalasia is a motility disorder in the LES [1]. Many drugs, neural, and humoral factors have been demonstrated to affect the LES [2]. It has been reported that gastrin increases the LESP [3]. In this study, we demonstrated that achalasia patients showed a hypersensitivity to gastrin, and this increased the LESP. This result is consistent with that of Cohen et al. [4].

Rattan et al. [5] reported that VIP reduced the LESP. Siegel et al. [6] investigated the effect of VIP on LES in the baboon and compared it with the

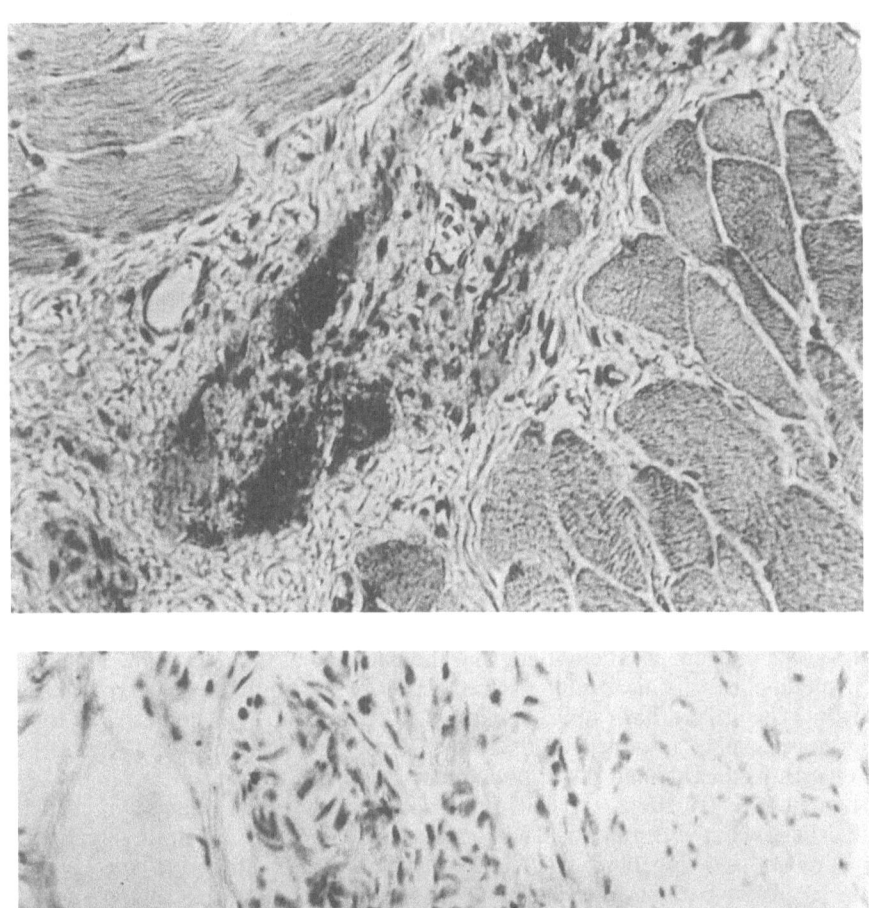

Fig. 9. Immunohistochemical study. Immunoreactive VIP nerve cells and fibers were observed in Auerbach's plexus in the LES in control patients (*upper*) and VIP nerves were rarely found in achalasia patients (*lower*)

effects of secretin and glucagon. They also reported that the effect of VIP was not influenced by tetrodotoxin and concluded that VIP affects the LES directly. Our previous results with dogs showed the effect of VIP on the resting LESP was five times greater than secretin and seven times greater than secretin on gastrin-stimulated LESP. Furthermore, reduction of the LESP was two times greater in achalasia model dogs compared to the controls [7]. In this study, secretin was used instead of VIP and the effect of secretin was examined in achalasia patients and normal volunteers and found secretin reduced LESP in both achalasia patients and normal controls, but the reduction rate was greater in achalasia patients. If we used VIP, the reduction rate might be greater. These results show that gastrin, secretin, and VIP may be useful indications for the diagnosis of achalasia.

As for treatment, there are controversies regarding the best method [8, 9]. Complications of esophagomyotomy include perforation, persistent dysphagia, and gastroesophageal reflux [8]. To prevent these complications, we employed a modified Jekler-Lhotka's operation. Different from the original method [10], we performed myectomy rather than myotomy to evaluate the deformity of Auerbach's plexus and to study pathophysiology of this disease. We also carry out intraoperative manometry to determine the adequate pressure after fundoplication. The results of gastroscintigraphy and follow-up study confirmed the efficacy of our operation. We found that gastroscintigraphy was excellent to test the grade of esophageal emptying and the outcome of the operation.

Immunohistochemical study showed that VIP immunoreactive nerve cells and fibers exist in Auerbach's plexus in normal LES. Fewer VIP nerves were found in the specimens from achalasia patients. This was consistent with the report of Aggestrup and Uddman [11]. Immunoreactivity in Auerbach's plexus in the LES suggests that VIP affects the LES directly. Lower levels of VIP immunoreactivity in achalasia patients may reflect incomplete relaxation of LES in these patients.

Kramer and Ingelfinger [12] reported a hypersensitivity to mecholyl in the achalasia patients and explained this phenomenon with Cannon's law of denervation [13]. Hypersensitivity to exogenous gastrin and secretin in achalasia patients may be explained by the denervation theory.

Jennewein et al. [14] reported that LESP increased in patients with achalasia, and also reported that administration of glucagon reduced LESP. Siewert and Fruh [15] suggested the clinical use of glucagon in achalasia patients with dysphagia. It is possible that secretin and VIP may aid in the diagnosis and treatment of achalasia of the esophagus.

References

1. Kramer P, Ingelfinger FJ (1949) II. Cardiospasm, a generalized disorder of esophageal motility. Am J Med 7:174–179
2. Goyal RK, Rattan S (1978) Neurohumoral, hormonal, and drug receptors for lower esophageal sphincter. Gastroenterology 74:598–619
3. Cohen S, Lipshutz W (1971) Hormonal regulation of human LES. J Clin Invest 50:449–454
4. Cohen S, Lipshutz W, Hughes W (1971) Role of gastrin supersensitivity in the pathogenesis of lower esophageal sphincter hypertension in achalasia. J Clin Invest 50:1241–1247
5. Rattan S, Said SI, Goyal RK (1977) Effect of vasoactive intestinal polypeptide on the lower esophageal sphincter pressure (LESP). Proc Soc Exp Biol Med 155:40–43

6. Siegel SR, Brown FC, Castell DO, Johnson LF, Said SI (1979) Effect of vasoactive intestinal polypeptide on lower esophageal sphincter in awake baboons: Comparison with glucagon and secretin. Dig Dis Sci 24:345–349
7. Tangoku A, Ishigami K, Murakami T (1988) Effect of vasoactive intestinal polypeptide on the cardiac closing mechanism and pathophysiology of achalasia of the esophagus. In: Siewert JR, Holscher AH (eds) Diseases of the esophagus. Springer, Berlin Heidelberg New York, pp 930–935
8. Donahue PH, Schlesinger PK, Bombeck CT, Samelson S, Nyhus LM (1986) Achalasia of the esophagus: Treatment, controversies, and method of choice. Ann Surg 203:505–510
9. Andreollo NA, Earlam RJ (1987) Heller's myotomy for achalasia: Is an added anti-reflux procedure necessary? Br J Surg 74:765–769
10. Jekler J, Lhotka J (1967) Modified Heller procedure to prevent postoperative reflux esophagitis in patients with achalasia. Am J Surg 113:251–254
11. Aggestrup S, Uddman R (1983) Lack of vasoactive intestinal polypeptide nerves in esophageal achalasia. Gastroenterology 84:924–927
12. Kramer P, Ingelfinger FJ (1951) Esophageal sensitivity to mecholyl in cardiospasm. Gastroenterology 19:242–253
13. Cannon WB (1939) A law of denervation. Am J Med Sci 198:737–750
14. Jennewein HM, Waldecke F, Siewert R, Weisen F, Thimm R (1973) The interaction of glucagon and pentagastrin on the lower esophageal sphincter in man and dog. Gut 14:861–864
15. Siewert R, Fruh E (1979) Senkung des Druckes im unteren Oesophagussphinkter bei der Achalasia durch Glucagon. Deutsch Med Sci 24:345–349

Endoscopic Ultrasonography for Esophageal Achalasia

HIRONOBU SATO, ISAO MURAYAMA, KIYOMI SUDA, JYOJI OHTSUKI, and
TAKASHI TANAKA[1]

Introduction

Although esophageal achalasia is a motor disorder, it is a fact that achalasia is
associated with obvious structual change such as the absence of ganglion cell,
atrophy or hypertrophy of the muscular layers [1]. Even at the operation, in
some cases of esophageal achalasia, esophageal wall thickening can be recognized. This esophageal wall thickening was evaluated by endoscopic ultrasonograph (EUS) preoperatively. This study was done to document the result
with the relations between the EUS findings and x-ray findings, and manometric
measurements of esophageal pressure.

Patients and Methods

In Japan, achalasia is classified by x-ray findings and manometric changes according to the Descriptive Rules for Achalasia of the Esophagus [2]. According to
rules which were made by the Japanese Society of Esophageal Diseases, achalasia
could be classified radiographically by type of esophageal dilatation which
included spindle type, flask type, and sigmoid type. The grade of esophageal
dilatation is also classified radiographically into three groups according to
maximal diameter of the esophageal width. Manometric change is classified as
either type A or B based on the positive pressure curve on swallowing: Type A
is characterized by a positive pressure curve on swallowing, and type B is
characterized by the absence of a positive pressure curve.

Between 1963 and 1991, 103 patients with esophageal achalasia were treated
at the Third Department of Surgery, Nihon University, School of Medicine. In

---
[1] Third Department of Surgery, Nihon University School of Medicine, 1-8-13, Kanda-Surugadai,
Chiyoda-ku, Tokyo, 101 Japan

Table 1. X-ray classification according to grade and type

Grade	Spindle	Flask	Sigmoid	Total
I	6	0	0	6
II	30	30	3	63
III	3	17	14	34
Total	39	47	17	103

all patients, the diagnosis of achalasia was based on symptoms and confirmed by manometry, barium roentgenograph and endoscopy. Of 103 patients, EUS was performed in 18 cases of achalasia. There were 3 males and 15 females, with a median age of 40 (range 18 to 72 years).

Endoscopic ultrasonography utilizes an optical system with an oblique orientation and a transducer with a mechanically rotating acoustic mirror in the distal tip. Ultrasound frequencies of 7.5 MHz and 12 MHz (Olympus GF-UM 2 and 3 radial type) were utilized. A balloon surrounding tranceducer at the tip is expanded by water in order to establish good contact with the esophageal wall. These instruments visualize the esophageal wall as five-layer sonographic pattern. The third layer, hyperechoic layer, corresponds to the submucosal layer, and the fourth layer also corresponds to muscuralis propria [3].

Results

Of 103 paitients, 39 were spindle type, 47 were flask type, and 17 were sigmoid type. Regarding the degree of dilatation, in grade I there were 6 paitients who were less than 3.5 cm in diameter of the esophagus by x-ray, and in grade II there were 63 patients who were between 3.5 cm and 6.0 cm (Table 1). By this classification, it is considered that the group of sigmoid type of achalasia was the most advanced type. There were many grade III cases in the sigmoid type.

Regarding the relation between the manometric classification and x-ray type, spindle type was predominantly type A on manometric testing and the sigmoid type was the only type B which did not demonstrate a positive pressure curve on swallowing in manometry (Fig. 1). This manometric classification showed a good correlation with x-ray type.

EUS was performed in 18 patients with esophageal achalasia. EUS findings were classified according to thickness of the fourth layer of the esophagus: 2 patients were under 4-mm-thick (mild group), 9 were between 4- and 7-mm-thick (moderate group), and 7 were over 7-mm-thick (severe group). The relation between EUS classification, x-ray type, and grade is shown in Table 2. In the mild group, there were no cases of flask or sigmoid type. In the severe group, there was no case of spindle type. There were more high grade cases (advanced) based on x-ray findings in the severe group. On the other hand, there was no case of grade III in the mild group. Of 18 patients, 8 were found to have low esophageal sphincter pressure using a triple-lumen catheter with microtranseducer tip (another 10 were measured by the open tip method). There was correlation between low esophageal sphincter pressure and the thickness of the fourth layer of the esophageal wall by EUS (Fig. 2).

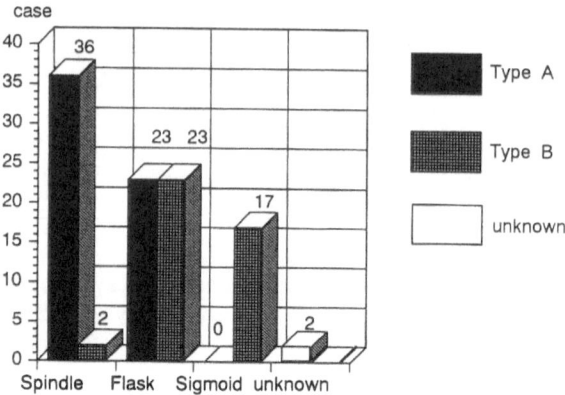

Fig. 1. Manometric classification and x-ray type

Table 2. Relationship between endoscopic ultrosonograph (*EUS*) and other achalasia classifications

EUS	X-ray type			Grade			Manometry	
	Spindle	Flask	Sigmoid	I	II	III	A	B
Mild	2				2		2	
Moderate	5	3	1		6	3	5	4
Severe		5	2		2	5	2	5
Total	7	8	3		10	8	9	9

Case Presentation

A 59-year-old female who had suffered from dysphagea for 5 years, was diagnosed as having flask type, grade III achalasia by x-ray. EUS showed the fourth layer of the esophageal wall to be 8-mm-thick (Fig. 3). Cardioplasty was then performed according to the modified Girald operation [4], which led to an improvement in symptoms. Pathologically, the smooth muscle of the esophageal wall which was taken at operation revealed the severe hypertrophy and degeneration of Auerbach's plexus.

Discussion

Previously, esophageal EUS has been used mainly for patients having malignant tumor or submucosal tumor since it provides a representation of the histologic components of the esophageal wall. However, functional disorders of the esophagus, such as esophageal achalasia and reflux esophagitis, also change the structure of the esophageal wall [5]. Therefore, morphological changes in the functional disorder of the esophagus can be obtained by EUS.

EUS was performed in 18 achalasia patients in this study and thickening of over 4 mm in the fourth layer of the esophagus was noted in 16. As the normal

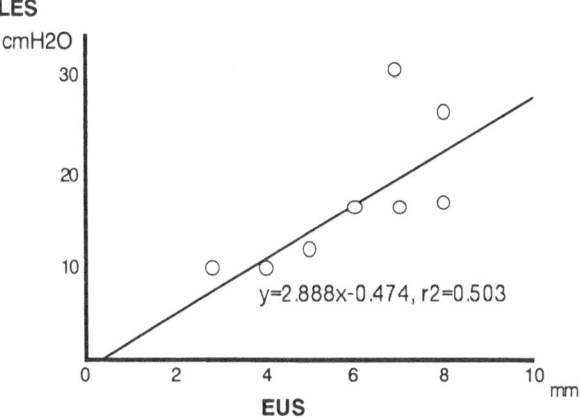

Fig. 2. Correlation between endoscopic ultrasonograph (*EUS*) and low esophageal sphincter pressure. *LES* low esophageal sphincter pressure

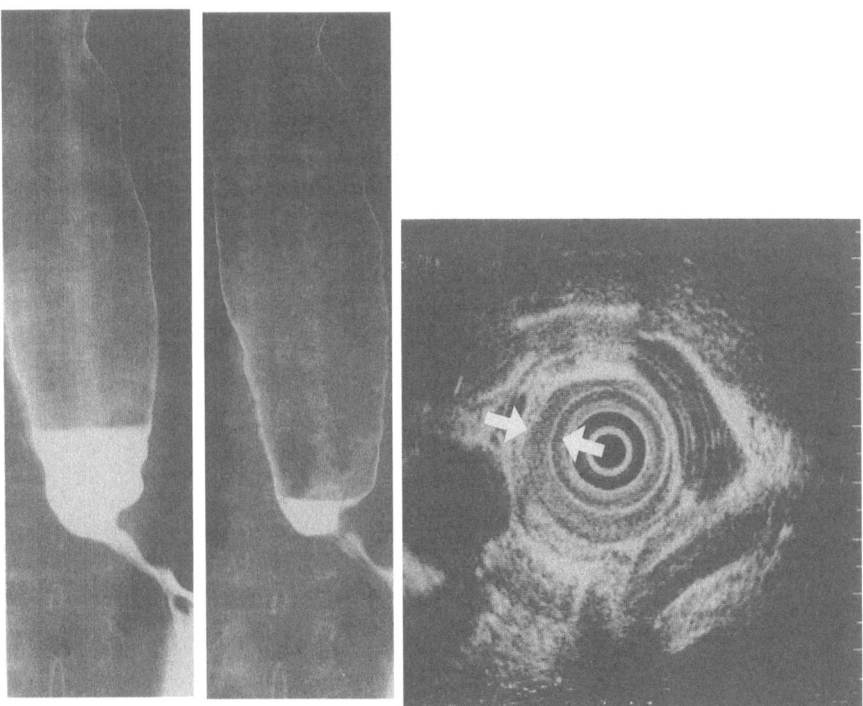

Fig. 3. X-ray showed the flask type, grade III achalasia. EUS showed the fourth layer of the esophagus wall to be 8-mm-thick (*arrows*)

esophageal fourth layer is less than 2-mm-thick by EUS observation, thickness of the fourth layer in achalasia can increase markedly. Since the fourth hypoechoic layer can be taken as representing the muscularis propria, EUS can obtain the degree of hypertrophic muscle layer in achalasia before operation. It is not known whether the thickening of the fourth layer is the cause or the result of the stricture of the esophagus, but it is important that the grade of esophageal hypertrophy be determined by EUS before the operation. The preoperative evaluation of esophageal wall thickening can help the surgeon select the operation method.

Manometric patterns and types in achalasia are reported by many authorities [6], but there is no study to date addressing the evaluation of achalasia by EUS. In this study, we introduced a method of classifying EUS features according to the degree of thickness of the fourth layer of the esophagus. This classification showed a good correlation between not only the x-ray type but also the manometric measurements. Recently, we have used EUS findings for determining the most appropriate operation technique. Therefore, we suggest that EUS is a useful examination method for achalasia.

References

1. Friesen DL, Henderson RD, Hanna W (1983) Ultrastructure of the esophageal muscle in achalasia and diffuse esophageal spasm. Am J Clin Pathol 79:319–325
2. Japanese Society of Esophageal Diseases (1983) Descriptive rules for achalasia of the esophagus 3rd edn. Kanehara, Tokyo
3. Sato H, Murayama I, Suda K, Takeya K, Tanaka T, Takeuchi K, Kohashi E (1992) Endoscopic ultrasonography for reflux esophagitis. Stomach and Intestine (Tokyo) 27: 1047–1051
4. Tanaka T, Sato H, Morikawa H, Matsushita T, Yoshida K, Sakabe T (1985) Modified Girard operation for esophageal achalasia. Dig Surg 2:73–78
5. Murayama I, Sato H, Tanaka T (1991) Endoscopic ultrasonography for esophageal achalasia and reflux esophagitis. Prog Dig End 39:152–156
6. Couturier D, Samama J (1991) Clinical aspects and manometric criteria in achalasia. Hepato-Gastroenterol 38:481–487

Clinical Use of Ambulatory 24-H Esophageal Motility Monitoring in the Evaluation of Patients with Primary Esophageal Motor Disorders

Hubert J. Stein[1] and Tom R. DeMeester[2]

Introduction

Motor abnormalities of the esophageal body are frequently implicated as the cause of dysphagia, regurgitation, or non-cardiac chest pain [1–4]. The diagnosis and classification of esophageal motor abnormalities and the proof of a causal relation between the abnormality and a symptom has, however, been difficult in the past for the following reasons: First, there usually is no reliable mucosal lesion that can be observed on endoscopy to indicate the presence of an esophageal motor disorder; second, roentgenographic signs of esophageal motor disorders occur only in advanced disease; third, the current "gold-standard" for the diagnosis of esophageal motor disorders, i.e., stationary esophageal manometry, has several shortcomings—it is performed in a laboratory environment with the patient in a supine position, the analysis is based on the motor response to ten wet or dry swallows only, and intermittent motor abnormalities may be missed; fourth, the current classification of motor disorders is controversial, and does not allow for the quantitation of the severity of the abnormality; fifth, spontaneous symptoms rarely occur during a short-term stationary motility study; and sixth, the use of provocative tests, i.e., acid perfusion, administration of tensilon, or balloon distention, to reproduce the patient's symptoms is not helpful since most of these tests have a low yield, symptoms are reproduced with unphysiologic stimuli, the endpoint is based on the patients symptom perception, and the results do not correlate with motility abnormalities associated with spontaneously occurring symptoms [4–6]. Consequently, the current diagnosis of esophageal motor abnormalities is inexact. This may account for some of the disappointing results of both pharmacologic and surgical therapy of the abnormalities [5, 7].

[1] Klinikum rechts der Isar der TU München, München, Germany
[2] University of Southern California School of Medicine, Department of Surgery, 1510 San Pablo Street, Suite 514, Los Angeles, CA 90033-4612, USA

197

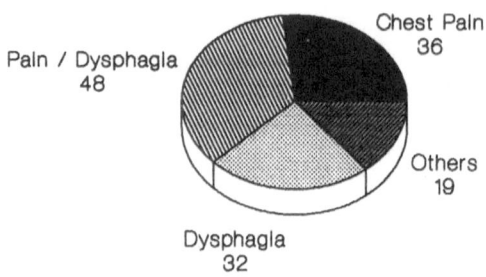

Fig. 1. Presenting symptoms of 135 patients who had ambulatory 24-h esophageal motility monitoring

The recently introduced technique of ambulatory 24-h esophageal motility monitoring overcomes the shortcomings of stationary manometry and provocative tests [8, 9]. It allows monitoring of esophageal motor activity over an entire circadian cycle in a variety of physiologic conditions. This multiplies the amount of data on which a diagnosis can be based, increases the probability of documenting an intermittent abnormality, and allows correlation of spontaneously occurring symptoms with abnormal esophageal motor function, provided the symptom occurs during the monitoring period. Furthermore, combination of this technique with esophageal and gastric pH monitoring allows integrated evaluation of esophageal body function, gastroesophageal reflux, and gastric secretory and motor function in a physiologic environment within one circadian cycle [8, 10]. We established normal values for 24-h ambulatory esophageal motility monitoring in asymptomatic volunteers (controls) and evaluated its clinical use in patients with symptoms suggestive of a primary esophageal motor disorder, i.e., non-obstructive dysphagia and/or non-cardiac chest pain.

Materials and Methods

Patient Population

The study populations consisted of 25 normal healthy volunteers, 135 patients referred to the senior author (DeMeester) for evaluation of symptoms suggestive of a primary esophageal motor disorder, and 9 patients who volunteered for follow-up studies 1–9 years (median 3 years) after a successful long esophageal myotomy performed for uncontrollable dysphagia and chest pain due to diffuse esophageal spasm. The major presenting symptoms of the patients are shown in Fig. 1. All normal subjects were screened by history, physical examination, and upper gastrointestinal barium roentgenography to exclude the presence of a foregut disorder. Similarly, all patients had an upper gastrointestinal endoscopy, barium roentgenography, and ambulatory 24-h esophageal pH monitoring. Patients with structural esophageal abnormalities, i.e., esophagitis, stricture, ring, web, or large hiatal hernia; and patients with increased esophageal exposure to gastric juice on 24-h esophageal pH monitoring were excluded. In all patients with chest pain, a cardiac or pulmonary cause of their symptoms had been excluded by the referring physician by chest roentgenography, ECG, stress ECG and, in selected cases, coronary angiography.

Stationary and Ambulatory 24-h Esophageal Manometry

Stationary and ambulatory 24-h esophageal manometry were performed after an overnight fast. All medications known to interfere with gastrointestinal secretory or motor function were discontinued at least 48 h prior to the study. Stationary manometry of the lower esophageal sphincter, esophageal body and upper esophageal sphincter were performed in a standard fashion as described in detail elsewhere [5].

Ambulatory 24-h monitoring of the motor activity in the esophageal body was performed with two electronic pressure transducers connected to a commercially available portable data recorder (Synectics Medical, Irving, Tex.). The subjects were encouraged to perform normal daily activity during the study. Pressure recordings of the ambulatory study were analyzed separately for the upright, supine, meal, and symptomatic periods as described previously [11]. The complete analysis of the 24-h ambulatory motility tracing was performed by a computer program which had been validated against manual analysis [9].

Esophageal motor disorders were diagnosed and classified according to the parameters shown in Table 1. The criteria used are based on the normal range of esophageal motility in our laboratory, and correlate well with those of other investigators [1, 12].

Results

Compared to stationary manometry, ambulatory 24-h esophageal motility monitoring provided a 100-fold larger database for the classification and quantitation of abnormal esophageal motor function. The diagnoses obtained by stationary and ambulatory 24-h esophageal manometry in the 116 patients with dysphagia and/or non-cardiac chest pain as their major symptom are classified and compared in Fig. 2. Stationary and 24-h ambulatory manometry resulted in the same diagnosis in 56/116 patients (48%). In 4/14 patients who had been diagnosed as having achalasia on stationary manometry, 24-h monitoring showed 5%, 7%, 11%, and 14% peristaltic contractions. Consequently, these 4 patients were classified as having diffuse esophageal spasm on 24-h monitoring. Similarly, 6/18 patients who met the criteria of diffuse esophageal spasm on stationary manometry had a normal frequency of simultaneous contractions on 24-h manometry and were classified as having a nutcracker esophagus ($n = 4$), a non-specific esophageal motility disorder ($n = 2$), or normal motor function ($n = 1$). A substantial degree of reclassification also occurred in patients who had the motor pattern of a nutcracker esophagus, a non-specific motor disorder, or normal esophageal motor function on stationary manometry.

Mean amplitude and duration of contractions in the esophageal body were not significantly different between volunteers, patients without dysphagia, and patients who had dysphagia but no evidence of obstruction on endoscopy or barium swallow. In all groups, the frequency of esophageal contractions increased from the supine, to the upright, and meal periods. Compared to volunteers and

Table 1. Diagnostic criteria for the classification of primary esophageal motor disorders based on esophageal body function

	Standard Manometry	Ambulatory 24-h Manometry
Achalasia	Complete absence of peristalsis	Complete absence of peristalsis
Diffuse esophageal spasm	>20% Simultaneous contractions[a]	>55% Simult. contractions (upright)[c] or >80%Simult. contractions (night)[c]
Nutcracker esophagus	Mean amplitude >180 mmHg[a]	Mean amplitude > 105 mmHg[c]
Non-specific motor disorder	>20% multi-peaked contractions[a], or >20% interrupted contractions[a], or >20% dropped contractions[a], or >20% not transmitted contractions[a], or Mean amplitude <30 mmHg[b]	>20% multi-peaked contract[c], or >20% isolated contractions[c], or Mean amplitude < 25 mmHg[d]

[a] >mean + 2 SD of 50 normal volunteers   [c] >mean + 2 SD of 25 normal volunteers
[b] <mean − 2 SD of 50 normal volunteers   [d] <mean − 2 SD of 25 normal volunteers

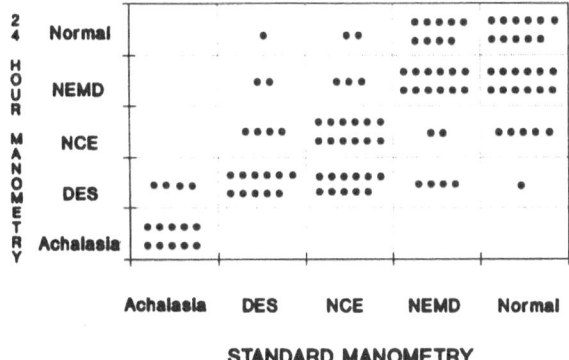

Fig. 2. Classification of esophageal motor disorders in 116 patients with dysphagia and/or non-cardiac chest pain according to the findings on standard or ambulatory 24-h manometry. *DES*, diffuse esophageal spasm; *NCE*, nutcracker esophagus; *NEMD*, non-specific esophageal motor disorder

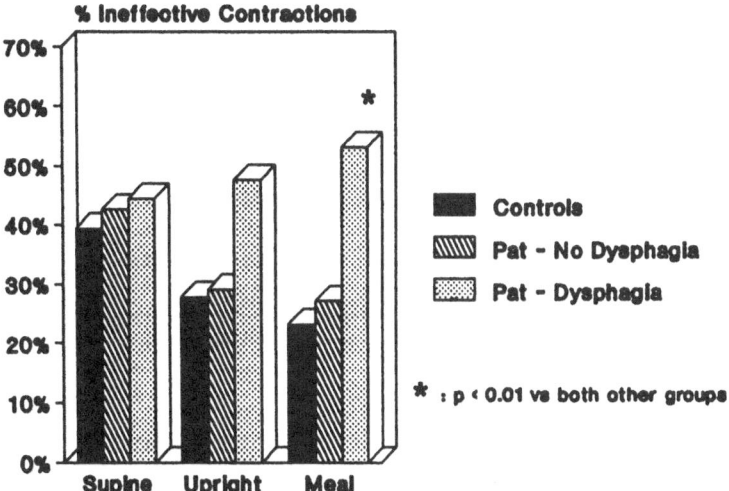

Fig. 3. Frequency of ineffective contractions, i.e., non-peristaltic contractions or contractions with an amplitude <30 mmHg, in volunteers, patients without dysphagia, and patients with non-obstructive dysphagia. *Pat*, patient

patients without dysphagia, patients with dysphagia, however, had a significantly increased frequency of ineffective contractions during meals, i.e., non-peristaltic contractions or contractions with an amplitude <30 mmHg (Fig. 3).

Of 84 patients, 26 (31%) with a history of non-cardiac chest pain experienced at least one pain episode during 24-h esophageal motility monitoring (Fig. 4). Spontaneous chest pain episodes did not occur during stationary manometry. Using each subject as his own control, spontaneous chest pain episodes were associated with abnormal esophageal motor activity in 13/26 patients who

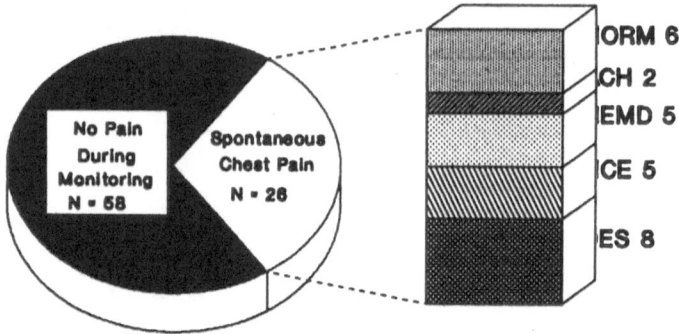

Fig. 4. Frequency of patients who experienced at least one episode of chest pain during ambulatory 24-h esophageal manometry and their underlying motor abnormality as diagnosed by 24-h manometry. *NORM*, normal; *DES*, diffuse esophageal spasm; *NCE*, nutcracker esophagus; *NEMD*, non-specific esophageal motor disorder; *ACH*, achalasia

experienced the symptom during 24-h monitoring. Chest pain was more frequently associated with abnormal esophageal motor activity in patients who, on ambulatory manometry, had a diffuse spasm or nutcracker esophagus (10/13 patients) as compared to those with a non-specific motor disorder or normal circadian esophageal motor activity (2/9 patients, $P < 0.05$).

The mean amplitude and duration of contractions associated with the chest pain episodes was not different from asymptomatic contractions during the supine episode. Compared to the recordings during the asymptomatic upright, supine, and meal periods, chest pain episodes were, however, associated with a significantly higher frequency of simultaneous contractions, contractions with two or multiple peaks, a higher number of contractions with an amplitude above 180 mmHg, and with a duration longer than 7 s ($P < 0.01$, Fig. 5).

The prevalence of abnormal esophageal contractions on 24-hour motility recording in patients with symptomatic diffuse esophageal spasm and patients who had successfully undergone a long esophageal myotomy for uncontrollable dysphagia and chest pain caused by diffuse spasm is shown in Fig. 6. Myotomy reduced the prevalence of simultaneous, double- or multi-peaked contractions, and contractions >180 mmHg and >7 s. This was associated with a marked decrease in the mean amplitude of contractions.

Discussion

The development of miniaturized electronic pressure transducers and the introduction of portable digital data recorders with large storage capacity has recently made prolonged monitoring of esophageal motor activity in an outpatient environment possible [8, 9]. We have previously shown that monitoring of esophageal motor activity over an entire circadian cycle allows quantitation of abnormal esophageal body function in patients with diffuse esophageal spasm or gastroesophageal reflux disease [9, 13]. Using standard criteria for the classification of esophageal motor disorders, the present study shows that ambulatory

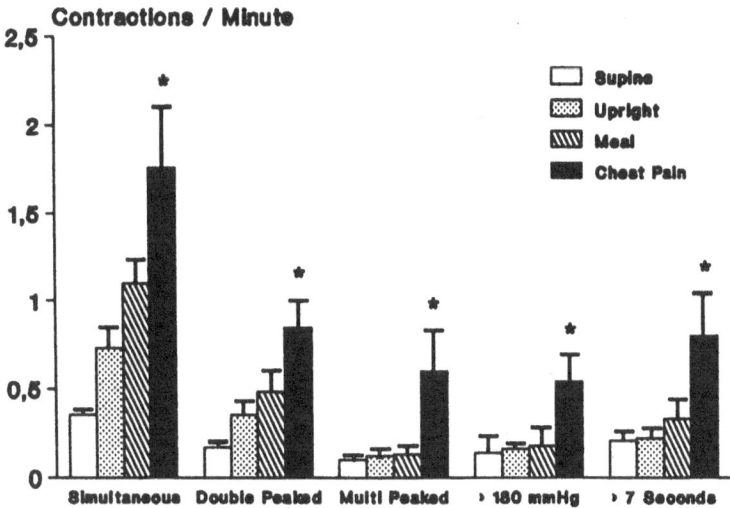

Fig. 5. Frequency of simultaneous, double-peaked, multi-peaked, high amplitude (>180 mmHg), and long-duration (>7 s) contractions during the supine, upright, meal, and chest pain episodes. *P < 0.01 vs all other periods

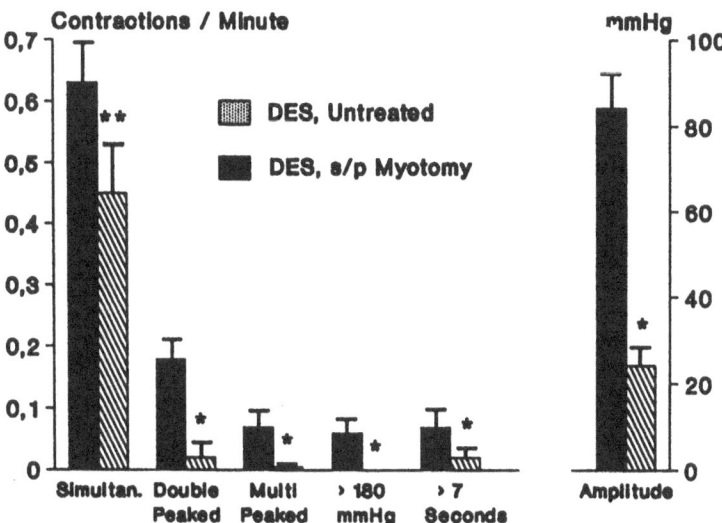

Fig. 6. Frequency of simultaneous, double-peaked, triple-peaked, high amplitude (>180 mmHg) and long-duration (>7 s) contractions and mean amplitude of contractions in patients with untreated diffuse esophageal spasm (*DES*) and patients who have undergone a long esophageal myotomy. *s/p*, status post. *P < 0.01 vs untreated DES; **P < 0.05 vs untreated DES

24-h esophageal manometry results in a more precise diagnosis than stationary manometry. Furthermore, ambulatory 24-h manometry provided the ability to document and characterize esophageal motor abnormalities associated with non-obstructive dysphagia and episodes of non-cardiac chest pain.

An increased frequency of abnormal contractions following ten wet swallows is currently considered the gold standard for the identification and classification of esophageal motor disorders [12]. Ambulatory 24-h esophageal manometry multiplies the number of esophageal contractions available for analysis and provides an opportunity to assess esophageal motor function in a variety of physiologic situations, thus increasing the accuracy and dependability of the measurement [14]. The comparison of the diagnoses obtained by stationary and ambulatory 24-h esophageal manometry showed surprisingly little agreement between the two techniques. The frequent underestimation of the severity of a motor disorder on stationary manometry appears to be due to the intermittent expression of esophageal motor abnormalities which can be easily missed on ten wet swallows, but are detected when motor activity is monitored over 24 h. On the other hand, ambulatory manometry also frequently showed normal or only mildly disordered circadian motor function in patients thought to have a more severe disorder on stationary manometry. The unphysiologic conditions under which stationary manometry is performed may trigger these abnormalities in patients known to have a low anxiety threshold [15].

Dysphagia in the absence of esophageal obstruction is a frequent symptom [2, 4] whose underlying pathophysiologic abnormality usually can not be determined on stationary manometry [4, 5]. Our study indicates that dysphagia in patients with no esophageal obstruction may be due to the inability to organize esophageal motor activity into peristaltic contractions during the meal periods. This is in accordance with the recent observation of an increased frequency of ineffective contractions during meal periods in patients with gastroesophageal reflux disease and non-obstructive dysphagia [16]. Only evaluation of the meal periods on an ambulatory 24-h esophageal motility record allows the identification of this abnormality.

Since its introduction in 1985, ambulatory esophageal manometry has been primarily used to assess esophageal motility abnormalities as the cause of non-cardiac chest pain [8, 17]. In the present study, only 31% of unselected patients with a history of non-cardiac chest pain actually experienced their symptom during 24-h monitoring. When a spontaneous episode of chest pain occurred during the monitored period, motor abnormalities were associated with the symptom in 50% of the patients. Contrary to our expectations, the mean amplitude and duration of esophageal contractions associated with chest pain episodes was similar to contractions during the asymptomatic recording. Esophageal chest pain episodes were, however, immediately preceded by a markedly increased frequency of contractions similar to that seen during meal periods. In contrast to meal periods, these contractions were mostly simultaneous, and double- or multi-peaked, as well as frequently having an amplitude >180 mmHg or a duration >7 s. Similar to the heart, esophageal blood supply may be interrupted during bursts of abnormal muscular contractions. This may become critical in situations where the resting blood flow to the esophagus is already compromised as has been shown for the hypertrophic esophageal muscle in patients with diffuse esophageal spasm [18]. A burst of disorganized motor activity in this situation may give rise to ischemic pain. Consequently an apt term for esophageal chest pain caused by a burst of uncoordinated motor activity under ischemic conditions would be "esophageal claudication" [19].

Ambulatory esophageal manometry in patients with diffuse esophageal spasm whose symptoms had been controlled by long esophageal myotomy showed a marked reduction in the mean contraction amplitude associated with a marked decrease or elimination of simultaneous, double-peaked, multi-peaked, high amplitude, and long-duration contractions. This would suggest that esophageal myotomy limits the ability of the esophagus to produce abnormal contractions, which, when occurring in bursts, may further decrease blood supply and cause chest pain in a relatively ischemic organ [20].

Based on this experience, we conclude that ambulatory esophageal motility monitoring allows for a more precise classification of esophageal motor disorders than stationary manometry and identifies abnormal esophageal motor pattern associated with non-obstructive dysphagia or non-cardiac chest pain. Ambulatory 24-h esophageal motility monitoring, therefore, has the potential to improve the diagnosis and management of patients with esophageal motor disorders and should replace stationary manometry in the evaluation of esophageal body function.

References

1. Vantrappen G, Janssens J, Hellemans J, et al (1979) Achalasia, diffuse esophageal spasm, and related motility disorders. Gastroenterology 76:450–457
2. Hennington JP, Burns TW, Balart LA (1984) Chest pain and dysphagia in patients with prolonged peristaltic contractile duration of the esophagus. Dig Dis Sci 29:134–140
3. Brand DL, Martin D, Pope CE (1977) Esophageal manometrics in patients with angina type chest pain. Am J Dig Dis 23:300–304
4. Katz PO, Dalton CB, Richter JE, et al (1987) Esophageal testing of patients with non-cardiac chest pain or dysphagia. Ann Int Med 106:593–597
5. Stein HJ, DeMeester TR, Hinder, RA (1992) Outpatient physiological testing and surgical management of foregut motor disorders. Current Problems Surg 29:415–555
6. Hewson EG, Dalton CB, Richter JE (1990) Comparison of esophageal manometry, provocative testing, and ambulatory monitoring in patients with unexplained chest pain. Dig Dis Sci 35:320–309
7. DeMeester TR (1982) Surgery for esophageal motor disorders. Ann Thorac Surg 34:225–229
8. Peters L, Maas L, Petty D, et al (1988) Spontaneous non-cardiac chest pain. Evaluation by 24-hour ambulatory esophageal motility and pH monitoring. Gastroenterology 94:878–886
9. Eypasch EP, Stein HJ, DeMeester TR, et al (1990) A new technique to define and clarify esophageal motor disorders. Am J Surg 159:144–151
10. Stein HJ, DeMeester TR (1992) Integrated 24-hour ambulatory foregut monitoring in patients with complex foregut symptoms. Surg Ann 24:161–180
11. Stein HJ, DeMeester TR, Eypasch EP, Klingman RP (1991) Ambulatory 24-hour esophageal manometry in the evaluation of esophageal motor disorders and non-cardiac chest pain. Surgery 110:753–763
12. Castell DO, Richter JE, Dalton CB (eds) (1987) Esophageal motility testing. Elsevier, New York
13. Stein HJ, Eypasch EP, DeMeester TR, Smyrk TC, Attwood SEA (1990) Circadian esophageal motor function in patients with gastroesophageal reflux disease. Surgery 108:769–778

14. Stein HJ, DeMeester TR (1991) Evaluation of esophageal motor disorders: 24-hour ambulatory esophageal motility monitoring. Gastroenterology International 4:60–64
15. Clouse RE, Lustman JJ (1983) Psychiatric illness and contraction abnormalities of the esophagus. N Engl J Med 309:1337–1342
16. Singh S, Stein HJ, DeMeester TR, Hinder RA (1992) Non-obstructive dysphagia in gastroesophageal reflux disease—A study with combined ambulatory pH and motility monitoring. Am J Gastroenter 87:562–567
17. Janssens J, Vantrappen G, Ghillebert G (1986) Twenty-four-hour recording of esophageal pressure and pH in patients with non-cardiac chest pain. Gastroenterology 90:1978–1984
18. MacKenzie J, Belch J, Land D, Park R, McKillop J (1988) Oesophageal ischaemia in motility disorders associated with chest pain. Lancet II 592–595
19. Stein HJ, Eypasch EP, DeMeester TR (1989) "Esophageal claudication" as the cause of chest pain in diffuse spasm and nutcracker esophagus? Gastroenterology 96:A491
20. Stein HJ, DeMeester TR (1992) Therapy of non-cardiac chest pain: Is there a role for surgery? Am J Med 92:122S–126S

Cricopharyngeal Myotomy and Stapling: Treatment of Choice for Zenker's Diverticulum

Luigi Bonavina, Fulvio Bettineschi, Valentino Fontebasso, Alberto Ruol, Attilio Nosadini, and Alberto Peracchia[1]

Introduction

The first successful excision of a pharyngoesophageal (Zenker's) diverticulum was performed by Wheeler in 1885 [1]. This procedure has been repeatedly criticized because of the potential incidence of leakage from the suture line and recurrent pouch formation [2]. The addition of a cricopharyngeal myotomy, first proposed by Aubin [3], has been more recently advocated by many authors [4–7], although no prospective studies have definitely shown that this approach results in a decreased leak or recurrence rate.

Stapling resection of a Zenker's diverticulum was reported for the first time in 1969 [8]. As for other sites of application, the use of stapling devices may prove useful and reliable to resect the pouch, but no large clinical series have been published that can support this assumption [9]. The aim of this study was to evaluate the long-term results of primary cricopharyngeal myotomy and stapling in our series of patients with Zenker's diverticulum.

Materials and Methods

From 1976 to 1990, 120 patients underwent surgery for symptomatic Zenker's diverticulum. Of these, 89 who were primarily treated by cricopharyngeal myotomy and stapled diverticulectomy form the study population.

There were 65 males and 24 females, with a median age of 62 years (range 30–83). Thirty-eight patients (43%) were older than 65 years. Symptoms consisted of cervical dysphagia in all patients, pharyngo-oral regurgitation in 44 (49%), and aspiration in 17 (19%). Fifteen patients (17%) also complained of

[1] Istituto di Clinica Chirurgica I, University of Padova Medical School, 35128 Padova, Italy

significant weight loss, and an additional 13 patients (15%) had symptoms of gastroesophageal reflux responsive to medical therapy.

The median size of the diverticula on standard barium roentgenograms was 4 cm (range 2.5–9 cm); the diameter of the diverticula measured less than 3 cm in 5 patients, between 3 and 5 cm in 66, and more than 5 cm in 18. Upper gastrointestinal endoscopy was attempted in the majority of the patients to rule out concomitant disease, but the examination was successfully carried out only in 40 individuals, 9 of whom had grade 1 esophagitis. In 12 patients, the endoscope also served as a guide to insert the manometric catheter in the esophageal body.

Esophageal manometry was performed in 65 patients using a low-compliance perfused system and a catheter assembly with 3 to 5 side-holes oriented 120° to 72° apart, placed at 5-cm intervals from the distal end of the catheter. Of these individuals, 29 (44.6%) showed either hypopharyngeal-upper esophageal sphincter (UES) incoordination ($n = 21$) or incomplete UES relaxation ($n = 8$) on swallowing. Manometric measurements of pharyngeal pressure, UES pressure, and UES length in patients with Zenker's diverticulum did not significantly differ from those obtained in a group of 26 healthy unrelated control subjects, except for a higher UES residual pressure (Table 1). Twenty four-hour esophageal pH monitoring showed an abnormal esophageal acid exposure in 3 of the 13 patients with reflux symptoms, 2 of whom had grade 1 esophagitis.

The operation was usually performed under general anesthesia. In 10 elderly individuals, a C5–C6 super-selective spinal anesthesia was used. A bougie was routinely inserted in the esophagus for use as a stent. The pharyngoesophageal junction was approached through an oblique left cervical incision, anteromedial to the sternocleidomastoid muscle, and centered at the level of the cricoid cartilage. The surgical procedure consisted of a posterior vertical myotomy over a length of 3 to 5 cm distal to the diverticulum neck, and resection of the mobilized pouch using a linear stapling device (TA 30 or 55). A nasogastric tube was then advanced under direct vision into the stomach, and the neck wound was closed leaving a Penrose drain. A gastrographin swallow study was routinely performed on the 4th postoperative day before the patient was started on a soft diet.

Table 1. Manometric measurements at the pharyngoesophageal junction in patients with Zenker's diverticulum and in control subjects (values are mean ± S.D.)

	Patients ($n = 65$)	Controls ($n = 26$)	P
Pharyngeal pressure (mmHg)	36.2 ± 18	33.4 ± 15.3	NS
UES resting pressure (mmHg)	39.1 ± 18	45.9 ± 14.4	NS
UES residual pressure (mmHg)	6.4 ± 9.7	0.8 ± 0.3	<0.02
UES length (cm)	3.1 ± 0.9	3.0 ± 1.1	NS

UES, upper esophageal sphincter

Table 2. Manometric measurements , before and after cricopharyngeal myotomy and stapled Zenker's diverticulectomy in 24 patients (values are mean ± S.D.)

	Pre	Post	P
Pharyngeal pressure (mmHg)	36.4 ± 10	34.3 ± 14	NS
UES resting pressure (mmHg)	38.0 ± 18	20 ± 8.3	<0.001
UES residual pressure (mmHg)	6.2 ± 8.8	0.7 ± 1.4	<0.02
UES length (cm)	3.1 ± 0.6	2.4 ± 0.4	<0.01

Patients were evaluated at 1 month, 6 months, and then at yearly intervals after surgery. A barium swallow study was performed within the 1st year of follow-up in all patients. Esophageal manometry was performed 1 to 30 months postoperatively in 24 patients who volunteered for the test (Table 2).

Results

One patient died from pulmonary embolism during the postoperative period (0.9% mortality rate). The overall morbidity rate was 4.4%: in 2 patients a leak from the stapled suture line occurred, and was treated conservatively with complete healing within 2 weeks; 1 patient had a transient palsy of the left recurrent nerve, and another patient required surgical revision for a wound hematoma. The mean hospital stay was 8 ± 3 days.

Eighty-eight patients were followed from 12 to 149 months (median 44 months). Overall, 83 patients (94.3%) were symptom-free and 4 (4.6%) demonstrated marked clinical improvement. The barium swallow study was normal in all but 1 patient (1.1%) who developed a symptomatic diverticulum 16 months after surgery and required reoperation. Esophageal manometry showed a significant reduction of UES resting tone ($P < 0.001$), residual tone ($P < 0.02$), and length ($P < 0.01$) over preoperative values, indicating a decrease in the outflow resistance at the pharyngoesophageal junction. Hypopharyngeal-UES incoordination persisted only in 2 of 14 patients in the absence of symptoms.

Discussion

Treatment of Zenker's diverticulum is always indicated to relieve the disabling symptoms of cervical dysphagia and pharyngo-oral regurgitation, and to prevent the life-threatening complication of aspiration pneumonia which is of special concern in elderly patients. It has been postulated that gastroesophageal reflux is common in patients with Zenker's diverticulum, and that priority should be given to its surgical correction to prevent postoperative aspiration [2]. Although this did not occur in our experience, we believe that a complete work-up including 24-hour esophageal pH monitoring should be performed to assess the pattern and the degree of exposure to gastric juice in patients with reflux symptoms. In most circumstances, medical treatment with H2 blockers or proton pump inhibitors is effective, allowing the surgeon to proceed primarily with the treatment of the diverticulum. If necessary, however, an antireflux repair can be performed during the same operative session.

During the past three decades, the treatment of Zenker's diverticulum has evolved through a better understanding of the underlying pathophysiology of this disease [10]. Most esophageal surgeons now believe that cricopharyngeal myotomy, alone or combined with diverticulum suspension [11, 12] or resection [5–7, 13], is the essential part of the operation.

The operation can be safely performed under local anesthesia, or, as in our experience, under super-selective spinal anesthesia to minimize the surgical risk in frail elderly patients. We believe that for small diverticular (2 cm or less) there is no need for resection and a simple cricopharyngeal myotomy will suffice to reduce the pouch and abate the symptoms. It has been demonstrated that a residual pouch up to 2 cm will not be evident on standard roentgenograms within 2 weeks of a cricopharyngeal myotomy [5].

The addition of a myotomy to resection or diverticulum suspension seems logical and useful, but no prospective studies have shown a significant advantage in reducing the incidence of leak or late recurrence of the pouch. In our opinion, myotomy should be routinely performed since it does not prolong operative time and does not increase morbidity. No complications due to the myotomy were recorded in our series: only a leak from the staple line occurred in 2 patients (2.2%), and resolved within 2 weeks of conservative treatment.

Manometric abnormalities are common in patients with Zenker's diverticula, justifying the addition of a cricopharyngeal myotomy [4, 14, 15]. This was confirmed in the present study, since about 45% of our patients showed abnormal findings on manometry and, as a group, the residual UES pressure was higher in the study population compared to control subjects. Changes in the morphology and contractility pattern of the cricopharyngeal muscle have been noted in patients with Zenker's diverticulum, supporting the use of myotomy as an essential step in the surgical treatment [16]. Recent studies have also demonstrated an incomplete sphincter opening, which is probably related to a decreased compliance of the proximal esophageal muscle [17]. This finding suggests an increased outflow resistance in these patients which may be underestimated by conventional manometry. Therefore, the myotomy can be effective in preventing pouch recurrence by creating a broader weak area in the muscle over which pharyngeal pressure can be distributed during swallowing.

We conclude that cricopharyngeal myotomy combined with stapling resection is a safe and effective procedure for medium- and large-sized Zenker's diverticula, providing low operative risk and excellent long-term results.

References

1. Wheeler WI (1886) Pharyngocele and dilation of pharynx, with existing diverticulum at lower portion of pharynx lying posterior to the oesophagus, cured by pharyngotomy, being the first case of the kind recorded. Dublin J Med Sci 82:349–357
2. Belsey R (1966) Functional disease of the esophagus. J Thorac Cardiovasc Surg 52:164–188

3. Aubin A (1936) Un cas de diverticule de pulsion de l'oesophage traite' par la resection de la poche associée a l'oesophagotomie extramuqueuse. Ann d'Otolaryngol 2:167–177

4. Ellis FH, Schlegel JF, Lynch VP, Payne WS (1969) Cricopharyngeal myotomy for pharyngoesophageal diverticulum. Ann Surg 170:340–349

5. Orringer M (1980) Extended cervical esophagomyotomy for cricopharyngeal dysfunction. J Thorac Cardiovasc Surg 80:669–678

6. Barthlen W, Feussner H, Hannig C, Holscher AH, Siewert JR (1990) Surgical therapy of Zenker's diverticulum: Low risk and high efficiency. Dysphagia 5:13–19

7. Moreno E, Rico P, Palomo JC, et al (1992) Surgical treatment of Zenker's diverticulum: Review of our experience. Gullet 2:19–23

8. Hoehn JG, Payne WS (1969) Resection of pharyngoesophageal diverticulum using stapling device. Mayo Clin Proc 44:738–741

9. Wolfensberger M, Simmen D (1991) Staple closure of the hypopharynx after diverticulectomy and total laryngectomy. Dysphagia 6:26–29

10. Ferguson MK (1991) Evolution of therapy for pharyngoesophageal (Zenker's) diverticulum. Ann Thorac Surg 51:848–852

11. Duranceau A, Rheault MJ, Jamieson GC (1983) Physiologic response to cricopharyngeal myotomy and diverticulum suspension. Surgery 94:655–662

12. Skinner DB, Altorki N, Ferguson M, Little AG (1988) Zenker's diverticulum: Clinical features and surgical management. Dis Esoph 1:19–22

13. Ribet M, Ghoch K, Pruvot F (1989) Traitement chirurgical du diverticule de Zenker. Lyon Chir 85:213–216

14. Ancona E, Frasson P, Peracchia A (1979) La myotomie du sphincter oesophagien superieur dans les diskinesies pharyngo-oesophagiennes. Ann Chir 33:467–473

15. Bonavina L, Kahn NA, DeMeester TR (1985) Pharyngoesophageal dysfunctions. The role of cricopharyngeal myotomy. Arch Surg 120:541–549

16. Lerut T, Guelinckx P, Done R, Geboes K, Gruwez J (1988) Does the musculus cricopharyngeus play a role in the genesis of Zenker's diverticulum? Enzyme histochemical and contractile properties. In: Siewert JR, Holscher AH (eds) Disease of the esophagus. Springer, Berlin Heidelberg New York, pp 1018–1023

17. Cook I, Gabb M, Panagopulos V, et al (1989) Zenker's diverticulum: A defect in upper oesophageal sphincter compliance? Gastroenterology 96:A-98

Should Modified Heller's Cardiomyotomy Be Combined with Antireflux Procedure?

PAWEŁ MISIUNA and GRZEGORZ WALLNER[1]

Introduction

Achalasia, one of the diffuse motor disorders, is characterized by the absence of the primary peristalsis of the esophagus. The response to normal deglutition is characterized by the absence of peristalsis in the body of the esophagus and the failure of the relaxation usually found in the hypertrophic lower sphincter [1]. The etiology is unknown. Pathologically, achalasia is confirmed by the lack or degeneration of Auerbach's plexus, and structural changes in the muscular layer of the lower esophagus [2, 3]. It leads to dilatation of the esophagus above a functional stricture with typical symptoms: dysphagia especially in emotional situations, vomiting, chest pain, weight loss, and broncho-pulmonary complications [1, 3, 4, 5].

The aim of this work was to give the answer to the question in the title. Particular attention was paid to the presence of gastroesophageal reflux and esophageal delayed emptying.

Methods and Material

Between 1973 and 1990 we operated on 62 patients for achalasia. There were 28 (45.2%) women and 34 (54.8%) men, aged 16 to 76, mean 41 years. The history of symptoms lasted from 3 months to 26 years. Up to 1981 only the modified Heller's operation—anterior cardiomyotomy—was carried out, in a total of 21 patients. Since 1982, in 41 patients we have used anterior cardiomyotomy combined with the antireflux procedure—Nissen Rossetti fundoplication. Only the patients with typical symptoms not responding to conservative treatment or simple dilatation were operated on, after thorough X-ray examination, endoscopy,

[1] Second Department of General Surgery, Medical Academy, Lublin Staszica 16, 20-081 Lublin, Poland

and biopsy. The diagnostic procedure was designed to evaluate the distal esophagus and also to exclude other causes of dysphagia.

In all cases the modified Heller's operation was carried out by thc abdominal approach. During the operation, attention was paid to radical anterior cardiomyotomy of the lower part of the esophagus, about 7–10 cm plus 0.5–1.0 cm of cardia, depending on the anatomical conditions. The trans-thoracic approach was used only for cases demanding reoperation.

The efficiency of cardia and the patients' conditions after the operation were evaluated on the grounds of anamnesis, physical examination, X-ray examination, endoscopy with biopsy, and isotopic scanning. Particular attention was paid to the presence of gastroesophageal reflux and esophageal delayed emptying. Postoperative complaints were estimated according to Visick's scale. X-ray examination as a rule was performed in supine and Trendelenburg positions. We observed the efficacy of the passage through the esophagus and the presence of gastroesophageal reflux. Similarly, in esophagoscopy we looked for endoscopic signs of reflux esophagitis. Specimens obtained during endoscopy were evaluated after hematoxylin and eosin staining. Isotopic scanning was carried out after a night fast. Patients received breakfast with a colloidal solution containing 1.0 mCi of technetium sulfide ^{99m}Tc. Measurements of the radiation from the gastric and esophageal fields were performed 1 h after administration.

As a sign of the delayed emptying of the esophagus, we found the persistence of high radiation levels in the esophagus during the period of investigation. With gastroesophageal reflux, characteristic changes of the radiation distribution between the stomach and esophagus were observed. The decrease of radiation in the stomach paralleled the increase of radiation in the esophagus at the same time.

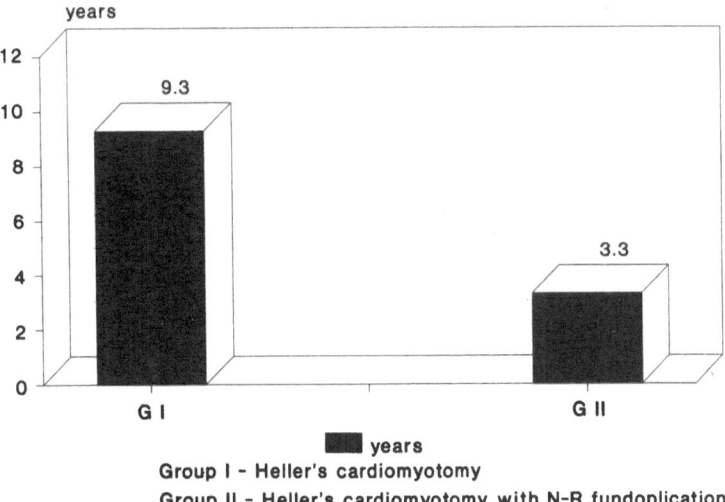

Fig. 1. Follow up. *N-R*, Nissen-Rossetti; *G*, group

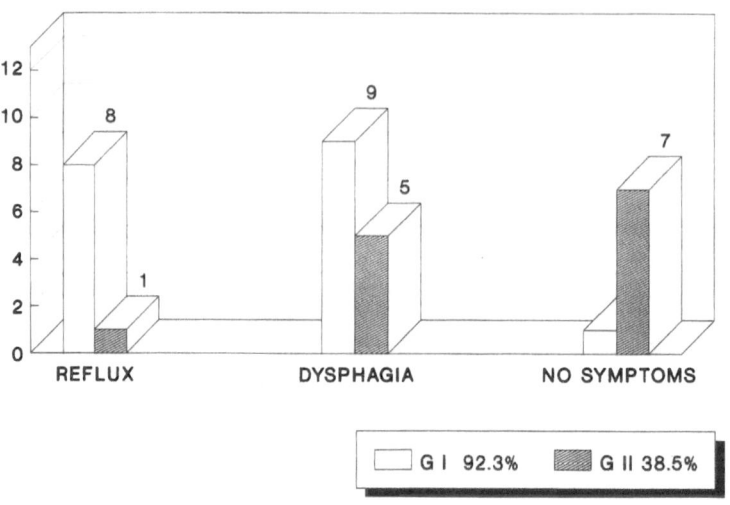

Fig. 2. Anamnesis (Visick's Scale)

Results

Long-term results were assessed in two groups (13 patients each): group I after the modified Heller's operation—simple anterior cardiomyotomy—and group II after cardiomyotomy with the antireflux procedure. The mean control time in group I was 9.3 years; in group II, 3.3 years (Fig. 1).

Analyzing the case-histories, we confirmed that all but one patient of group I had suffered complaints of varying intensity. In group II, only one patient had reflux symptoms, and five patients experienced persistent dysphagia (Fig. 2). Similarly, X-ray examination showed worse results in group I. In group I as well as group II, delayed emptying predominated (Fig. 3). On examination by endoscopy, patients of group I also had more pathological abnormality than group II, mainly inflammation (Fig. 4). With isotopic scanning, reflux was detected at almost the same high level in both groups; however, in this examination we did not observe delayed emptying of the esophagus (Fig. 5). The microscopic studies revealed pathological changes in all of the group I cases, but only four (about 31%) of group II (Fig. 6). These patients were found to have abnormal hyperplasia with keratosis and squamous esophagitis.

Discussion

Surgeons generally agree that the operation of choice in treatment of typical achalasia is modified Heller's cardiomyotomy. However, the question arises whether or not antireflux procedure is needed. After operation for achalasia, we have three possible options. The first is to perform optimal cardiomyotomy. In this situation, the physiological conditions in the lower part of the esophagus are

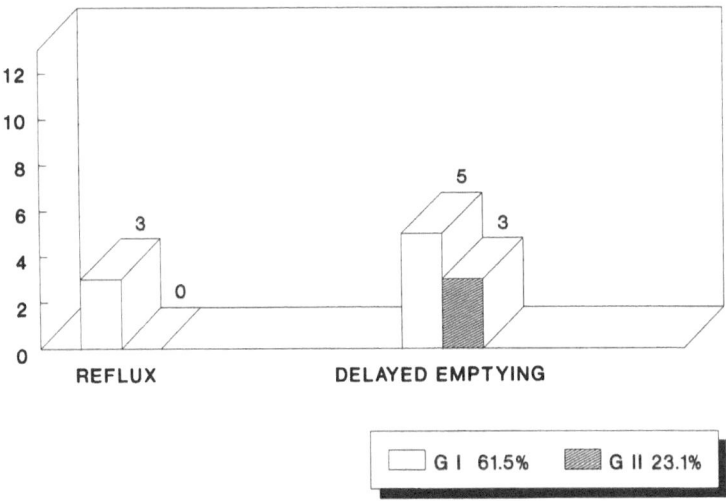

Fig. 3. X-ray examination

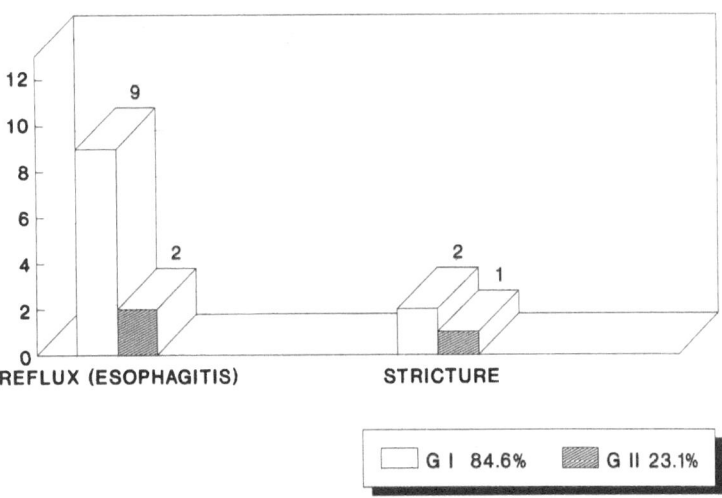

Fig. 4. Endoscopy

preserved and long-term results are excellent. The second option is to perform incomplete cardiomyotomy. This leads to incomplete relaxation of the lower esophageal sphincter. Persistent high pressure in the lower esophagus with dismotility gives dysphagia, and the long-term results are bad. The third situation is when a surgeon performs excessive cardiomyotomy that reduces the pressure in the lower esophageal sphincter to below the normal level. Excessive cardiomyotomy destroys the antireflux mechanism, with all the consequences. The

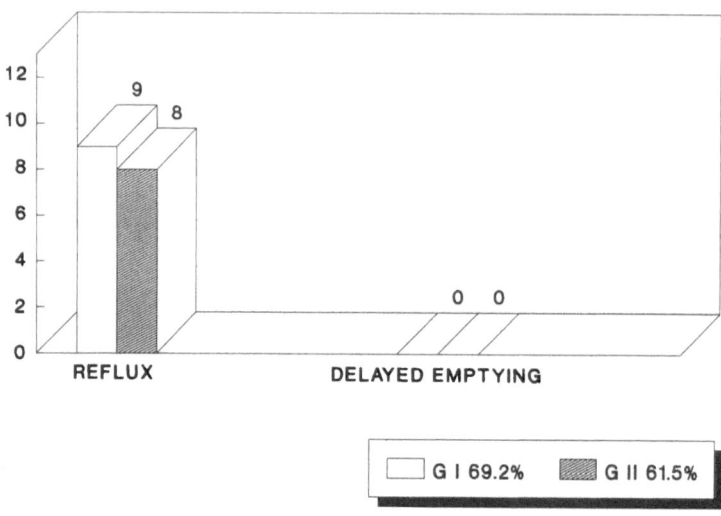

Fig. 5. ^{99m}Tc-scanning

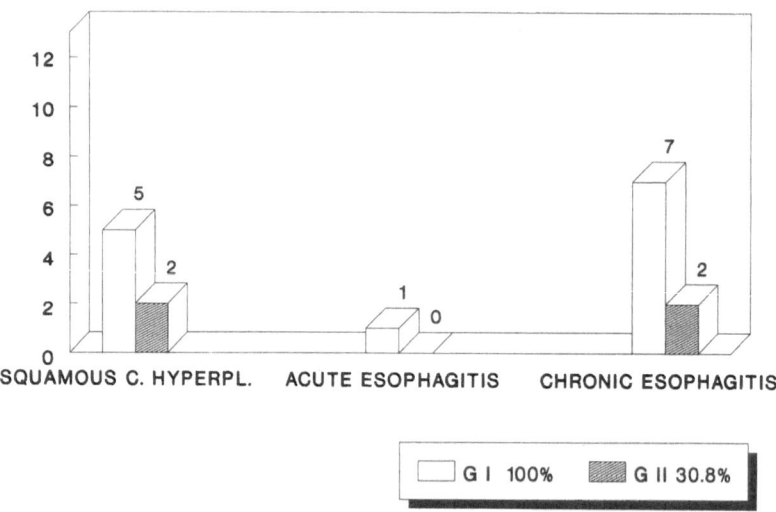

Fig. 6. Histopathology. *C. HYPERPL*, cell hyperplasia

results are bad because of long-term irritation by harmful factors. Patients have pyrosis and chest pain due to reflux esophagitis.

We compared the long-term results in both groups and we conclude that group II gave statistically better results in all diagnostic procedures (Fig. 7). Our results demonstrate that antireflux procedure is indispensable when performing Heller's cardiomyotomy.

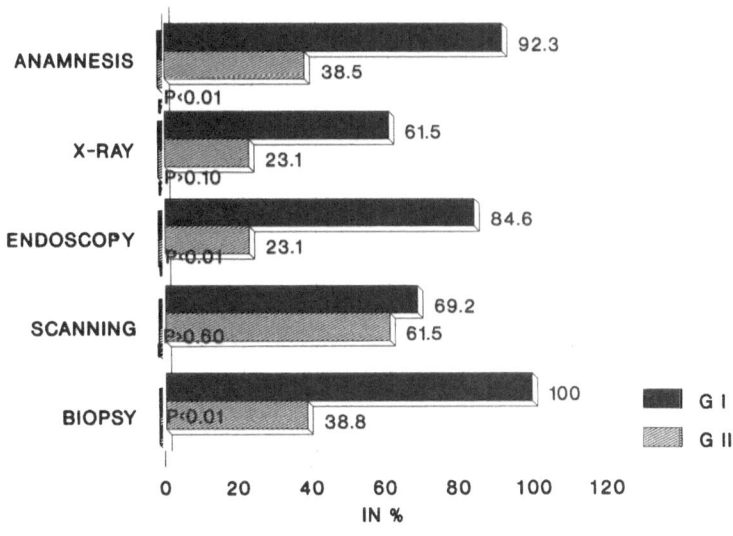

Fig. 7. Statistical data (pathology)

Conclusions

1. After the modified Heller's cardiomyotomy, histopathological changes persist in all patients operated on.
2. Heller's operation should be combined with the antireflux procedure.

References

1. Baunack AR, Weihrauch TR (1988) Classification and diagnosis of esophageal motility disorders. Esophagus 88, Danish Esophagus Club: 165–170
2. Davis JH (1987) Esophagus. In: Van Schaik Th, Manning TA, Clinical surgery. CV Mosby, pp 1398–1402
3. Ellis FH Jr (1984) Esophageal achalasia—is simple esophageal myotomy the treatment of choice? In: Doody DJ, Advances in gastrointestinal surgery. Year Book Medical Publishers, pp 47–55
4. Farmer RG, Achkar E, Flesher B (1983) Motor disorders of the esophagus. In: Farmer RG, Achkar E, Flesher B, Clinical gastroenterology. Raven, pp 157–164
5. Vantrappen G, Hellemens J (1983) Esophageal motility disorders. In: Chey WY, Functional disorders of the digestive tract. Raven, pp 117–124

Megaesophagus in Experimental Chagas' Disease

Masayuki Okumura, Mitsunori Matsuda, Toshiyasu Fujioka, and Kiyoshi Iriya[1,2]

Introduction

Chagas' disease is a parasitosis and its etiological agent is the flagellate protozoa *Trypanosoma cruzi* [1]. The parasite is a hemoflagellate, Phylum Protozoa, subphylum Mastigophora, order Kinetoplastida, suborder Trypanosomatidae, and section Stercoraria. Described for the first time by the Brazilian scientist Carlos Chagas when, during the construction of the Brazilian Central Railway and a malaria prevention program in the town of Lassance in northern Minas Gerais state, his attention was drawn to an hematophagous insect found in the region and known in Brazil by the common name "barbeiro" (barber bug), *Conorhinus megistus*, *Triatoma megistus* and presently *Panstrongylus megistus*. He examined the content of the caudal portion of the insect's intestine and succeeded in isolating a *Trypanosoma* flagellate with "critidia" characteristics.

Some samples of "*Triatomineos*" were sent to Oswaldo Cruz of the Manguinhos Institute in Rio de Janeiro who let them bite a saguin monkey and then isolated the. *T. cruzi*.

Later on, upon examining a sick cat in a home highly infested by the barber bug, he found the *T. cruzi* parasite in the animal's circulation. About 20 days later, in this same house, he came across a feverish child and many insects biting the residents. Previously, the child had been perfectly healthy. Evidence of the flagellate *Trypanosoma cruzi* was found in her circulation [1].

We must admit this is a rare occurrence in the history of medicine: a doctor by himself discovering the etiological agent, the carrier, the sensitive agents (humans and animals) the reservoirs of the viral agent of the disease, with the complete clinical picture, pathologic anatomy and its prevention. All we do not know is whether Chagas prescribed any medication. Ironically, up to the present time, an effective treatment for the chronic stage of the disease is still unknown.

[1] University of S. Paulo Medical School, Av. Dr. Arnaldo 455 (01246 903), S. Paulo, Brazil
[2] Hospital Santa Cruz, Ruá Santa Cruz 398, Vila Mariana, S. Paulo, Caixa Postal 2976, Brazil

Chagasic Megaesophagus

This includes all forms of dilatation, elongation and hypertrophy of the muscle layer of the esophagus, with degeneration of Meissner's and Auerbach's plexuses, with motor changes, without organic or mechanical obstruction of the cardia (achalasia). Until the year 1957, Professor Corrêa Netto's Center emerged as one of the most experienced in dealing with acquired megacolon—megaesophagus. At this time, their hypothesis of "chronic and incomplete deficiency of vitamin B1, was the most generally accepted.

In April 1958 at a meeting of the "Associação Paulista de Medicina", Professor Fritz Koberle, of the University of São Paulo (U.S.P.) Medical School in Ribeirão Preto, Brazil announced his chagasic theory regarding acquired megaesophagus and megacolon. He pointed out the histologic similarity between esophageal and chagasic heart disease. The speaker stated that unfortunately when staining the histologic section to prove his thesis by confirming the presence of the parasite (nest of leishmanias) in the esophagus, it had been destroyed. On the day after the conference, manifesting his noble scientific spirit, professor Alipio Correa Netto, who had been present at the meeting, invited us to investigate the association of Chagas' disease with the "megas" of the digestive tract.

The literature on the subject was sparse. We were familiar only with the studies of Carlos Chagas [1–3] and his colleagues. They included Gaspar Vianna [4] and Neiva and Penna [5] concerning acquired megaesophagus and megacolon associated with Chagas' disease. The finding by Mazza and Jorg [6], of a nest of leishmanias in the esophagus of a naturally infected dog during the acute stage and later confirmed by Alvarenga [7] during the chronic stage.

Laranja, a collaborator of Carlos Chagas in the Manguinhos Institute, studied chagasic heart disease in a Rhesus monkey (F.S. Laranja, 1989, personal communication). Ten years later, this monkey died of pulmonary tuberculosis, and at autopsy Guimarães and Miranda [8] observed a nest of leishmanias in the esophageal muscles.

Koberle [9] was the first to link megaesophagus with Chagas' disease, when he reported finding megaesophagus, megacolon and megabladder in naturally infected dogs. A year after beginning the study, we and Correa Netto were already convinced of the accuracy of the chagasic theory, confirming that the inoculation of *Trypanosoma cruzi* in laboratory animals could produce "megas". In January of 1960, the first reports on the subject were published by the Correa Netto Center. In 1961, Okumura and Correa Netto [10] confirmed the production of "megas" in the digestive tract. It was the first time megaesophagus, megastomach, megacolon and megabladder had been reproduced in experimental Chagas' disease. At the request of Koberle himself, who was anxious to see his theory confirmed, an incomplete preliminary report was published. It is interesting to note that Correa Netto's Center whose pathogenetic theory had been undermined was now supporting and confirming the new hypothesis.

The injury to both the central and peripheral nervous systems by the parasitic infection of the neurons and plexuses by the *Trypanosoma cruzi*, emphasized by Correa Netto's Center and confirmed by Tafuri [11] (ganglionitis and periganglionitis), placed a check on Koberle's neurotoxin theory explaining neuronal destruction in Chagas' disease.

Using the same line of study, in 1976 Marsden et al. [12] were able to produce megaesophagus in Rhesus monkey.

Materials and Methods

Four hundred white male mice (*Mus musculus-L.*) weighing from 20 to 25 g were utilized. They were kept in individual cages for the study of the acute stage of Chagas' disease and in group boxes for the chronic stage. The animals were fed standard rations furnished by the "Bioterio Central" of the U.S.P Medical School. Four hundred mice were also utilized in a second experiment. They were kept in group boxes for the study of the chronic stage of the disease, a total of 800 animals.

At the same time, three 3-month-old puppies from the same litter were inoculated.

Parasite

Trypanosoma cruzi (Y strains) isolated by Silva and Nussenzweig [13] from a patient in the acute stage of Chagas' disease and utilized in the parasitolgy laboratory of the U.S.P. It demonstrated a constant pathogenicity, with marked parasitemia and tissue parasitism in several animal species. Blood specimens (1000) or cultured specimens (10^6) were used for the white mice and 6×10^6 blood specimens were used for the puppies, and they were inoculated either subcutaneously or peritoneally.

The etiologic agent of *Trypanosoma cruzi* is different from that of sleeping sickness (*Trypanosoma gambiense* and *Trypanosoma rhodesiense*) because in the latter, the trypanosome is the only and definitive form since it reproduces in the peripheral blood and lymph nodes and it is also the infecting form. In Chagas' disease, the *Trypanosoma cruzi* has two essential forms: the Trypanosome form which circulates in the peripheral blood and is infectious, and the oval-shaped leishmania which reproduces in the tissues.

The characteristic of the trypanosome of Chagas' disease, is that it circulates in the peripheral blood in the flagellate fusiform shape. It possesses a nucleus, basal body, and kinetoplast. The latter communicates with a flagellus enveloped by the undulating membrane, responsible for its active motion. Upon penetrating a cell, it loses its flagellus and is transformed into an oval leishmania or amastigote with a nucleus and basal body (its reproductive form). By consecutive binary fission, it forms a pseudocyst or nest of leishmanias.

Parasitemia

In order to diagnose the acute stage of Chagas' disease, a specimen of peripheral blood is taken from the inoculated animals and examined for the parasite in the form of a flagellate *Trypanosome*. During the early days after the inoculation, blood is utilized to investigate the parasites because they are rare. After the 5th to 10th day, a Neubauer counting chamber is used. Approximately 5 days after inoculation, the parasitemia increases, achieving its maximum on the 20th day, when it decreases. Minimum values are reached around the 30th day, disappearing from the circulation at 90 days, when the disease enters the chronic stage. The parasites do not disappear completely, they are merely undetectable by ordinary means. They can be isolated by xenodiagnosis or by injecting blood into young sensitive animals.

Histology

The animals were sacrificed using ether inhalation. The chest and abdomen were opened the specimens fixed in a 10% formaldehyde solution for 4 days. The five micro histologic sections were stained with hematoxylin and eosin and other specific stains.

Radiologic Study

Intestinal transit or opaque enema studies were accomplished on mice and adult dogs during the acute stage of the disease (before the 30th day), subacute stage (30th to 90th day) and chronic stage (365 days) after inoculation.

Results

Clinical Picture

Presenting symptoms during the acute stage included paleness around the mouth, nose, ears and tail, and some animals displayed diarrhea, shaggy coats, and listlessness. In the chronic stage, they were smaller in size, with paralysis of the posterior limbs (medular involvement of the disease) and epileptiform attacks, dyspnea and ascitis in some. During the acute stage, the dogs exhibited neurologic changes characterized by nervous tic, tonico-clonic convulsive crises and changes in gait, with a tendency to deviate toward one side during ambulation.

After 1 year, of the 800 mice inoculated with *T. cruzi*, only 105 survived the chronic stage of Chagas' disease. The distribution of the "megas" was as follows: a) bronchiectasis—2 (1.9%); b) megaesophagus—8 (7.8%); c) megastomach—7 (6.7%); d) megaintestine—4 (3.8%); e) megacolon—15 (14.3%); f) megagallbladder—2 (1.9%); g) megabladder—11 (10.5%) and cardiomegaly—12 (11.4%) for a total of 81 (58.1%) types of "megas".

The results of the study utilizing the three dogs from the same litter inoculated with *T. cruzi* at the age of 3 months were as follows: one dog died on the 90th day, his progress was marked by convulsions and megaesophagus was confirmed at autopsy; the second dog died on the 170th day with evidence of cerebellar injury, tonico-clonic convulsions, and nervous tics, with evidence of mega-esophagus. The third animal progressed normally.

Pathogenesis

The trypanosome circulating in the bloodstream penetrates a cell of the reticulo-endothelial system (SRE) or muscle, nerve, adipose, or glandular tissue and is changed into an oval leishmania by losing its flagellum and fusiform shape.

Reproducing intensely by binary fission, the leishmania forms a parasitic nest or pseudocyst. Initially, the nest is compact but becomes loose and increases in volume. With the progression of the leishmanias to the chritidial and trypanosomal (flagellate) stage and due to their active movements, the cellular membrane swells and breaks. The parasites escape together with the cytoplasm and products of cellular breakdown and metabolites into the intersticial space. While the nest (or pseudocyst) is whole, there is no tissue reaction. After the cell ruptures, an inflamatory response, especially lympho-histo-plasmocytic, is initiated, and includes the presence of mastocytes.

Ten days after rupture of the leishmanias nest, the multiplication of fibroblasts that attempt to circumscribe the injured area is evident. A granuloma is outlined and later, with the disappearance of the parasites and cellular debris, is changes into a fibrotic scar.

The thickening of the interstitium of the muscle fibers responsible for the "hypertrophy of the muscle layer" is unleashed by the initial multiplication of the mastocytes [11]. Hypertrophy or hypotrophy of the muscle fibers was found, but not hyperplasy. Tafuri [11] called attention to the extensive fibroplasy dependent on the mastocytosis as the fundamental element explaining the thickening of the muscle layer in the chronic stage of Chagas' disease. When this reaction reaches the region of the nervous plexuses, both the submucosal (Meissner's) and the intermuscular (Auerbach's) plexuses, the neurons are destroyed, causing them to disappear. This reaction is interspersed so that not all the plexuses are affected. Therefore, areas with intact plexuses and neurons are present next to ones with plexular injury and decreased or absent neurons. Besides the intramural autonomous nervous system, the sympathetic ganglia, the nerves and the elements of the central nervous system can be infected by the leishmanias and their respective tissue reaction (glial). Together with the neurons, the satellite cells, Schwann's sheath and fibroblasts of the capsule of the plexus may be infected by the leishmanias.

The vascular reaction is also significant in Chagas' disease. During the acute stage, the perivascular reaction predominates with inflammatory infiltrate causing periarteritis. Subsequently they progress to arteritis with the possibility of thrombosis and at a later stage, necrotizing arteritis. Parasitic infection by leishmanias can be observed both in the endothelium, as well as in the muscle layer and adventitia.

References

1. Chagas C (1909) New human trypanosomiasis (in Portuguese). Mem Inst Oswal do Cruz 1: 159–218
2. Chagas C (1916) Symptoms of American trypanosomiasis (in Portuguese). Mem Inst Oswaldo Cruz 8:5–37
3. Chagas C (1916) American trypanosomiasis (acute type of disease) (in Portuguese). Mem Inst Oswaldo Cruz 8:37–59
4. Vianna G (1911) An anatomopathologic study of "Carlos Chagas' Disease" (in Portuguese). Mem Inst Oswaldo Cruz 3:276–294
5. Neiva A, Penna B (1919) Scientific travels through the Brazilian states of northern Bahia, southern Piauhy and northern and southern Goiaz (in Portuguese). Mem Inst Oswaldo Cruz 8:74–224
6. Mazza S, Jorg ME (1936) Natural fatal infection by S. cruzi in a dog "Pila" Jujuy (in Portuguese), Publ MEPRA 365:411

7. Alvarenga RJ (1960) Histopathology of Chagas' disease and kala-azar in naturally infected dogs (in Portuguese). Hospital (RJ) 57:35–54
8. Guimaräes JP, Miranda A (1959) Megaesophagus in a Rhcsus monkey 10 years after chagasic infection (in Portuguese). An Congr Inter Chagas' Disease (Rio de Janeiro) 2:657–671
9. Koberle F (1957) Pathogenesis of Chagas' Disease (in Portuguese). Rev Goiana Med 3:155–180
10. Okumura M, Correa Netto A (1961) Experimental production of "megas" in animals innoculated with T. cruzi (in Portuguses). Rev Hosp Clin Fac Med S. Paulo 16:338–341
11. Tafuri WL (1974) Ultrastructural changes of the muscle interstitial and nervous structures of the heart, esophagus and intestines in experimental Chagas' disease (in Portuguese). Thesis Belo Horizonte
12. Marsden PD, Seah SKK, Draper CC, Pettitt LE, Miles MA, Voller A (1976) Experimental T. cruzi infections in Rhesus monkeys. II The early chronic phase. Trans R Soc Trop Med Hyg 70:247–251
13. Silva LHP, Nussenzweig V (1953) A strain of T. cruzi highly virulent for white mice (in Portuguese). Folia Clin Ciol S. Paulo 20:191–208

Quantitation of Eosinophils and Mast Cells in Diffuse Oesophageal Spasm

J.P. Duffy[1], I.P. Adams[2], S.J. Darnton[1], and H.R. Matthews[3]

Introduction

It is over 100 years since Osgood, in his paper "a peculiar form of oesophagismus", described the clinical features of the condition we know as diffuse oesophageal spasm (DOS) [1]. However, the aetiology of the disease is still unknown and reports of its pathological features are scant.

The intramural nerve plexus of the oesophagus (Auerbach's plexus) plays a major role in the control and coordination of normal oesophageal contraction. In diffuse oesophageal spasm, ganglion cells and nerves are still present when examined under light microscopy but there are conflicting reports of neural damage when tissue is examined with the electron microscope [2, 3]. It is of interest that in some instances a cellular infiltrate (lymphocytic and in some cases eosinophilic) in the region of Auerbach's plexus has been found [4, 5].

The role of the eosinophil in tissue inflammation has recently received much attention particularly in relationship to bronchial asthma. The role of the mast cell in the early asthmatic reaction is well established. The later asthmatic reaction occurring some 6 to 12 h after antigen challenge is characterised by a cellular infiltrate containing eosinophils. Initially, it was believed these eosinophils were present to modulate the allergic response by detoxifying mast cell products, but it has been shown that eosinophils contain several cytotoxic proteins in their cytoplasmic granules (eosinophilic cationic protein, major basic protein, eosinophil-derived neurotoxin, and eosinophil peroxidase). These proteins and other mediators released by eosinophils are believed to be responsible for the pathological changes of epithelial damage, basement membrane thicken-

[1] Oesophageal Research Laboratory, [2] Oesophageal Function Laboratory and [3] Department of Thoracic Surgery, East Birmingham Hospital NHS Trust, Bordesley Green East, Birmingham, B9 5ST, UK

ing and smooth muscle hypertrophy which result in the smooth muscle spasm and bronchial hyperreactivity that are seen clinically [6].

This study was undertaken to stain and quantify eosinophils and mast cells in Auerbach's plexus in patients with symptomatic diffuse oesophageal spasm to assess whether these cells might be involved in the pathogenesis of this disease (also characterised by disordered smooth muscle contraction).

Methods

Biopsies of the muscular wall of the oesophagus (including both layers of the muscularis propria and the intervening plexus) 1–2 cm above the gastro-esophageal junction were taken at the time of long myotomy for symptomatic diffuse oesophageal spasm. As a control group, biopsies were taken at a similar site from the oesophagus in patients undergoing hiatus hernia repair. The study had local ethical committee approval and patients gave informed consent. There were 9 patients in the DOS group (6 male, 3 female) and 11 patients in the hiatus hernia group (9 male, 2 female). None of the DOS patients had a history of atopy whilst 3 of the hiatus hernia patients did.

The manometric technique was standard throughout the period of study. A 4-lumen manometry catheter (Portex Ltd., UK; modified) was used with each lumen separately perfused with water 0.6 ml/min from a pneumohydraulic infusion pump (Arndorfer, Medical Specialities, Inc., Wis) with separate transducers for pressure measurement. A throat microphone which recorded voluntary swallows and respiration was monitored with a belt pneumograph. All the information was recorded simultaneously on a multichannel pen recorder (Lectromed UK, Ltd., UK). A station pull-through technique was used with the response to at least one dry swallow assessed at each 1-cm interval at a mean of 45 s between each swallow. In those patients diagnosed with DOS, at least 50% of the contractions were simultaneous. Other features present included frequent spontaneous and/or repetetive contractions. Twenty four-hour oesophageal pH testing revealed significant acid reflux in those patients with hiatus hernia but not in those with DOS.

The biopsies were all fixed in buffered formaldehyde for 20–24 h, embedded in paraffin wax, and subsequently sectioned at 3 μm. Sections were stained with a combined histochemical stain, astra blue, and vital new red [7], so that both eosinophils and mast cells could be stained on the same tissue section. Monoclonal antibodies against activated ECP (EG2; Pharmacia, Uppsala, Sweden) were used in an avidin-biotin peroxidase technique to stain activated eosinophils.

A video camera attached to the viewing microscope allowed the image from the microscope to be digitised and displayed on a computer screen. It was possible to manipulate this image with a software package (Revelation 2, Longman Logotron, Cambridge, U.K.) which allowed accurate measurements of areas of the microscope slide. Manual counting of cells within a measured area allowed the number of cells/mm^2 to be expressed.

In ten patients with hiatus hernia and in ten patients with diffuse oesophageal spasm, peripheral blood eosinophil counts were measured using a VCS Coulter counter. All data were statistically analysed using a Mann-Whitney U-test.

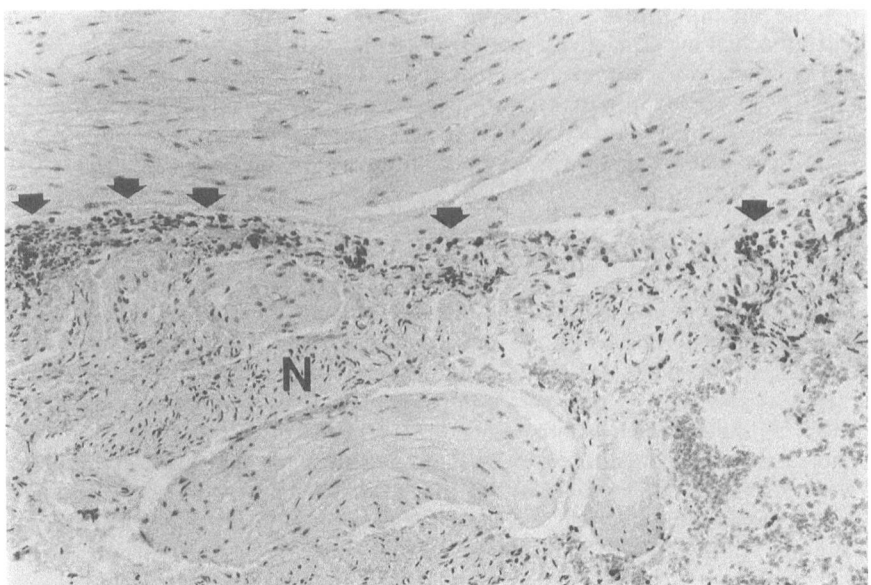

Fig. 1. Eosinophil infiltrate, stained with astra blue/vital new red, in region of Auerbach's plexus in a patient with diffuse oesophageal spasm. (Original magnification 100) A nerve (*N*) is clearly seen. An infiltrate of dark staining eosinophils is indicated with the *arrows*

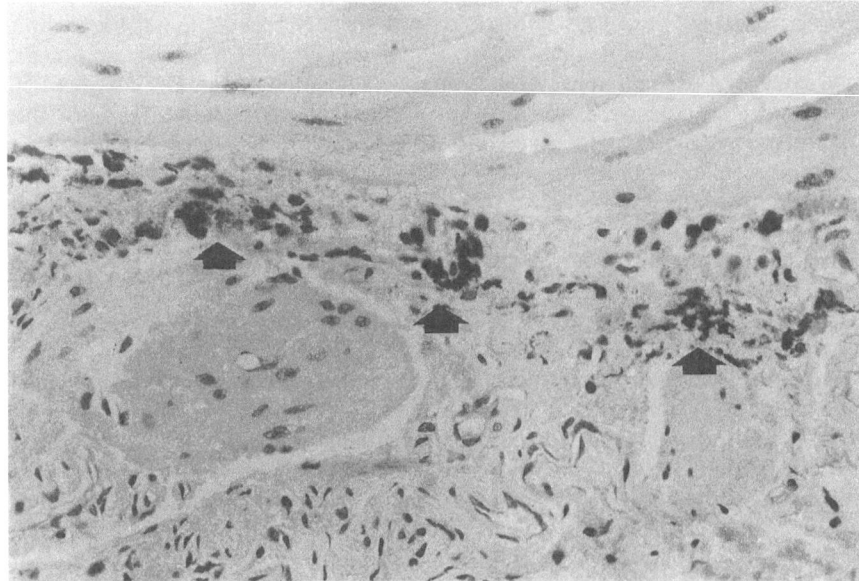

Fig. 2. Eosinophil infiltrate stained with astra blue/vital new red stain in region of Auerbach's plexus in a patient with diffuse oesophageal spasm. Many degranulating eosinophils can be seen (*arrows*). (Original magnification 400)

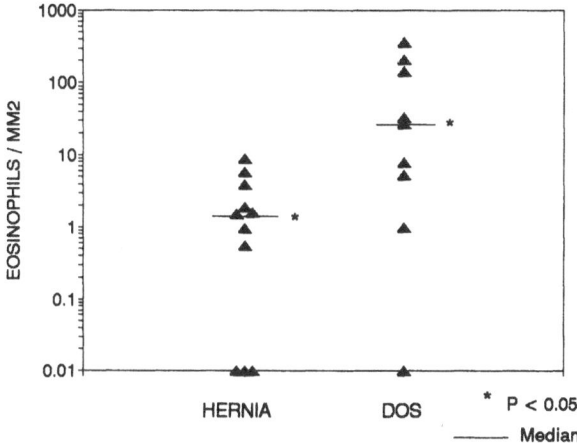

Fig. 3. Counts of eosinophils/mm^2 in region of Auerbach's plexus in biopsies from patients with DOS compared with counts from biopsies taken at time of hiatus hernia repair

Results

In five of the biopsies from patients with DOS, there was an eosinophil infiltrate in the region of Auerbach's plexus. In three cases, this was a very dense infiltrate (Fig. 1). At high power, eosinophils were seen to be degranulating (Fig. 2), and they stained positively with EG2 antibodies suggesting they were activated. This was not seen in any hiatus hernia biopsy.

In all cases of DOS and hiatus hernia, ganglion cells and nerves could still be identified. Mast cells were scattered throughout the intermuscular connective tissue and there were no dense collections.

Quantitation revealed a median of 1.6 eosinophils/mm^2 in the hiatus hernia biopsies compared to 27 cells/mm^2 in those from patients with DOS. This was statistically significant ($P < 0.05$) (Fig. 3).

In contrast, there was no significant difference in mast cell counts between the two groups: a median of 75 cells/mm^2 in hiatus hernia compared to 65 cells/mm^2 in DOS ($P > 0.05$).

Comparison of peripheral blood eosinophil counts revealed no significant difference between hiatus hernia and DOS patients, both groups having results within the normal range for our laboratory ($<0.44 \times 10^9$/l).

Discussion

Diffuse oesophageal spasm only rarely is treated surgically, and therefore the opportunity to study pathological changes within the muscle wall of the oesophagus is limited. This is the first study to stain for eosinophils and mast cells specifically and to perform quantitative analysis.

Nicks et al. [4] studied muscle biopsies taken from patients with manometrically proven DOS at the time of myotomy. Although eosinophils were neither stained for specifically nor quantified, they were noted in varying numbers. Their presence was thought to be a nonspecific response to operative trauma.

Studies of idiopathic muscular hypertrophy of the oesophagus, a condition where a thickened oesophagus is found at postmortem in patients who have often had no oesophageal symptoms during life, have shown an inflammatory infiltrate in less than half the cases and an eosinophilic infiltrate in some [8]. Although these cases are of interest, their relationship to symptomatic diffuse oesophageal spasm is unclear and the underlying disease process could be different.

We used hiatus hernia patients as controls since biopsies could be taken and processed in a similar way to those from patients with DOS. It is known that eosinophils may be found in the mucosa in reflux disease but we found very few in Auerbach's plexus. This is in keeping with studies we have done of resected oesophagus where intense infiltration of the lamina propria, when it occurred, was not associated with an infiltrate in Auerbach's plexus.

Our evidence suggests that DOS is associated with a significant infiltrate of activated eosinophils in the region of Auerbach's plexus, although the stimulus for eosinophil accumulation is unknown. In asthma, the disease is often associated with a clearly defined allergen and may be associated with a peripheral eosinophilia. In our patients, there was no suggestion of associated allergy and the eosinophil counts were within the normal range. In asthma, where mast cells have a significant role in the disease, there is often no increase in the numbers of mast cells seen in the tissues despite evidence for mast cell degranulation [9]. Thus, although we did not find an increase in mast cell numbers in DOS, this does not necessarily mean they are not involved in the inflammatory response.

The clinical implication of this eosinophil infiltrate in DOS is that treatment directed against the eosinophil, as used in asthma with some success, might also be effective in diffuse oesophageal spasm. This is a subject that will be part of our future research.

Acknowledgements. JPD and SJD are funded by OCRA (Oesophageal Cancer Research Appeal, Birmingham, UK)

References

1. Osgood H (1989) A peculiar form of oesophagismus. Boston Med Surg J 120:401–405
2. Friesen DL, Henderson RD, Hanna W (1983) Ultrastructure of the esophageal muscle in achalasia and diffuse esophageal spasm. Am J Clin Pathol 79:319–325
3. Cassella RR, Ellis FH, Brown AL (1965) Diffuse spasm of the lower part of the esophagus. Fine structure of esophageal smooth muscle and nerve. JAMA 191:379–382
4. Nicks R, Gillies M, Skyring A (1968) Diffuse musclar spasm (Diffuse muscular hypertrophy of the oesophagus). Bull Soc Int Chir 6:637–649
5. Marston EL, Bradshaw HH (1959) Idiopathic muscular hypertrophy of the esophagus. J Thorac Cardiovasc Surg 38:248–252
6. Johnston SL, Holgate ST (1991) The inflammatory response in asthma. Br J Hosp Med 46:84–90

7. Duffy JP, Smith PJ, Crocker J (to be published) Combined staining method for the demonstration of tissue eosinophils and mast cells. J. Histotechnol
8. Sloper JC (1954) Idiopathic diffuse muscular hypertrophy of the lower oesophagus. Thorax 9:136–146
9. Jeffrey PK (1992) Pathology of asthma. Br Med Bull 48:23–29

Achalasia: The Length of the Esophagus and the Response to Treatment

RODNEY JOHN MASON and CEDRIC GORDON BREMNER[1]

Introduction

Achalasia of the esophagus is a disease of unknown etiology, characterized by increased esophageal outflow resistance and absent body peristalsis. These two factors gradually lead to a progressive decompensation in function and a progressive increase in diameter. Whether the increase in diameter is related to functional decompensation or outflow, obstruction is conjectural. The decompensation is manifest clinically by increasing dysphagia and regurgitation, radiologically by an increase in the diameter and tortuosity of the esophagus, and manometrically by a decrease in swallow response amplitude. The lower esophageal sphincter pressure is increased in some achalasic patients, and whether the high pressure is related to simultaneous increases in length and diameter of the esophagus as well as a decrease in function is also not established. We measured the esophageal length in normal adults and achalasic patients manometrically, and correlated the results with the patients height. The aim was to determine if esophageal length could be used as a measure of esophageal decompensation. In a separate group, we assessed the changes in length following pneumatic dilatation or surgical myotomy.

Material and Methods

Between 1976 and 1992, 146 consecutive achalasia patients were seen in consultation or treated at the Johannesburg Hospital's esophageal clinic. There were 78 female and 68 male patients ranging in age from 9 to 86 years (average age 42 years). The average duration of symptoms was 49 months and the

[1] Department of Surgery, University of the Witwatersrand, 7 York Road, Parktown, 2193, Johannesburg, South Africa

diagnosis was usually based on a combination of radiographic, endoscopic and motility findings. Esophageal motility studies were performed in each patient using open-tipped perfused catheters (Arndorfer system) [1, 2] and a station pull-through technique. Patients' height in stockinged feet was assessed before each test. The length of the esophagus was assessed by measuring the distance between the distal border of the cricopharyngeal sphincter and the proximal border of the lower esophageal high pressure zone. For each patient, the mean distance of the various channels of the manometry catheter was used. The lower esophageal sphincter pressure was measured in mmHg, and was referenced relative to the end inspiratory gastric pressure. The barium studies were also reviewed and evaluated with regard to grade of tortuosity, maximum diameter of the esophagus and by calculating the ratio of the esophagus measured at its largest diameter, to the height of a mid-thoracic vertebra [3].

Nine patients (four males, five females, average age 51 years old) were also studied following pneumatic dilatation and a further nine patients (six males, three females, average age 43 years) after surgical myotomy. Follow-up manometric evaluation was performed after a mean of 31 months following myotomy and after a mean of 32 months following pneumatic dilatation. Comparisons were made with the esophageal length in 42 normal volunteer patients who had no history of any foregut disorders and esophageal symptoms and had no previous surgery.

Description of Procedures Employed

Pneumatic Dilatation

A Regiflex TTS (Microvasive) balloon (35 to 40 mm) was employed for the dilatations which were performed under sedation and radiological screening. The balloon was placed across the gastroesophageal junction and inflated to a pressure of 18–20 pounds per square inch for 1 min. After dilatation, a water soluble contrast study was performed.

Esophagomyotomy

A modified (Ellis) limited myotomy technique [3] was employed via an abdominal incision. The esophagus was identified and mobilized taking care to avoid the vagus nerve. The narrowed lower esophageal segment was identified, and a longitudinal incision of the longitudinal and circular muscle of the esophagus was performed. The gastric extension of the incision was limited to a few millimeters onto the stomach. No antireflux procedures were performed.

Statistical Methods

The differences between the patients and controls was determined using unpaired t-tests and ANOVA. The correlation between height and esophageal length was performed using a simple linear regression model. The differences post-treatment were determined using paired t-tests.

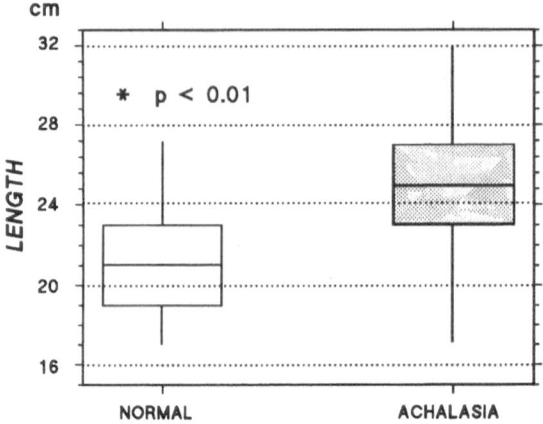

Fig. 1. Box whisker plot of esophageal length in normal adults and untreated achalasic patients

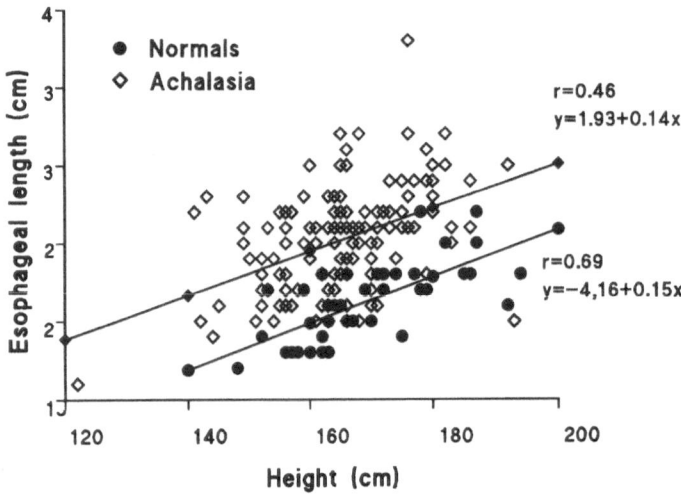

Fig. 2. Correlation between esophageal length and patients' height (cm) in normal adults and in untreated achalasic patients

Results

There were no perforations or deaths in the treated patients. The normal length of the esophagus is demonstrated in Figs. 1 and 2. A significant increase ($P < 0.01$) in esophageal length in achalasic patients was demonstrated. The length of the esophagus following pneumatic dilatation and surgical myotomy are summarized in Fig. 3. Note the significant ($P < 0.05$) decrease in length follow-

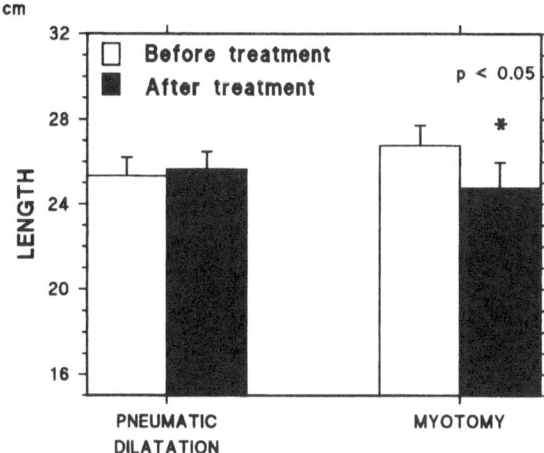

Fig. 3. Bar graph depicting effect of treatment on esophageal length in achalasic patients treated by pneumatic dilatation versus myotomy

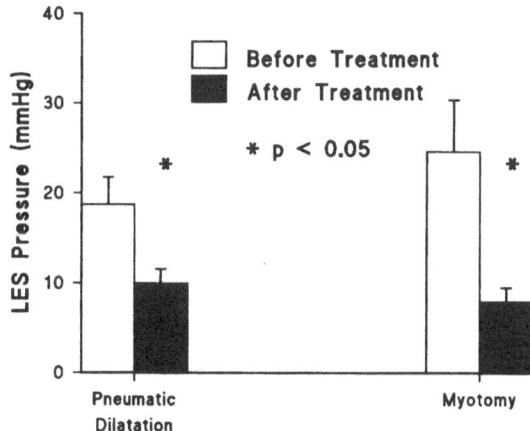

Fig. 4. Lower esophageal sphincter pressure before and after treatment in achalasic patients treated by pneumatic dilatation versus myotomy. *LES*, lower esophageal sphincter

ing myotomy but no change following pneumatic dilatation. The lower esophageal sphincter pressure decreased significantly following both procedures (Fig. 4).

The average lower sphincter pressure following pneumatic dilatation was 12 mmHg and following myotomy was 8 mmHg. The average duration of symptoms for the pneumatically treated group was 45 months and for the myotomy group was 48 months. The average diameter of the esophagus for the pneumatically treated group was 40 mm and 47 mm for the myotomy group. The average age of the pneumatic dilatation group was older than the myotomy group. None of these differences were statistically significant.

Discussion

The length of the esophagus in achalasia is increased significantly when compared to normal adults. The length decreased significantly following surgical myotomy, but not after pneumatic dilatation. A decrease in length may be an indicator of a more complete relief of outflow obstruction. Lower esophageal sphincter pressure was reduced to a greater extent following myotomy than after pneumatic dilatation. These results are in keeping with a previous report in which the diameter of the esophagus following myotomy was more reduced than in the series which were dilated [5, 6]. The ability of the esophagus to shorten after relief of outflow obstruction may depend on the denervation and degree of decompensation. The average age of the patients pneumatically treated was older than the myotomy group. However, this reflects our unit's policy of treating older patients with pneumatic dilatation rather than myotomy and does not indicate that these patients had a greater degree of decompensation initially. The duration of symptoms in the two groups was similar and the maximum diameter of the esophagus was the same in both groups, indicating a comparable degree of esophageal decompensation.

There is considerable debate regarding the treatment of the totally decompensated esophagus. Orringer and Stirling [7] and Ellis [8] advocate esophageal resection in megaesophagus or failed treatment by pneumatic dilatation or myotomy. Orringer's definition of a megaesophagus is one in which the diameter exceeds 8 cm. Richter, [9] however advocates dilatation even in megaesophagus. Certainly, objective evaluation of the pathophysiology of esophageal decompensation is warranted in an effort to define which patients are more likely to respond to conservative management. We feel that esophageal length is a more objective measure of decompensation than conventionally used history and maximum esophageal diameter. History is subjective and maximum diameter of the oesophagus depends on too many variables, namely the amount of barium swallowed, the timing of the x-ray, the orientation of the x-ray plate, phase of respiration and distance of the patient from the x-ray plate, etc. It is for these reasons we advocate using esophageal length as a more objective evaluation of decompensation.

Our hypothesis is that failure of reduction of esophageal length following treatment is an indicator of either irreversible decompensation or inadequate treatment. This would possibly indicate that alternative treatment options should be considered. We also feel that esophageal length could also be a useful tool in the follow up of treated achalasics, and we feel that this modality should be used in the follow-up of all achalasics whether treated medically or surgically. Our results with a limited series suggest that PD is less effective than myotomy because the length does not shorten after dilatation (Fig. 3).

References

1. Arndorfer RC, Stef JJ, Dodds WJ, Linehan ME, Hogan WJ (1977) Improved infusion system for intraluminal esophageal manometry. Gastroenterology 73:23–27
2. Dodds WJ, Hogan WJ, Arndorfer RC, Dent J (1978) Efficient manometric technique for accurate regional measurement of esophageal body motor activity. Am J Gastroenterolol 70:21–24

3. Goldenberg SP, Burrell M, Fette GG, Vos C, Traube M (1991) Classic and Vigorous Achalasia: A comparison of manometric, radiographic, and clinical findings. Gastroenterol 101:743–748

4. Ellis FH Jr, Gibb SP, et al (1980) Esophagomyotomy for achalasia of the esophagus. Ann Surg. 192:157–161

5. Csendes A, Braghetto I, Henriquez A, Cortes C (1989) Late results of a prospective randomised study comparing forceful dilatation and oesophagomyotomy in patients with achalasia. Gut 30:299–304

6. Parilla Paricio P, Martinez de Haro L, Ortiz A, Aquayo JL (1990) Achalasia of the cardia: long term results of oesophagomyotomy and posterior fundoplication. Br J Surg 77: 1371–1374

7. Orringer MB, Stirling MC (1989) Esophageal Resection for Achalasia: Indications and Results. Ann Thorac Surg 47:340–5

8. Ellis FH Jr (1989) Esophagectomy for Achalasia: Who, When, and How Much? Ann Thorac Surg 47:334–5

9. Richter JE (1991) Achalasia: Whether the knife or balloon? Not such a difficult question. Am J Gastroenterol 86: 7:810–811

Primary Heller's Myotomy and Belsey Repair for Achalasia of the Esophagus

C. Iascone, A. Moraldi, P. Addario Chieco, S. Moscetti, M. Barreca, and S. Stipa[1]

Introduction

Esophageal myotomy is a widely accepted treatment in patients with achalasia. However, a definite incidence of reflux and peptic strictures has been described after simple myotomy [1, 2]. Therefore, in the last few decades, several types of antireflux procedure have been added to esophageal myotomy to prevent these complications [3–5]. At the First Department of Surgery of the University of Rome "La Sapienza," the modified Belsey repair has been added to myotomy on a routine basis since 1972.

The aim of this study was to evaluate the long-term clinical results of this procedure in 88 consecutive patients with achalasia, proved on manometry, who were operated upon from 1972 through December 1991.

Methods

The group for this study consisted of 62 males and 26 females, with a mean age of 44 years. In six patients the myotomy and Belsey repair was the second or third procedure after failure of previous operations performed elsewhere. During the follow-up all patients but three, who were lost, underwent repeated roentgenographic and clinical evaluations based on a specific questionnaire. Instrumental work-up, consisting of upper gastrointestinal endoscopy, esophageal manometry, and 24-h pH monitoring of the esophagus, was not routinely performed, except in symptomatic patients.

Seventy-nine patients with primary operations were eligible for long-term evaluation (lost patients and patients with failed previous procedures were

[1] First Department of Surgery, University of Rome "La Sapienza," Via Maurolico 3, 00146 Rome, Italy

excluded). Mean follow-up time was 92 months (range 6–228 months), with fifty patients having 5 years' minimum follow-up. This latter group was broken down into two subsets; the results of surgical treatment of 23 subjects with follow-up ranging between 5 and 10 years, were compared to those of 27 patients with follow-up ranging from 10 to 18 years.

Results

Short-Term Results

There were no operative deaths. Five patients (5.7%) experienced complications (two pneumonitis, one rib osteomyelitis, one superficial wound infection, and one postoperative respiratory distress requiring 48-h intubation) that did not affect the patients' discharge.

Long-Term Results

Good to excellent results (absent or occasional esophageal symptoms) were achieved in 63 patients (80%), and fair results in 8 patients (10%) (patients who, although improved, showed esophageal symptoms more than occasionally or required medical treatment). Surgical failures were observed in 8 patients (10%), due to recurrent dysphagia in 4 cases or to a combination of reflux and obstructive symptoms in the remaining 4 cases. No patient developed peptic strictures; erosive esophagitis was observed in two subjects and healed with medical therapy.

When asked for a personal assessment on operative results, 30 patients (38%) declared themselves to be cured, 22 patients greatly improved (28%), 20 patients improved (25%), and one was unchanged. In six cases, the patient's personal judgement was unknown.

When results of surgical therapy were compared in subsets with different lengths of follow-up, good to excellent results were achieved in 19 out of 23 patients (83%) with follow-up ranging from 5 to 10 years and in 19 out of 27 patients (70%) with follow-up ranging from 10 to 18 years. The corresponding numbers for fair results were 2 (8.7%) and 4 (15%) respectively. Similarly, failures totalled 2 (8.7%) in the former group and 4 (15%) in the latter.

Esophageal complaints were analyzed in detail in all symptomatic subjects (patients with good results, fair results, or failures): heartburn was observed in 5 patients with follow-up from 5 to 10 years (22%) and in 16 patients with follow-up from 10 to 18 years (59%) ($P < 0.02$); regurgitation was found in 1 patient (4%) and 8 patients (30%) respectively ($P < 0.02$).

Fifteen patients (65%) in the group with follow-up from 5 to 10 years and 15 patients (56%) in the group with follow-up from 10 to 18 years complained of dysphagia (P = n.s.). Retrosternal pain was observed in one patient (4%) and five patients (18%) respectively (P = n.s.). In the majority of patients, the above-mentioned symptoms were only occasionally present, as moderate heartburn was reported by 9% of patients with follow-up between 5 and 10 years and by 14% of patients with follow-up of 10 to 18 years. The frequency of moderate regurgitation was 0% and 15% respectively. Finally, moderate dysphagic problems were present in 13% of patients with follow-up between 5 and 10 years and in 19% of those with follow-up longer than 10 years.

Discussion

The treatment of choice for achalasia of the esophagus is still controversial [6, 7]. As etiologic factors of this disease are still unknown, palliative treatment of symptoms is the current goal of therapy, the restoration of the swallowing function being the major target, avoiding as well the onset of new symptoms over the long-term.

However, simple myotomy is associated with gastroesophageal reflux which increases in the long-term follow-up [1] and is complicated by peptic strictures in 5%–20% of patients [1, 8, 9]. Therefore, the association of myotomy with one of several antireflux procedures is presently the approach performed in more than 80% of patients undergoing surgery for achalasia [10]. In this regard, our experience shows that left thoracotomy is a safe procedure without mortality and with negligible morbidity. Furthermore, the modified Belsey repair is able to prevent reflux complications without interfering with palliative treatment of dysphagia, as suggested by 80% relief of dysphagia and 2.5% incidence of erosive esophagitis after a mean follow-up of 10 years. However, it must be stressed that achalasic patients, submitted to myotomy and Belsey repair, become more symptomatic with the years, as indicated by comparative results of subsets of patients with different lengths of follow-up. Heartburn and regurgitation were significantly more frequently observed in subjects with longer follow-up than in patients with shorter follow-up. However, these symptoms were occasional in most patients. These data suggest a slight deterioration of the antireflux ability of the fundoplication and a progressive derangement of the motor activity of the esophageal body, as shown by absent motor response to swallows, in seven out of seven patients with unsatisfactory results, who had volunteered for manometric tests several years after surgery. In spite of these findings, 10 or more years after the initial operation, 70% of patients have objectively satisfactory palliation of their symptoms, and 98% report themselves to be cured or improved by the operative procedure performed.

References

1. Jara FM, Toledo Pereira LH, Lewis JW, Magilligan DJ Jr (1979) Long-term results of esophagomyotomy for achalasia of the esophagus. Arch Surg 114:935
2. Scott HW Jr, Delozier JB III, Sawjers JL, Adkins RB Jr (1985) Surgical management of esophageal achalasia. South MED J 78:1309
3. Hiebert CA (1988) Long-term follow-up of patients with achalasia treated by myotomy and partial fundoplication. In: Siewert JR, Hoelsher AH (eds) Diseases of the esophagus: Pathophysiology, diagnosis, conservative and surgical treatment. Springer Berlin Heidelberg, p 962
4. Stipa S, Fegiz G, Iascone C, Paolini A, De Marchi C, Addario Chieco P (1990) Heller-Belsey and Heller-Nissen operations for achalasia of the esophagus. Surg Gynecol Obstet 170:212
5. Csendes A, Braghetto I, Mascaro G, Henriquez A (1988) Later subjective and objective evaluation of the result of esophagomyotomy in 100 patients with achalasia of the esophagus. Surgery 104:489
6. Csendes A, Braghetto I, Henriquez A, Cortes C (1989) Late results of prospective randomized study comparing forceful dilatation and esophagomyotomy in patients with achalasia. Gut 30:299

7. Barki JS, Guelrud M, Reiner DK (1990) Forceful balloon dilatation: An outpatient procedure for achalasia. Gastrointest Endosc 36(2):123
8. Tomlinson P, Grant A (1981) A review of 74 patients with esophageal achalasia. Aust N Z J Surg 51:48
9. Menzies-Gown J, Gunner JWP, Edwards DAW (1978) Results of Heller's operation for achalasia of the cardia. Br J Surg 65:483
10. Moreno Gonzales E, Garcia Alvarez A, Landa Garcia I, Gomez Gutierrez M, Rico Selas P, Garcia Garcia I, Jouer Navalon JM, Arias Diaz J (1988) Results of surgical treatment of esophageal achalasia. Multicenter retrospective study of 1856 cases. Int Surg 73:69

Long-Term Follow-Up of Heller Myotomy for Achalasia After Thoracic, Abdominal, and Thoracoabdominal Approach

C. Ricci[1], F. Francioni[1], P. Trentino[2], R. Basile[1], T. De Giacomo[1], F. Venuta[1], and F. Silvestri[2]

Introduction

The objective of therapy for achalasia of the esophagus is to relieve the functional obstruction at the esophagogastric junction avoiding at the same time gastroesophageal reflux (GER).

There are two effective means of treating achalasia: forceful dilatation and surgical esophagomyotomy. Surgical treatment may provide satisfactory results in more than 90% of patient; however, the best surgical approach for the performance of myotomy and whether an antireflux procedure (AP) should be performed at the time of myotomy are still controversial. In our study, we report the results of 202 patients who underwent Heller's myotomy through three different surgical approaches with or without antireflux procedures.

Subjects and Methods

From 1960 to 1991, we experienced 262 patients with esophageal achalasia. The mean age was 43 ± 18 years and the M/F ratio was 0.6 (97 male and 165 female). Clinical data obtained in this series were typical of achalasia, and symptoms varied from 2 months to 25 years in duration with a median of 5 years. The stage of the disease determined by the degree of esophageal dilatation on Rx esophagogram was classified as stage I, <3.5 cm ($n = 88$, 34%); stage II, 3.5–6 cm ($n = 119$, 45%); stage III, >6 cm ($n = 45$, 17%); and stage IV, a sigmoid esophagus ($n = 10$, 4%).

Two hundred and twenty-seven patients underwent Heller's myotomy performed through a thoracic approach from 1960 to 1974 ($n = 129$), and after 1974

Department of Thoracic Surgery[1], Surgical Endoscopic Unit[2], Second Surgical Clinic, University "La Sapienza" Viale del Policlinico 161 0016 Rome Italy

we performed the myotomy through an abdominal approach with an antireflux procedure ($n = 50$), or through a combined (thoracic-abdominal) approach ($n = 48$).

Surgical Techniques

Thoracic Approach

Between 1960 and 1974, 129 patients were operated on through a left thoracotomy (T group). The lower esophagus, after incision of the mediastinal pleura, was gently elevated without disruption of hiatal attachments. The myotomy is deepened through circular muscle until the mucosa and extended 5–7 cm in length, several millimeters onto the stomach wall and continued up the esophageal wall for 6–7 cm.

Abdominal Approach

Since 1974, 50 patients were operated on by Heller's myotomy through an abdominal approach (A group). The length of the myotomy was from the dilated portion of the esophagus onto the stomach for 2 cm. An antireflux procedure was associated with the myotomy in all cases. In 12 cases, a Lortat-Jacob procedure was chosen, in 4 cases a Nissen operation, and in 34, as we do today, a Dor anterior hemifundoplication. In the latter procedure the apex of the fundus was secured to the superior limit of the myotomy and the two margins of myotomy were sutured to the fundus.

Thoraco-Abdominal Approach

In the T-A group, a left posterolateral thoracotomy, in the seventh intercostal space, was performed to reach the middle and lower esophagus as far as the lower pulmonary vein. The diaphragmatic hiatus was opened by a radial incision no more than 4 cm, and mobilization of gastroesophageal junction was not carried out. The myotomy was extended from the lower pulmonary vein to the cardial muscle fibers of the so-called Helvetius' collar. In this approach, it is very important to respect all anatomic structures which fix the esophagus and the stomach to the diaphragm and to the posterior wall of the abdomen, and also to respect the angle of His. The edges of myotomy are sutured to the borders of the hiatus, fixing the diaphragm as high as possible, which prevents the myotomy scar. The myotomy incision tends to remain open due to pressure created by diaphragmatic action.

Results

There were no postoperative deaths in the three different groups. Four postoperative complications due to left pleural empyema were observed: All patients recovered completely with chest drain. A follow-up from 6 to 29 years was possible in 202 cases. It was possible to control 115 patients in the T group, 43 in the A group, and 44 in the T-A group.

The symptomatic assessment of results took into account dysphagia and gastroesophageal reflux symptoms. Dysphagia results were classified as follows: excellent, free of symptoms; good, dysphagia once a week; fair, dysphagia more than once a week and no weight loss or regurgitation; and poor, dysphagia, regurgitation, and weight loss.

Improvement of symptoms was obtained in 86% of the cases. The thoracic approach, with the longest follow-up (18–29 years), allowed an improvement of achalasic symptoms in 80% of the cases. Poor results were observed in 16 cases (14%) due to an incomplete myotomy, in 4 cases (3.50%) due to severe peptic stenosis, and in two other cases (2.0%) to esophageal carcinomas which were demonstrated after 16 and 23 years from primary surgical treatment. In one case, we performed a transhiatal esophagectomy with isoperistaltic gastric tube reconstruction for a sigmoid esophagus with severe stasis esophagitis after 5 years from the esophagomyotomy.

The long-term follow-up of transabdominal myotomy showed an improvement of symptoms in 93% of patients. In this group, poor results were due to an inadequate myotomy in one case only, while in two other cases reoperation was necessary for a hiatal hernia.

No reoperations were performed in the group of patients who underwent myotomy with a Dor antireflux procedure. Follow-up of T-A group revealed improvement in 95% of all cases in this group. A poor result was demonstrated in only two patients.

Clinical symptoms of gastroesophageal reflux were obtained from 47 patients (23%). One hundred and fifteen operated patients did not have the antireflux procedure: in these, GER was more frequent (30%). Only four required reoperation for peptic stenosis, and all other patients were easily controlled by medical antireflux treatment. In groups A ($n = 43$) and T-A, ($n = 44$) the percentage of GER symptoms was 14% and 11%, respectively; but if we consider only the group which underwent a Dor procedure, the percentage of GER symptomatology is only 10%. In all these patients, an antireflux medical therapy completely controlled their symptomatology.

In 119 cases taken from all three groups, it was possible to compare the esophagography before and at time of follow-up. In stage I, II, and III, it was possible to demonstrate a significant reduction of the maximum diameter of esophageal body, while in cases of sigmoid esophagus no significant reduction was found.

In 38 patients, it was possible to compare the pre- and postoperative pH-manometric findings; in one patient esophageal peristalsis reappeared, and lower esophageal sphincter inhibition was present in seven patients (18%). The 24-h pH-metry showed GER in ten patients (26%), but four of them were completely asymptomatic.

Discussion

Esophagomyotomy is the operation of choice for treatment of achalasia. The myotomy may be performed transabdominally or transthoracically with or without an antireflux procedure. The mortality for Heller's myotomy has been reported as 0.2% [1], although in our series we had no postoperative mortality. Our study

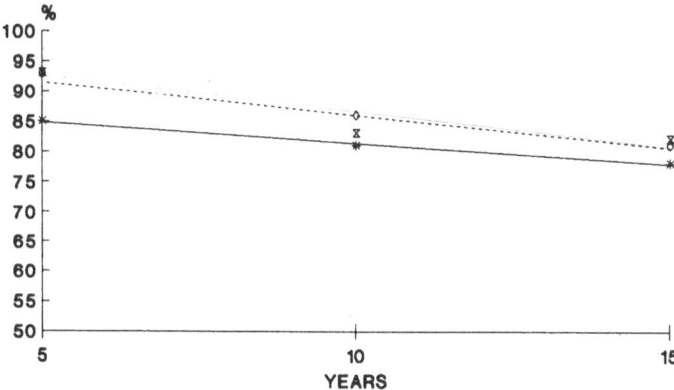

Fig. 1. Long-term symptomatic results—trend of improvement in 202 cases. Follow-up: 5–29 years. *Solid line*, T group (*n* = 115); *dotted line*, A group (*n* = 43); *dashed line*, T-A group (*n* = 44)

is based on clinical results, but it is very difficult to perform a comprehensive long-term follow-up study of the esophagus due to refusal of asymptomatic patients to undergo testing. Nevertheless, in our experience, the clinical results after Heller's myotomy performed by three different approaches are not significantly different. We found that improvement of symptomatology decreases with time and the trend in improvement showed no difference at 15 years from operation using different surgical techniques (Fig. 1).

In our experience, the poor results after a transthoracic myotomy (14%) was related to an incomplete myotomy on the gastric wall, but it is important to note that the largest number of this type of complication was observed at the beginnig of our experience.

Only in one case operated on through an abdominal approach was there an incomplete myotomy, while this complication was not present in any of the thoracoabdominal approach cases.

Hiatal haernia can occur in 5%–10% of patients following esophagomyotomy [2] and its incidence is lower when esophagodiaphragmatic attachments are respected or if an antireflux procedure is performed [1, 3]. This value is higher when the diaphragm is incised to aid the performance of the myotomy [4]. In our experience, we have seen this complication in two cases who underwent an abdominal approach with a Lortat-Jacob antireflux procedure.

Incidence of esophageal peptic stricture following esophagomyotomy ranges from 0% to 7% (5–7). In our experience, it was only 2% and in all cases the myotomy performed with a thoracic approach without an antireflux procedure.

Gastroesophageal reflux is the most important cause of failure (i.e. reoperation required) of Heller's myotomy (3%–53%) [8]; we maintain that GER is not due so much to compromise of the esophagocardial muscle, but to the division of the hiatal structures. Based upon this assumption, from 1974 we started to perform the esophagomyotomy through either an abdominal or a thoracoabdominal approach. The basic difference between abdominal and thoracoabdominal approach is that in the first the disruption of hiatal structrues is mandatory for a good myotomy. Consequently, an antireflux procedure is necessary. The latter approach allows us to respect all anatomic structures connected with the gastroesophageal region to the greatest extent possible, and an antireflux procedure is not necessary.

Conclusions

Long-term follow-up of the T, A, and T-A groups showed no statistically significant differences concerning symptomatic results in patients operated on for achalasia. At present, we prefer an abdominal approach with a Dor antireflux procedure, as it seems the easiest and least traumatizing operation. Future treatment of these patients include a laparoscopic approach, but this technique needs at least the same length of follow-up to compare results with traditional surgery.

Bibliography

1. Andreollo NA, Earlam RJ (1987) Heller's myotomy for achalasia: Is an added antireflux procedure necessary? Br J Surg 74:765–769
2. Ellis FH, Olsen AM (1969) Achalasia of the esophagus. Major problems in clinical surgery, vol IX. WB Saunders, Philadelphia, p 221
3. Castrini G, Pappalardo G, Mobarhan S (1982) New approach to esophagocardiomyotomy: Report of 40 cases. J Thor Cardiovasc Surg 84:575–578
4. Drake EH (1982) Surgical treatment of cardiospasm. N Engl J Med 266:173–179
5. Okike N, Payne WS, Neufeld DM, et al (1979) Esophagomyotomy versus forceful dilation for achalasia of the esophagus: Results in 899 patients. Ann Thorac Surg 28:119–125
6. Ferguson MK (1991) Achalasia: Current evaluation and therapy. Ann Thorac Surg 52:336–342
7. Csendes A, Braghetto I, Henriquez A, Cortes C (1989) Late results of a prospective randomized study comparing forceful dilatation and oesophagomyotomy in patients with achalasia. Gut 30:299–304
8. Castrini G, Pappalardo G, Correnti S, Toccaceli S, Trentino P, Pitasi F (1983) A new technique of esophagocardiomyotomy for achalasia without fundoplication. In: Castrini G, Pappalardo G, Trentino P (eds) Proceedings of the second international congress of ISDE. La Porziuncola, Rome, pp 85–92

Long-Term Prognosis of Pneumatic Bag Dilatation Therapy in Esophageal Achalasia

Fumiaki Sugimura and Yutaka Matsuo[1]

Subjects and Methods

Cardial dilatation was performed using the Matsuo pneumatic bag dilator during the 26 year period from 1964 to 1989. The long-term efficacy of the method was assessed in 163 cases of esophageal achalasia after more than 1 year had elapsed since therapy. Of these cases, 54 (33.1%) were male and 109 (66.9%) were female.

Using only local anesthesia of the throat with lidocaine hydrochloride, a Matsuo pneumatic bag dilator was inserted orally in the same way as a gastric tube while monitoring the procedure with fluoroscopy. By observing the two lead pieces attached to either end of the rubber balloon, and the image of the air injected into the balloon with a sphygmomanometer connected to the dilator via a polyethylene tube (Fig. 1), the dilator was finally positioned so that the balloon extended from the lower esophagus to the upper stomach centered on the lower esophageal sphincter (LES). The balloon was then inflated by the hand bulb to a pressure of approximately 200 mmHg. This pressure was maintained for about 3 min, at which time the balloon was deflated and the patient was allowed to rest for a few minutes. The same procedure was repeated about 3–4 times. Normally, the therapy was carried out about 1–3 times at a frequency of once a week.

To complete clinical charts and to examine recent symptoms of patients, a questionnaire was sent to patients in December 1990.

---

[1] Third Department of Internal Medicine, Nihon University School of Medicine, 30 Oyaguchikami-machi, Itabashi-ku, Tokyo, 173 Japan

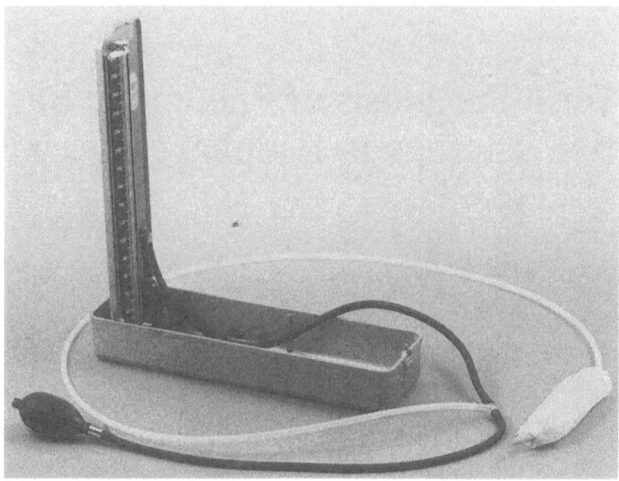

Fig. 1. Matsuo-type pneumatic bag dilator (Nogami Medical Instruments, Tokyo, Japan) connected to a mercury sphygmomanometer

Results

Grade of Esophageal Dilatation and Prognosis

The relation between grade of esophageal dilatation prior to cardial dilatation therapy and the prognosis after dilatation therapy was studied. The therapy was deemed "highly effective" if patients had either no symptoms or almost none, and "effective" if patients had only slight symptoms or symptoms which did not interfere with daily life. The therapy was deemed "slightly effective" if the patient did not often vomit, could manage his daily life even if symptoms were present, and was in better condition after therapy. The therapy was deemed "ineffective" if the patient was liable to vomit, suffered from pain, and if their condition did not improve following therapy. It cannot be said, therefore, that any correlation necessarily exists between the grade of esophageal dilatation prior to therapy and the long-term therapeutic prognosis.

Duration of Symptoms and Prognosis

Considering the time interval between the onset of symptoms and cardial dilatation therapy in relation to prognosis, it can be said that the efficacy of therapy was unrelated to the duration of symptomatic distress.

Number of Dilatations Performed and Efficiency of Therapy

Increasing the number of cardial dilatations does not necessarily improve efficacy.

Table 1. Clinical efficacy judged by increase in body weight (n = 163)

Increase in body weight		
	1–5 kg	59
	6–10 kg	48
	11–15 kg	7
	16–20 kg	6
	21–30 kg	1
No change		42

Table 2. Long-term efficacy of treatment (1–26 years later, n = 163)

	No. of cases	Efficacy
Highly effective	61	37.4% ⎫ 74.2%
Effective	60	36.8% ⎭
Slightly effective	26	16.0%
Ineffective	16 (7)	9.8% (4.3%)

( ) No. of cases operated

Efficacy of Therapy as Judged from Increase in Body Weight

It appears that the efficacy of the therapy is best reflected in increase in body weight. An increase of 1–5 kg was observed in 59 patients (36.2%) and 6–10 kg in 48 (29.4%) (Table 1).

Long-Term Prognosis

As of December 1990, of 163 cases treated by cardial dilatation therapy using a Matsuo pneumatic bag dilator were "highly effective" in 61 patients (37.4%) and "effective" in 60 (36.8%), i.e., a total of 121 cases (74.2%). The therapy was "ineffective" in 16 patients (9.8%) of which 7 (4.3%) underwent a surgical operation after cardial dilatation therapy (Table 2).

Esophageal Intraluminal Pressure Prior to Cardial Dilatation Therapy

Finally, esophageal intraluminal pressure was measured using an infusion catheter system in 14 patients prior to cardial dilatation therapy, and in 5 subsequent to therapy. In all 14 cases, a rise of esophageal resting pressure was noted prior to therapy, and high values of LES pressure were noted in about half of these (n = 6). In all of the five patients examined after therapy, there was a decrease of esophageal resting pressure compared to the pressure before therapy, and the LES pressure also fell in three of these.

Discussion

From these results, it emerged that there were no clear correlations between the efficacy of cardial dilatation therapy and the grade of esophageal dilatation caused by achalasia, the time between onset of symptoms and cardial dilatation therapy, or the number of dilatations performed.

It seems therefore impossible to judge whether cardial dilatation therapy or surgery should be chosen based on grade of esophageal dilatation, duration of symptomatic distress, or number of dilatations performed. Cardial dilatation therapy using a pneumatic bag dilator is a highly effective technique even from a long-term viewpoint. Thus, it would appear expedient to first attempt dilatation therapy several times, and then have recourse to surgery in those cases which do not show a long-term improvement.

Conclusions

Cardial dilatation therapy was performed using a Matsuo type pneumatic bag dilator. The long-term efficacy of treatment was evaluated in 163 cases of esophageal achalasia 1 year or more after therapy, with the following conclusions arrived at:

1. There is almost no relation between the efficacy of cardial dilatation therapy and grade of esophageal dilatation, previous duration of symptomatic distress, or the number of dilatations performed.
2. The efficacy of cardial dilatation therapy is best correlated with the increase in body weight. An increase of 1–5 kg was seen in 59 patients (36.2%), and an increase of 6–10 kg in 48 (29.4%).
3. Therapy was effective in a total of 121 patients (74.2%): "highly effective" in 61 (37.4%) and "effective" in 60 (36.8%).
4. Therapy was ineffective in 16 patients (9.8%), of which 7 (4.3%) had previously undergone a surgical operation.
5. In patients where therapy was ineffective despite repeated application, surgical operation of esophageal achalasia should be performed.

Characteristics of Esophageal Peristaltic Motor Activity After Distal Partial Gastrectomy

YOSHIYUKI FURUKAWA, NOBUYOSHI HANYU, TETSUYA KAJIMOTO, HIROSHI AOKI, SADANOBU ABE, and TERUAKI AOKI[1]

Introduction

Postoperative disorders after gastrectomy have been attracting attention due to the improvement in the operative results of gastric cancer. Gastroesophageal reflux disease is one of the postgastrectomy complications which affects the quality of life of the patient. The incidence of reflux esophagitis after gastrectomy is high and it tends to be refractory once it occurs [1]. There are many reports about alkaline reflux esophagitis after total gastrectomy, but only a few papers report on esophagitis after distal partial gastrectomy. Understanding the pathophysiology of reflux esophagitis after distal partial gastrectomy is important for therapy. The aim of the study presented here was to determine the mechanisms of reflux esophagitis following distal partial gastrectomy.

Subjects and Method

Patients with gastric cancer on whom distal partial gastrectomy was indicated were included in this study. Billroth I method was used for gastric reconstruction.

Radiological Study

Postoperative contrasting radiograms for upper gastrointestinal tracts were compared to preoperative ones in 60 patients. Anatomical changes were evaluated and the incidence of postoperative hiatus hernia was determined.

---

[1] The Second Department of Surgery, Jikei University School of Medicine, 3-25-8, Nishi-Shinbashi, Minato-ku, Tokyo, 105 Japan

249

250   Y. Furukawa et al.

Manometric Study

Preoperative and postoperative (4 weeks following operation) intraesophageal pressure was measured using an eight-channel manometric catheter with a Dent sleeve in 15 patients with gastric cancer. Of the 15 patients, 10 were male and 5 were female with the average age of 57.4. Sideholes were spaced at 3-cm intervals and each lumen was perfused at 0.3 ml/min with water by a low compliance pneumohydraulic system. The catheter was inserted through the nostril and then the sleeve was fixed at the lower esophageal sphincter (LES) to determine the resting pressure of the LES, the peristaltic pressure of the esophagus and the LES, the transmission velocity of peristalsis, and the period of relaxation of the LES at the time of swallowing. The results before and after the operation were compared. Peristaltic pressure was determined based on the gastric pulsion, and swallowing was done by both the dry swallow (DS) and 5-ml water swallow (WS) methods. The sideholes at 6 cm, 9 cm, and 12 cm above the sleeve were equivalent to the upper, middle, and lower parts of the esophagus.

The paired t-test was performed to test difference between before and after distal partial gastrectomy.

Results

Radiological Study

Postoperative contrasting radiograms revealed 48% of the 60 patients had complications of newly developed esophageal hiatus hernia.

Manometric Study

The resting pressure of the LES significantly decreased after operation compared with that before operation (21.2 ± 3.2 mmHg before operation and 14.6 ± 4.3 mmHg after operation) ($P < 0.05$) as shown in Fig. 1.

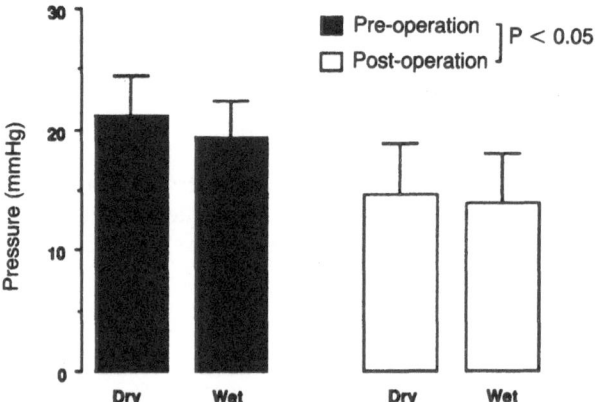

Fig. 1. Difference of basal LES (lower esophageal sphincter) pressure. Basal LES pressure was significantly lower after gastrectomy than before ($P < 0.05$)

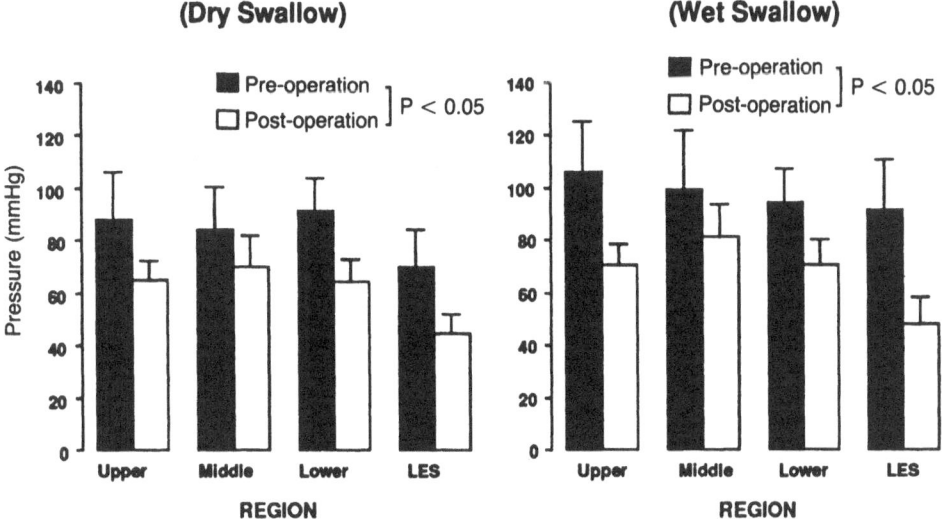

Fig. 2. Amplitudes of esophageal peristaltic pressure waves at each part of the esophagus were significantly lower after gastrectomy than before in both dry and wet swallows ($P < 0.05$)

The postoperative peristaltic pressure at various parts of the esophagus significantly decreased compared to that before operation both at DS and WS throughout the upper, middle, lower esophagus and the LES, as shown in Fig. 2 ($P < 0.05$). The peristaltic pressure both before and after operation had higher values at WS than that at DS ($P < 0.05$).

Similarly the transmission velocities of the esophageal peristaltic wave at the upper, middle, and lower part of the esophagus were significantly lower at DS after operation ($P < 0.05$). However, as shown in Fig. 3, no significant decrease of the velocity was demonstrated at WS after operation. The transmission velocities were higher at the upper, middle, and the lower part of esophagus, in descending order.

Measurements during relaxation demonstrated no significant difference between before and after operation (at DS: preoperative, 5.2 ± 0.6 s, and postoperative, 5.3 ± 0.6 s and at WS: preoperative, 5.7 ± 0.9 s and postoperative, 6.1 ± 0.9 s).

·There was a characteristic change in the peristaltic wave of the esophagus after operation. The peristaltic pressure markedly decreased or ceased before it reached the LES at the time of both DS and WS. This was observed in about 9% of all the swallowings.

Discussion

Anatomical and physiological changes induced by gastric surgery result in post-gastrectomy syndromes [2]. However, we demonstrated that not only remnant gastric motor dysfunction but also esophageal motor dysfunction occurred after distal partial gastrectomy.

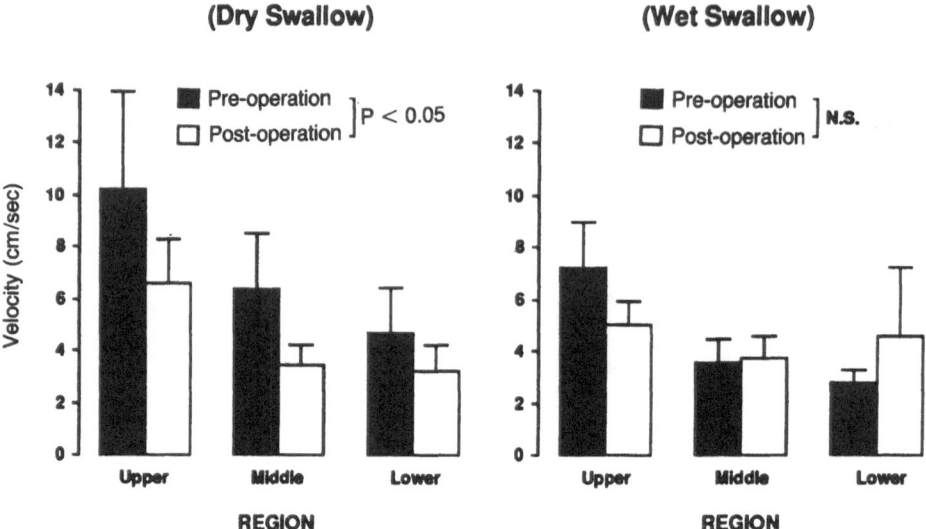

Fig. 3. Velocity of esophageal peristaltic pressure waves at each part of the esophagus was significantly faster after gastrectomy than before in dry swallows ($P < 0.05$), but not significant in wet swallows

The present study revealed postoperative anatomical changes of the esophagogastric junction and lowering of the resting pressure of the LES, as well as damage throughout esophageal peristalsis after distal partial gastrectomy. This lowering of the esophageal peristalsis was considered to cause a decrease in esophageal clearance. In addition, retention of refluxate caused by the lowered resting pressure of the LES is increased. These conditions were supposed to be the causative factor of reflux esophagitis. Therefore, it was suggested that improvement of esophageal peristalsis, together with maintenance of the LES resting pressure should be considered in the postoperative therapy of reflux esophagitis.

On the other hand, newly developed hiatus hernia was observed in 37.5% of the post-gastrectomy patients by endoscopic study [1]. This incidence was quite high, resembling our results.

The operative procedures to maintain esophageal competency are naturally effective in controlling symptoms of esophageal reflux. However, a re-operation after hiatal repair treated by gastrectomy with Roux-en-Y gastrojejunostomy gives better results than the Nissen procedure [3]. The same is reported in cases of severe gastroesophageal reflux diseases [4]. The refluxate after distal partial gastrectomy is mainly composed of alkaline material. This esophageal alkaline exposure was related to duodenogastric reflux. Roux-en-Y reconstruction is more useful than Billroth I method in the prevention of alkaline reflux esophagitis [5]. Therefore, it is suggested that Roux-en-Y anstomosis for reconstruction after distal partial gastrectomy might be the better method.

Conclusion

Basal LES pressure and amplitude of peristaltic pressure waves are impaired by gastrectomy. Newly developed esophageal hiatus hernia was seen in gastrectomized patients. The hypofunction of LES and esophagus after distal partial gastrectomy may cause reflux esophagitis.

References

1. Sodeyama H, Ishizaka K, Takahashi C, Kuroda T, Iida F, Kusama J (1990) Endoscopic and manometric study of the cardia in post-gastrectomy patients. Jpn J Surg 20:64–69
2. Eagon JC, Miedema BW, Kelly KA (1992) Post-gastrectomy syndrome. Surg Clin North Am 72(2):445–465
3. Washer GF, Gear MWL, Dowling BL, Gillison EW, Royston CMS, Spencer J (1984) Randomized prospective trial of Roux-en-Y duodenal diversion versus fundoplication for severe reflux esophagitis. Br J Surg 71:181–184
4. Herrington JL, Mody B (1976) Total duodenal diversion for the treatment of reflux esophagitis uncontrolled by repeated antireflux procedure. Ann Surg 183:636–644
5. Perniceni T, Gayet B, Fekete F (1988) Total duodenal diversion in the treatment of complicated peptic esophagitis. Br J Surg 75:1108–1111

Esophageal Varices

Pathological Changes of Esophagogastric Varices After Endoscopic Sclerotherapy

Susumu Shibuya, Yasuhiro Takase, and Niranjan Sharma[1]

Introduction

In cases where gastric varices are contiguous with esophageal varices, it has been reported that most of the feeders of the esophagogastric varices are the left gastric vein and/or the short gastric veins [1, 2]. It was thought that the gastric varices are residual varices that sometimes become larger after the treatment of esophageal varices alone by injection sclerotherapy. Simultaneous obliteration of the gastric and the esophageal varices were obtained, when the sclerosant was intravariceally injected into their feeders during treatment for esophageal varices. At times, a histopathological study of esophagogastric variceal changes is not enough to predict the final outcome of the sclerotherapy. Therefore, the present study was carried out in an attempt to elucidate the pathological course of the esophagogastric varices after injection sclerotherapy.

Materials and Method

In order to evaluate the course of esophagogastric varices, we examined 19 autopsy patients that had undergone endoscopic embolization [3] for esophagogastric varices at the Tsukuba University Hospital and its related hospitals from October, 1977 to May, 1992 (Table 1). Hepatocellular carcinoma with liver cirrhosis was seen in 10 patients and liver cirrhosis in 9. Causes of death were hepatic failure in 13 patients, hepatoma in 2, upper and lower gastrointestinal bleeding in 3, and operative death for cholecystolithiasis in 1, without proven esophageal variceal bleeding. The esophagus and the stomach of the autopsy specimens were serially and vertically sectioned, which sections were then

[1] Department of Surgery, Institute of Clinical Medicine, University of Tsukuba, 1-1-1 Tennoudai, Tsukuba, 305 Japan

Table 1. Patients and results

Case No.	Age/Sex	Pathological diagnosis of the liver	Cause of death	Duration after therapy	Stomach				Esophagus			
					T	G	O	R	T	G	O	R
1	69 F	HCC with LC	Hepatic failure	6 days	+	−	−	−	+	−	−	−
2	70 M	LC	Hepatic failure	9 days	+	−	−	−	+	−	−	−
3	44 M	HCC with LC	Hepatic failure	14 days	+	+	−	−	+	+	−	−
4	43 M	HCC with LC	Hepatic failure	25 days	+	+	−	−	+	+	−	−
5	50 M	HCC with LC	HCC	29 days	+	+	−	−	+	+	−	−
6	70 M	LC	Operation death after cholecystectomy and splenectomy	51 days	+	+	+	+	+	+	+	+
7	64 M	HCC with LC	Hapatic failure	2.5 months	−	−	+	+	−	−	+	+
8	45 M	LC	Ileal bleeding	3 months	−	−	+	+	+	−	+	+
9	55 M	HCC with LC	Hepatic failure	3 months	−	−	+	+	−	−	+	+
10	52 M	HCC with LC	HCC	3 months	−	−	+	+	−	−	+	+
11	62 F	HCC with LC	Bleeding from the stomach	6 months	−	−	+	+	−	−	+	+
12	47 M	LC	Hepatic failure	7 months	−	−	+	+	−	−	+	+
13	57 M	HCC with LC	Jejunal bleeding	11 months	−	−	+	+	−	−	+	+
14	59 M	LC	Hepatic failure	17 months	−	−	+	+	−	−	+	+
15	50 M	HCC with LC	Hepatic failure	29 months	−	−	+	+	−	−	+	+
16	5 M	LC	Hepatic failure	44 months	−	−	+	+	−	−	+	+
17	51 M	LC	Hepatic failure	55 months	−	−	+	+	−	−	+	+
18	56 M	LC	Hepatic failure	61 months	−	−	+	+	−	−	+	+
19	53 M	HCC with LC	Hepatic failure	88 months	−	−	+	+	+	−	+	+

HCC, Hepatocellular carcinoma; *LC*, Liver cirrhosis; *T*, Thrombus; *G*, Granulation; *O*, Organization; *R*, Recanalization

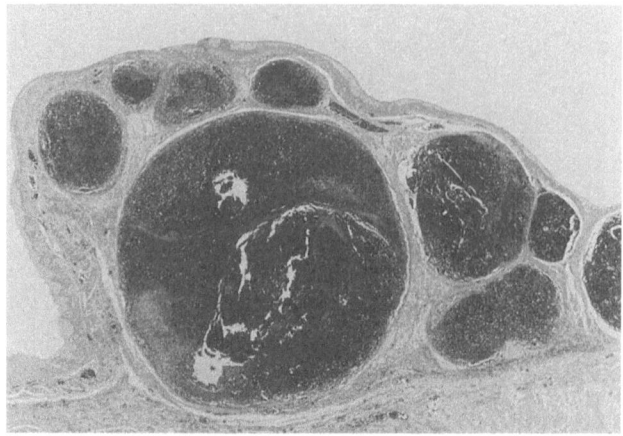

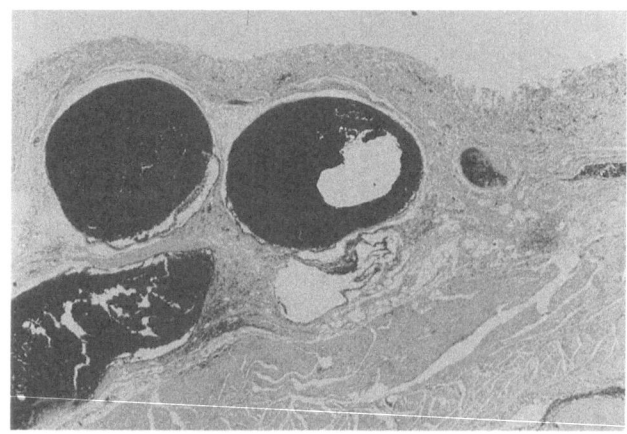

Fig. 1a,b. This patient died due to hepatic failure 6 days after sclerotherapy. **a** Microscopic findings of the thrombosed esophageal varices (H&E). **b** Gastric varices were thrombosed

stained with hematoxylin-eosin, Masson-trichrome, and Elastica von Gieson for thrombus formation, granulation, organization, and recanalization of the esophageal and gastric varices after treatment.

Results

The esophageal varices were found thrombosed within 3 months after treatment and gastric varices were found within 51 days (Table 1, Fig. 1). Granulation of the esophageal and gastric varices was found from 14 to 51 days after treatment, respectively (Table 1, Fig. 2). Esophagogastric varices were organized after 51 days. Recanalization was observed in organized varices (Table 1, Fig. 3).

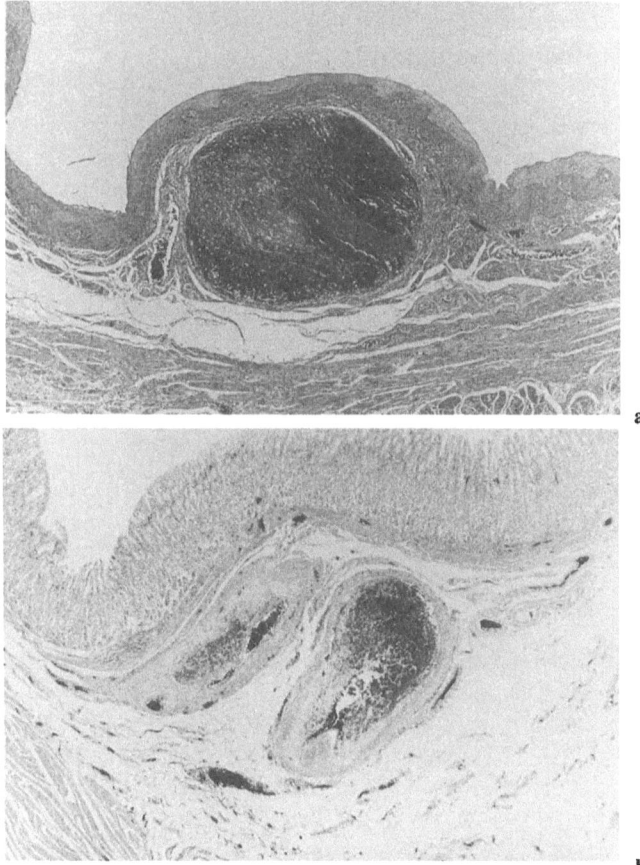

Fig. 2a,b. This patient died due to hepatic failure 14 days after therapy. Microscopic findings of **a** the esophageal varices and **b** the gastric varices. The esophagogastric varices were simultaneously granulated with thrombosis (H&E)

Discussion

Smith-Laing et al. [1], based on their study on percutaneous transhepatic portography, reported that the feeders of the esophageal varices were left gastric vein and/or short gastric veins in 62 of 64 cases with variceal bleeding. It was reported that most of the feeders of the esophageal varices and/or gastric varices in 230 cases with portal hypertension were left gastric vein and short gastric veins [2]. Therefore, gastric varices were thought to be residual; when they were contiguous with esophageal varices, sometimes they became larger after the treatment of esophageal varices alone by injection sclerotherapy for the esophagogastric varices. Moersch [4] reported that 2 of 16 patients, in whom splenectomy was performed before sclerotherapy for esophageal varices, died due to gastric fundic variceal bleeding after sclerotherapy. MacDougall et al.

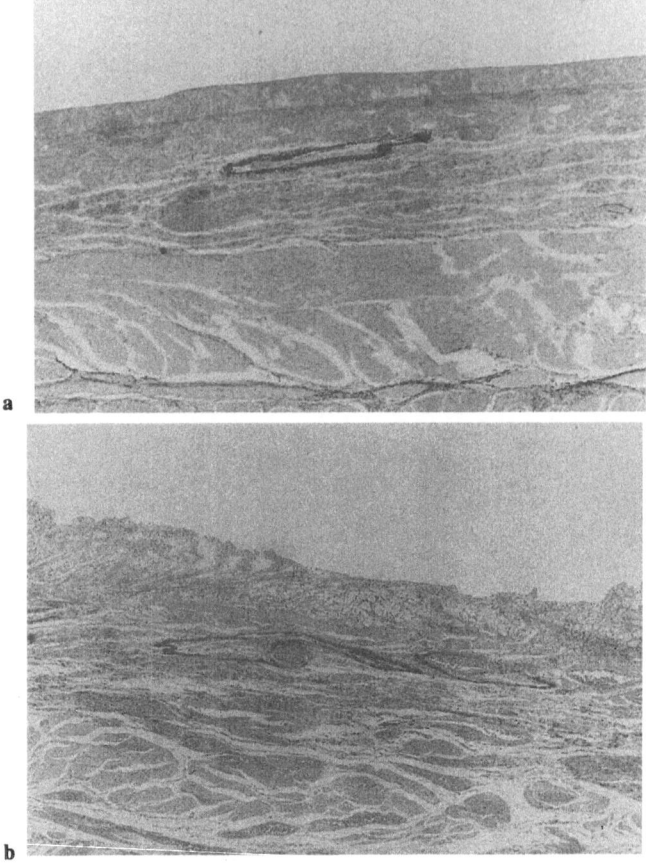

Fig. 3a,b. This patient died due to hepatic failure 44 months after sclerotherapy. After operation for primary biliary atresia, sclerotherapy for esophagogastric varices associated with liver cirrhosis was performed at 1 year and 8 months of age. Organization of **a** esophageal varices and **b** gastric varices. (Elastica von Gieson stain)

[5] reported 2 patients with gastric variceal bleeding with esophageal varices out of 42 patients with esophageal varices which had disappeared following sclerotherapy for the esophageal varices. Hennessy et al. [6] reported 1 patient with gastric variceal bleeding out of 25 patients with long-term follow-up after emergency sclerotherapy for esophageal varices. Soderlund et al. [7] reported the death of three patients due to gastric variceal bleeding which was considered to be a complication of the sclerotherapy carried out for the treatment of esophageal varices. Shemesh et al. [8] reported the complications and the causes of death in 84 patients after sclerotherapy for esophageal variceal bleeding; the cause of death in 3 patients was reportedly due to gastric variceal bleeding.

Our technique for injection sclerotherapy [3] is to embolize esophageal varices, and their feeders as well, by injecting a sclerosant intravariceally. Thus, simulta-neous obliteration of the gastric varices, which are also the feeders of the esophageal varices, and the esophageal varices themselves was obtained. Histopathological study also showed these varices to be thrombosed, granulated, and organized. Therefore, gastric variceal bleeding after sclerotherapy for esophageal varices was thought to be a complication of sclerotherapy.

References

1. Smith-Laing G, Camil E, Dick R, Sherlick S (1980) Percutaneous transhepatic portography in the assessment of portal hypertension. Gastroenterology 78:197–205
2. Watanabe K, Kimura K, Matsutani S, Ohto M, Okuda K (1988) Portal hemodynamics in patients with gastric varices. Gastroenterology 95:434–440
3. Takase Y, Ozaki A, Orii K, Nagoshi K, Okamura T, Iwasaki Y (1982) Injection sclerotherapy of esophageal varices for patients undergoing emergency and elective surgery. Surgery 92:474–479
4. Moersch HJ (1947) Treatment of esophageal varices by injection of a sclerosing solution. JAMA 135:754–746
5. MacDougall BRD, Westaby D, Theodossi A, Dawson JL, Williams R (1982) Increased long-term survival in variceal haemorrhage using injection sclerotherapy. Lancet I:124–127
6. Hennessy TPJ, Stephen RB, Kaene FB (1982) Acute and chronic management of esophageal varices by injection sclerotherapy. Surg Gynecol Obstet 154:374–377
7. Soderlund C, Ihre T (1985) Endoscopic sclerotherapy V: Conservative management of bleeding oesophageal varices. Acta Chir Scand 151:449–456
8. Shemesh E, Czerniak A, Klein E, Pines A, Bat L (1990) A comparison between emergency and delayed endoscopic injection sclerotherapy of esophageal varices in non-alcoholic portal hypertension. J Clin Gastroenterol 12:5–9

Overview of Endoscopic Injection Sclerotherapy in 1200 Patients with Esophageal Varices

Makoto Hashizume, Seigo Kitano, Masayuki Ohta, Kiichiro Ueno, Morimasa Tomikawa, and Keizo Sugimachi[1]

Introduction

Endoscopic injection sclerotherapy is the treatment of choice worldwide for actively bleeding esophageal varices [1]. Long-term, repeated sclerotherapy eradicates varices in most patients and reduces the rate of subsequent hemorrhage. However, in recent prospective randomized trials, the frequency of episodes of bleeding was significantly greater among patients undergoing variceal sclerotherapy and mortality did not differ in the two study and control groups [2, 3]. The differences in those studies seem to be due to the different techniques used and to the follow-up system.

The objective of this study is to examine the overall clinical results of injection sclerotherapy in our institution.

Patients and Methods

Patients

From January 1982 to June 1992, 1200 patients with esophageal varices who were admitted to the Department of Surgery II, Kyushu University Hospital, were treated with endoscopic injection sclerotherapy. The clinical data of these patients are shown in Table 1. Under acute conditions, 267 underwent initial injection of the sclerosant, and 244 cases were elective. According to our criteria, 689 patients were given prophylactic injections [4]. Acutely bleeding patients were electively treated by repeated sclerotherapy even after variceal bleeding was brought under control. Severity of liver disease was classified into

[1] Department of Surgery II, Faculty of Medicine, Kyushu University, 3-1-1 Maidashi, Higashi-ku, Fukuoka, 812 Japan

Table 1. Clinical data of patients

No. of patients	1200
Mean age (years)	56.3 ± 10.3
Sex (M/F)	868/332
Liver disease	
Cirrhosis	1167
IPH	18
Other	15
Hepatoma	360
Child's grade	
A	289
B	551
C	360

IPH, Idiopathic Portal Hypertension

three grades according to the modified Child classification [5]: Child grade A in 289 patients, Child grade B in 551 patients, and Child grade C in 360 patients.

Sclerotherapy

The techniques of injection sclerotherapy have been described in detail elsewhere [6, 7]. The sclerosant used most often was 5% ethanolamine oleate. The first sclerotherapy session was performed using a tansparent overtube (ST-E1). Subsequent sessions were performed using the free-hand technique. Sclerotherapy was repeated once a week until all esophageal varices had been eradicated. Endoscopy was performed at 3-month intervals. Additional sclerotherapy was performed whenever new, small, dilated venous vessels appeared.

Statistical Analysis

The entry point of the study was the date of the initial session of sclerotherapy. All values were expressed as mean $\pm$ S.D. Survival curves were plotted as Kaplan-Meier estimates and compared by means of the log-rank test. The variables of interest were compared by the χ^2-test or Student's t-test.

Results

Acute variceal bleeding was controlled in 262 of 267 patients (98.1%). In the remaining five patients, repeat bleeding was controlled by additional sclerotherapy. Patients underwent a mean of 4.2 sessions of sclerotherapy. Esophageal varices were completely eradicated in 944 patients (78.6%). In the remaining 256 patients, esophageal varices were not completely eradicated: 73 patients died within 1 month, hepatic deterioration was noted in 18 patients, and 41 patients dropped out of the study. Heavy bleeding from the upper gastrointestinal tract occurred in 110 patients (9.2%) after entry into the study: in 65 patients, bleeding was from the esophagus and in 45 patients it was from the stomach.

Complications included the development of transient strictures in 149 patients (12.4%), for whom two or three sessions of dilatation treatments with a Maloney tube had to be performed. Acute renal failure occurred in seven patients. Aspiration pneumonia and pulmonary edema occurred in one patient each and both died.

Small dilated venous vessels that required additional sclerotherapy appeared in 244 of 944 patients (25.8%) in whom esophageal varices had been eradicated. Of 944 patients, 36 (3.8%) bled from small dilated vessels after eradication of varices by sclerotherapy. The cumulative non-bleeding rate at 5 years was 93.8%. The incidence of appearance of small, dilated venous vessels was reduced with time after sclerotherapy, but the cumulative rate of appearance was 46.1% at 5 years.

Four hundred and fifty-four patients died (37.8%). Upper gastrointestinal bleeding accounted for 2.9% of deaths (13 patients), whereas the rates in case of liver failure and hepatoma were 41.0% (186 patients) and 45.4% (206 patients), respectively. The mean follow-up for all patients was 1866.6 ± 64.0 days. The 5-year cumulative survival rate was 57.7% in patients without hepatoma and 11.7% for patients with hepatoma. When the patients without concomitant hepatoma were classified according to Child's grade, those patients in Child grades A and B had longer survival times than did those in Child grade C for acute, elective, and prophylactic treatments (Fig. 1).

Discussion

In controlled trials [8, 9] the frequency of repeat bleeding in sclerotherapy patients was reduced; however, as many as 50% of the patients experienced repeat bleeding before complete eradication of the varices had been achieved. In contrast, the rate of cumulative non-bleeding was 93.8% at 5 years. We attribute the differences in these studies to the different techniques used [7] and to the follow-up system. We follow the patients closely and add one or two sessions of sclerotherapy to obliterate the newly developed, small-sized, dilated vessels in the lower esophagus. The bleeding from the small vessels occurred in 36 patients (3.8%). Bleeding from these small vessels probably could have been prevented had additional sclerotherapy been given with regular follow-up endoscopy at 3-month intervals. Therefore, the lower esophagus is kept free of varices for the patient's lifetime. This close follow-up is a key factor.

The influence of repeated sclerotherapy on long-term survival has limitations. Hepatic reserve and concomitant hepatoma are the main determinants of survival time in Japanese patients with cirrhosis [7]. In the Japanese patients, survival seems to be greatly influenced by the complications associated with hepatoma [10]. However, upper gastrointestinal bleeding accounted for only 2.6% of all deaths, whereas 75% of all deaths were related to bleeding in the sclerotherapy group treated by Santangelo et al. [2]. It is clear that their quality of life was improved by sclerotherapy and a life-threatening situation was removed.

The main complication of sclerotherapy was esophageal stenosis, but this was easily managed with bougienage using a Maloney tube. Acute renal failure is a serious complication requiring intensive care [11]. Hemolysis and functional

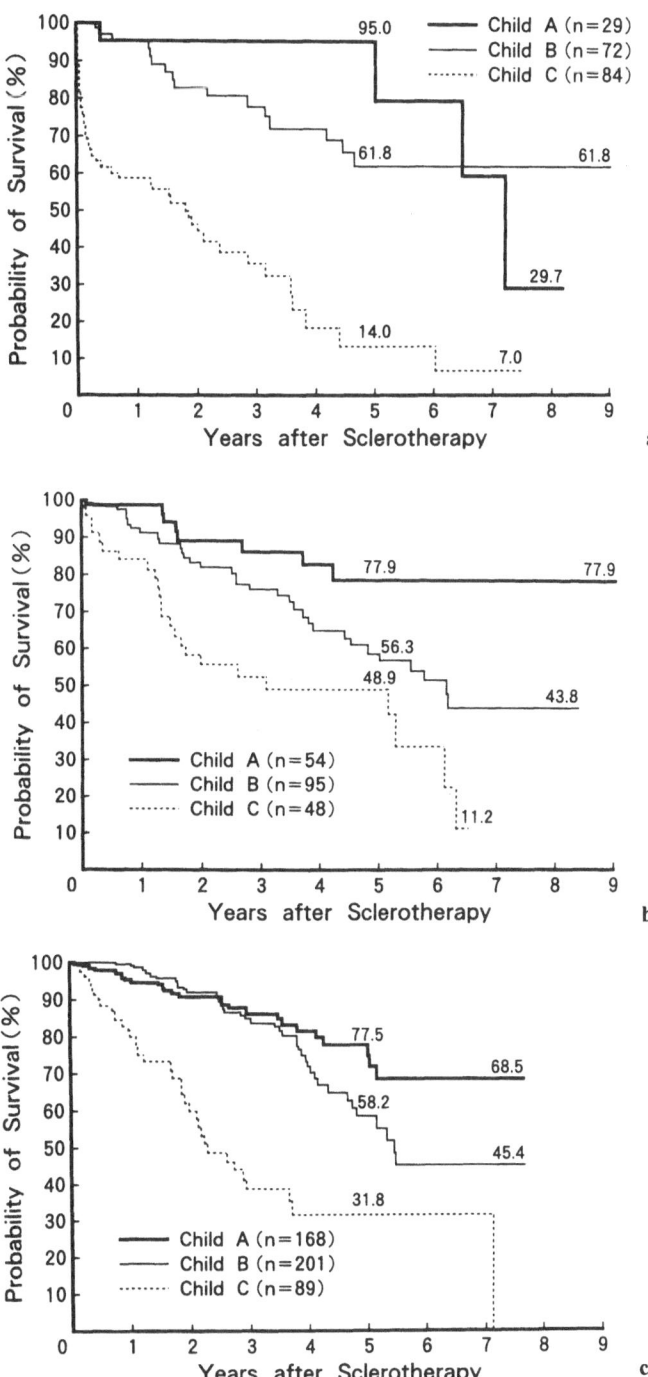

Fig. 1a–c. Cumulative survival curves. **a** acute cases, **b** elective cases, and **c** prophylactic cases. ($P < 0.001$ between Child class A and B, and Child class C)

ischemia of the renal artery can lead to an acute tubular necrosis. The dose of sclerosant used should be carefully controlled in high-risk patients [12]. In some patients, the varices are difficult to eradicate, and for those patients with giant bar-type esophageal varices, devascularization of the upper stomach and lower esophagus with splenectomy is useful to eradicate the varices [13, 14]. Preoperative portography facilitates a prediction of patients in whom sclerotherapy is likely to ultimately fail at an early stage of management and surgical treatment can be given [15].

References

1. Terblanche J (1990) Has sclerotherapy altered management of patients with variceal bleeding? Am J Surg 160:37–42
2. Santangelo WG, Dueno MI, Estes BL, Krejs GJ (1988) Prophylactic sclerotherapy of large esophageal varices. N Engl J Med 318:814–818
3. Sauerbruch T, Wotzka R, Kopcke W, Harlin M, Heldwein W, Bayerdorffer E, Sander R, et al (1988) Prophylactic sclerotherapy before the first episode of variceal hemorrhage in patients with cirrhosis. N Engl J Med 319:8–15
4. Beppu K, Inokuchi K, Koyanagi N, Nakayama S, Sakata H, Kitano S, Kobayashi M (1981) Predictions of variceal hemorrhage by esophageal endoscopy. Gastrointest Endosc 27:213–218
5. Pugh RNH, Murray-Lyon IM, Dawson JL, Pietroni MC, Williams R (1973) Transection of the oesophagus for bleeding oesophageal varices. Br J Surg 60:646–649
6. Kitano S, Koyanagi N, Iso N, Higashi H, Sugimachi K (1987) Prevention of recurrence of esophageal varices after endoscopic injection sclerotherapy with ethanolamine oleate. Hepatology 7:810–815
7. Hashizume M, Kitano S, Koyanagi N, Tanoue K, Ohta M, Wada H, Yamaga H, Higashi H, Iso Y, Iwanaga T, Sugimachi K (1992) Endoscopic injection sclerotherapy for 1000 patients with esophageal varices: A nine-year prospective study. Hepatology 15:69–75
8. Westaby D, Macdougall BRD, Williams R (1985) Improved survival following injection sclerotherapy for esophageal varices: Final analysis of a controlled trial. Hepatology 5:827–830
9. The Copenhagen Esophageal Varices Sclerotherapy Project (1984) Sclerotherapy after first variceal hemorrhage in cirrhosis: A randomized multicenter trial. N Engl J Med 311:1594–1600
10. Hashizume M, Inokuchi K, Beppu K, Koyanagi N, Nagamine K, Sugimachi K, Hirose S (1984) The natural history of non-alcoholic cirrhosis. Gastroenterol Jpn 19:430–435
11. Hashizume M, Kitano S, Yamaga H, Sugimachi K (1988) Haptoglobin to protect against renal damage from ethanolamine oleate sclerosant. Lancet II:340–341
12. Wada H, Hashizume M, Yamaga H, Kitano S, Sugimachi K (1990) Hemodynamic and morphological changes in the dog kidney after injection of 5% ethanolamine oleate into the superior vena cava. Eur Surg Res 22:63–70
13. Hashizume M, Tanoue K, Kitano S, Ohta M, Sugimachi K (1991) Giant bar type esophageal varices non-eradicated by repeated injection sclerotherapy. Gastrointest Endosc 37:187–189
14. Hashizume M, Kitano S, Sugimachi K, Sueishi K (1988) Three-dimensional view of the vascular structure of the lower esophagus in clinical portal hypertension. Hepatology 8:1482–1487
15. Hashizume M, Kitano S, Yamaga H, Higashi H, Sugimachi K (1989) Angioarchitectural classification of esophageal varices and paraesophageal veins in selective left gastric venography. Arch Surg 124:961–966

Limitation of Non-Shunting Operation and Endoscopic Injection Sclerotherapy for Esophageal Varices and the Role of Combined Treatment

Kiyoaki Ouchi, Shuji Matsubara, Tsuyoshi Tominaga, Taisei Muto, and Seiki Matsuno[1]

Introduction

Formerly, the purpose of the non-shunting operation was to eradicate esophageal varices completely. Although most patients who received the complete operation of transthoracic esophageal transection and gastric devascularization (the Sugiura procedure) could achieve eradication of esophageal varices, patients who only received esophageal transection or gastric devascularization because of limited hepatic functional reserve showed a higher chance of residual or recurrent varices [1]. After induction of endoscopic injection sclerotherapy (EIS) treatment strategy for esophageal varices varied dramatically. Although some authors reported that EIS is more than palliative treatment for esophageal varices, some reported high incidence of re-bleeding following EIS [2, 3]. There may be a place for combined therapy employing non-shunting operation and EIS for the treatment of esophageal varices. Based on our clinical experience with 132 non-shunting operations and 80 EISs for esophageal varices due to liver cirrhosis, the significance of combined therapy of both methods was studied referring the limitation of those two kinds of treatment.

Patients and Methods

Non-shunting operation was carried out in 132 patients with liver cirrhosis during past 20 years (operated group). The mean age of patients was 49 years. The patients were comprised of 108 men and 24 women. Fifty-four patients belonged to Child's grade A, 58 to grade B, and 20 to grade C. Eighteen patients received emergent operation, 81 elective operation, and

[1] First Department of Surgery, Tohoku University School of Medicine, 1-1 Seiryocho, Aoba-ku, Sendai, 980 Japan

33 prophylactic operation. Operations performed were two-stage operations of transthoracic esophageal transection and splenectomy with devascularization (the Sugiura procedure) in 71 patients, one-stage operation of transabdominal esophageal transection using end-to-end stapled anastomosis (EEA) and splenectomy with devascularization in 16, esophageal transection alone in 31, devascularization alone in 8, and proximal gastrectomy in 6.

EIS was performed in 80 cirrhotic patients during past 10 years (EIS group). The mean age of patients was 56 years. The patients were comprised of 55 men and 25 women. Thirty patients belonged Child's grade A, 32 to grade B, and 18 to grade C. Emergent treatment was undergone in 14 patients, elective treatment in 32, and prophylactic treatment in 34. Patients were routinely sclerosed using 5% ethanolamine oleate into varices. EIS was repeated every week until the red color disappeared. Hepatoma was associated in 6 patients (5%) in the operated group and in 10 patients (13%) in the EIS group. There was one patient older than 70 years in the operated group (0.7%), and eight patients in the EIS group (10%).

Studies were made to elucidate the limitations of these two kinds of treatment modalities, and to find the best combination of operation and EIS. EIS was performed in eight patients who showed a recurrence of varices after a non-shunting operation, and operation was additionally performed following EIS in four patients. Cumulative survival rates of patients were obtained by use of the Kaplan-Meier method.

Results

In the operated group, hospital death occurred in 13 patients (9.8%). No patients died during the admitted period after 1981. The hospital mortality rate was 6% in Child's grade A, 7% in grade B, and 30% in grade C. The 5-year survival rate was 57% in the operated group; 66% in Child's grade A, 58% in grade B, and only 23% in grade C (Fig. 1, left). The hospital mortality rate was 7% in elective, 6% in prophylactic, and 28% in emergent cases. The 5-year survival rate was 62% in prophylactic, 60% in elective, and 43% in emergent cases (Fig. 2, left). Rebleeding from varices was found in eight patients (7%) among patients discharged from the hospital. The rebleeding rate was only 6% after the Sugiura procedure, but it was 23% after esophageal transection alone.

In the EIS group, hospital death occurred in 11 out of 80 patients (14%). The hospital mortality rate was 7% in Child's grade A, 6% in grade B, and 41% in grade C. The 5-year survival rate was only 28% in the EIS group; 50% in Child's grade A, 0% in grade B, and 20% in grade C (Fig. 1, right). The hospital mortality rate was 54% in emergent cases, and 6% in both elective and prophylactic cases. The 5-year survival rate was 12% in emergent cases, and 40% in both elective and prophylactic cases (Fig. 2, right). Rebleeding after EIS was found in 20 cases (25%) and most rebleeding occurred within a year after the first EIS treatment.

Eight patients underwent EIS for recurrent varices following operation: three after esophageal transection (14%), three after the Sugiura procedure (6%), and two after one-stage transabdominal esophageal transection with devascularization (13%). Intervals between operation and EIS were 6–64 months (mean 36 ± 20

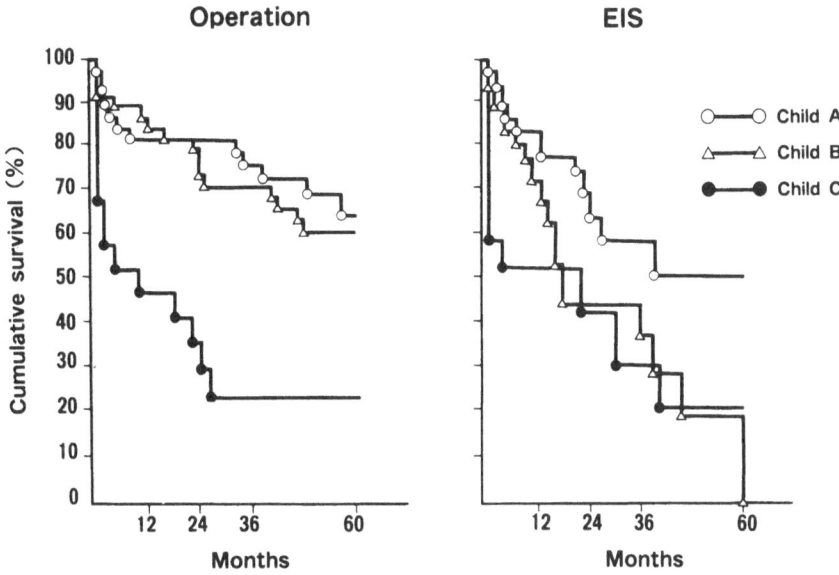

Fig. 1. Survival curves of patients undergoing non-shunting operation and endoscopic injection sclerotherapy (*EIS*) by Child's classification

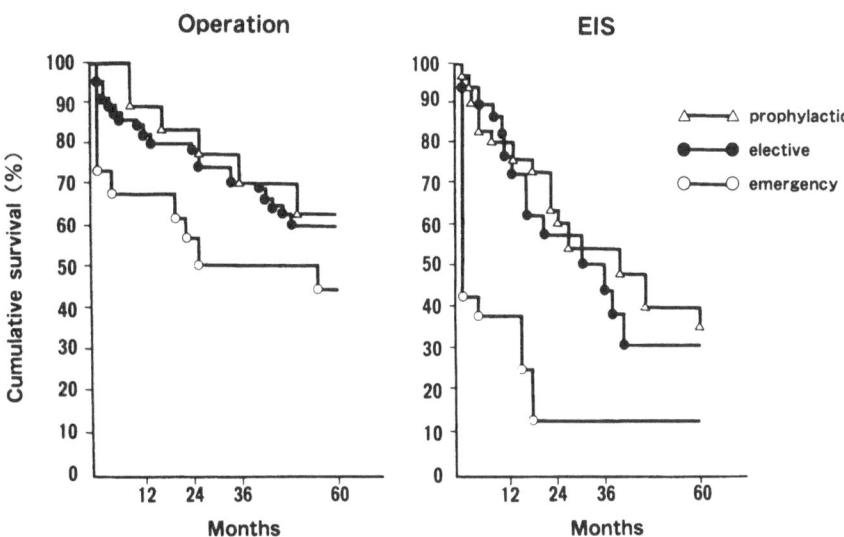

Fig. 2. Survival curves of patients undergoing non-shunting operation and endoscopic injection sclerotherapy (*EIS*) by urgency of treatment

months). Conversely, non-shunting operations were carried out following EIS in 4 patients whose liver function improved after EIS. Two cases underwent esophageal transection and 2 proximal gastrectomy. Intervals between EIS and operation were 10–25 months (mean 15 ± 6 months) which were significantly shorter than intervals between operation and subsequent EIS ($P < 0.05$). Twelve patients who received combined treatment of operation and EIS showed no variceal bleeding in an average follow-up period of 4.7 years after the final treatment.

Discussion

The non-shunting operation has been the most widely applied among surgical treatments of esophageal varices in Japan. Satisfactory results have been reported in terms of both operative mortality and incidence of recurrent bleeding. Less than 10% of both operative mortality and recurrent bleeding was reported following non-shunting operation [4, 5]. As demonstrated in our series of patients, however, Child's grade C patients or patients undergoing emergent operation had extremely poor short-term as well as long-term outcome. Spence [6] also reported that emergent esophageal transection gave hospital mortality rate of 27% compared to a 12% mortality in patients undergoing elective surgery, and operative mortality in Child's grade A patients was 10%; in grade B mortality was 8%, and mortality in grade C patients was 28.5%. The 5-year survival rate of Child's grade A was 59.3%, grade B was 62.4%, and grade C significantly worse at 24%. In Child's grade A or B, the non-shunting procedure should be performed aggressively, while in Child's grade C patients the procedure should be performed selectively.

EIS has been carried out mainly in patients who had severely deteriorated hepatic function, emergent situation, old age (over 70 years), or associated unresectable hepatoma. Both the short-term and long-term outcome of patients with Child's grade B or C and patients treated with emergent situation were extremely poor. The results of the non-shunting operation seem to be superior to results of EIS in these patients, though the background of patients in both groups was different. Although EIS during emergency endoscopy has been reported to be established as a primary therapeutic mode to successfully control bleeding varices [7], there may be no long-term efficacy on patients survival. Operation should possibly be performed after controlling variceal bleeding with emergent EIS and improving hepatic dysfunction. Even in patients who underwent prophylactic or elective EIS, it is recommended that operation should be added in cases achieving improvement of hepatic function. In order to avoid rebleeding from varices during the interval between EIS and operation, meticulous follow-up of the patients must be recommended.

Rebleeding from esophageal varices was more frequent in patients who underwent a lesser extent of devascularization. Patients undergoing the Sugiura procedure had lower incidence of recurrent varices than those who received transabdominal esophageal transection with devascularization, esophageal transection alone, or devascularization alone. In patients who are considered capable of tolerating the procedure, the Sugiura procedure which has long-term hemostatic efficacy for varices, is the best procedure of choice. However, in patients who have some risk factors for the Sugiura procedure, esophageal transection or devascularization should be selected in order to reduce hospital mortality. At that time frequency of rebleeding from varices might be high, and EIS should be added to treat residual or recurrent varices. Combined therapy employing nonshunting operation and EIS would be widely applied for future treatment of esophageal varices.

References

1. Ouchi K, Abe M, Sato T (1987) Prediction of outcome following Sugiura's procedure in patients with liver cirrhosis: A multiple linear regression analysis and scoring system. Dig Surg 4:93–97
2. Chung RS, Dearlove J (1988) The sources of recurrent hemorrhage during long-term sclerotherapy. Surgery 104:687–696
3. Söderlund C, Ihre T (1985) Endoscopic sclerotherapy vs conservative management of bleeding esophageal varices. A 5-year prospective controlled trial of emergency and long-term treatment. Acta Chir Scand 151:449–456
4. Inokuchi K (1985) Present status of surgical treatment of esophageal varices in Japan: A nationwide survey of 3588 patients. World J Surg 9:171–180
5. Sugiura M, Futagawa S, Fukasawa M, Kinoshita E, Nakanishi R, Nishimura Y (1988) Experience with non-shunting operation for esophageal varices, 1980–87. In: Idezuki Y (ed) Treatment of esophageal varices. Elsevier, Amsterdam, pp 149–159
6. Spence RAJ (1988) Oesophageal transection for varices: Rationale, indications, technique and results. In: Idezuki Y (ed) Treatment of esophageal varices. Elsevier, Amsterdam, pp 123–139
7. Paquet K-J, Feussner H (1985) Endoscopic sclerosis and esophageal balloon tamponade in acute hemorrhage from esophageal varices: A prospective controlled randomized trial. Hepatology 5:580–583

Esophageal Perforation

Esophageal Perforation in the People's Republic of China

LIAN-QIAN ZENG, YI-FENG ZENG, and CHUN-SHENG NIU[1]

Introduction

Perforation of the esophagus remains a challenge to the thoracic surgeon [1]. Despite modern forms of therapy, the use of hyperalimentation, antibiotics, and better postoperative care, esophageal perforation or rupture continue to be associated with high mortality and morbitity. While the esophagus is infrequently injured as a result of external penetrating trauma in the neck, perforation due to surgical instrumentation, foreign body, or spontaneous rupture were the most common causes in the thoracic esophagus. We review here the data of esophageal perforation in the People's Republic of China. The purpose of this study is to analyze the causes, surgical treatment, and outcome of esophageal perforation. This paper does not address the issue of postoperative leaks developing in esophageal anastomosis.

Material and Methods

Incidence

Between 1971 and 1990, 1611 cases of benign esophageal disease were reported in China. The incidence of esophageal perforation was 7.8%; it was the fifth most common of the conditions in this classification. (Fig. 1).

Patient Population

Between 1971 and 1990, the diagnosis of esophageal perforation was confirmed in 511 patients from the Chinese literature reported and investigated by letters [2–20]. Three hundred and sixty-seven (71.8%) were men, and 144 (28.2%)

---
[1] Department of Thoracic Cardiovascular Surgery, Second Affiliated Hospital, The Medical University of Henan, No. 2 Jingba road, Zhengzhou, Henan 450003 People's Republic of China

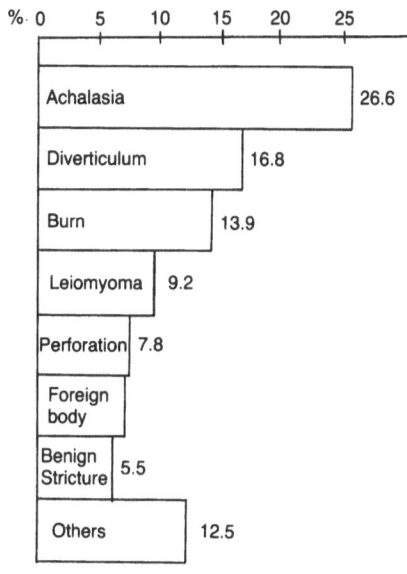

Fig. 1. Incidence of esophageal perforation in 1611 cases of benign esophageal disease

Table 1. Characteristics of LCH and CH groups

Variable	LCH (n = 343)	CH (n = 168)	P Value
Age (Years)			
Mean	38.4	32.2	NS
Sex			
Male	70.6	74.4	NS
Female	29.4	25.6	NS
Location			
Cervical	11.1	20.8	0.014
Thoracic	86.0	75.6	0.001
Abdominal	2.9	3.6	NS

NS, not significant; LCH, large city hospital; CH, county hospital

patients were women. The age ranged from 2 to 74 years with a mean age of 35.3 years. Seventy-three perforations (14.3%) occurred in the neck, 422 (82.6%) were intrathoracic, and 16 (3.1%) were abdominal.

Groups

The patients were divided into two groups: Group A consisted of 343 patients (67.1%) from large city hospitals (LCH group), including thirty-six patients from the department of the thoracic surgery of Henan Medical University. Group B consisted of 168 patients (32.9%) from county hospitals (CH group). The characteristics of each group are summarized in Table 1.

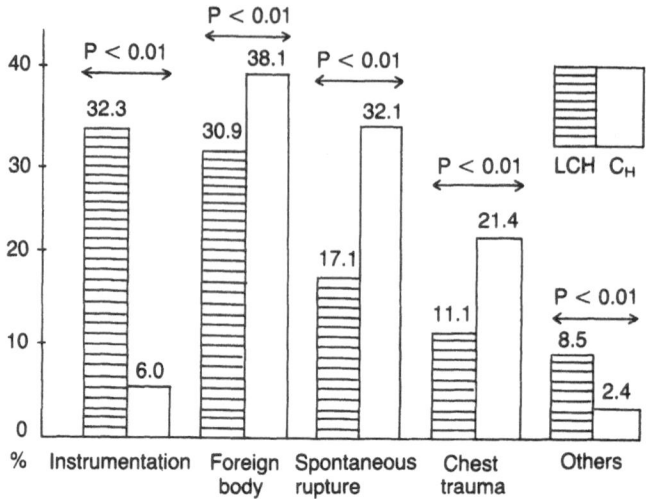

Fig. 2. Causes of esophageal perforation

Causes

We classified the causes of esophageal perforation into five types: (1) iatrogenic instrumentation injury, 121 cases, 23.7%; (2) spontaneous rupture (Boerhaave's Syndrome), 113 cases, 22.1%; (3) foreign body, 170 cases, 33.3%; (4) chest trauma, 74 cases, 14.5%; and (5) others, 33 cases, 6.4%.

The comparative study of causes of esophageal perforation in the LCH and CH groups is shown in Fig. 2. The etiology of the two groups is quite different. The P value <0.001 was selected as the level of statistical significance. In the 36 patients with esophageal perforation at Henan Medical University, the causes were foreign body (30.6%), spontaneous (25.0%), chest trauma (25.0%), surgical instrumentation (13.9%), and others (5.5%).

Perforation by a foreign body is the leading cause. By chi-square analysis, the distributions of the various foreign bodies in the two groups (Fig. 3) were significantly different ($P < 0.001$). Other foreign bodies included firewood, jujube-pits, and water chestnuts.

Treatment and Results

The selection of the operative procedure is dependent on the clinical condition of the patient after the esophageal perforation. This, in turn, is dependent on the time interval elapsed between the perforation and the initiation of therapy. If the perforation is cervical, suture and drainage can be performed through an incision along the sternocleidomastoid, but there were many methods of treatment for thoracic perforations. The purpose of this paper is not to address them all, but only to summarize the treatments available for thoracic perforation.

Four hundred and twenty-two patients were included and the effect of various therapies on the eventual outcome was determined (Table 2). The most favorable

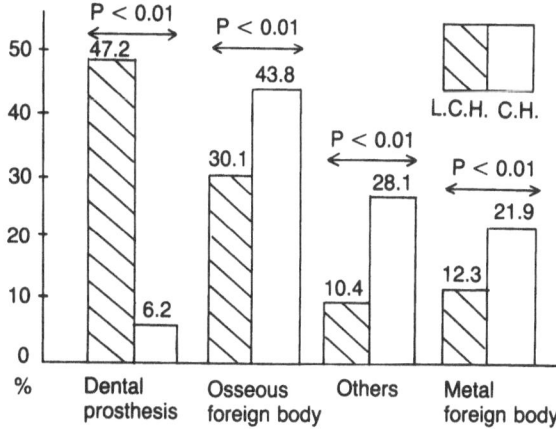

Fig. 3. Distribution of causes of esophageal perforation with foreign bodies

outcome, with an 88.2% survival rate, was seen following simple drainage ($P < 0.01$). The mortality of the total group, the operative mortality of the thoracic esophageal perforation group, and the mortality of the drainage group in both the LCH and CH groups were compared and the results are shown in Table 3. The most favorable outcome was use of drainage to treat the thoracic esophageal perforation. The mortality for both groups combined was 11.8%. Especially of note, the mortality in the CH group was 9.5%. The difference was very significant ($P < 0.01$).

The treatment of 36 patients with esophageal perforation in Henan Medical University hospital was initiated more than 24 h after perforation in 91.7% and more than 48 h afterward in 72.2%. So only two patients underwent esophageal resection and four patients were primary repair, none of whom died. Of the 30 patients who underwent thoracic drainage, 5 patients died. The hospital mortality (LCH group) was 13.9%.

Discussion

The esophagus, lacking a serosal layer and being surrounded by loose areolar tissue, allows bacteria and digestive enzymes easy access to the mediastinum, and this can lead to the development of severe mediastinitis, empyema, sepsis, and ultimately multiple organ failure. Prompt recognition and proper treatment may avert death of minimize a prolonged and difficult convalescense. Delay in diagnosis appears to be a major factor contributing to morbitity and mortality. The etiologic factors were different from various Chinese Large City Hospital reports. The most common cause varied with each report: 62.0%, 67.3%, and 85.2% were iatrogenic instrumental injuries according to references [15], [9], and [5], respectively, and 51.1% and 81.0% were foreign bodies according to references [3] and [4], respectively. Included among foreign bodies were artificial teeth (44.4%) [5]. In this series, the most common cause was surgical instrumentation in the LCH group, and foreign bodies in the CH group. The dif-

Table 2. Surgical treatment and cure rate of thoracic esophageal perforation

Variable	LCH (n = 295)	CH (n = 127)	P Value
Drainage			
No.	141	105	
Percent	47.8	82.7	<0.01
Cure rate (%)	86.5	90.5	NS
Primary repair			
No.	103	9.0	
Percent	34.9	7.1	<0.01
Cure rate (%)	77.7	66.7	NS
Esophageal resection			
No.	40	9.0	
Percent	13.6	7.1	NS
Cure rate (%)	60.0	44.4	<0.01
Repair of aortic perforation			
No.	11	4	
Percent	3.7	3.7	NS
Cure rate (%)	37.0	0	<0.01

NS, not significant

Table 3. Comparison of mortality

Variable	Patients No.	Mortality No.	%
Total	511	105	20.6
LCH	343	73	21.3
CH	168	32	19.1
Thoracic Perforation	422	87	20.6
LCH	295	65	22.0
CH	127	22	17.3
Drainage of Thoracic Perforation	246	29	11.8
LCH	141	19	13.5
CH	105	10	9.5

ference of causes between the two groups was significant. It probably represents differences in medical conditions, living, and diet habits. The higher incidence of spontaneous rupture of the esophagus in rural populations in China is related to alcohol consumption. Perforations resulting from traumatic injuries or penetrating wounds have been reported with increasing frequency in recent years.

Surgical closure or esophagectomy for esophageal perforation has been advocated [21, 22]. The key to a successful outcome is diagnosis and treatment early, within 24 h. The primary esophagectomy and esophagogastrectomy should be performed within a few hours after perforation, because with greater delay and the presence of more severe infection, the resection would be made in badly contaminated tissues with potential risks to the esophageal anastomosis [23]. As for the management of thoracic perforation with delayed diagnosis (more than 24 h) various modalities of therapy have been recommended.

The mortality of esophageal perforations was 20.0% 28.5% in most Chinese reports [3, 9, 10, 24, 25]. The mode of treatment remains controversial. If the patient is diagnosed within 24 h, primary suture repair and adequate drainage is preferable. It is advantageous if operative trauma is less than that caused by esophagectomy. Wide drainage of the mediastium and direct debridement and irrigation of the pleural cavity may be of benefit, as may the use of autogenous tissue buttresses with pleural or intercostal muscle, or omentum or fundoplication [4, 26]. One drainage or multiple drainages are useful if performed correctly with feeding-jejunectomy. If the patient perforation occurred more than 24 h previously, most older more traditional, doctors emphasize "not to operate", but most young doctors opt "to operate" in China. In these data, there is an important fact which has been considered, that the treatment of drainage alone with thoracic esophageal perforation has a lower mortality. It has been shown that adequate thoracic drainage and feeding-jejunectomy was the one of best methods of management for many patients with esophageal perforations.

References

1. Attar S, Hankins JR, Suter CM (1990) Esophageal perforation: A therapeutic challenge. Ann Thorac Surg 50:45–51
2. Zeng IQ (1986) Injury of esophagus. In: Zeng LQ (ed) Mediastinum surgery. Henan Science Skill Publishing, Zhengzhou, pp 175–186
3. Chen J, Tang HS (1985) Emergency management of traumatic esophageal rupture: Analyses of 45 cases. Chinese J Thorac Cardiovasc Surg 1:164–166
4. Cheng BC, Gao SZ, Tu ZF (1989) Choice of surgical treatment for spontaneous rupture of the esophagus among various surgical procedures. Chinese J Thorac Cardiovasc Surg 5:160–161
5. Chen SQ, Liu K (1990) Diagnosis and management of esophageal perforation: 34 cases reported. Chinese J Thorac Cardovasc Surg 6:39–42
6. Chen LK (1989) Spontaneous rupture of esophagus. Chinese J Thorac Cardiovasc Surg 5:220–221
7. Lee CM, Yu YX, Gent DS (1982) Esophageal rupture due to high-pressure gas ejection. Chinese J Surg 20:594–595
8. Liu YG (1980) Mechanical perforation of esophagus. Chinese J Surg 18:526–531
9. Wu SC, Huang OL, Zhou YZ (1985) Operative management of esophageal perforation. Chinese J Surg 230–232
10. Yan JH, Zheng SD, Du XQ (1980) Spontaneous rupture of esophagus: Report of 35 cases. Chinese J Surg 18:526–529
11. Guo SQ (1988) Treatment of traumatic esophageal perforation. Symposium of the Second National Meeting on Thoracic and Cardiovascular Surgery. Chinese Med Assocn, Hian, p 56
12. Zhan LH (1991) Esophageal rupture and perforation. National symposum on disease of benign esophagus. A book of Symposium, May 18–21, 1991, Nanjing, China, pp 17–20

13. Lee WQ, Wang QZ, Chen DH (1991) Esophageal rupture and perforation: report of 69 cases. National symposium on disease of benign esophagus. A book of Symposium, May 18–21, 1991, Nanjing, China, pp 87–89

14. Cui NH (1991) Esophageal perforations: Analysis of 80 cases. National symposium on disease of benign esophagus. A book of Symposium, May 18–21, 1991, Nanjing, China, pp 89–90

15. Zhou SM, Lee GC, Ren GL (1991) Surgical treatment of esophageal perforation. National symposium on disease of benign esophagus. A book of Symposium, May 18–21, 1991, Nanjing, China, pp 85–86

16. Ma WK, Shong QY, Zhu YR (1991) Experience of surgical treatment for spontaneous esophageal rupture. National symposum on disease of benign esophagus. A book of Symposium, May 18–21, 1991, Nanjing, China, pp 83–84

17. Lee W, Wu XL, Yang QW (1991) Diagnosis and treatment of spontaneous esophageal rupture. National symposum on disease of benign esophagus. A book of Symposium, May 18–21, 1991, Nanjing, China, pp 93–94

18. Lee ZZ, Quan XL, Yang QW (1991) Experience of diagnosis and treatment for esophageal rupture. National symposium on disease of benign esophagus. A book of Symposium, May 18–21, 1991, Nanjing, China, pp 95–96

19. Wang LY, Lee HG, Ren GH (1991) Clinical report of 13 cases of spontaneous rupture of esophagus. National symposum on disease of benign esophagus. A book of Symposium, May 18–21, 1991, Nanjing, China, pp 97–98

20. Giang CQ, Xu SG, Fan ZH (1991) Surgical treatment of esophageal rupture. National symposium on disease of benign esophagus. A book of Symposium, May 18–21, 1991, Nanjing, China, pp 100–101

21. Skinner DB, Little AG, DeMeester TR (1980) Management of esophageal perforation. Am J Surg 139:760–764

22. Orringer MB, Stirling MC (1990) Esophagectomy for esophageal disruption. Ann Thorac Surg 49:35–43

23. Johnson J, Schwegman CW, Macvaugh H (1968) Early esophagogastostomy in the treatment of iatrogenic perforation of the distal esophagus. J Thorac Cardiovasc Surg 55:24–27

24. Zhang TS, Zhou JH, Yan LY. Experience of diagnosis and treatment for esophageal rupture. Symposium of the Third National Meeting on Thoracic and Cardiovascular Surgery. Chinese Med Assocn, Beijing, pp 58–59

25. Qin JW, Lee QQ, Fang SQ. Diagnosis and treatment of esophageal perforation: report of 42 cases. Symposium of the third national meeting on thoracic and cardiovascular surgery. Chinese Med Assocn Beijing, pp 54–55

26. Nashef SAM, Pagliero KM (1987) Instrumental perforation of the esophagus in benign disease. Ann Thorac Surg 44:360–362

Esophageal Perforations

Amadeu Pimenta, Valdemar Cardoso, Joaquim Rodrigues, and Diogo Ayres-De-Campos[1]

Introduction

Esophageal perforations, regardless of their etiology or location, are the most life-threatening of all digestive perforations [1, 2]. The spilling of air, food particles, digestive, and nasopharyngeal secretions into the neighboring tissues, caused by the rupture of the esophagus, provokes a fast and dangerous bacterial dissemination, frequently leading to a mediastinal abscess [1, 3].

With this review of 23 cases of esophageal perforations operated in the last 25 years in our department, we hope to stress the importance of early diagnosis and treatment of this condition and help clarify the indications for the various therapeutic options available in a situation where it is difficult to accumulate experience.

Materials and Methods

Between November 1966 and the end of October 1991, a total of 23 patients were treated for esophageal perforation at the Cirurgia (Surgery) 4 Department of the S. João Hospital in Porto. The group included 14 female and 9 male patients, whose ages varied between 29 and 78 years (mean 53 years).

There were 8 cervical, 9 thoracic and 6 abdominal esophageal perforations. The etiology and anatomic location are shown in Fig. 1.

One of the cervical perforations was caused by the patient himself, trying to remove a piece of meat caught in his oropharynx with the handle of a spoon. Another patient had a double cervical perforation caused by a gunshot wound. One of the iatrogenic perforations not caused by endoscopy, occurred in the abdominal esophagus and was due to a traumatic intubation with a gastric washing tube.

---

[1] Cirurgia 4, S. João Hospital, Porto Medical School, 4200 Porto, Portugal

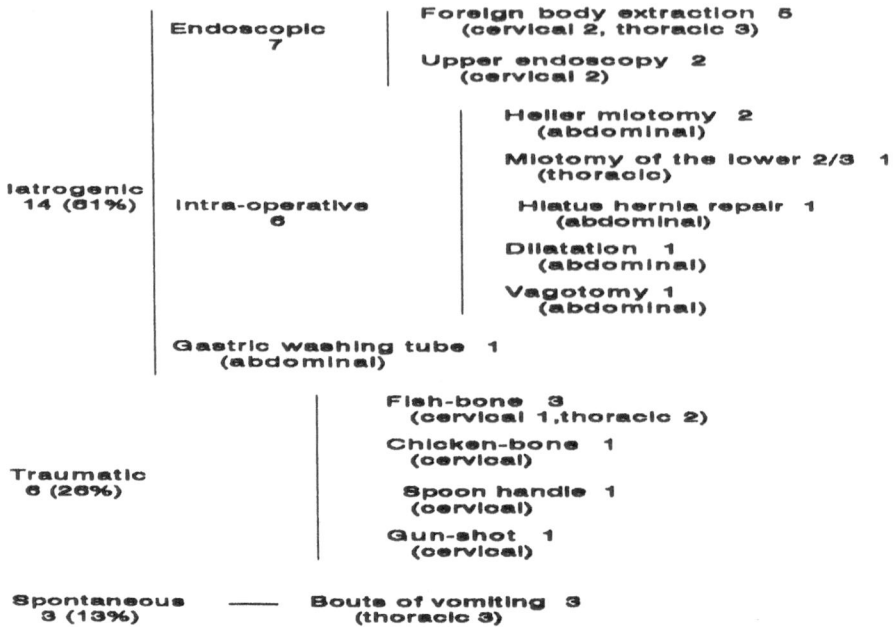

Fig. 1. Relation between etiology and site of perforation

The most common symptom was pain. It was usually intense, sometimes dramatic, and varied in localization from the cervical to the thoracic or epigastric regions, radiating to the sternum or to the neck. Various other symptoms and signs were found in these patients, but it was the presence of a subcutaneous or mediastinal emphysema, pleural effusion, or free air in the abdomen that led us to suspect the perforation. The drainage of a pleural effusion led to the diagnosis of perforation in two patients. In one, food particles were obtained, while in the other, the liquid smelt characteristically of wine.

The diagnosis, suspected by clinical background and plain x-ray of the cervical, thoracic or abdominal regions, was confirmed by contrast roentgenography (with water-soluble contrast). The latter demonstrated the site of perforation in 15 of 16 patients studied. As a diagnostic technique, endoscopy was considered dispensable, not only because contrast roentgenography gave more detailed information on the site of perforation, but also because it involved a certain risk to the patient. In one patient with a cervical perforation, methylene blue was given orally in order to help locate the site of perforation at surgery. Abdominal ultrasonography and computed tomography were only used in the diagnosis of complications and their follow-up.

All patients were surgically treated, although in four patients with cervical perforations, a "conservative" approach had previously been attempted in other departments, for periods of 4, 5, 16 and 33 days respectively. None showed improvement with this treatment. Drainage alone was used in four patients, two with cervical perforations and two with iatrogenic perforations (one in the abdomen and the other in the thorax). Seventeen patients were treated with suture of the perforation and drainage of the site. Two thoracic perforations were treated more aggressively by excluding the esophagus. One of these, however, was only a temporary exclusion, carried out by tying the cervical esophagus with the help of a Dacron prothesis according to the technique described by Ergin et al. [4]. In addition to this, we performed the suture of the perforation, drainage of the site, gastrostomy for drainage of gastric secretions, feeding jejunostomy and a lateral cervical esophageal stoma for drainage of oropharyngeal secretions.

Results

The morbidity rate was 38% in cervical perforations, 89% in thoracic and 33% in abdominal perforations. The overall mortality rate was 17%: three deaths occurred in patients with thoracic perforations and one in a patient with a cervical perforation. The latter died as a result of septicaemia (he was operated on 5 days after perforation). Two of the patients with thoracic perforations died as a result of esophageal fistulae and the third due to a pyothorax and cardiac arrythmia.

Thirteen patients (56%) were operated in the first 24 h after perforation (9 of these in the first 8 h). There was only one death in this group. The other ten patients (43%) were operated on only days after perforation (2 to 33 days) and three died.

Of the four patients with thoracic perforations operated on after 48 h, the only survivors were those submitted to more aggressive surgery (temporary or definitive exclusion of the esophagus).

Discussion

Morbidity and mortality rates associated with esophageal perforations are significant and unquestionably higher in patients operated on more than 24 h after the incident [1, 5, 6]. In patients operated on after 48 h, the mortality rate is in the range of 50% [1, 5, 6]. The fact that, in our patients, mortality was much higher in the group whose delay to surgery exceeded 48 h and that 75% of deaths occurred in thoracic perforations, stresses the importance of early diagnosis and treatment in esophageal perforations, especially those located in the thoracic segment.

At the slightest clinical suspicion of esophageal perforation, a contrast x-ray should be performed, introducing a water-soluble contrast through an endogastric tube that is progressively withdrawn from the esophagus. This procedure is simple, non-toxic and perfectly tolerable for the patient. It allows the visualization of the site of perforation with more precision than when contrast is given orally.

Is it advisable to treat a patient with an esophageal perforation solely with a "conservative" approach? In four of our patients, all without previous lesions of the esophagus and with cervical perforations, a "conservative" approach had previously been attempted without success. The toxic and infectious process was difficult to control and the general health state was greatly deteriorated. As the vast majority of authors, we advocate against this procedure as the sole method of treatment in the previously healthy esophagus. In the few successful cases reported, treatment is usually long and accompanied by a high rate of complications, leading to a prolonged and hazardous in-hospital stay [1, 5, 6]. In the case of therapeutic failure, surgical approach will be delayed hours or even days, the surgeon will be faced with a patient whose general state is more deteriorated than at the time of perforation, requiring a more complex and usually less successful operation.

Because of these reasons, we believe that "conservative" therapy alone should only be tried for a period of 24 hours in patients with very small perforations, which evolve without rupture into the pleural space, with mild infectious syndromes and in an esophagus with previous chronic inflammatory lesions. In the opinion of some authors [6] the cellulitis already present in these cases would limit the diffusion of the infectious process.

In accordance with our results, the selection of the most appropriate surgical interventions should be based on the previous state of the esophagus, the site of perforation and the time elapsed between perforation and surgery. Thus, in the previously nonpathologic esophagus, if no more than 24 h have elapsed, the perforation should be closed independent of its location, together with the drainage of the periesophageal space next to the suture. In thoracic and abdominal esophageal perforations, it is advisable to buttress the closure with gastric fundus, omentum or with a vascularized flap of pleura, pericardium, muscle or diaphragm [1, 5, 7].

If a longer period of time has elapsed after perforation, if the borders of the esophageal wound are friable or if infection of the surrounding tissues is intense, then ideal conditions for primary healing of the wound are no longer present. We believe that in thoracic perforations in these conditions, in addition to closure of the wound after debridement of necrotic-infected tissues [7], a more aggressive surgical approach should be associated, with the exclusion of the esophagus. The temporary exclusion of the cervical esophagus, as described by Ergin et al. [4] seems to us the most reasonable approach.

In perforations of the cervical esophagus, even if time elapsed has exceeded 24 h, our results suggest that primary suture should be tried. The most important measure, however, is drainage of the site.

Perforations of the abdominal esophagus operated on more than 24 h after the incident should be managed with surgical suture of the perforation, reinforced with a flap from the gastric fundus, and drainage of the site.

Acknowledgments. The authors would like to thank Drs. Pereira Cernadas, Costa Santos, Moreira Dias, Goes Pinheiro, and M. Graça Loureiro for their expert support in the diagnosis and treatment of the patients studied.

References

1. Nesbitt JC, Sawyers JL (1987) Surgical management of esophageal perforation. Am Surgeon 53:183–190
2. Skinner DB, Little AG, DeMeester TR (1980) Management of esophageal perforation. Am J Surg 139:760–764

3. Andreassian B, Breil PH, Fékété F, Laisne MJ (1986) Les infections du médiastin. Encyclo-pédie Médico-Chirurgicale. Techniques Chirurgicales Vol 1. Poumon, Paris, p 16
4. Ergin MA, Wetstein L, Griepp RB (1980) Temporary diverting cervical esophagostomy. Surg Gynecol Obstet 151:97–98
5. Baulieux J, Balique JG, Boulez J, Peix JL, Maillet P (1979) Possibilité d'un traitement chirurgical conservateur des ruptures spontanées de l'oesophage vues a un stade tardif. Lyon Chir 75:358–363
6. Couraud L, Dumas PJ, Martigne C, Houdelette P (1978) Les perforations oesophagiennes non tumorales. Lyon Chir 74:110–113
7. Brewer L, Carter R, Mulder GA, Stiles QR (1986) Options in the management of perfora-tions of the Esophagus. Am J Surg 152:62–69

Esophageal Trauma: A Modern Perspective

Daniel Kirgan, Arjun Pennathur, and Alex G. Little[1]

Introduction

Esophageal trauma remains a diagnostic and therapeutic challenge. This is reflected by reported mortality rates of 15%–20% which have remained unchanged for several decades. Outcome is clearly influenced by several factors, such as the mechanism of injury, extent of associated injuries, age, anatomic location, and timing of operation [1]. Historically, early aggressive surgical intervention has been the mainstay of therapy. Conservative treatment is only appropriate for carefully selected cases of chronic contained perforations [2].

Except for iatrogenic trauma during endoscopic maneuvers, isolated injuries to the esophagus are rare. Due to its proximity to other organs, associated injuries leading to the patient's death diminishes the numbers of patients with external trauma being treated. For these reasons, it has been difficult to accumulate a large enough series of patients with esophageal injuries without reviewing extensive time periods spanning several decades. This often results in heterogeneous patient populations for study which compromises the ability to form definite conclusions regarding diagnostic and clinical intervention. We therefore reviewed a recent experience at a single institution in an attempt to identify current trends in etiology, diagnosis, and management of this injury.

Patient Population

A review of admissions from 1982–1992 to the University of Nevada Hospitals identified 23 patients with esophageal injuries. Full thickness injuries were identified in 19 of these patients, with 4 having only partial thickness injuries. Of

[1]Department of Surgery University of Nevada School of Medicine, 2040 W. Charleston Boulevard, Las Vegas, NV 89102, USA

Table 1. Esophageal trauma: etiology in 19 patients

External trauma	15	(79%)	Patients
Penetrating	14		
Stab	9		
Gunshot	5		
Blunt	1		
Iatrogenic	2	(11%)	Patients
Boerhaave's	2	(11%)	Patients

Table 2. Esophageal trauma: operative treatment of 19 patients

External trauma	
Drainage only	2 Patients
Primary closure	13 Patients
Single-layer	8
Double-layer	4
Indeterminate	1
With drainage	12
Iatrogenic	
Primary closure and drainage	2 Patients
Spontaneous	
Primary closure with pleural buttress and drainage	1 Patient
Esophageal exclusion	1 Patient

these 19 patients with full thickness injuries, 12 were male and 7 were female. The age range was 7 months to 73 years.

The anatomic distribution of these injuries was as follows: 16 of the 19 injuries were to the cervical esophagus or pharyngoesophageal junction, 2 were located in the thoracic esophagus, and 1 was to the abdominal esophagus. The etiologic distribution is shown in Table 1. There is a preponderance (15/19) of patients with esophageal injuries as a result of external trauma. Only two patients had an iatrogenic or instrumental injury, and two had spontaneous rupture, Boerhaave's syndrome.

In terms of diagnosis, the esophageal injury was identified by barium or gastrografin swallow x-ray in each of the four patients with instrumental perforation or spontaneous rupture. Of the 15 patients with external trauma, in contrast, 14 had the esophageal injury identified during surgical exploration. Intraoperative endoscopy was utilized in two patients and helped locate a suspected cervical esophageal injury.

The operative approaches are summarized in Table 2. Primary closure and drainage was utilized in the majority of cases. Two patients had sump tube drainage of the neck without closure of the injuries; both injuries eventually healed although drainage persisted for 2 weeks in one patient.

Seventeen of the 19 patients survived, giving an overall survival rate of 90%. However, patients operated on more than 24 h after diagnosis had a higher mortality (one of three or 33%) than patients operated or within 24 h (one of 16 or 6.2%). Both deaths occurred in patients in shock at their initial presentation.

Of the nine patients with an unbuttressed, drained, single-layer closure, there was one postoperative leak which healed with continued drainage and conservative management. None of the four with a double-layer closure leaked, but one developed a stricture.

Discussion

Etiologic causes of esophageal injury are in transition. Historically, iatrogenic perforation, predominately during endoscopic manipulation, was the most common etiologic factor. The iatrogenic esophageal injury rate was reported to be as high as 60%–70% of all esophageal injuries [3] with more recent series reporting 30% to 40% [3]. This change in the etiology of esophageal trauma which is present in our series in large part reflects improvements in endoscopic techniques and routine use of flexible endoscopy, reducing the frequency of iatrogenic perforation. In addition, this trend reflects an increasing incidence of external trauma as a major cause of esophageal injury.

Expeditious surgical intervention remains the mainstay of treatment of eso- phageal perforation as mortality is still influenced by the timing of operation. Operative technique is also important. With injury to the thoracic esophagus, the use of a pleural buttress with primary closure has been shown to improve results even in instances where operation is delayed beyond 24 h [4, 5].

In cases of cervical esophageal injuries, pleural buttressing is not realistic. Our experience suggests that drainage of the neck, following closure of pharyngoes- ophageal injuries or even alone, gives good results as well drained esophageal leaks, either from the original injury or following breakdown of a repair, will eventually resolve. Both morbidity and mortality are reduced compared to earlier experiences.

In conclusion, there is clearly a trend toward external trauma as the primary cause of esophageal injuries, rather than iatrogenic perforation. Surgery remains the mainstay of therapy. Primary closure of the injury with buttressing of thoracic injuries and drainage of cervical injuries provides satisfactory results.

References

1. Flynn AE, Verrier ED, Way LW, Thomas AN, Pelegrini CA (1989) Esophageal Perforation. Arch Surg 124:1211–1215
2. Cameron JL, Kieffer RF, Hendrix TR, Mehigan DG, Bala RR (1978) Selective nonoperative management of contained intrathoracic esophageal disruption. Ann Thorac Surg 27(5):404–408
3. Nesbitt JC, Sawyers JL (1987) Surgical management of esophageal perforation. Am Surg 53:183–191
4. Michel L, Grillo HC, Malt R (1982) Esophageal perforations. Ann Thorac Surg 33(2): 203–209
5. Gouge TH, Depan HJ, Spencer FC (1989) Experience with the Grillo pleural wrap procedure in 18 patients with perforation of the thoracic esophagus. Ann Surg 209(5):612– 619

Multimodal Strategy for the Management of Esophageal Perforations and Ruptures

L. Kotsis[1]

Introduction

Worse outcome following traditional treatment of esophageal disruptions [1]—including even primary closure without reinforcement—led us in 1981 to introduce a more varied management in this major emergency.

The value of this selective approach in 4 spontaneous esophageal ruptures and 23, mostly intrathoracic (88.9%), esophageal perforations: 10 instrumental, 7 traumatic, 4 foreign bodies, and 2 postoperative, was investigated.

Patients and Methods

From 1981 to 1991, 27 patients with ruptures or perforations of the esophagus, intrathoracic in 25 and cervical in 2, were treated at the Thoracic Surgical Clinic in Budapest.

Among the patients with preexisting obstructive esophageal diseases, suture plus myotomy and Dor or Hatafuku + Belsey fundoplication were carried out in early perforated achalasia ($n = 4$). Traction intubation with a personal, cuffed funnel tube—providing a watertight and reflux free exclusion—was used in five inoperable malignancies and in an instrumental perforation of a caustic stricture that had occurred 10 days previously. In instances of a lower mediastinal abscess of similar etiology and origin, transhiatal mediastinal [2] suction-lavage (plus gastrostomy) was performed. In a 7-day-old peptic stricure perforation, in spite of localized empyema, breakdown of the closure was avoided by reinforcement of the suture line with a pedicled diaphragmatic flap.

[1] Postgraduate Medical University Thoracic Surgical Clinic, H-1529 Budapest, Pihenö ut 1, Hungary

Table 1. Perforations of the intact esophagus ($n = 9$)

	No	Treatment	Recurrent leak	Alive
Cervical	2	Conservative	—	2
Early intramediastinal	1	S + diaphragmatic	—	1
12 h		flap buttress		
48 h	1	S + Grillo Flp (modified)	—	1
Late intrathoracic				
48 h	1	Woodward op.	—	1
7 days	1	S + Grillo flp.	—	—
9 days	1	S + diversion (Urschel)	—	1
7 days	1	Diversion (Johson)	—	—
6 weeks	1	Diversion (Urschel—Ergin)	—	1

S, suture; *Flp*, flap; *op*, operation

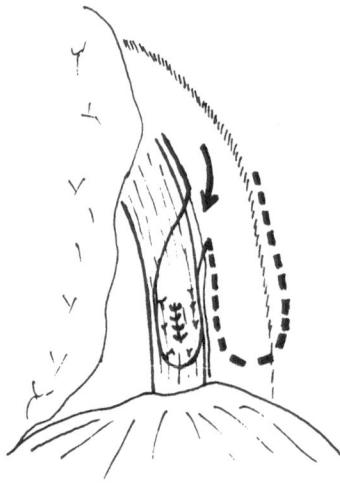

Fig. 1. Modified, vertical fashioned, better vascularized Grillo flap

Mediastinal decompression and two-layer closure were performed within 24 h to 5 days in 4 spontaneous esophageal ruptures. If the repair had been supported by fundoplication or diaphragmatic flap, postoperative development would probably have been free from breakdown of the closure. Only a nasogastric tube was used for gastrointestinal decompression.

The following treatment was adopted in perforation of the esophagus without preexisting disease. (Table 1). Nonoperative treatment was used in two early, small cervical perforations. In the case of lower third intramediastinal lesions (24–48 h after occurrence), the suture was covered either with a diaphragmatic or with a modified, better vascularized, vertical fashioned Grillo flap (Fig. 1). In late (48 h, 7 days, and 6 weeks after occurrence) intrathoracic traumatic perforations, recovery was obtained by Woodward operation or suture and Urschel type diversion [3]. In a 6-week-old perforation with right side empyema (Fig. 2)

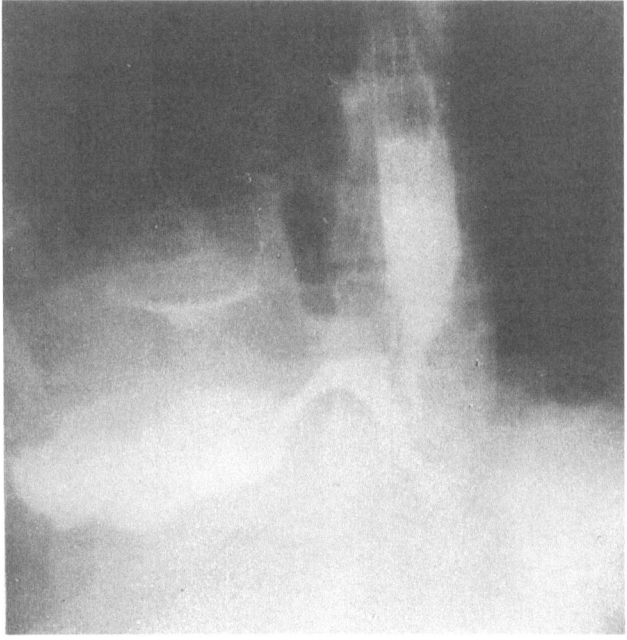

Fig. 2. Six-week-old esophageal perforation with right side empyema

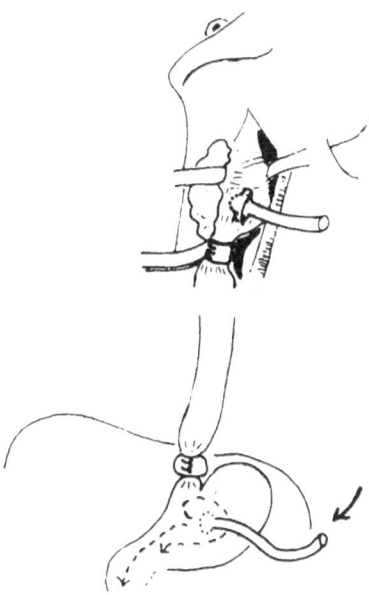

Fig. 3. Urschel-Ergin type esophageal exclusion and diversion used in this case

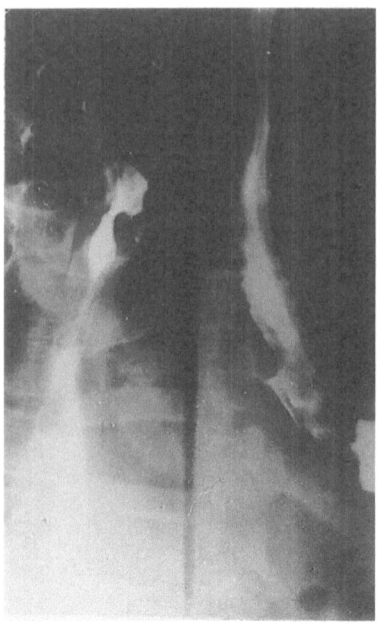

Fig. 4. Final aspect after removal of the bandings

a similar distal and also a cervical banding [4] (Fig. 3) plus tube thoracostomy with suction lavage was successful (Fig. 4).

In the two patients with small postoperative (intramediastinal) disruption, discovered 4 and 7 days after transthoracic diverticulectomy or enterocyst resection, conservative treatment was instituted.

Results

Although these operations were used in 62.9% of the late (24 h to 6 weeks) perforations, in all instances the leakage was controlled. Only patients with major complications such as contralateral aspiration, lung abscess, purulent pericarditis, renal failure, and duodenal perforation, were lost due to delayed recognition before admission ($n = 5$). The overall hospital mortality was 18.5%.

Neither stricture nor the need for a late dilatation was noted after subsequent removal of the bandings at 10 and 21 days, respectively, after esophageal diversion by the Urschel technique.

Discussion

Once the diagnosis of esophageal disruption is made, the most critical decision is to select the type of the management.

The presence of surrounding mediastinal fibrosis in caustic strictures creates a unique set of conditions in cases of instrumental perforations. The injury and also the contamination often remain intramediastinal. Nonoperative treatment

Table 2. Perforated caustic strictures

Cervical, intramural		nonop. treatment
Early intrathoracic	Distal 1/3	Resection + Roux-en-Y interposition
	Higher	Torek op. (conventional or transmediastinal)
	Lye perf.	Stripping (Akiyama technique)
Intramediastinal + −		Intubation + −
Intrapleural		Mediastinal, + pleural D
Late intrathoracic		Transhiatal mediastinal D
		+ − pleural D + G

D, drainage; *G*, gastrostomy; *nonop.*, nonoperative; *perf*, perforation

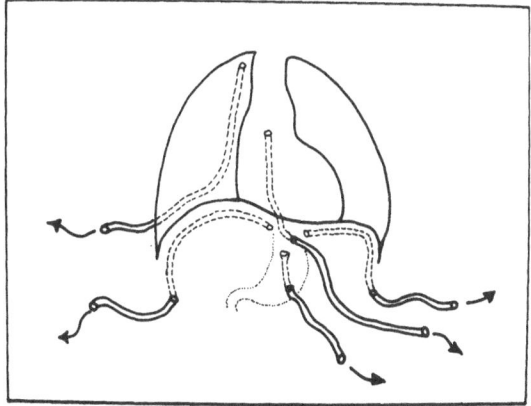

Fig. 5. Illustration of the transhiatal mediastinal drainage

or gastrostomy (to combat gastroesophageal reflux) should be used in early small cervical or intramural perforations, and in early mediastinitis (Table 2). For intrathoracic instrumental perforation within 24 h, primary (conventional) resection, with or without replacement, should be recommended. Endoprosthesis insertion [5] proved to control the intramediastinal perforation (48 h). Transhiatal mediastinal drainage (Fig. 5) with or without suction-lavage (with gastrostomy plus tube thoracostomy for associated empyema) is the most useful type of mediastinal drainage for lower or middle mediastinal abscesses [2].

Underlying, stenosing, distal esophageal diseases compromises healing of suture repair of the perforation. As a rule, the obstruction should be relieved together with the suturing and support the closure (Table 3). The antireflux procedures buttress both the suture line and the formal operation. In late cases, diversion [6] or intubation should be instituted.

Conservative treatment [7] may be sufficient in small intramediastinal spontaneous ruptures (Table 4). Recovery even after primary closure of these ruptures within 24 h has been described by many authors [8–10]. The patch procedures with the gastric fundus [3, 9] or diaphragmatic flap [10] ensure a more secure healing of the closure than other (pleural, intercostal muscle) applied flaps. Large lacerations at the characteristic level should be repaired

Table 3. Management of preexisting esophageal diseases with perforations

Early cases <24 h		
Achalasia	→	S + Heller op + FPL
Hiatal hernia	→	S + FPL
	↗	Dilatation + S + FPL
Peptic strict	→	Woodward or Thal op
	↝	Resection + interposition with Γ loop
Tu resectable	→	Resection (blunt)
unresectable	→	Intubation
Late cases	→	Intubation, resection, diversion (Urschel)

S, suture; *FPL*, fundoplication; *strict*, stricture; *op*, operation; *Tu*, tumor

Table 4. Management of spontaneous ruptures

Small, intramediastinal	Conservative
Characteristic, early <24 h and late >24 h	Mediastinal decompression + S + reinforcement with fundoplication or diaphragmatic flap
Major laceration (characteristic site)	Thal or Woodward operation Resection (blunt)
Late cases with sepsis, recurrence	Urschel operation + pleural drainage

S, suture

using a Woodward operation or resection. Failure after initial repair or severe sepsis calls for diversion (Urschel type [6]).

Injuries of the healthy esophagus demand complex procedures to salvage the organ (Table 1). In early cases, primary closure with reinforcement (pleural, diaphragmatic, extrathoracic muscular flaps) and in late intrathoracic tears, Woodward and especially the organ-preserving Urschel type diversion [6, 11] performed either simultaneously with the primary repair or after the failure of the initial attempt of the esophageal closure, has clinical value.

In esophageal disruptions due to operation (vagotomy, hiatal hernia repair, Heller myotomy, pneumonectomy, etc.), suture closure supported by fundoplication (Dor or Belsey type) or muscle flap should be performed. Extrathoracic muscular flap is advised for postpulmonectomy esophageal perforation.

This experience suggests that the key to improvement of the prognosis in this type of emergency is more selective management that takes into account the close connection between the procedure used and underlying esophageal diseases, the time factor, and the site and type of the perforation.

References

1. Postlethwait RW (1979) Surgery of the esophagus. Appleton Century Crofts, New York, pp. 152–176
2. Krisár Z, Kotsis L, Dobjanschy S (1969) 25 perforations of caustic esophageal strictures. Orv Hetil 110:178–180.

3. Kotsis L, Gondos T, Pénzes T, Botsos A (1983) Modern treatment of the spontaneous rupture of the esophagus. Orv Hetil 124:1755–1759
4. Ergin AM, Wetstein L, Griepp RB (1980) Temporary diverting cervical esophagostomy. Surg Gynecol Obstet 151:97–98
5. Imre J (1973) Plastic tube prosthesis for the surgical treatment of perforations in esophageal strictures. Ann Thorac Surg 15:275–278
6. Urschel HC, Razzuk MA, Wood RE, Galbraith N, Pockey M, Paulson DL (1974) Improved management of esophageal perforation: exclusion and diversion in continuity. Ann Surg 179:587–591
7. Cameron JL, Kieffer RF, Hendrix TR, Hehigan DE, Baker RR (1979) Selective nonoperative management of contained intrathoracic esophageal disruptions. Ann Thorac Surg 27:404–408
8. Symbas PN, Hatcher ChR, Harlafist N (1978) Spontaneous rupture of the esophagus. Ann Surg 187:634–640
9. Finley RJ, Pearson G, Weisel RD, Todd RJ, Ilves R, Cooper J (1980) The management of nonmalignant intrathoracic esophageal perforation. Ann Thorac Surg 30:575–581
10. Westaby S, Shepard MP, Nohl-Oser HC (1982) The use of diaphragmatic pedicle grafts for reconstructive procedures in the esophagus and tracheobronchial tree. Ann Thorac Surg 33:486–490
11. Kotsis L, Szabadi G, Kostic SZ (1983) Successful treatment of a 9-day-old iatrogenic esophageal perforation by suture and Urschel type exclusion. Magy Seb 36:358–363

A Case of Esophageal Rupture After Gastrectomy

Masatoshi Isogai, Kitao Hachisuka, Akihiro Yamaguchi, and Akihiro Hori[1]

Introduction

We report here a case of esophageal rupture which occurred immediately after gastrectomy. An unusual postoperative course confused the diagnosis. The aim of this report is to heighten awareness of this catastrophic complication and to discuss the etiology, diagnosis, and treatment of rupture of the esophagus after surgery.

Case Report

A 58-year-old man was referred to our hospital for resection of a gastric carcinoma. He had a history of hypertension, alcoholic liver disease, and duodenal ulcer. He had occasionally complained of heartburn.

On September 7, 1987, he underwent surgery. Partial distal gastrectomy with lymph node dissection and Billroth I reconstruction were performed. A nasogastric tube was placed preoperatively without difficulties. There were no particular troubles during surgery. Microscopic examination of the stomach revealed that the tumor was 1.5 cm × 1.5 cm in size, limited to the mucosa, and there was no evidence of regional lymph node involvement.

After surgery, he was extubated and was in stable condition. Early the next day, September 8, he retched at 1:00 a.m. and complained of wound pain which was relieved by epidural anesthesia of 30 mg of morphine. He retched again at 2:40 a.m. At 6:05 a.m., he suddenly complained of severe pain and restlessness. After that, his general condition deteriorated and he developed a high fever, tachycardia, and tachypnea. His blood gases also deteriorated and he was reintubated at 4:30 a.m. on September 9.

[1] Department of Surgery, Ogaki Municipal Hospital, 4-86, Minaminokawa, Ogaki, 503 Japan

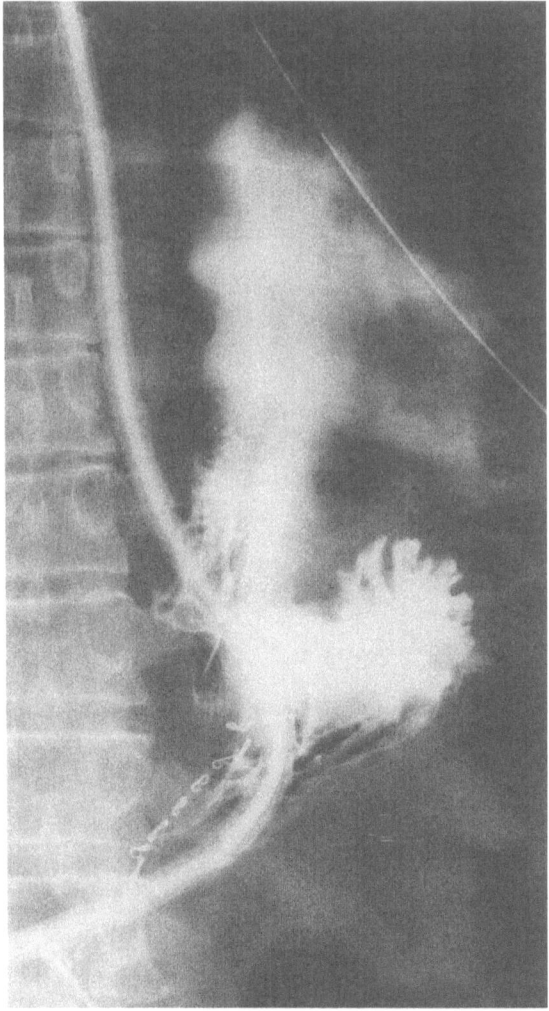

Fig. 1. A Gastrografin study 7 days after gastrectomy demonstrated marked extravasation of contrast from the distal esophagus to the left pleural space

A chest x-ray the same day revealed massive left pleural effusion. A left chest tube was inserted, which drained 1400 ml of a serosanguinous fluid. Aspiration pneumonia was considered responsible for the blood gas deterioration and pleural effusion was considered to be secondary to a leak at the suture line of the gastroduodenostomy. Nutritional and respiratory support and antibiotic therapy were started. Meanwhile, the chest tube continued to drain approximately 500–1000 ml of a serosanguinous fluid daily. On September 14, 7 days after gastrectomy, the pleural fluid contained a very high amylase level of 16920 IU. At this time, the diagnosis of esophageal rupture was advanced. Then a

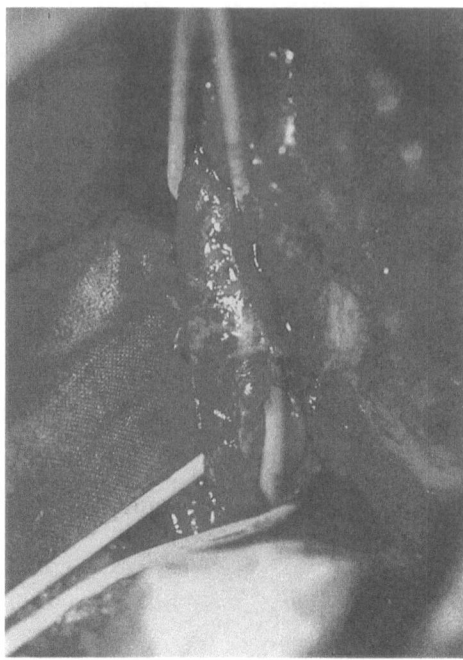

Fig. 2. A left thoracotomy 8 days after gastrectomy showed a longitudinal rupture of the left lateral distal esophagus, approximately 2.5 cm in length and just above the diaphragm. Two Nelaton catheters were placed around the esophagus just below and above the rupture. A nasogastric tube was seen from the tear in the esophagus

Gastrografin study was performed which demonstrated marked extravasation of contrast from the distal esophagus to the left pleural space (Fig. 1), and the diagnosis of esophageal rupture was confirmed.

He underwent a left thoracotomy on September 15, 8 days after gastrectomy. A small amount of brownish fluid was present in the left pleural cavity with a marked pleural and mediastinal inflammatory reaction. Upon opening the mediastinum, a longitudinal rupture of the left lateral distal esophagus, approximately 2.5 cm in length and just above the diaphragm, was discovered (Fig. 2). The inner aspect of the esophagus was inspected, and the presence of other esophageal disease was excluded. The rupture was repaired primarily with a two-layer closure. The mediastinum and pleural spaces were irrigated with saline and drained with three chest tubes. The histological findings of the esophageal specimen obtained by debridement of the edges of the rupture was inflammatory granulation.

His postoperative course was complicated by a suture line leak and then a esophago-broncheal fistula, necessitating left lobectomy of the lung together with closure of the esophageal fistula. With prolonged drainage as well as enteral and intravenous nutrition, the fistula closed gradually. He was discharged 245 days after the initial gastrectomy.

Discussion

Postlethwait [1] classified rupture of the esophagus after surgery as rupture under conditions of abnormal stress. Three types of esophageal rupture are placed in this category: (1) rupture associated with neurologic lesions, (2) rupture after surgery, and (3) rupture after burns.

We were able to find 15 reported cases of esophageal rupture after surgery in the English literature [2-14]. Age ranged from 44 to 79 years with a mean of 56; there were ten males and five females. Many kinds of procedures were described as the initial surgery. In the majority of cases (12 out of 15, 80%), vomiting occurred as a precipitating factor early in the postoperative period. Rupture occurred in the distal esophagus in the majority of cases (13 out of 15, 87%). In spontaneous rupture of the esophagus, Boerhaave's syndrome, which connotes that the rupture is not due to direct trauma, foreign body, or instrumentation, there is a predisposing or precipitating factor and is never purely spontaneous [15]. Esophagitis may well be a prediaposing factor [1]. The major factor in production of spontaneous rupture appears to be vomiting and retching [1, 15]. In approximately 80%-90% of spontaneous ruptures of the esophagus, the tear is in the distal esophagus on the left [1, 15]. Accordingly, the clinical picture of esophageal rupture following surgery is almost the same as that seen in spontaneous rupture, and some confusion exists with regard to spontaneous rupture and those ruptures that occur under conditions of abnormal stress [1]. Kinsella [16] reported that some spontaneous ruptures of the esophagus occurred after recurrent postoperative vomiting or postoperative severe continuous retching after the stomach has apparently been emptied. Meagher et al. [12] reviewed the literature and reported that 25 (8.8%) out of 283 spontaneous ruptures of the esophagus occurred following postoperative vomiting, but details were not given.

The etiology specific to rupture of the esophagus after surgery is not clear. Motility studies of the esophagus in vivo have demonstrated that in 80% of instances, there is a functioning inferior esophageal sphincter contracting with sympathetic stimulation and relaxing with vagal stimulation. This inferior sphincter mechanism is located 1-2 cm above the diaphragm which coincides with the area most vulnerable to rupture [12]. Incoordination of the vomiting center may arise from a variety of postoperative conditions such as heavy sedation and the anesthetic recovery period [1, 12]. Should the markedly increased intra-abdominal pressure be released suddenly into the esophagus against the closed sphincter or spasm, the intraesophageal pressure might then exceed the tensile strength of the wall of the esophagus [1, 12]. Several factors during surgery and in the postoperative period have been shown to contribute to lower esophageal ulceration [11, 17].

In the present case, recurrent postoperative retching may have initiated the series of events that resulted in the esophageal rupture. Predisposing factors may have included his history of duodenal ulcer and alcoholism, with possible weakning of the esophageal wall due to reflux and esophagitis. He had epidural anesthesia for relief of postoperative wound pain, which may have caused incoordination of the vomiting center. He had a nasogastric tube in place, which may be considered in the possible etiology [3, 11]. Jackson et al. [18] have reported several factors which may predispose adult patients to esophageal perforation during nasogastric intubation. In our patient, no difficulties were encountered during nasogastric intubation, and these risk factors were not present. The remaining possibility might be injury to the esophagus during gastrectomy. Wichern [19] reported 19 cases of esophageal perforation after paraesophageal surgery: 3 were perforation of the lower thoracic esophagus after transthoracic vagotomy, 12 abdominal esophagus after transabdominal vagotomy, and the remaining 4 perforations occurred at the abdominal eso-phagus during repair of a hiatal hernia. Tilanus et al. [20] reported 7 cases (11.9%) among 59 esophageal perforations, the cause of which were surgery: one accidental perforation of the cervical esophagus occurred during thyroid-ectomy, five occurred accidentally during surgery at the intra-abdominal esophagus and the remaining perforation occurred at the intrathoracic eso-phagus (the details of which were not given). Accordingly, all except one perforartion of the intrathoracic esophagus after surgery in two series were caused by intrathoracic paraesophageal surgery. In our case, no particular troubles were encountered during partial distal gastrectomy and the rupture occurred in the lower thoracic esophagus. The possible role which the surgical maneuver may have played is small.

Careful consideration of the onset of the illness with careful attention to characteristic symptoms, signs, and repeated x-ray studies with a high index of suspicion will lead to better diagnosis [7]. Since vomiting or retching, however, is often considered an innocent and normal physiological process in the imme-diate postoperative or postanesthetic period [12] and chest x-ray abnormality is often considered a postoperative chest complication, the diagnosis is difficult. In the 15 reported cases of esophageal rupture after surgery, the provisional diagnosis included bronchopneumonia [2, 6], pulmonary embolism [3, 4, 11], pulmonary infarction [11], perforated peptic ulcer [13], myocardial infarct [13], and postoperative pancreatitis [14]. In the definite diagnosis of esophageal rupture, an esophagogram with water-soluble contrast material such as Gastro-grafin is usuful [15]. High amylase level of the pleural effusion might be a useful indicator [1, 14, 15].

Treatment for esophageal rupture consists of thoractomy, exploration of the pleural space and mediastinum, closure of the rupture, and proper drainage [1, 7]. However, leak of the esophageal closure with subsequent esophagocutaneous fistula, a situation encountered in late repairs as shown in our case, is the most common complication [15]. The poor blood supply, absence of a protective omentum, lack of a serosal layer, and friable submucosa lead to breakdown of the suture line. For this reason, many surgeons have suggested buttressing the primary repair [15] with a flap or graft of pericardium, pleura, diaphragm, intercostal muscle, lung or gastric fundus [14, 21]. The technique of exclusion and diversion is advocated by Urschel et al. [22] for late cases, large perfora-tions, or after failure of standard repair [15]. Extirpation may be indicated in some cases [21]. Intensive medical treatment including proper antibiotic therapy and respiratory and nutritional support are also mandatory.

Summary

A case of esophageal rupture after gastrectomy is described. The disease is uncommon and may be missed because other postoperative complications may initially be thought to be the cause of the symptoms. It is emphasized that, for postoperative patients who deteriorate following an episode of retching or vomiting and develop chest complications, rupture of the esophagus should be suspected and an early esophagogram obtained [6].

References

1. Postlethwait RW (1979) Perforation and rupture. In: Postlethwait RW, Sealy WC (eds) Surgery of the esophagus. Appleton-Century-Crofts, pp 152–176
2. Gott R (1933) Spontaneous rupture of the esophagus with a report of four cases. Am J Med Sci 186:400–409
3. Eliason WL, Welrty RF (1946) Spontaneous rupture of the esophagus. SGO 83:234–238
4. Barrett NR (1947) Report of a case of spontaneous perforation of the oesophagus successfully treated by operation. Br J Surg 35:216–218
5. Higginson JF, Clagett OT (1948) Complete disruption of the esophagus. J Thorac Surg 17:846–848
6. Muendel HJ, Levinson W. (1953) Spontaneous rupture of the esophagus. Arch Surg. 67:943–946
7. Hayes DW (1953) Spontaneous rupture of the esophagus. South Med J. 46:962–965
8. Arata JA, Zwick H. (1955) Spontaneous rupture of the esophagus. Dis Chest 27:685–690
9. Cummins CFA, Wedgewood J. (1958) Spontaneous rupture of the oesophagus. Br J Surg. 12:33–36
10. Pate JW, Hughes AH, Patton TB (1958) Spontaneous rupture of the esophagus. Am Surg. 24:385–394
11. Gould EA, Philbin PH, Kerr HH (1959) Spontaneous rupture of the esophagus complicating major abdominal surgery. Am Surg. 25:744–747
12. Meagher RP, Lupien J, Albert SN (1962) Postoperative rupture of the esophagus. SGO. 115:677–681
13. Vatashsky E, Haskel Y, Aronson HB (1983) Esophageal rupture and spinal anesthesia. Anesth Analg. 62:606–608
14. Nooten GV, Azagra JS, Alle JL, Deuvaert FE, Paepe JD, Jacobs D., Osmani A, Primo G. (1987) Spontaneous rupture of the esophagus after coronary artery bypass. Acta Chir Belg 87:367–370
15. Curci JJ, Horman MJ (1976) Boerhaave's syndrome: The importance of early diagnosis and treatment. Ann Surg. 183:401–408
16. Kinsella TJ (1951) Spontaneous perforation of the esophagus. Am Surg. 17:584–597
17. Brooker RM (1956) Spontaneous perforation of the esophagus with report of a case. Am Surg. 22:129–134
18. Jackson RH, Payne DK, Bacon BR (1990) Esophageal perforation due to nasogastric intubation. Am J Gastroenterol 85:439–442
19. Wichern WA (1970) Perforation of the esophagus. Am J Surg. 119:534–536
20. Tilanus HW, Bossuyt P, Schattenkerk ME, Obertop H. (1991) Treatment of oesophageal perforation: A multivariate analysis. Br J Surg. 78:582–585
21. Goldstein LA, Thompson WR (1982) Esophageal perforations: A 15-year experience. Am J Surg. 143:495–503
22. Urschel HC, Razzuk MA, Wood RE, Gaebraith N, Pockey M., Paulson DL (1974) Improved management of esophageal perforation. Ann Surg. 179:587–591

Treatment of Boerhaave's Syndrome According to Its Clinical Manifestations

U. Kania, P. Decker, C.H. Siebert, D. Decker, and A. Hirner[1]

Introduction

Since Boerhaave first described the spontaneous rupture of a healthy esophagus in 1772, case reports describing this illness have repeatedly appeared in the literature. Reports of large patient groups or prospective studies regarding the most effective treatment forms do not seem to exist. The untreated rupture of the esophagus has a mortality rate of nearly 100%. The elapsed time between the rupture and the onset of treatment has the greatest influence on the survival rate. The choice of treatment is also of critical importance and must be made in regard to the general health of the patient, the location of the rupture, and the intraoperative findings, which change depending on the elapsed time.

Case Reports

Case No. 1

A 20-year-old patient presented in the emergency room of an outlying hospital complaining of severe epigastric pain following an episode of strained emesis. He was referred to surgery and a diagnostic laparotomy was carried out without discovery of a lesion.

Upon developing a septicemic shock, the patient was transferred to our department. The initial chest roentgenography revealed a mediastinal emphysema. A left thoracotomy was performed 72 h after the esophageal rupture and the mediastimum was opened. Intraoperatively an advanced case of mediastinal inflammation and a partial necrosis of the esophagus was discovered. The necrotic tissue was resected and a diverting cervical esophagostomy, ligation of the distal

[1] Department of Surgery, University of Bonn, Sigmund-Freud-Str. 25, D-5300 Bonn 1, Germany

esophagus and a gastrostomy were carried out. The patient survived and underwent a successful reconstruction in form of a substernal esophagogastrostomy 2 months later.

Case No. 2

A 61-year-old patient was admitted to our hospital with the typical symptoms of a Boerhaave's syndrome. The Gastrografin swallow showed a dorsolateral rupture just above the diaphragm. Additionally, a high-grade distal gastric obstruction was diagnosed. A laparotomy waš carried out 18 h after the rupture and the distal esophagus was explored transabdominally through the hiatus. Due to the fact that the esophageal wall was still viable and amenable to primary closure, a single layer suture repair of the tear was carried out and reinforced with a modified semifundoplication as described by Thal [1]. An extensive lavage and closed drainage was performed. Because of the distal obstruction, a longitudinal pylorotomy was carried out. Intraoperatively, no ulcer or scarring was found but rather a generalized thickening of the pylorus, so that a Heineke-Mikulicz pyloroplasty was performed. The patient recovered quickly and was discharged 18 days postoperatively.

Discussion

Boerhaave's syndrome is associated with classical clinical manifestations (severe epigastric or substernal pain preceded by episodes of vomiting; frequently associated with alcohol abuse) and the diagnosis (chest X-ray, Fig. 1; Gastrografin swallow, Fig. 2) is relatively simple [2]. Still, a spontaneous esophageal rupture is frequently not recognized due to a lack of awareness of this disease. As a result, the prognosis of this dramatic condition is quite poor.

Due to the fact that the Boerhaave's syndrome is a rare condition, no prospective, randomized studies exist to document the ideal treatment regimen. Still, surgeons agree that Boerhaave's syndrome needs to be treated surgically. It is also general knowledge that the rate of morbidity and mortality is directly related to the lapse of time between rupture of the esophagus and its treatment. Therefore, a prompt and correct diagnosis and early surgical intervention are vital [3].

The location of the perforation should determine the surgical approach. In light of the fact that 91% [4] of all esophageal ruptures are located in the distal third (Fig. 3), a transabdominal, transhiatal approach can frequently be used. This represents a good approach, once the diaphragm has been incised, to the left- as well as right-sided distal ruptures. Additionally, it is then easier to carry out the reinforcing fundoplication and the treatment of other causal intraabdominal lesions, as described in the second case report, is possible during the same procedure. In the literature review published by Hafer et al. [5], patients treated by means of a laparotomy have the lowest postoperative mortality rate. In case of rupture in the mid-third of the esophagus we prefer the left thoracotomy, while cervical ruptures are approached through a left cervical incision (Table 1) [6]. A great variety of recommendations for the treatment of Boerhaave's syndrome have been published in the past [7–11]. A strictly conservative treatment regimen including intravenous fluids, parenteral nutrition, antibiotics,

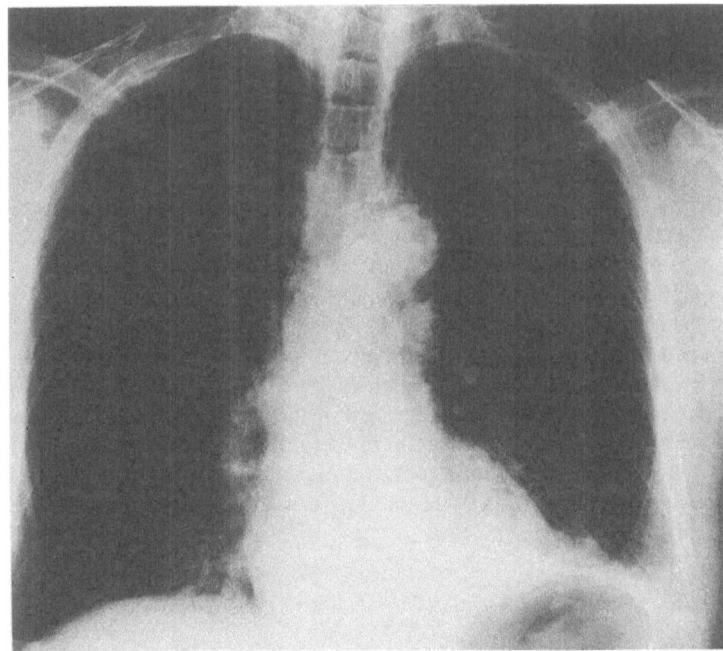

Fig. 1. Mediastinal emphysema and pleural effusion following a spontaneous esophageal rupture

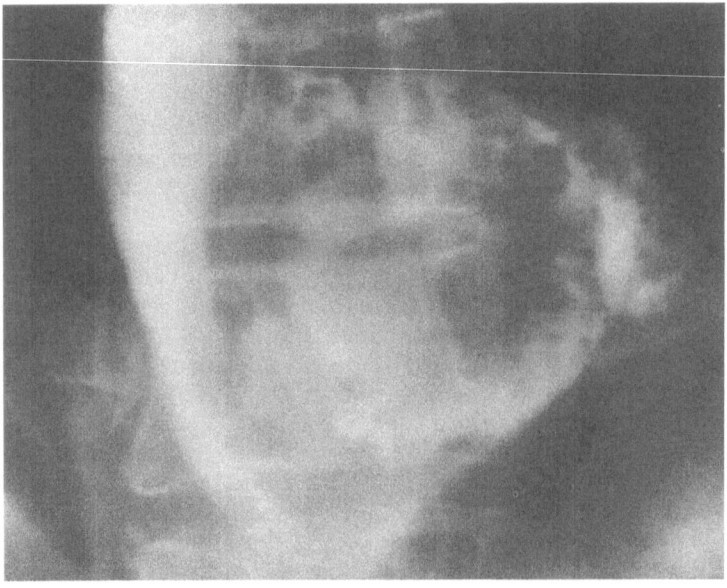

Fig. 2. Esophageal rupture with dorsal leak to the left side

Fig. 3. Location distribution of esophageal ruptures

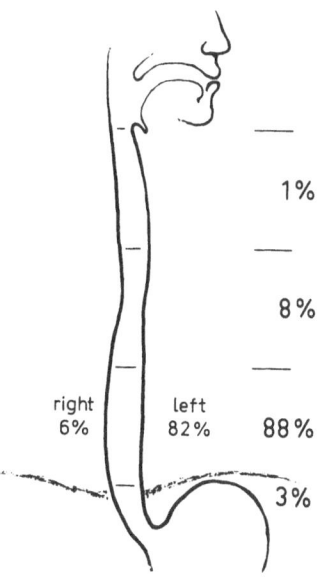

1%

8%

right   left
6%   82%   88%

3%

Table 1. Approach, depending on the rupture location

Height of the rupture	Approach
Upper third	Left-cervical
Mid third	Left-thoracical
Lower third	Abdomino-transhiatal

Table 2. Operative strategy, depending on the intraoperative situation

Condition of the esophagus	Therapy
Vital, suture possible	Rinse + primary suture secured by semifundoplication or a pleuraflap
Vital, no suture possible	Rinse + extensive drainage
Necrotic	Resection of the necrosis + cervical esophagostoma + Witzel's fistula + extensive drainage; esophagogastric anastomosis in a second operation

drainage of pleural effusion, and tubus implantation has been reported [12]. Due to the high complication rates, this treatment regimen should be reserved for those rare patients with limited clinical manifestation, a small transmural defect and free drainage into the esophageal lumen [5].

Surgical intervention is generally viewed as the treatment of choice for this lesion. The treatment must be adjusted to the intraoperative findings of the esophagus (Table 2). In cases in which the tissue is viable and amenable to primary suture, the tear should be closed with a single row suture. If the esophageal wall is still viable but markedly edematous and therefore not amenable to suture, the intervention should be restricted to an extensive drainage. If the tissue is already necrotic, it should be resected, and a diverting cervical esophagostomy, ligation of the distal esophagus, and a gastrostomy performed. Once the patient has survived the procedure and been adequately stabilized, a secondary substernal esophagogastrostomy is carried out, as described in the first case report. The substernal reconstruction is advisable, due to the severe scarring and inflammatory changes in the original esophageal bed.

In addition to any surgical treatment, broad antibiotic coverage as well as extensive drainage should be carried out. Intravenous fluids should also be administered promptly.

Considering that the prognosis of this disease is less influenced by the form of the surgical intervention than by the time interval between the occurrence of the rupture and the beginning of treatment [13, 14], our goal must be to increase the awareness of this illness and to thereby achieve an early diagnosis.

References

1. Thal AP, Hatfuku T (1964) Improved operation for esophageal rupture. JAMA 188:826–831
2. Gaa J, Deininger HK (1989) Die spontane Ösophagusruptur—Boerhaave-Syndrom. Radiologe 29:371–376
3. Schwarz JA, Turnbull TL, Dymowski J, Uehara DT (1986) Boerhaave's Syndrome: An elusive diagnosis. Am J Emerg Med 4:532–536
4. Hirner A, Häring R (1981) Pathophysiologie und Klinik der spontanen Ösophagusruptur (Boerhaave-Syndrom). In: Häring R (1981) (ed) Ösophaguschirurgie. IV. Symposium "Aktuelle Chirurgie" Edition Medizin Weinheim, pp 257–277
5. Hafer G, Haunhorst WH, Stallkamp B (1990) Die atraumatische Ruptur des Ösophagus (Boerhaave-Syndrom). Zent. bl. Chir 115:729–735
6. Wagner HE, Schroeder R (1985) Zur Behandlung der intrathorakalen Ösophagusperforation. Helv Chir Acta 52:647–650
7. Bradley SL, Pairolero PC, Payne WS, Gracey DR (1981) Spontaneous rupture of the esophagus. Arch Surg 116:755–758
8. Graeber GM, Niezgoda JA, Albus RA, Burton NA, Collins GJ, Lough FC, Zajtchuk R (1987) A comparison of patients with endoscopic esophageal perforations and patients with Boerhaave's syndrome. Chest 92:995–998
9. Pate JW, Walkre WA, Cole FH, Owen EW, Johnson WH (1989) Spontaneuos rupture of the esophagus: A 30-year experience. Ann Thorac Surg 47:689–692
10. Walker WS, Cameron, EW, Walbaum PR (1985) Diagnosis and management of spontaneus transmural rupture of the oesophagus (Boerhaave's-syndrome). Br J Surg 72:204–207
11. Fabian W (1990) Das Boerhaave-Syndrom. Fortschr. Med. 108:134–137
12. Asplund CM, Hill LD (1985) Delayed lower esophageal perforation: Management with Celestin tube. Ann Otol Rhinol Laryngol 94:114–116
13. Saario I, Kostiainen S, Salo J, Meurala H, Eerola S (1983) Treatment of spontaneous rupture of the esophagus. Acta Chir Scand 149:771–774
14. Yellin A, Schachter P, Lieberman Y (1989) Spontaneous transmural rupture of the esophagus—Boerhaave's syndrome. Acta Chir Scand 155:337–340

Esophagectomy for Esophageal Disruption

ÁRON ALTORJAY, JÁNOS KISS, and ATTILA VÖRÖS[1]

Introduction

In thoracic surgical practice, there are just a few acute conditions which have sequelae as serious as perforation of the thoracic segment of the esophagus. Its mortality is almost three times that of lesions to the cervical esophagus [1].

Prolonged leakage of saliva, gastric digestive enzymes, oropharyngeal bacteria, and bile into the mediastinum is often fatal. In the majority of patients, a close correlation can be demonstrated between the time from onset of symptoms to treatment and mortality [5, 8, 9]. A sometimes desperate adherence to saving the esophagus has brought about a wide variety of methods for exclusion and techniques to control esophago-cutaneous fistulas. In sharp contrast is the method whereby resection and repair are performed at the same time; this method was preferred as early as 1968 by Hedren and Henderson [3]. In the present paper, our results achieved with resections of perforations of the esophagus are evaluated.

Methods

At the Department of Surgery, Postgraduate Medical University of Budapest, Hungary, we have performed esophagectomies for perforations of the esophagus in 22 patients in the period 1985 to 1992. In 21 patients, repair was also carried out in the same sitting. Of these, continuity of the alimentary tract was restored with jejunal interpositum in 9 patients and with stomach in 12. In one of the patients, a neo-esophagus was created from the left half of the colon 4 months after subtotal esophagectomy. The neo-esophagus made of stomach was pulled into the cervical area retrosternally in eight patients and via the posterior mediastinum in four.

---

[1] Department of Surgery, Postgraduate Medical University, Budapest, H-1135 Szabolcs u. 33–35, Hungary

We have treated 10 male and 12 female patients with an average age of 55.5 years. In 36% (8/22) the lesion was in the middle third of the esophagus, while in 64% (14/22) it was in the lower third. As regards causes of perforation, iatrogenic causes were the most common at 13 (59.1%), followed by lesions caused by foreign bodies (27.3%). In three patients, spontaneous perforation was observed (13.6%), and in three (13.6%), perforation took place in intact, not diseased esophagus.

The interval between rupture and treatment was less than 24 h in ten patients (45.5%), 24–48 h in one (4.5%), 48–72 h in four (18.2%), while it was longer than 72 h in seven (31.8%).

The diagnosis could be established by means of swallowing radiography in all but one of the patients, which means a 94.5% success rate. In two patients, gastrografin (9.1%), and in three (13.6%) barium was also required.

Postoperative surgical complications were observed in three patients (13.6%): one was failure of the cervical anastomosis, and two were wound purulences. Non-surgical complications occurred in six (27.3%): respiratory failure in three and pulmonary embolism, renal failure, and multisystemic organ failure in one case each. We lost one patient (a mortality rate of 4.5%). He was 74 years old, had a tumorous perforation of the esophagus, and died of pulmonary embolism on the 12th postoperative day when he had been ingesting liquids. At autopsy, a green nut-sized secondary deposit was found in segment VII of the liver. In his history, there was also evidence of myocardial infarction 2 years prior to the present illness. The mean duration of hospital stay was 17 days, with 12 days the shortest and 22 the longest. On an average, peroral nutrition could be begun on the 10th day. The longest clearance lasted 18 days. The anastomosis had to be dilated in two patients, at 4 and 5.5 months after operation; jejunal interposition was performed in one and retrosternal gastric repair in the other.

Discussion

In 1968, Hendren and Henderson described in their report their successful operations, curing perforation of the thoracic esophagus by resection and substitution performed at the same time [5]. However, even though 20 years have passed, this method is still not universally accepted. Some surgeons claim it to be justified exclusively in the treatment of perforated esophageal tumours and prohibit its use in any other case [6]. According to Imre [7], resection of a non-tumorous esophagus may be justified when we find on the esophageal wall multiple lesions which are not reparable by suturing or covering. Resections performed because of intrathoracic esophageal perforations have been analyzed by Orringer and Stirling [8] in 24 and Matthews and Mitchell [9] in 9 cases. They claim that resection is less hazardous than attempting primary closure, drainage, or diversions.

In selecting the method of treatment, Skinner et al. expressed the view [4] that no success can be anticipated with esophageal sutures placed above the obstructive esophageal change or in the presence of acid-peptic reflux. An esophageal perforation above a stricture with reflux that is diagnosed quickly can be successfully treated by intraoperative bougienage, closure of the perforation, and covering the suture line with intercostal muscular flap, or pericardiac or omental tissue patch. Similarly, when the perforation in an achalasiac esophagus is caused by pneumatic dilatation, esophagomyotomy and suturing the perforation are very likely successful. Michel and Grillo [2] described a death rate of 23% in cases of perforation associated with intrinsic esophageal disease; in sharp contrast to the 4% mortality rate of perforations occurring in otherwise normal esophagus.

In our opinion, resection appears to be more reliable and safer in advanced perforations of the thoracic esophagus, although it represents a major primary therapeutic intervention. It eliminates once and for all the source of intrathoracic sepsis, the hole in the esophagus, and removes the affected esophagus.

We think it is best to avoid any form of esophageal exclusion, since such methods merely complicate the reconstructive procedures required later on. Orringer and Stirling [8] voiced a similar view when emphasizing that in a patient in a very serious condition due to thoracic esophageal disruption closure and exclusion will not fulfill the hopes attached to them because they cannot control sepsis adequately. Therefore he advocates resection.

Whether the transthoracic or the transhiatal approach is be used for resection of a perforated esophagus depends on how much the lesion has been neglected, how serious the concomitant mediastinitis are, and pleural contamination. Transhiatal esophagectomy is an excellent method in cases of esophageal rupture, especially when performed early, when pleural contamination is minimal, or when the hole is localized to the mediastinum only. After extraction of the esophagus, intraoperative mediastinal and pleural irrigation through the hiatus diaphragmaticus and cervical incision will effectively cleanse the infected areas. When a rupture is present for a longer time, when there has been previous thoracic surgery, and in the presence of pleural contamination, the transthoracic approach is preferred since at the same time the resection is carried out we can also cleanse the thoracic cavity or even decorticate it when necessary.

During the past 7 years at the Department of Surgery, Postgraduate Medical University, Budapest, Hungary we have performed resection of the esophagus for thoracic esophageal perforation in 22 patients. One patient was lost due to non-surgical complications. In view of our results, we attribute significance to the following points in the indication of this radical operation.

We perform primary resection with simultaneous repair:

1. In perforation of the thoracic esophagus with concomitant obstructive esophageal disease
2. In cases of thoracic perforation treated within 24 h
   - When the lesion is extensive, and there is serious mediastinal or intrapleural contamination.
   - When the viability of the wound lips is even slightly questionable and no adequate stemmed tissue flap can be created to cover the suture line.
   - When the primary suture would cause a 50% narrowing of the esophageal lumen.
3. In the presence of diffuse extravasation or free flow of contrast medium towards the adjacent body cavities for more than 24 h.
4. In advanced spontaneous perforation.
5. When there is a circumscribed extravasation caused by foreign body impaction for more than 24 h (especially when there is a low epidermal growth factor level in diabetes mellitus [10]).

6. In the presence of serious septicemia with severe changes in physiological functions.
7. When the human and material resources required for high level intensive care are available.
8. When adequate thoracic and esophageal surgical skills are available.

As regards surgical approach and method of repair our views are as follows:

1. Left-sided thoracolaparotomy
   - Lesion in the lower third or abdominal area, or
   - When a coexistent esophageal disease involves the lower third only.
2. Transhiatal approach
   - In cases of thoracic esophageal perforation, when the size of the lesion or the nature of the esophageal disease (tumor) or the length of the change (stricture) would abovo rule out anything but subtotal esophagectomy.
   - When there has been a previous thoracic operation.
   - It should be taken into consideration also when the patient is old and is in poor general condition.
3. Transthoracic approach
   - In mid-third segment lesions.
   - In the presence of marked contamination of the thoracic cavity (correct decortacation is required).
   - When we plan an intrapleural esophagogastrostomy.

In addition, the following should also be taken into consideration when selecting the method of operation:

1. Following resection in the lower third jejunal interposition is recommended, even when there has been a previous resection.
2. Repair with stomach is feasible when there has been a two-thirds esophagus resection or subtotal esophagectomy.
3. We recommand the Torek operation only when a distal gastric resection was performed earlier, or when the stomach or the jejunum is not fit for immediate repair. In such cases, a colon substitution is carried out 6 weeks later.

It is believed that in light of our operative success, it is correct to say that primary resection with immediate substitution may be the method of choice in the treatment of perforation or rupture of the esophagus and the field of indications for this method may be expanded with careful considerations.

References

1. Sandrasagra FA, English TA (1978b) Esophageal intubation in the management of perforated esophagus with stricture. Ann Thorac Surg 25:399–401
2. Michel L, Grillo HC (1981) Operative and nonoperative management of esophageal perforations. Ann Surg 194:57–63
3. Sandrasagra FA, English TA (1978b) The management and prognosis of oesophageal perforation. Br J Surg 65:629–32
4. Skinner DB, Little AG, DeMeester TR (1980) Management of esophageal perforation. Am J Surg 139:760–64
5. Hendren WH, Henderson BM (1968) Immediate esophagectomy for instrumental perforation of the thoracic esophagus. Ann Surg 168:192–94

6. Finley RJ, Pearson FG (1980) The management of nonmalignant intrathoracic esophageal perforation. Ann Thorac Surg 30:575–583

7. Imre J (1973) Plastic tube prothesis for the surgical treatment of perforations in esophageal strictures. Ann Thorac Surg 15:275–78

8. Orringer MB, Stirling MC (1990) Esophagectomy for esophageal disruption. Ann Thorac Surg 49:35–43

9. Matthews HR, Mitchell IM (1989) Emergency subtotal esophagectomy. Br J Surg 76:918–20

10. Gray MR, Donnelly RJ (1991) Role of salivary epidermal growth factor in the pathogenesis of Barret's columnar lined esophagus. Br J Surg 78:1461–66

Clinical Evaluation of Esophageal Perforation

Hitoshi Irie, Teruo Kakegawa, Hideaki Yamana, Hiromasa Fujita, and Hiroshi Rikitake[1]

Introduction

Esophageal perforation is a rare condition but it often results in a severe course [1], and delayed diagnosis can result in prognosis [2].

The purpose of this paper is to evaluate the clinical courses and surgical results in 12 patients with esophageal perforation.

Patients

Between 1980 and 1992, we evaluated 12 patients with esophageal perforation. Their age ranged from 21 to 86 years old, 10 males and 2 females.

Causes of the esophageal perforation are indicated in Table 1. Seven patients had mechanical injuries and the other five patients developed spontaneous perforation.

The location of the perforation was the upper third of the thoracic esophagus in five cases, the middle third in three cases, and the lower third in four. Mechanical injuries were caused by endoscopic examination, endotracheal intubation, and foreign body in three, two, and two patients respectively (Table 1).

Clinical Symptoms

Clinically, subcutaneous emphysema was noted in all patients and a majority of them had severe chest and/or abdominal pain. Dyspnea was recognized in five cases, and only two cases with spontaneous rupture had a history of vomiting. Hematomesis was found in one case who had a major rupture of the esophagus (Table 2).

---

[1] First Department of Surgery, Kurume University School of Medicine, Kurume, 830 Japan

Table 1. Causes of esophageal perforation in 12 patients

Case	Age	Sex	Cause of perforation	Location
1	47	F	Endotracheal intubation	Upper third
2	52	M	Endoscopic examination	Middle third
3	39	M	Endoscopic examination	Lower third
4	44	M	Foreign body	Upper third
5	46	M	Spontaneous	Lower third
6	47	M	Spontaneous	Lower third
7	46	M	Spontaneous	Lower third
8	81	F	Spontaneous	Middle third
9	42	M	Foreign body (false teeth)	Upper third
10	86	M	Endotracheal intubation	Upper third
11	21	M	Endoscopic examination	Upper third
12	54	M	Spontaneous	Middle third

Table 2. Clinical symptoms in 12 patients with esophageal perforation

Symptom	No. patients (%)
Subcutaneous emphysema	12 (100%)
Chest pain	7 (58%)
Dyspnea	5 (41%)
Abdominal pain	4 (33%)
Cervical discomfort	3 (25%)
Vomiting	2 (17%)
Hematemesis	1 (8%)

Diagnosis

Esophagography is a useful examination to diagnose esophageal perforation however, there was one false negative case who was finally diagnosed by endoscopic examination. Endoscopic examination is a useful procedure to avoid a missdiagnosis, and then we usually determine the surgical procedure based on the endoscopic findings such as extent of perforation, bleeding, necrosis of the wall, and so on.

Chest X-ray showed mediastinal and/or subcutaneous emphysema in all of the 12 patients and effusions of the intrathorax and/or pneumothorax was also recognized in 8 patients.

Recently, computed tomography (CT) examination was often used for diagnosis because CT indicates exact situation of the intrathorax and mediastinum (Table 3).

Surgical Procedures

Surgical procedures for those patients were shown in Table 4. We performed primary suture and thoracomediastinal drainage. Only one patient underwent subtotal esophagectomy due to major spontaneous rupture with massive bleeding,

Table 3. Diagnosis of 12 patients with esphageal perforation. A *double circle* indicates a final diagnosis, a *closed triangle* indicates negative findings, an *open circle* indicates positive findings, and an *open square* indicates no examination was performed

Case No.	Esophagography/Endoscopy	Chest X-ray		CT scan
		Hemo/Pneumo-Thorax	Emphysema	
1	◎/○	○	○	□
2	□/◎	▲	○	□
3	◎/□	○	○	□
4	◎/○	▲	○	□
5	▲/◎	○	○	○
6	◎/○	○	○	○
7	○/○	○	○	□
8	◎/◎	○	○	○
9	○/○	○	○	○
10	○/○	▲	○	○
11	◎/○	▲	○	○
12	◎/○	○	○	○

Table 4. Surgical procedure in 12 patients with esophageal perforation

Case	Surgical procedure	Condition
1	Drainage alone	Small rupture
2	Drainage alone	Severe mediastinitis
3	Primary suture + drainage	Small rupture
4	Drainage alone	Poor risk
5	Primary suture + drainage	Early diagnosis
6	Subtotal esophagectomy + drainage	Esophageal necrosis
7	Primary suture + drainage	Early diagnosis
8	Primary suture + drainage	Small rupture
9	Drainage alone	Preop. complication
10	Drainage alone	Early diagnosis
11	Drainage alone	Unknown leak
12	Primary suture + drainage	Early diagnosis

7 cm in length. Drainage alone was performed in 6 cases with the following indications: small rupture ($n = 3$), severe mediastinitis with sepsis ($n = 1$), poor risk ($n = 1$), preoperative complication ($n = 1$), and a leak of unknown source ($n = 1$). Three of four patients with early diagnosis underwent primary suture of the injured esophagus (Table 4).

Surgical Results

Only one case, who underwent drainage alone, died of severe mediastinitis followed by sepsis. The reason for this death may have been due to the long time (43 h) from onset.

In our cases, severe postoperative complications were not recognized except for the one postoperative mortality. All four patients with early diagnosis had a good prognosis after surgery (Table 5).

Table 5. Surgical results and prognosis in 12 patients with esophageal perforation

Case	Time from onset	Surgical procedure	Result	Survival
1	72 h	Drainage	Alive	3.5 years
2	43	Drainage	Dead	40 days
3	72	Primary suture	Alive	2.0 years
4	24	Drainage	Alive	4.0 years
5	10	Primary suture	Alive	3.0 years
6	30	Esophagectomy	Alive	6.5 years
7	12	Primary suture	Alive	2.0 years
8	30	Primary suture	Alive	3.5 years
9	Unknown	Drainage	Alive	3.0 years
10	10	Drainage	Alive	2.0 years
11	18	Drainage	Alive	2.0 years
12	12	Primary suture	Alive	6 months

Discussion

The most important factor in the treatment of this disease is making an early and accurate diagnosis so that the most appropriate modality can be selected. Generally, motality rises sharply with delayed diagnosis, and the best time lag between onset and diagnosis and treatment is less than 24 h [3]. In diagnostic examination, endoscopic findings are useful for the investigation of injured status.

In the surgical treatment, primary suture and drainage are basic procedures for this condition, while esophagectomy is also indicated for the case with major perforation, massive bleeding and/or necrosis of the esophageal wall.

From our experience in 12 patients with esophageal perforation, relatively good surgical results were obtained in 11 patients. One case died of severe sepsis.

References

1. Berry BE, Ochsner JL (1973) Perforation of the esophagus: A 30-year review. J Thorac Cardiovasc Surg 65:1
2. Nealon TF, Templeton JY, Cuddy VD, et al (1961) Instrumental perforation of the esophagus. J Thorac Cardiovasc Surg 19:233
3. Skinner DB, Little AG, DeMeester TR (1980) Management of esophageal perforation. Am J Surg 139:760

Clinical Studies of Spontaneous Rupture of the Esophagus

Hiroyuki Komoriyama, Yoshiaki Kataba, Kaname Shimizu,
Syouhei Imaki, Yukihiro Adachi, Kazuyuki Mizutami, Ichirou Tanaka,
Hiroyoshi Ikezawa, Kazuo Kanasugi, Susumu Yamaguchi[1],
and Kenji Katayama[2]

Introduction

The incidence of spontaneous rupture of the esophagus (Boerhaave's syndrome) is rare, and identification of the disease is considered to be the first step in early treatment. In Japan, the site is the left wall of the lower esophagus in 90% of cases of esophageal rupture. We have experienced five patients (including one autopsied case) with this disease; two of the patients had a rupture on the right side. Three of these patients were cured by resection of the ruptured esophagus.

We studied four operated patients with spontaneous rupture of the esophagus. The hospital course of each patient was analyzed with emphasis on the cause and location of rupture, clinical manifestation, presence of underlying esophageal and nonesophageal disease, duration of period from rupture to treatment, method of treatment, complications, and prognosis.

Patients and Methods

From January 1985 to December 1991, a total of five patients (one was an autopsied case) with spontaneous rupture of the esophagus were treated in St. Marianna University Hospital (three patients), Kawasaki City and St. Marianna University Yokohama City Seibu Hospital (two patients), Yokohama City, Japan. They comprised four males and one female (mean age 52 years; range 40–71 years).

---

[1] Department of Surgery, St. Marianna University School of Medicine, Yokohama City Seibu Hospital, 1197-1 Yasashi, Asahi-ku, Yokohama, 241 Japan
[2] First Department of Surgery, St. Marianna University School of Medicine, 2-16-1 Sugao, Miyamae-ku, Kawasaki, 213 Japan

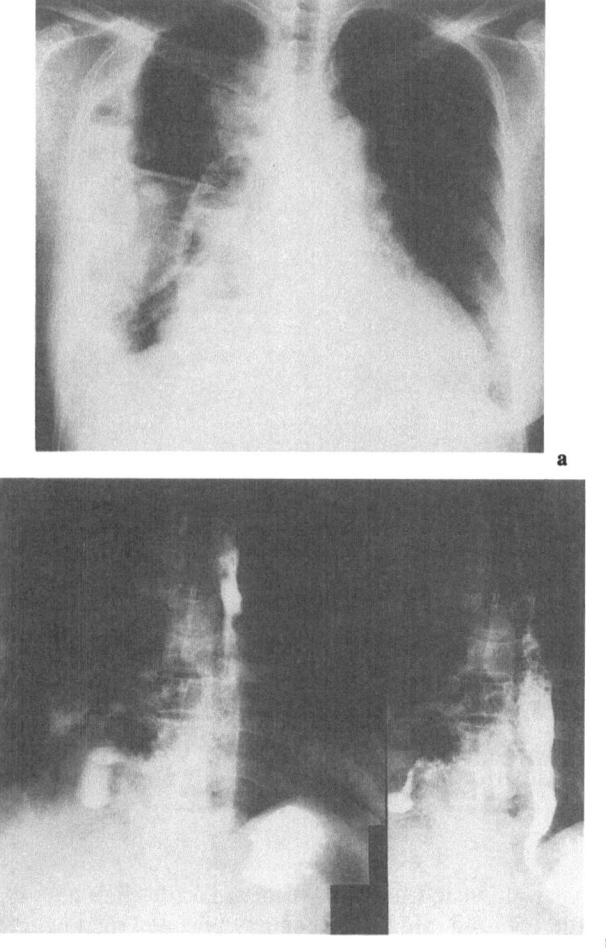

Fig. 1a,b. Case 1: 52 year-old female. **a** Chest X-ray examination revealed a right hydro-pneumopyothorax. **b** Esophagogram revealed a leakage of contrast medium from esophagus to right thoracic cavity

Case 1

A 52-year-old woman presented with an episode of epigastric pain and hem-atemesis of 48-h duration. Cholecystolithiasis and cholecystitis were diagnosed by ultrasonography. A course of antibiotics was started for the cholecystitis. Forty hours after admission, right hydropneumo-pyothorax was found. This indicated esophageal rupture, which was confirmed by esophagography. The chest X-ray and esophagogram showed spontaneous rupture (Fig. 1). Right thoracotomy was performed 98 h after the onset of epigastric pain and a 7-cm rupture of the middle esophagus was seen under the azygos vein. Extroversion and severe necrosis of the mucosa were observed and then the thoracic esophagus

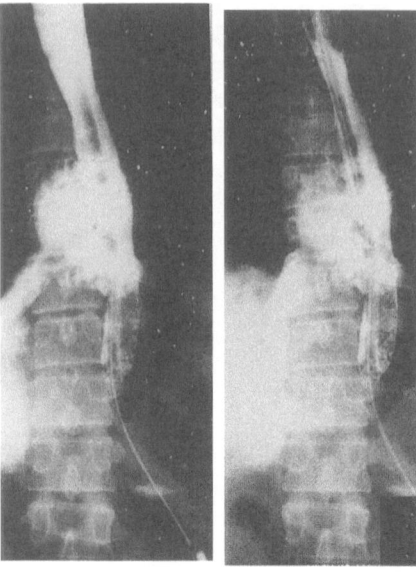
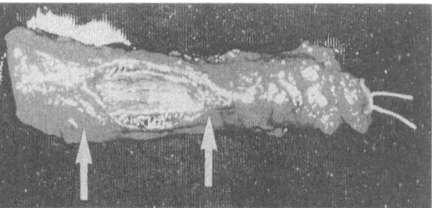

a   b

Fig. 2a,b. Case 2: 40 year-old male. **a** Esophagogram revealed a leakage of contrast medium from esophagus to right thoracic cavity. **b** The specimen showed no pathological change except tear

was resected. On the 59th day esophagectomy, with surgical construction using a gastric tube, was performed in the second stage.

Case 2

He was a 40-year-old male with a 4-h history of acute chest and upper abdominal pain on ingestion of food. Mediastinal emphysema and right hydropneumothorax were found on chest X-ray examination and confirmed by esophagography and computed tomography (CT). Right thoracotomy was performed 5h after the onset of pain and a 5-cm rupture was found in the right wall of the middle thoracic esophagus. Extroversion of the thoracic esophagus and severe inflammation of the mucosa were observed and a thoracic esophagectomy was performed. Microscopic examination of the specimen showed no pathological change except partial esophageal rupture (Fig. 2). On the 67th day after diagnosis, surgical construction with a gastric tube was performed in thhe second stage.

Case 3

A 51-year-old male presented with a 3-h history of hematemesis while consuming alcohol. On chest X-ray examination, left hydrothorax was found and the fluid level was reduced by aspiration of gastric juice using gastric endoscopy. A gastric perforation with a diaphragmatic rupture was diagnosed in the initial clinic. The patient was transferred to our hospital and emergency laparotomy was performed 67h after the onset of hematemesis. No abnormalities were found in the intraperitoneal cavity. Then, thoracotomy was performed and a 4-cm rupture was found in the left wall of the lower esophagus. As it was considered to be too difficult to perform primary suture, the thoracic esophagus was resected. On the 129th day after diagnosis, surgical construction with ascending colon was performed because of severe adhesion. Leakage at the cervical esophago-colonic anastomosis was recognized but the patient was discharged on the 170th day.

Case 4

He was a 46-year-old male with a 1-h history of vomiting while consuming alcohol, with acute, severe upper abdominal and back pain experienced immediately. A chest X-ray film showed left hydrothorax and the patient was placed under conservative therapy in another hospital. On the following day, the left hydrothorax increased. The patient was transferred to our hospital with shock: a blood pressure of 58 mmHg, pulse rate 134/min, and liver dysfunction. Preoperative laboratory studies disclosed: total bilirubin 3.3 mg/dl, glutamic oxaloacetic transaminase (GOT) 240 IU/l, glutamic puruvic transaminase (GPT) 73 IU/l, γ-glutamil transpeptidase (γ-GTP) 518 IU/l, creatine kinase (CK) 373 IU/l, C-reactive protein (CRP) 9.2 mg/dl, white blood cell count 3300/μl, platelets 3.5×10^4/ml, and activated partial thromboplastin time 54%. The chest X-rays showed mediastinal emphysema and left hydropneumothorax: these were confirmed by esophagography and CT. Left thoracotomy was performed 26 h after the onset of symptoms, and a 6-cm rupture in the left wall of the lower esophagus was found; simple suturing was performed (Fig. 3). The patient died 23 h after the operation from disseminated intravascular coagulopathy.

Table 1 summarizes the clinical course in these patients and one autopsied case. The autopsied patient's chest X-ray showed findings such as mediastinal emphysema, subcutaneous emphysema, and hydropneumothorax, typical of Boerhaave's syndrome (Fig. 4).

Discussion

The etiology of esophageal perforation may be conveniently grouped into iatrogenic (endoscopy, esophageal dilations, passage of tubes, major thoracotomy) and noniatrogenic (missiles, foreign bodies, spontaneous rupture, blunt trauma, caustic injury) [1]. Spontaneous rupture of the esophagus (Boerhaave's syndrome) is characterized by its dramatic onset, diagnostic difficulty, high mortality rate, high morbidity, and rare incidence. Nesbitt et al. [2] reported 22 cases of Boerhaave's syndrome, spanning a 50-year period.

Identification of the esophageal rupture is considered to be the first step in early diagnosis and treatment. The second step is chest X-ray findings. The radiologic studies are particularly important. The roentgenologic manifestations are as follows: mediastinal emphysema, which is a relatively early sign; subcutaneous emphysema, particularly following the presence of mediastinal air, and first seen deep in the supraclavicular and suprasternal regions; and hydrothorax, hydropneumothorax, or pneumothorax, usually on the left, less often on the right, and infrequently bilateral.

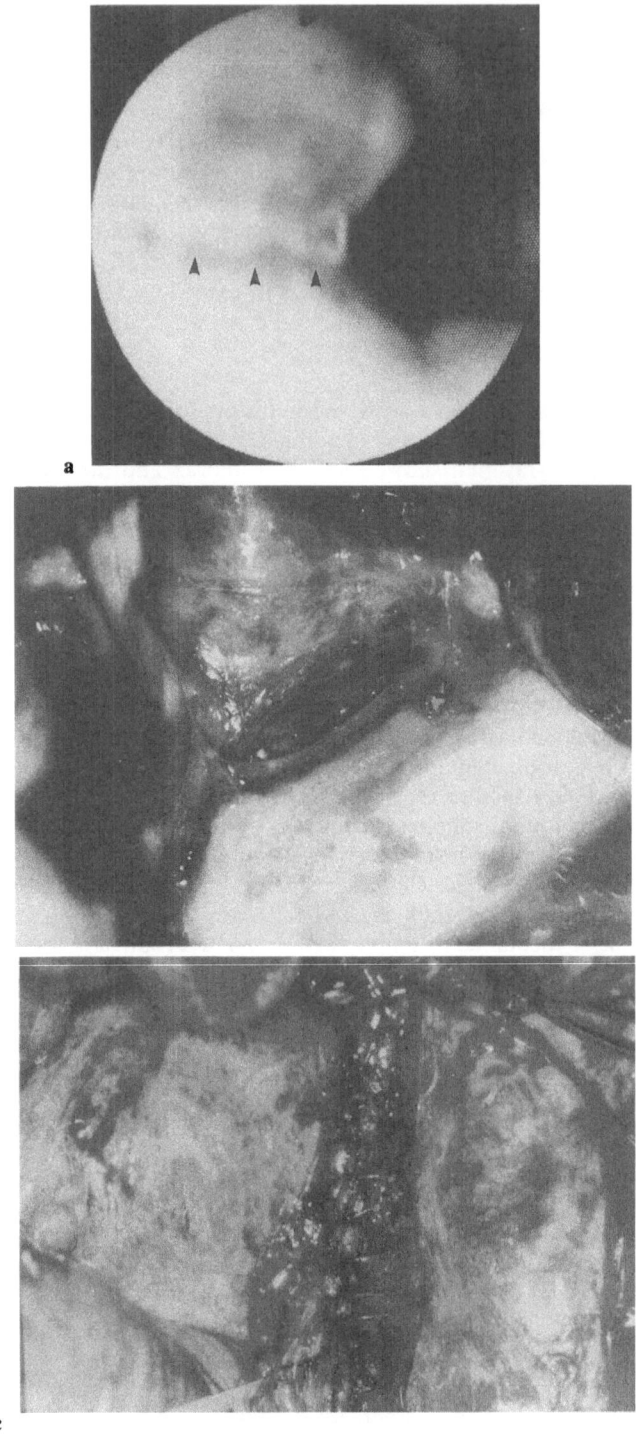

Fig. 3a–c. Case 4: 46 year-old male. **a** Longitudinal ulcer at the left side (*arrowheads*) of the lower esophagus was recognized but it was not confirmed by endoscopy. **b,c** Simple suturing was performed

Table 1. The five cases of the Boerhaave's syndrome

Case No	Age	Sex	Basic ailment	Inducement	Chief complaint	Initial diagnosis (referring hospital)	Chest X-ray findings	Diagnosis method	Preoperative diagnosis	Duration to operation from onset	Position of rupture size	Operation	Prognosis
1.	52	F	(−)	Drinking Vomiting	Epigastralgia Hematemesis	Cholecystitis	Rt. hydro-pneumothorax Pyothorax	Esophagography CT	Boerhaave's syndrome	98 h	Rt. side under the azygos vein 7 cm	Rt. thoracotomy Esophagectomy	Alive Construction by a gastric tube
2.	40	M	(−)	Swallowing food	Dyspnea Upper abdominal pain	GI tract perforation	Mediastinal emphysema Rt. hydro-pneumothorax	Esophagography CT	Boerhaave's syndrome	5 h	Rt. side middle esophagus 5 cm	Rt. thoracotomy Esophagectomy	Alive Construction by a gastric tube
3.	51	M	Live dysfunction	Drinking Vomiting	Dyspnea Hematemesis Abdominal pain	GI tract perforation Rupture of diaphragma	Lt. hydrothorax	Thoracotomy (No abnormalities in the peritoneal cavity)	Gastric perforation Rupture of diaphragma	67 h	Lt. side lower esophagus 4 cm	Laparotomy Lt. thoracotomy Esophagectomy	Alive Construction by a large intestine
4.	46	M	Liver cirrhosis	Drinking Vomiting	Dyspnea Back pain	Aneurysm Shock	Lt. hydrothorax Mediastinal emphysema	Esophagography CT	Boerhaave's syndrome	26 h	Lt. side lower esophagus 6cm	Lt. thoracotomy Simple suturing	DIC Death
Autopsy													
5.	71	M	(−)	Strain of defecation	Hematemesis Back pain	Melena Shock	Mediastinal emphysema Lt. hydrothorax Subcutaneous emphysema	(−)	Death 8 h after admission		Lt. side lower esophagus 13 cm	Final diagnosis ○ Boerhaave's syndrome ○ Gastric ulcer (ul-II) destruction of arterial wall ○ Renal cancer (3.7 cm)	

Rt, right; *Lt*, left; *DIC*, disseminated intravascular coagulation

321

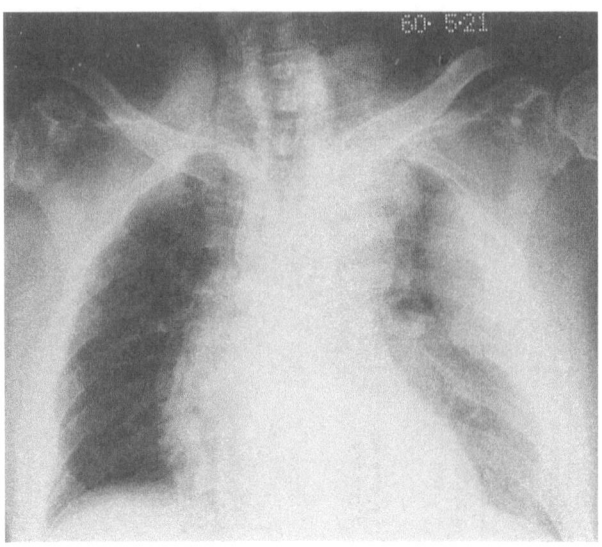

Fig. 4. 71 year-old male. Mediastinal emphysema, subcutaneous emphysema, and hydro-pneumothorax were observed

If diagnosis by chest X-ray examination is not conclusive, definitive diagnosis should be obtained by esophagography; correct diagnosis by endoscopy has not been possible in our case. Contrast studies in our hospitals showed communication with the right or left pleural space. The use of esophagoscopy was reported by Keighley et al. [3], who were able to define the site and extent of the tear in four of six cases. Esophagoscopy is usually not performed for the diagnosis of spontaneous rupture, as this diagnosis is usually made on the basis of clinical and radiologic findings.

The review by Larsen et al. [4] of 1787 patients from the world literature revealed a strong correlation between delay in treatment and mortality rate in iatrogenic perforation; their personal experience with Boerhaave's syndrome showed no effect on mortality rate between patients operated on in less than 24 h (43%) and those operated on more than 24 h (38%) after onset. According to Pate et al. [5], their patients having operations less than 24 h after onset had a mortality rate of 33%; those diagnosed and operated on later than 24 h after onset also had a mortality rate of 33%. Delay in diagnosis was correlated with complication rates.

The ruptures showed various macroscopic conditions irrespective of the time elapsed before thoracotomy, and there was no correlation between prognosis and the duration from onset of symptoms to time of operation: the prognosis appeared to depend on the underlying disease and general condition of the patient.

Generally, early operations after definite diagnosis are recommended for esophageal ruptures. However, if the patient's systemic condition is poor, conservative treatment including pleural drainage, control of infection, and nutritional management should be performed first to improve the patient's general condition before a further treatment strategy is decided.

Nonoperative treatment of thoracoabdominal perforation is more controversial. Cameron et al. [6] recommended strict guidelines for patients who should be considered for nonoperative treatment: disruption contained in the mediastinum or between the mediastinal and visceral pleura, drainage of the cavity back into the esophagus, minimal symptoms, and minimal signs of clinical sepsis.

Surgery is probably indicated in almost all cases of Boerhaave's syndrome because this type of rupture is associated with a very high incidence of respiratory failure and septic shock. Many operative methods (simple suturing, closure with free pericardial patch graft, or a vascularized pedicle flap constructed from pleura, diaphragma, intercostal muscle, gastric fundus, omentum, T-tube drainage from laceration, esophagectomy, etc.) have been reported with a variety of treatment modalities.

Esophagectomy may seem excessively invasive, but the method used should aim at complete removal of the source of contamination with an early cure.

References

1. Lyons WS, Serementir MG, deGuzman VC, Peabody JW (1978) Rupture and perforation of the esophagus: The case for conservative supportive management. Ann Thorac Surg 25:346–350
2. Nesbitt JC, Sawyers JL (1987) Surgical management of esophageal perforation. Am Surg 53:183–191
3. Keighley MRB, Gridwood RW, Ionescu MI, Wooler GH (1972) Spontaneous rupture of the esophagus. Br J Surg 59:649–651
4. Larsen K, Jensen BS, Axelsen F (1983) Perforation and rupture of the esophagus. Scand J Thorac Cardiovasc Surg 17:311–316
5. Pate JW, Walker WA, Core FH Jr, Owen EW, Jonson WH (1989) Spontaneous rupture of the esophagus: A 30-year experience. Ann Thorac Surg 47:689–692
6. Cameron JL, Kieffer RF, Hendrix TR, Mehigan DG, Baker RR (1981) Selective nonoperative management of contained intrathoracic esophageal disruptions. Ann Thorac Surg 194:57–63

Other Diseases and Strictures

Surfactant-Like Material in Human Esophageal Mucosa: An Ultrastructural Study

R.T. Spychal, S.Y. Kwun, and A. Watson[1]

Introduction

Phospholipid structures, closely resembling those present in pulmonary surfactant, have been found in the mucosa of the stomach and small intestine
[1–4]. Gastric surfactant is believed to represent an important component of the
defence of the epithelium against luminal aggression [4–6].

The ultrastructural features of human oesophageal epithelium have been
described by several groups [7–10]. Although phospholipids have been demonstrated at a light microscopic level using histochemical methods [11], no study
has addressed the ultrastructure of the human oesophagus with reference to the
existence, distribution, and morphology of surface-active phospholipid. Several
techniques have been described to improve the identification of phospholipid-
rich layers in various tissues [1, 3, 4, 12–14]. These structures can be identified
ultrastructurally through their osmiophilic, lamellar forms between or within
cells. In this ultrastructural study, we used fixation techniques that enabled the
morphology and distribution of surfactant-like structures to be identified in the
normal human oesophageal epithelium.

Materials and Methods

Biopsy specimens of normal distal oesophageal mucosa were obtained from
patients undergoing upper gastrointestinal endoscopy. Full-thickness specimens
were also obtained from normal segments of oesophagus following resection for
oesophageal carcinoma. Specimens were immediately fixed in ice-cold fixative,
and processed for light and electron microscopy.

---

[1] Department of Surgery, Wallace Freeborn Block, Royal North Shore Hospital, St. Leonards
NSW 2065, Australia

Specimens were placed in a mixture of 4% paraformaldehyde, 1% glutaraldehyde, and 2.5% tannic acid (Sigma Chemical Co. St. Louis, MO, USA) in 0.1 M cacodylate buffer at pH 7.4 (320 mOsm) and 4°C. During primary fixation, the specimens were carefully diced into pieces suitable for proper orientation and embedding under a stereomicroscope and were then left in cold fixative overnight. Tissue blocks were then rinsed extensively (over 30 min) in cacodylate buffer, postfixed in 1% buffered osmium tetroxide for 1 h at 4°C, rinsed in water, and stained en bloc with uranyl acetate. The tissue blocks were dehydrated through ascending grades of ethanol and propylene oxide, embedded in Spurr's resin, and polymerized at 68°C overnight. Semi-thin plastic sections (0.5 μm) were cut, stained with 1% methylene blue/1% azure II mixture and examined with an Olympus (Tokyo, Japan) BH-2 light microscope. Ultra-thin sections (60–80 nm) were mounted on grids and double-stained with uranyl acetate and lead citrate, and were examined in a JEOL (Tokyo, Japan) 100-S electron microscope at 60 or 80 kv.

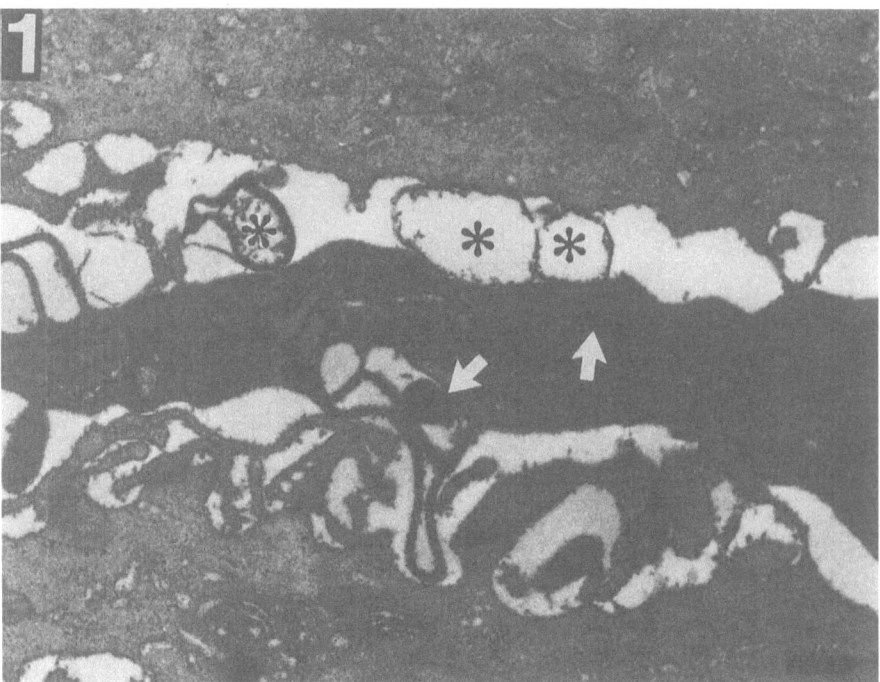

Fig. 1. Transmission electron micrograph (*TEM*) of dendritic cells in the functional layer. These cells contain various forms of extracellular and intracellular lamellar bodies (*arrows*). Electron-dense, multilayers of coiled structures are seen (*asterisks*). Surfactant-like membranous particles are possibly in various stages of uncoiling above irregular cell processes. *Bar* = 1 μm

Results

Several cell layers were distinguished at light microscopic level and classification of the epithelium into basal, prickle cell, functional, and superficial layers is relatively easy because well-defined strata are present. Potential surfactant-like structures were identified by their electron density (osmiophilic) and as myelin forms.

The material coating the surface of the luminal cells was sparse. Occasionally, variably coiled lamellar structures were present on the surface. In the functional layer, the amount of surfactant-like material increased. The intercellular space of the functional layer contained osmiophilic structures which often took the form of whorl-like myelin figures. The intercellular form of lamellar bodies had varied morphologies. In some areas, the lamellar bodies appeared to form a continuous barrier over the microvillous processes of cells. In the functional layer of the mucosa, several dendritic cells were identified containing various forms of intracellular lamellar bodies (Fig. 1). At higher magnifications, these cells contained an intracellular form of the lamellar body located within the matrix of membrane-bound cytoplasmic organelles (Fig. 2).

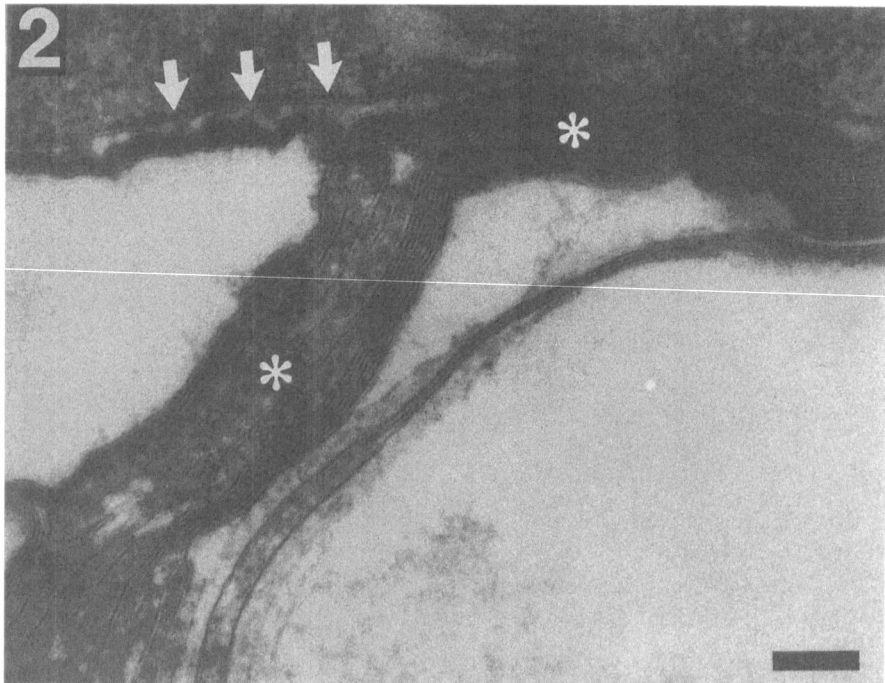

Fig. 2. TEM of the dendritic cell in the functional layer. An intracellular form of the lamellar body (*asterisks*) located within the matrix of membrane-bound cytoplasmic organnelles is recognisable. The lamellar body consists of several bilayers of phospholipid with regular interlaminar spacing. A remarkably uniform lining consists of multilayers of phospholipid with almost the same interlaminar spacing as the intracellular membrane (*arrows*). *Bar* = 0.1 μm

Surfactant-like material was also found to be abundant in the intercellular space of the prickle cell layer of the oesophageal mucosa. These polygonal cells had wide intercellular spaces and the cell membranes possessed numerous irregular small processes which occasionally branched. Various forms of coiled and uncoiled membrane particles were identified and some of the lamellar lining appeared to coat surfaces outside the oesophageal cell membranes. These structures showed stacks of osmiophilic lamellae, the periodicity of which was about 40 Å. In the basal cell layer, intercellular lamellar bodies were often found in a tightly coiled granular form.

Discussion

We have been able to demonstrate the presence of surfactant-like material in the mucosa of the human oesophagus. Surfactant-like material forming multi-layers were abundantly present in the intercellular space throughout the mucosa. Lamellar materials were also found within dendritic cells in the functional layer and within prickle cells. The structure of the lamellar bodies within the squamous epithelium of the human oesophagus as described in this study, is likely to represent phospholipid-rich material. Their morphology, when fixation is performed with a tannic acid-containing fixative, correspond to the observations obtained on pulmonary and gastric surfactant-like material [5, 7, 8].

Tannic acid has been used previously with great success to increase membrane contrast in conventionally fixed tissue [15, 16] and has an affinity for saturated phospholipids in general, and phosphatidyl choline (PC) in particular in the lung [15]. It has been shown that tannic acid interacts with the choline component of PC to form a complex which is then stabilized by treatment with osmium tetroxide [15, 16].

The mechanism by which the oesophageal lining is protected against a potentially noxious luminal environment is not fully understood. A "gastric mucosal barrier" is generally accepted as the intrinsic mechanism by which the stomach is protected against ulceration. It has been proposed that a layer of phospholipid adsorbed to the mucosal surface may provide the biophysical basis of the gastric mucosal barrier [5], by providing a non-wettable lining which has been shown experimentally to reduce the rate of transition of hydrogen ions [6]. Ueda et al. [1], using an electron microscopic fixation method containing tannic acid, demonstrated the presence of multilamellar bodies on the luminal surface of rat stomach. Hills [4] confirmed Ueda's findings in the rat stomach and demonstrated that experimental ulcerogenesis is associated with absence of these structures. He proposed that oligolamellar phospholipid may provide a ubiquitous system for barrier formation. Since the oesophagus is susceptible to damage through reflux of gastroduodenal contents and ingestion of noxious substances, it is conceivable that a similar barrier mechanism might exist in the oesophageal epithelium.

It is tempting to speculate that this study has identified an "oesophageal mucosal barrier" which may have many of the same properties as the "gastric mucosal barrier". Further studies are in progress to examine the presence and distribution of surface-active phospholipid in patients with erosive oesophagitis, reflux-induced stricture, and Barrett's columnar-lined oesophagus. These studies may make a further contribution to our understanding of the mechanism of oesophageal mucosal damage in patients with gastro-oesophageal reflux and may have potential therapeutic implications.

Acknowledgement. Dr. S.Y. Kwun was supported by a research grant from the Northern Sydney Area Health Service.

References

1. Ueda S, Kawamura K, Ishii N, Matsumoto S, Hayashi K, Okayasu M, Saito M, Sakura I (1986) Morphological studies on the surface lining layer of the lungs (Part IV)—Surfactant-like substance in other organs (pleural cavity, vascular lumen, and gastric lumen) than lungs (1). J Jpn Med Soc Biol Interface 17:132–156
2. Eliakim R, Becich J, Green K, Alpers DH (1991) Developmental expression of intestinal surfactant-like particles in rats. Am J Physiol 261:G269–279
3. Kao Y-C J, Lichtenberger LM (1991) Phospholipid and neural lipid containing organellels of rat gastroduodenal cells. Gastroenterology 101:7–21
4. Hills BA (1990) A physical identity for the gastric mucosal barrier. Med J Aust 153(2): 76–81
5. Hills BA, Butler BD, Lichtenberger LM (1983) Gastric mucosal barrier: hydrophobic lining to the lumen of the stomach. Am J Physiol 244:G561–G568
6. Hills BA, Kirkwood CA (1992) Gastric mucosal barrier: barrier to hydrogen ions imparted by gastric surfactant in vitro. Gut 33:1039–1041
7. Gebos K, Mebis J, Desmet V (1988) The oesophagus: Normal ultrastructure and patho-logical patterns. In: Motta PM, Fujita H, Correr S (eds) Ultrastructure of the Digestive Tract. Martinus Nijhoff, Boston, pp 17–34
8. Al Yassin TM, Toner PG (1977) Fine structure of squamous epithelium and submucosal glands of human oesophagus. J Anat 123(3):705–721
9. Hopwood D, Logan KR, Bouchier IAD (1978) The electron microscopy of normal human oesophageal epithelium. Virchows Arch [B] 26:345–358
10. Ferey L, Herlin P, Marnay J, Jacob JH, De Raucourt, Gignoux M, Segol P, Oliver JM, Mandard AM (1985) Histology and ultrastructure of the human esophageal epithelium. I. Normal and parakeratotic epithelium. J Submicrosc Cytol 17(4):651–665
11. Hopwood D, Logan KR, Coghill G, Bouchier IAD (1977) Histochemical studies of mucosubstances and lipids in normal human oesophageal epithelium. Histochem J 9: 153–161
12. Dierichs R, Incezedy-Marseck M (1976) Iodoplatinate as a marker of quaternary ammonium compounds in electron microscopy. J Histochem Cytochem 14:962–964
13. Voorhout WF (1990) Freeze-substitution and immuno-gold labelling. In: Busing WM (ed) Cryo-electron Microscopy. Electron Optics Bull 129:7–9
14. Girod S, Fuchey C, Galabert C, Lebonvallet S, Bonnet N, Ploton D, Puchelle E (1991) Identification of phospholipids in secretory granules of human submucosal gland respiratory cells. J Histochem Cytochem 39(2):193–198
15. Kalina M, Pease DC (1977) The preservation of ultrastructure in saturated phosphatidyl cholines by tannic acid in model systems and type II pneumocytes. J Cell Biol 74:726–741
16. Kalina M, Pease DC (1977) The probable role of phosphatidyl cholines in the tannic acid enhancement of cytomembrane electron contrast. J Cell Biol 74:742–760

Twenty-Four-Hour pH Monitoring Study of Gastric Tube Used for Reconstruction After Esophagectomy for Esophageal Carcinoma

Mitsuaki Hashimoto, Masayuki Imamura, Yutaka Shimada, and Takayoshi Tobe[1]

Introduction

The gastric tube has often been used as a replacement for the esophagus after the resection of an esophageal carcinoma. The acidity of a completely vagotomized stomach has been estimated to be not high enough to cause a peptic ulcer. However, we experienced a few cases of peptic ulcer of the postoperative gastric tube or duodenum. In this study, we assessed the dynamics of gastric acid secretion in patients with esophageal carcinoma before and after esophagectomy.

Subjects and Methods

Thirty-eight patients with esophageal carcinoma were studied. There were 33 males and 5 females ranging in age from 50 to 78 years. Twenty-four-h pH monitoring was performed on the 38 patients postoperatively. Seventeen of these patients had also been monitored preoperatively. Resection of the eso-phageal carcinoma and reconstruction with the retrosternally shifted stomach were performed by the same surgeon (the second author). The gastric tube was prepared as previously described [1]. Two-channel Monocrystant pH catheters (distance between each electrode was 15 cm; Mod 91-0215, Synectics Medical, Stockholm, Sweden) were passed transnasally into the preoperative stomach or the gastric tube. Then the electrodes were fluoroscopically placed at the fundus (5 cm below the cardia or the esophagogastrostomy) and the antrum (20 cm below the cardia or the esophagogastrostomy). Measurements of pH were obtained and recorded with an ambulatory apparatus (Digitrapper MK II gold, Synectics Medical). Meals and daily behavior were unrestricted except that the

[1] First Department of Surgery, Faculty of Medicine, Kyoto University, 54-Shogoin Kawara-cho, Sakyo-ku, Kyoto, 606 Japan

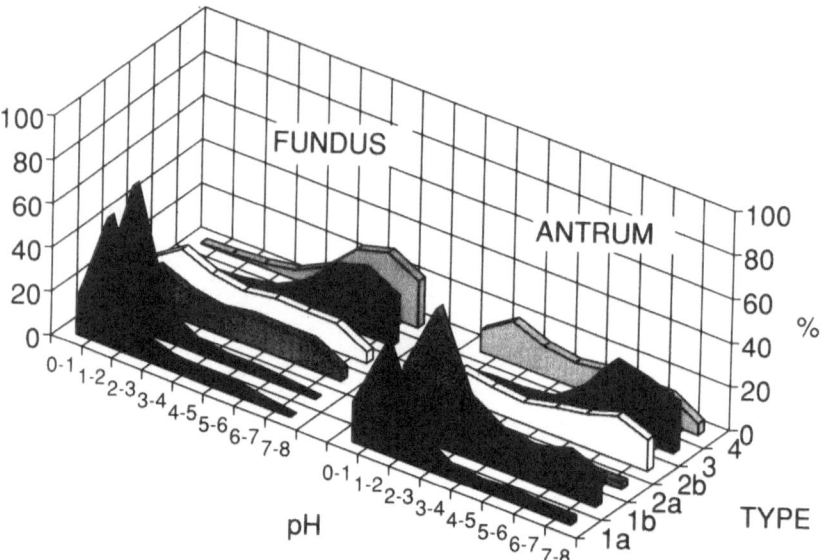

Fig. 1. Classification of the patients according to their pH frequency distribution. *Type 1*, high acidity type; the fundic pH distribution curve shows a single peak below pH 2 (the fundic pH is below 2 40% or more of the time). *Type 2*, intermediate type; the fundic pH distribution curve shows a plateau or two peaks, one below and one above pH 2 (the fundic pH is below 2 from 10% to 40% of the time). *Type 3*, low acidity type; the fundic and antral pHs rarely drop below 2 (the fundic, as well as the antral pH is below 2 less than 10% of the time). *Type 4*, antral high acidity type; the antral pH is lower than the fundic pH (the fundic pH is below 2 less than 10% of the time but the antral pH is below 2 more than 10% of the time). *Subtype a*, the antral pH is below 2 40% or more of the time. *Subtype b*, the antral pH is below 2 less than 40% of the time

patients were asked not to take baths. Night was defined as the period from midnight to 6 a.m. when the patients were generally fasting and in the recumbent position. Since different trends in pH levels were observed, we divided the patients into four types and two subtypes using a modified classification that has been described elsewhere [2] (Fig. 1).

Results

In the postoperative study, 4 patients were classified as type 1a, 10 as type 1b, 3 as type 2a, 6 as type 2b, 11 as type 3, and 4 as type 4. There were no significant differences in age among these groups. Figure 2 shows median pH values in these patients. In type 1a patients, pH values were low all day and night at the fundus and the antrum. In type 1b patients, pH values were low all day and night at the fundus. In type 2a patients, pH values were low all day and night at the antrum and also low during the night at the fundus. The mean proportion of time over 24 h that the fundic pH remained below 2 in type 1a and 1b patients was 52.6 ± 12.7% and 55.0 ± 10.1%, respectively. The mean proportion of time

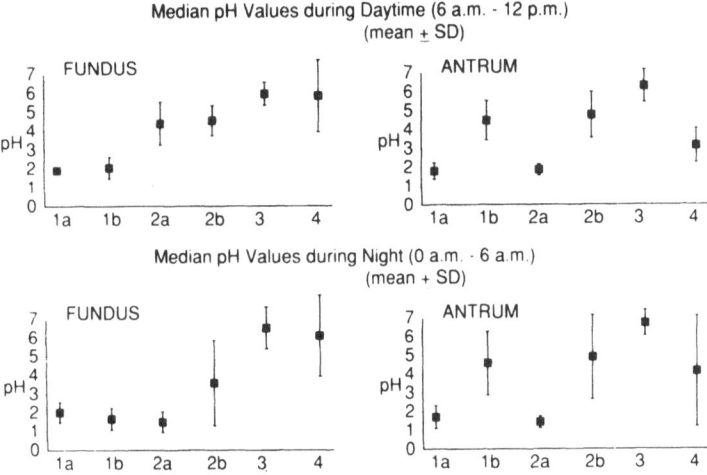

Fig. 2. Median pH values during the day and at night

over 24 hours that the antral pH remained below 2 in type 1a and 2a patients was 63.0 ± 21.3% and 63.7 ± 14.4%, respectively.

Shifts in the pH frequency distribution caused by the operation were analyzed in a total of 17 patients (Table 1). In eight patients (47%) the pH frequency distribution type was unchanged. In four patients (24%) a shift to a more acidic type was noted. In four patients (24%) a shift to a less acidic type was recorded. In another patient, a shift from type 1a to type 4 was observed. In type 3 patients, no shifts were noted. Figure 3 shows correlations between the preoperative and the postoperative proportions of time over 24 h that the pH remained below 2 in these 17 patients. A significant correlation existed at the antrum and these proportions tended to be maintained even after surgery.

Discussion

We have experienced a few cases of peptic ulcer of the stomach or duodenum after esophagectomy for esophageal carcinoma. To our knowledge, there have been no reports on the pathogenesis of the postoperative peptic ulcer in patients who had undergone esophagectomy for esophageal carcinoma. Our experience prompted us to estimate the acid secretion of the gastric tube more precisely. Some investigators have reported a reduction in gastric acid output in studies utilizing the aspiration of gastric juices [3] or using the Congo-red method [4]. Domergue et al. reported that acidity, as evaluated by 24-h pH monitoring, was lower in a group that had undergone gastroplasty than in a control group [5]. The obvious advantage of 24-h intragastric pH monitoring, which we took advantage of in this study, is the ability to measure the acidity over long periods and under conditions which approximate daily living [6]. The procedure is also useful in the investigation of the effects of diet and drugs on gastric acidity in ulcer patients.

Table 1. pH frequency distriction shifts caused by the operation

Type after surgery	Type before surgery					
	1a	1b	2a	2b	3	4
1a	2			1		
1b				2		
2a	1			1		
2b		1		1		
3		1		1	4	
4	1					1

$n = 17$

For an explanation of the types, see legend to Fig. 1

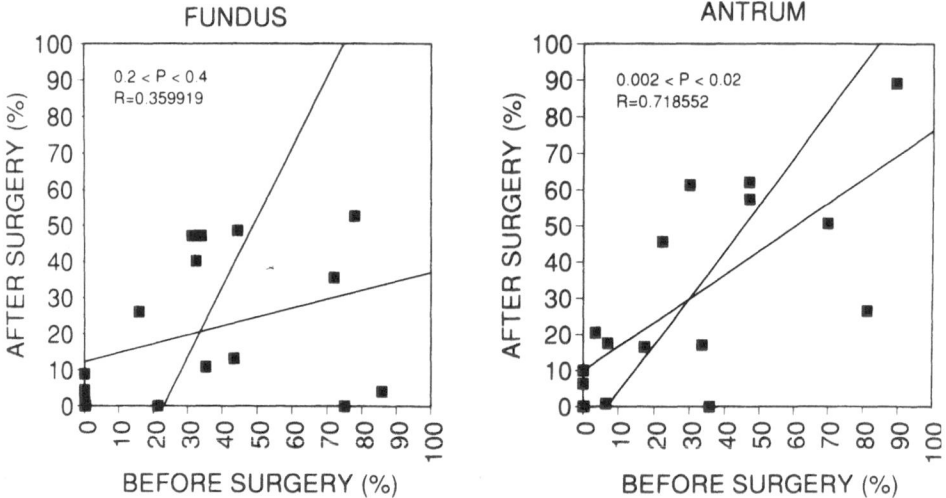

Fig. 3. Changes in the proportion of time that the pH remained below 2 during the total measurement period

In this study, we analyzed the results of 24-h pH monitoring and classified patients into four groups according to the proportion of time their pH remained below 2. The proportion of time the intraluminal pH remains below 2 could be an index of the risk of mucosal injury, because pepsin activity is thought to be maximized at pHs below 2. Patients of type 1a, 1b, and 2a (45% of all subjects) and especially type 1a patients (11% of all subjects) showed low pHs over long periods. Furthermore, intraluminal pH remained relatively constant, especially at the antrum, in a study comparing preoperative and postoperative conditions. These results indicate that the gastric luminal pH was low enough to cause peptic ulcers in the postoperative stomach or duodenum. It is concluded that the administration of an antacid is important in preventing peptic ulcers of the gastric tube in patients showing high preoperative acidity levels.

References

1. Imamura M, Ohishi K, Tobe T (1987) Retrosternal esophagogastrostomy with the EEA stapler. Surg Gynecol Obstet 164:368–371
2. Hashimoto M, Imamura M, Shimada Y, Tobe T (1992) Acid secretion ability of gastric tube used for reconstruction after esophagectomy for esophageal carcinoma: 24-hour pH monitoring study (in Japanese; summary in English). Jpn J Gastroenterol Surg 25(7):1924–1929
3. Lam KH, Lim STK, Wong J, Lam SK, Ong GB (1979) Gastric history and function in patients with intrathoracic stomach replacement after esophagectomy. Surgery 85:283–290
4. Okada N, Sakurai T, Tsuchihashi S, Nishimura O, Juhri M (1986) Gastric functions in patients with the intrathoracic stomach after esophageal surgery. Ann Surg 204:114–120
5. Domergue J, Veyrac M, Huin-Yan S, Rouanet P, Collet H, Michel H, Pujol H (1990) pH monitoring for 24 hours of gastroesophageal reflux and gastric function after intrathoracic gastroplasty after esophagectomy. Surg Gynecol Obstet 171:107–110
6. Walt R (1986) Twenty-four-hour intragastric acidity analysis for the future. Gut 27:1–9

Is There a Relationship Between an Area of Muscular Deficiency and the Vascularisation of the Dorsal Wall of the Hypopharynx and Zenker's Diverticulum?

J. Mebis, K. Geboes, and V. Desmet[1]

Introduction

A previous study on the human pharyngo-esophageal sphincter revealed the micro-anatomical organization of its motor innervation and arterial supply [1]. During the vascular injection studies it became evident that not only the arterial supply, but also the venous drainage of the sphincter area is highly characteristic. It turned out that the intramural venous bed is drained by veins traversing the upper part of the cricopharyngeus muscle. Unfortunately, few studies provide detailed data on the micro-anatomical organization of the venous drainage of the sphincter area [2–4].

The upper part of the sphincter muscle anatomically corresponds to "Kilian's dehiscence", and has been poorly defined as an area of "muscular deficiency". Within this area, Zenker's diverticulum may develop. It represents a typical example of a pulsion diverticulum of the hypopharyngeal wall. It is formed by a protrusion of epithelium and corium trough "so-called" weak spots in the dorsal pharyngo-esophageal muscular wall. This mostly occurs in the upper part of the cricopharyngeus muscle [5].

We performed a micro-anatomical study on the human pharyngo-esophagus to reveal its arterial blood supply together with its venous drainage. Special attention was given to the arrangements in the muscular wall and the relationship with blood vessels.

[1] Laboratorium voor Histochemie en Cytochemie Department Medical Research, Minderbroedersstraat 12, B-3000 Leuven, Belgium

Materials and Methods

This study was performed on pharyngo-esophageal specimens obtained at autopsy from ten patients with a mean age of 73 years. Patient's death was caused by diseases not involving the upper alimentary tract.

Unfixed specimens were anterogradely injected with liquid Microfil (Flow Tek Boulder, Colo. USA) by the inferior and superior thyroid artery (red silicone rubber), and retrogradely by the superficial pharyngeal venous plexus (blue silicone rubber). On overnight fixation (Pearson's fixative: 100 ml formalin-36%, 10 ml ammonia d: 0.885, 150 g sucrose, water added to 1000 ml) [6] the injected specimens were microdissected under stereomicroscopic control. Stereomicroscopic observations were performed under a Wild M3C stereomicroscope equipped with Leitz Orthomat photographic devices. Incident light for stereomicroscopy was obtained from an Intralux 5000 (Volpi) light source equipped with flexible double fiber optic light guides, or with a fiber optic ring illumination. The specimen was lengthwise opened along its ventral midline, and after removal of the laryngeal cartilage, it was pinned flat. The corium/submucosa with the overlaying epithelium was dissected free from the muscular wall. From the latter the prevertebral fascia and adventitia of the cervical esophagus were carefully removed to reveal the external vascular supply of the muscular wall. The connective tissue and pharyngeal aponeurosis were carefully removed to reveal the vascular bed ensheated in the hypopharyngeal corium and esophageal submucosa. So, we could obtain an "en face" view of the external supply and intramural distribution of vascular structures, and of their relationship with the muscle bundles of the pharyngo-esophageal wall.

"Pharyngo-esophageal segment" is commonly used as a general term for that part of the alimentary tract forming the cavity of the hypopharynx and lumen of the cervical esophagus, both of which are separated by the pharyngo-esophageal sphincter (upper esophageal sphincter). In our descriptions of the pharyngo-esophagus we consequently differentiate among three parts: its cranial hypopharyngeal wall, its sphincter area, and the cervical part of the esophageal body.

Results

The results are shown in detail in Figs. 1 to 4.

Muscular Wall

The inferior thyroid artery raises a special branch that supplies the muscular wall of the laryngo-pharynx along its dorsal aspect: the laryngo-pharyngeal artery (Figs. 1 and 4). In its inferior part, the laryngo-pharyngeal artery supplies the cricopharyngeus muscle by numerous transverse branches: the inferior laryngopharyngeal artery and its cricopharyngeal branches. In its superior part, the laryngo-pharyngeal artery supplies the thyropharyngeus muscle, and anastomoses with a descending branch of the superior thyroid artery: the superior laryngopharyngeal artery and its thyropharyngeal branches.

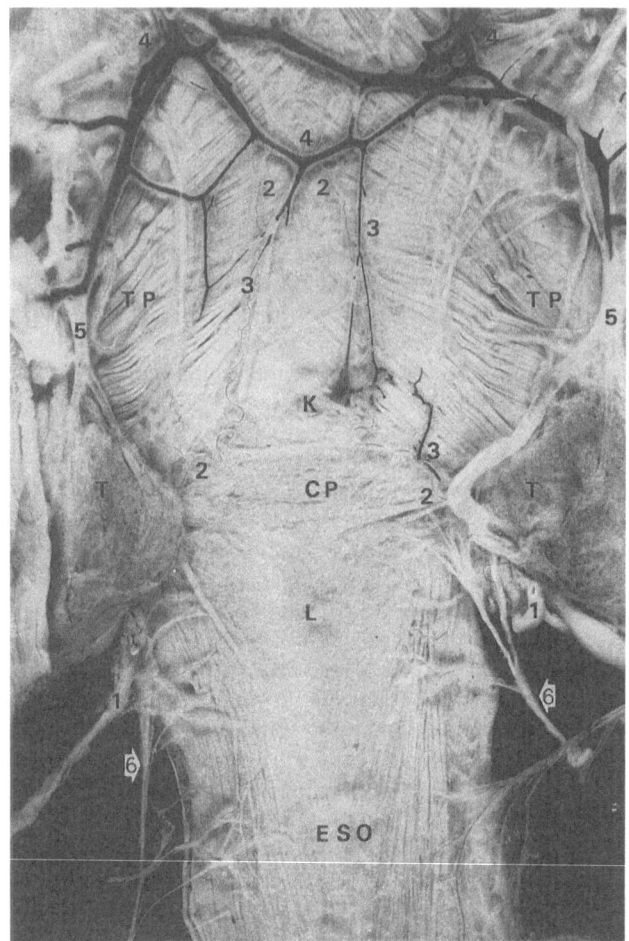

Fig. 1.

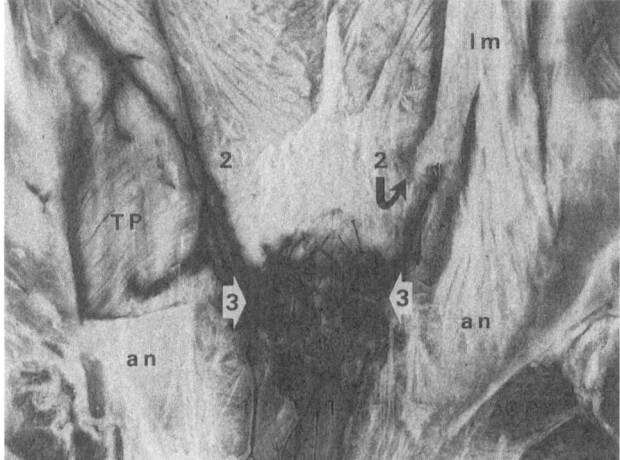

Fig. 2.

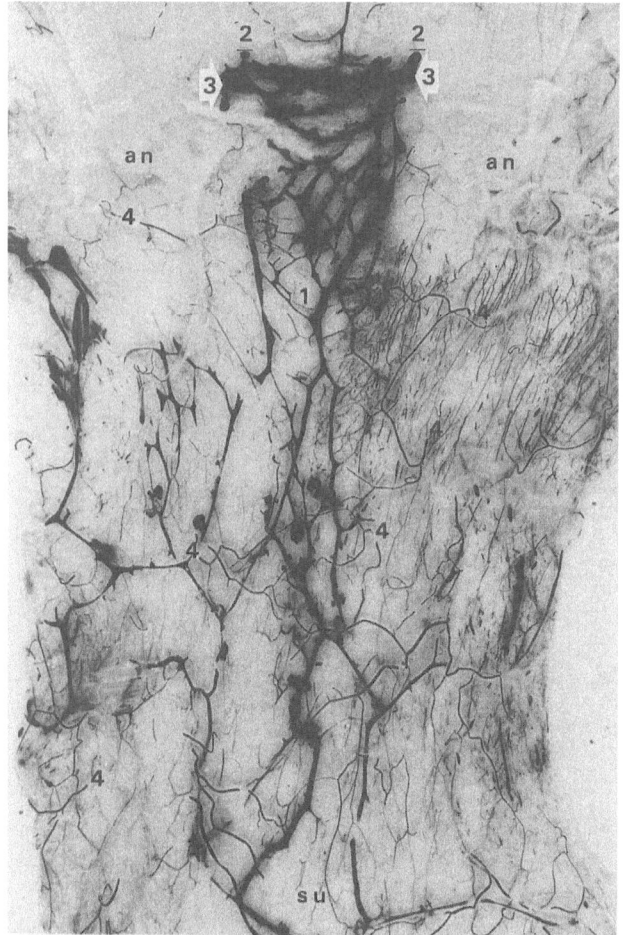

Fig. 3. Intramural vascular supply in the corium/submucosa of the human pharyngo-esophagus (dorsal view at the abluminal face). The intramural pharyngo-esophageal venous plexus in the sphincter area is seen as a prominent labyrinth of thin-walled venous cavities. *1*, aboral contacts with veins of the esophageal submucosa, *2*, cut end of oral extension towards the hypopharynx (cf. Fig. 2), *3*, cut end of dorsal extension towards a vein perforating the muscular wall in the upper part of the cricopharyngeus (cf. Fig. 4), *4*, cut end of the general vascular supply as in the remainder of the digestive tract; *an*, hypopharyngeal aponeurosis; *su*, esophageal submucosa

---

Fig. 1. External vascular supply of the human pharyngo-esophagus (dorsal view at the muscular wall). *1* Inferior thyroid artery (with esophageal branches), *2* laryngo-pharyngeal artery (with cricopharyngeal and thyropharyngeal branches), *3* laryngo-pharyngeal vein (left vein not filled), *4* superficial pharyngeal venous plexus, *5* branching superior thyroid vein, and *6* recurrent laryngeal nerve (with esophageal branches). *TP*, thyropharyngeus; *CP*, cricopharyngeus; *K*, Kilian's dehiscence; *L*, Laimer's triangle; *ESO*, esophagus; *T*, thyroid

Fig. 2. Intramural pharyngo-esophageal venous plexus (ventral view at the luminal face of the muscular wall). Epithelium, corium and submucosa are removed; the longitudinal muscle (*lm*) layer and aponeurosis (*an*) of the dorsal hypopharyngeal wall is wholly removed at the right side and dorsal midline, but only partly at the left side (*black arrow*). The labyrinth of venous cavities in the sphincter area aborally (*1*) communicates with esophageal submucosal veins, and orally (*2*) with veins ascending between the longitudinal muscle of the hypopharynx and the thyropharyngeus (*TP*). At the abluminal face of the venous labyrinth a small draining vein bilaterally perforates (*3*) the muscular wall in the upper part of the cricopharyngeus (*CP*)

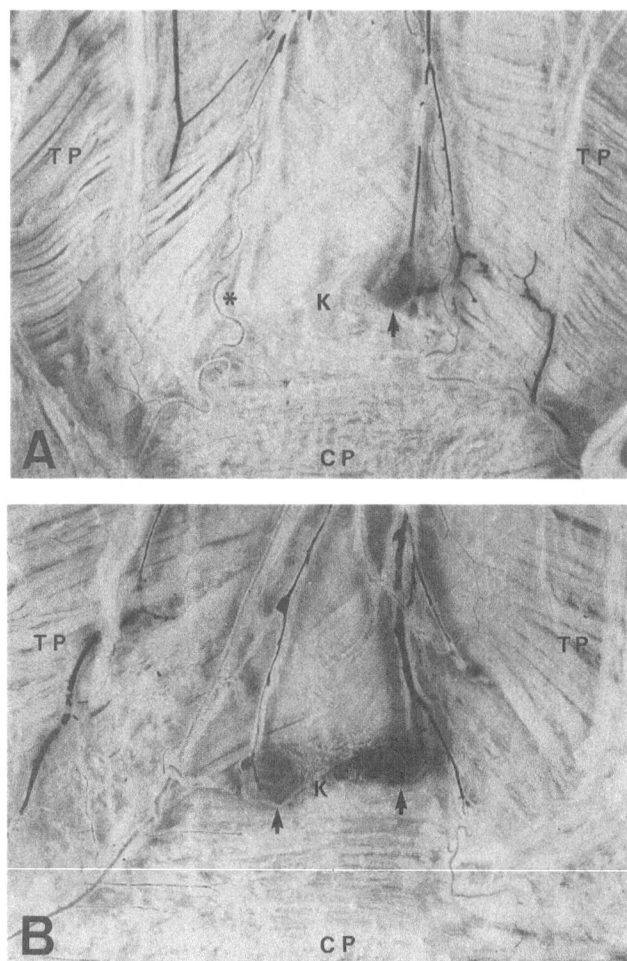

Fig. 4a,b. External vascular supply of the human pharyngo-esophagus (dorsal view at the muscular wall of the sphincter area). **a** Unlike in the normal case (*), a prominent varicose-like structure (*arrow*) perforates the muscular wall at the right side. **b** Unlike in the normal case, prominent varicose-like structures (*arrows*) bilaterally perforate the muscular wall. *TP*, thyropharyngeus; *CP*, cricopharyngeus; *K*, Kilian's dehiscence

The laryngo-pharyngeal vein runs parallel to the branching laryngo-pharyngeal artery. Its inferior part flows into the inferior thyroid vein. Its superior part merges with the prominent dorsal venous plexus of the pharyngeal wall.

Corium and Submucosa

The hypopharyngeal corium and esophageal submucosa are supplied by vascular branches in the same manner as for the general vascularisation of the gut.

A special, intramural venous plexus is found in the corium of the sphincter area (Figs. 2 and 3). It is present at the abluminal face of the aponeurosis of the pharyngeal longitudinal muscles. In the dorsal wall of the sphincter area, this venous plexus is seen as a prominent labyrinth of thin-walled venous cavities. The size of the cavities is strikingly increased when compared with general vascular structures of the pharyngo-esophageal wall (Fig. 3). At three main sites, this venous labyrinth communicates with the surrounding tissue (Fig. 2). Aborally, several extensions descend into the esophageal submucosa. Orally, other extensions bilaterally ascend between the longitudinal muscles of the hypopharynx and the oblique thyropharyngeus muscle fibres. At the upper dorsal aspect of the venous labyrinth, two small veins perforate the muscular wall in the upper part of the cricopharyngeus, ascend along the dorsal thyropharyngeal wall, and constitute a part of the external pharyngeal venous plexus. In six out of ten cases, a prominent varicose-like structure perforated the muscular wall (Fig. 4). In one case, this only occurred on the right side, in three cases only at the left side, and in two cases it was present bilaterally.

Discussion

The human pharyngo-esophageal sphincter receives arterial blood by branches that originate from an arterial loop between the inferior and superior thyroid artery (laryngo-pharyngeal artery). The latter bilaterally ascends along the dorsal aspect of the laryngo-pharynx, while transverse branches supply the cricopharyngeal and thyropharyngeal muscles. Venous blood is drained by the laryngo-pharyngeal vein [7].

Specific for the sphincter area is an additional and separate venous drainage, continuous with the external pharyngeal venous plexus of the dorsal hypopharynx: the intramural pharyngo-esophageal venous plexus. It is located in between the aponeurosis of the longitudinal hypopharyngeal muscle and the cricopharyngeal muscle. This venous labyrinth orally merges with veins of the hypopharyngeal wall and aborally with submucosal veins of the esophageal wall. At its abluminal face, this venous labyrinth is bilaterally drained by veins perforating the dorsal wall of the pharyngo-esophagus in the upper part of the cricopharyngeus muscle. The venous drainage of the sphincter area is highly characteristic in all cases examined, and quite distinct from the general vascularisation of the pharyngo-esophagus.

Zenker's diverticulum presents as a diverticulum of the hypopharyngeal wall [8]. The average age of patients with Zenker's diverticulum in many series is over 60 years. For its pathogenesis, it is generally believed that the protrusion is caused by a combination of two factors: a disturbance in intrapharyngeal pressure and an anatomical weak area in the posterior muscular wall of the hypopharynx. In a dissection study on 40 cadavers, weak spots were found in at least five different area's of the pharyngo-esophageal wall. The commonest site of origin of the diverticulum appeared to be in the upper part of the cricopharyngeus, where muscle fibers showed their highest incidence and degree of variation [5].

The mean age of autopsy patients in our study was 73 years, well above the mean age of patients with Zenker's diverticulum. In 40% of our cases, the draining veins, perforating the dorsal wall of the pharyngo-esophagus in the upper part of the cricopharyngeus muscle, were varicose-like widened. Consequently, they were filling a muscular slit in the upper part of the cricopharyngeus, and thus created a weak spot in the dorsal pharyngo-esophageal muscular wall within the confines of Kilian's dehiscence. A small plexus of veins found at the superior border of the neck of the diverticular sac [9] supports the hypothesis that in its early stage the pulsion diverticulum indeed may protrude through a muscular slit largely filled by a varicose venous structure. These varicose veins, therefore, may be a factor of predisposition for progressive pathological changes: a local or general disturbance of the venous drainage in this area may lead to tissue damage and muscular atrophy. The latter may create an area of muscular deficiency and allow the formation of Zenker's diverticulum.

References

1. Mebis J, Ramaekers K, Geboes K, Desmet V, Vantrappen G (1991) The human pharyngo-esophageal sphincter has a characteristic neural and vascular supply. Gastroenterology 100:A468
2. Elze C (1918) Die venösen Wundernetze der Pars laryngea pharyngis. Anat Anz 51:205–207
3. Butler H (1951) The veins of the esophagus. Thorax 6:276–296
4. Tose D, Rodrigues H, Didio LJA (1984) The venous architecture of the human pharyngo-esophageal transition. Arch Ital Anat Embriol 89:157–165
5. Perrott JW (1962) Anatomical aspects of hypopharyngeal diverticula. Aust NZ J Surg 31:307–317
6. Pearse AGE (1968) Histochemistry. Theoretical and applied. 3rd edn Churchill, London, p 98
7. Ramaekers D, Mebis J, Geboes K, Desmet V (1990) De vascularisatie van de faryngo-oesofageale transitiezone. Acta Gastro-Enterol Belg 53:376–385
8. Vantrappen G, Deloof W (1974) Esophageal diverticula. In: Vantrappen G, Hellemans J (eds) Diseases of the esophagus. Handbuch der inneren Medizin. Dritter Band: Verdauungsorgane. Teil 1 Esophagus. Springer, Berlin, pp 591–613
9. Coburn DE (1951) The treatment of esophageal diverticulum by inversion. N Engl J Med 244:791–795

Lye Stricture of the Esophagus and Gastric Antrum

ARILDO DE TOLEDO VIANA[1]

Introduction

The purpose of this work is to demonstrate how to diagnose antro-pyloric stenosis in patients with esophageal lesions due to ingestion of caustic or corrosive substances, as well as to emphasize the possibility of creating a standard for surgical therapy of gastric injuries which takes into consideration the physiopathological elements of such a condition.

Caustic and corrosive substances cause lesions on all organic tissue when they come into direct contact with them. When ingested, they produce perioral injuries on the lips, tongue, oral cavity, pharynx; often in the larynx, esophagus, and stomach; rarely in the duodenum, and only exceptionally in the jejunum.

Injuries caused by these kinds of chemicals must be evaluated for extent as well as depth.

Spasmodic contractions of both the skeletal and flat musculature are the leading factors which restrict alterations to the highest segments of the digestive tract, up to the esophagus.

Nevertheless, in many cases, more distal lesions of the stomach tract occur which are associated with the highest segments.

Once the acute phase of the insult is past, biological reaction is somewhat different in each type of injured tissue: in the skin, lesions develop into scabs and then into epithelia. This does not occur in either the esophagus or the stomach mucosa, where epithelialization is restricted by the contiguity of the walls, where light is minimal. Because of this, in the esophagus, the scab is followed by collagenous proliferation which can lead to stenosis. In the stomach, caustic and corrosive substances run through the small curve—just as food does—and are prevented from passing through the antrum by pyloric spasms. This course was well proven by experimental studies on dogs which were given a

---

[1] Department of Surgery Faculdade de Ciências Médicas, Santa Casa de São Paulo, Brazil

barium diet mixed with sodium hydroxiyde, all under radioscopic monitoring [1, 2].

In the antrum, caustic or corrosive substances produce tissue necrosis which may affect all layers of the gastric wall, eventually perforating it. Most of the time, though, necrosis is limited to the mucosa and sub-mucosa due to the smaller quantity of caustics and corrosives that reaches the stomach.

In necrotized areas, glands will be destroyed and intense collagenous proliferation will occur in the sub-mucosa, extending to the muscle tissue [3].

In the gastric antrum, the ensuing cicatricial shrinkage generates anular stenosis that will lead to occlusion and sub-occlusion. Therefore, during the chronic phase, esophageal and gastric injuries may co-exist. This condition was described by Goñi Moreno [4] as a "double lesion". Esophageal lesions are not difficult to diagnose, although their presence may hamper the clinical evaluation of the stomach both by endoscopy and contrast radiology, and possible gastric alterations will thus not be detected. Treatment of esophageal stenosis post caustic or corrosive ingestion is usually done through gastrostomy by retrogressive dilation.

The stoma also has the purpose of feeding patients who are unable to take food per os.

Treatment structured in such a way—focusing on esophageal conditions—will be successful most of the time, since the incidence of "double lesion" ranges from 23.6% to 37.5% [5]. Should antral stenosis occur, though, gastrostomy will lead to the serious problem of reflux of food and gastric juice itself. The stoma expands progressively and reflux of acid contents will damage neighboring epithelium. This damaged condition impedes preventive dilations because of pain.

Yet, if the treatment is successful, the patient will be able to orally ingest, and there will be an overflow through the gastrostomy which can become a bona fide gastric fistula.

Such complications were described by several authors who generally blame them on the lack of diagnosing gastric lesions associated with esophageal stenosis. Some authors even consider reflux through the stoma to be an indication of antral stenosis.

Such diagnosis is rather late if made based on gastrostomy reflux which is a complication of a procedure that is presumed to be therapeutic. It is mandatory to establish ab initio the presence of gastric involvement.

Classification

Twenty-two (22) patients with lye stricture of the esophagus and gastric antrum were treated and followed-up from 1981 through 1991.

Methods

The main diagnostic features of the antro-pyloric stenosis were obtained after diluted barium x-ray studies of the stomach were carried out in nine patients (Fig. 1). In the other 13 patients, the diagnosis was confirmed through laparotomy.

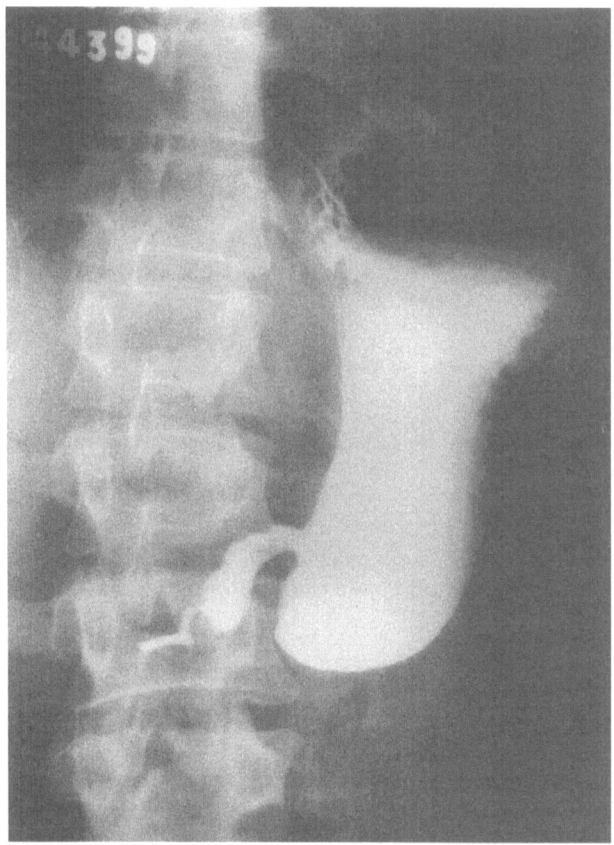

Fig. 1. Pronounced antral stenosis and gastric content of the contrast medium (diluted barium meal)

The pattern of treatment adopted for antral stenosis was resection of the injured gastric segment, usually through antrectomy, with the removal of 1–2 cm of normal gastric and duodenal tissues both proximally and distally. A "Billroth I" gastroduodenostomy was then performed for digestive tract reconstruction. Also, at the same time, gastrostomy was done for feeding purposes, as well as for esophageal bougienage (Fig. 2). Figure 3 shows a macroscopic view of the resected antrum.

Results

Good results were observed in the short- and long-term postoperative period with this combined pattern of treatment in 19 patients. Of the remaining patients, two needed esophagocoloplasty, and one developed stenosis adjacent to of the gastroduodenal stoma, but had a good result after vagotomy and gastro-

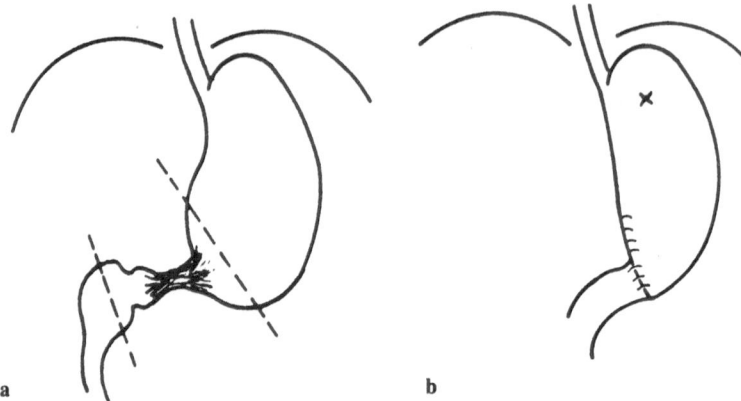

Fig. 2. a Resected area (*dotted lines*). **b** Gastroduodenoanastomosis and gastrostomy (marked by *X*)

jejunostomy. There were no other complications, or deaths. All patients were given psychiatric support during and after hospitalization.

Discussion

Diagnostis

Diagnosis of esophageal stenosis resulting from either caustic or corrosive elements is not difficult. It is easily done by taking the clinical history, by contrast radiology, and by endoscopy. Gastric stenosis is just as easily identified by the same means when the esophagus is not affected.

On the other hand, diagnosis of gastric stenosis in patients already affected by esophageal stricture is quite difficult, so much so that bibliographic research has shown that in early records such diagnoses were confirmed only by necropsy. More recently, it has been identified by complications following inadequate treatment.

In 1925, Vinson and Hartman [6] published the case of a patient who developed esophageal stenosis following lye ingestion. This patient underwent anterograde dilations, which improved his dysphagia but produced vomiting problems. He died 6 months later and necropsy revealed pyloric stenosis, in addition to the esophageal injuries previously diagnosed. McLanahan [7] emphasized how difficult it was to identify pyloric obstruction when all attention was focused on the treatment of esophageal stenosis. Goñi Moreno [4] taught us that it is difficult to distinguish caustic esophagitis from esophagogastritis because the agent continues its action inside inside the stomach, and frequently we are bound to face a double lesion. In spite of this reasoning, he made no specific reference to the ways to diagnose what he called "double lesion". There are reports in the literature of cases where gastrostomy reflux was the first sign of distal obstruction of the stomach.

Fanganiello et al. [8], who were the first in Brazil to study stomach caustic stenosis, reviewed 24 cases in which diagnosis was reached 11 times based on

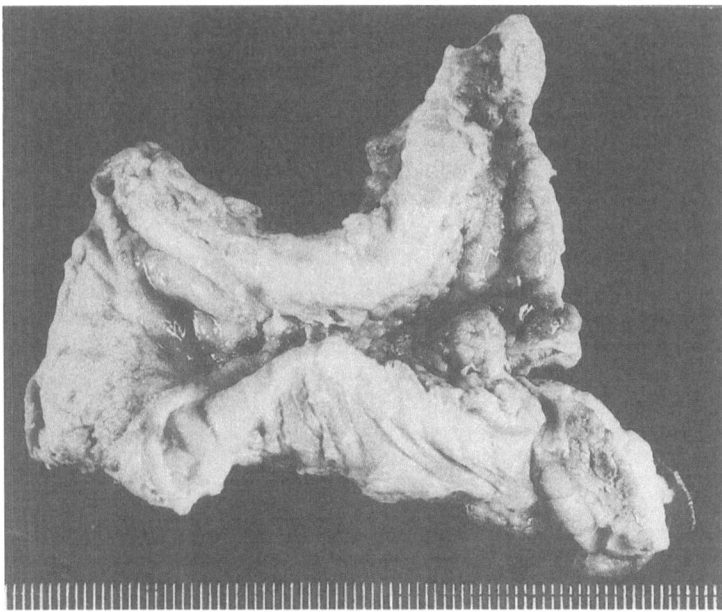

Fig. 3. Macroscopic view of resected antrum

reflux of gastric juices and food through the gastric stoma. All this shows that diagnosis proved difficult to all authors and that they started worrying about it only after complications arose in their patients.

Our criteria—adopted to confirm the diagnosis—enabled us to establish a correct therapeutic strategy. Contrast radiological study and laparotomy are, in effect, the most useful diagnostic tests. Contrast radiology of the stomach, though, is rarely feasible due to the conditions of esophageal stenosis.

Using correctly diluted contrast and sometimes inserting a haso-gastric tube pulled through the esophageal stenosis may help in obtaining gastric images. Radiographic images showed the areas of the small and large antral curves affected by cicatricial shrinkage that lead to stenosis, letting the contrast through an irregular small passage.

There will be gastric stasis and slowness in deflation delaying the opacity of the duodenum and of the jejunal proximal loops. Endoscopy is not helpful to diagnose gastric stenosis in patients already suffering from esophageal stenosis. Most of the time we reached a diagnosis only through laparotomy prior to gastrostomy.

Treatment

Dilations of the antrum have been reported historically only for unsatisfactory results [7]. Jejunostomies [9–11] may be performed on patients needing nutritional improvement. Pyloroplasties [12, 13] are inadequate because they must be performed on injured areas, which is technically incorrect. Until 1950 [14, 15] and afterwards [16, 17] gastroenteroanastomosis was the surgical treatment of choice to treat gastric stenosis caused by caustic and corrosive ingestion. The efficacy of this procedure is well known in severe case's of stenosis; in duodenal ulcerations, whether or not they are associated with different types of vagotomy; in distal gastric obstructions produced by non-resectable carcinomas; and in cases of duodenal or bile-pancreatic fistulae. The histological development of lesions in gastric lye stricture shows that collagen may proliferate progressively, causing cicatricial shrinkage, leading to injury of the anastomosis.

On the other hand, diversion of the digestive flow, allowing gastric secretion to directly reach the jejunum without being neutralized by the duodeno-bileo-pancreatic juices, may cause marginal ulcers to be formed. In addition to this, we risk malignant neoplasia in the lesion itself [18]. Therefore, patients with lye stricture of the gastric antrum should not undergo gastroenteroanastomosis.

Gastric stenosis caused by caustics and corrosives must be unequivocally considered—as McLanahan [7] and Bosch Del Marco [13] put it—as a pathologic entity of its own, demanding treatment suitable to its own physiopathology. Most modern authors have recommended stomach resection to treat gastric stenosis produced by caustics and corrosives. Bosch Del Marco [3], in his 1949 thesis, presented a case in which he had performed subtotal gastrectomy and gastroenteroanastomosis by the Hoffmeister-Finsferer technique; in his conclusion he ended by recommending gastric resection. Two cases described by Strode and Dean [17] were treated by gastric resection: in one by applying "Polya" reconstruction, in the other by gastrogastroanastomosis. Herrington [19], in a case of antro-pyloro-duodenal stenosis, where the gastric body itself was injured, performed a resection, saving 30% of the proximal stomach; he reconstructed the transit by the "Poth" method, which allows a larger stomach reservoir capacity. Fanganiello et al. [8] also emphasized the advantage of such resection in preventing neoplasia in the lesion area [18].

After a general review of all such authors who practice gastric resections, it is striking to not how varied is the extent of resection and reconstruction. Regarding the extent of resection, most authors adopt the same resection as the or they are familiar with in gastroduodenal ulcer, and do not concern themselves with the larger or smaller extent of injury produced by the ingestion of caustics or corrosives. It so happens that in most cases of gastric stenosis of such origin, the injured areas are either restricted to the antrum or are antro-pyloric [14, 20–22].

Reconstruction by Billroth II often presents clinical complications such as "dumping", macrocytic anemia, and non-absorbant syndrome. Also, we must not forget the inconvenience of Billroth II when there is a need to connect a loop of the large intestine to the thorax to perform esophagoplastia. This eventuality occurred in two of our patients and we had no difficulty with colon mobility because we had performed a Billroth I beforehand. Two-thirds partial resection and the Billroth II reconstruction technique—which are usually performed to treat gastroduodenal ulcers—are not acceptable when dealing with stomach stenosis produced by corrosives and caustics, because the physiopathology of this condition is completely different from the etiology and pathology of gastroduodenal peptic ulcer.

The use of sub-total gastrectomy as a routine treatment for gastric stenosis caused by caustics and corrosives has three important disadvantages:

– Resection unnecessarily reduces the capacity of the gastric reservoir.
– Reconstruction by Billroth II may exacerbate clinical complications.
– Colon mobility—if needed—may be reduced.

Therefore, gastric stenosis produced by caustics and corrosives, a specific entity with its own characteristics, must have a specific therapy, adequate for its particular physiopathogenic peculiarities. Despite the gravity of the injury in some cases, in general, gastric stenosis injuries produced by caustics and corrosives are simpler than ulcerative injuries.

Treatment should therefore follow a much simpler pattern; however two conditions should be strictly adhered to:

– Resection should be limited to injured areas (safety edges of 1.0–2.0 cm).
– Transit reconstruction should be carried out
  by gastroduodenoanastomosis.

Adherence to the first guideline the injury, maintains stomach capacity, and prevents the development of carcinoma; adherence to the second produces physiological reconstruction the transit.

Conclusions

1. Lye stricture of the stomach must be always considered in patients showing esophageal stenosis caused by ingestion of caustic or corrosive substances.
2. Always attempt a radiological study of the stomach, using a contrast medium of properly diluted barium or sodium diatrizoate, administered either by ingestion or by injection in a naso-gastric tube pulled through the esophageal stenosis.
3. Should gastrostomy be necessary for feeding purposes or to expand esophageal stenosis, extensive laparotomy must be performed in order to inspect and diagnose possible lye stricture of the antrum.
4. The safest procedure, for treating lye stricture of the gastric antrum with the best results in both the short- and long-term, is resection limited to the injured area, with a safety edge of 1.0–2.0 and transit reconstruction by the Billroth I technique.

References

1. Hodgson JH (1959) Corrosive stricture of the stomach: Case report and review of literature. Br J Surg 46:358–361
2. Maggi AL, Meeroff M. (1953) Stenosis of the stomach caused by corrosive gastrits. Gastroenterology 24:573–578
3. Bosch del Marco LM (1949) Contribuición al estudio de la gastrits corrosiva; estudio clinico y experimental. An Fac Med Montevideo 34:891–1010
4. Moreno IG (1964) Esofagitis caustica. In: Moreno IG (ed) Cirurgia del esófago y hernias por el hiato esofágico. Editorial Universitária, Buenus Aires, pp 201–214
5. Viana AT (1981) Stricture of the esophagus and gastric antrum caused by ingestion of caustic or corrosive substances: Diagnosis and treatment (in Portuguese). Doctoral thesis, University of Sorta Casa, Sao Paul

6. Vinson PP, Hartman HR (1925) Pyloric obstruction due to swallowing a solution of concentred lye. Med Clin North Am 8:1037–1040
7. McLanhan S (1934) Pyloric occlusions following the ingestion of corrosive liquids. JAMA 102:735–739
8. Fanganiello M, Oliveira MR, Branco PD (1956) Estenose cáustica do estômago: estudo de 24 casos. Rev Paul Med 49:93–105
9. Gonzalez LL, Zinninger MM, Altemeier WA (1962) Cicatricial gastric stenosis caused by ingestion of corrosive substance. Ann Surg 156:84–89
10. Povici Z (1977) Attitude chirurgicale dans les stenoses prepyloriqus post-caustiques antrectomie segmentaire intravasculaire en Y-V: considérations sur 80 cas. J Chir 113:181–190
11. Ragheb MI, Ramadan AA, Khalia MA (1976) Management of corrosive esophagitis. Surgery 79:494–498
12. Arena JM (1936) Pyloric stricture following the ingestion of muriatic acid. South Med J 29:331–332
13. Bosch del Marco çLM (1963) Gastritis corrosiva: cinco observaiones de evolución esclerosa y estrechez pilórica. An Fac Med Montevideo 48:42–51
14. Boikan WS, Singer HA (1930) Gastric sequelae of corrosive poisoning Arch Intern Med 46:342–57
15. Schulemburg CAR (1941) Corrosive stricture of the stomach: Without involvement of the oesophagus. Lancet II:367–368
16. Jalundhwala JM, Shan RC (1967) Corrosive stricture of the stomach. Am J Surg 114:461–463
17. Strode EC, Dean ML (1950) Acid burns of the stomach: Report of two cases. Ann Surg 131:801–811
18. O'donnell CH, Abbott WE, Hirshfeld JW (1949) Surgical tretment of corrosive gastrits. Am J Surg 78:251–255
19. Herrington JL (1964) Stenosis of the gastric antrum and proximal duodenum resulting from the ingestion of a corrosive agent. Am J Surg 104:580–585
20. Gatta R (1936) Su un caso di stenosi pilorica da ingestione di acido clorídrico. Arch Ital Mall Apo Diger 5:593–601
21. Gray HK, Holmes CL (1948) Pyloric stenosis caused by ingestion of corrosive substance: Report of a case. Surg Clin North Am 28:1041–1056
22. Harris VJ (1968) Pyloric stenosis: An usual complication of alkaline corrosive poisoning. Am J Roentgenol 104:594–597

Caustic Esophageal Stricture: Bypass Versus Resection

JÁNOS KISS, ATTILA VÖRÖS, and ÁRON ALTORJAY[1]

Introduction

Just 60 years ago, in 1932, Oshawa reported the first successful resection with esophagogastrostomy. Thereafter, the earlier extrathoracic methods of esophagoplasty with skin tubes—which was a bypass procedure—were largely abandoned in favor of newer retrosternal or transthoracic esophagoplasty.

Nowadays, there are two topics of debate in surgery of the corrosive esophageal strictures. The first question is whether to perform a bypass or a resection, and the second is the choice of organ to be used for substitution (stomach or a colonic segment).

Subjects and Methods

In the past 15 years, 51 esophageal replacements have been performed on patients suffering from corrosive esophageal injuries (Table 1, Fig. 1). We have used large and small bowel and stomach in these operations. In cases of strictures in the lower third of the esophagus ($n = 10$), esophageal resection was performed through a left thoracolaparotomy with jejunal interposition. With strictures in the middle third or in the whole of the esophagus, a new esophagus was made from colon ($n = 28$) or stomach ($n = 13$) in an intrapleural or retrosternal route. Three patients died in the esophagocolo-gastrostomy group (Fig. 2). Generally, colon has been the preferred method of replacement or bypass because of associated gastric involvement.

[1] Postgraduate Medical University, Department of Surgery, H-1135 Budapest Szabolcs u. 35. Hungary

Table 1. Esophageal resection (1973–1990)

	n	%	Deaths	
			n	%
Total resections	834	100.0	66	8.1
Malignant	722	86.5	69	9.5
Benign	112	13.5	3	3.3
Alkaline reflux	30	26.8	—	—
Corrosive stricture	51	45.5	3	5.9
Eso. perforation	17	15.1	—	—
Failed Heller's operation	14	12.5	—	—

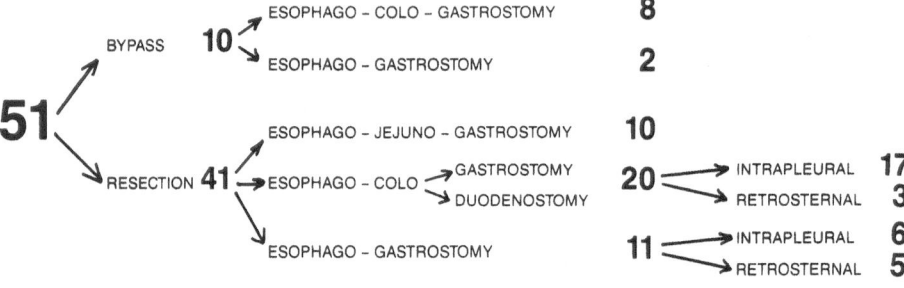

Fig. 1. Caustic Esophageal Stricture. Bypass versus resection

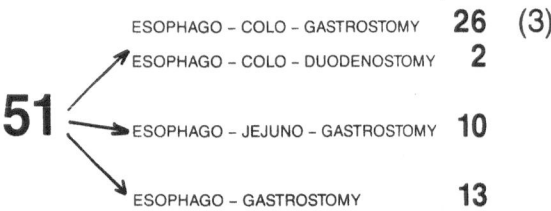

Fig. 2. Caustic Esophageal Stricture. Bypass versus resection; types of surgery

Discussion

Some surgeons deliberately avoid stomach as a substitute in cases of benign disease, even though the initial risk factors for colon are higher. We agree with Orringer and Stirling [1] that the stomach appears to be a good visceral esophageal substitute, because it allows a technically easier operation and good long-term functional results. However, it is not always possible to use stomach because of associated gastric involvement.

There is still some controversy concerning bypass or resection. Because of the risk of carcinoma in caustic strictures, there is a theoretical advantage in performing prophylactic excision of the organ. Because of the hazard of dissection due to adherence and fibrosis, some surgeons prefer the bypass procedure.

Bremner [2] states that the incidence is low (1%–2%) and the time interval is long before a carcinoma develops, there is little argument in favor of resection as opposed to bypass. The added morbidity of resection means that resection has little advantage, if any, over bypass procedure. According to Siewert and Bartels [3], some of the patients suffering from corrosive stricture will develop scar cancer, but this number corresponds to the average death rate from esophageal resection. There is, therefore, no use in performing preventive total esophagectomy.

On the other hand, the most hazardous part of esophageal reconstruction is the anastomosis to the esophagus, as stated by Horvath [4], esophagectomy does not vitally increase this risk, so it wise to perform esophageal resection if surgical intervention is necessary to restore the swallowing capability of the patient.

However, esophageal resection will not provide full safety for the two patients in whom scar cancer developed in the remnant part of esophagus 14 and 4 years after resection. Our standpoint has been formed during the past 15 year-period. Summarizing our present practice and opinion in this field, it is our opinion that A bypass procedure be carried out:

- In postperforational conditions, after thoracotomy, and after serious mediastinitis.
- With an operation performed in an early phase of a transmural (but not perforated) injury. We believe that malignant malformation develops only in patients who have had repeated dilatation besides regular per oral feeding for a long time.
- With operations performed in elderly patients.

A resection is preferred:

- If the patient's condition has been chronic for many years after the injury, in cases of less serious transmural esophageal injuries.
- If the corrosive stricture is combined with a traction type hiatal hernia with gastroesophageal reflux.
- In case a scar carcinoma exits or is localized in the distal part of the esophagus.
- As an emergency procedure when the esophagus is necrotic or at an iatrogenic perforation if a primary resection and replacement is possible. (Twelve of our patients fell into this category and all of them were successful.)

References

1. Orringer MB, Stirling MC (1988) Cervical esophagogastric anastomosis for benign disease. Functional results. J Thorac Cardiovasc Surg 96:887–893
2. Bremner CG (1982) Caustic strictures. In: Bremner, CG (ed) Benign strictures of the esophagus. Curr Prob Surg XIX:450–460
3. Siewert JR, Bartels H (1985) Oesophagus veratzung—"prophylaktische" Oesophagectomie? Langenbecks Arch Chir 365:227–229
4. Horváth ÖP (1987) Surgical management of caustic injuries to the upper gastrointestinal tract—discussion. In: DeMeester TR, Matthews HR (eds) International trends in general thoracic surgery, vol 3. Benign esophageal disease C.V. Mosby, pp 266–268
5. Csikos M; Horváth ÖP, Petri A, Petri I, Imre J (1985) Late malignant transformation of chronic corrosive oesophageal strictures. Langenbecks Arch Chir 365:231–238

A Case of Funnel-Type Benign Esophageal Stricture Due to Foreign Body

Hitoshi Ohtaka, Shigenao Kan, Fumio Suzuki, Mitsuo Nakayama, Hidefumi Baba, Fujio Nishibori, Takao Moriya, and Takatsugu Satoh[1]

Introduction

Since a foreign body lodged in the esophagus produces acute symptoms, urgent treatment is essential to prevent fatal complications such as mediastinitis and perforation of the aorta [1]. We encountered an exceptional case who had chronic symptoms due to an esophageal foreign body which resulted in a funnel-type esophageal stricture.

Case Report

The patient, a 65-year-old Japanese female who had been in the hospital due to schizophrenia since being diagnosed at 20 years of age, presented a progressive swallowing disturbance 3 months prior to her admission to our hospital. An esophagogram taken in January 1991 at a prior hospital showed a circumferential stricture at the middle portion of the esophagus causing severe dysphagia even for a liquid diet (Fig. 1, left). As she refused to eat, intravenous hyperalimentation was applied for nutritional support. During her clinical course at the prior hospital, no remarkable episode was noted such as swallowing caustic agents, chest pain, and fever.

Because of the necessity for a surgical procedure, she was transferred to our hospital in February 1991. A barium esophagogram taken at our hospital showed a funnel-type stricture featuring a narrower stenosis of about 2 mm in diameter and 3 cm in length, although the margin of the stenosis was not very stiff and was smoothly tapered (Fig. 1, right). Both a blood panel and a chest computed tomography (CT) scan were normal. Endoscopic examination of the lesion

[1] Department of Surgery, Tachikawa Hospital, 4-22-2 Nishiki-cho, Tachikawa, Tokyo, 190 Japan

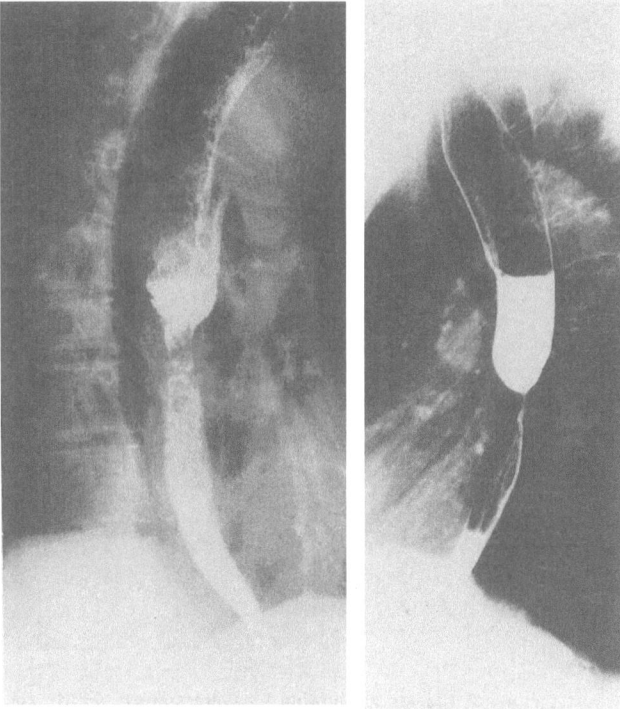

Fig. 1. Esophagogram taken at the former hospital (*left*) and at our hospital (*right*) showing a circumferential stricture at the middle portion of the esophagus. Note that the stricture is not so narrow on the left but it is narrower and smoothly tapered on the right

revealed a severe stenosis of an approximately 1 mm in diameter 26 cm below the incisors. The stenosis was covered with normal esophageal epithelium shown by iodine staining technique (Fig. 2). Although malignancy was not seen in the biopsy specimen; under a tentative diagnosis of esophageal cancer, an operation consisting of intrathoracic esophagectomy and reconstruction using a stomach roll was performed to relieve the patient from dysphagia. After the operation, the patient has been in good condition physically, and is able to eat normal Japanese foods.

The resected specimen showed a severe stenosis without ulceration. The esophageal wall surrounding the stenosis was very thick and was very similar to that of scirrhous type of a cancer (Fig. 3). Histological examination showed marked fibrosis in the esophageal wall, hemosiderin deposition, and a foreign body such as a splinter or part of a toothpick at the lesion (Fig. 4). No evidence of malignancy was seen in the specimen.

Discussion

The patient reported here subsequently disclosed that the esophageal stricture resulted from chronic inflammation due to a foreign body in spite of the preoperative diagnosis of esophageal cancer.

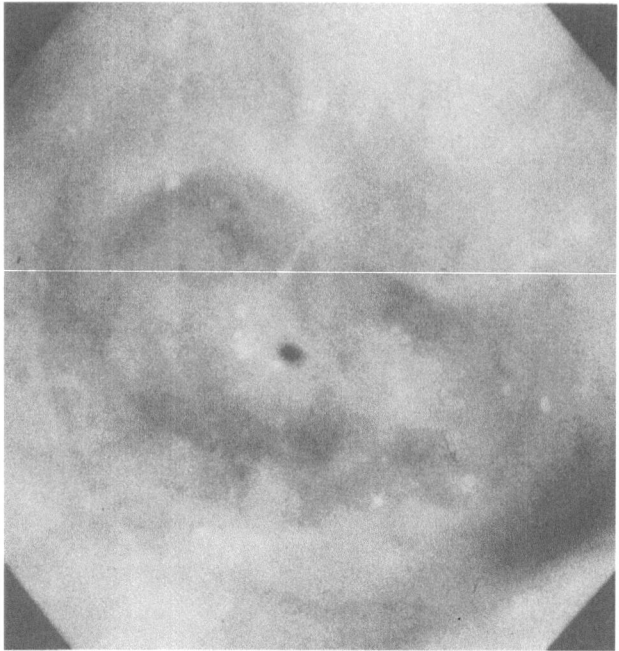

Fig. 2. Endoscopic picture of the lesion showing a severe stenosis which was covered with normal esophageal epithelium shown by iodine staining technique

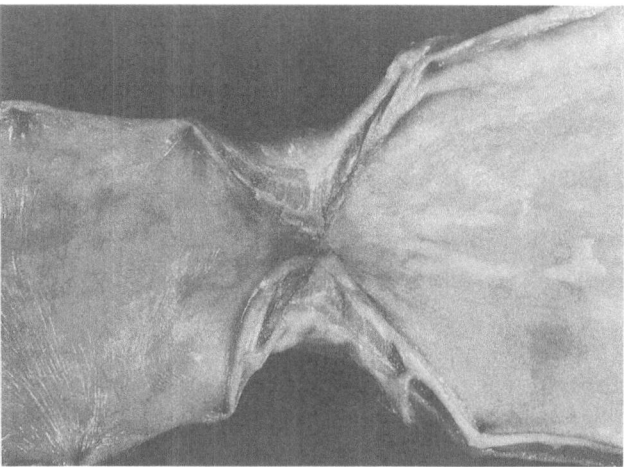

Fig. 3. Macroscopic findings of the resected specimen. The stenotic lesion was covered with iodine-stained epithelium and surrounded with thickened tissue

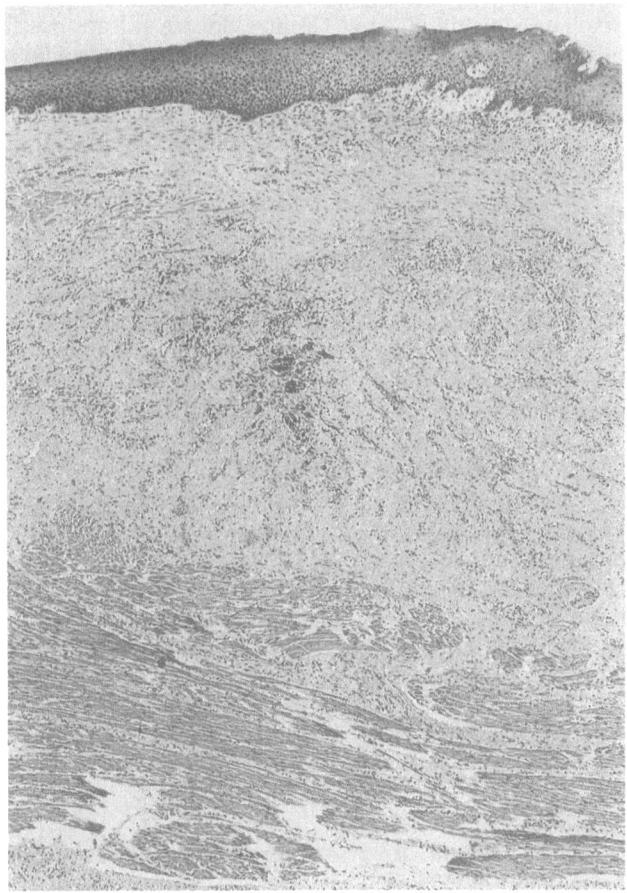

Fig. 4. Microscopic picture showing severe fibrosis in the esophageal wall, hemosiderin deposition, and a foreign body in submucosal layer. No evidence of malignancy was seen in the specimen

The stenosis was so severe and progressively worse within a month that we still could not exclude esophageal cancer as a possible diagnosis. Although the biopsy specimen obtained endoscopically did not present malignancy, it is rather common in patients with esophageal cancer to be funnel-type strictures. Therefore, before the operation, we were convinced that the complaints of the patient could have resulted from esophageal cancer and that the operation was indispensable since the physical findings indicated the operation. Even if we had diagnosed the lesion as being benign stricture of the esophagus, we could not have applied a conservative dilation method [2] to her because of her mental condition.

Among the causes of benign esophageal strictures in elderly people, abnormal gastroesophageal reflux and lye ingestion are easily diagnosed. Besides these two causes, iron deficiency anemia [3], dermatoses [4], viral [5] and fungal [6] infections, dysphagia lusoria [7], and Crohn's disease [8] are possible but rare causes of benign esophageal strictures. As far as the authors could tell from the literature, there are no reports indicating that a foreign body could induce a stricture of the esophagus without having an apparent inflammation such as perforation of the esophageal wall and periesophageal abscess formation.

Location of a foreign body in the normal esophagus has been reported that the cervical portion of physiological narrow segments is most common [9]. It is unlikely that a foreign body remains at the same position in the normal esophagus other than in physiological narrow segments. Diverticula or tumor sites may trap foreign bodies, but esophageal cancer rarely is manifested by a foreign body [9]. Relatively large or sharp-edged foreign bodies are easily lodged in the esophagus and they require urgent treatment because of the abruptly occurring dysphagia. In our case, on the contrary, the foreign body was located at the middle portion of the esophagus which did not correspond to physiological narrow segments. The foreign body shown histologically was too small to cause acute symptoms. As histology showed hemosiderin deposition in the esophageal wall, the foreign body anyhow stuck into the esophageal wall and remained there as a stimulus of chronic periesophagitis. Therefore, the patient did not take notice of the lesion until it became symptomatic.

Since the histology clearly showed a foreign body, obviously of woody fiber, and hemosiderin deposition in the esophageal wall in this case, we speculate that accidental swallowing of a foreign body which stuck into the esophageal wall may have caused chronic periesophagitis which resulted in funnel-type esophageal stricture.

References

1. Cavo JW, Koops HJ, Gryboski RA (1977) Use of enzymes for meat impactions in the esophgus. Laryngoscope 87:630–634
2. London RL, Trotman BW, Dimarino AJ Jr, Olega A, Friman DB, Reng EJ, Rosato EF (1981) Dilatation of severe esophageal strictures by inflatable balloon catheter. Gastroenterology 80:173–175
3. Chisholm M, Ardran GM, Callender ST, Wright R (1971) Iron defficiency and autoimmunity in post-cricoid webs. Q J Med 40:421–433
4. Farooq PA, Raji MR (1982) Esophageal involvement in pemphigoid: Clinical and roentgen manifestaions. Gastrointest Radiol 7:109
5. Sethumadhavan VS, Rashmi P (1982) Herpes esophagitis. Am J Gastroenterol 77:48–50
6. Orringer MB, Sloan H (1978) Monilial esophagitis: An increasingly frequent cause of esophageal stenosis. Ann Thorac Surg 26:364
7. Terracol J, Sweet RH (1958) Diseases of the esophagus, 1st edn. WB Saunders, Philadelphia
8. Haggitt RC, Meissner WA (1972) Crohn's disease of the upper gastrointestinal tract. Am J Clin Pathol 59:613–622
9. Giordano A, Adams G, Boies L, Meyerhoff W (1981) Current management of esophageal foreign bodies. Arch Otolaryngol 107:249–251

Assessment of the Surgical Treatment of Reflux Esophagitis Complicated by Esophageal Stricture

Nobuyoshi Hanyu, Shigeo Morita, Yoshiyuki Furukawa, Yoichi Ohira, Sadanobu Abe, Yoshihiro Hashimoto, Tetsuya Kajimoto, and Teruaki Aoki[1]

Introduction

It was some 40 years ago that acid reflux esophagitis associated with hiatus hernia was first reported by Allison et al. [1] in 1951. Since then, reflux esophagitis has been common in the American and European countries, with cases in Japan occurring infrequently. Recently, however, increasing numbers of cases have been diagnosed as reflux esophagitis in Japan due to demographic reasons associated with the aging of society and the westernization of life styles in particular with respect to diet and advances in diagnostic techniques such as esophageal manometry [2], pH monitoring [3], and esophageal scintigraphy [4]. This change of circumstances has caused treatment of the disease to be notably improved: Good results have been reported with histamine H_2 receptor antagonists and proton pump inhibitors [5, 6]. However, some cases of reflux esophagitis are resistant to these treatments and develop esophageal stricture during the course of the disease.

We have retrospectively studied the cases of reflux esophagitis experienced by us and discussed the pathophysiology and treatment of esophageal stricture.

Subjects and Methods

Four cases of esophageal stricture associated with reflux esophagitis were experienced at our hospital (Table 1). The patients were two men and two women of ranging in age from 54 to 75 years. Dysphagia and heartburn were primary clinical symptoms of the four cases. Three of them underwent surgery, and

[1] Second Department of Surgery, Jikei University School of Medicine, 3-25-28 Nishi-Shinbashi, Minato-ku, Tokyo, 105 Japan

Table 1. Cases of reflux esophagitis accompanied by esophageal stricture

Case	Age (years)	Sex	Symptoms	Surgical procedures
1	75	F	Dysphagia Heartburn	Surgical enlargement of stricture + Nissen's fundoplication
2	56	M	Heartburn Dysphagia	Surgical enlargement of stricture + fundic patch operation
3	68	F	Dysphagia	Nissen's fundoplication
4	54	M	Dysphagia Heartburn	Endoscopic dilatation with balloon

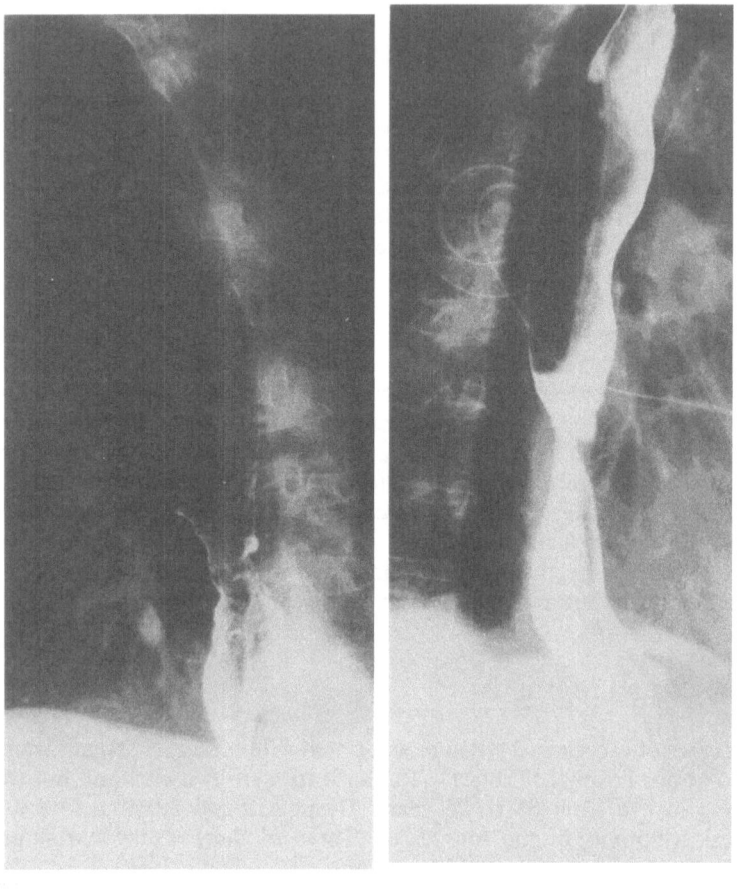

(October 1989)   (June 1990)

Fig. 1. Preoperative esophagograph of case 1

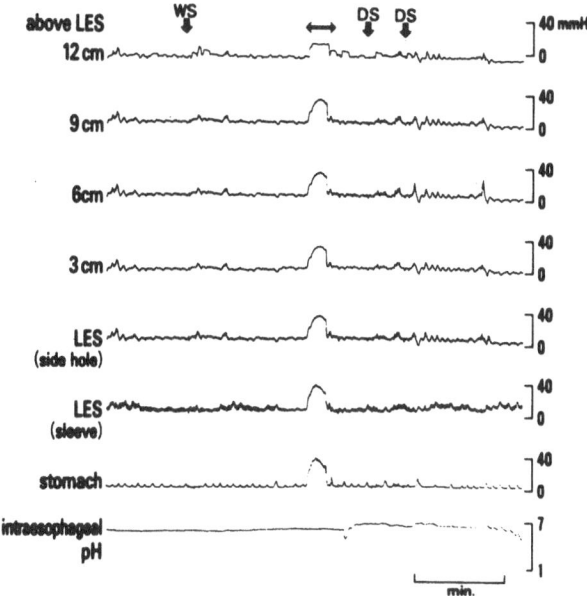

Fig. 2. Postoperative esophageal manometry of case 1. Gastroesophageal reflux caused by heightened abdominal pressure (*horizontal arrow*, abdominal pressure) observed before operation was improved, but swallowing-induced esophageal peristalsis was not observed. *LES*, Lower esophageal sphincter; *DS*, dry swallow; *WS*, wet swallow

the remaining case underwent endoscopic dilatation with balloon. Esophageal manometry was conducted with Dent Sleeve [7] catheter and Arndorfer's infusion pump [8] before and after surgery.

Results

Case 1 is a 75-year-old female patient who developed esophageal stricture in the progressive course of reflux esophagitis. A preoperative esophagography revealed an ulcer with non-symmetric borders in the lower esophagus. Another esophagography taken 8 months later revealed advancement of stricture and short esophagus (Fig. 1). The patient underwent Nissen's fundoplication [9] after the esophageal stricture was surgically enlarged. This surgical treatment brought about some improvement in the esophaged stricture. Postoperative esophageal manometry revealed improvement of gastroesophageal reflux due to heightened abdominal pressure observed before operation, but swallowing-induced esophageal peristalsis was not observed (Fig. 2). The patient has a favorable prognosis, gaining 7 kg body weight, though mild dysphagia still remains.

Case 2 is a 56-year-old male patient who complained of severe heartburn and dysphagia. Preoperative esophagography revealed stricture in the lower esophagus (Fig. 3), and hemorrhagic circular stricture was observed endoscopically. Preoperative esophageal manometry demonstrated low amplitude of contractile waves

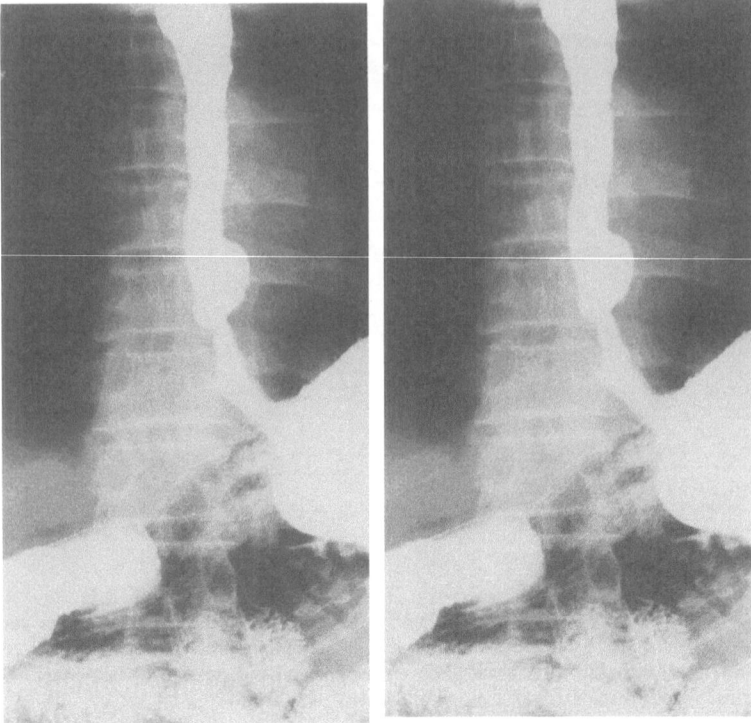

Fig. 3. Esophagograph of case 2. The lower portion of the esophagus presented lead pipe-shaped stricture

and the presence of simultaneous contractile waves and gastroesophageal reflux (Fig. 4). Esophagomyotomy was performed on the stricture followed by a fundic patch operation. This operation resolved the heartburn, but it failed to improve the esophageal motility as indicated by the esophageal manometry after operation, with mild dysphagia remaining.

Case 3 is a 68-year-old female patient who was diagnosed with reflux esophagitis and has been treated with drugs for 2 years. The patient eventually underwent operation since the treatment with drugs has not been effective in improving clinical symptoms. Preoperative esophagography and endoscopy revealed circular stricture on the upper side of the hernial sac (Fig. 5). While the only surgical procedure carried out was a Nissen's fundoplication, this patient showed complete resolution of esophagitis after operation both in subjective symptoms and endoscopic findings.

Case 4 is a 54-year-old male patient with several decades' history of alcohol consumption who experienced deterioration of his esophagitis as a result. Esophagography revealed a shortened esophagus and hiatus hernia (Fig. 6). The patient is presently under treatment with frequent endoscopic dilatations with balloon, since he elected not to undergo the recommended operative procedure.

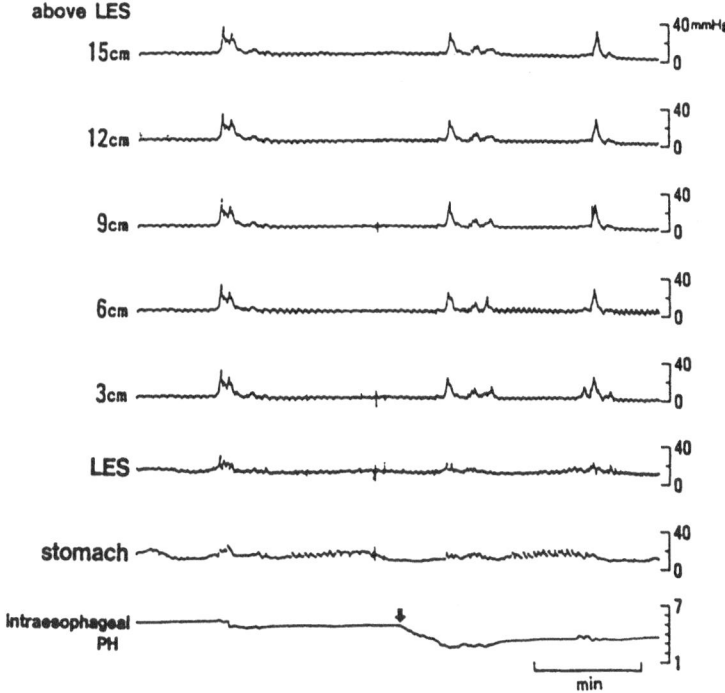

Fig. 4. Esophageal manometry in case 5. The esophagus presented simultaneous contractile waves with low amplitude and gastroesophageal reflux (*arrow*). *LES*, lower esophageal sphincter

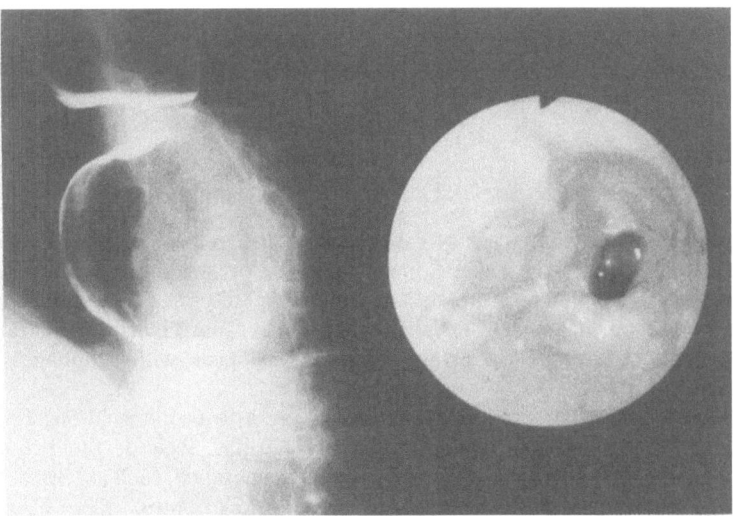

Fig. 5. Esophagograph and endoscopic findings of case 3. Circular stricture was observed on the upper side of the hernial sac

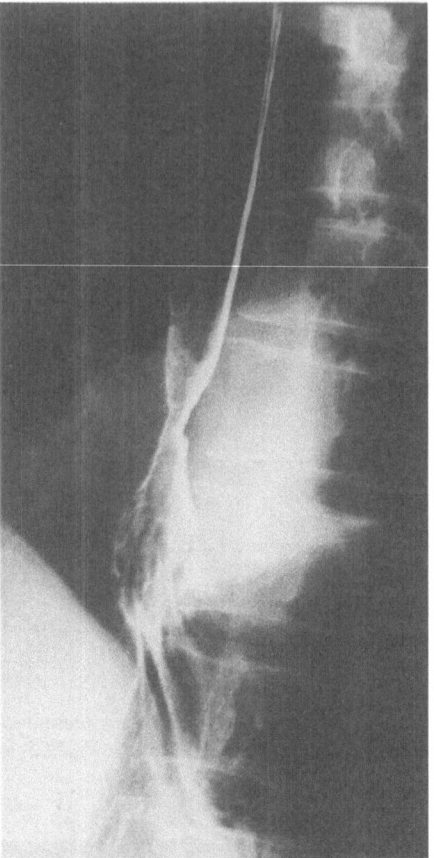

Fig. 6. Esophagograph of case 4. Hiatal hernia and esophageal stricture were observed

Discussion

It is still unknown what types of cases tend to progress to esophageal stricture, as indicated in our experience. Some cases develop stricture after repetition or recurrence of esophagitis due to an underlying diseases, but others do not. Three of our four cases were esophageal stricture caused by sliding hiatal hernia and the other developed after treatment of achalasia with esophageal motor disorder.

The most important preconditions for progress to esophageal stricture seem to be, first, the presence of sliding hiatal hernia. Second, the presence of esophageal motor disorder with severly reduced clearance, such as with achalasia, seems to be involved in the progress to esophageal stricture.

The following three surgical treatments are possible for esophageal stricture: (1) preservative treatment of the stricture followed by operation only for the purpose of prevention of reflux [10], (2) esophagoplasty at the stricture [11], or (3) esophagectomy of the stricture. The most effective surgical treatment of esophageal stricture is esophagectomy. We recommend, however, as the procedure of first choice, to open up the esophageal stricture to prevent regurgitation since esophagectomy is rather invasive and also because the disease is usually benign [12]. Esophagectomy should also be considered in patients with severe esophageal motor disorders like achalasia.

References

1. Allison PR (1951) Reflux esophagitis, sliding hiatal hernia, and the anatomy of repair. Surg Gynecol Obstet 92:419
2. Morita S, Hanyu N, Aoki T (1991) LES pressure and surgical treatment of achalasia and reflux esophagitis. J Smooth Muscle Res 27:163–164
3. Robertson D (1987) Patterns of acid reflux in complicated oesophagitis. Gut 28:1483–1488
4. Fisher RS, Malmud LS, Robert GS. Gastroesophageal (GE) scintiscanning to detect GE reflux. Gastroenterology (1976);70:301–308
5. Wesdorp ICE (1982) Treatment of reflux oesophagitis. Scand J Gastroenterol 17 [Suppl 79]:106–13
6. Kishi S (1992) Pharmacotherapy of reflux esophagitis. Monthly Book Gastro 3:65–71.
7. Dent J, Chir B (1976) A new technique for continuous sphincter pressure measurement. Gastroenterology 71:263–267.
8. Arndorfer RC, Steff JJ, Dodds WJ (1977) Improved infusion system for intraluminal esophageal manometry. Gastroenterology 73:23–27.
9. Nissen R (1961) Gastropexy and fundoplication in surgical treatment of hiatus hernia. Am J Dig Dis 6:954
10. Aoki T, Hanyu N (1990) Surgical treatment of reflux esophagitis and its timing. Current Therapy 18:70–73.
11. Thal AP (1968) A unified approach to surgical problems of the esophagogastric junction. Ann Surg 168:542–550.
12. Aoki T, Hanyu N (1991) Limitations of preservative treatment of reflux esophagitis and application of surgical treatment. Gastroenterol Endosc 3:49–55.

Treatment of Benign Esophageal Stricture

Kenji Kobayashi, Hitoshi Shiozaki, Masatoshi Inoue, Shigeyuki Tamura, Toshimasa Tujinaka, Atsuo Murata, Jun-ichi Nishijima, Takatoshi Kadowaki, Shigeo Matsui, Yoshihiro Kido, and Takesada Mori[1]

Introduction

Benign esophageal stricture is caused by a variety of conditions. Considering its benign character, conservative management should be attempted first, using various dilatation instruments, such as a Celestin dilator [1, 2] and a baloon catheter [3, 4]. If the conservative management is not successful, surgical treatment is required to relieve the stricture. This retrospective study was attempted to clarify the limitation of conservative management and the indications for surgical treatment for benign esophageal strictures.

Subjects

From January 1978 to December 1991, 96 patients with benign esophageal strictures were treated in our department. All patients suffered from dysphagia. The esophageal stricture was diagnosed when an ordinary endoscope could not pass through the stenotic lesion. Among these 96 patients, good improvement was obtained with conservative treatment in 90 cases, and in the other resistant 6 patients from the conservative treatments subsequently underwent various surgical procedures.

Results

Causes of Strictures

Postoperative anastomotic strictures developed after surgery for esophageal carcinomas ($n = 62$), gastric carcinomas ($n = 11$), esophageal varices ($n = 4$), and other diseases ($n = 4$) (Table 1). Strictures due to severe reflux esophagitis

[1] Department of Surgery II, Osaka University Medical School, 1-1-50 Fukushima, Fukushima-ku, Osaka, 553 Japan

Table 1. Causes of benign esophageal strictures

Postoperative anastomotic stricture	81
Esophageal cancer	62
Gastric cancer	11
Esophagaeal varices	4
Thyroid cancer	2
Pharyngeal cancer	1
Achalasia	1
Reflux esophagitis	8
Corrosive esophagitis	5
Idiopathic esophageal stricture	1
Progressive systemic sclerosis	1
Total	96

Table 2. Methods of treatment for benign esophageal stricture

	Bougie, baloon	Electric incision	Operation	Total
Anastomotic stricture	63 (77.8%)	17 (21.0%)	1 (1.2%)	81
Reflux esophagitis	3 (37.5%)	2 (25.0%)	3 (37.5%)	8
Corrosive esophagitis	3 (60.0%)	2 (40.0%)	0	5
Others	0	0	2 (100%)	2
Total	69 (71.9%)	21 (21.9%)	6 (6.2%)	96
	90 (93.8%)			

occurred in eight patients, corrosive esophagitis in five, and progressive systemic sclerosis in one. Idiopathic stricture was diagnosed in one patient.

Endoscopic Treatments

Methods of treatment for benign esophageal stricture are shown in Table 2. A dilatation procedure by balooning or bougienaging is as follows: After a guide wire was endoscopically passed through a stenotic region, a baloon catheter or a bougie tube (Celestin dilator [1, 2]) was then introduced to dilatate the stricture. When the site of esophageal stricture located in the upper or middle esophagus, a bougienage with a Celestin dilator was applied. Figure 1 shows a patient with middle esophageal stricture by corrosive esophagitis. After successive dilatation by Celestin dilator, the stricture was almost completely resolved. A baloon catheter was applied for dilatation of the lower esophageal stricture. Using these methods, satisfactory food intake was restored in 69 patients. In the other 21 patients, the combination of these two dilatation methods were not effective, since either the diameters of the strictures at x-ray film were less than 10 mm or the stenotic lesion was too hard to dilatate by balooning or bougienaging. In these circumstances, dilatation was effectively accomplished by an endoscopic incision with an electric knife. Moreover, to obtain a sufficient dilatation of stricture, repeated endoscopic treatments with a combination of these methods

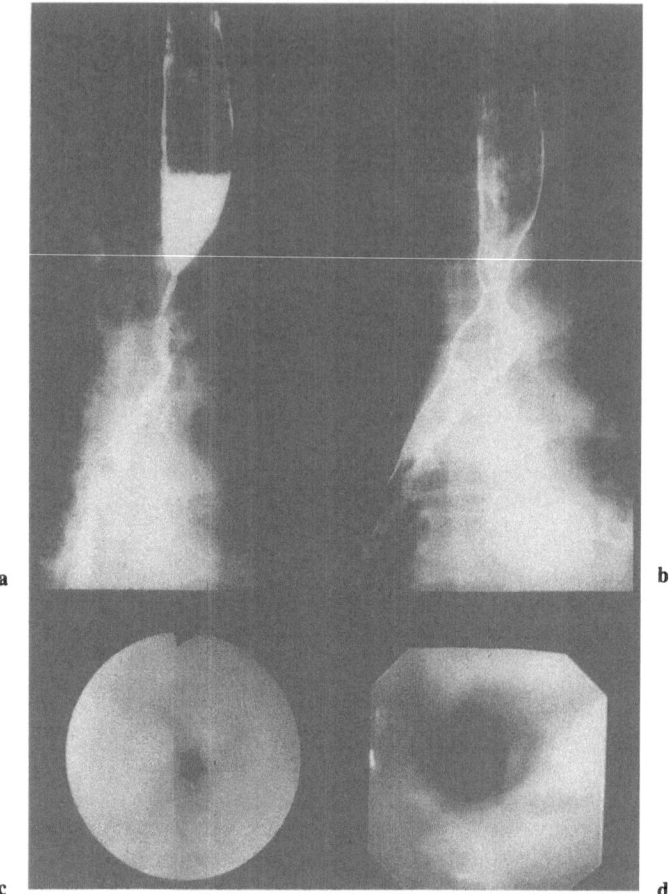

Fig. 1a–d. Middle esophageal stricture due to corrosive esophagitis. **a,c** before dilatation, **b,d** after dilatation by a Celestin dilator

were necessary. The success rate of the conservative endoscopic dilatation was 93.8% (90/96).

Surgical Treatments

Six (6.2%) of the 96 patients were refractory to various endoscopic treatments, whose stenotic lesions were very long in length (mean length about 3 cm) and hard, or accompanied with bleeding ulceration. Finally, these patients underwent surgical operations as follows.

Case 1

A 50-year-old male, diagnosed with idiopathic cervical esophageal stricture. The stricture was very hard. Resection of cervical esophagus was carried out with a reconstruction by a skin tube.

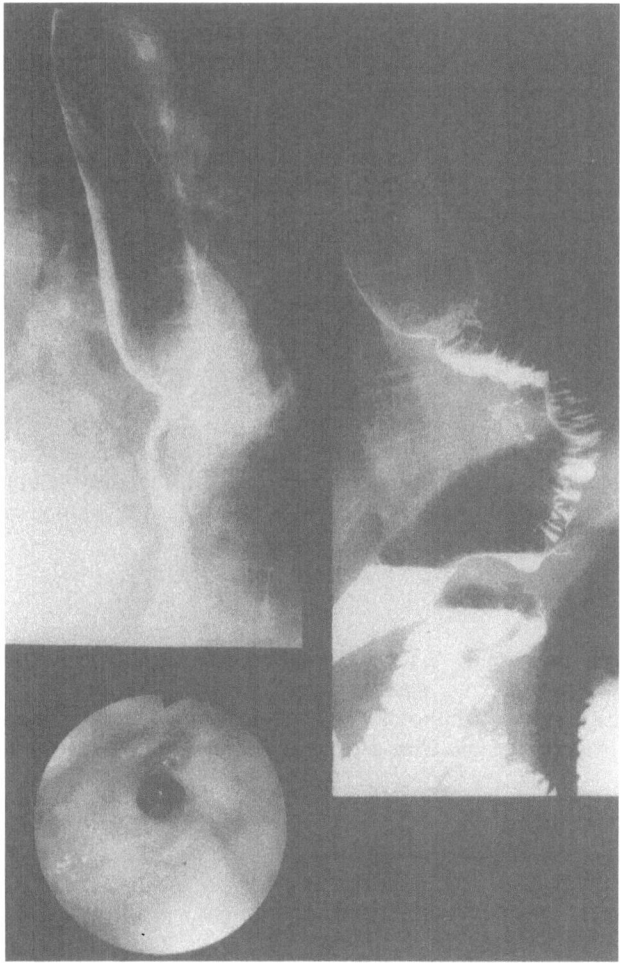

Fig. 2. Lower esophageal stricture due to progressive systemic sclerosis (patient 2)

Case 2

A 58-year-old female (Fig. 2.) developed lower esophageal stricture which was caused by progressive systemic sclerosis. Bleeding ulcers were found around the area of the stricture. Resection of lower esophagus, with reconstruction of jejunal interposition.

Case 3

A 63-year-old female with middle-lower esophageal stricture caused by severe reflux esophagitis with multiple endocrine neoplasm (type 2a). The stricture was very long in length (5 cm) and hard. Subtotal esophagectomy through right thoracotomy was performed with a jejunal reconstruction of Roux-Y anastomosis.

Case 4

A 43-year-old male with postoperative esophagojejunal anastomotic stricture which developed following total gastrectomy and jejunal interposition. The patient repeated endoscopic treatments for 7 years to relieve his symptoms. Consequently, the patient underwent elective surgical treatment for his condition: Resection of site of stricture, with a reconstruction of the second jejunal interposition.

Case 5

A 54-year-old male with lower esophageal stricture caused by reflux esophagitis after distal gastrectomy for gastric ulcer. The stricture was very long in length (7 cm) and hard. Resection of lower esophagus and total gastrectomy of residual stomach through left thoracotomy and laparotomy, with jejunal reconstruction of Roux-Y anastomosis.

Case 6

A 64-year-old male (Fig. 3.) with middle-lower esophageal stricture caused by reflux esophagitis with gastric sliding hernia. The stricture was long in length (3 cm) and hard. Subtotal esophagectomy through left thoracotomy and laparotomy was performed with a retromediastinal reconstruction of the gastric tube.

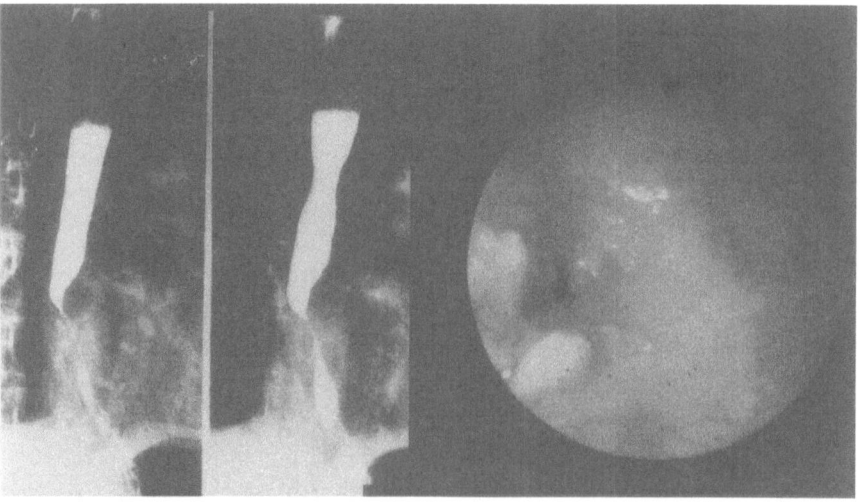

Fig. 3. Middle-lower esophageal stricture caused by reflux esophagitis with gastric sliding hernia. A surgical treatment was required (patient 6)

Discussion and Conclusion

Treatment of benign esophageal stricture should be planned and performed considering safely and palliation. Therefore, most patients are first treated by various conservative methods, such as a Celestin dilator, a baloon catheter, and incision by an electric knife using endoscopy. By these procedures, 93.8% of all 96 patients were effectively and safely treated. However, in six patients (6.2%), these endoscopic treatments were not effective because stenotic lesions were very long in length and hard or accompanied with bleeding ulceration. In these patients, surgical treatment is necessary to correct the stricture.

References

1. Celestin LR, Campbell WB (1981) A new and safe system for oesophageal dilatation. Lancet 1:74–75
2. Fellows IW, Raina S, Holmes GKT (1986) Celestin dilatation benign esophageal strictures: A review of 100 patients. Am J Gastroenterol 81(11):1052–1054
3. Satou M, Hamachi J, Tanaka K, Nomura S, Maeda C, Mitsuzane K, Matsuoka T, Kawabata M, Mishima T, Yamada R (1985) Treatment of benign esophageal strictures by means of baloon catheter dilatation. Jpn J Radiol 45(8):1095–1103
4. Kawano T, Yoshino K, Takiguchi T, Yamazaki S, Taenaka T, Shimoju K, Menjo M (1985) Use of the Medi-Tech catheter and surgical treatment for benign esophageal stricture (in Japanese). J Jpn Soc Clin Surg 46:1320–1326

Esophageal Cancer

Early Carcinoma of the Esophagus

KIN-ICHI NABEYA[1]

Introduction

Early esophageal cancer first attracted attention in 1966. Yamagata discovered a superficial cancer by cytology, and Nakayama accurately diagnosed a polypoid cancer with endoscopy. Both detected cases underwent operation. Following this, many reports were made on radiologic examinations [1–3], on endoscopic examinations [4, 5], and on cytology [6–8]. Much discussion has followed on the concepts of early esophageal cancer and the definition thereof. In Japan, the definition of early esophageal cancer [9] is a cancer located within the submucosa and without metastasis. From a clinical standpoint, a cancer located within the submucosa, regardless of metastasis, is defined as a superficial cancer. In accordance with this definition, diagnosis and treatment on early esophageal cancer, including superfical cancer, in Japan will be presented. Particularly, the studies on diagnosis and treatment methods in our department will be discussed.

Materials and Methods

In cooperation with the Japanese members of the I.S.D.E., 2517 cases of resected superficial esophageal cancer in Japan were recorded at 127 hospitals from 1966 to 1990. From 1973 to 1991, there were 45 cases of superficial cancer and 38 cases of early cancer experienced in our department. Studies were made of clinical factors, pathologic finding, and prognoses in these cases.

Classifications of endoscopic types were made following the "Guidelines for the Clinical and Pathologic Studies on Carcinoma of the Esophagus" [9]: Superficial and protruding type is classified as 0–I, superficial and flat type as 0–II,

[1] Second Department of Surgery, Kyorin University School of Medicine, 6-20-2 Shinkawa, Mitaka, Tokyo, 181 Japan

and superficial and distinctly depressed type as 0–III. The doubling-time definitions were made according to:

$$D = \frac{1}{3} \cdot \frac{\log 1}{\log d_2 - \log d_1}$$

d_1: initial tumor diameter
d_2: secondary tumor diameter
T : time interval for d_1 to develop to d_2

Statistical significance was evaluated using the χ^2 test.

Results

Present Status and Clinical Factors

Of the 2517 cases of superficial cancer, there were 1826 cases of early cancer
[n(−)] and 691 cases of superficial cancer [n(+)]. By depth of invasion of
cancer, there were 287 cases of epithelial (ep) cancer and all were n(−); there
were 439 cases of muscularis mucosae (mm) cancer and 91.3% were n(−); and
1791 cases of submucosal (sm) cancer and 63.5% were n(−) (Fig. 1).

Clinically, 45% of all cases were asymptomatic, whereas slight dysplagia and
retrosternal pain were experienced in 25%. Small cancers, those measuring less
than 3 cm, comprised 70%, and cancers measuring over 3 cm comprised 30%,
the latter of which were mainly superficial spreading types. Those cancers that
were diagnosed preoperatively by either X-ray or endoscopy to be other than
the superficial type were thought to be advanced types (Table 1).

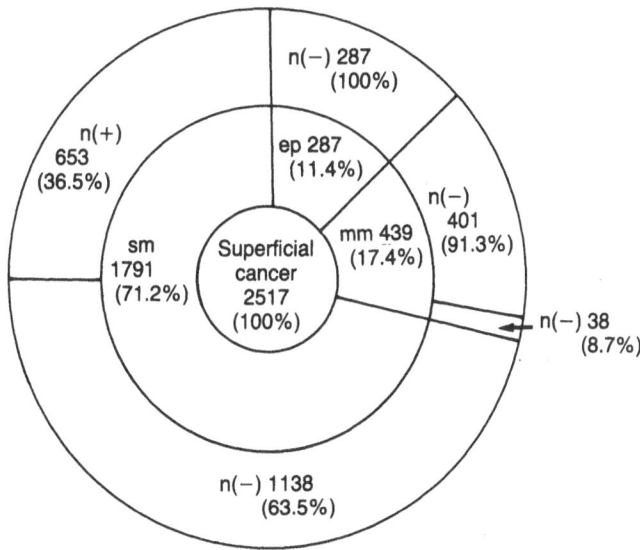

Fig. 1. Superificial cancer in Japan (127 Hospitals, 1966–1990). *ep*, Epithelial; *mm*, muscularis
mucosae; *sm*, submucosal; *n*(+), lymph node metastasis; *n*(−), no lymph node metastasis

Table 1. Clinical matters on superficial esophageal cancer (2517 cases from 127 hospitals, 1966–1990)

Sex:	Male vs. female	5.5 : 1
Age:	Above 50 years of age	93%
Symptoms:	Asymptomatic	45%
Size:	Less than 3 cm	60%
	Less than 1 cm	10%
Location:	Middle third	60%
X-ray type:	Superficial elevated	35%
	Superficial depressed	20%
	Superficial flat	15%
Endoscopic type:	0–II	55%
	0–I	15%
	0–III	5%
Histologic type:	Squamous cell ca.	95%

ca., Carcinoma

Table 2. Doubling time of digestive tract cancers (KUSM[a], 1992)

	Early	Advanced
Esophageal cancer	11.97 months	4.67 months
	(6.02)	
Gastric cancer (After [11])	25–77	3.5–10
Colon cancer (After [12])	51.7	11.7

[a] *KUSM*, Kyorin University School of Medicine

Doubling Time

The doubling time of 22 lesions of 21 esophageal cancer cases in our department ranged from a short 0.54 months to as long as 25.4 months, with a mean of 6.02 months. The mean doubling time of 4 cases of superficial cancer was 11.97 months, and in advanced cancer the doubling time was 4.67 months. Comparisons with gastric and colon cancer show that the doubling time of esophageal cancer was shorter in both early and advanced cases (Table 2) [10–12].

Detection Method

In 1983, 352 cases of early esophageal cancer were investigated to determine how they were detected. In ep cancer, physical check-up or mass screening accounted for 44%; in mm cancer, 42% were detected through esophageal symptoms; and in sm cancer, 62% were detected by esophageal symptoms. The initial detection method in early esophageal cancer was evaluated. In ep cancer, 91% were detected by endoscopy; in mm, 64% were detected with endoscopy and 32% with X-ray. However, in sm cancer, 76% were detected with X-ray and those detected by endoscopy comprised a mere 15%.

Table 3. Diagnostic rate of radiologic examinations for superficial esophageal cancer by depth of invasion (KUSM, 1991)

Depth of invasion	Cases	Longitudinal dia. lesion (mm)	Diagnostic rate	
			Initial X-ray exam.	Close X-ray exam.
ep	7	8–45 (20.9 ± 11.8)	0 (0.0%)	3 (42.9%)
mm	11	10–57 (26.5 ± 14.2)	3 (27.3%)	7 (63.6%)
sm	27	8–115 (33.9 ± 21.1)	22 (81.5%)	27 (100.0%)
Total	45		25 (55.6%)	37 (82.2%)

ep, Epithelial; *mm*, muscularis mucosae; *sm*, submucosal

Table 4. Diagnostic rate of capsulated brushing cytology for esophageal cancer by radiologic types (KUSM, 1991)

Radiologic type	Cases	Class					Diagnostic rate (%)
		I	II	III	IV	V	
Superficial	41	0	8	7	16	10	80.1
Tumorous	24	0	1	3	12	8	95.8
Serrated	30	0	0	3	11	16	100.0
Spiral	108	0	4	23	53	28	96.3
Funnelled	15	0	0	7	5	3	100.0
Total	218	0	13	43	97	65	94.0

The diagnostic rate of X-ray examination by depth of invasion was studied in our department. In ep cancer, the diagnostic rate with close examination was 42.9%; in mm, 63.6%; and in sm, 100% were detected (Table 3).

The accuracy of brushing cytology was studied by comparing the results with X-ray findings. The overall diagnostic rate was 94%, 80% in superficial cancer (Table 4).

The detection process of superficial esophageal cancer in our department was evaluated (Fig. 2). Lugol-staining was performed in all patients who underwent biopsy. Types 0–I and 0–III were chiefly detected with the initial X-ray examination. Detection of type 0–II endoscopically with Lugol staining was excellent; while only eight lesions were detected with Lugol-staining endoscopy, all were ep cancers. One ep lesion of a double lesion went undetected preoperatively and was detected after operation.

Consequently, we performed the Lugol-staining esophageal endoscopy to evaluate out-patients over 50 years of age, regardless of symptoms. As a result, we detected 5 cases (0.61%) of 0–II type cancer out of 824 out-patients. Three cases underwent resection and their histological depth of invasion was ep. The remaining two patients rejected operation, and therefore, were given radiation therapy. At present, their courses are satisfactory.

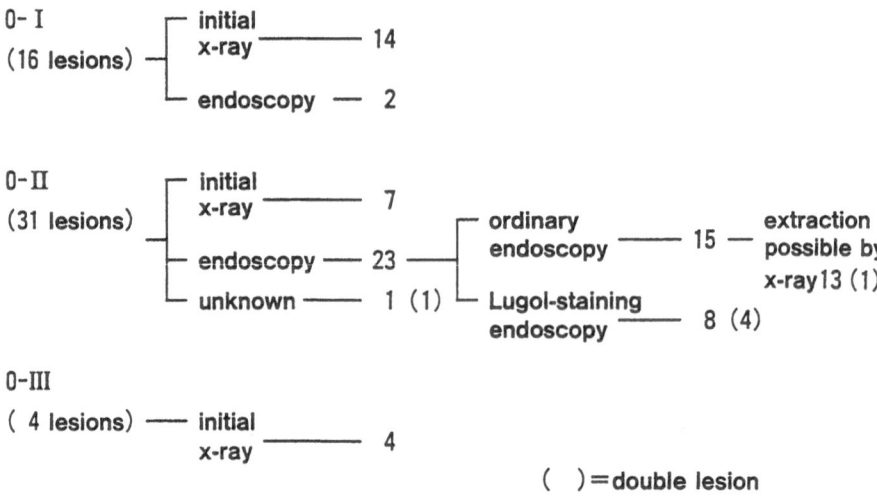

Fig. 2. Methods of detection of superficial esophageal cancer (51 lesions of 45 cases, KUSM 1991)

Treatment Results

The treatment results of superficial cancer in Japan were analysed. The 5-year survival rate was 94.5% for ep cancer. For early mm cancer, the rate was 89.1%; and for early sm cancer, the rate was 75.2%. However, when metastasis was positive, the rate dropped to approximately 40% to 50% (Table 5).

In Japan, as a nonsurgical treatment, we perform radiation therapy. The 5-year survival rate for the 117 cases of early cancer was 29.0%. In 14 cases of ep cancer, the 5-year survival rate was 54.5%. Laser therapy is also applied to ep cancers in Japan. In 22 patients who received laser therapy, the 5-year survival rate was 60%. Recently, endoscopic mucosectomy is being applied to early

Table 5. Follow-up results of superficial esophageal cancer after surgery (127 Hospitals 1966–1990)

Depth of invasion	Cases		Lymph nodes	5-Year survival[a] rates		
ep	287 (11.4%)	n(−)	287 (100%)	94.5		
		n(+)	—			
mm	439 (17.5%)	n(−)	401 (91.3%)	89.1]*]	87.6	]**]*
		n(+)	38 (8.7%)	50.0		
sm	1791 (71.2%)	n(−)	1138 (63.5%)	75.3]*]	63.6%	
		n(+)	653 (36.5%)	43.6		
Total	2517 (100.0%)	n(−)	1825 (72.5%)			
		n(+)	691 (27.5%)			

* $P < 0.001$; ** $P < 0.01$
[a] Excluding death due to natural causes or other diseases

cancer and 72 patients have received this type of therapy, but the follow-up period is still too short to comment on this.

Discussion

Approximately 25 years have elapsed since the first report on early esophageal cancer was made. Viewing the cancer treatment results of esophageal cancer, it is apparent that early detection plays a most important role in the improvement of treatment in this disease [12, 13]. From a statistical viewpoint, those in the high-risk group are male patients over 50 years of age. Since esophageal symptoms are rare in the early stage, physical check-up or mass screening should be carried out. The doubling time of esophageal cancer [14], in comparison with gastric cancer and colon cancer, is short and it is desirable that the patient undergo physical examinations at least once every 6 months.

In detection methods, the diagnostic rate of ep cancer with X-ray was unsatisfactory at 42.9%. In brushing cytology, the diagnostic rate of superficial cancer was much improved at 80%. However, minute cancers measuring less than 1 cm often have false negative results, and this size may be considered to be the limit of cytologic detection. From the detection process of superficial esophageal cancer in our department, the Lugol-staining endoscopy is most effective, but X-ray and cytologic examinations are simple and easy methods to follow through and it is desirable that these three methods are utilized in combination. The detection of ep cancer, in particular Type 0-II, is quite difficult and examinations should be made repeatedly. As can be observed from the data of our department, the people in the high-risk group should undergo periodic examination.

The ideal treatment policies, not only in early cancer but also in other cancers, are: (1) long-term survival potential, (2) minimum complications, (3) quality of life, and (4) inexpensive treatment. From the follow-up results of superficial esophageal cancer in Japan, the treatment plans should take into consideration the depth of cancer invasion and the presence or absence of lymph node metastasis. In ep and mm cancer, reduced surgery without lymphadenectomy is possible and nonsurgical treatment such as irradiation [15], laser therapy [16], and endoscopic mucosectomy can be considered as well. On the other hand, in sm cancer, radical surgery corresponding to that of advanced cancer is desired; and if lymph node metastasis is positive, a combined radio-chemotherapy should be applied.

References

1. Yamada A, Kobayashi S, Kakumae Y, et al (1975) Study on X-ray findings of superficial esophageal cancer. Jpn J Gastroenterol Surg 8:334–342
2. Zernoza J, Lindell MM Jr (1980) Radiologic evaluation of small esophageal carcinoma. Gastrointest Radiol 5:107–111
3. Nabeya K, Okura S, Hanaoka T, et al (1988) Radiological studies of esophageal cancer development with emphasis on serial esophagography and Fuji Computed Radiography. Dis Esoph 1:23–33
4. Endo M, Kobayashi S, Suzuki H, et al (1971) Diagnosis of early esophageal cancer. Endoscopy 3:61–66

5. Toriie S, Kohli Y, Akasaka Y, et al (1975) New trial for endoscopical observation of esophagus by dye scattering method. Endoscopy 7:75–79
6. Chinese Academy of Medical Sciences and Honan Province (1973) The Coordinating Group for the Research of Esophageal Carcinoma: The early detection of carcinoma of the esophagus. Sci Sin 16:457–463
7. Bishop D, Lushpian A, Louis C (1977) The cytology of carcinoma in situ and early invasive carcinoma of the esophagus. Acta Cytol 21:298–300
8. Nabeya K, Onozawa K, Ri S (1979) Brushing cytology with capsule for esophageal cancer. Chir Gastroenterol 13:101–107
9. Japanese Society for Esophageal Diseases (1992) Guidelines for the Clinical and Pathologic Studies on Carcinoma of the Esophagus, 8th edn. Kanehara, Tokyo
10. Koori Y, Yamashita S, Shimamoto K, et al (1969) (in Japanese) Proliferation and growth of gastric cancer in the human body. The Saishin Igaku 24:471–481
11. Ushio K, Shima Y, Goto, et al (1985) Growth and progression of colorectal cancer: Retrospective study based on roentgenologic findings. I to Cho (Stomach and Intestine) Vol 20 No. 8:843–858
12. Nabeya K (1983) Markers of cancer risk in the esophagus and surveillance of high-risk groups. In: Sherlock P, Morson BC, Barbara L, Veronesi U (eds) Precancerous lesions of the gastrointestinal tract. Raven, New York, pp 71–80
13. Iizuka T, Isono K, Kakegawa T. Watanabe H (1989) Parameters linked to 10-year survival in Japan of resected esophageal carcinoma. Chest 96:1005–1011
14. Nabeya K, Hanaoka T, Onozawa K, Ri S, Nyumura T, Kaku C (1990) Early diagnosis of esophageal cancer. Hepato gastroenterology 37:368–370
15. Hishikawa Y, Tanaka S, Miura T (1983) Early esophageal carcinoma treated with intra-cavitary irradiation. Radiology 156:519–522
16. Fujimaki M, Nakayama K (1986) Endoscopic laser treatment of superficial esophageal cancer. Semin Surg Oncol 2:248–256

Epidemiology and Biology

Risk Factors for Squamous Cell Carcinoma of the Esophagus in Southern Thailand

Apinop Chanvitan[1], Alan F Geater[1], Verasak Chongsuvivatwong[2], and Siwaporn Ubolcholket[3]

Introduction

Data on the incidence of oesophageal cancer in Thailand place this country among the low incidence regions of the world. Crude annual incidence in 1982 was reported to be 0.85 per 100 000 [1]. Within the southern region however, the provincial incidences increase the further south the location. Overall annual age-adjusted incidences per hundred thousand in the lower south subregion (7 provinces) in 1989 were 5.4 in males and 1.5 in females, compared with 4.1 and 1.1, respectively, in the more northerly 7 southern provinces [2].

In several low and intermediate incidence regions of the world, the main risk factors for oesophageal cancer have been shown to be alcohol consumption and smoking, with low socioeconomic status also being associated with increased risk [3]. Alcohol consumption and smoking have previously been shown to act as risk factors among the population of southern Thailand [4], but whether the elevated incidence of oesophageal carcinoma in this region is due to increased levels of exposure to each of these factors has not been investigated. The fact that at least four of the lower southern provinces have predominantly Muslim populations, who do not consume alcohol, suggests that drinking habits at least are unlikely to account for the elevated incidence, and, if anything, would tend to skew the figures in the other direction.

However, the traditional foods and beverages of the southern region differ considerably from those of other regions. Several of these are consumed almost exclusively by southerners and most commonly in the lower south, which has until recently been less subject to the influence of central Thai living habits. In view of the possibility of direct action of tumour-inducing and/or promoting substances on the oesophageal epithelium in the aetiology of this malignancy,

---

[1] Department of Surgery, [2] Epidemiology Unit, [3] Department of Community Medicine, Faculty of Medicine, Prince of Songkla University, Hat Yai, Songkla, Thailand

the hypothesis that consumption of certain traditional southern foods and beverages might increase the risk of oesophageal cancer, and be responsible for the locally elevated incidence, has been postulated.

Local traditional foods considered as potential risk factors include several types of fermented fish, which are commonly stored in open bowls and rapidly become mold-infested, cooked and raw beans of the genera Parkia and Archidendron, and an alcoholic beverage produced from fermented sugar-palm syrup.

This case-control study was designed to examine the associations of such exposures with oesophageal cancer and to explore the roles of known risk factors, including total alcohol consumption, smoking, betel chewing and tobacco chewing.

Methods

During the period October 1988 to October 1989, all patients with suspected oesophageal carcinoma admitted to one university, and one regional and four provincial hospitals in the southern region of Thailand were considered for inclusion in the study. Cases were interviewed and accepted into the study only if they were symptomatic, had a histologically confirmed diagnosis of squamous cell carcinoma, were free of lesions of the oesophagogastric junction, and had no evidence of adenocarcinoma.

Controls, which were matched to each case by hospital of admission, sex and age (± 5 years of case age), were interviewed. Two controls for each case were accepted into the study on the basis of satisfying all of the following conditions: hospitalized at the same time or up to no more than 2 months after the case with which they were matched; free of any disease related to alcohol consumption or smoking; no malignant disease of the upper aero-digestive tract.

Two hundred and two cases and 2 controls matched to each case were selected for inclusion. This number was chosen to provide the study with a power of 90% of detecting an odds ratio for exposure versus non-exposure of 2.0 at two-sided significance level of 0.05, given an exposure rate among controls of between 20% and 70% [5].

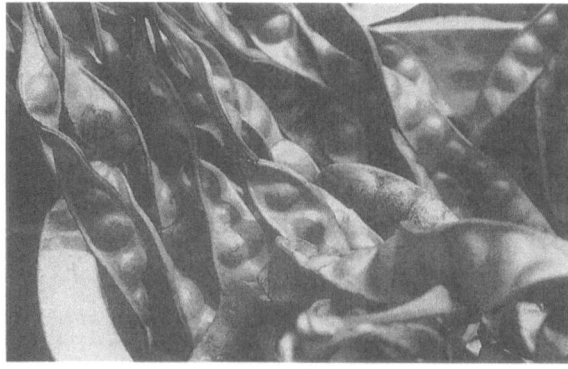

Fig. 1. *Parkia speciosa* (sataw)

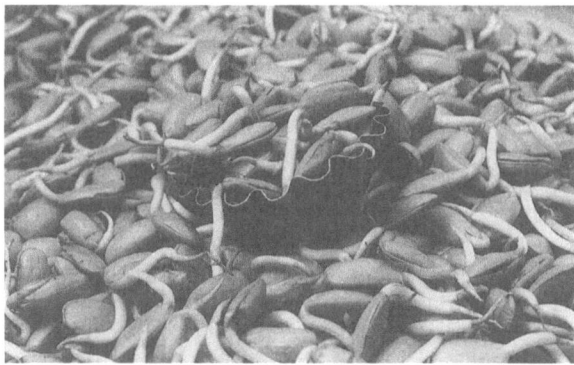

Fig. 2. *Parkia timoriana* (luk rieng)

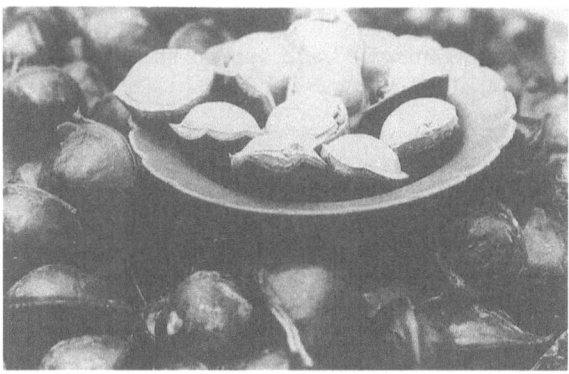

Fig. 3. *Archidendron jiringa* (luk nieng)

Questionnaires were completed using trained non-medical interviewers. Fields of enquiry were: demography and social background; present and past frequency of consumption of local and general foods, and of use of cooking additives, cooking fuels and water supplies; frequency, amounts and periods during lifetime of various kinds of smoking, various kinds of alcohol consumption, various kinds of coffee and tea drinking, betel chewing and tobacco chewing. Interviewees were asked to consider the last 3 years as "present" and a similar period about 10 years prior as "past".

Local foods about which information was sought included the fermented fish dishes bu-du, tai pla and kao yam, the leguminous beans sataw (*Parkia speciosa*; Fig. 1), luk rieng (*Parkia timoriana*; Fig. 2), luk nieng (*Archidendron jiringa*; Fig. 3), and luk nieng nok (*Archidendron bubalinum*), and the alcoholic beverage wahk, the product of fermented syrup of the sugar palm (*Borassus flabellifer*), containing approximately 6 g ethanol per 100 ml.

Data were analyzed for the most part by conditional logistic modelling. Relative risks of disease were approximated by the odds ratios for exposure between cases and controls.

The crude associations of disease with exposure status, mean dose and duration of exposure to smoking, alcohol consumption, and betel chewing and tobacco chewing were initially explored in a univariate analysis, and the variable or variables best accounting for the association of disease with each of these exposures selected for incorporation into a multivariate model. Odds ratios for these exposures were calculated after adjustment for each other and for those variables of socioeconomic status and demography which had significant confounding effects in the data set.

Associations of disease with dietary components, including local foods and beverages of primary interest, were investigated after adjustment for main risk factor and socioeconomic/demographic variables already found to be significantly associated with disease.

Information regarding the joint effects of smoking, alcohol consumption and betel chewing was explored after breaking the matching and applying a stratified analysis.

Two-sided tests of significance were applied and 95% confidence intervals determined for all variables.

Results

All 202 sets consisted of one case and two controls. Forty three sets (21.3%) were female. Approximately 70% of both male and female cases were admitted at the one University hospital included in the study.

Cases were more generally of lower socioeconomic status, as revealed by the rate of occupations, involving physical labor, especially among females, and lower per capita income. Among males, a greater proportion of cases smoked and drank alcohol. Prevalence of smoking and/or drinking among women was low. Wahk was drunk almost exclusively by males but only by about 4% among controls. Both male and female cases were more commonly betel and/or tobacco chewers than were controls. Most of the traditional foods were reported to be consumed by a greater proportion of cases than controls, with little difference between males and females.

Smoking, Total Alcohol Consumption and Betel and Tobacco Chewing

Among females, only seven controls and two cases had ever drunk alcohol, and less than 10% of controls had smoked. Among male controls, only 15% were non-smokers and 35% non-drinkers.

Because of these major differences in exposure to smoking and alcohol between males and females, the associations of these habits with disease were explored separately for the two sexes.

Almost all smokers smoked cigarettes, but these included both commercially produced and hand-rolled cigarettes. In this report, the differences between the two types are not explored, and rates of exposure are based on numbers of cigarettes per day. Rates of alcohol consumption are expressed in grams of ethanol per day.

Among males, there was a strong association between current smoking and disease. Ex-smokers, having given up the habit for 2 or more years, were at substantially lower risk than were current smokers. Drinkers of alcohol were also at increased risk but with a reduction in risk associated with stopping only after more than 10 years.

The risk of disease associated with either smoking or alcohol consumption increased with higher mean rates of exposure. Increasing durations of exposure

Table 1. Odds ratios adjusted for the independent variables, smoking, alcohol consumption, and betel chewing and socioeconomic and demographic variables. Males and females. Conditional logistic regression

	Male		Females	
	Adjusted OR[e]	P[a]	Adjusted OR[e]	P[a]
Smoking:				
Mean daily dose				
(No. of cigarettes/				
day):[d]				
0	1	0.00015[b]	1	0.06243
1 to 5	4.23 (0.71–25.35)	)		
6 to 10	10.64 (2.00–56.72)	)		
11 to 15	12.88 (2.52–65.91)	)		
16 to 20	15.95 (2.74–92.99)	)	8.29 (0.64–107.10)	
>20	17.78 (2.81–112.78)	)		
Ex-smoker:				
(>2 years)	0.35 (0.16–0.79)	0.00763[c]		
Alcohol consumption:				
Mean daily dose				
(g EtOH/day):[d]				
0	1	0.00000	1	0.31496
>0 to 20	2.32 (0.97–5.56)	)		
>20 to 40	5.59 (1.45–21.56)	)	0.24 (0.01–4.76)	
>40 to 80	31.48 (8.49–116.74)	)		
>80	11.86 (3.71–39.90)	)		
Betel Chewing:				
Mean daily dose				
(No. of quids/day):[d]				
0	1	0.00000	1	0.00007
1	1.78 (0.65–4.91)			
2 to 3	2.62 (0.78–8.84)		) 8.22 (1.16–57.98)	
4 to 5	6.89 (2.34–20.28)		) 25.19 (3.77–168.32)	
>5	17.56 (5.76–53.58)			

Numbers in parentheses are 95% confidence limits

OR, odds ratios

[a] Chi square for inclusion of exposure in the model

[b] Includes number of smokes per day and current/ex-smoker status

[c] Effect of ex-smoker status alone

[d] Mean daily dose lifetime intake (number of years in which habit was practised ×365.25)

to smoking up to more than 40 years were associated with increasing risks, but alcohol consumption for periods of longer than 39 years appeared not to incur any further increase in risk, as compared to smoking.

Since the proportion of heavy drinkers was higher among those groups with heavier smoking habits, the disease-exposure relationships were re-examined after adjusting for confounding factors among these exposures. Exposures to smoking, alcohol, and betel were represented by mean rate, current/ex-status and duration, while that to tobacco chewing was represented by daily dose alone. The measures of exposure which retained significance after controlling for confounding were mean exposure rates for alcohol and betel, and mean exposure rate together with current/ex-status for smoking. Risks associated with tobacco chewing were reduced to non-significant levels after adjustment. Table 1 shows the odds ratios for these exposures after a further adjustment for confounding effects of socioeconomic and demographic variables.

It appears that the relative risks related to alcohol consumption and to betel chewing increase more rapidly at higher than at lower levels of exposure, in contrast to risks related to smoking, which rise more rapidly at lower levels of exposure and thereafter increase only slowly.

Joint effects of exposure to smoking, alcohol consumption and betel chewing were explored in males after breaking the matching and applying a stratified analysis. Because so few males were non-smokers, the referent category for smoking was set at 0–5 cigarettes per day. Although 35% of male controls were non-drinkers, the odds ratio associated with consuming low daily doses of alcohol was not significantly different from unity, so that 0–20 g/day was chosen as the referent category for alcohol consumption.

The data suggest that the effects of heavy smoking may be considerably greater among heavy chewers of betel than among light chewers, although the interaction in this data set is not statistically significant. There is no evidence of interaction between smoking and alcohol consumption.

Common Food Types

Risk related to past and present consumption of common food types were evaluated after controlling for mean rates of smoking, alcohol consumption and betel chewing, for stopping smoking and for socioeconomic and demographic variables.

No significant association with disease status was evident among past frequencies of consumption of any food type.

Among current frequencies, a convincing association occurred only with green vegetables and fruit, in each of which there was a significant trend of increasing risk with lower frequency of intake (Table 2).

Traditional Foods

All of the traditional foods included in the study were consumed by a larger proportion of cases and controls 10 years previously than at the time of the study. Since the focus of attention of this study was the hypothesis that traditional dietary factors might increase risk of oesophageal carcinoma, and the onset of oesophageal cancer in diagnosed cases was likely to have occurred several years

Table 2. Odds ratios associated with present consumption frequencies of common foodstuffs, each separately adjusted for smoking, alcohol consumption, betel chewing, and socioeconomic and demographic variables. Males and females combined. Conditional logistic regression

Food	Present frequency of consumption					Trend	
	Daily or almost daily	1–3 times /week	1–3 times /month	Less than once/month	Never	chi-sq	P
Meat	1	1.7 (0.7–4.3)	1.9 (0.7–5.2)	5.4 (1.8–16.0)	1.3 (0.4–4.2)	2.91	0.088
Poultry	1	0.87 (0.4–2.2)	1.1 (0.4–2.7)	1.7 (0.6–4.7)	0.81 0.2–3.0	0.48	0.490
Freshwater fish	1	1.4 (0.6–3.4)	1.5 (0.6–3.5)	1.2 (0.5–3.0)	1.0 0.2–3.8	0.03	0.852
Sea fish	1	1.2 (0.6–2.4)	1.9 (0.8–4.8)	2.2 (0.9–5.4)	1.5 (0.2–14.6)	3.21	0.073
Eggs	1	0.71 (0.3–1.9)	1.2 (0.5–2.8)	1.0 (0.4–2.5)	1.5 (0.2–8.9)	0.60	0.438
Milk	1	3.1 (0.8–12.0)	2.1 (0.6–7.9)	1.7 (0.7–4.0)	1.0 (0.4–2.3)	0.43	0.511
Green vegetables	1	0.92 (0.5–1.8)	1.5 (0.6–3.7)	3.2 (1.2–8.4)		4.45	0.035
Fruit	1	0.82 (0.3–2.2)	1.3 (0.5–3.4)	2.1 (0.8–5.9)		4.47	0.034

Numbers in parentheses are 95% confidence limits

Table 3. Odds ratios adjusted for local dietary components[a] and for smoking, alcohol consumption, betel chewing, and socioeconomic and demographic variables. Males and females combined. Conditional logistic regression

	No. of controls	No. of cases	Adjusted OR (95% c/l.)	P[b]	Trend	
					Chi-sq	P
Luk rieng (cooked):						
None	301	110	1	0.00209	11.69	0.00063
Less than once/month	77	60	2.19 (0.98–4.89)			
At least once/month	26	32	6.36 (2.04–19.83)			
Luk nieng (raw):						
Less than once/month	189	53	1	0.01667	8.98	0.00272
1–3 times per month	112	55	1.92 (0.81–4.54)			
At least once/week	103	94	3.92 (1.44–10.65)			
Sataw (raw):						
Less than once/month	91	44	1	0.00670	9.96	0.00160
1–3 times per month	131	59	0.36 (0.14–0.90)			
At least once/week	182	99	0.21 (0.07–0.60)			

[a] Frequency of consumption when in season
[b] Chi square for inclusion of exposure in model

previously, the analysis concerning these foods was confined to past frequencies of exposure.

After adjustment for the independent variables, smoking, alcohol consumption, and betel chewing, and for socioeconomic and demographic variables, a clear frequency-response relationship was evident for each of the legumes, luk rieng (cooked) and luk nieng (raw), whereas a clear frequency-related protective effect was found for a third legume, sataw (raw) (Table 3). Consumption of fermented fish dishes was not significantly associated with disease.

Differences in effect of cooked vs. raw sataw were examined. Consumption of cooked sataw was almost as common as that of raw sataw and the consumption frequencies were moderately correlated ($r = 0.55$ for controls, $r = 0.79$ for cases). Cooked sataw, however, showed only a weak and statistically non-significant protective effect.

Among both controls and cases, there was a moderate correlation ($r = 0.63$ for controls $r = 0.77$ for cases) between the frequencies of eating raw sataw and raw luk nieng, leading to negative confounding. Only about one fifth of either controls or cases seldom ate sataw. Of the remainder, who consumed sataw regularly, about 90% of cases but only 66% of controls also ate luk nieng regularly. The relative risk for the joint effects of luk nieng and sataw show no evidence of interaction on the basis of a multiplicative model.

Effect modifications between each of these traditional foods and other risk factors were explored but no significant statistical interactions were found.

When the effects of these traditional foods was controlled for, the protective effect of frequent fruit consumption was reduced and no longer showed a significant association with disease. The relative risk of frequent consumption of green vegetables, however, was virtually unaltered.

"Wahk" and Other Types of Alcohol

Several types of alcohol were consumed. The four commonest were: lao kao (a spirit distilled from rice wine, 28 g EtOH/100 ml), Mekong (referring to a number of similar proprietary products—a rum prepared from molasses, 28 to 32 g EtOH/100 ml), Wahk (fermented palm sugar syrup, approximately 6 g EtOH/100 ml) and beer (approximately 9 g EtOH/100 ml).

As total alcohol consumption had been accounted for by daily dose, the effects of different types of alcohol were examined by including a variable for long-term duration of exposure to each type. More than 20 years' exposure to alcohol of any type, or to lao kao or Mekong showed no alteration in the overall risk associated with alcohol consumption. A similar long-term exposure to Wahk however, appears to carry a threefold risk compared with shorter-term duration of Wahk exposure and/or exposures to other alcohol types of whatever duration. With the small numbers of cases and controls in this catregory, the value of chi-square cannot be expected to be large. The numbers of cases and controls with long-term exposure to beer are even smaller and the odds ratio of 2.4 is not statistically significant.

Discussion

The acceptance of 202 patients into this study in a period of 1 year from a population with a reported annual incidence of about 3 per 100 000 suggests a catchment population of almost 7 million. This approximates the population of the entire south of Thailand, and suggests that close to 100% of diagnosed incident cases of oesophageal carcinoma in the southern region within the study period were included in the study. The data thus indicate that the disease occurs in a male to female ratio of 3.7 : 1 and that over 80% of cases are diagnosed over the age of 55.

The study confirmed that the known risk factors for oesophageal carcinoma in other populations—smoking, alcohol consumption and betel chewing—are also linked with increased risk of disease among the southern Thailand population. In addition, the hypothesis that the risk is increased also by consumption of certain local traditional foods is supported.

With respect to the risks of oesophageal carcinoma associated with smoking and alcohol consumption, the southern region of Thailand shows similarities to several developed countries. Smoking and alcohol have been shown to be major risk factors among populations in North and South America, Europe, South Africa and Japan, though not among those of the high incidence regions of China and Central Asia or the Singapore Chinese [6, 7]. Furthermore, the difference in shape of the dose-response curves for alcohol consumption and smoking among southern Thailand males is similar to that for populations in France [8] although the overall range of daily dose of ethanol among cases in southern Thailand is much narrower. Only 23% of male cases (26% of male drinkers) had a daily intake of ethanol in excess of 80 g.

The relative effects of different types of alcohol have been a matter of some dispute. Although reports have suggested that consumption of spirits may pose a greater risk than that of beer or wine [9] or that apple cider and its distillates display a stronger association with oesophageal cancer than do wine and beer [10] other studies have stressed the lack of convincing evidence for different risks when considered on the basis of dose of ethanol [11]. It is to be expected that in most populations few people consume significant amounts of the less common drinks. This was the case of wahk-drinking in the current study. Because of its illegal status, this activity is largely confined to the areas where sugar-palm tapping is practised, which form only a small part of the total area of the southern region. The practice was reported by only 4% of male controls (mean daily dose 5.6 g EtOH) and 21% of male cases (mean daily dose 16.6 g EtOH), compared with any forms of alcohol drunk by 65% of male controls (mean daily dose 14.2 g EtOH) and 86% of male cases (mean daily dose 43.2 g EtOH). It is of interest in this male population which consumes mainly the spirits, lao kao and Mekong with an ethanol content of at least 28 g/100 ml, that after controlling for mean daily dose of ethanol, relative risks well in excess of unity were obtained for long term consumption of wahk and beer, with ethanol contents of only about 6 and 9 g/100 ml, respectively. This suggests that some component other than ethanol might be responsible. A similar finding has been reported by Graham et al. [12] in which the risk associated with beer-drinking among residents of New York was threefold higher than that of spirit drinking.

The prevalence of betel chewing among the adult population appears to be high. Among the controls in this series, 31% of males and 40% of females reported the habit. The apparently increased relative risk associated with betel chewing among females compared with males is in contrast to a higher risk in males reported by Jussawalla and Deshpande [13] among an Indian population. A satisfactory explanation has not yet been found. The difference could be partly accounted for by the use of dose-range categories in the analysis. Nevertheless, in a trend model based on actual daily dose, the odds ratio for an increase of one quid/day was still higher among females (2.2) than among males (1.9), although the difference does not reach statistical significance.

Among the three classes of local food and beverage investigated for association with oesophageal carcinoma, two—beans and sugar palm spirit—include exposures associated with increased risk of the disease independently of other risk factors. The analysis indicated that consumption of fermented fish dishes did not increase risk of disease.

Exposure to alcohol, smoking and betel, and a decreased intake of fruit over the previous 10 years were also identified as risk factors in this region, with physical labor occupation, especially among females, and marital separation also associated with increased risk.

The proportions of cases in the population which might be due to each of these local risk factors, assuming exposure rates of controls reflect those in the population and equal effects in both sexes, are 32.4% for consumption of luk rieng more than three times a month, 32.4% for consumption of cooked luk rieng at least once a month, and 8.7% for 20 or more years of wahk consumption [14].

Among controls, there was a significant tendency for regular past consumers of luk nieng to be also regular present consumers of sataw (about 25% for more than expected consumed both, $P = 0.005$, chi square), so that the true aetiological fraction for luk nieng consumption might be higher than indicated.

However, there was no evidence among the control group that frequent consumers of luk nieng were also frequent consumers of luk rieng. Wahk consumption was almost entirely confined to males and its long term use was not associated with either frequent luk nieng or luk rieng consumption. If consumption of these two beans is in fact confined to the southern provinces, as believed, then this dietary feature could account for a large part of the elevated incidence of oesophageal carcinoma in this region.

Summary. The southern region of Thailand has an incidence of oesophageal cancer more than threefold that of the whole country. This hospital-based case-control study investigated the hypothesis that consumption of traditional foods and beverage peculiar to southern Thailand contributes to the risk of oesophageal carcinoma. Foods and drink investigated included fermented fish, four species of bean of the genera *Parkia* and *Archidendron*, and wahk, a beverage made from fermented syrup of the sugar palm, *Borassus flabellifer*. Effects of known risk factors were also explored. Two hundred and two case-control sets were used, each matched in a ratio of 1:2 on sex, age and hospital of admission with controls. Smoking, betel chewing and total alcohol consumption were shown to be major risk factors, and there was also an association of disease with low socioeconomic status and low frequencies of fruit and green vegetable intake. A greater proportion of patients than of controls reported high frequency of consumption of most traditional foods and beverage. After adjusting for major risk factors and socioeconomic status, and for independent variables, in a conditional logistic regression, significant frequency-related risks were found to be associated with past consumption of the beans *A. Jiringa* [luk nieng] (OR for at least once a week/less than once a month = 3.9) and *P. timoriana* [luk rieng] (OR for at least once a month/none = 6.4). By contrast, consumption of raw beans of *P. speciosa* [sataw] was associated with a significant frequency-related protective effect (OR for at least once a week/less than once a month = 0.21). Considering the quite high prevalences of past consumption of *A. jiringa* and *P.*

timoriana, it is suggested that these dietary habits may have some role in elevating the incidence of oesophageal carcinoma in southern Thailand.

References

1. National Cancer Institute, Cancer Statistics 1982, Ministry of Public Health, Bangkok, 1987
2. Chanvitan A, Geater AF (1990) Incidence and mortality In: Chanvitan A (ed) Oesophageal cancer. Studies In Southern Thailand. Medical Media, Bangkok, pp 3–13
3. Day NE, Munoz N, Esophagus (1982) In: Schottenjeld D, Fraumeni JF (eds) Cancer epidemiology and prevention. Saunders, Philadelphia, pp 526–623
4. Chongsuvivatwong V (1990) Case-Control study on oesophageal cancer in southern Thailand. J Gastroenterol Hepatol 5:391–394
5. Schlesselman JJ (1982) Case-Control studies. Oxford University Press, Oxford, p 168
6. IARC (1986) Monographs on the evaluation of the carcinogenic risk of chemicals to humans, vol 38. Tobacco smoking. International Agency for Research on Cancer, Lyon
7. IARC (1988) Monographs on the evaluation of the carcinogenic risk of chemicals to humans, vol 44. Alcohol drinking. International Agency for Research on Cancer, Lyon
8. Tuyns AJ, Pequignot G, Jensen OM (1977b) Le cancer del'oesophage en Jlle-et-Vilaine en fonction des niveaux de consommation d'alcohol et de tabac. Des risques qui se multiplient. Bull Cancer (Paris) 64:45–60
9. Wynder EL, Bross IJ (1961) A study of etiological factors in cancers of the esophagus. Cancer 14:389–413
10. Tuyns AJ, Pequignot G, Abbatucci JS (1979) Oesophageal cancer and alcohol consumption; importance of type of beverage. Int J Cancer 23:443–447
11. Breslow NE, Day NE (1980) Statistical methods in cancer research. The analysis of case-control studies (IARC Scientific Publications No. 32). International Agency for Research on Cancer, Lyon
12. Graham S, Marshall J, Haughey B, Brasure J (1990) Nutritional epidemiology of cancer of the esophagus. Am J Epidemiol 131:454–466
13. Jussawalla DJ, Deshpande VA (1971) Evaluation of cancer risk in tobacco chewers and smokers: An epidemiological assessment. Cancer 28:244–252
14. Walter SD (1976) The estimation and interpretation of attributable risk in health research. Biometrics 32:829–49

Patterns of Presentation of Carcinoma of the Esophagus and Cardia in Patients Less Than 50 Years Old

MARK K. FERGUSON[1], MARIO ALBERTUCCI[1], RUDY P. LACKNER[1], PHILIP C. HOFFMAN[2], and HARVEY M. GOLOMB[2]

Introduction

Squamous cell carcinomas of the esophagus in the Western hemisphere are epidemiologically related to tobacco use and alcohol consumption. In the past 10 years, there has been a striking increase in the incidence of adenocarcinomas of the distal esophagus and cardia, many of which do not arise from Barrett's mucosa. Coincident with this rise in the incidence of adenocarcinomas has been an apparent shift to involvement in younger patients, most of whom do not share the risk factors associated with squamous cell cancers. We reviewed our recent experience with carcinoma of the esophagus and cardia to address several questions. Is the prevalence of cancer among young people increasing? Do young people develop a different type of cancer than that seen in older individuals, and, if so, do their prognoses differ? Can risk factors be identified that facilitate earlier diagnosis in young people?

Methods

We retrospectively reviewed the records of all patients with carcinoma of the esophagus and cardia seen at the University of Chicago from 1980 through 1990. Data were collected regarding patient demographics, prior reflux symptoms and their treatment, family history of cancer, risk factors for cancer including tobacco use and alcohol consumption, results of staging tests (computed tomography of the chest and abdomen; endoscopy; chest radiograph; scintigraphic bone scan; and surgical exploration in most patients) and pathology reports, type of therapy, and survival from the time of diagnosis. Adenocarcinomas

[1] Section of Thoracic Surgery, Department of Surgery and [2] Section of Hematology/Oncology, Department of Medicine, The University of Chicago, 5841 South Maryland Avenue, MC5035 Chicago, IL 60637 USA

arising from the distal esophagus or cardia were divided into two groups. Barrett's adenocarcinoma was defined as a cancer developing in a patient with Barrett's mucosa, regardless of the presence or absence of dysplastic changes. The remaining adenocarcinomas had no endoscopic or pathological evidence for Barrett's mucosa. Statistical comparisons were performed using the t-test and chi-square analysis, and Kaplan-Meier survival curves were constructed.

Results

Records of 299 patients were reviewed, of whom 232 were male and 67 were female; 227 were white, 65 were black, and 7 were members of other racial groups. The median age was 61.2 years, with a range of 29–89 years. A total of 43 patients were less than 50 years old (younger patients). During the 5-year period 1980–1984, 13% of patients were less than 50 years old, compared to 16% during 1985–1989. This difference was not statistically significant.

Squamous cell cancers were most common, comprising 150 (50%) of all tumors, followed in frequency by adenocarcinoma (92, or 31%), Barrett's adenocarcinoma (48, or 16%) and other cell types (9, or 3%). Adenocarcinomas and Barrett's adenocarcinomas were more common during the second half of the study period than during the first half (59% versus 41%; $P < 0.02$). Squamous cancers were equally divided among white and black patients (57% versus 45%) while adenocarcinomas and Barrett's adenocarcinomas were much more prevalent in white individuals (96% and 100%, respectively). Adenocarcinomas were more common among younger patients compared with older patients (45% versus 30%), while the prevalence of squamous cell cancers was lower (35% versus 55%) and that of Barrett's adenocarcinoma was similar (19% versus 15%; $P = 0.07$).

The stage at presentation was usually advanced, as is common in esophageal cancers. Younger patients had somewhat worse stage at diagnosis than did older patients (Table 1; $P < 0.03$). There was no apparent relationship between cell type and stage at presentation.

Evaluation of risk factors demonstrated that younger patients were more likely than older patients to have a history of cancer in a family member (55% versus 31%; $P < 0.01$) and were more likely to have had reflux symptoms

Table 1. Tumor stage according to age group

	Number of patients (%)	
	Age < 50 years	Age ≥ 50 years
Stage		
I	2 (4.7)	14 (5.9)
IIa + b	5 (11.6)	56 (23.6)
III	15 (34.9)	89 (37.6)
IV	21 (48.8)	78 (32.9)
Total	43 (100)	237 (100)[a]

[a] Staging information not available in 19 patients

Table 2. Risk factor incidence according to cell type (Percentage of patients by histology)

	Adenocarcinoma	Squamous Cell Cancer	Barrett's Adenocarcinoma	P
Reflux symptoms	39	10	59	<0.005
Antireflux therapy	22	9	52	<0.005
Tobacco use	75	84	71	N.S.
Alcohol use	46	60	32	<0.01
Family history for cancer	47	27	31	<0.03

(49% versus 24%; $P < 0.005$). Risk factors were also strongly correlated with cell type. A positive family history for cancer was more common in patients with adenocarcinoma, while the likelihoods of a history of reflux symptoms, medical antireflux therapy, and alcohol use in adenocarcinoma patients were intermediate between those of patients with squamous cancers and Barrett's adenocarcinoma (Table 2). All the groups shared a similarly high incidence of tobacco use.

Treatment was based on tumor stage and patient physiologic status. Resection with or without chemotherapy and/or radiation therapy was performed in 173 patients, 75 received chemotherapy and radiotherapy, 35 underwent radiotherapy alone, 10 had chemotherapy only, and 6 patients received no antitumor therapy. Survival was related to stage at the time of diagnosis (Fig. 1), and was not related to patient age group or cell type. Median survival for stages I through IIb was 13 months in younger patients and 7 months in older patients, while for stages III and IV it was 10 months and 5 months in younger and older patients, respectively.

Discussion

Cancers of the esophagus and cardia are a continuing challenge to physicians because they are typically diagnosed at a late stage and, as a result, have a poor prognosis. Although squamous cell cancer has not changed in incidence in the past 15 years [1], the frequency of adenocarcinoma of the distal esophagus and cardia has risen dramatically [1, 2], increasing in men at a rate of 4%–10% per year, faster than any other type of cancer [3]. The increase in incidence, along with the overall poor prognosis, make efforts at earlier diagnosis to improve therapy and survival imperative. Our impression prior to performing this retrospective study was that the rate of carcinoma was increasing among younger patients. We found that, over the 11-year period from 1980 to 1990, there was no change in the percentage of those affected by these cancers made up by younger patients. However, since younger patients are more likely to have adenocarcinoma, and because the overall incidence of adenocarcinomas has increased, the absolute number of young patients encountered rose by more than 25%. We, therefore, focused our efforts at identifying risk factors related to the development of adenocarcinomas in general and in younger patients specifically.

The etiologic factor most strongly related to the development of squamous cell carcinoma of the esophagus in Western civilization is alcohol consumption,

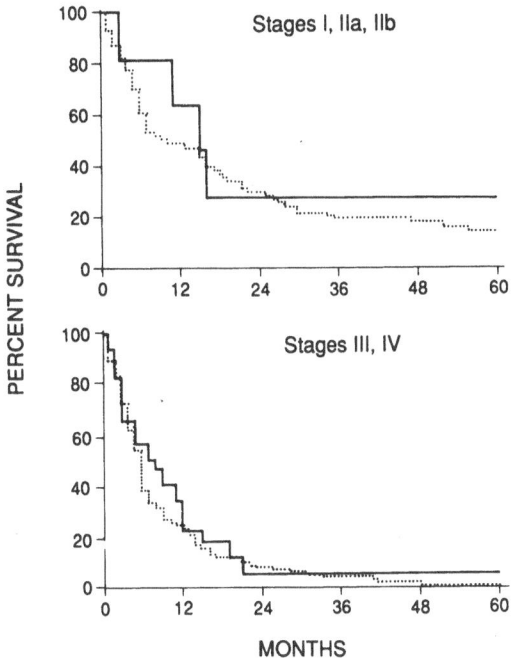

Fig. 1. Survival from time of diagnosis for patients with cancer of the esophagus and cardia. *Solid lines* depict patients less than 50 years old; *broken lines* depict patients 50 years old and greater. *Upper graph* combines stages I, IIa and IIb, while *lower graph* combines stages III and IV

which increases the risk by 10- to 25-fold [4]. This risk is further enhanced by tobacco use, while tobacco use in the absence of alcohol consumption increases the risk of squamous cell cancer of the esophagus only marginally. We found that adenocarcinomas had some unique risk factors that suggest different etiologies for this histology. In younger patients, common risk factors included a history of cancer in a family member and a history of reflux symptoms. Among all patients with adenocarcinoma, risk factors included a positive family history for cancer, prior reflux symptoms, and previous medical antireflux therapy. Alcohol use among adenocarcinoma patients was less frequent than among squamous cell cancer victims, while the incidence of tobacco use did not differ significantly between these two groups.

It is sometimes problematic to differentiate between adenocarcinomas arising de novo in the distal esophagus and cardia and those developing in dysplastic Barrett's mucosa. Certainly our definition of Barrett's adenocarcinoma, requiring the contemporaneous presence of benign Barrett's epithelium, may underestimate the actual incidence of this cancer as compared to ordinary adenocarcinomas, but it is our impression that the degree of underestimation is probably small. It is interesting to note that these two types of adenocarcinoma, while sharing similar locations within the esophagus and a strong predominance for affecting white males, findings that have also been noted by others [5], differ in terms of other risk factors. We confirmed previous findings that Barrett's adenocarcinomas are strongly related to a history of reflux symptoms and prior antireflux therapy [5–8], and identified a lower incidence of these factors in the other adenocarcinoma patients. Alcohol consumption in Barrett's adenocarcinoma patients was less frequent than in the group of other adenocarcinomas, while the incidence of tobacco use was high in both groups. The relationship between tobacco use and the development of either type of adenocarcinoma has been previously reported [6, 7, 9]. Of interest, the incidence of a family history of cancer was much higher in the adenocarcinoma patients than in those with Barrett's adenocarcinoma. The epidemiologic data provide support that adenocarcinoma and Barrett's adenocarcinoma are distinct clinical entities. Other evidence that these two cancers differ histologically [10] further suggests that these are indeed separate and distinct types of cancer.

The identification of a high incidence of prior antireflux therapy associated with adenocarcinoma and Barrett's adenocarcinoma suggests that there may be an etiologic relationship between alterations in the acid-base milieu of the stomach and the development of these cancers. This speculation has been shared by others, but remains unproven at this time. Further epidemiologic data and experimental work will be necessary to determine whether such a relationship really exists.

We found that survival among the three types of cancer was related to disease stage at the time of diagnosis and was not affected by patient age at diagnosis or histologic type. It has been shown previously that younger age at diagnosis does not affect outcome [11]. This suggests that, as with squamous cell cancers, early diagnosis of adenocarcinomas is the key to improving prognosis. In our review, tumor stage was more advanced among the younger patients than among those in the older group, perhaps because younger patients were less likely to seek medical attention or because the possibility of cancer was not entertained early enough by the treating physician. The identification of risk factors for adenocarcinoma, including male gender, Caucasian race, younger age, history of reflux disease, and a family history of cancer, may aid in the earlier diagnosis of cancer in these individuals. Patients who are seen with symptoms of reflux and a family history of cancer warrant endoscopy and frequent follow-up rather than empiric and prolonged trials of medical antireflux therapy alone.

References

1. Blot WJ, Devesa SS, Kneller RW, Fraumeni JF Jr (1991) Rising incidence of adenocarcinoma of the esophagus and gastric cardia. JAMA 265:1287–1289
2. Yang PC, Davis S (1988) Incidence of cancer of the esophagus in the US by histologic type. Cancer 61:612–617
3. Hesketh PJ, Clapp RW, Doos WG, Spechler SJ (1989) The increasing frequency of adenocarcinoma of the esophagus. Cancer 64:526–530
4. Sons HU (1987) Etiologic and epidemiologic factors of carcinoma of the esophagus. Surg Gynecol Obstet 165:183–190
5. Duhaylongsod FG, Wolfe WG (1991) Barrett's esophagus and adenocarcinoma of the esophagus and gastroesophageal junction. J Thorac Cardiovasc Surg 102:36–42
6. Skinner DB, Walther BC, Riddell RH, Schmidt H, Iascone C, DeMeester TR (1983) Barrett's esophagus. Ann Surg 198:554–566

7. MacDonald WC, MacDonald JB (1987) Adenocarcinoma of the esophagus and/or gastric cardia. Cancer 60:1094–1098
8. Streitz JM Jr, Ellis FH Jr, Gibb SP, Balogh K, Watkins E Jr (1991) Adenocarcinoma in Barrett's esophagus. Ann Surg 213:122–125
9. Mathisen DJ, Wilkins EW, Grillo HC, Moncure AC (1988) Adenocarcinoma in columnar lined esophagus (Barrett's esophagus). In: Siewert JR, Holscher AH (eds) Diseases of the esophagus. Springer, Berlin Heidelberg New York, pp 559–561
10. Nogami H, Stephens JK, Ferguson MK, Nabeya K-I (1990) Glycoprotein alterations in Barrett's esophagus, adenocarcinoma arising in Barrett's epithelium and adenocarcinoma of the gastroesophageal junction. In: Ferguson MK, Little AG, Skinner DB (eds) Diseases of the esophagus, vol I: Malignant diseases. Mount Kisco, New York, pp 17–23
11. Mori M, Ohno S, Tsutsui S, Matsuura H, Kuwano H, Sugimachi K (1990) Esophageal carcinoma in young patients. Ann Thorac Surg 49:284–286

Interaction Between Epidermal Growth Factor and Its Receptor in the Progression of Human Esophageal Carcinoma

AKIRA KAWAGUCHI, JYUNSUKE SHIBATA, HIROYUKI NAITO
and MASASHI KODAMA[1]

Introduction

Epidermal growth factor (EGF) is known to stimulate the growth and proliferation of various cells through interaction with its receptors (EGFR) [1–3].
In esophageal carcinoma, it has been reported that many squamous cell carcinomas express a large number of EGF receptors [4–7]. Furthermore, it has
been suggested that the patients with EGF receptor-positive tumor has a worse
prognosis than those with EGF receptor-negative tumors [6–7]. Thus, the expression of EGF receptors have been a focus of attention to be a significant
prognostic indicator for esophageal carcinoma. However, as for the EGF, there
had been no agreement regarding the effect of EGF on the progression of
esophageal carcinoma in vivo and in vitro [3–9].

In this study, we examined the effect of EGF/EGFR system upon the
proliferative activity of esophageal carcinoma by staining the EGF, its receptor,
and proliferative cell nuclear antigen (PCNA) of esophageal carcinoma immunohistochemically.

Materials and Methods

This study was based on 48 patients with esophageal carcinoma who received a
curative operation in the First Department of Surgery, Shiga University of
Medical Science, from 1980 to 1991.

Each resected specimen was fixed in 10% formalin and embedded in paraffin.
After a 4 µm thin section was made, EGF, EGFR, and PCNA were detected by
the avidin-biotin-peroxidase complex method. Monoclonal antibody to human

[1] First Department of Surgery, Shiga University of Medical Science, Tsukinowa-cho, Seta,
Otsu, Shiga, 520–21 Japan

EGF and EGFR were purchased from Wakunaga Parmaceutical Co., Ltd. (Tokyo), and Oncogene Science, Inc. (Manhasset, NY), respectively. PCNA was purchased from DAKO (Denmark). Vectastain ABC kits (PK-4002) were obtained from Vector Labs, Inc. (Burlingame, CA). Deparaffinized thin sections were incubated in 0.3% H_2O_2 in methanol for 15 min to block the endogenous peroxidase activities. After being washed in phosphate buffer saline (PBS), the sections were incubated with diluted normal serum for 30 min and then incubated successively with primary antibody for 48 h, diluted in biotinylated antibody solution for 30 min and avidin-biotin-peroxidase complex for 50 min each at room temperature. After each step, sections were washed with PBS, and were stained by incubation with a solution of 20 mg 3,3'-diaminobenzidine-4HCl in 100 ml of 50 mM Tris-HCl (pH 7.6) containing 0.02% hydrogen peroxidase. The sections were then washed in water, counterstained, dehydrated, and mounted. As a negative control, mouse IgG was used for primary antibodies.

The difference between the means of continuous variables was calculated with the unpaired Student's t-test. The relationship between discrete variables was tested using the chi-square test. Follow-up survival was analyzed by the Kaplan-Meier method.

The histopathological findings and cancer staging were made according to the criteria of the Japanese Society for Esophageal Diseases.

Results

Immunohistochemical Staining of EGF and Its Receptor

In the cancer nest, EGF was stained in the cytoplasm and EGFR was stained on the cell membrane. The distribution of EGF- and EGFR-stained tumor cells among the tissues appeared to be heterogenous, and the staining patterns varied from focal or mosaic to diffuse type. Twenty-five (55.6%) of 45 primary tumors

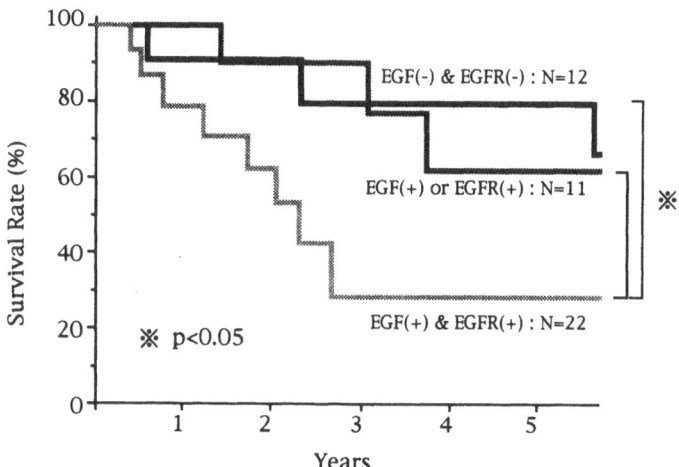

Fig. 1. Survival curves with epidermal growth factor (*EGF*) and epidermal growth factor receptor (*EGFR*) expression

and 10 (38.5%) of 26 metastatic lymph nodes were EGF-positive, and 30 (66.7%) of 45 primary tumors and 13 (50%) of 26 metastatic lymph nodes were EGFR-positive.

Prognosis

When follow-up study was made, the patients with synchronous expression of EGF and EGFR showed the poorest prognosis, and a significant difference was observed between subgroups with synchronous expression of EGF and EGFR and with neither expressed. However, there was no difference between subgroup with expression of neither EGF nor EGFR and with either EGF or EGFR expression (Fig. 1).

As for the disease-free interval (DFI) after operation, the mean DFI of patients with synchronous expression of both EGF and EGFR was 1.2 years, while the mean DFI of patients with expression of neither EGF nor EGFR was 4.4 years. There was a significant difference between the two groups.

Correlation Between the Depth of Tumor Invasion and the Incidence of EGF and Its Receptor Immunoreactivity

EGF was expressed in 33.3% including superficial carcinomas, and the incidence of EGF expression increased as the tumor invaded more deeply. However, there was no significant correlation between EGF or EGFR expression and the depth of tumor invasion statistically.

Labelling Index of PCNA

The mean labelling index of the group with neither EGF nor EGFR expression was 64.7% (Fig. 2), while the mean labelling index of the group in which both were positive was 67%. Thus, there was no relationship between the labelling index and the expression of EGF or EGFR.

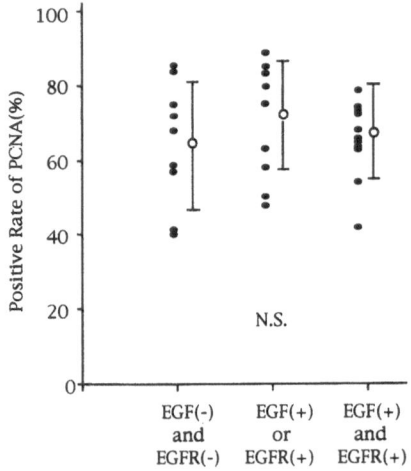

Fig. 2. Labelling index of proliferative cell nuclear antigen (*PCNA*)

Table 1. Relationship between EGF/EGFR expression and lymph node metastases

	n(−)	n(+)
*EGF(−)	11	9
(+)	6	18
EGFR(−)	8	7
(+)	9	20

* P < 0.05
LN, Lymph node; EGF, epidermal growth factor; EGFR, epidermal growth factor receptors

Table 2. Relationship of EGF/EGFR expression between primary lesion and lymph nodes

LN ＼ Primary	EGF(−)	EGF(+)	LN ＼ Primary	EGFR(−)	EGFR(+)
EGF(−)	9	0 ⎫ *	EGFR(−)	7	0 ⎫ *
EGF(+)	7	10 ⎭	EGFR(+)	6	13 ⎭

* P < 0.05

Correlation Between the Expression of EGF/EGFR and Lymph Node Metastasis

Lymph node metastases were observed in 75% of the EGF-positive patients, and a significant correlation was observed between EGF expression and lymph node metastasis (Table 1). Similarly, EGFR-positive tumor or tumor with synchronous expression of EGF and EGFR had a tendency to metastasize to the lymph nodes.

A comparison of the expression of EGF and EGFR between the primary lesion and the metastatic lymph nodes revealed that all of the tumors not expressing EGF or EGFR in primary lesions also showed no expression of EGF or EGFR in metastatic lymph nodes. On the other hand, 59% of the tumors which expressed EGF in primary lesions also showed EGF expression in metastatic lymph nodes, and 68% of the tumors expressing EGFR in primary lesions showed EGFR expression in metastatic lymph nodes (Table 2).

Discussion

In this study, we examined the expression of EGF, EGFR, and PCNA in 45 esophageal carcinomas.

Depalo and Das [9] has reported that EGF increases synthesis of its receptor. In our study, 88% of EGF-positive tumors expressed EGFR synchronously.

Furthermore considering the data of follow up of the survival rate and DFI, EGF and its receptor might act as autocrine growth factors and the malignant potential of esophageal carcinoma may depend on the interaction between EGF and its receptor.

Singletary et al. [3] demonstrated that EGF could increase tumor growth in a wide variety of human tumors and this enhanced growth induced by EGF was related to accelerated cellular division. In esophageal carcinoma, it has been reported that stimulation of growth of squamous cell carcinoma by EGF has been seen in vivo [9] and the growth rates of the tumor were shown to depend on the EGFR levels using human esophageal cancer xenografts in nude mice [6]. Conversely, it has been also reported that the growth of squamous cell carcinoma cell lines was inhibited partially by EGF in vivo and the sensitivity to the inhibitory effect of EGF correlated well with the level of EGFR [4]. Thus, there is no agreement as to the effect of EGF/EGFR is on the progression of esophageal carcinoma. In order to reveal the effect of EGF and EGFR on esophageal carcinoma, we estimated the proliferative activity of tumor cells based on the labelling index of PCNA. However, there was no relationship between the labelling index and the expression of EGF or EGFR. Hence, especially in human esophageal carcinoma, EGF and EGFR may or may not regulate proliferative activity.

The grade of lymph node metastasis is an important prognostic factor. In expression of EGF/EGFR and lymphatic invasion, a tumor which expresses EGF has a relatively high incidence of lymph node metastases. So, there may be a possibility that the interaction of EGF and EGFR may regulate the malignant potential of esophageal carcinoma, not by accelerating proliferative activity but by elevating the metastatic potential. Niedbala et al. [10] reported that EGF and the over-expression of its receptor in tumor cells has a potential regulatory role in plasminogen activator (PA)-mediated extracellular proteolysis. Yoshida et al. [11] has also reported that EGF induces the mRNA for collagenase and stromelysin. Furthermore, these extracellular degenerative enzymes are assumed to play an important role in tumor invasion and metastasis. In our study, the metastatic cells in lymph nodes are not always EGF- or EGFR-positive cells. These data suggest that EGF might affect the extracellular matrix and provide a suitable environment for metastasis. Hence, further examination is needed to elucidate the relation between the expression of EGF/EGFR and the mechanism of metastases.

References

1. Cohen S (1962) Isolation of a mouse submaxillary gland protein accelerating incisor eruption and eyelid opening in the newborn animal. J Biol Chem 237:1555–1562
2. Carpenter G, Cohen S (1979) Epidermal growth factor. Ann Rev Biochem 48:193–216
3. Singletary SE, Baker FL, Spitzer G, Tucker SL, Tomasovic B, Brock WA, Ajani JA, Kelly AM (1987) Biological effect of epidermal growth factor on the in vitro growth of human tumors. Cancer Res 47:403–406
4. Kamata N, Chida K, Horikoshi M, Enomoto S, Kuroki T (1986) Growthinhibitory effect of epidermal growth factor and overexpression of its receptors on human squamous cell carcinoma in culture. Cancer Res 46:1648–1653

5. Banks-Schlegel Sp, Quintero J (1986) Human esophageal carcinoma cells have fewer, but higher affinity epidermal growth factor receptors. J Biol Chem 261:4359–4362
6. Mukaida H, Hirai T, Nakamura T, Yamashita Y, Kawano K, Toge T, Niimoto M, Hattori T (1988) Measurement of epidermal growth factor receptor and its effect on growth of human esophageal cancer xenografts implanted into nude mice. Oncologia 21:55–60
7. Ozawa S, Ueda M, Ando, Shimizu N, Abe O (1989) Prognostic significance of epidermal growth factor in esophageal squamous cell carcinomas. Cancer 63:2169–2173
8. Ozawa S, Ueda M, Ando, Abe O, Hirai M, Shimizu N (1987) Stimulation by EGF of the growth of EGF receptor-hyperproducing tumor cells in athymic mice. Int J Cancer 40:706–710
9. Depalo L, Das M (1988) Epidermal growth factor-induced stimulation of epidermal growth factor receptor synthesis in human cytotrophoblasts and A431 carcinoma cells. Cancer Res 48:1105–1109
10. Niedbala MJ, Bajetta S, Carbone R, Sartorelli AC (1990) Regulation of human squamous cell carcinoma plasma membrane-associated urokinase plasminogen activator by epidermal growth factor. Cancer Commun 2:317–324
11. Yoshida K, Tsujino T, Yasui W, Kameda T, Sano T, Nakayama H, Toge T, Rahara E (1990) Induction of growth factor receptor and metalloproteinase genes by epidermal growth factor and/or transforming growth factor-a in human gastric carcinoma cell line MKN-28. Jpn J Cancer Res 81:793–798

Cell Kinetics and Epidermal Growth Factor Receptor Expression: Useful Guides in Esophageal Cancer?

K. Haustermans[1], K. Geboes[2], T. Lerut[4], J. Van Thillo[1],
W. Coosemans[4], M. Waer[3], and E. Van Der Schueren[1]

Introduction

Radiotherapy and chemotherapy both cause cell death in tumors as well as in normal tissues. As soon as a certain level of damage is reached in the tissue, repopulation starts via feedback mechanisms. In fast proliferating tissues like skin and intestinal epithelia, this compensatory proliferation starts within 2–3 weeks. Compensatory proliferation is not linear but increases exponentially as a function of the overall treatment time [1, 2]. This repopulation can influence the effect of protracted irradiation to a large extent. When the overall treatment time is shortened from 7 to 2 weeks, the tolerance of the acutely responding tissues decreases to such a degree that the total dose must be reduced from 70 to 50 Gy. Probably similar effects occur in fast proliferating tumors. By this mechanism the therapeutic effect of extremely protracted irradiation is jeopardized [3, 4]. It has been described in head and neck cancer that local tumor control did decrease from 86% to 32% when treatment was protracted from 35 days to 50 days or more [5]. Hence the rationale for shortening overall treatment time for fast proliferating tumors to counteract repopulation. Preliminary results of the European Organization for Research and Treatment of Cancer (EORTC) trial for head and neck tumors indeed show that local tumor control in fast proliferating tumors is higher after accelerated radiotherapy (70 Gy/5 weeks) compared to conventional irradiation (70 Gy/7 weeks) [6]. This remains to be assessed for esophageal tumors, especially for squamous esophageal cancer which is histologically comparable with head and neck cancer.

Thanks to recently developed monoclonal antibodies against IUdR (iododeoxyuridine), it is now possible to measure cell kinetics in vivo in patients.

Departments of [1] Radiation Oncology, [2] Pathology, [3] Immunology, and [4] Thoracic Surgery, University Hospital, Capucijnenvoer 33, 3000 Leuven, Belgium

IUdR is a thymidine analogue that is incorporated in the DNA of the cell during S-phase. This incorporated IUdR is recognized by fluorescent monoclonal antibodies and quantitated by flow cytometry. Compared to the traditional application of tritiated thymidine, halogenated thymidine analogues have the following advantages: no radioactivity involved, rapid measurement (thousands of cells per second) and the possibility to measure DNA content and IUdR uptake independently in the same cell. T_{pot} values (potential doubling time of a population) are determined by the growth fraction as well as by the cell cycle time. The term potential doubling time (Steel [7]) represents the time for the population to double without cell loss. T_{pot} is considered as the most relevant parameter for the assessment of growth-kinetics [8–11], although it is only one of the parameters determining growth rate. Cell loss for instance is not assessed by T_{pot} measurements. T_{pot} measurements also do not detect differences between cell populations. Nevertheless, T_{pot} can be very important but more data on intratumor variability need to be gathered as it is unknown whether one biopsy is representative of the whole tumor. Until now, it was difficult to measure on a large scale the kinetics of proliferation of tumors before treatment but the development of new techniques nowadays allows an in vivo approach. Besides information on the cell kinetic status of a tumor (T_{pot}) it is also important to examine other prognostic factors like the expression of growth factors. It has been known for a long time that the absence of estradiol and progesterone receptors in breast cancer is associated with a poor prognosis [12]. Recent studies have suggested that growth factors such as epidermal growth factor (EGF) may have an important influence. In most studies, a high level of epidermal growth factor receptor (EGFr) expression in the tumor cells is associated with a poor prognosis [13–16]. Probably growth is controlled by these receptors and thus tumors with a high level of EGFr expression may be more stimulated to proliferation. Therefore the aims of this study were to assess T_{pot} in esophageal cancer, to study intratumor variability, and to assess the correlation between EGFr expression and cell kinetics.

Materials and Methods

Sixty patients with cancer of the esophagus and cardia were studied. The majority of patients had an advanced stage at diagnosis: 26 had squamous cell carcinomas, 32 patients suffered from adenocarcinomas of the distal part of the esophagus and cardia, and the remaining 2 patients had signet ring cell carcinomas. The primary treatment was surgery.

IUdR was injected 6–8 h before surgery. Following surgery, the specimen was immediately recovered and brought to the laboratory. After the specimen was opened and gently washed with tap water, five biopsies were taken from the tumor: one central and four peripheral from the left, right, upper, and lower part of the tumor. For a circular tumor, three central and two peripheral biopsies were taken. Each biopsy was cut into two pieces. One piece was fixed in ethanol and used for flow cytometry, and the second biopsy was divided in two parts: One part was fixed in B5, a mercury-based fixative allowing immunohistochemical staining, and used for the detection of IUdR-positive cells; the second part was frozen in isopentane-cooled liquid nitrogen and stored at −70°C until further use. Cryostat sections of this biopsy were used for immunohistochemical detection of EGFr.

Cell kinetics on 287 biopsies were measured using flow cytometry and microscopically using IUdR staining (immunoperoxidase technique after DNA denaturation). IUdR staining was performed only on biopsies from squamous cancer. The percentage of stained cells (nuclei) was counted to yield the S-phase labelling index. The labelling index (LI) is the ratio between the labelled cells and the labelled + unlabelled cells, expressed as a percentage after counting 500 cells. EGFr expression was assessed microscopically. Cryostat sections of squamous tumors were stained with monoclonal antibodies directed against EGFr1 (Amersham International; dilution 1/10) using an immunoperoxidase technique. EGFr1 recognizes an epitope on the external domain of the EGFr. Staining intensity was assessed in a semiquantitative method, by a pathologist unaware of the other results. In addition, the type (adenocarcinoma, squamous carcinoma), grade (poorly, moderately, well differentiated) of the tumor and the distribution of the staining pattern (focal, patchy, diffuse) were noted.

Statistical analysis of the results was done using Student's t-test, analysis of variance (ANOVA) and Spearman rank correlation.

Results

Cell Kinetic Measurements

Flow Cytometry

In Fig. 1, the differences between the different tumors are shown. Almost all tumors are fast proliferating with a mean T_{pot} value of 4.97 days ± 3.71 days. For squamous cell carcinomas, the mean T_{pot} value is 4.4 days. For adenocarcinomas the mean T_{pot} value is 5.56 days.

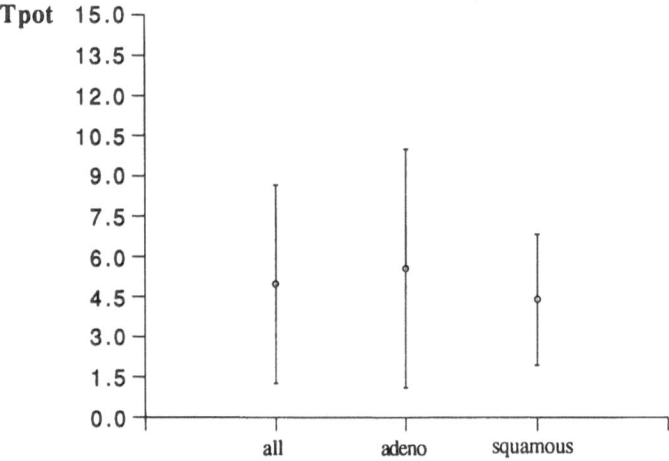

Fig. 1. This figure represents the mean T_{pot} ± 1 SD for all tumors and for adenocarcinomas and squamous cell carcinomas separately

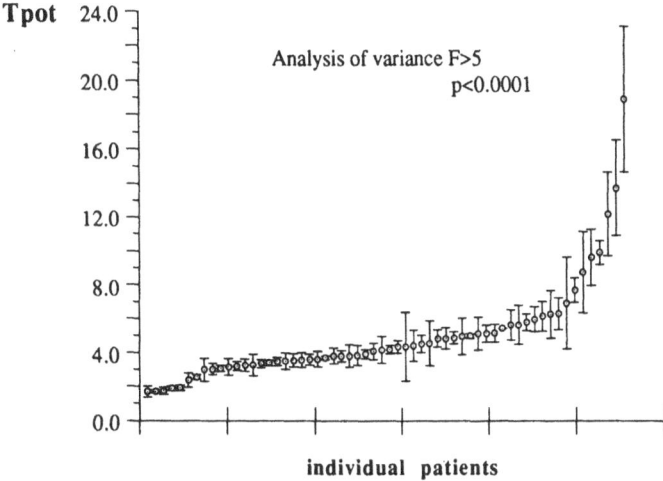

Fig. 2. The differences between the different tumors are larger than the differences within each tumor. On the X-axis, the individual patients are shown and on the Y-axis the T_{pot} values ± 1 SEM are represented

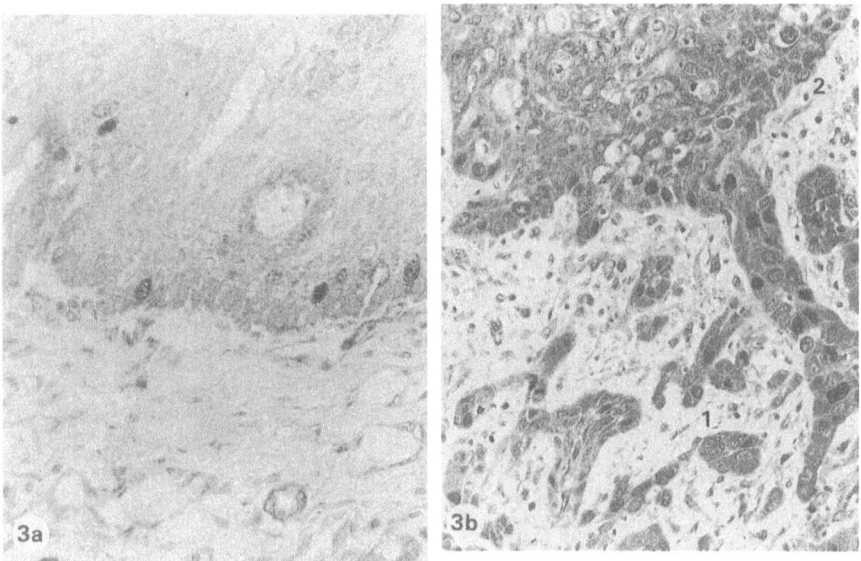

Fig. 3a,b. Microphotograph of human esophageal biopsies stained with monoclonal antibodies directed against iododeoxyuridine (*IUdR*). **a** Normal mucosa with the presence of cells with positively staining nuclei in the basal layer and along the papillae (immunohistochemistry ×150). **b** Biopsy from a squamous carcinoma, with small tumor sheets containing numerous positive cells (*1*) and a larger area with only a few positive cells (*2*). (Immunohistochemistry ×125)

In Fig. 2, the variability between the tumors, compared with the variability within each tumor, assessed by analysis of variance, is shown. The variability between the different tumors is larger than the variability within each different tumor.

The mean values of T_{pot}, LI, and T_s (T_s = duration of S-phase) of peripheral and central biopsies were not significantly different. We found no significant difference between adenocarcinomas and squamous cell carcinomas (Student's t-tests). With our results, we could detect differences of 1.17 days with 90% power, accepting type I error of 1%.

IUdR Staining

The labelling index is 8.7% for the normal proliferative layer in the normal esophageal squamous mucosa and 0.95% for the entire mucosa. For squamous cancer, the LI shows a mean value of 18.51% (range 7.86%–33.57%). In 12 cases, focal areas with high LI were observed (Fig. 3). Figure 3 shows a picture from a biopsy obtained in a moderately well differentiated squamous cell carcinoma stained with a monoclonal antibody directed against IUdR. Staining positivity is characterized by a dark (brownish) coloration of nuclei in the

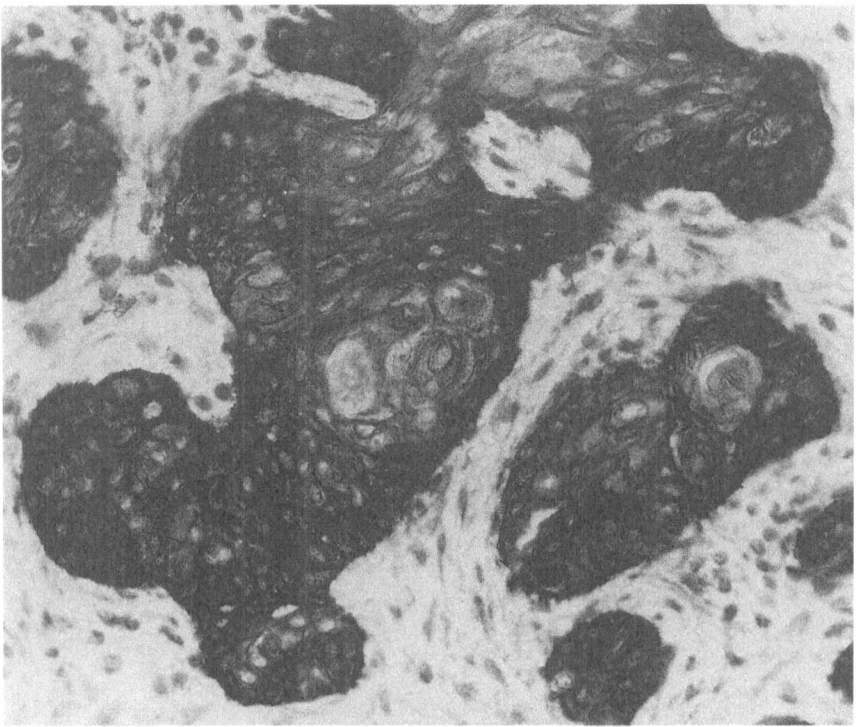

Fig. 4. Epidermal growth factor receptor (*EGFr*) staining in a squamous carcinoma. Intense positive membranous staining is observed in the periphery of the tumor strands, while a better differentiated area in the center is only weakly positive. (Immunohistochemistry ×125)

positive cells. Several cells with positively staining nuclei are present in the small extensions of the tumor, while in the larger tumoral areas no positively staining cells are seen.

EGFr Staining on the Squamous Cell Carcinomas

Ninety-four biopsies of 26 squamous cell carcinomas stained weakly to strongly positive for EGFr. In 73 cases, the EGFr expression was clearly membranous, while in 21 cases additional cytoplasmic staining was observed. Fifty-four cases expressed the EGFr diffusely over the whole tumor, while in 40 biopsies only the periphery of the tumor strands stained positively. In the cases where only periphery stained positively, the tumor showed variable degrees of differentiation with usually a well differentiated area characterized by keratinization in the center.

Figure 4 shows a moderately well differentiated squamous cell carcinoma stained for EGFr. The periphery and less well differentiated areas are intensely positive while more differentiated areas are stained weakly or not at all.

Relation Between T_{pot}, EGFr, and Pathology

The correlation between differentiation grade and intensity of staining was assessed using the Spearman rank correlation. There was a significant correlation between the intensity of staining and grade (Fig. 5).

There was no correlation between T_{pot} and stage as assessed by Spearman rank and no correlation between T_{pot} and tumor differentiation grade. Finally,

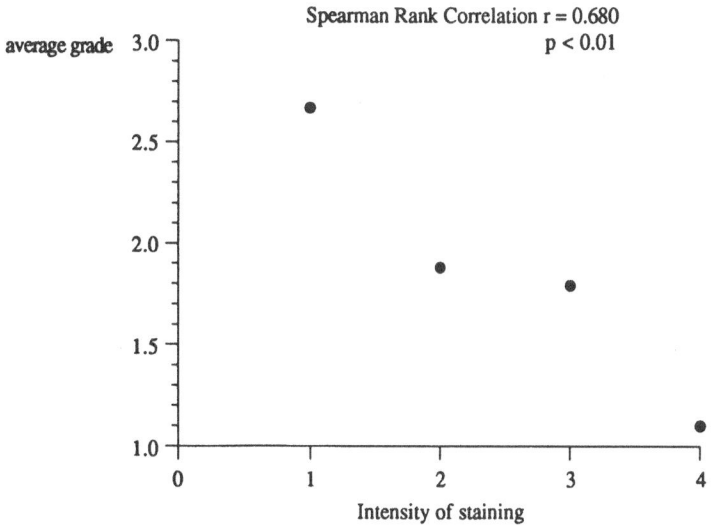

Fig. 5. The intensity of EGFr staining was positively correlated to differentiation grade. On the Y-axis, the average grade is represented, with 1 being poorly differentiated; 2, moderately differentiated; and 3, well differentiated. On the X-axis, the intensity of staining is shown, with 1, weakly positive and 4, strongly positive

there was no correlation between T_{pot} and EGFr expression as assessed by Spearman rank.

Discussion

From these studies, it appears that cell kinetics, assessed by T_{pot} measurements and by microscopy on sections stained with antibodies directed against IUdR, can be evaluated reliably in patients. EGFr expression can equally be assessed. The T_{pot} measurements indicate that the intratumor differences are smaller than the intertumor differences and that biopsy site, central or peripheral, is not critical. However, whether one biopsy is enough to characterize the tumor is currently under investigation. In vivo evaluation of tumor cell kinetics using endoscopic biopsies is certainly feasible. On the other hand, we did not find any correlation between tumor extension or stage, tumor grade, and cell kinetics. Also no correlation was found between EGFr expression assessed histologically and T_{pot} measurements. The lack of correlation has also been observed in other studies on other types of tumors. So probably, T_{pot} will give additional independent prognostic information.

Overall, squamous cancer of the esophagus showed intense positive staining for EGFr, although not always in a diffuse pattern. The high level of staining intensity correlates well with the fast proliferating character of these tumors as assessed by T_{pot}.

Analysis of split-course radiotherapy schedules has shown that clonogenic cells repopulate at a rate similar to T_{pot} as measured by flow cytometry. The local control of fast proliferating tumors is higher when irradiated in an accelerated way [7]. As T_{pot} gives information on repopulation, its value is very important in deciding upon the optimal treatment time for an individual patient. Therefore, it can be concluded that T_{pot} measurements give additional, independent prognostic information and can be considered as a useful guide for determining optimal radiotherapy schedules, either in association with surgery or when used alone.

References

1. Ang KK, Xu FX, Vanuytsel L, et al (1985) Repopulation kinetics in untreated mouse lip mucosa: The relative importance of treatment protraction and time distribution of irradiations. Radiat Res 101:162–169
2. Ang KK, Landuyt W, Rijnders A, et al (1984) Differences in repopulation kinetics in mouse skin during split course multiple fractions per day (MFD) or daily fractionated irradiations. Int J Radiat Oncol Biol Phys 10:95–99
3. Withers HR, Taylor JMG, Mackiejewski B (1988) The hazard of accelerated tumor clonogen repopulation during radiotherapy. Acta Oncol 27:131–146
4. Peters LJ, Ang KK, Thames HD (1988) Accelerated fractionation in the radiation treatment of head and neck cancer: A critical comparison of different strategies. Acta Oncol 27:185–194
5. Bataini JP, Asselain B, Janlerry C, et al (1989) A multivariate primary tumor control analysis in 465 patients treated by radical radiotherapy for cancer of the tonsillar region: Clinical and treatment parameters as prognostic factors. Radiother Oncol 14:265–277
6. Begg AC, Hofland I, Moonen L, et al (1985) The predictive value of the cell kinetic measurements in a European Trial of Accelerated Fractionation in advanced head and neck tumors: An interim report. Cytometry 6:620

7. Steel GG (1977) Growth kinetics of tumors. Clarendon, Oxford
8. Begg AC, McNally NJ, Shrieve DC, et al (1990) A method to measure the duration of DNA synthesis and the potential doubling time from a single sample. Int J Radiat Oncol Biol Phys 19:620–626
9. Fowler JF (1986) Potential for increasing the differential response between tumors and normal tissues: Can proliferation rate be used?. Int J Radiat Oncol Biol Phys 12:641–645
10. Fowler JF, Tanner MA, Bataini JP, et al (1990) Futher analysis of the time factor in squamous cell carcinoma of the tonsillar region. Radiother Oncol 19:237–244
11. Wilson GD (1991) Assessment of human tumor proliferation using bromodeoxyuridine: Current status. Acta Oncol 30:903–910
12. Henderson IC, Harris JR, Kinne DW, et al (1989) Breast cancer. In: Cancer, principles and practice of oncology, 3rd edn. JB Lippincott, Philadelphia, pp. 1197–1268
13. Travers MT, Barrett-Lee PJ, Berger U. et al (1988) Growth factor expression in normal, benign and malignant breast tissue. Br Med J 296:1621–1624
14. Horwitz KB, Mc Guire WL (1978) Estrogen control of progesterone receptor in human breast cancer. Correlation with nuclear processing of estrogen receptor. J Biol Chem 253:2223–2228
15. Nicholson S, Halcrow P, Gavinsburg JR, et al (1988) EGFr status associated with failure of primary endocrine therapy in eldery postmenopausal patients with breast cancer. Br J Cancer 58:810–814
16. Neal DE, Sharples L, Smith K, et al (1990) The epidermal growth factor receptor and prognosis of bladder cancer. Cancer 65:1619–1625

Epidermal Growth Factor Receptor (EGF-R) and HER-2/NEU p185 Protein Expression in Esophageal Cancer

A. Ruol[1], R. Dittadi[2], M. Gion[2], A. Segalin[4], M. Panozzo[3],
A. Brazzale[2], S. Meo[2], and A. Peracchia[4]

Introduction

Epidermal Growth Factor receptor (EGF-R) and p185 protein, encoded by oncogene *neu*, are structurally related proteins of the *erb*-B family involved in the growth control of several cancer types. Overexpression of both EGF-R and p185 seems to be related to malignant transformation in several cancer types [1].

To date, there are few and conflicting results concerning EGF-R and p185 expression in cancer of the esophagus [2–10].

Since 1989, we have been evaluating prospectively the expression of EGF-R and p185 in fresh esophageal tissue to investigate the expression of these proteins in normal and cancer tissue, and to evaluate the possible relationships with well-known clinico-pathologic prognostic parameters and with overall survival.

Material and Methods

Thirty one samples of cancer and 31 of normal mucosa, 1 each from 31 operative specimens, were evaluated. During surgery, the samples of normal mucosa and cancer were taken from the operative specimen and immediately frozen and stored at −85°C until processing.

---

[1] Second Department of General Surgery, University of Padova, Via Giustiniani, 2; 35128 Padova, Italy

[2] Center for the Study of Biological Markers of Malignancy, Ospedale Civile S. Giovannic Paolo, Castello 6776; 30100 Venezia, Italy

[3] IST Biotechnology Section, and Institute of Oncology, University of Padua, Via Gattamelata, 64; 35128 Padova, Italy

[4] Department of General Surgery, University of Milan, Hospital Policlinico, Monteggia, Via F. Sporza, 35; 20122 Milano, Italy

Processing of Esophageal Tissue

Tissue samples were pulverized and homogenized in phosphate buffer. Fifty μl of the crude homogenate were used for p185 determination. The homogenate was centrifuged at $800 \times g$ for 10 min at 4°C. The pellet was washed twice and the supernatants pooled and centrifuged at $100\,000 \times g$ for 1 h at 4°C. The membrane pellet was homogenized and collected for EGF-R determination.

EGF-R Determination

EGF-R determination was performed by Scatchard analysis according to EORTC Receptor Study Group [11]. Briefly, the membrane fraction was incubated with human 125-I-EGF (8 points with final concentrations from 1.5 to 0.1 nM). The non-specific binding was determined using cold human EGF at a concentration 100 nM. The mixture was incubated for 20 h at 22°C and a HAP slurry was added. The reaction mixture was incubated for another 60 min at room temperature and centrifuged at $1000 \times g$ for 2 min. The supernatant was decanted, washed twice, and the pellet was counted in a gamma-counter.

p185 Assay

p185 was determined using a commercially available enzyme immunoassay (Oncogene Science, Uniondale, New York) that uses two monoclonal antibodies (TA1 and NB3) raised against the extracellular domain of p185. Homogenates of esophageal normal mucosa and esophageal cancer tissue were solubilized, centrifuged at $10\,000\,g$ for 30 s and diluted with PBS (10 mM). The optimal dilution factor was 1:300 for cancer specimens and 1:50 for non-malignant specimens. The results were expressed as U/mg of homogenate proteins.

Results

The binding affinity of EGF-R was similar in cancer tissue and in normal mucosa (Table 1).

EGF-R concentration in normal mucosa and in cancer tissue was not statistically different, although higher values were found in cancer tissue (Table 2).

Table 1. EGF-R binding affinity in normal and esophageal cancer tissue (nM/l)

	Normal mucosa	Cancer tissue
Mean	0.44	0.36
Median	0.29	0.24
Range	0.05–1.3	0.06–0.60
n	27	18

P NS

EGF-R, epidermal growth factor receptor

Table 2. EGF-R concentration (Fmol/mg of protein) in esophageal tissue

	Normal mucosa	Cancer tissue
Mean	32.3	51.5
Median	2.7	16.7
Range	0–186	0–400
Positive samples	18/31	27/31

P NS

Table 3. p185 concentration (U/mg of protein) in esophageal tissue

	Normal mucosa	Cancer tissue
Mean	1965	2733
Median	1855	1766
Range	597–3258	500–11 185

P NS

Table 4. EGF-R and p185 correlations with clinico-pathological parameters

	EGF-R	p185
Histologic type		
(squamous cell vs adenoca.)	*P* NS	*P* 0.016
Histologic grading	*P* NS	*P* NS
T pattern	*P* NS	*P* NS
N status	*P* NS	*P* NS
TNM stage	*P* NS	*P* NS
Flow-cytometric DNA pattern		
(euploid vs aneuploid)	*P* NS	*P* NS
Type of resection		
(curative vs palliative)	*P* NS	*P* NS

T, primary tumor bulk; *N*, lymph node status; *TNM*, tumor node metastasis; *adenoca.*, adenocarcinoma

The median concentration in normal mucosa and in cancer tissue was 2.7 and 16.7 FMol/mg of protein, respectively.

p185 concentration in normal mucosa and in cancer tissue was not statistically different, although higher values up to more than 11 000 U/mg of protein were found in cancer tissue (Table 3).

No relationship was found between EGF-R or p185 expression and the following clinico-pathologic parameters (Table 4): histologic grading, primary tumor bulk (T), lymph node status (N), pathologic TNM stage, flow cytometric DNA pattern (euploid vs aneuploid), and the type of surgical resection which was possible to perform (curative or R0 vs palliative or R1–2).

The only statistically significant finding was that p185 expression was greater in adenocarcinomas than in squamous cell carcinomas (Table 5).

Table 5. Correlation between p185 concentrations (U/mg of protein) and histologic type

	Adenocarcinoma	Squamous cell carcinoma
Mean	3990	1688
Median	3179	1190
Range	1160–11 185	500–5085
n	11	12

P 0.016

As far as prognosis is concerned, no relationship was found between EGF-R or p185 expression and the short-term survival after surgery. The considered cut-off values were both the median values and the ratio cancer/normal (>1 vs <1).

Discussion

EGF-R has been shown to be involved in cellular proliferation and differentiation. In several cancer types, it also participates in oncogenesis when the former process becomes abnormal due to increased expression or increased ligand affinity [1, 2].

In the literature, it is still unclear whether increased EGF-R levels have significant correlation with pathologic caracteristics and prognosis.

Mukaida et al. [3, 4] reported that the average content of EGF-R of esophageal cancer is significantly higher than that of normal esophageal mucosa. Meirowitz et al. [5] reported that the mean density of EGF-R is significantly higher in esophageal squamous cell carcinoma tissue than in controls, and also that the affinity for EGF is greater. On the other hand, Francois et al. [6] reported that EGF-R affinity binding is similar in tumoral and non-tumoral tissue.

Jankowski et al. [7] reported that inflamed esophageal mucosa has significantly greater density of EGF-R expression than normal mucosa, which may be related to the increased cellular proliferation in esophagitis. Jankowski et al. [8] also reported an increased expression of EGF-R in Barrett's mucosa and adenocarcinoma arising in Barrett's mucosa.

According to Yano et al. [9], patients with greater EGF-R expression are more likely to have lymph node metastases, and therefore also a poorer prognosis. Mukaida et al. [3, 4] found no correlation between EGF-R and pathologic findings such as primary tumor bulk (T), lymph node status (N), and pathologic stage, with the only exception of the histologic degree of differentiation of esophageal squamous cell carcinoma. Francois et al. [6] and Ozawa et al. [10] found no difference between patients with high and low EGF-R according to sex, age, location of cancer, histology, histological grading, T pattern, N status, staging, and type of treatment.

Mukaida et al. [3, 4] and Ozawa et al. [10] showed that an elevated EGF-R level is a significant prognostic indicator for esophageal squamous cell carcinoma.

The conflicting results obtained to date could be due to the different and non-standardized methods used for EGF-R determination. A method that offers the best characteristics of precision and accuracy for the determination of EGF-R has been recently developed by the EORTC Receptor Study Group [11]. Using this standardized method, we found a wide distribution of EGF-R in esophageal tissue. Although cancer tissue shows a trend towards higher expression in comparison with normal tissue, no significant differences were found. A malignant transformation seems to cause variations in EGF-R activity which are independent of EGF-R levels in the corresponding normal tissue and without any apparent relationship with clinico-pathologic parameters.

As for the p185 expression, we evaluated for the first time, to our knowledge, its distribution in esophageal tissue. No significant differences were found between normal and cancer tissue. In the cases evaluated, we did not find correlations to the clinico-pathologic parameters except a higher expression of p185 in adenocarcinoma with respect to squamous cell carcinoma.

In conclusion, EGF-R and p185 are expressed in esophageal tissue, probably independent of malignant transformation. The possible prognostic role of EGF-R and p185 in cancers of the esophagus and cardia is currently being evaluated in more patients with longer follow-up.

References

1. Gullick WJ (1990) The role of epidermal growth factor receptor and the c-erbB2 protein in breast cancer. Int J Cancer 5:55–61
2. Mufti SJ, Zirvi KA, Garewal HS (1991) Precancerous lesions and biologic markers in esophageal cancer. Cancer Detect Prev 15:291–301
3. Mukaida H, Yamamoto T, Hirai T, Toi M, Nakamura T, Wada T, Yamashita Y, Kawano K, Niimoto M (1990) Expression of human EGF and its receptor in esophageal cancer. Jpn J Surg 20:275–282
4. Mukaida H, Toi M, Hirai T, Yamashita Y, Toge T (1991) Clinical significance of the expression of EGF and its receptor in esophageal cancer. Cancer 68:142–148
5. Meirowitz RF, Dutta SK, Vengurlekar S, Resau J (1990) Expression of EGF-R in squamous cell carcinoma of the esophagus. Gastroenterol 98:A297
6. Francois E, Formento JL, Mouroux J, Francoual M, Birtwisle-Peyrottes I, Ferrero JM, Ettore F, Lagrange JL, Milano G (1992) Characterization and quantification of EGF-R in epidermoid esophageal carcinoma. Proceedings of the International Conference on Biology and Treatment of Gastrointestinal Malignancies, Frankfurt, p 94
7. Jankowski J, Murphy S, Coghill G, Grant A, Wormsley KG, Sanders DSA, Kerr M, Hopwood D (1992) EGF-Receptors in the esophagus. Gut 33:439–443
8. Jankowski J, Hopwood D, Wormsley KG (1992) Flow-cytometric analysis of growth-regulatory peptides and their receptors in Barrett's esophagus and esophageal adenocarcinoma. Scand J Gastroenterol 27:147–154
9. Yano H, Shiozaki H, Kobayashi K, Yano T, Tahara H, Tamura S, Mori T (1991) Immunohistologic detection of the EGF-R in human esophageal squamous cell carcinoma. Cancer 67:91–98
10. Ozawa S, Masakazu U, Ando N, Shimizu N, Abe O (1989) Prognostic significance of EGF-R in esophageal squamous cell carcinoma. Cancer 63:2169–2173
11. Benraad TJ, Foekens JA (1990) Hydroxyapatite assay to measure epidermal growth factor receptor in human primary breast tumors. Ann Clin Biochem 27:272–273

New Strategy of Treatment for Esophageal Squamous Cell Carcinoma Using Immunotoxin Which Reacts to Epidermal Growth Factor Receptor

Soji Ozawa, Masakazu Ueda, Norifumi Hirota, Nobutoshi Ando, and Masaki Kitajima[1]

Introduction

Squamous cell carcinoma is by far the most common neoplasm of the esophagus and the survival rate of its patients is generally low [1]. To treat this cancer more effectively, it is necessary to develop a strategy of targeted cancer therapy. Most squamous carcinoma cells hyperproduce epidermal growth factor (EGF) receptor [2, 3], and EGF in turn promotes the growth of EGF receptor-hyperproducing squamous carcinoma cells in vivo [4]. Moreover, an elevated EGF receptor level is a significant prognostic factor for patients with esophageal squamous cell carcinoma [5]. Therefore, since EGF and its receptor system play an important role in the growth of this cancer, EGF receptor is an ideal cell surface object for targeted therapy. We synthesized an immunotoxin consisting of murine monoclonal antibody (B4G7) against human EGF receptor and gelonin, a 60s ribosome-inactivating protein. We studied the cytotoxic effects of the immunotoxin on squamous carcinoma cells and tumors, and investigated the possibility of it as a new treatment for squamous cell carcinoma.

Materials and Methods

Human squamous carcinoma cells, TE5, A431, NA, and Ca9-22, are from tumor of the esophagus, vulva, tongue, and gingiva. H69 cells are from human small cell lung cancer. Toxin gelonin was conjugated to monoclonal antibody B4G7 as described previously [6]. Briefly, sulfhydryl groups were incorporated into gelonin by treatment with 2-iminothiolane. Dithiopyridyl groups were incorporated into B4G7 with N-succinimidyl-3-(2-pyridyldithio) propionate.

[1] Department of Surgery, Keio University School of Medicine, 35 Shinanomachi, Shinjuku-ku, Tokyo, 160 Japan

417

Modified gelonin and B4G7 were mixed and the reaction was stopped with iodoacetamide. Non-conjugated gelonin was removed by passage of the solution through a Sephacryl S-200 column. Non-conjugated B4G7 was removed by passage of the solution through a CM-cellulose column (CM-52). The purified conjugate was sterilized by filtration through a 0.22-μm membrane.

The cytotoxic effects of the immunotoxin was analyzed. Exponentially growing cancer cells (2×10^4) were transferred to 24-well plates. The next day, the medium was replaced with fresh medium containing various concentrations of the immunotoxin. After 3 days quadriplicate dishes were washed with PBS and trypsinized. The surviving cells were counted using trypan blue exclusion.

Next, antitumor effects of the immunotoxin were analyzed as described previously [7]. A431 or H69 cells (10^7/site) were injected subcutaneously into 6-week-old female BALB/c nude mice. After each solid tumor formed, 10 μg of the conjugate or the unconjugated mixture of B4G7 and gelonin was administered intraperitoneally into nude mice for 5 days. Two weeks after the first injection, the animals were sacrificed and the tumors were removed and weighed.

Results

The cytotoxic effects of the immunotoxin: IC_{50} of the immunotoxin for NA, A431, Ca9-22, and TE5 were 0.13 nM, 0.22 nM, 0.37 nM, and 22.5 nM, respectively. The IC_{50} for H69 was well over 100 nM. The number of EGF receptors of these five cells decreased in the above order (Table 1). Therefore, the cytotoxic effects of the immunotoxin correlated to the number of EGF receptors.

The antitumor effects of the immunotoxin: It took 5 or 10 days for A431 or H69 cells to form solid tumor, respectively. Two weeks after the first injection of the immunotoxin or the mixture, the weight of A431 tumors in treated mice was 77.5% less than that in control mice. The weight of H69 tumors in the treated

Table 1. The cytotoxic effect of the immunotoxin

cells	IC_{50} (nM)	EGF receptor number (sites/cell)
NA	0.13	3×10^6
A431	0.22	3×10^6
Ca9–22	0.37	1.3×10^6
TE5	22.5	1×10^5
H69	>100	Not detected

Table 2. The anti-tumor effect of the immunotoxin

Tumor type	Tumor weight (g)		
	Immunotoxin	Control	
A431 tumor	0.9 ± 0.1	4.0 ± 0.5	$P < 0.01$
H69 tumor	0.9 ± 0.4	0.9 ± 0.5	NS

NS, not significant

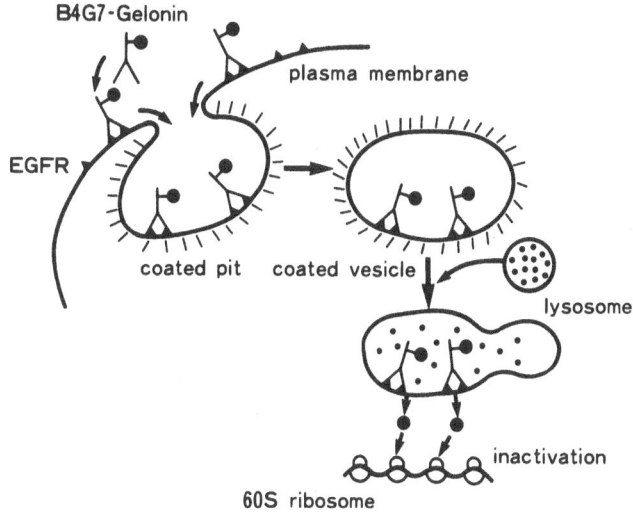

Fig. 1. Steps in immunotoxin action on cancer cells. Immunotoxin binds to cell surface epidermal growth factor receptor (*EGFR*), moves to coated pits, enters coated vesicles, splits into gelonin and B4G7, and finally gelonin inactivates protein synthesis

mice showed no difference from that in the control mice. The immunotoxin inhibited the growth of A431 tumor which had many EGF receptors, but not the growth of H69 tumor which lacked EGF receptors (Table 2). There was no difference in tissue weight of heart, kidney, liver, lung, and spleen between the treated and control mice. No toxic change in these tissues from the treated mice was detected microscopically.

Discussion

The immunotoxin action is explained in Fig. 1. The immunotoxin, B4G7 and gelonin conjugate, binds to cell surface EGF receptors, and is incorporated into the cancer cells through coated pits. The coated vesicles including the immunotoxin are attacked by lysosomes, and B4G7 and gelonin are split from each other. The gelonin released from the vesicle reaches 60s ribosome and inactivates it, leading to cell death.

We studied the possibility of this immunotoxin being a targeted therapy for squamous cell carcinoma. It showed cytotoxic and antitumor effects on the cells according to the EGF receptor number. EGF receptor is a product of proto-oncogene c-*erb* B [8] which is overexpressed in squamous cell cancer including esophageal cancer [3]. The monoclonal antibody (B4G7) reacts to the low affinity type of cell surface EGF receptors, which usually overexpress in cancer tissues. EGF receptor does not circulate systemically or form an immune complex in the blood. Moreover, EGF receptor is easily internalized into cells. Therefore, EGF receptor is an ideal object for targeted immunotoxin therapy. Gelonin is a 30 kDa-polypeptide plant hemitoxin, which is stable and non-toxic to intact cells because it lacks a membrane transport chain like ricin B chain. It is also a good substance for use in preparing immunotoxins.

There may be several problems associated with clinical trials of gelonin immunotoxin. General toxicities were reported with ricin A chain immunotoxin and *Pseudomonas* exotoxin A immunotoxin [9]. Ricin A chain immunotoxin produces a capillary leak syndrome with low serum albumin, edema, and weight gain, and rarely, pulmonary edema. *Pseudomonas* exotoxin A immunotoxin complicates significant liver toxicity. Administration of steroids and short treatment schedules may overcome these toxicities. The gelonin immunotoxin showed a good anti-tumor effects and could be a useful agent for targeting esophageal squamous carcinoma with traditionally poor prognoses. While our animal studies did not reveal any severe toxicity, further basic in vivo studies, in terms of both toxicity and efficiency, are necessary before clincal trials.

References

1. Adkins PC (1981) Tumors of the esophagus. In: Sabiston DC (ed) Textbook of surgery: The biological basis of modern surgical practice, vol 1, edn 12. WB Saunders, Philadelphia, pp 841–855
2. Hunts J, Ueda M, Ozawa S, Abe O, Pastan I, Shimizu N (1985) Hyperproduction and gene amplification of the epidermal growth factor receptor in squamous cell carcinomas. Jpn J Cancer Res (Gann) 76:663–666
3. Ozawa S, Ueda M, Ando N, Abe O, Shimizu N (1988) Epidermal growth factor receptors in cancer tissues of esophagus, lung, pancreas, colorectum, breast, and stomach. Jpn J Cancer Res (Gann) 79:1201–1207
4. Ozawa S, Ueda M, Ando N, Abe O, Hirai M, Shimizu N (1987) Stimulation by EGF of the growth EGF receptor-hyperproducing tumor cells in athymic mice. Int J Cancer 40:706–710
5. Ozawa S, Ueda M, Ando N, Shimizu N, Abe O (1989) Prognostic significance of epidermal growth factor receptor in esophageal squamous cell carcinomas. Cancer 63:2169–2173
6. Ozawa S, Ueda M, Ando N, Abe O, Minoshima S, Shimizu N (1989) Selective killing of squamous carcinoma cells by an immunotoxin that recognizes the EGF receptor. Int J Cancer 43:152–157
7. Hirota N, Ueda M, Ozawa S, Abe O, Shimizu N (1989) Suppression of an epidermal growth factor receptor-hyperproducing tumor by an immunotoxin conjugate of gelonin and a monoclonal anti-epidermal growth factor receptor antibody. Cancer Res 49:7106–7109
8. Downward J, Yarden Y, Mayes E, Scrace G, Totty N, Stockwell P, Ullrich A, Schlessinger J, Waterfield MD (1984) Close similarity of epidermal growth factor receptor and v-*erb* B oncogene protein sequences. Nature 307:521–527
9. Hertler AA, Frankel AE (1989) Immunotoxins: A clinical review of their use in the treatment of malignancies. J Clin Oncol 7:1932–1942

Two Types of Monoclonal Antibodies Against Human Esophageal Squamous Cell Carcinoma

YUSUKE TOMITA, HIDEAKI YAMANA, and TERUO KAKEGAWA[1]

Introduction

In this paper, we summarized our preliminary results using two types of murine monoclonal antibodies (mAb) against human squamous cell carcinoma of the esophagus for quantitative diagnosis and selection of the optimum therapy.

Materials and Methods

Production of Monoclonal Antibody [1]

Male BALB/c mice, 8- to 10-weeks old, were immunized i.p. with 1×10^7 cells (KE-1 or KE-2 tumor cell lines) of esophageal squamous cell carcinomas. The BALB/c mice spleens were harvested under sterile conditions and fused with NS-1 murine myeloma line, using polyethylene glycol 1000, by a modified method of Gefter et al. [2]. All hybrids were selected in hypoxanthine amino-pterine thymicline (HAT) medium. About 2 weeks after fusion, supernatants from growth positive cells were screened for frozen sections of KE-1 or KE-2 tumor by immunohistochemical staining. Subsequently, hybrids with high reactivity were cloned.

Human Cell Lines

The following cell lines were used for screening of mAb: Epidermoid carcinoma, A-431; tongue carcinoma, SCC-9; lung adenocarcinoma, PC-3; gastric aden-ocarcinoma, KATO-III; colon cancer, COLO-205; leukemia cell, K-562 and Daudi; esophageal carcinoma, KE-1, KE-2, TE-10, TE-11, YES-2, and YES-6.

---

[1] The First Department of Surgery, Kurume University School of Medicine, 67 Asahimachi, Kurume, Fukuoka, 830 Japan

Immunohistochemical Staining

The avidine-biotin-peroxidase complex (ABC) method [3] was used to study the phenotypic expression of squamous cell carcinoma of the esophagus. Several normal tissues and malignant tumor tissues were also used in the immunohistochemical study.

Isotyping and Purification of mAb

To determine the isotype of mAb monospecific rabbit antisera to mouse immunoglobulin isotypes (Mouse Monoclonal Typing Kit, BDS (Birmingham, UK)) were used. A large amount of mAb was purified from ascitic fluid by 50% ammonium sulfate precipitation and gel chromatography using Sephacryl S-300 (Pharmacia Fine Chemicals; Uppsala, Sweden) or Protein-A MAPS kit (Bio-Rad Laboratories; Richmond, Calif.).

SDS-PAGE and Immunoblotting

The cell extracts were separated on 10% sodium dodecyl sulfate (SDS) gel and transferred electrophoretically to nitrocellulose membrane (Western blotting). The nitrocellulose membrane was incubated with diluted culture supernatant of mAb and immunoperoxidase staining was done by using an ABC kit, followed by 3'3-diaminobenzidine HCl (DAB) used as a chromogen.

Radioiodination of mAb and In Vivo Radioimmuno Precipitation

Purified mAb was radiolabeled with ^{125}I with limiting amounts of chloramine-T, followed by gel filtration on PD-10 column in bovine serum albumin-phosphate buffered saline (BSA-PBS).

   Iodinated antibodies with specific activities ranged from 10 to $15 \mu Ci/ml$.

   About $10 \mu Ci$ radiolabeled mAb was injected i.p. into nude mice with KE-1 or KE-2 tumor to investigate in vivo distribution of the antibodies. The nude mice were sacrificed at 3, 5, and 7 days after the injection and the percentage of injected dose per g of tissue weight was calculated by using a scintillation counter.

Results

Production of mAbs

Only two clones, KYSM-1 and KIS-1, were selected for detailed studies. KYSM-1 and KIS-1 were produced by KE-1 and KE-2 cells as a antigen, respectively.

Reactivity Against Human Cells, Normal Tissues, and Malignant Tumors

Both mAbs reacted with six esophageal squamous cancer cell lines, the KATO-III gastric cancer cell line, and SCC-9 tongue cancer cell lines (Table 1).

Table 1. Immunohistochemical reactivity of KYSM-1 and KIS-1 with various human cell lines

Monoclonal antibodies		KYSM-1	KIS-1
Human cell lines		Reactivity	
Epidermoid carcinoma:	A-431	−	−
Tongue carcinoma:	SCC-9	+	+
Lung adenocarcinoma:	PC-3	−	−
Esophageal carcinoma:	KE-1, KE-2	+	+
(Squamous cell carcinoma)	TE-10, TE-11	+	+
	YES-2, YES-6	+	+
Gastric adenocarcinoma:	KATO-III	+	±
Colon adenocarcinoma:	COLO-205	−	−
Leukemia cell:	K-562, Daudi	−	−

Table 2. Immunohistochemical reactivity of KYSM-1 and KIS-1 with various normal tissues

mAbs	KYSM-1	KIS-1
Normal Organ	Reactivity	
Skin	−	−
Mammary gland	−	−
Lung	−	−
Esophagus	+[a]	+[b]
Stomach	−	−
Liver	−	−
Spleen	−	−
Pancreas	−	−
Colon	−	−
Kidney	−	−
Lymph node	−	−

[a] Basal cells were weakly stained; [b] Basal and prickle cells were stained

KYSM-1 and KIS-1 had no reactivity with various normal tissues, excluding normal esophageal epithelium (Table 2). In the immunohistochemical staining of the normal esophageal epithelium, KYSM-1 weakly reacted with basement cells alone, while KIS-1 also reacted with basal and prickle cells. On the other hand, both mAbs strongly reacted with human squamous cell carcinomas with slightly different reactivities between the two mAbs (Table 3).

Isotyping of mAb

The isotypes of KYSM-1 and KIS-1 were IgM and IgG_1, respectively.

SDS-Polyacrylamide Gel Electrophoresis (PAGE) Analysis

For biochemical characterization of antigen, SDS-PAGE analysis of KYSM-1 was performed (Fig. 1). In Western blot analysis of the KE-1 cell lysate, antigen

Table 3. Immunohistochemical reactivity of KYSM-1 and KIS-1 with various human malignant tumors

Monoclonal Antibodies	KYSM-1		KIS-1	
Malignant tumor	Reactivity (%)			
Esophageal carcinoma (Squamous cell ca)	58/63	(92%)	28/30	(93%)
Gastric carcinoma (Adenocarcinoma)	1/12	(8%)	1/15	(7%)
Colon carcinoma (Adenocarcinoma)	0/10	(0%)	0/5	(0%)
Lung carcinoma				
(Squamous cell ca)	4/4	(100%)	6/7	(86%)
(Adenocarcinoma)	0/6	(0%)	2/5	(40%)
(Large cell ca)	0/1	(0%)	0/1	(0%)
(Small cell ca)	0/1	(0%)	0/1	(0%)

ca, Carcinoma

reacting with KYSM-1 showed a single band with a molecular weight of about 60 000; antigen reacting with KIS-1 is now being analyzed.

Radioiodination of mAb and In Vivo Distribution

Immunoreactivity of iodinate mAb was studied by enzyme-linked immunosorbent assay (ELISA) analysis. Both of radiolabeled KYSM-1 and KIS-1 showed a high binding to KE-1 and KE-2 cells. Regarding in vivo accumulation of ^{125}I-labeled antibodies, however, KIS-1 alone showed significantly high values in the tumor at 5 and 7 days after the injection (Fig. 2). Furthermore, the value was significantly higher than that of the ^{125}I-labeled control IgG$_1$.

Discussion

In this study, we present the characterization of two mAbs which seem to recognize different protein antigen of esophageal squamous cell carcinomas. The results showed that KYSM-1 and KIS-1 antibodies strongly reacted with several cell lines and tissues of esophageal squamous cell carcinoma. These two mAbs were also weakly reactive with non-cancerous esophageal epithelium; however, some differences of binding with the tissue specimens were recognized between them. KYSM-1 reacted with basal cells alone and KIS-1 reacted with peribasal cells in the non-cancerous esophageal epithelium. This suggests that each antibody recognized what may be classified as growth antigens of the squamous cell carcinomas. It may be hypothesized from these data that expression of antigen reacting with the two mAb undergoes amplification after cell proliferation during tumor growth.

The molecular weight of KYSM-1 and tissue distribution of target antigens indicate that our mAbs are distinct from anti-EGF receptor antibody and anti-CEA antibody. Therefore, it seems as though our mAbs recognized new antigenic specificities.

Fig. 1. Western blot sodium dodecyl sulfate-polyacrylamide gel electroptoresis (*SDS-PAGE*; 10% gel) analysis of the KE-1 cell lysate. Immunostained with KYSM-1 (lane 1), and with normal mouse IgM (lane 2)

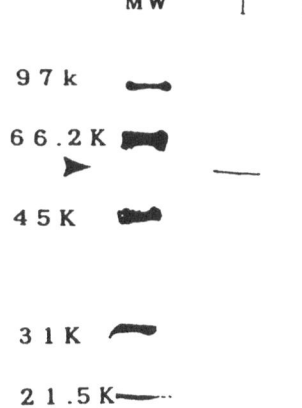

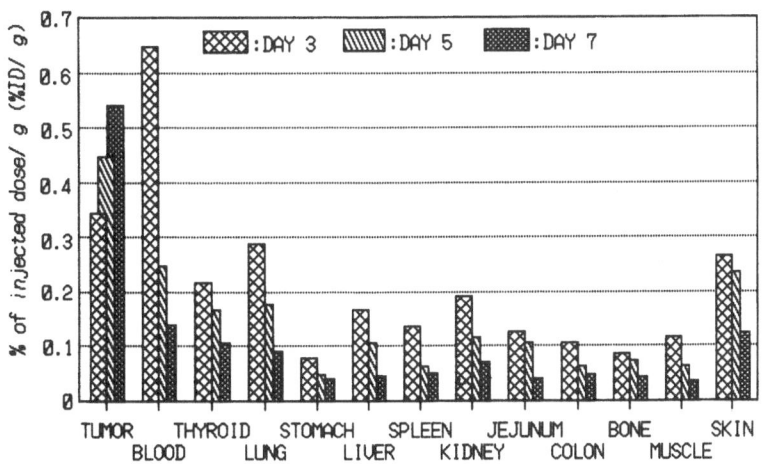

Fig. 2. In vivo distribution of ^{125}I-labeled KIS-1 in nude mice with KE-1 tumor

On the other hand, the result of in vivo distribution of the labelled KIS-1 antibody suggested the possibility of quantitative diagnosis and selection of the optimum therapy for esophageal squamous cell carcinomas, although tumor accumulation of ^{125}I-labeled KYSM-1 antibody had a low value because its subclass was IgM with high molecular weight. Therefore, we are now producing mAb fragment F(ab')2 and/or Fab.

These results suggest that the efficacy of the KIS-1 antibody in quantitative diagnosis and therapy of the esophageal squamous cell carcinomas should be the subject of a subsequent study.

Acknowledgments. TE cells were provided by the Second Department of Surgery, Tohoku University School of Medicine, Sendai, Japan, and YES cells were provided by the Second Department of Surgery, Yamaguchi University School of Medicine, Yamaguchi, Japan.

References

1. Köhler G, Milstein C (1975) Continuous cultures of fused cells secreting antibody of predefined specificity. Nature 256:495–497
2. Gefter ML, Margulies DH, Scharff MD (1977) A simple method for polyethylene glycol-promoted hybridization of mouse myeloma cell. Somat Cell Genet 3:231–236
3. Hus SM, Raine L, Fanger H (1981) Use of avidine-biotin-peroxidase complex (ABC) in immunoperoxidase techniques. J Histochem Cytochem 29:577–580

Statistical Study of Second Primary Malignancies After Esophagectomy for Esophageal Cancer

Toshiyuki Kabuto and Takeshi Iwanaga[1]

Introduction

Along with improvements in the prognosis of esophageal cancer patients, the risk of a patient developing a second primary cancer may have increased. Although double cancer is not rare [1, 2], there have been no statistical studies on whether the incidence of double cancer, involving the esophagus and another organ, is high compared with the estimated incidence based on the morbidity of the general population. We studied the risk of patients developing second primary cancers after esophagectomy for esophageal cancer, using the morbidity rates of malignant neoplasms in our prefecture in Japan.

Materials and Methods

The present study was based on 420 patients who had undergone esophagectomy for primary esophageal cancer in our institute during the years 1962–1990. Age-sex distributions of these patients at the time of esophagectomy are given in Table 1. Thirty-nine patients among them had other organ malignancies which were pathologically confirmed. Ten patients with other primary malignancies preceding esophageal cancer were omitted in this study. Table 2 shows the sites and time of detection of second primary cancers after esophagectomy. Eighteen out of these 39 patients were found to have other organ malignancies simultaneously or less than 1 year after esophagectomy, and 21 patients developed second primary cancers more than 1 year after esophagectomy. The expected incidence of other malignant neoplasms in these 420 patients was calculated by using the person-year method with the morbidity data from our Osaka prefecture,

[1] Department of Surgery, The Center for Adult Diseases, Osaka, 1-3-3 Nakamichi Higashinari-ku, Osaka, 537 Japan

Table 1. Age-sex distribution of study subjects

Age (years)	Male	(%)	Female	(%)	Total	(%)
35–	2	0.6	0	0.0	2	0.5
40–	11	3.3	4	4.9	15	3.6
45–	17	5.0	5	6.1	22	5.2
50–	46	13.6	10	12.2	56	13.3
55–	85	25.1	12	14.6	97	23.1
60–	74	21.9	16	19.5	90	21.4
65–	55	16.3	26	31.7	81	19.3
70–	31	9.2	7	8.5	38	9.0
75–	14	4.1	2	2.4	16	3.8
80–	3	0.9	0	0.0	3	0.7
Total	338	100.0	82	100.0	420	100.0
Mean	60.8 years		61.4 years		61.0 years	

35–, 35–40 years old

Table 2. Second primary cancers after esophagectomy for esophageal cancer by time of occurrence of secondary malignancies

Site	Period after esophagectomy											Total
	<1	1–	2–	3–	4–	5–	6–	7–	8–	9–	10< (years)	
Head and neck	6	1							1	1	1	10
Stomach	10	1	1			1			1			14
Colon		1	1	1		1					1	5
Lung		1				1						2
Gall bladder	1					1						2
Liver									1			1
Uterus	1											1
Breast				1								1
Urinary bladder												1
Leukemia						1						1
Soft tissues						1						1
Subtotal	18	4	2	2	0	6	0	0	3	1	2	
Total	18						21					39

1–, from 1 to 2 years after esophagectomy

in Japan. Calculations were made from the morbidity data to give the site-specific sex, 5-year age, and 5-year calendar period incidence rates for each cancer among Osaka residents. The statistical methods used were based on the assumption that the observed number of cancers in any specific category follows a Poisson distribution.

Table 3. Observed (O) and expected (E) numbers of second primary cancers after esophagectomy for esophageal cancer, by site

Site	Observed (O)	Expected (E)	O/E
Head and neck	10	0.43	23.26**
Stomach	14	3.79	3.69**
Colon	5	0.76	6.58*
Lung	2	2.19	0.91
Gall bladder	2	0.36	5.56
Liver	1	1.74	0.57
Uterus	1	0.19	5.26
Breast	1	0.19	5.26
Urinary bladder	1	0.40	2.50
Leukemia	1	0.15	6.67
Soft tissues	1	0.14	7.14
All malignancies	39	13.38	2.91**

** $P < 0.01$, * $P < 0.05$

Table 4. Observed (O) and expected (E) numbers of second primary cancers after esophagectomy for esophageal cancer, by sex

Site	Males (338)			Females (82)		
	Observed (O)	Expected (E)	O/E	Observed (O)	Expected (E)	O/E
Head and neck	9	0.40	22.50**	1	0.03	33.33
Stomach	12	3.21	3.74**	2	0.58	3.45
Colon	4	0.60	6.67*	1	0.16	6.25
Lung	2	1.96	1.02	—	—	—
Gall bladder	1	0.26	3.85	1	0.10	10.00
Liver	1	1.57	0.64	—	—	—
Uterus	—	—	—	1	0.19	5.26
Breast	—	—	—	1	0.19	5.26
Urinary bladder	1	0.36	2.78	—	—	—
Leukemia	1	0.12	8.33	—	—	—
Soft tissues	—	—	—	1	0.13	7.69
All malignancies	31	11.03	2.81**	8	2.35	3.40*

** $P < 0.01$, * $P < 0.05$

Results

In Table 3, the observed and expected numbers of second primary cancers after esophagectomy are shown. Overall, the observed number of 39 patients with other organ malignancies was significantly higher than the expected number, which was 13.38 (observed/expected (O/E) ratio = 2.91). Considering the specific organs, significant elevations of the O/E ratio were noticed in the head and neck, stomach, and colon, for which the O/E ratios were 23.38, 3.69, and 6.58, respectively. In Table 4, these data are further analyzed according to sex. O/E ratios in all malignancies in both sexes were also significantly greater than 1.

Table 5. Observed (O) and expected (E) numbers of second primary cancers in 239 patients surviving more than 1 year after esophagectomy for esophageal cancer

Site	Observed (O)	Expected (E)	O/E
Head and neck	4	0.23	17.39**
Stomach	4	3.59	1.11
Colon	5	0.72	6.94*
Lung	2	2.08	0.96
Gall bladder	1	0.35	2.86
Liver	1	1.65	0.61
Uterus	0	—	—
Breast	1	0.18	5.56
Urinary bladder	1	0.39	2.56
Leukemia	1	0.15	6.67
Soft tissues	1	0.13	7.69
All malignancies	21	12.72	1.65*

** $P < 0.01$, * $P < 0.05$

However, in relation to specific organs, significant elevations of the O/E ratio for head and neck, stomach, and colon cancers were demonstrable only in males. Table 5 shows data on second primary cancers detected in surviving patients more than 1 year after esophagectomy. The O/E ratio for all malignancies was also significantly elevated, and among specific organs, significant elevation was seen in the head and neck and in the colon O/E ratios.

Discussion

Multiple primary cancers in patients with esophageal cancer are not rare. Goodner and Watson [1] reported an incidence of 9.5% for multiple primary cancer in 1315 cases of cancer of the esophagus. In their series, the majority of second cancers were found in the head and neck, an incidence of 53.9% among double cancers. In Japan, Abo et al. [2] reported 387 cases of double primary cancers of esophagus and other organs among 11 732 cases collected from all over Japan, an incidence of 3.6%. In their series, the majority of double cancers were associated with stomach cancer, an incidence of 76.5% among double cancers.

In our studies, double cancers involving the esophagus and other organs were detected in 39 cases out of 420 with esophageal cancer, an incidence of 9.3%. (If 10 cases with a primary cancer preceding esophageal cancer are included, the incidence was 11.7%). About one-third of the second cancers in our series were in the head and neck and in the stomach, the incidences being 23.8% and 33.3% respectively. In the two previously reported series, the incidence of metachronous second malignancies after esophageal cancer was 0.4% in both cases. In contrast, the incidence was 5% in our present studies. These differences could be due to differences between nations, materials, or periods of studies. Anyway, the incidence of malignancies associated with esophageal cancer was very high. This study revealed that the coexistence of esophageal cancer and other organ malignancies was not a coincidence. Patients with esophageal cancer had a predisposition to other organ malignancies 2.91 times greater than would be expected from the morbidity rate of malignant neoplasms if these patients had the same rates as were prevailing in the corresponding general population. According to sex, significant elevation of the O/E ratio was demonstrable in males, but not in females, because of the small number of the latter. However, essential differences between the sexes cannot be ruled out. In males, significantly elevated O/E ratios were noticed for malignancies in the head and neck, the stomach, and the colon. The close association of cancers in the head and neck and in the stomach with esophageal cancer was suspected, as the same predisposing factors might be involved. However, such a association has not been suspected for colon cancer until now. Further studies on this will be needed.

Our results have revealed such a high incidence of second primary malignancies that careful following up is needed for esophageal cancer patients with this factor in mind.

References

1. Goodner JT, Watson WL (1956) Cancer of the esophagus. Its association with other primary cancers. Cancer 9:1248–1252
2. Abo S, Miura H, Kudo T, Tooma H, Ikeda T, Nakamura M (1980) Concurrent cancer of the esophagus and other organ in Japan (in Japanese). Jpn J Gastroenterol Surg 13:377–381

Clinical Study of Superficial Esophageal Cancer

HIROSHI KUSANAGI, TAKUO MURAKAMI, AKIRA TANGOKU, HIROTO HAYASHI,
HIROYUKI UCHISAKO, and TAKASHI SUZUKI[1]

Summary. Esophagectomy was performed in 31 cases of esophageal cancer in our hospital over the past 16 years. We conducted a retrospective study on superficial esophageal cancer concerning treatment and prognosis, and the therapeutic policy based on the depth of invasion was evaluated. As a result, endoscopic mucosectomy or blunt dissection was found to be suitable for cancer which invaded as far as the epithelium. For cancer, which reached the mucosal layer, esophagectomy with level III node dissection should be performed. However, radical esophagectomy with nodal dissection in three areas (cervical, mediastinal, and abdominal), and postoperative adjuvant therapy should be performed for cancer that involves the submucosa.

Introduction

In Japan, superficial esophageal cancer is defined as carcinoma with a depth of invasion limited to the submucosal layer of the esophageal wall [1]. Recently, endoscopic mucosectomy or extraction of the esophagus without thoractomy is recomended for treatment of superficial esophageal cancer [2, 3]. We studied the treatment and prognosis of superficial esophageal cancer, and evaluated the therapeutic policy based on the depth of invasion.

Patients and Methods

Between January 1975 and January 1991, 31 cases with superficial esophageal cancer were treated by esophagectomy in our hospital. The mean patient age

[1] Department of Surgery II, Yamaguchi University School of Medicine, 1144 Kogushi, Ube, Yamaguchi, 755 Japan

was 60.4 years (range 44–84 years). There were 26 men (84%) and 5 women (16%). The clinicopathological findings, treatment, and prognosis were evaluated.

Results

Table 1 shows the chief complaint of the patients at the time of diagnosis. Seven patients had chest pain or substernal pain. Dysphagia is the most common symptom in patients with advanced cancer. However, 14 cases (45.2%) had no symptoms with regard to the esophagus in superficial cases. Therefore, early diagnosis of esophageal cancer is seldom achieved.

Table 2 shows the location of cancer. This is classified as the cervical, upper thoracic, middle thoracic, and lower thoracic esophagus. Middle thoracic lesions were the most common. This result was similar to advance cancer. The lesion invaded as far as the epithelium (EP) in 3 cases, up to the level of mucosal muscle (MM) in 4 cases, and the submucosal layer (SM) in 24 cases histologically (Table 3).

As shown in Table 4, longitudinal diameter of cancer increases with the depth of invasion. However, eight SM cases of under 20 mm in diameter were found. Of 29 cases, 1 was 8 mm and 7 were 11–20 mm. Table 5 shows the incidence of lymph node metastasis and permeation of lymphatic or vascular vessels. No evidence of lymph node metastasis and permeation of vessels was found in EP cases. Of the 4 MM cases, lymph node metastasis and lymphatic infiltration were observed in 1 case. Of the 31 cases of SM cancer, 7 cases (29%) had lymph node metastasis, 7 had lymphatic infiltration, and 3 had vascular infiltration. EP and MM cases underwent radical resection (lymph node dissection to level III) [1] without any radiochemotherapy, and SM cases were treated by radio-chemotherapy after operation.

Table 6 shows the prognosis of 22 cases (excluding 9 cases with a different other cause of death and intraoperative death). Eight cases died from primary

Table 1. Chief complaint

Chief complaint	No. of patients
Chest pain or substernal pain	7
Dysphagia	6
Vague discomfort	4
Others	6
No complaints	8

Table 2. Location of cancer

Location	No. of patients
Cervical esophagus	3
Upper thoracic esophagus	5
Middle thoracic esophagus	14
Lower thoracic esophagus	9

Table 3. Depth of invasion

Depth of invasion	No. of patients
EP	3
MM	4
SM	24

EP, epithelium; *MM*, muscularis mucosae; *SM*, submucosa

Table 4. Longitudinal diameter of cancer (mm)

	6–10	11–20	21–30	31–40	>41	Mean (mm)
EP	0	3	0	0	0	15
MM	1	2	1	0	0	20
SM	1	7	10	1	5	29

Table 5. Incidence of lymph node metastasis [n(+)], permeation of lymphatic vessels [ly(+)], and permeation of vascular vessels [v(+)]

	n(+)	ly(+)	v(+)
EP	0 (0%)	0 (0%)	0 (0%)
MM	1 (25%)	1 (25%)	0 (0%)
SM	7 (29%)	7 (29%)	3 (14%)

Table 6. Prognosis of 22 patients (except for 9 with other causes of death and intraoperative death)

	Total	Survivals	Death
EP	2	2	0
MM	4	3	1[a]
SM	16	9	7[b]

[a] Radical node dissection was not performed due to cardiac disease
[b] Five patients died from recurrence in the cervical and upper mediastinal lymph nodes

cancer. The relapse in the cervical and upper mediastinal lymph nodes were recognized in five of eight cases. Figure 1 shows cumulative survival curve according to the Kaplan-Meier method. The 5-year survival rate for SM cancer was 56.5%.

Discussion

Recently the rate of detection of superficial esophageal cancer has been increasing by advances in endoscopic diagnosis and chromoendoscopy. In EP cancer, neither the evidence of metastasis involving the lymphatic or vascular vessels, nor lymph node metastasis, has been reported at the present time. Therefore, we emphasize that a limited operation such as endoscopic mucosectomy provides not only radical surgical cure but also satisfactory quality of life after surgery.

The rate of lymph node metastasis in MM cancer is 5.3%–8.3% [4–6]. Of 4 cases of MM cancer, 1 case had lymph node metastasis in our study. In this case, radical node dissection was not performed due to cardiac disease, and he died from recurrence in the lymph nodes. Therefore, the esophagectomy with lymph node dissection is needed for MM cancer. However, it is reported that in most cases of MM cancer, cancer cells invaded close to the mucosal muscle histopathologically [7]. The lesion of MM cancer with lymph node metastasis in our study deeply invaded the mucosal muscle.

If we can precisely evaluate the depth of invasion into the mucosal layer preoperatively indication of limited esophagectomy for MM cancer will be extended. Hence, endoscopic mucosectomy is recommend for mucosal cancer, as not only treatment but also as a diagnostic procedure.

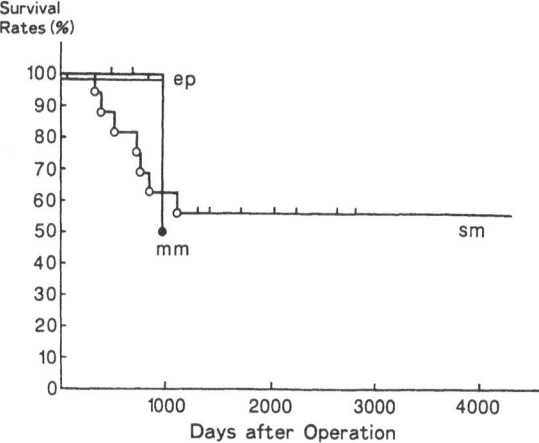

Fig. 1. Survival curve according to Kaplan-Meier, *ep*, epithelium; *mm*, muscularis mucosae; *sm*, Submucosa

In SM cancer, the incidence of lymph node metastasis is approximately 30%–40% [4, 5], and 5-year survival rates for SM cancer have been reported to be approximately 50% to 70% [5, 7, 8]. In our study, of 24 lesion of SM cancer, 7 cases were found to have lymph node metastasis and the 5-year survival rate was 56.5% (Fig. 1). Five of 7 recurrent cases died from the relapse in the cervical and upper mediastinal lymph nodes. In these cases, removal of the lymph node in these area was inadequate. Thus, radical esophagectomy with nodal dissection in the three areas should be done for SM cancer, as in advanced cases.

References

1. Esophageal Disease Research Society (1992) Guidelines for the Clinical and Pathologic Studies on Carcinoma of the Esophagus, 8th edn (in Japanese). Kanehara, Tokyo
2. Makuuchi H, et al. (1991) Endoscopic mucosectomy for mucosal carcinomas in the esophagus (in Japanese with English abstract). Jpn J Gastroenterol 24:2599–2603
3. Momma K, Yoshida M (1991) Indications and results of endoscopic mucosectomy for intraepithelial and mucosal cancer of the esophagus (in Japanese with English abstract). Jpn J Gastroenterol 24:2604–2609
4. Bogomoletz WV, et al (1989) Superficial squamous cell carcinoma of the esophagus. A report of 76 cases and review of literature. Am J Surg Pathol 13:535–546
5. Mitomi T, Makuuchi H, et al (1992) Strategy of treatment for superficial esophageal cancer (in Japanese with English abstract). Based on its clinicopathological features. 15:1729–1739
6. Goseki N, Koike M, Yoshida M (1992) Histopathologic characteristics of early stage esophageal cancer. Cancer 69:1088–1093
7. Endo M, Yoshino K, et al (1992) Modalities of surgical treatment in superficial esophageal cancer (in Japanese). Gastroenterol Surg 15:1741–1747
8. Watanabe H, et al (1992) Surgical treatment for superficial esophageal carcinoma (in Japanese). Gastroenterol Surg 15:1749–1755

Heparin-Binding (Fibroblast) Growth Factors are Potential Autocrine Regulators of Esophageal Epithelial Cell Proliferation

Masafumi Katayama[1] and Mikio Kan[2]

Introduction

We previously established a serum-free culture system for normal human esophageal epithelial cells [1, 2] and reported that crude bovine neural tissue extracts were an effective growth stimulant of normal human esophageal epithelial cells. Neural extracts are a widely used source of heparin-binding (fibroblast) growth factors (HBGF) [3]. Esophageal cell lines also respond to and express epidermal growth factor (EGF) and transforming growth factor (TGF-α) [4]. These results prompted us to establish and examine the role of both the EGF and HBGF families in nonmalignant and malignant esophageal epithelial cell lines. The same culture system used for normal human esophageal cell culture was applied to establish an immortal nonmalignant epithelial cell line from normal esophageal epithelium from the BALB/c mouse (MEE). In the absence of neural extract, a malignant cloned cell line (MEE/C8) was selected from the MEE cells. Here, we compare the growth kinetics of MEE, MEE/C8, and cell lines derived from human esophageal cancer, and their response to EGF and HBGF-1 (acidic fibroblast growth factor, FGF). We show that an HBGF-like activity may play a growth cycle-dependent autocrine role in nonmalignant esophageal epithelial cell proliferation and a constitutive role in support of the malignant cell line.

Materials and Methods

Methods for primary culture of mouse esophageal epithelial (MEE) cells were a modification of previously described procedures [1, 2]. Basal medium (MEE

---

[1] The Second Department of Surgery, Tohoku University School of Medicine, 1-1 Seiryo-machi, Aoba-ku, Sendai, 980 Japan
[2] W. Alton Jones Cell Science Center, Inc., 10 Old Barn Road, Lake Placid, NY 12946, USA

basal medium) consisted of hormone-free, Ca^{2+}-free medium RITC 80-7 containing $CaCl_2$ $(30 \mu M)$, insulin $(1 \mu g/ml)$, transferrin $(10 \mu g/ml)$, L-proline $(175 \mu g/ml)$, and bovine serum albumin (BSA) $(5 mg/ml)$. HBGF-1, EGF, and bovine hypothalamic extract (H-Neurext) (BHE) were from Upstate Biotechnology (Lake Placid, New York). To prepare crude cell extracts, cells were scraped from culture surfaces, suspended in phosphate-buffered saline (PBS), centrifuged and washed twice with PBS, and the cell pellets were stored at $-70°C$ until used. The cell pellets were homogenized with a Potter's homogenizer in $0.5 M$ NaCl, $25 mM$ Tris-HCl (pH 7.1), $1 mM$ EDTA, $0.25 mM$ phenyl methyl sulfonyl fluoride (PMSF), and $1 \mu g/ml$ each of leupeptin and pepstatin, and centrifuged for $30 min$ at $20 000 \times g$ at $4°C$.

Results

Establishment of Mouse Esophageal Cell Lines (MEE and MEE/C8)

The previously reported serum-free culture system for normal human esophageal epithelial cells [1, 2] was applied to normal mouse esophageal epithelium. Rapidly growing colonies of cells (MEE) with apparently normal epithelial cell morphology were observed within several days, and these were subcultured after 20–30 days. Neural tissue extract was absolutely required for colony formation in the primary culture. MEE cells have been maintained for over 1 year (100 passages). We selected a cloned cell line (MEE/C8) from the MEE cultures that grew independently of neural extract at clonal densities. The epithelial character of both MEE cells and MEE/C8 cells was evident under phase contrast microscopy and confirmed by immunochemical staining for keratin antigen (data not shown). Karyotype analysis indicated that MEE cells (92%) were subtetraploid with a modal number of 73 (67–78). However, 97% of MEE/C8 cells exhibited a slightly lower modal number of 68 with a range of 65 to 72 chromosomes. The malignant potential of MEE cells and MEE/C8 cells was compared by inoculation into syngeneic BALB/c mice. MEE cells formed small cysts, and MEE/C8 cells formed solid tumors. Histologic examination revealed only cystic structures that consisted of keratinized squamous epithelium in animals inoculated with MEE cells (data not shown). In contrast, tumors resulting from MEE/C8 cells exhibited an invasive pattern of cell growth (data not shown). MEE/C8 cells clearly exhibited a more malignant phenotype than the MEE cells.

Response of MEE Cells, MEE/C8 Cells, and Human Esophageal Cancer Cell Lines to Growth Factors

A preliminary screen of the activity of single members of major growth factor families on MEE cells in BHE-free medium indicated that EGF/ (TGF-α) and HBGFs were most active. HBGF-1 exhibited about a twofold higher specific activity than that of HBGF-2 (basic FGF) (data not shown); therefore, HBGF-1 was utilized for further study. Dose-responses of MEE cells, MEE/C8 cells, and human esophageal cancer cell lines, TE9 and TE11, to HBGF-1 and EGF are compared in Fig. 1. HBGF-1 or EGF significantly stimulated growth of MEE cells, but had no effect or a slight inhibitory effect on MEE/C8, TE9, or TE11 cells.

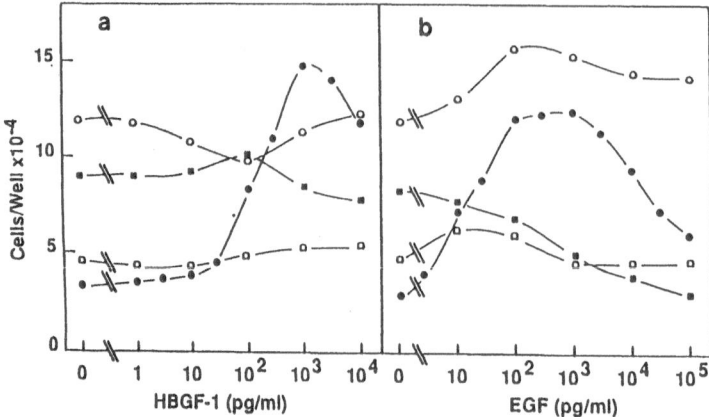

Fig. 1. Effects of heparin-binding growth factor 1 (*HBGF-1*) (**a**) or epidermal growth factor (*EGF*) (**b**) on growth of MEE cells (*solid circles*), MEE/C8 cells (*open circles*), TE9 (*solid squares*) and TE11 (*open squares*). Cells were cultured in MEE basal medium in the presence of the indicated amounts of HBGF-1 (**a**) or EGF (**b**). Cells from subconfluent cultures were harvested and counted

Comparison of Growth-Promoting Activities in Medium and Extracts of MEE Cells, MEE/C8 Cells, and Human Esophageal Cancer Cell Lines

We tested the growth-promoting activity of the medium and extracts of growing MEE cells on quiescent, confluent MEE cells. The crude condition medium of growing MEE cells exhibited only inhibitory effects on confluent MEE cells; however, crude cell extracts exhibited significant stimulatory effects (Fig. 2). Crude extracts of quiescent, confluent MEE cells exhibited no detectable effects (Fig. 2). Extracts from MEE cells, MEE/C8, TE9, and TE11 cells in various media or culture conditions were also tested for effect on DNA synthesis of quiescent, confluent MEE cells (Table 1). The activity in extracts of growing, subconfluent MEE cells was independent of medium components. Growth-promoting activity in extracts of growing and confluent MEE/C8 cells was about the same as that from growing, subconfluent MEE cells. Activity of crude extracts from confluent TE9 or TE11 on DNA synthesis of resting MEE cells was significant, but lower than that of both growing MEE and MEE/C8 cells.

Partial Characterization of the Growth-Promoting Activity in Extracts of MEE/C8 Cells

Because of the ease of scale-up, rapid growth rates, and constitutive expression of activity at high cell densities, we first performed a partial characterization of the activity in extracts of MEE/C8 cells. Crude cell extracts were applied to heparin-agarose [5], and fractions were eluted at different NaCl concentrations and tested for mitogenic activity on quiescent, confluent, nonmalignant MEE cells. Fractions that eluted from the column between 0.7 and 1.0 M NaCl yielded significant growth-promoting activity (data not shown). The fractions from the MEE/C8 cells which were eluted between 0.6 and 1.0 M NaCl from heparin-

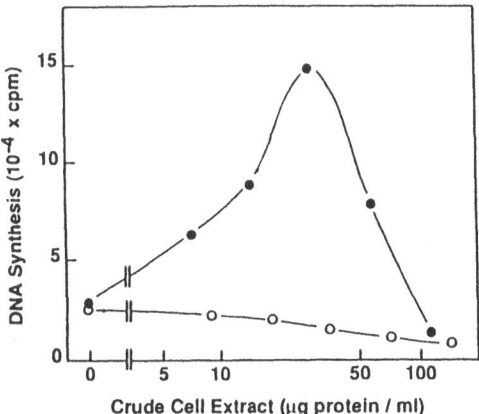

Fig. 2. Activity of crude extracts of proliferating and quiescent MEE cells on DNA synthesis of quiescent MEE cells. Crude cell extracts were prepared from growing, subconfluent MEE cells in MEE basal medium (*solid circles*) or quiescent, confluent MEE cells in MEE basal medium minus insulin (*open circles*). Increasing concentrations of crude cell extracts were added to quiescent, confluent MEE cells, and DNA synthesis was determined

Table 1. Activity of extracts of various mouse esophageal epithelial cell lines on nontumorigenic cells (MEE)[a]

Cells	Medium	Growth stage	ED_{50} (µg/ml)
MEE cells	Serum-free	Quiescent, confluent	Not detectable
	Serum-free + I	Quiescent, confluent	Not detectable
	Serum-free + I	Growing, subconfluent	14.5
	Serum-free + I + EGF	Growing, subconfluent	12.9
	Serum-free + I + BHE	Growing, subconfluent	16.8
	$CaCl_2$ + I + 1% FBS	Growing, subconfluent	16.0
MEE/C8 cells	$CaCl_2$ + I + 1% FBS	Confluent	14.7
TE9	$CaCl_2$ + I + 1% FBS	Confluent	31.2
TE11	$CaCl_2$ + I + 1% FBS	Confluent	50.4

[a] Crude cell extracts were prepared from MEE cells, MEE/C8 cells, TE9, and TE11, cultured in the media and cell growth stages indicated. Increasing concentrations of crude cell extracts were added to quiescent, confluent MEE cells and DNA synthesis was determined. The amount of protein required for half-maximal effect (ED_{50}) on DNA synthesis was determined from dose-response curves similar to those in Fig. 2. "Serum-free" medium consisted of medium RITC 80-7 (HF) containing transferrin (10 µg/ml). Where indicated insulin (I), epidermal growth factor (EGF), bovine hypothalamic extract (BHE), and $CaCl_2$ were added at 1 µg/ml, 1 ng/ml, 75 µg/ml, and 1.8 mM, respectively. *FBS*, fetal bovine serum

agarose chromatography were further purified by reverse-phase HPLC by published procedures established for purification of HBGF-1 [5]. The major growth-promoting activity eluted between 36% and 38% acetonitrile (data not shown). The active HPLC fractions were subjected to immunoblot analysis.

Antibodies against bovine HBGF-1 and HBGF-2 failed to detect specific immun-oreactive bands in fractions exhibiting amounts of activity equal to or greater than easily detectable standard bovine HBGF-1 and HBGF-2 (data not shown).

Discussion

Preliminary characterization of growth factor activity from both proliferating, nonmalignant MEE cells and malignant MEE/C8 cells indicated that the pre-dominant growth factor activity had properties very similar to HBGF-1. However, we were unable to demonstrate clearly the presence of authentic HBGF-1 antigen, although expressor cells exhibit HGBF-1 mRNA (data not shown). Therefore, one or more active factors expressed by esophageal epithelial cells may be HBGF-1 or a homologue. Resolution of this question requires structural identification of the HBGF in the extracts.

Acknowledgments. We thank Dr. Wallace L. McKeehan, in whose laboratory this work was carried out, for support and help in writing the manuscript. The work was supported in part by NCI grants CA37589 and DK35310 to Dr. McKeehan.

References

1. Katayama M, Akaishi T, Nishihira T, Kasai M, Kan M, Yamane I (1984) Primary culture of human esophageal epithelial cells. Tohoku J Exp Med 143:129–140
2. Katayama M, Akaishi T, Nishihira T, Kasai M, Kan M, Yamane I (1986) Primary cultures and serial passages of normal human esophageal epithelial cells in a serum-free medium. In: Kasai M (ed) Esophageal cancer. Excerpta Medica Tokyo, pp 31–34
3. Burgess WH, Maciag T (1989) The heparin-binding (fibroblast) growth factor family of proteins. Annu Rev Biochem 58:575–606
4. Yoshida K, Kyo E, Tsuda T, Tsujino T, Ito M, Niimoto M, Tahara E (1990) EGF and TGF-α, the ligands of hyperproduced EGFR in human esophageal carcinoma cells, act as autocrine growth factors. Int J Cancer 45:131–135
5. McKeehan WL, Crabb JW (1987) Isolation and characterization of different molecular and chromatographic forms of heparin-binding growth factor 1 from bovine brain. Anal Biochem 164:563–569

Association of *hst-1* Gene Amplification with Poor Postoperative Prognosis of Esophageal Carcinoma

Kiyone Chikuba, Takao Saito, Shinya Uchino, Kouich Sato,
Katsuhiro Shimoda, Masaki Miyahara, and Michio Kobayashi[1]

Introduction

In esophageal carcinoma, amplification of epidermal growth factor receptor and *c-myc* gene [1], and coamplification of *hst-1* and *int-2* genes [2, 3] have been reported. The incidence of coamplification of the *hst-1* and *int-2* genes was reported at 30%–50% and was correlated with poor prognosis and high incidence of postoperative recurrence in distal organs of esophageal carcinoma [4]. In this study, we examined whether or not the intensity of *hst-1* amplification is associated with the grade of malignant potential, especially organ metastasis, of esophageal carcinoma.

Subjects and Methods

Subjects

A total of 73 patients with esophageal carcinoma who underwent eso-phagectomy in our clinic between January 1982 and September 1991 were examined. There were 62 men and 11 women ranging in age from 41 to 83 years (mean 63.9 ± 9.12 years). The clinical and pathologic evaluations were made according to the guidelines established by the Japanese Society of Esophageal Diseases [5]. Patients were followed by a periodic check-up in our outpatient clinic.

DNA Extraction

Samples for DNA extraction were obtained from formalin-fixed, paraffin-mbedded blocks of the primary tumors, metastatic lymph nodes, and normal

---
[1] First Department of Surgery, Oita Medical University, Hasama-machi, Oita, 879-55 Japan

tissues adjacent to tumors for controls. The blocks were cut into sections 75 μm thick using a microtome and were removed with a scalpel blade. DNA was extracted following the method of Goelz et al. [6]. After deparaffinization by 100% xylene, the tissue was suspended in TE buffer (500 mM Tris, 20 mM EDTA, 10 mM NaCl, pH 9.0) containing 1% sodium dodecyl sulfate (SDS) and 500 mg/ml proteinase K (Merck Inc.) which were incubated for 24 h at 48°C. Additional SDS and proteinase K were added and incubated for 48 h. Then DNA was extracted by phenol and chlorophoform, two times each.

Dot Blot Analysis

Ten micrograms of DNA were applied to a BAS85 nitrocellulose filter with a Minifold-II apparatus (Schleicher and Schuell Inc.). Filters were baked at 80°C for 2 h in a vacuum. Probes were labeled with [^{32}P] d-CTP using the oligolabeling system [7]. Filters were prehybridized and hybridized to the probes. Filters were washed twice and exposed to Kodak XAR5 film at −80°C using intensifying screens. The probes were removed from the filters, and the filters were rehybridized in turn with the other probes. Autoradiograms were evaluated quantitatively in reference to the signals of serially diluted standards dotted on the same filters. Ten micrograms of DNA were diluted from ×1 to ×1/32 by TE solution and dot hybridized to probes. A copy number over 3-fold was considered to represent amplification.

Probes

Probe C, a 0.59-kilobase pair *AvaII-AvaII* fragment of the *hst-1* gene was kindly provided by Dr Sakamoto [8]; and probe pHIND6.0 gene was obtained from the Japanese Cancer Research Resources Bank (JCRB). pHIND6.0 probe was used as an internal control probe of chromosome 11.

Statistical Analysis

Patient groups were compared using the χ^2-test. The cumulative survival curves for patient groups were calculated by the Kaplan-Meier method, and were compared using general wilcoxon test (two-side test).

Results

Amplification of *hst-1* gene more than 3-fold was observed in 33 of the 73 cases (45%). The degree of amplification evaluated by dot blot analysis with serially diluted DNA samples ranged from 3- to 32-fold. According to the intensity of amplification, patients were divided into three groups: group A, patients with negative amplification (the intensity of amplification, 2-fold or less); group B, those with low-grade amplification (3- to 6-fold); and group C, those with high-grade amplification (7-fold and above). The number of patients was 40, 16, and 17 in groups A, B, and C, respectively.

We then compared demographic features and clinicopathological data among those three groups. The degree of *hst-1* amplification was positively associated with the extent of blood vessel invasion but not with other factors. In 49 patients who underwent curative surgery, the 5-year survival rate was 29% in group A, 15% in group B, 0% in group C, with significant differences between group A and group B, and between group A and group C. The 5-year desease-free rate for recurrent organ metastasis was lower in group C than in groups A and B, and there was a significant difference between groups A and C.

Discussion

The *hst-1* gene, first isolated from gastric carcinoma by NIH3T3 transfection assay [8], is frequently amplified in human cancer of the esophagus or other organs [2]. We have detected *hst-1* gene amplification in 45% of esophageal carcinoma, and an intensity of 7-fold or higher was seen in 23% of patients (group C). This group showed significantly poorer prognosis and more frequent recurrent organ metastasis compared with the other two groups. These results suggest that *hst-1* gene amplification above 7-fold is associated with a higher malignant potential, especially postoperative recurrent organ metastasis, of esophageal carcinoma.

Acknowledgments. The authors would like to thank Dr. S. Hirohashi and Dr. H. Tsuda (Pathology Division, National Cancer Center Research Institute) for their expert technical direction.

References

1. Lu SH, Hsieh LL, Luo FC, Weinstein IB (1988) Amplification of the EGF receptor and *c-myc* genes in human esophageal cancers. Int J Cancer 42:502–505
2. Tsutsumi M, Sakamoto H, Yoshida T, Kakizoe T, Koiso K, Sugimura T, Terada M (1988) Coamplification of the *hst-1* and *int-2* genes in human cancers. Jpn J Cancer Res (Gann) 79:428–432
3. Tsuda T, Tahara E, Kajiyama G, Sakamoto H, Terada M, Sugimura T (1989) High incidence of coamplification of *hst-1* and *int-2* genes in human esophageal carcinoma. Cancer Res 49:5505–5508
4. Kitagawa Y, Ueda M, Ando N, Shinozawa Y, Shimizu N, Abe O (1991) Significance of *int-2/hst-1* coamplification as a prognostic factor in patients with esophageal squamous carcinoma. Cancer Res 51:1504–1508
5. Japanese Society for Esophageal Disease (1992) Guidelines for the Clinical and Pathologic Studies on Carcinoma of the Esophagus, 8th ed. Kanehara, Tokyo
6. Goelz SE, Hamilton SR, Vogelstein B (1985) Purification of DNA formaldehyde-fixed and paraffin-embedded human tissue. Biochem Biophys Res Commun 130:118–126
7. Feinberg AP, Vogelstein B (1983) A technique for radiolabeling DNA restriction endonuclease fragments to high specific activity. Anal Biochem 132:6–13
8. Sakamoto H, Mori M, Taira M, Yoshida T, Matsukawa S, Shimizu K, Sekiguchi M, Terada M, Sugimura T (1986) Transforming gene from human stomach cancers and a noncancerous portion of stomach mucosa. Proc Natl Acad Sci USA 83:3997–4001

Amplification of *hst-1* and *int-2* Genes as a Biological Marker of High Malignancy for Human Esophageal Carcinomas

Kazuhiro Yoshida[1], Hiroki Kuniyasu[2], Toshihiro Hirai[1], Tetsuya Toge[1], and Eiichi Tahara[2]

Introduction

We have previously demonstrated that esophageal carcinomas have some genetic abnormalities and abnormal expression of growth factor-receptor systems. That is, expression of epidermal growth factor (EGF) and EGF receptor (EGFR) genes are expressed in about 40% of esophageal carcinomas and also EGF and transforming growth factor (TGF)-alpha, the ligands of hyperproduced EGFR in human esophageal carcinoma cells act as autocrine growth factors [1, 2]. Moreover, the prognosis of patients with positive expression is poorer than those without expression [3]. We have also reported that coamplification of *hst-1* and *int-2* genes occurs in human esophageal carcinomas [4]. In the present study, we examined whether the amplification of these gene might be a good prognostic marker of high malignancy for human esophageal carcinomas.

Materials and Methods

Materials

A total of 100 primary esophageal squamous cell carcinomas resected in the Department of Surgery in the Research Institute for Nuclear Medicine and Biology were used to extract DNAs from formalin-fixed paraffin-embedded tissues, and 18 metastatic carcinomas of esophageal carcinomas were taken at autopsy. The clinicopathological studies were estimated according to the classification of the Japanese Society for Esophageal Disease.

---

[1]Department of Surgery, Research Institute for Nuclear Medicine and Biology and [2]First Department of Pathology, School of Medicine, Hiroshima University, 1-2-3, Kasumi, Minami-ku, Hiroshima, 734 Japan

DNA Extraction and Slot and Southern Blot Hybridization

DNAs were extracted from formalin-fixed paraffin-embedded tissues as we have described previously [5]. We extracted DNAs from primary tumors and non-neoplastic lesions in the same section and we confirmed the histology at the same time. High molecular DNAs were extracted from fresh samples taken at autopsy and Southern blot analysis was performed. *Hst-1* and the 0.79 kb restriction endonuclease EcoR1 was provided by Dr. M. Terada, the 0.9 kb *int-2* probe from Dr. G. Peters, and the progesterone receptor probe was provided by Dr. G.L. Greene.

Results

The amplification of *hst-1* and *int-2* genes were examined in 18 dysplastic lesions and 100 primary esophageal carcinomas. Figure 1 shows the representative results of slot blot analysis. Although we could not detect any amplification of these genes in dysplastic lesions of the esophagus (Fig. 1A), the amplification of *hst-1* and *int-2* genes were detected in case 11 and case 12. The degree of amplification was 16- and 32-fold, respectively. The progesterone receptor gene, which is located on chromosome 11q, was not amplified. Among 100 primary esophageal carcinomas, coamplification of these genes was detected in 41 cases (41%). Although it was not correlated to patient age and histology of the tumor,

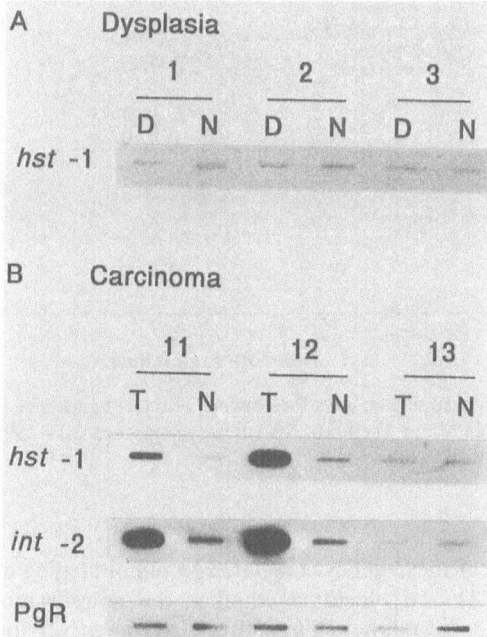

Fig. 1A,B. Coamplification of *hst-1* and *int-2* genes in esophageal carcinomas of case 11 and case 12. Ten μg of DNA from dysplastic lesion (*D*) and carcinomas (*T*) and their adjacent normal tissue (*N*) was used for slot blot analysis. *PgR*, progesterone receptor

Table 1. Correlation of *hst-1* and *int-2* gene coamplification with clinicopathological data

	Cases	Positive cases
LN metastasis		
+	63	27 (42.9%)
−	37	14 (37.8%)
Stage		
0,I	19	3 (15.8%)
II	12	5 (41.7%)
III	36	17 (47.2%)
IV	33	16 (48.5%)
Depth of invasion		
ep-sm	22	3 (13.6%)
mp	18	4 (22.2%)
a_1	20	9 (45.0%)
a_2, a_3	40	25 (62.5%)

LN, lymph node; *ep*, epithelium; *sm*, submucosal; *mp*, muscularis propria; a_1–a_3, adventitia

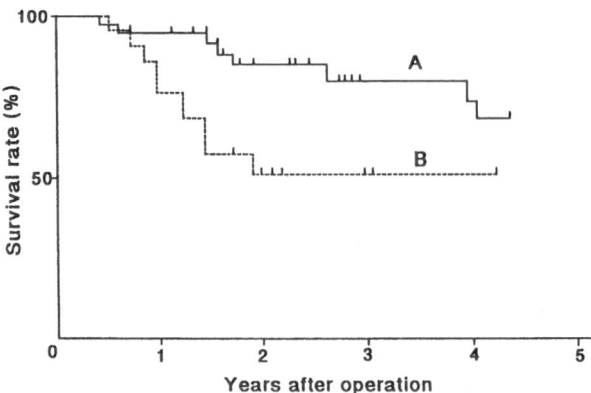

Fig. 2. The cumulative survival curves for patients with (*A*) or without (*B*) gene amplification calculated by Kaplan-Meier method. Statistical significance was observed between gene amplification and patient prognosis ($P < 0.05$)

the amplification of these genes correlated to tumor staging and depth of tumor invasion (Table 1). To elucidate whether the amplification of these genes might be a prognostic marker, cumulative survival curves for the patients with and without gene coamplification were calculated by the Kaplan-Meier method among patients of stage 0 to III and those who underwent curative operation. The prognosis of patients with gene amplification was poorer than those without gene amplification (Fig. 2). Moreover, coamplification of these genes was detected in all the metastatic tumors examined (data not shown). These results indicate that the amplification of these genes might play an important role for tumor progression and patient prognosis for human esophageal carcinomas.

Discussion

Although *hst-1* and *int-2* genes were amplified in 41% of primary esophageal carcinomas, the expression of mRNA has not yet been detected. Recently, the gene which codes for cyclin D which is located on chromosome 11q13 has been isolated [6]. Jiang et al. [7] reported that the coamplification of cyclin D and *hst-1* genes was detected in 20% of primary esophageal carcinomas and expression of mRNA for cyclin D gene was detected in cell lines. Cyclin D is a cell cycle regulatory protein that is found at high levels during G_1 phase of the cell cycle and amplification and overexpression of the gene might lead to uncontrollable tumor cell proliferation. This could play a crucial role in multistep carcinogenesis of esophageal carcinomas. We should further examine the expression of the cyclin D gene in primary and metastatic esophageal carcinomas.

References

1. Yoshida K, Yasui W, Ito H, Tahara E (1991) Growth factors in progression of human esophageal and gastric carcinomas. Exp Pathol 40:291–300
2. Yoshida K, Kyo E, Tsuda T, Tsujino T, Ito M, Niimoto M, Tahara E (1990) EGF and TGF-alpha, the ligands of hyperproduced EGFR in human esophageal carcinoma cells, act as autocrine growth factors. Int J Cancer 45:131–135
3. Mukaida H, Toi M, Hirai T, Ysmashita Y, Toge T (1991) Clinical significance of the expression of epidermal growth factor and its receptor in esophageal cancer. Cancer 68:142–148
4. Tsuda T, Tahara E, Kajiyama G, Sakamoto H, Terada M, Sugimura T (1989) High incidence of coamplification of *hst-1* and *int-2* genes in human esophageal carcinomas. Cancer Res 49:5505–5508
5. Tsujino T, Yoshida K, Nakayama H, Ito H, Shimosato T, Tahata E (1990) Alterations of oncogenes in metastatic tumors of human gastric carcinomas. Br J Cancer 62:226–230
6. Kiyokawa H, Busquets X, Powell CT, Ngo L, Rifkind RA, Marks PA (1992) Cloning of a D-type cyclin from murine erythro-leukemia cells. Proc Natl Acad Sci USA 89:2444–2447
7. Jiang W, Kahn SM, Tomita N, Zhang Y-J, Lu S-H, Weinstein B (1992) Amplification and expression of human cyclin D gene in esophageal cancer. Cancer Res 52:2980–2983

Analysis of Gene Amplification in Human Esophageal Cancer

Hiroyuki Suzuki[1], Shichisaburo Abo[1], Michihiko Kitamura[1], Masaji Hashimoto[1], Keiichi Izumi[1], Kunihiko Terada[2], and Toshihiro Sugiyama[2]

Introduction

The "multistep" of genetic alterations is necessary for cancer formation [1], but there are few reports dealing with both oncogenes and tumor suppressor genes in human esophageal cancer. To investigate the correlation between oncogenes and esophageal cancer, we examined gene amplification of the *int-2* and *erbB* genes, and the p53 and DCC tumor suppressor genes by Southern blot analysis.

Methods

Tissues

From 23 patients with esophageal carcinoma, 23 primary tumors, 23 normal esophageal mucosas, and 4 metastatic tumors, including 3 lymph node and 1 liver tumor, were collected at surgical operation or autopsy. There were 22 squamous cell carcinoma and 1 adenosquamous carcinoma of the esophagus.

DNA Extraction

Genomic DNA was extracted with phenol-chloroform method [2] after treatment with sodium dodecyl sulfate (SDS) and proteinase K.

Southern Blot Analysis

DNA was digested with a 10-fold excess of restriction endonuclease (*EcoRI* to detect the amplification of *erbB*, p53 and DCC, *BamHI* to detect the amplification

[1] Second Department of Surgery, [2] Department of Biochemistry, Akita University School of Medicine, 1-1-1 Hondo, Akita, 010 Japan

of *int-2*) and 10 µg of completely digested DNA was electrophoresed in 0.8% agarose gel. Gels were transferred to nylon filters (Gene Screen Plus, Dupont) using the Southern blot technique [3], and hybridized with probes labeled to specific activity of 10^8–10^9 cpm/µg, by [α-^{32}P]-dCTP using random primers. After hybridization, the filters were washed for 2 h at 65°C in 1 mM EDTA, 40 mM $NaHPO_4$, 1% SDS, changing the buffer every 30 min, and then exposed to x-ray films at −80°C.

Probes

The probes used were: SS6, a 0.9 kb *SacI* fragment of the *int-2* gene [4]; pE7, a 2.4 kb cDNA fragment of the *erbB* gene [5]; p53-176, a 1.35 kb cDNA fragment of the p53 gene [6]; and DCC, a cDNA fragment of the DCC gene. SS6, pE7, and p53-176 were obtained from JCRB (Japanese Cancer Research Resources Bank-Gene), and DCC was provided by Dr. Akiyama.

Statistical Analysis

Patient groups were compared using the Chi-square test with the criterion of $P < 0.05$. The cumulative survival curves for patient groups were calculated by the Kaplan-Meier method and were compared using the generalized Wilcoxon test.

Results and Discussion

As it has become possible to identify the molecular events that underlie carcino-genesis, we focused our attention on "multistep carcinogenesis". We examined 23 esophageal tumors for amplification of oncogenes and tumor suppressor genes by Southern blot analysis. Our results reinforce several observations from prior studies [7]–[10]. Figure 1 shows examples of Southern blot analysis with the SS6 probe, which is a part of the *int-2* gene. Primary tumor tissues sampled from cases 2, 6, 7, 8, 9, and 10 and metastatic tissues sampled from case 10

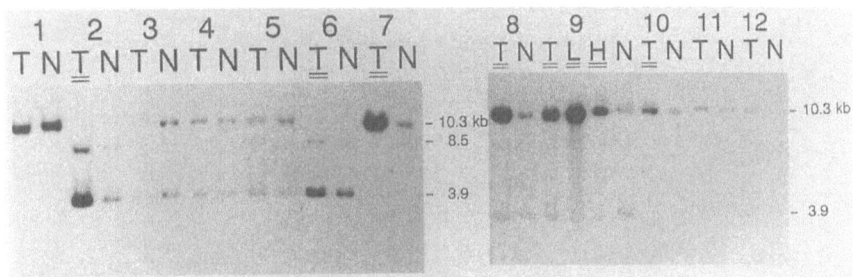

Fig. 1. Southern blot analysis with the SS6 probe which is specific for the *int-2* gene. *Top abscissa numbers*, patient number; *Right ordinate number*, size of gene. *T*, primary tumor tissue; *L*, metastatic lymph node; *H*, metastatic tumor of the liver; *N*, normal adjacent esophageal mucosa. = indicates *int-2* gene amplification

Table 1. Analysis of gene amplifications in human esophageal cancer

No.	int-2	erbB	p53	stage	Prognosis	month
1	—	—	—	IV	DEAD	12
2	●	●	○	III	RECUR	22
3	—	—	—	IV	alive	21
4	—	—	—	IV	dead	8
5	—	—	—	0	alive	19
6	●	—	—	IV	RECUR	18
7	●	—	—	IV	DEAD	8
8	●	—	NP	IV	dead	0
9	●	NP	NP	IV	DEAD	4
10	—	—	NP	III	alive	18
11	—	—	NP	III	alive	18
12	—	—	NP	III	DEAD	10
13	●	—	NP	IV	alive	17
14	NP	NP	NP	III	alive	16
15	●	—	NP	III	alive	13
16	●	—	NP	IV	alive	13
17	NP	NP	NP	III	alive	13
18	●	●	NP	III	alive	12
19	—	—	NP	IV	RECUR	11
20	●	—	NP	IV	DEAD	9
21	NP	NP	NP	IV	DEAD	4
22	NP	NP	NP	III	alive	11
23	NP	NP	NP	III	alive	10

●, Amplification; ○, Rearrangement; *NP*, not performed; *DEAD*, Death caused cancer; *dead*, Death caused other disease; *RECUR*, Recurrence; *alive*, Disease free state

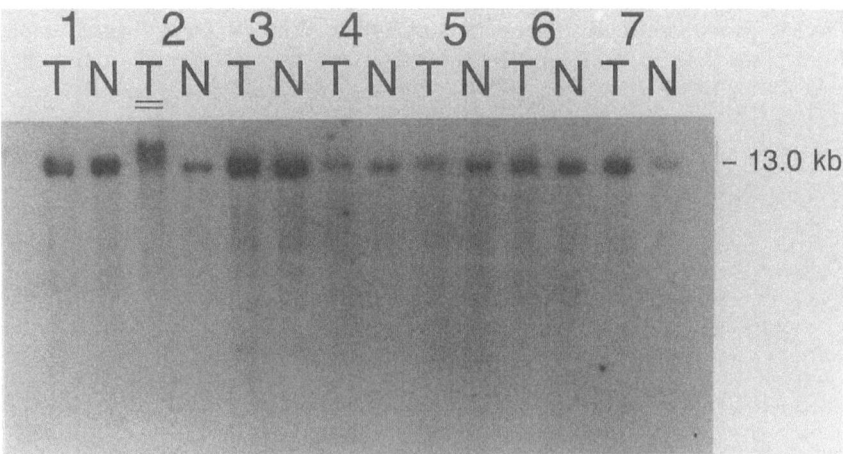

Fig. 2. Southern blot analysis with the p53-176 probe which is specific for the p53 gene. *Top abscissa numbers*, patient number; *Right ordinate number*, size of gene; *T*, primary tumor tissue; *N*, normal adjacent esophageal mucosa. = indicates p53 gene rearrangement

showed amplification of the *int-2* gene. Overall, amplification of the *int-2* gene was observed in ten primary tumor tissues in 17 cases (58.8%). Previously, amplification of the *int-2* gene, mostly coamplifying with the *hst-1* gene, was reported in breast carcinoma [11], carcinoma of the head and neck [12], bladder cancer [13], melanoma [14], gastric carcinoma [15], and hepatocellular carcinoma [16]. Comparing these reports, the frequency of *int-2* gene amplification in esophageal carcinoma was higher than that in the other tumors. However, the incidence of amplification in the four metastatic tumors in our series was 100%.

Table 2. Correlation of *int-2* amplification with clinicopathological data

Parameter[a]	Number	amplification (%)
Age years		
50–60	5	4 (80)
60–70	8	4 (50)
>70	5	2 (40)
Location		
Ce	1	0 (0)
Iu	2	2 (100)
Im	9	7 (78)
Ei	6	1 (17)
Histologic type		
Well differentiated	5	4 (80)
Moderately differentiated	8	3 (38)
Poorly differentiated	4	2 (50)
Adenosquamous	1	1 (100)
Invasion to the adventitia		
a_0	4	1 (25)
a_1	2	0 (0)
a_2	7	5 (71)
a_3	5	3 (60)
Lymph node metastasis		
$n_{(-)}$	4	2 (50)
$n_{1(+)}$	0	
$n_{2(+)}$	7	4 (57)
$n_{3(+)}$	3	2 (67)
$n_{4(+)}$	4	2 (50)
Histological stage		
0	1	0 (0)
I	0	
II	0	
III	7	4 (57)
IV	10	6 (60)
Recurrence		
Positive	8	5 (63)
Negative	8	4 (50)

[a] According to the classification of the Japanese Society for Esophageal Disease. *Ce*, cervical esophagus; *Iu*, upper intra-thoracic esophagus; *Im*, middle intra-thoracic esophagus; *Ei*, lower intra-thoracic esophagus

This result suggests that amplification of the *int-2* gene plays a role in the progression or metastasis of esophageal cancer.

Two of 17 cases (11.8%) of esophageal carcinomas showed amplification of the *erbB* gene (Table 1). The incidence of *erbB* gene amplification was similar to that in another report [7].

Concerning the tumor suppressor genes in esophageal cancer, we could detect the amplification of neither the p53 gene nor the DCC gene. However, we found rearrangement of the p53 gene in primary esophageal carcinoma (Fig. 2). Although numerous studies have reported on the mutation of the p53 gene [17] and on the loss of heterozygosity involving the p53 gene [18] in esophageal cancer, there are few reports which describe the rearrangement of the p53 gene in human neoplasms [19].

The clinicopathological data for each case are summarized in Table 2. We did not find a significant correlation between amplification of the *int-2* gene and any of a variety of clinicopathological backgrounds, although the location of the primary tumor tended to correlate with amplification of the *int-2* gene.

In addition, we found a patient with esophageal cancer (case 2) with three different types of genetic alterations in oncogenes and a tumor suppressor gene, i.e., amplification of the *int-2* and *erbB* gene and rearrangement of the p53 gene. This is the first report of a case with such genetic alterations in esophageal cancer. Further studies of this case may reveal the mechanisms of multistep carcinogenesis in esophageal cancer.

References

1. Fearon ER, Vogelstein B (1990) A genetic model for colorectal tumorigenesis. Cell 61:759–767
2. Maniatis T, Fritsch EF, Sambrook J (1982) Molecular cloning: A laboratory manual. Cold Spring Harbor, NY: Cold Spring Harbor Laboratories
3. Southern EM (1975) Detection of specific sequences among DNA fragments separated by gel electrophoresis. J Mol Biol 98:503–517
4. Casey G, Smith R, McGillivray D, Peters G, Dickson C (1986) Characterization and chromosome assignment of the human homolog of int-2, a potential proto-oncogene. Mol Cell Biol 6:502–510
5. Xu Y-H, Richert N, Ito S, Merlino G, Pastan I (1984) Characterization of epidermal growth factor receptor gene expression in malignant and normal human cells. Proc Natl Acad Sci USA 81:7308–7312
6. Zakut-Houri R, Bienz-Tadmor B, Givol D, Oren M (1985) Human p53 cellular tumor antigen: cDNA sequence and expression in COS cells. Embo J 4:1251–1255
7. Hollstein MC, Smits AM, Galiana C, Yamasaki H, Bos JL, Mandard A, Partensky C, Montesano R (1988) Amplification of epidermal growth factor receptor gene but no evidence of *ras* mutations in primary human esophageal cancers. Cancer Res 48:5119–5123
8. Toshitaka Tsuda, Eiichi Tahara, Goro Kajiyama, Hiromi Sakamoto, Masaaki Terada, Takashi Sugimura (1989) High incidence of coamplification of *hst*-1 and *int*-2 genes in human esophageal carcinomas. Cancer Res 49:5505–5508
9. Takashi Wagata, Kanji Ishizaki, Masayuki Imamura, Yutaka Shimada, Mituo Ikenaga, Takayoshi Tobe (1991) Detection of 17p and amplification of the *int*-2 gene in esophageal carcinomas. Cancer Res 51:2113–2117
10. Yuhkoh Kitagawa, Masakazu Ueda, Nobutoshi Ando, Yohtaro Shinozawa, Nobuyoshi Shimizu, Osahiko Abe (1991) Significance of *int-2/hst-1* coamplification as a prognostic factor in patients with esophageal squamous carcinoma. Cancer Res 51:1504–1508

11. Ali IU, Merlo G, Callahan R, Lidereau R (1989) The amplification unit on chromosome 11q13 in aggressive primary human breast tumors entails the *bcl-1*, *int-2* and hst loci. Oncogene 4:89–92
12. Zhou DJ, Casey G, Cline MJ (1988) Amplification of *int-2* gene in breast cancers and squamous cell carcinomas. Oncogene 2:279–282
13. Tsutsumi M, Sakamoto H, Yoshida T, Kakizoe T, Koiso K, Sugimura T, Terada M (1988) Coamplification of the *hst-1* and *int-2* genes in human cancers. Jpn J Cancer Res 79:428–432
14. Adelaide J, Mattei MG, Marics I, Raybaund F, Planche J, Lapeyriere OD, Brinbaum D (1988) Chromosomal localization of the *hst* oncogene and its coamplification with the *int2* oncogene in human melanoma. Oncogene 2:413–416
15. Yoshida MC, Wada M, Satoh H, Yoshida T, Sakamoto H, Miyagawa K, Yokota J, Koda T, Kakinuma M, Sugimura T, Terada M (1988) Human *HST-1* (*HSTF1*) gene maps to chromosome band 11q13 and coamplifies with the *INT2* gene in human cancer. Proc Natl Acad Sci USA 85:4861–4864
16. Hatada I, Tokino T, Ochiya T, Matsubara K (1988) Coamplification of integrated hepatitis B virus DNA and transforming gene *hst-1* in a hepatocellular carcinoma. Oncogene 3:537–540
17. Hollstein MC, Metcalf RA, Welsh JA, Montesano R, Harris CC (1990) Frequent mutation of the p53 gene in human esophageal cancer. Proc Natl Acad Sci USA 87:9958–9961
18. Meltzer SJ, Jing Yin, Ying Huang, McDaniel TK, Newkirk C, Iseri O, Vogelstein B, Resau JH (1991) Reduction to homozygosity involving p53 in esophageal cancers demonstrated by polymerase chain reaction. Proc Natl Acad Sci USA 88:4976–4980
19. Masuda H, Miller C, Koeffler HP, Battifora H, Cline MJ (1987) Rearrangement of the p53 gene in human osteosarcomas. Proc Natl Acad Sci USA 84:7716–7719

pH Monitoring of Gastric Tube After Esophagectomy

Masahiro Nishikawa, Takuo Murakami, Akira Tangoku,
Hiroto Hayashi, Hiroyuki Uchisako, Hiroshi Kusanagi,
Masashi Tsurumi, and Takashi Suzuki[1]

Introduction

Recently, an increasing number of patients with esophageal cancer who were not considered successfully treated have survived for prolonged periods. Proper selection of the tissue to be reconstructed as well as the reconstruction route is important for proper postoperative functioning. However, there have been few reports concerning acidity in the reconstructed gastric tube after esophagectomy combined with bilateral truncal vagotomy. In this study, we used pH monitoring to examine acid secretion in the reconstructed gastric tube.

Subjects and Methods

The patients were divided into an acute group which was observed immediately after surgery and a chronic group which was observed only during the period of oral digestion.

Acute Phase

Sixteen patients (14 males and 2 females; median age of 62.2 years) received reconstructed gastric tubes by a retrosternal reconstruction route in 14 cases and posterior mediastinal route in 2 cases. Eight patients had a pyloroplasty and eight had a pyloromyotomy which ruptured the pylorus with gradual pressure between the externally applied thumb and forefinger. The gastric tube was 4 cm wide and made using the greater curvature of the stomach (Fig. 1). A miniature glass electrode pH sensor (diameter 2.4 mm; PH-3110, KR-5010, Kuraray) was

[1] Department of Surgery II, Yamaguchi University School of Medicine, 1144 Kogushi, Ube, Yamaguchi, 755 Japan

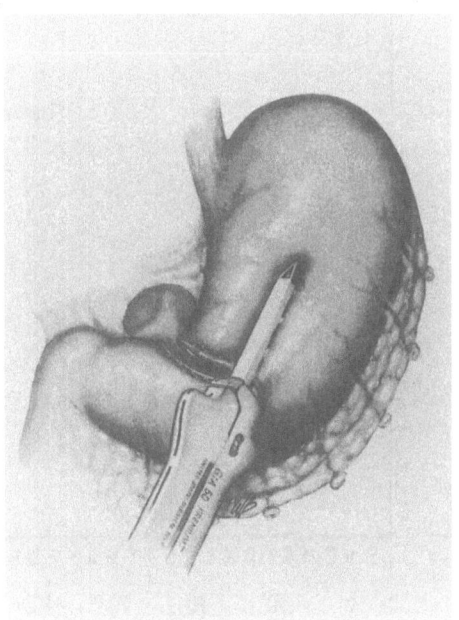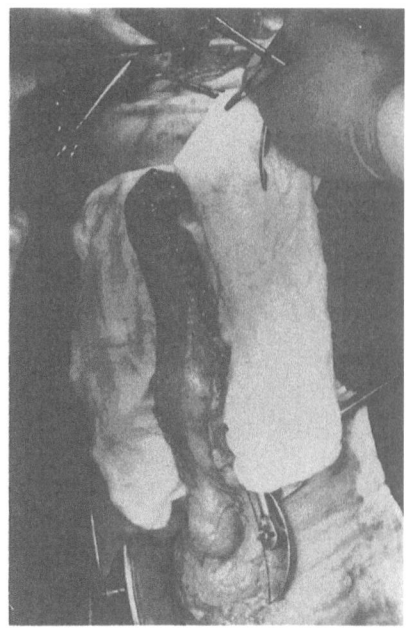

b

Fig. 1. a The gastric tube being made with auto suture "GIA," and **b** completed, with a width of 4 cm

calibrated at 20°C with standard buffers (pH 7.2 and 3.8) and then during surgery, it was inserted in the gastric tube about 10 cm in the rectal direction from the position of esophagogastroanastomosis. The patients were kept in the intensive care unit with tracheal cannulation and monitored for periods up to 10 days. All patients received H2 blocker intravenously (20 mg, twice a day).

Chronic Phase

Fifteen patients (11 males and 4 females; median age of 58.0 years) received gastric tubes by the retrosternal route in 11 cases, intrathoracic route in 3 cases, and posterior mediastinal route in 1 case. All cases were subjected to digital pyloromyotomy. They were observed for periods from 1 month to 28 months. A pH sensor similar to that used in the acute phase was cannulated nasally under fluoroscopic observation, and the tip of the sensor was placed in the gastric tube about 10 cm in the rectal direction from the position of esophagogastroanastomosis, and monitored for 24 h. The placement of the sensor was similar to that in the acute group.

Data were accumulated every 15 min, and stored on a floppy disc via an NEC computer. Analysis was performed using software available from Kuraray to obtain average pH and pH holding time (ratio of the time period of pH 3 or higher, to the entire continuous monitoring period).

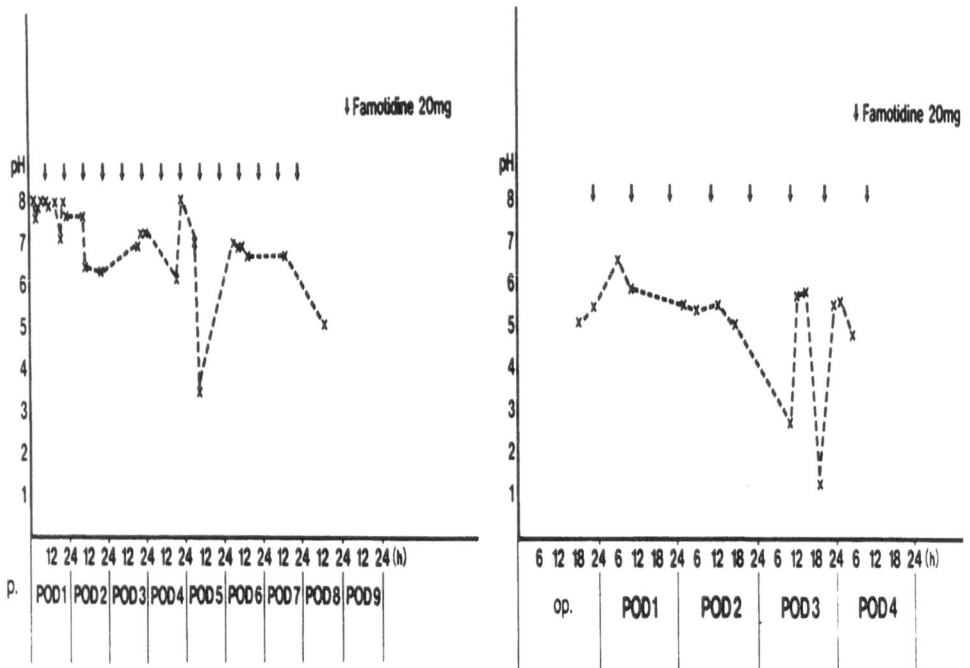

Fig. 2. The pH profiles of intragastric tubes of two cases in the acute phase after esophagectomy. *OP*, operation; *POD*, postoperative day

Results

Acute Phase

All cases exhibited pH 3 or lower on the 5th postoperative day. pH increased temporarily when H2 blocker was given intravenously (Fig. 2).

Chronic Phase

The average pH over 24 h was 3.9 ± 1.5, while the holding time was 52.2%.

Discussion

Acid secretion ability of the reconstructed gastric tube combined with bilateral truncal vagotomy for esophageal cancer is not well understood.

Using pH monitoring, acid secretion ability was observed immediately after surgery and sustained well even 3 months after surgery when the effects of vagotomy began to appear. In fact, no significant difference was observed in average pH or in pH holding time between patients with reconstructed gastric tubes and healthy volunteers without a history of ulcers (14 males; median age of 50.2) (Fig. 3, pH: 3.9 ± 1.5 vs 3.3 ± 1.9, pH holding time: 52.2% vs 57.1%).

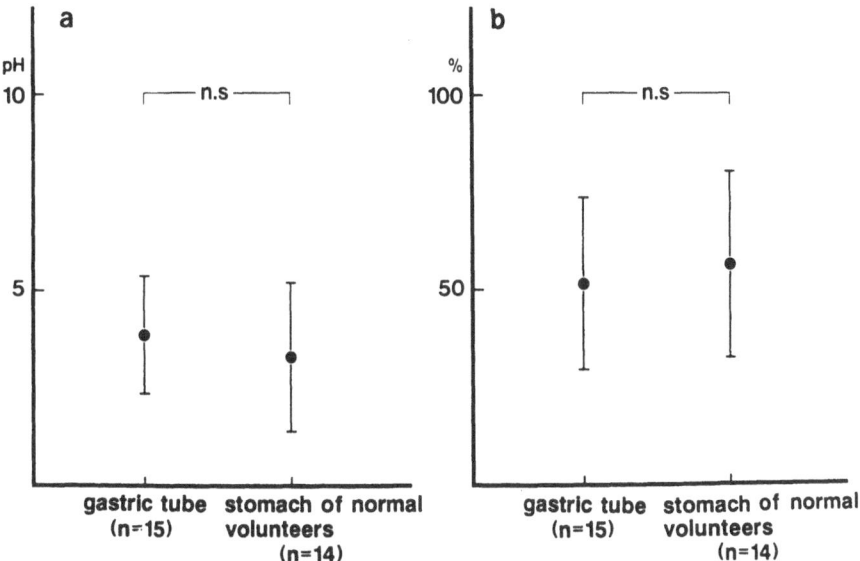

Fig. 3. a Average pH value and **b** pH-3 holding time of reconstructed gastric tubes compared with stomach of normal volunteers. *n.s.*, nonsignificant; *Bars*, mean ± standard error

pH monitoring of the reconstructed gastric tube was also reported by Bouchucha et al. [1]. We reported the present monitoring study at the Japanese Chest Surgery Society meeting in 1990 in Japan, and suggested the presence of acid secretion ability. Then, similar reports were made from other facilities, with the secreted acid being emphasized as the reason for ulceration at the site of anastomosis in cases of reconstructed gastric tube. However, no quantitative factor of acid secretion was observed in pH monitoring. Gastric emptying, on which pyloroplasty has an effect, and humoral factors such as gastrin, may also be involved to some degree, depending on the case. As the number of patients surviving esophageal cancer surgery increases, ulceration in the reconstructed gastric tube becomes a more serious complication. Further investigation of individual cases is required to understand and utilize protective factors such as enhancing blood flow in the reconstructed gastric tube, rather than long-term administration of a drug with an inhibitory effect on acid secretion such as an H2 blocker or a proton pump inhibitor.

References

1. Bouchoucha M, Cugnenc PH, Drevillon C, Faye A, Boboc B, Arphan P, Barbier JPh (1989) Functional evaluation of gastric transplants used in esophageal reconstruction. Dysphagia 4:53–57

Experimental and Clinical Study of Blood Flow in the Tracheal Mucosa

HIROYUKI UCHISAKO, TAKUO MURAKAMI, AKIRA TANGOKU,
HIROTO HAYASHI, HIROSHI KUSANAGI, and TAKASHI SUZUKI[1]

Introduction

We investigated the relationship between prevention of pulmonary complications after surgery for esophageal cancer and preservation of the right bronchial artery and the vagus nerve during surgery experimentally in dogs, and clinically. Changes in the bronchial mucosal blood flow (BMBF) were studied using Laser Doppler velocimetry.

Animal Study

Method

Endotracheal intubation was done and right thoracotomy was performed on adult mongrel dogs under general anesthesia (GOE). The dogs were divided into the following groups:

Group 1: Thoracotomy
Group 2: Divided right bronchial artery
Group 3: Divided vagal nerve
Group 4: Divided right bronchial artery and vagal nerve, and extensive mobilization of the trachea

Changes in blood flow (ml/min/100 g) in the bronchial mucosa were observed and compared among these groups. For determination of the blood flow in the tracheal mucosa, Laserflo (Vasa Medics, St Paul, Minn.) was attached to a spiral tube equipped with a Fome-Cuf (Bivona, Gary, Ind.) so that pressure could be monitored.

[1] Department of Surgery II, Yamaguchi University School of Medicine, 1144 Kogushi, Ube, Yamaguchi, 755 Japan

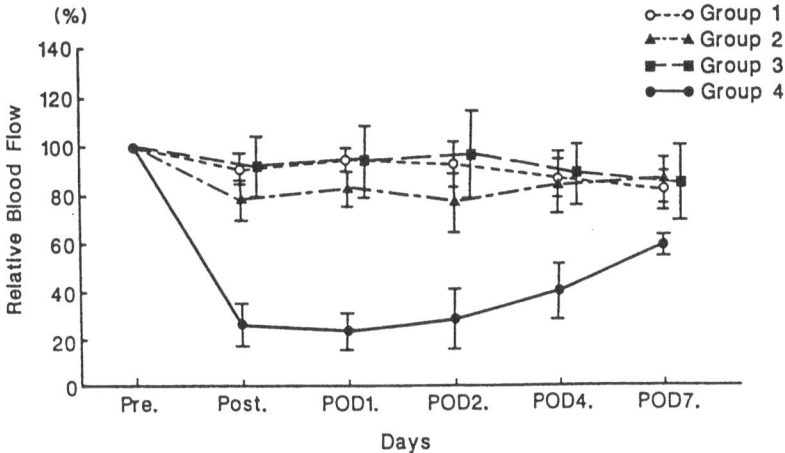

Fig. 1. Postoperative change of mucosal blood flow in each group in the animal study. *Group 1*, thoracotomy; *group 2*, divided right bronchial artery; *group 3*, divided vagal nerve; *group 4*, divided right bronchial artery and vagal nerve, and extensive mobilization of the trachea. *POD*; postoperative day

Results

There was no significant difference in blood flow between groups 1 and 3. In group 2, the blood flow was significantly decreased postoperatively as compared with the values in group 1, but revealed no differences at the 7th day post-operatively. In group 4, the blood flow decreased to one-fifth of the pre-surgical value immediately after surgery. The time course observation showed a tendency for recovery of the decreased blood flow from the 2nd day postoperatively, but the value did not return to the pre-surgical level (Fig. 1).

Clinical Study

Methods

Seven patients with thoracic esophageal carcinoma who underwent esophageal resection and reconstruction in one stage were included in the study. The patients were classified into three groups:

Group 1: Preserved bronchial artery and vagal nerve ($n = 3$)
Group 2: Preserved vagal nerve and divided bronchial artery ($n = 3$)
Group 3: Divided bronchial artery and vagal nerve ($n = 1$)

In each group, blood flow was measured at the 1st, 2nd, and 3rd postoperative days. The flowmeter was introduced through a bronchofiberscope channel and was slightly pressed perpendicular to the bronchial mucosa.

Results

As shown in Fig. 2, mucosal blood flow immediately decreased to about three-fifths of control value upon transient clamp of the bronchial artery during

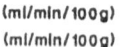

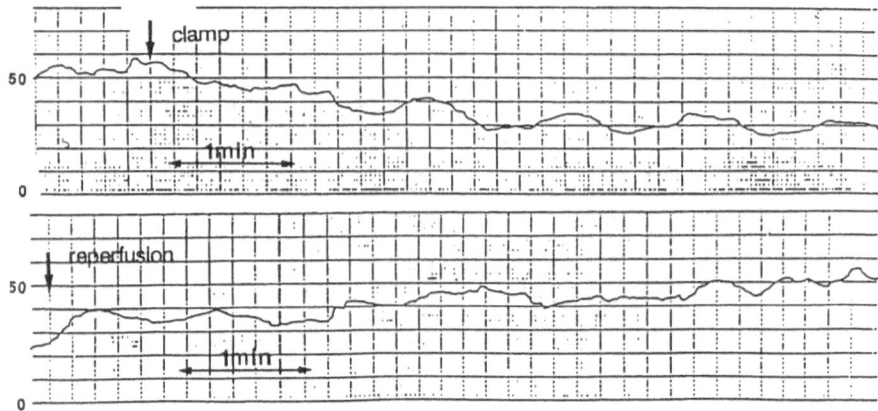

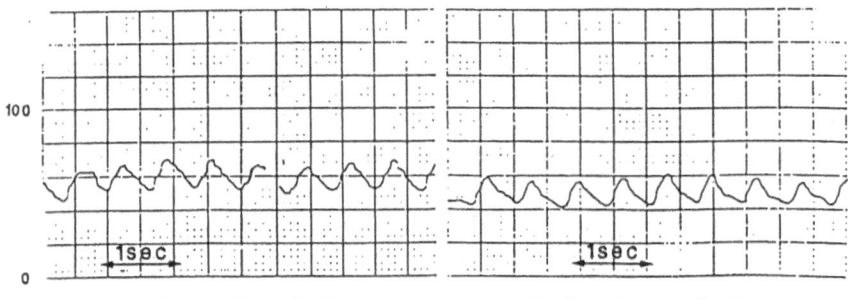

pre–dissected mediastinum   post–dissected mediastinum

Fig. 2. Intraoperative change of mucosal blood flow in the clinical study

operation, and immediately returned to the previous value upon release of the clamp. In group 1, the blood flow after mediastinal lymph node dissection decreased to about four-fifths of the presurgical value, while that in groups 2 and 3 was preserved in comparison with that in group 1. In group 3, with extensive mobilization of the trachea and lymph node dissection, mucosal flow was markedly decreased (Fig. 3).

Conclusions

These results suggest that preservation of the right bronchial artery and proper tracheal sheath significantly reduced the risk of ischemic disorder in the tracheal mucosa, thus preventing pulmonary complications after surgery for thoracic esophageal carcinoma.

The Laser Doppler method for the measurement of the bronchial mucosal blood flow seemed to be useful in determining the extent of tracheal ischemic disturbance [1–3].

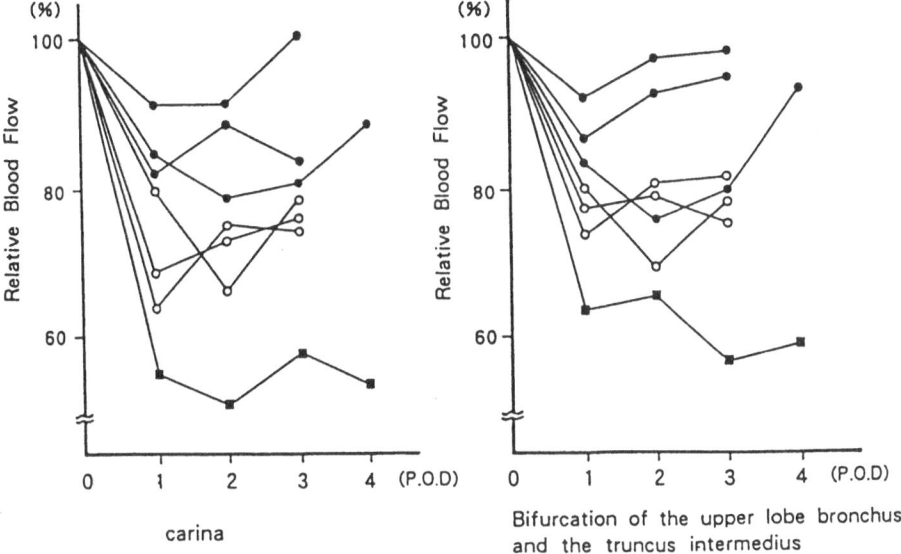

Fig. 3. Postoperative change of blood flow: Clinical study. *Closed circles* indicate group 1 (preserved bronchial artery and vagal nerve); *open circles*, group 2 (preserved vagal nerve and divided bronchial artery); *closed squares*, group 3 (divided bronchial artery and vagal nerve)

References

1. Fujino S, et al (1986) Analysis of bronchial mucosal hemodynamics by electrochemically generated hydrogen gas clearance method. J Jpn Soc Bronchology 8(4):606–612
2. Kobayashi M, et al (1986) The application of hydrogen gas clearance method with bronchoscopy for the measurement of bronchial mucosal blood flow. JJSB 8(4):613–621
3. Aoki M, et al (1986) Measurement of bronchial mucosal blood flow by Laser Doppler velocimetry in the dog. JJSB 8(4):622–629

Pathology

Prognostic Factors for T1 Carcinoma of the Esophagus

HIROKO IDE, REIKI EGUCHI, TSUTOMU NAKAMURA, KAZUHIKO HAYASHI, KAZUNARI YOSHIDA, ATARU KOBAYASHI, AKIYOSHI YAMADA, and FUJIO HANYU[1]

Introduction

While most cases of T1 carcinoma of the esophagus have a good prognosis, some cases show poor results. This study analyzed clinicopathological factors to evaluate prognostic factors of T1 esophageal carcinoma.

Materials and Methods

From 1965 to 1991, we resected 182 cases of T1 esophageal carcinoma (37 mucosal, 145 submucosal) without any preoperative therapy. Ages ranged from 39 to 84 (ave. 64). Of these, 158 were male and 24 were female. Fourteen cases were located in the upper, 125 cases in the middle, and 43 cases in the lower thoracic esophagus.

Concerning the approach, we performed 131 right thoracotomies, 30 left thoracotomies, and 21 blunt dissections. The blunt dissections were mainly performed in case of curative operation for mucosal carcinoma and limited operation for high risk cases.

Results

Operative Results and Staging Factors

Subtotal esophagectomy was performed in 92% of all cases, and reconstruction with the stomach was performed in 89%. The operative mortality rate was 1.6%.

[1] Department of Surgery, The Institute of Gastroenterology, Tokyo Women's Medical College, 8-1 Kawada-cho, Shinjuku-ku, Tokyo, 162 Japan

Table 1. Background factors of pT1 carcinoma of the esophagus

Operative results	
Subtotal esophagectomy	167 (92%)
Reconstruction with stomach	161 (89%)
Operative mortality	3 (1.6%)
Palliative resection (R2)	6 (3.3%)
[Double cancer 1 case, LYM 5 cases]	
TNM-Staging	
Stage I [T1, N0, M0]	128 (70%)
II B[T1, N1, M0]	45 (25%)
IV [T1, N1, M1(LYM)]	9 (5%)
Rate of lymph node metastasis	
Mucosal carcinoma	3/37 (8%)
Submucosal carcinoma	51/145 (35%)

TWMC, Tokyo Womens Medical College (1965–1991)

Table 2. Macroscopic types of pT1 carcinoma and depth of invasion

	Mucosal ca.	Submucosal ca.
Protruding type (0-I)[a]	1 (3%)	80 (55%)
Flat type (0-II)	36 (97%)	38 (26%)
Depressed type (0-III)		26 (18%)
Unclassified		1 (1%)
Total	37 (100%)	145 (100%)

TWMC (1965–1991)
[a] Japanese macroscopic classification
ca., cancer

Palliative resection was performed in 6 cases, in 1 case due to double cancer, and in 5 due to lymph node metastasis. Stage I cases accounted for 70% of resected cases, while 25% were stage IIB, and 5% were stage IV.

The resected stage IV cases included those with only distant lymph node metastasis. (no organ metastasis). Lymph node metastasis was seen 8% in mucosal carcinomas and 35% in submucosal carcinomas (Table 1).

Table 2 shows the macroscopic type of resected pT1 carcinoma of the esophagus. Almost all mucosal carcinomas were flat erosive lesions, while 56% of submucosal carcinomas were protruding lesions, 26% were flat, and 18% were depressed lesions.

The overwhelming majority (89%) of resected pT1 carcinomas were squamous cell carcinoma, 5% were adenosquamous cell carcinoma, and 6% consisted of other carcinoma such as adenocarcinoma, carcinosarcoma, and undifferentiated carcinoma. Lymphatic invasion was observed chiefly in the lamina propria mucosae while lymph node metastases were seen mostly in distant nodes without regional nodes as skip metastasis.

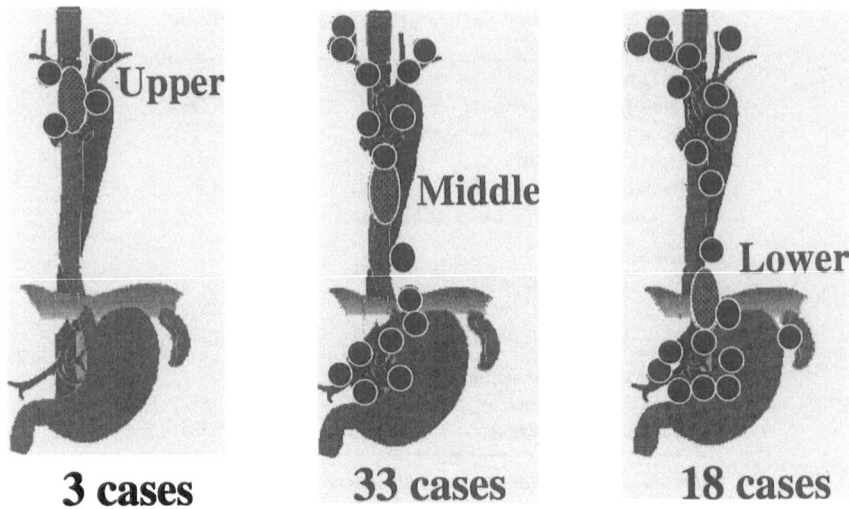

Fig. 1. Areas of lymph node metastasis in pT1 carcinoma of the esophagus

Figure 1 shows the areas of lymph node metastases in pT1 carcinomas. Upper-mediastinal and abdominal node metastasis were seen in many cases as the initial single metastasis.

Clinical Prognostic Factors

The 5-year survival rate of all resected cases was 61%. The survival rate of patients aged 59 or younger was slightly higher than those aged 70 or more, but the survival rate was not significantly in terms of sex, tumor location, or surgical approach (Table 3).

There were 79 fatalities among resected pT1 cases, the causes of which are shown in Table 4. Deaths due to recurrence were 9 at 1 year, 13 at 1–2 years, 15 at 2–5 years, and 2 after 5 years.

The causes of death unrelated to the original carcinoma consisted of 68% of the fatalities within 1 year and 87% after 5 years. The causes of death were due to postoperative complications and pneumonia within 1 year and aging and metachronous primary cancers after 5 years.

Pathologic Prognostic Factors

To obtain the prognostic factors of primary carcinoma, we calculated the cumulative survival rate, excluding direct death and other causes of death, by Kaplan-Meier's method.

Figure 2 shows the survival curves for each stage of pT1 carcinoma. The 5-year survival rate of stage I with no metastasis was significantly better than that of IIB and IV cases with lymph node metastasis ($P < 0.001$).

The 5-year survival rate for mucosal carcinoma was 97.1%, which was extremely good. In contrast, that of submucosal carcinoma was 69.1% (Fig. 3).

Table 3. Clinical prgonostic factors and survival rate

		1-year	3-year	5-year	
Sex					
Male	$n = 158$	83%	68%	60%	NS
Female	$n = 26$	88%	74%	68%	
Age					
−59 years	$n = 62$	92%	82%	68%	
60–69 years	$n = 79$	83%	66%	64%	NS *
70– years	$n = 41$	73%	56%	52%	
Location					
Upper	$n = 14$	79%	63%	63%	
Middle	$n = 125$	86%	72%	60%	NS
Lower	$n = 43$	79%	64%	60%	
Approach					
Right thoracotomy	$n = 131$	85%	69%	61%	
Left thoracotomy	$n = 30$	77%	70%	61%	NS
Blunt dissection	$n = 21$	91%	73%	65%	

* $P < 0.05$
TWMC (June 1992)

Table 4. The causes of death in pT1 esophageal carcinoma

Survival term (months)	−12	13–24	25–60	61–
Died with recurrence	9	13	15	2
	(32%)	(87%)	(71%)	(13%)
Died without recurrence	19	2	6	13
	(68%)	(13%)	(28%)	(87%)
Double cancer	2	2	1	3
Old age			1	8
Complication	9			
Others	8		4	2
Total	28	15	21	15

TWMC (June 1992)

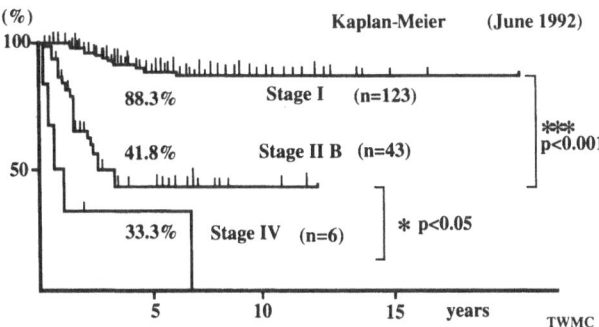

Fig. 2. Cumulative survival curves of pT1 esophageal carcinoma according to TNM-staging

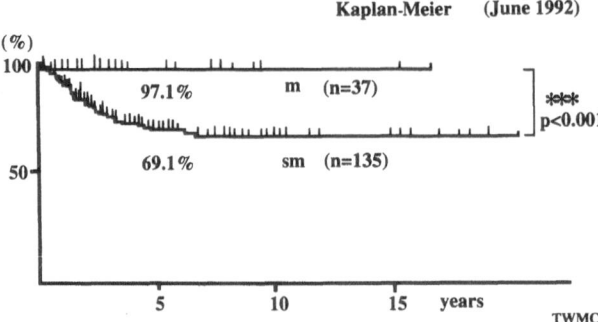

Fig. 3. Cumulative survival curves of pT1 esophageal carcinoma according to depth of invasion

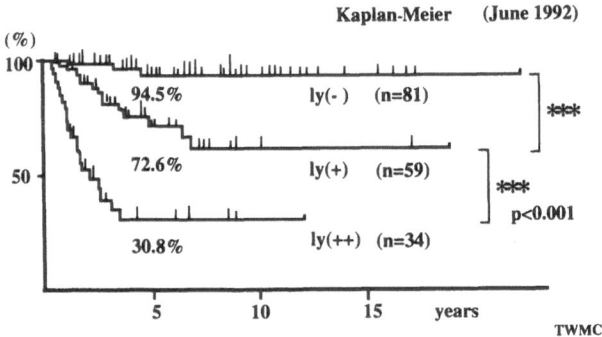

Fig. 4. Cumulative survival curves of pT1 esophageal carcinoma according to lymphatic involvement

In pT1 carcinoma of the esophagus, the survival rate was closely related to the degree of lymphatic invasion (Fig. 4).

Since the prognosis of pT1 carcinoma appeared to be related to the degree of depth of invasion and lymphatic invasion, we classifed the depth of invasion of pT1 carcinima into 4 categories (Fig. 5): from sm-0 (mucosal carcinoma without sm-invasion) to sm-3 (markedly deep invasion).

Table 5 shows the relationships of every depth of invasion, vascular invasion, and node metastasis in terms of survival rates. The rates of vascular invasion and lymph node metastasis of sm-1 carcinomas were low and the survival rate of this category was similar to that of mucosal carcinoma. However in sm-2 and sm-3 carcinomas, vascular invasion and lymph node metastasis were frequently observed, and some of these showed poor courses similar to advanced cancer.

Concerning the macroscopic type of pT1 carcinoma, flat type lesions (0-II type) generally showed only shallow sm invasion and had a good prognosis compared to 0-I or 0-III types ($P < 0.001$), while obviously protruding 0-I or depressed type 0-III lesions tended to show moderate or deep sm-invasion and displayed poor courses.

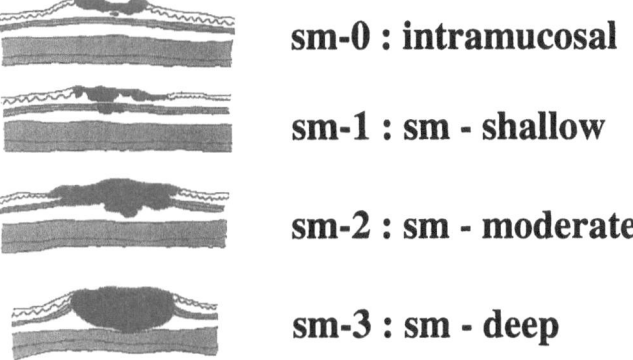

sm-0 : intramucosal

sm-1 : sm - shallow

sm-2 : sm - moderate

sm-3 : sm - deep

Fig. 5. Depth of invasion in pT1 carcinoma of the esophagus

Table 5. Vascular invasion, lymph node metastasis, and survival rate according to pathologic findings

		ly(+)	v(+)	LN(+)	5-year survival rate (Kaplan-Meier)
Depth of invasion					
sm-0	$n = 37$	11%	0%	8%	97.1%
sm-1	$n = 26$	26%	0%	4%	89.5%
sm-2	$n = 75$	65%	31%	37%	71.8%
sm-3	$n = 44$	84%	45%	50%	53.1%
Macroscopic type					
0-I	$n = 81$	69%	32%	38%	64.2%
0-II	$n = 74$	28%	7%	14%	90.4%
0-III	$n = 26$	77%	42%	46%	56.5%

* $P < 0.05$, ** $P < 0.001$
TWMC (June 1992)
ly, lymphatic invasion; *v*, vessel invasion; *LN*, lymph node metastasis

Discussion

Endoscopic staining using a spray of Lugol's solution is extremely effective for the detection of superficial esophageal carcinoma. With this approach, T1 cases comprised 20%–25% of resected cases, with resultant improvement of the long-term survival rate [1–3].

While some T1 cases succumbed within a short period due to recurrence and postoperative complications, the overall 5-year survival rate was 61%. Since the major clinical factor affecting prognosis was age, care is required to operative indications in elderly high-risk cases.

Among resected T1 carcinoma cases, positive the lymph nodes were seen in 39%, primary in the upper mediastinal and perigastric fields chiefly but also occasionally in the cervical field.

The 5-year survival rate of mucosal and sm-1 carcinoma were good. However, sm-2 and sm-3 carcinomas showed vascular invasion in 65%–84% and the 5-year survival rate was low. Therefore, such are thought to require extended lymph node dissection.

Makuuchi [4] reported 88% accuracy in endoscopic evaluation of submucosal invasion. Murata [5–6] reported 80% accuracy of esophageal ultrasonography (EUS) evaluation of depth of invasion in T1 cancer and more than 90% accuracy of diagnosis of lymph node metastasis with preoperative US and EUS. Some T1 cases require lymph node dissection, while others do not, therefore preoperative staging with endoscopy, US, and EUS is essential to determine the appropriate extent of dissection.

Conclusions

Among 182 pT1 esophageal carcinoma, the initial lymph node metastasis occured mainly in the upper mediastinum and perigastric region.

The prognosis of pT1 esophageal carcinoma correlated with the degree of lymphatic invasion and lymph node metastasis. Cases of mucosal carcinoma and sm-1 showed low rates of vascular invasion and good prognoses.

In moderately or deeply invading sm carcinoma (sm-2, sm-3), vascular invasion and lymph node metastasis were frequently observed and they showed relatively poor prognoses similarly to advanced carcinoma.

In pT1 esophageal carcinoma with sm invasion, mediastinal and abdominal lymph node dissection was required for curative resection and preoperative US and EUS examinations were useful in determining the dissection field.

References

1. Endo M, Ide H (eds) (1992) Endoscopic staining in the early diagnosis of esophageal cancer. Japan Scientific Societies Press, Tokyo
2. Ide H, Nogami A, Hanashi T, Endo T, Nakamura T, Muroi M, Eguchi R, Kobayashi A, Hanyu F, Yamada A, Murata Y (1990) A Clinical Study on Prognosis of Submucosal Esophageal Cancer (in Japanese). I to Cho (Stomach and Intestine) 25:1067–1074
3. Ide H, Eguchi R, Nakamura T, Hayashi K, Yoshida K, Endo T, Hanashi T (1992) Early esophageal carcinoma. Clin Gastroenterol 7:1683–1693
4. Makuuchi H, Machimura T, Sugihara T, Sasaki T, Mitomi T, Shiina Y, Miwa T, Itakura M, Matuzaki S, Shigeta H, Ohomori T, Kumagaya Y (1990) Endoscopic diagnosis and treatment of mucosal carcinoma of the esophagus. Endoscopia Digestiva 2:447–452
5. Murata Y (1989) Evaluation of endoscopic ultrasonography and conventional ultrasonography for staging in superficial esophageal cancer—Assessment by histological findings and clinical course. Jpn J Gastroenterol Surg 22:195–204
6. Murata Y, Muroi M, Yoshida M, Ide H, Hanyu F (1987) Endoscopic ultrasonography in diagnosis of esophageal carcinoma. Surg Endoscopy 1:11–16
7. Murata Y, Ide H (1992) Staging of esophageal cancer by ultrasonography (EUS, US) and CT. Jpn J Cancer of the Digest Organ 2:43–45

Esophageal Cancer Associated with Multiple Primary or Intramural Metastatic Lesions

Michio Maeta, Akira Kondo, Syunsuke Shibata, Hiroshi Yamashiro, and Nobuaki Kaibara[1]

Introduction

The presence of multiple primary [1] or intramural skip metastatic lesions [2], in addition to the main tumor are well recognized as specific features of invasive esophageal cancer. A detailed histological examination by serial blocks and subserial sections of the entire resected esophagus, as a routine procedure enabled us to detect the associated minute lesions that were barely identifiable macroscopically on the resected specimen. In the present study, we analyzed the clinicopathological findings of esophageal cancers associated with multiple cancerous lesions, apart from the main lesions, and we compared clinical features between multiple primary lesions (MPLs) and intramural metastatic lesions (IMLs).

Methods

Between 1975 and 1989, 111 patients with esophageal squamous cell carcinoma underwent esophagectomy in our clinic. Fifty-three patients received preoperative radiotherapy, up to a total dose of 30–40 Gy. Clinical and histological findings were evaluated according to the "Guidelines for the clinical and pathologic studies on carcinoma of the esophagus [3]".

Histologic criteria of MPL and IML have been defined as follows [3, 4]:

MPL: 1. The multiple lesions are distant from one another and are not continuous, regardless of vascular or lymphatic invasions.
   2. The lesions are fully exposed to the esophageal lumen.
   3. The largest tumor is taken as the main lesion and smaller one is taken

[1] First Department of Surgery, Tottori University School of Medicine, 36-1 Nishimachi Yonago, 683 Japan

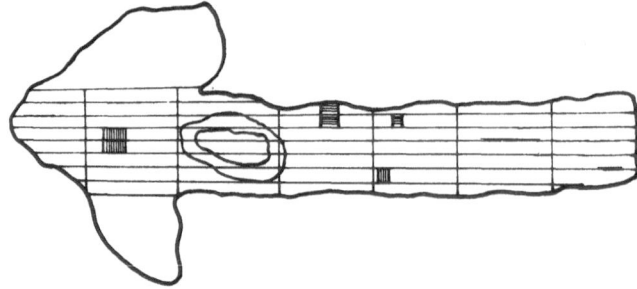

Fig. 1. Serial and subserial sections of an entire resected specimen showing two multiple primary lesions (*horizontal lines*) and two intramural metastatic lesions (*vertical lines*) simultaneously, apart from the main tumor of the lower thoracic esophagus

as an associated lesion, or if they are the same size, the deeper tumor of the cancer invasion is taken as the main lesion.

IML: 1. The histologic type of carcinoma is the same in all the lesions, regardless of the grade of differentiation.
2. The lesions are distant from one another and are not continuous, regardless of vascular or lymphatic invasions.
3. The lesions are not exposed to the esophageal lumen, or if they are exposed, the center of the tumor is in the submucosal layer of the wall.
4. The lesions are not continuous with metastatic lesions around the esophagus.

Student's *t*-test was used for statistical analysis.

Results

Overall, MPLs were found in 23 (20.7%) patients (27 lesions), who ranged in age from 45 to 79 years (mean 63 years; males 22, females 1); IMLs were found in 10 (9.0%) patients (11 lesions), who ranged in age from 46 to 70 years (mean 66 years; males, 10). Three patients had both MPLs and IMLs simultaneously, as shown in Fig. 1.

The incidence of MPL was 18.9% (10/53) for pre-operatively irradiated and 22.4% (13/58) for non-irradiated patients, as shown in Table 1. The incidence of IML for irradiated and non-irradiated patients was 11.3% (6/53) and 6.9% (4/58), respectively. Among the 27 MPLs, all were of the superficial type; 23 of which were of the superficial flat type that were barely identifiable macroscopically. While all 11 IMLs were of the protruding or superficial elevated type, the majority were identifiable macroscopically on the resected specimens. The mean maximum diameters of each MPL and IML were 0.7 ± 0.5 cm and 1.7 ± 0.9 cm, respectively; there was a significant difference between the two groups ($P < 0.01$).

With respect to the depth of invasion by the cancer in the main lesions, 4 of 23 patients with MPLs had superficial cancer confined within the submucosal layer, while none of the patients with IMLs had superficial cancer. With respect to the associated lesions, there were great differences in the depth of invasion of

Table 1. Incidence of MPL and IML analyzed in terms of the presence or absence of pre-operative radiotherapy

Associated lesions	Irradiated ($n = 53$)	Non-irradiated ($n = 58$)
MPL	10 (18.9%)	13 (22.4%)
IML	6 (11.3%)	4 (6.9%)

MPL, multiple primary lesion; *IML*, intramural metastatic lesion

the cancer between MPLs and IMLs. All 27 MPLs were confined within the submucosal layer (superficial cancer), the IMLs varied in depth from the submucosa to adventitia, although the center of the IMLs was in the submucosal layer. The incidence of lymph node involvement was significantly higher for IMLs (10/10, 100%) than for MPLs (11/23, 47.8%) ($P < 0.05$); metastatic lymph nodes were more widely distributed in patients with IMLs than in those with MPLs. Furthermore, the incidence of lymphatic vessel invasion by the cancer within the esophageal wall in patients with MPLs and IMLs was 65.2% (15/23) and 90% (9/10), respectively.

Histologically, the transition between 27 MPLs and the noncancerous epithelium was abrupt in 20 lesions. Seven MPLs showed a gradual transition to slight or moderate dysplasia of the esophageal epithelium, but none showed a gradual transition to severe dysplasia.

Thirteen and 14 MPLs were detected on the proximal and distal sides, respectively, of the main tumor with the same mean distance (2.6 cm). Eight of the 11 IMLs were distributed on the distal side of the main tumor (4.6 cm) and 3 IMLs were detected on the proximal side (3.4 cm).

Discussion

In this series of serial blocks and subserial sections of the entire surgically resected esophagus, MPLs were shown to be associated not only with invasive cancer but also with superficial cancer as main tumors. A possible relationship between various degrees of epithelial dysplasia and carcinoma has been suggested [5, 6]. This is because some intra-epithelial esophageal carcinomas are frequently surrounded by severe dysplasia and occasionally show a gradual transition to dysplasia, and it seems that dysplasia plays an important role in carcinogenesis of the esophagus, as a precursor lesion. This high incidence of MPLs may indicate a possible increased multicentric carcinogenic potential in the noncancerous epithelium of patients who have had an antecedent esophageal cancer. In this series, no MPL was surrounded by severe dysplasia, while IMLs were detected in patients with invasive esophageal cancer and not in patients with superficial cancer as main tumors. Patients with IMLs exhibited pathologic characteristics: These were a high incidence of both lymphatic vessel invasion by the cancer and lymph node involvement, and the low incidence of blood vessel invasion by the cancer. These findings may indicate that IMLs are developed not by hematogenous dissemination but by intramural lymphatic spread from the primary esophageal cancer.

In the surgical treatment of esophageal cancer, the preoperative diagnosis of any associated lesions has important implications for the planning of surgery. Although these associated lesions may be easily overlooked during routine radiographic and endoscopic examinations, endoscopic staining with Lugol's solution has been reported to be useful for the preoperative detection of such fine superficial epithelial changes of the esophagus [7].

In esophageal surgery, surgeons are required to undertake the complete removal of both the main tumor and associated MPLs or IMLs. Our data indicate a mean distance of 2.6 cm between the main tumor and associated MPLs and an even longer distance in the case of IMLs, especially on the distal side of the main tumor (4.6 cm). Careful attention must be paid to the choice of surgical margins during resection of the esophagus.

References

1. Steiner PE (1956) Etiology and histogenesis of carcinoma of esophagus. Cancer 9:436–452
2. Akiyama H, Ushiyama T, Kogure T (1969) Intraepithelial carcinoma associated with esophageal carcinoma (in Japanese). Geka 31:1287–1297
3. Japanese Society for Esophageal Diseases (1976) Guidelines for the clinical and pathologic studies on carcinoma of the esophagus. Jpn J Surg 6:69–78
4. Saito T, Iizuka T, Kato H, Watanabe H (1985) Esophageal carcinoma metastatic to the stomach. A clinicopathologic study of 35 cases. Cancer 56:2235–2241
5. Ushigome S, Spjut HJ, Noon GP (1967) Extensive dysplasia and carcinoma in situ of esophageal epithelium. Cancer 20:1023–1029
6. Kuwano H, Morita M, Matsuda H, Mori M, Sugimachi K (1991) Histopathologic findings of minute foci of squamous cell carcinoma in the human esophagus. Cancer 68:2617–2620
7. Endo M, Takemoto T, Shirakabe H (1986) Minute lesions of esophageal cancer. Semin Surg Oncol 2:177–186

Histopathologic Investigation of Squamous Epithelial Dysplasia and Carcinoma of the Esophagus

Hiroyuki Kuwano, Masahiko Ikebe, Kaoru Kitamura, Kinya Baba, Yasushi Toh, Yosuke Adachi, and Keizo Sugimachi[1]

Introduction

Squamous epithelial dysplasia is frequently encountered in the esophagus with squamous cell carcinoma, and several studies have suggested its significance as a precancerous lesion.

In the current study, we performed a serial histopathologic investigation of esophageal squamous cell carcinoma, on the basis of continuity and coexistence with several degrees of epithelial dysplasia. Attention was directed to the histopathologic significance of epithelial dysplasia.

Materials and Methods

A total of 149 patients with primary esophageal carcinoma, who underwent esophageal resection without preoperative treatment in the Second Department of Surgery, Kyushu University, Fukuoka, Japan from 1965 to 1991, were reviewed.

Microscopic sections of the whole resected esophagus were prepared from step-sectioned blocks 0.5 cm wide and were stained with hematoxylin and eosin.

Histopathologic Criteria for Diagnosis of Squamous Epithelial Dysplasia

For the histologic diagnosis of squamous epithelial dysplasia, we used the criteria defined by the World Health Organization's International Histological Classification of Tumors in 1990 [1]: the nuclei of the lesion are enlarged and hyperchromatic, and they show increased mitotic activity. In the case of a mild dysplasia, such atypical nuclei are limited to the basal zone, and there is evidence

[1] Department of Surgery II, Faculty of Medicine, Kyushu University, 3-1-1, Maidashi, Higashi-ku, Fukuoka, 812 Japan

of cytoplasmic maturation superficially. With increasing grades of dysplasia there is a progressive increase in the proportion of atypical basal cells until the entire thickness of the epithelium is replaced. Therefore, moderate dysplasia was diagnosed when an intraepithelial lesion similar to mild dysplasia with an atypical proliferative zone, expanding up to one-half the thickness of the epithelium, was found. Severe dysplasia was defined as an intraepithelial lesion with an atypical proliferative zone encompassing up to three-quarters of the epithelium.

In addition, a diagnosis of intraepithelial carcinoma was made when an epithelium was either completely or almost completely composed of atypical immature cells but lacked invasive growth.

The numbers of various lesions were counted by a histologic diagram, mapping their extent in two dimensions, and these lesions were then investigated with regard to either the presence or absence of continuity to areas of carcinoma. Clinicopathologic factors were compared between the cases with and without areas of squamous epithelial dysplasia, and a chi-square test was used for the statistical analysis.

Results

A serial histologic review of 149 specimens from patients with squamous cell carcinoma revealed 69 dysplastic lesions in 29 cases (19.5%). In three cases of intraepithelial carcinoma, there was no lesion of dysplasia, while areas of dysplasia in the esophagus were found in 7 of 12 cases (58.3%) with mucosal cancer, 10 (34.5%) of 29 with submucosal carcinoma, 4 (18.2%) of 22 cases with carcinoma which had invaded to the muscularis externa, and 8 (9.6%) of 83 tumors which had reached the adventitia. Thus, excluding the cases of intraepithelial carcinoma, the less the cancer has invaded, the greater the frequency of the coexistence of dysplasia. In the cases of mucosal cancer, there were 17 lesions of dysplasia, of which 5 had mild degrees of dysplasia, 7 moderate, and 5 severe. In 23 dysplastic lesions associated with submucosal cancer, dysplasia was adjudged as mild in one, moderate in 10, and severe in 12. The corresponding numbers for cancer which had invaded to the muscular layer proper and to the adventitia, respectively were (mild to severe) 3, 7, and 7; and 3, 4, and 5. Thus, there were a total of 12, 28, and 29 lesions of mild, moderate, and severe dysplasia, respectively (Table 1). The relationship between the grade of dysplasia and the continuity to areas of carcinoma is shown in Table 2. Although the frequency of continuity of the dysplasia to the carcinoma was not high (47.8%), the more severe the grade of dysplasia, the higher the frequency of continuity to the areas of carcinoma.

Clinicopathologic features of early stage esophageal cancer both with and without dysplasia were also analyzed. There was no difference between the groups regarding age, sex distribution, location and depth of the invasion of the main lesion, frequencies of lymph node metastasis, intraepithelial spread of the main lesion of esophageal cancer, or lymphatic vessel and vascular permeation of the carcinoma. However, the incidences of multiplicity of squamous cell carcinoma within the esophagus and the intraepithelial spread of the main

Table 1. Coexistence of various degrees of squamous epithelial dysplasia and carcinoma

Depth of invasion of main lesion	Number of specimens	Dysplasia			
		Cases Number (%)	Number of lesions		Total
Epithelium	[3]	0 (0)			
Mucosal layer	[12]	7 (58.3)	Mild	5	
			Moderate	7	17
			Severe	5	
Submucosal layer	[29]	10 (34.5)	Mild	1	
			Moderate	10	23
			Severe	12	
Proper muscular layer	[22]	4 (18.2)	Mild	3	
			Moderate	7	17
			Severe	7	
Adventitia	[83]	8 (9.6)	Mild	3	
			Moderate	4	12
			Severe	5	
Total	[149]	29 (19.5)	Mild	12	
			Moderate	28	69
			Severe	29	

Table 2. Continuity between carcinoma and various degrees of dysplasia

Degrees of dysplasia	[lesions]	Continuity	
		(+) Number (%)	(−) Number (%)
Mild	[12]	3 (25.0)	9 (75.0)
Moderate	[28]	13 (46.4)	15 (53.6)
Severe	[29]	17 (58.6)	12 (41.4)
Total	[69]	33 (47.8)	36 (52.1)

lesion were significantly higher in the group with dysplasia than in that without it ($P < 0.001$) (Table 3).

Discussion

To investigate the histogenesis of esophageal cancer, we demonstrated the high incidence of glandular or mucus-secreting components in esophageal squamous cell carcinoma [2], frequent coexistence of intraepithelial carcinoma contiguous to the main squamous cell carcinoma in early esophageal cancer [3], a close relationship between multiplicity and the existence of intraepithelial carcinoma with squamous cell carcinoma [4], and a high incidence of the coexistence of intraepithelial carcinoma and glandular differentiation, particularly in early

Table 3. Clinicopathologic features of esophageal cancer with and without dysplasia

	Dysplasia	
	(−) Number (%) n = 120	(+) Number (%) n = 29
Age (years old)	63.1 ± 9.7	62.7 ± 12.4
Sex (M/F)	100/20	25/4
Location		
Upper	15 (12.5)	4 (13.8)
Middle	62 (51.7)	17 (58.6)
Lower	43 (35.8)	8 (27.6)
Depth of invasion of main lesion		
Epithelium	3 (2.5)	0
Mucosa	5 (4.2)	7 (24.1)
Submucosa	19 (15.8)	10 (34.5)
Proper muscular	18 (15.0)	4 (13.8)
Adventitia	75 (62.5)	8 (27.6)
Lymph node metastasis**		
(−)	52 (43.3)	22 (75.9)
(+)	68 (56.7)	7 (24.1)
Multiplicity of squamous cell carcinoma*		
(−)	112 (93.3)	20 (69.0)
(+)	8 (6.7)	9 (31.0)
[a] Intraepithelial spread of main lesion*		
(−)	68 (58.1)	2 (6.9)
(+)	49 (41.9)	27 (93.1)
[a] Lymphatic vessel permeation		
(−)	53 (45.3)	21 (72.4)
(+)	64 (54.7)	8 (27.6)
[a] Vascular permeation		
(−)	84 (71.8)	20 (69.0)
(+)	33 (28.2)	9 (31.0)

* $P < 0.001$ ** $P < 0.01$
[a] Excluding three with intraepithelial carcinoma

cancers [5]. These results were thought to support the possibility of the concept of multicentric or field carcinogenesis of esophageal cancer.

In the study of intraepithelial carcinoma concomitant with esophageal squamous cell carcinoma, we analyzed the incidence of intraepithelial carcinoma in each group, divided according to the depth of invasion of the main lesion, and demonstrated that the greater the invasion of the main lesion, the lower were the incidences of intraepithelial carcinoma [3]. In the current study, it was evident that the less advanced the main lesion, the higher the incidence of coexistence of dysplasia, excluding the three cases of intraepithelial carcinoma. Therefore, it could be assumed that a dysplastic lesion, as well as intraepithelial carcinoma contiguous to the main lesion, would have become involved during the progression of the invasive cancer.

To investigate the pathologic significance of dysplasia as a precancerous lesion, a careful chronological observation of the lesion will be essential. However, it is very difficult to investigate the chronological change using biopsy specimens of human materials. Therefore, the serial histopathologic observation of the relationship between carcinoma and dysplasia in the resected esophagus would be useful, and from this viewpoint, continuity of both lesions could be important. From the current study as well as our recent investigation of esophageal dysplasia [6–8] it was demonstrated that the continuity of dysplastic lesions to the areas of carcinoma was often encountered in severe dysplasia rather than in moderate or mild dysplasia, though it was not frequent. We also performed cytophotometric DNA analysis of chemically-induced esophageal carcinoma in rats and demonstrated that, biologically, the lesion of the severe dysplasia might be considered as serious as cancer [9]. Although the dysplasia to the carcinoma sequence could not be disproved, the possibility exists that severe dysplasia contiguous to the carcinoma would already have malignant characteristics and that various degrees of dysplasia would occur in the esophagus containing carcinoma.

The current study also demonstrated that the multiplicity of squamous cell carcinoma and intraepithelial spread of the main lesion of carcinoma were greater in cases with dysplasia than in those without it. If it is assumed that an intraepithelial lesion contiguous to the invasive cancer originated by the field effect, various degrees of lesions such as dysplasia and carcinoma may occur multicentrically or with field effect in the same esophagus, especially one which contains dysplastic lesions.

References

1. Watanabe H, Jass JR, Solin L (1990) Histological typing of oesophageal and gastric tumour, 2nd edn. Springer, Berlin
2. Kuwano H, Ueo H, Sugimachi K, Inokuchi K, Toyoshima S, Enjoji M (1985) Glandular or mucus secreting components in squamous cell carcinoma of the esophagus. Cancer 56: 514–518
3. Kuwano H, Matsuda H, Matsuoka H, Kai H, Okudaira Y, Sugimachi K (1987) Intraepithelial carcinoma concomitant with esophageal squamous cell carcinoma. Cancer 59: 783–787
4. Kuwano H, Ohno S, Matsuda H, Mori M, Sigimachi K (1988) Serial histologic evaluation of multiple primary squamous cell carcinoma of the esophagus. Cancer 61:1635–1638
5. Kuwano H, Nagamatsu M, Ohno S, Matsuda H, Mori M, Sugimachi K (1988) Coexistence of intraepithelial carcinoma and glandular differentiation in esophageal squamous cell carcinoma. Cancer 62:1568–1572
6. Nagamatsu M, Mori M, Kuwano H, Sugimachi K, Akiyoshi T (to be published) Serial histologic investigation of squamous epithelial dysplasia associated with carcinoma of the esophagus. Cancer
7. Kuwano H, Morita M, Matsuda H, Mori M, Sugimachi K (1991) Histopathologic findings of minute foci of squamous cell carcinoma in the human esophagus. Cancer 68:2617–2620
8. Kuwano H, Baba K, Ikebe M, Adachi Y, Toh Y, Sugimachi K (to be published) Histopathology of early esophageal carcinoma and squamous epithelial dysplasia. Hepatogastroenterology
9. Koga Y, Sugimachi K, Kuwano H, Mori M, Matsufuji H (1988) Cytophotometric DNA analysis of esophageal dysplasia and carcinoma induced in rats by N-methyl-N-amylnitrosamine. Eur J Cancer Clin Oncol 24:643–651

A Clinico-Pathological Study on Esophageal Carcinoma Associated with Dysplasia

W. Takiyama[1], S. Moriwaki[2], K. Mandai[2], and S. Takashima[1]

Introduction

Epithelial dysplasia of the cervix uteri and esophagus are considered to be common sites of origin of cancer development. However, there are few reports on the histogenesis of esophageal carcinoma compared to carcinogenesis in the cervix uteri. This study reviewed the histological findings of the epithelium in 96 cases with squamous cell carcinoma of the esophagus.

Materials and Methods

One hundred and seventeen patients with primary esophageal carcinoma underwent esophageal resection from 1983 to 1992 at the Shikoku Cancer Center Hospital, and 113 of these underwent surgery without preoperative radiotherapy. Specimens of 96 squamous cell carcinomas from these 113 patients were available for study. After fixation in 10% formalin solution, each entire esophagus was sectioned longitudinally in widths of 5 mm and embedded in paraffin. A histologic section made from each block was stained with hematoxylin and eosin for histological examination. The histologic criteria used for diagnosis of squamous cell carcinoma in situ (CIS) were: (1) increased cellularity of the entire thickness of the epithelium, (2) the cells appeared to be of basal origin, hyperchromatic, with some pleomorphism and increased mitotic activity, and (3) no evidence of invasion through the basement membrane. Dysplasia was classified as mild, moderate, or severe, depending on the degree of cellular and structural alterations between normal esophageal tissue and CIS.

[1] The Departments of Surgery and [2] Pathology, Shikoku Cancer Center Hospital, 13 Horinouchi, Matsuyama, Ehime, 790 Japan

Table 1. Number of lesions in 96 esophageal carcinoma patients

	Male $n = 83$	Female $n = 13$	Total $n = 96$
Dysplasia			
Mild	52 (62.7)	4 (30.8)	56 (58.3)
Moderate	47 (56.6)	3 (23.1)	50 (52.0)
Severe	15 (18.1)	0 (0.0)	15 (15.6)
Total	65 (78.3)	6 (46.1)	71 (74.0)
Carcinoma in situ	22 (26.5)	0 (0.0)	22 (22.9)

Numbers in parentheses indicate percentages

Table 2. Number of lesions in 71 esophageal carcinoma patients with dysplastic lesions

	Male $n = 65$	Female $n = 6$	Total $n = 71$
Dysplasia			
Mild	287 (4.4)	8 (1.3)	295 (4.2)
Moderate	147 (2.3)	5 (0.8)	152 (2.1)
Severe	42 (0.7)	0 (0.0)	42 (0.6)
Total	476 (7.3)	13 (2.2)	489 (6.9)
Carcinoma in situ	59 (1.0)	0 (0.0)	59 (0.9)

Numbers in parentheses indicate mean value of the number of dysplastic lesions in each esophagus

In all 96 cases, smoking and drinking habits were examined in the patient records. The patients were divided into two groups: those who had three or less lesions of dysplasia (group A), and those who had four or more (group B). Differences between each group were analyzed by the Chi-square test or Student's *t*-test.

Results

The mean age of the 96 patients at operation was 64 years. All sections of each esophagus were examined by microscopy (Tables 1, 2). Four hundred and eighty nine lesions of dysplasia were observed in 71 patients (74.0%) (Table 2), and CIS was observed in 22 of the 96 patients (22.9%) (Table 1). These lesions were usually small and multicentric and, occasionally, a continuity between carcinoma and dysplasia was observed. The rates of each grade of dysplasia and CIS was higher in men than in women.

As shown in Tables 3 and 4, there were significant differences in the male to female ratio, Brinkman index, incidence of multiple primary carcinoma of the esophagus, and incidence of primary carcinoma of the oropharynx between the two groups. There was no significant difference in survival rate between them.

Table 3. Characteristics of the groups A and B

	Group A	Group B	P value
No. of dysplasia lesions	0–3	$4 \leqq$	
No. of patients	55	41	
Age (mean ± SD)	63 ± 9	64 ± 8	0.451
Sex (male/female)	43/12	40/1	0.015
T-factor			
T_{is-1}	9	12	0.206
T_2	5	4	
T_3	27	13	
T_4	14	12	
N-factor			0.150
N_0	14	17	
N_1	41	24	
M-factor			0.957
M_0	47	34	
M_1	8	7	
Brinkman index			
Mean ± SD	668 ± 434	944 ± 478	0.003
Alcohol index[a]			
Mean ± SD	90 ± 105	115 ± 82	0.145

[a] Volume of Japanese wine (Gou: 180 ml) consumed per day, period one continue to drink every day (years)

Table 4. Characteristics of groups A and B

	Group A	Group B	P value
No. of dysplasia lesions	0–3	$4 \leqq$	
No. of patients	55	41	
No. of primary carcinomas in each esophagus			
1	48	23	0.001
2–4	7	14	
$\geqq 5$	0	4	
Separate primary carcinomas of Other organs			
Oropharynx	4	13	0.046
Larynx	1	1	
Lung	1	0	
Stomach	5	1	
Colo-rectal	0	1	
Liver	1	0	
Others	2	1	

Discussion

The frequent association of esophageal infiltrative carcinoma with dysplasia and/or CIS has suggested that there is a progression from dysplasia to CIS and to invasive carcinoma [1, 2]. Nagamatsu et al. histologically examined the surgical specimens obtained from 41 patients with esophageal carcinoma and found a low frequency of CIS with continuity to dysplasia, that might suggest the possibility of de novo carcinogenesis [3]. In this study, four or more lesions of dysplasia were seen in specimens from 57% of the patients with squamous cell carcinoma of the esophagus, while few such lesions were found in those from other patients. This finding might suggest that more than half of squamous cell carcinomas of the esophagus are preceded by dysplasia, while some of them have developed de novo.

It is well known that the incidence of esophageal carcinoma is much lower in women than in men, and the survival rate of female patients with esophageal carcinoma is significantly higher than that of male patients. That might suggest the possibility of different carcinogenesis between women and men. The finding that the incidence of multicentric dysplasia in female patients with esophageal carcinoma reported here was much lower than in male patients suggests that hormonal influences seem to play a major role in neoplastic development.

In the present study, there were significant correlations between tobacco consumption and incidence of multiple lesions of esophageal dysplasia, and they were frequently observed in patients with oropharyngeal carcinoma and multiple primary carcinoma of the esophagus. In relation to the etiology of esophageal carcinoma, Auerbach et al. emphasized striking histological changes of the esophageal mucosa among cigarette smokers [4]. Epithelial cells with disintegrated nuclei, basal cell hyperplasia, hyperactive glands, and cellular infiltration of the wall were more frequent and more pronounced among cigarette smokers than among non-smokers. All these changes are similar to dysplasia of the esophagus. Goldstein and Zornoza reported that esophageal carcinoma was frequently associated with squamous cell carcinoma of the head and neck region [5]. They also speculated that tobacco was a causative factor in these two primary cancer groups. These studies and ours support the possibility that the progress of dysplasia to squamous cell carcinoma is accelerated by tobacco consumption.

Our results show that the risk factors of esophageal squamous cell carcinoma associated with dysplasia are gender, smoking, oropharyngeal cancer, and multicentric carcinoma of the esophagus.

Acknowledgments. The authors are grateful to Mr. M. Yamauchi and Ms. Y. Yamamoto for their technical assistance. The present study was supported, in part, by a Grant-in-Aid for Cancer Research (2S-1) from the Ministry of Health and Welfare of Japan.

References

1. Ushigome S, Spjut HJ, Noon GP (1967) Extensive dysplasia and carcinoma in situ of esophageal epithelium. Cancer 20:1023–1029

2. Mandard AM, Marnay J, Gignoux M, Segol P, Blanc L, Ollivier JM, Borel B, Mandard JC (1984) Cancer of the esophagus and associated lesions: Detailed pathologic study of 100 esophagectomy specimens. Hum Pathol 15:660–669
3. Nagamatsu M, Mori M, Kuwano H, Sugimachi K, Akiyoshi T (1992) Serial histologic investigation of squamous epithelial dysplasia associated with carcinoma of the esophagus. Cancer 69:1094–1098
4. Auerbach O, Stout AP, Hammond EC, Garfinkel L (1965) Histologic changes in esophagus in relation to smoking habits. Arch Environ Health 11:4–15
5. Goldstein HM, Zornoza J (1978) Association of squamous cell carcinoma of the head and neck with cancer of the esophagus. Am J Roentgenol 131:791–794

Factors Influencing the Prognosis of Mucosal Carcinoma of the Esophagus

SHIN-ICHI MURAKAMI, YUZO UCHIDA, NOBUHIRO KUBO, TSUYOSHI NOGUCHI, KATSUHIKO MATSUMOTO, and TETSUO HADAMA[1]

Introduction

In recent years, an increasing number of cases of esophageal carcinoma have been diagnosed and resected curatively at the stage of mucosal carcinoma because of technical advances in endoscopic diagnosis. However, one such patient in our department died of recurrent carcinoma 13 months after resection. We observed a group of patients who underwent resection and investigated the factors which influenced the prognosis of mucosal esophageal carcinoma.

Patients and Methods

A total of 149 patients underwent resection of esophageal carcinoma in our department during the 11 years from 1981 to 1992; 126 were male and 23 female. The age distribution showed a peak in the 50s and 60s. These 149 cases included 13 cases of mucosal carcinoma, all in men. The locations of the main lesion in these 13 patients were classified and compared with those of the total population. In the mucosal carcinoma group, the main lesion was most frequently found in the middle intrathoracic esophagus (Im) region ($n = 6$), followed by the lower intrathoracic esophagus (Ei) region ($n = 4$), the upper intrathoracic esophagus (Iu) region ($n = 2$), and then the abdominal esophagus (Ea) region ($n = 1$). This distribution was similar to that of the total population.

We further classified the type of carcinoma as a function of the location of the main lesion according to the depth of invasion. We also observed the presence of lymph node metastasis, and studied the relationship between metastasis in each type of carcinoma and the findings from macroscopic observation.

[1] The Second Department of Surgery, Oita Medical University, 1-Idaigaoka, Hasama-machi, Oita, 879-55 Japan

Results

The types of mucosal carcinoma in the 13 patients were classified by the depth of carcinoma invasion. There were eight cases of ep (epithelial layer) carcinoma and five cases of mm (mucosal layer) carcinoma.

Next, we investigated the relationship between the lymph node metastasis and the depth of invasion and the macroscopic type. The classification of carcinoma by macroscopic observation was done in accordance with the *Guide lines for the Clinical and Pathologic Studies on Carcinoma of the Esophagus* [1] for macroscopic classification of mucosal carcinoma.

We further investigated tumors macroscopically. One case of ep-carcinoma belonged to a slightly elevated type (0-II$_a$), seven cases were a flat type (0-II$_b$), and five cases of mm-carcinoma were a slightly depressed type (0-II$_c$). Only one case involved lymph node metastasis.

We studied vascular invasion as a function of the depth of carcinoma. No lymphatic invasion of ep-carcinoma was found and there was no lymph node metastasis. Furthermore, lymphatic invasion was detected in only one out of five cases of mm-carcinoma, and lymph node metastasis was found in this case (Table 1). However, blood vessel invasion was not detected in any of these cases.

Among the 13 patients, 11 underwent high intrathoracic suture, while the other 2 patients underwent esophageal reconstruction through the antethoracic or retrosternal route. The one patient who had lymphatic invasion died because of recurrence in the upper thoracic paraesophageal lymph node 13 months after resection. The main lesion of the carcinoma was located in the middle intrathoracic esophagus (Fig. 1A,B). Histologically, the carcinoma was limited to the lamina propria mucosae (Fig. 2). Carcinoma cells were noticed in lymphatic vessels of the mucosal layer (Fig. 3). The other patients ($n = 12$) are alive without recurrence.

Table 1. Lymphatic invasion and lymph node metastasis in mucosal carcinoma

Lymph node metastasis	Depth of tumor invasion			Total
	ep	mm		
	n (−)	n (−)	n (+)	
ly (+)	0	0	1	1
ly (−)	8	4	0	12
Total	8	5		13

ep, invasion limited to the epithelium; *mm*, invasion confined to the lamina muscularis mucosae; *ly*, lymphatic vessels; *n*, regional lymph node; (+), positive for carcinoma invasion; (−), negative for carcinoma invasion

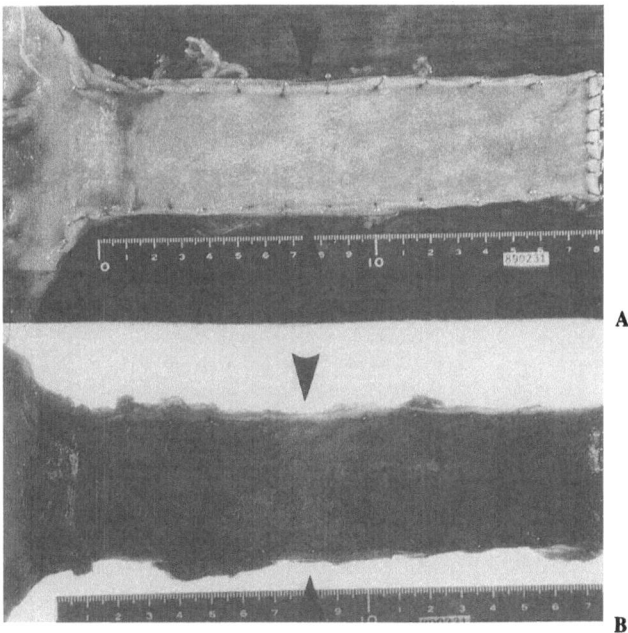

Fig. 1A,B. The resected specimen before (**A**), and after (**B**) dying with Lugol solution. **A** *Arrows* indicate an irregular depressed lesion with a granular or nodular surface in the middle intrathoracic esophagus. **B** An irregular unstained area is seen at the same site

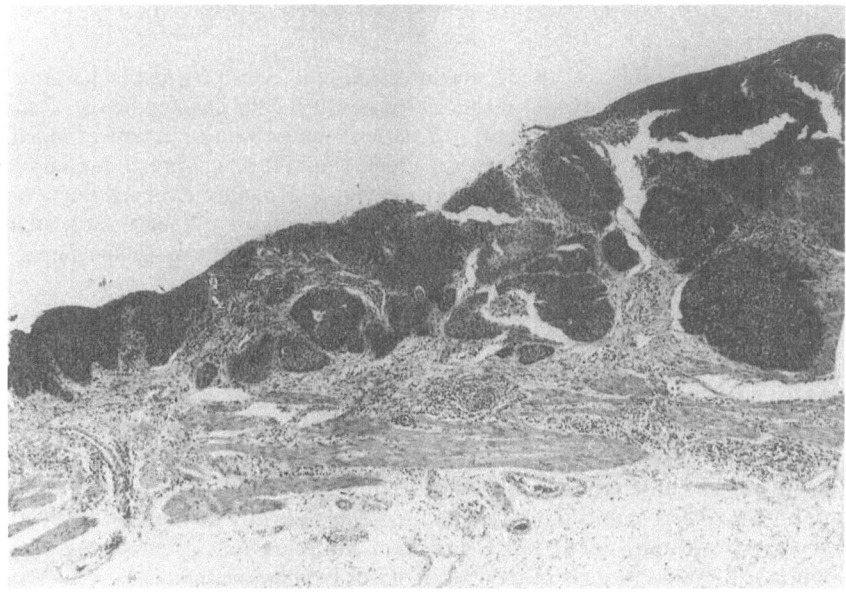

Fig. 2. Low magnification view of the depressed lesion. Moderately differentiated squamous cell carcinoma is seen in the deep lamina propria mucosae

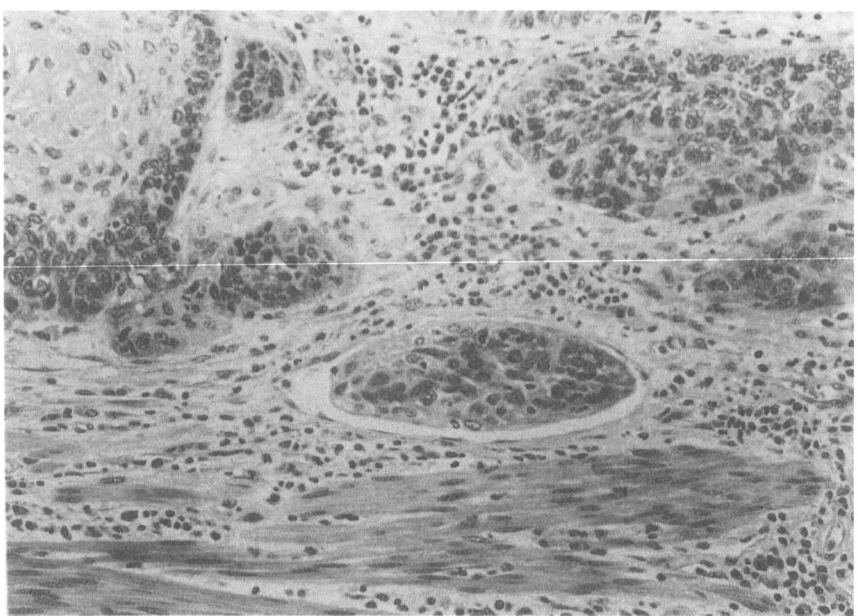

Fig. 3. Histologically, the carcinoma is limited to the lamina propria mucosae. Carcinoma cells are seen in lymphatic vessels of the lamina propria mucosae

Discussion

Mucosal esophageal carcinomas are increasing in recorded number because of improvements in endoscopic diagnosis, especially with developments in chro-moendoscopy [2–5]. In this study, 13 patients underwent resection of mucosal esophageal carcinoma. This number is greater than that in a previous study [3].

No special features in the incidence of mucosal esophageal carcinoma were observed, when comparing with the total population of esophageal carcinoma cases in terms of the male-to-female ratio, age distribution, or incidence by region.

Early detection and treatment are of great importance because the 5-year survival rate of patients undergoing resection of ep-carcinoma and mm-carcinoma is reported to be nearly 100% [4, 5]. Chromoendoscopy with iodine staining is very useful because it allows easier detection of minute or mucosal carcinoma [2, 3].

Among five cases of mm-carcinoma, one case (20%) had lymph node metastasis and lymphatic infiltration. Other institutions have reported lower percentages [4, 6]. The macroscopic finding of this case was a slightly depressed type (0-II$_c$). Therefore, we may need to pay particular attention to mm-carcinoma with a depressed lesion, because of the possibility of lymph node metastasis.

Acknowledgment. The authors thank Dr S. Yokoyama for pathological advice, and Dr K. Ono for critical reading of the manuscript.

References

1. Japanese Society for Esophageal Diseases (1992) Guide lines for the clinical and pathologic studies on carcinoma of the esophagus. Kanehara, Tokyo
2. Sugimachi K, Ohno S, Matsuda H, Mori M, Kuwano H (1988) Lugol-combined endoscopic detection of minute malignant lesions of the thoracic esophagus. Ann Surg 208:179–183
3. Misumi A, Harada K, Murakami A, Arima K, Kondo H, Akagi M, Yagi Y, Ikeda T, Kobori Y, Matsukane H, Baba K (1989) Early diagnosis of esophageal cancer. Ann Surg 210:732–739
4. Endo M, Kawano T (1992) Clinical evaluation of mucosal cancer of the esophagus: Analysis of 500 cases resected in Japan (in Japanese). Surgical Therapy 66:248–251
5. Makuuchi H, Machimura T, Soh Y, Mizutani K, Shimada H, Sugihara T, Tokuda Y, Sasaki T, Tajima T, Mitomi T, Ohmori T, Miyoshi H (1991) Endoscopic mucosectomy for mucosal carcinomas in the esophagus (in Japanese). Jpn J Gastroenterol Surg 24:2599–2603
6. Gaseki N, Koike M, Yoshida M (1992) Histopathologic characteristics of early stage esophageal carcinoma. Cancer 69:1088–1093

Cytokeratin 14, 18, and 19 Expression in Normal Epithelium and in Squamous Cancer of the Esophagus

K. Geboes, K. Haustermans, T. Lerut, and M. Van der Schueren[1]

Introduction

The normal esophagus is lined by a tough non-keratinizing stratified squamous epithelium, except for a short segment of columnar epithelium at the gastroesophageal junction. Different cell layers have classically been described in this epithelium. The basal or germinative layer is made up of cylindrical, basophilic cells and is covered by several intermediate layers of polyhedral cells. The layers adjacent to the lumen are flattened and form the superficial compartment [1–2]. The proliferative compartment in the squamous epithelium of the esophagus resides in the basal layer of cells. The basal cells can be divided in two topographically different but contiguous compartments both forming the junction with the lamina propria connective tissue: One is a flat layer lying parallel with the longitudinal axis of the esophagus and the second is lining the stromal papillae and lying perpendicular to the luminal axis of the esophagus. The connective tissue of the stromal papillae is highly vascularized [3]. Random mitotic figures can be observed by routine microscopy in both compartments of the basal cell layer. Immunohistochemistry using antibodies directed against BRDU (bromodeoxyuridine), a compound which is incorporated in the nucleus, can demonstrate the presence of S-phase cells in the same layer. For the normal proliferative layer, the labelling index, indicating the ratio between the number of cells showing a positive staining for BRDU and the sum of the labelled and the unlabelled cells is 8.7%. For the entire mucosa, we found a labelling index of 0.95%. This indicates a slow rate of cell renewal.

The properties of shape, internal organization, and tissue organization of eukaryotic cells depend on a complex network of protein filaments in the

[1] Laboratory of Histo and Cytochemistry, University Hospital St. Rafael KUL, Minderbroedersstraat 12, B-3000 Leuven, Belgium

cytoplasm of the cells that serve as a "cytoskeleton". Cytokeratins constitute the largest group of intermediate filaments, one of the three families of cytoskeletal proteins (microtubules, microfilaments, and intermediate filaments). Cytokeratins are characteristic of epithelial cells. The 19 different (epithelial) cytokeratin polypeptides identified can be divided into two families according to their charges, immunoreactivity, and other characteristics. One family comprises relatively acidic polypeptides (numbers 9–19) while the other consists of neutral to basic cytokeratins (numbers 1–8). Individual epithelial cells express a limited number of cytokeratins consisting of pairs of one type I and one type II cytokeratin [4]. Acidic type I cytokeratins 17, 18, and 19 occur in simple epithelia. Acidic type I cytokeratins 14 and 16 occur in stratified epithelia. Acidic type I cytokeratin 13 is associated with esophageal type differentiation. In the esophagus, the pairs of keratins vary in the different compartments with the degree of differentiation of the epithelial cells. Keratin types 4 and 13 have been demonstrated in the cells of the basal compartment and types 1 and 10 have been found in the parabasal cells [5].

Epidermal growth factor (EGF) receptor is a plasma membrane glycoprotein which binds EGF [6]. EGF is a mitogenic polypeptide which plays an important role in the maintenance of tissue integrity, healing, and maturation [7]. EGF receptors are normally expressed in normal squamous epithelium of the esophagus. The expression is observed as a membranous staining and is limited to the basal cell layers (including the proliferative compartment and some layers of the stratum spinosum). The superficial functional layer of the esophageal epithelium adjacent to the lumen is normally negative for EGF receptors [6].

Aim of the Study

The aim of the study was to further examine the expression of cytokeratins in the normal esophagus and in squamous cancer of the esophagus, and to correlate the expression with the presence of EGF receptors.

Materials and Methods

Biopsies from 15 patients (8 male and 7 female, mean age 60 years) operated for advanced squamous cell carcinoma were studied. The biopsies were obtained from the resection specimen which was transferred to the laboratory immediately after surgery. The biopsies were taken from normal mucosa ($n = 15$), from different areas of the tumor (center and periphery) ($n = 60$), and from dysplastic areas either adjacent to the tumor ($n = 5$) or at a distance ($n = 3$). Dysplasia was defined according to internationally accepted criteria [8]. The specimens were snap-frozen in liquid nitrogen-cooled isopentane and stored at $-70°C$ until further use. Cryostat sections were used for routine staining and for immunohistochemistry.

Cryostat sections of the biopsies were stained with haematoxylin and eosin for routine microscopy and with monoclonal antibodies directed against cytokeratins 14 (Ramaekers/Van Eyken, Leuven) and 18 and 19 (Amersham International,

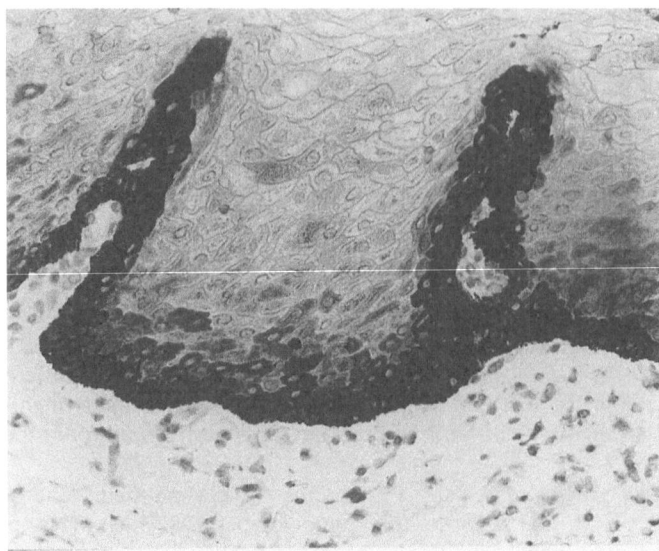

Fig. 1. Normal squamous epithelium of the human esophagus stained with a monoclonal antibody directed against cytokeratin 14 showing positive staining in the basal cell layer lining the stromal papillae and the flat basal cell layer parallel with the longitudinal axis of the esophagus. (×125)

England) and a monoclonal antibody directed against EGF receptor (Amersham) following an indirect immunoperoxidase method. Acidic types 18 and 19 were chosen because they are common in simple epithelia. Controls, which were invariably negative, consisted of omission of the primary antibody.

Results

Normal Squamous Epithelium

EGF receptor was expressed on the basal and immediately suprabasal cells as a peripheral membranous staining. No differences were observed between the basal cells lining the stromal papillae and the basal cells in the flat layer lying parallel to the longitudinal axis of the esophagus.

Cytokeratin 14 was expressed diffusely in the cells of the basal layer of both compartments and in some cells lying in a suprabasal position. A more extensive staining of suprabasal cells was observed in 9/15 biopsies of normal mucosa (Fig. 1).

Cytokeratin 19 was mainly expressed in the basal cells lining the stromal papillae and, to a certain extent, also in basal cells of the flat layer. In the latter position, positivity could be observed in single cells or in groups of cells in contiguity with the stromal papillae (Fig. 2). Cytokeratin 18 was not expressed in the esophageal epithelium.

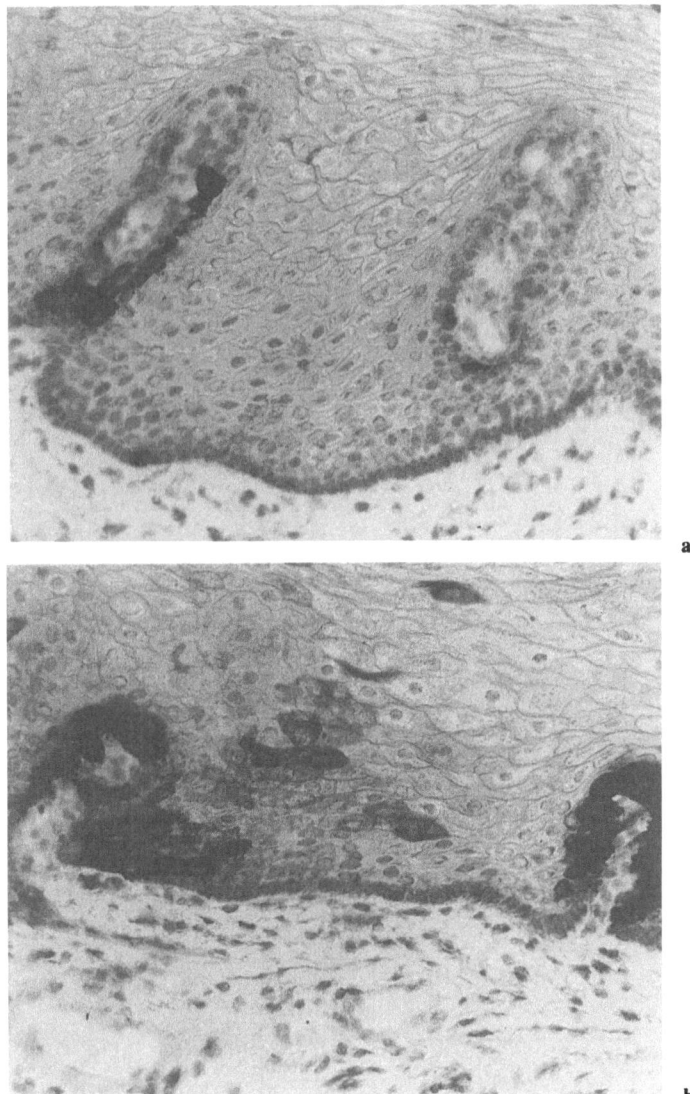

Fig. 2a,b. Normal squamous epithelium of the human esophagus stained with a monoclonal antibody directed against cytokeratin 19. **a** is a serial section of Fig. 1 and shows positive staining in the basal cells lining the stromal papillae and in a solitary cell in the flat basal layer. **b** Positivity in some suprabasal cells and in cells of the basal layer. (×125)

Dysplasia

In areas of dysplasia, an increased expression of EGF receptor was present in all layers of the esophageal epithelium, including the superficial layers adjacent to the lumen. For cytokeratin 14, the expression was also increased and present in

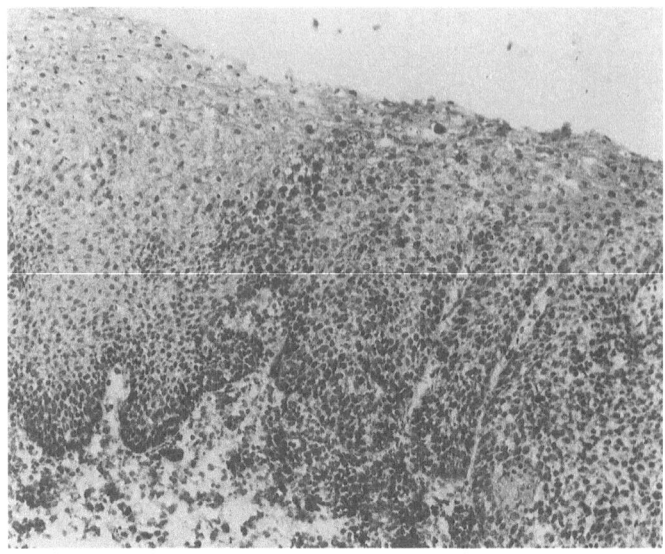

Fig. 3. Squamous epithelium of the human esophagus showing on the *left* normal epithelium and on the *right* half an area of dysplasia. (H&E, ×50)

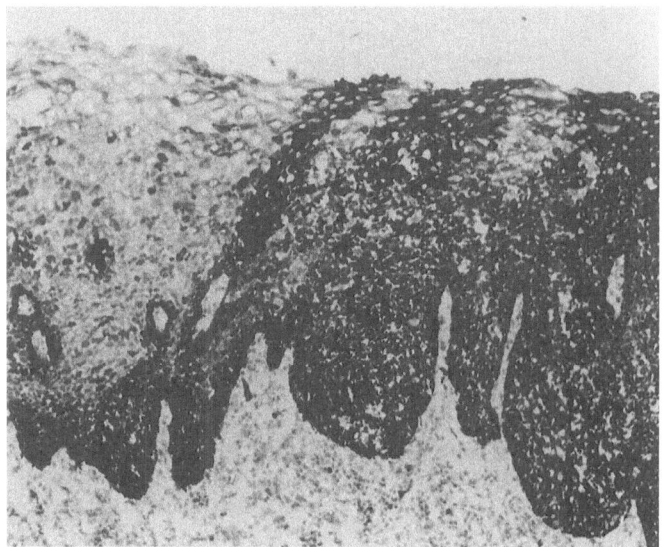

Fig. 4. Serial section of Fig. 3 stained with a monoclonal antibody directed against cytokeratin 14 showing widespread and intense staining in the area of dysplasia. (×50)

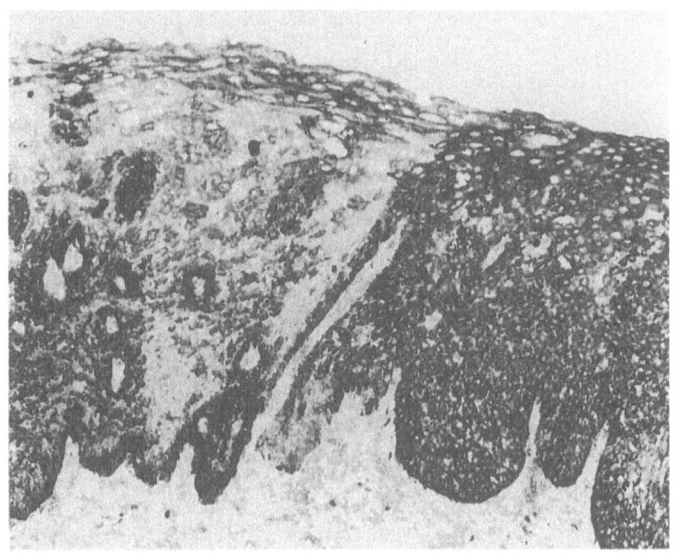

Fig. 5. Serial section of Figs. 3 and 4 stained with a monoclonal antibody directed against cytokeratin 19 showing widespread and intense staining in the area of dysplasia, but also in the normal-appearing adjacent epithelium. (×50)

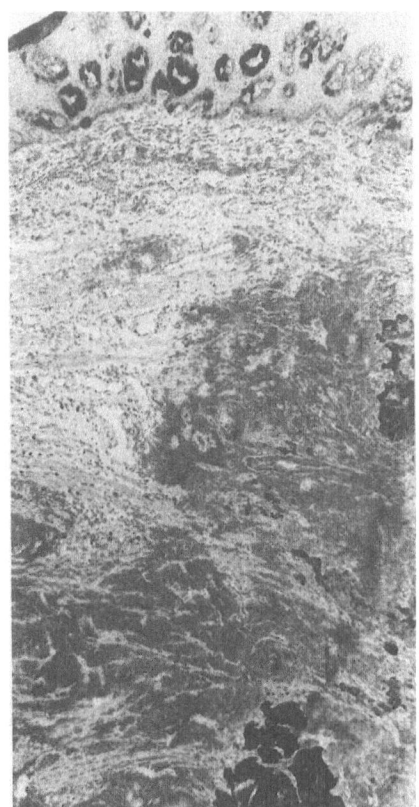

Fig. 6. Human esophageal biopsy stained with antibodies directed against cytokeratin 19 showing, at the *top*, a positive staining for the cells in the basal layer lining the stromal papillae and positively-staining tumor nodules in the deeply situated muscularis. (×20)

all cell layers (Figs. 3, 4). A similar pattern was observed for cytokeratin 19, while cytokeratin 18 staining remained negative (Fig. 5).

Squamous Carcinoma

EGF receptor expression was widely increased in tumor nodules. For cytokeratins 14 and 19, an increased expression was also observed in tumor areas. In carcinomas, the expression was most pronounced in moderately or poorly differentiated areas and this correlated well with the localization of the expression of EGF receptor. Intratumoral variation was minimal. Cytokeratin 18 expression remained negative (Fig. 6).

Conclusion

Our findings show that staining for cytokeratins makes it possible to distinguish between various compartments of cells in the normal squamous epithelium of the esophagus. Cytokeratin 14 is more intensely expressed in basal cells lining the stromal papillae than in the basal cells forming the flat layer. Whether this difference is functionally important cannot be concluded from this type of study. Such a difference might well be possible and might be related to differences in vascularization, as the stromal papillae are highly vascularized. The expression of cytokeratins 14 and 19 is limited to basal cells and to cells in an immediately suprabasal position, and hence to cells of the proliferative compartment and young cells. The expression of EGF receptor is more widely present than for cytokeratins 14 and 19. The greatest intensity of epidermal growth factor receptor correlates well with the presence of cytokeratin 14- and 19-positive cells. EGF receptor staining does, however, not show any difference between the basal cells lining the stromal papillae and those forming the flat layer. The expression of cytokeratins 14 and 19 and of EGF is greatly increased in areas of dysplasia and of squamous carcinoma. Staining with antibodies directed against cytokeratins 14 and 19 can therefore serve as a biomarker for the identification of early epithelial abnormalities with increased predisposition to esophageal malignancy, especially when a diagnosis of dysplasia is difficult on routine microscopy. Technically, it is easier to perform than morphometry and therefore immunohistochemical coloration may be more acceptable in general pathology laboratories.

References

1. Geboes K, Desmet V (1978) Histology of the esophagus. Front Gastrointest Res 3:1–17
2. Geboes K, Mebis J, Desmet V (1988) The esophagus: Normal ultrastructure and pathological patterns. In: Motta PM, Fujita H (eds) Ultrastructure of the digestive tract. Martinus Nijhoff, Boston, pp 17–34
3. Geboes K, Janssens J, Vantrappen G (1992) Basic lesions in inflammatory disorders of the esophagus. Dig Dis Pathol 3:2–34
4. Van Eyken P (1990) Phenotypic modulation of hepatocytes: A cytokeratin-immunohisto-chemical study. Acco, Leuven, pp 11–54

5. Moll R, Franke WW, Schiller DA, Geiger B, Krepler R (1982) The catalog of human cytokeratins: Patterns of expression in normal epithelia, tumors and cultured cells. Cell 31:11–24
6. Jankowski J, Murphy S, Coghill G, Grant A, Wormsley KG, Sanders DSA, Kerr M, Hopwood D (1992) Epidermal growth factor receptors in the oesophagus. Gut 33:439–443
7. Hirayama D, Fujimori T, Satonaka K, Nakamura T, Kitazawa S, Horio M, Maeda S, Nagasako K (1992) Immunohistochemical study of epidermal growth factor and transforming growth factor-beta in the penetrating type of early gastric cancer. Hum Pathol 23:681–685
8. Lindholm J, Rubio CA, Kato Y, Hata J (1989) A morphometric method to discriminate normal from dysplastic/carcinoma in situ squamous epithelium in the human esophagus. Path Res Pract 184:297–305

Studies on the Relationship Between Desmosomes and Metastasis and Prognosis of Esophageal Cancer

Takashi Koyama, Masayuki Matsumori, Toshihiro Omori,
Satoru Hayashi, Tetsuya Hattori, Nobuhisa Watanabe,
Masayoshi Okada[1], and Sakan Maeda[2]

Introduction

Desmosomes are intercellular junctions, particularly characteristic of epithelial cells, and they are major contributors to cell-cell adhesion in many epithelial cells. Decreased intercellular adhesion has been reported for many carcinomas, and it has been suggested that in part, such alterations in adhesion may be due to changes in adhering junctions, such as the desmosome [1]. In the human urinary bladder, a correlation between decreased numbers of desmosomes and aggressiveness of transitional cell carcinomas has been reported [2]. To define highly malignant esophageal squamous cell carcinoma (SCC) we have investigated the relationship of desmosome numbers to tumor invasiveness and metastasis in esophageal SCCs in a quantitative electron microscopic study [3]. We have also studied this structure with reference to outcome, because all cases studied had been followed for at least 5 years.

Material and Methods

Twenty-five esophageal SCCs treated in the Second Department of Surgery at Kobe University Hospital from 1985 to 1987 were analyzed electron microscopically. Five normal esophageal biopsy specimens were used as normal controls. In each case, four specimens were obtained endoscopically before treatment. Each specimen was thinly sliced into five sections, and 20 Epon blocks were prepared for electron microscopy in conventional fashion [3]. Four blocks were selected at random and thin-sectioned. With standard morphometric intercept

[1] Department of Surgery, Division II, and [2] Department of Pathology, Division II, Kobe University School of Medicine, 7 Kusunoki-cho, Chuo-ku, Kobe, 650 Japan

counting techniques, as described in detail by Wiebel et al. [4], we determined the percentage of tumor cell surface occupied by desmosomes (%DES). In brief, five electron micrographs were taken from each of the four blocks at a constant direct magnification of 10000×. The images were projected onto a screen with a double-lattice test system and we calculated the surface-to-volume ratio of desmosomes. This system is useful for studying the volumetric density of scarce components, such as desmosomes, in the cytoplasm.

Statistical comparisons between the various groups were performed with the unpaired Student's t-test. The level of significance was determined at $P < 0.05$.

Results

Comparison of Non-Cancerous and Cancerous Stratified Squamous Epithelial Cells

The percentages of tumor cell surface occupied by desmosomes (%DES) in noncancerous cells, and in well, moderately, and poorly differentiated cancer cells were 6.82% ± 0.83%, 5.06% ± 1.97%, 3.70% ± 1.14%, and 1.22% ± 0.66%, respectively, with half of the well-differentiated cells showing approximately the same %DES as noncancerous cells (Fig. 1a). In general, %DES clearly decreased in cancer cells, among which %DES decreased with decreasing degree of differentiation.

Growth Pattern

We classified the growth patterns of esophageal SCCs into four groups, according to the classification by Crissman et al. [5], as follows: α: well-defined borderline;

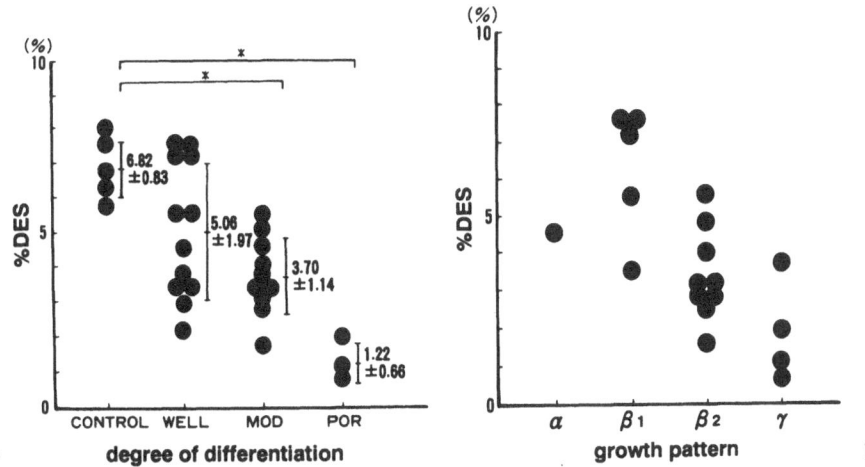

Fig. 1. a Percentage of cell surface occupied by desmosomes (%DES) for noncancerous stratified squamous epithelial cells and for cancerous ones *$P < 0.01$. b %DES of various growth patterns of squamous cell carcinomas (SCCs)

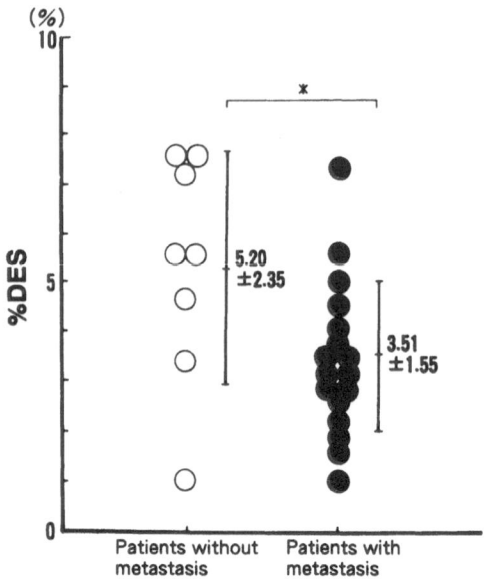

Fig. 2. %DES of esophageal SCCs with and without lymph node metastasis. *$P < 0.05$

β1: cords, less-marked borderline; β2: groups of cells, no distinct borderline; γ: diffuse invasion as thin irregular cords or single cells. The cells with only a few desmosomes showed an invasive growth pattern while those with many desmosomes tended to show an expansive growth pattern (Fig. 1b).

Lymph Node Metastasis

In the group without metastasis, %DES was 5.20% ± 2.35%, while %DES was significantly lower, 3.51% ± 1.55%, in the group with metastasis (Fig. 2).

Patients' Outcome

The patients who died from other diseases were excluded from the group of patients who underwent radical surgery, and the resulting 18 patients were divided into two groups, one with %DES of 5.0% or higher and the other with %DES of lower than 5.0%. Most patients in both groups were stage III or IV, and there was no difference in stage between these two groups. However, there was a significant difference in survival rates between these groups: 1-year survival rates were 76% and 37%, respectively, and 2-year survival rates were 76% and 8%, respectively (Fig. 3a). The %DES in stage III and IV patients who died within 6 months was compared with that in patients who survived for more than 2 years after surgery. The latter group showed a significantly higher %DES (Fig. 3b). Of three patients with %DES higher than 5.0%, two survived more than 5 years without recurrence.

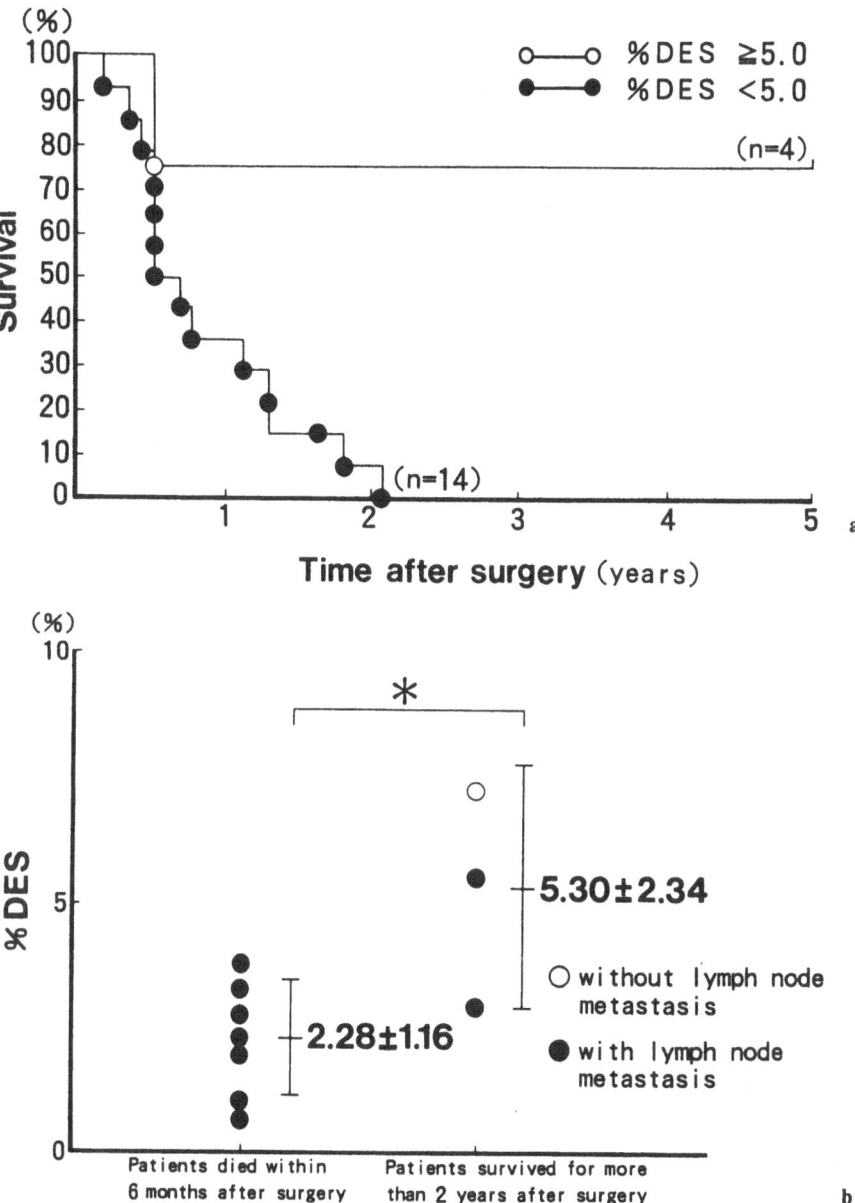

Fig. 3. a Comparison of survival rates between patients with %DES more than 5.0 and those with %DES less than 5.0. There was a significant difference between these two groups ($P < 0.01$). b %DES in stage III and IV patients who died within 6 months after surgery and those who survived for more than 2 years. $*P < 0.05$

Discussion

Whether cancer cells possess the ability to metastasize is important to the choice of cancer therapy. Based on the biological behavior of cancer, patients with potentially highly metastatic cancer should undergo extended surgery, whereas those with a low metastatic potential may undergo modified surgery. Therefore, it is important to evaluate the grade of malignancy before treatment. Histologic evaluation of malignancy by light microscope, for instance by degree of differentiation, is not sufficient to predict the possibility of metastasis, or the patient outcome. Recently, the malignancy of cancer cells was quantitatively determined, by measuring the nuclear DNA level [6, 7] or the immunoreactivity of epidermal growth factor [8] as indices, for assessing the treatment of esophageal cancer. In order to evaluate the metastatic potential of esophageal cancer, we attempted to examine the desmosome, which contributes to cell-cell adhesion. It has been proposed that decreased intercellular adhesion is a general property of carcinomas [9]. In fact, cancer cells express fewer specialized cell-cell contacts such as communication ("gap") junctions [10] and desmosomes [2, 11–13]. Such decreases in intercellular adhesion may explain certain patterns of tumor growth and may be prerequisites for the occurrence of tumor invasion and dissemination [14]. Low desmosome counts were generally reported in oral and urinary SCCs experimentally induced in animals [12, 13] and in transitional cell carcinomas of the human bladder, in which a correlation between decreased numbers of desmosomes and the aggressiveness of transitional cell carcinomas has been reported [2]. We have also demonstrated a negative correlation between desmosome numbers and the grade of lymph node metastasis in esophageal carcinoma in a previous report [3]. In the present study, we calculated the percentage of tumor cell surface occupied by desmosomes with standard morphometric intercept counting techniques and obtained essentially the same results as in the previous study.

Our results demonstrated a positive correlation between degree of differentiation and desmosome numbers, as previously reported. Even among similarly well differentiated SCCs, some showed numerous desmosomes, while others showed only a few. In biological behavior of esophageal SCCs, there was a significant difference between these two groups. All five patients with %DES less than 4.0% had lymph node metastasis and died within 15 months (mean 7 months), whereas three of four patients with %DES more than 7.0% had no metastasis. All patients in this study had been followed for at least 5 years. Only 3 of 25 patients survived for more than 5 years, and the %DES of these three patients was more than 5%. As shown in Fig. 3, there is a close correlation between desmosome numbers and survival. These findings suggest that desmosome numbers have a prognostic value in patients with esophageal SCCs. Early in our research, desmosome numbers had been considered a good parameter of metastatic potential. As our research advanced, we found that desmosome number is a useful parameter of malignancy rather than metastatic potential, because metastases are the result of a complex process that is characterized by a sequence of steps [15] and detachment from the primary tumor alone does not constitute metastasis. Although in this first step, decreased adhesiveness may promote detachment from the primary tumor, many factors, including the immune response of the host, subsequently influence the metastasis. In an ultrastructual study of colon cancer cell lines, which were treated with *N,N*-dimethylformamide (DMF) to reduce tumorigenicity in nude mice, Christensen and co-workers [16] demonstrated that cytoplasmic organelles in these cells were essentially unchanged except for an increase in tonofilaments and associated desmosomes. They concluded that whether the supernumerary desmosomes in DMF-treated cells contribute to the reduction in the malignant behavior of these cells in vivo remains to be determined. However, the mechanism of the DMF-induced increase in desmosomes is unknown and the reduction in tumorigenicity may or may not be due to an increase in the number of desmosomes.

Based on these results, we conclude that desmosome numbers are a good parameter for grading the malignant potential in esophageal SCC.

References

1. Pauli BU, Alroy J, Weinstein RS (1983) In: Bryan GT, Cohen SM (eds) The pathology of bladder cancer, vol 2. CRC, Boca Raton, pp 41–140
2. Alroy J, Pauli BU, Weinstein RS (1981) Correlation between numbers of desmosomes and the aggressiveness of transitional cell carcinoma in human urinary bladder. Cancer 47:104–112
3. Koyama T (1989) Studies on the relationship between desmosomes and the mode of infiltration and metastasis of esophageal cancer (in Japanese with English abstract). Nippon Geka Gakkai Zasshi (J Jpn Surg Soc) 90:1–10
4. Weibel ER, Kistler GS, Scherle WF (1966) Practical stereological methods for morphometric cytology. J Cell Biol 30:23–38
5. Crissman JD, Makuch R, Budhraja M (1985) Histopathologic grading of squamous cell carcinoma of the uterine cervix—an evaluation of 70 Stage Ib patients. Cancer 55:1590–1596
6. Hasegawa M (1990) Cytodynamic evaluation on the relationship between the mode of intracellular DNA content and the prognosis of esophageal cancer patients (in Japanese with English abstract). Nippon Geka Gakkai Zasshi (J Jpn Surg Soc) 91:191–199
7. Rikitake H (1990) Studies on DNA content in ploidy patterns of esophageal cancer (in Japanese with English abstract). Nippon Geka Gakkai Zasshi (J Jpn Surg Soc) 91:564–574
8. Mukaida H, Yamamoto T, Hirai T, Toi M, Nakamura T, Wada T, Yamashita Y, Kawano K, Niimoto M (1990) Expression of human epidermal growth factor and its receptor in esophageal cancer. Jpn J Surg 20:275–282
9. Coman DR (1944) Decreased mutual adhesiveness, a property of cells from squamous cell carcinoma. Cancer Res 4:625–629
10. Kocher O, Amaudruz M, Schindler AM, Gabbiani G (1981) Desmosomes and gap junctions in precarcinomatous and carcinomatous conditions of squamous epithelia. J Submicrosc Cytol 13:267–281
11. McNutt NS, Hershberg RA, Weinstein RS (1971) Further observation on the occurrence of nexuses in benign and malignant human cervical epithelium. J Cell Biol 51:805–825
12. Tachikawa T, Yamura T, Yoshiki S (1984) Changes occurring in plasma membranes and intercellular junctions during the process of carcinogenesis and in squamous cell carcinoma. Virchows Arch [B] 47:1–15
13. Pauli BU, Cohen SM, Alroy J, Weinstein R (1978) Desmosome ultrastructure and biological behavior of carcinogen-induced urinary bladder carcinomas. Cancer Res 38:3276–3285
14. McNutt NS, Weinstein RS (1969) Carcinoma of the cervix: Deficiency of nexus intercellular junctions. Science 165:597–599
15. Brodland DG, Zitelli JA (1992) Mechanisms of metastasis. J Am Acad Dermatol 27:1–8
16. Christensen TG, Burke B, Dexter DL, Zamcheck N (1985) Ultrastructural evidence of dimethylformamide-induced differentiation of cultured human colon carcinoma cells. Cancer 56:1559–1565

Immunohistochemical Study of Esophageal Carcinomas Other Than Squamous Cell Carcinoma

YOSHIHISA MORISAKI, SHINGO SHIMA, YUTAKA YOSHIZUMI, YOSHIAKI SUGIURA, and SUSUMU TANAKA[1]

Introduction

It was previously thought that esophageal carcinomas other than squamous cell carcinoma were very rare; for example, Suzuki and Nagayo found 256 (2.1%) of 11,932 resected cases and 360 (7.2%) of 4995 autopsied cases of the esophagus [1]. However, recently some authors have indicated that these tumors were not so rare [2, 3]. We found 29 cases (12.7%) of these carcinomas among 229 resected cases of esophageal carcinoma from 1978 to 1991, we interested the histological origins of the 29 cases (12.7%) of non-squamous cell carcinoma. These tumors were immunohistochemically stained for the purpose of determination of their histological origin and/or differentiation.

Materials and Methods

Materials

Eighteen resected specimens of primary esophageal carcinoma were collected from the National Defense Medical College, Saitama, Japan. All these specimens were diagnosed as primary esophageal carcinomas other than squamous cell carcinoma, according to the histological classification of esophageal cancer of the Japanese Society for Esophageal Disease [4]. These specimens consisted of adenosquamous carcinoma (9 cases), basaloid-squamous carcinoma (4 cases), adenoid cystic carcinoma (one case), and so-called carcinosarcoma (4 cases). One normal esophageal specimen was used for the control material. All specimens were fixed with 10% buffered formalin and embedded in paraffin.

---

[1] Department of Surgery II, National Defense Medical College, 3-2 Namiki, Tokorozawa, Saitama, 359 Japan

Antibodies

Antibodies to: (1) three different classes of human keratin, (2) secretory component (SC, polyclonal), (3) vimentin (monoclonal), (4) desmin (polyclonal), (5) myoglobin (polyclonal), (6) muscle actin (monoclonal), and (7) S-100 protein (S-100, polyclonal) were used. These three anti-keratin antibodies were two monoclonal, PKK-1 and KL-1, and one polyclonal (Poly). PKK-1 was obtained from Labsystem Oy (Helsinki, Finland), KL-1 from Immunotech S.A. (Marseille, France), and all other antibodies from DAKO Co Ltd (Copenhagen, Denmark).

Immunohistochemistry

Formalin-fixed, paraffin-embedded tissues were stained using the streptavidin-biotin peroxidase complex method [5]. Tissues were cut into 4-μm sections, and deparaffinized in xylene and then rehydrated in graded alcohol and water. Before the tissues were incubated with primary antibodies, 0.3% H_2O_2 and normal rabbit or gout serum were used to eliminate endogenous enzyme and cut non-specific background staining, respectively. The tissues were allowed to react with each primary of the antibodies for 2 h at room temperature. After being washed with phosphate-buffered saline (PBS), the tissues were allowed to react with biotinylated rabbit anti-mouse or gout anti-rabbit immunoglobulin as secondary antibodies for 1 h at room temperature. Subsequently, they were reacted with streptavidin-biotin peroxidase complex for 30 min at room temperature. After being washed with PBS, the slides were developed in 0.02% 3- 3'diaminobenzidine then counter stained with hematoxylin, dehydrated in graded alcohol, cleared in xylene and mounted.

Results

Normal Esophageal Specimens (Table 1)

In normal mucosal epithelium, basal cells did not react with any keratin, but most of the cells in suprabasal layer reacted with keratin excepting PKK-1. On the other side, ductal cells in esophageal glands proper reacted with SC and PKK-1.

Table 1. Immunohistochemical staining in normal esophageal specimens

	Poly	KL-1	PKK-1	SC
Epithelia				
Suprabasal	+	+	−	−
Basal	−	−	−	−
Gland proper				
Ductal cell	+	+	+	+
Mucous cell	+	+/−	−	−

+, All cells positive; +/−, some cells positive; −, negative; *SC*, secretory component; *Poly*, polyclonal anti-Keratin antibody; *KL-1 and PKK-1*, monoclonal anti-Keratin antibodies

Table 2. Immunohistochemical staining in adenomatous components of adenosquamous carcinoma

	Poly	KL-1	PKK-1	SC
Glandular type				
Case 1	+	+	−	−
2	+	+	−	−
3	+	+	+	+
4	+	+	+	+
5	+	+	−	−
6[a]	+	+	−	−
7[a]	+	+	−	−
8[a]	+	+	−	−
Mucous cell type				
Case 6[a]	+	+	−	−
7[a]	+	+	−	−
8[a]	+	+	−	−
9	+	+	−	−

[a] Combined type; +, positive; −, negative

Table 3. Immunohistochemical staining in basaloid-squamous and adenoid cystic carcinoma

	Poly	KL-1	PKK-1	SC	S-100
Basaloid-squamous ca.					
Case 1	−	−	−	−	−
Case 2	−	−	−	−	−
Case 3	−	−	−	−	−
Case 4	−	−	−	−	−
Adenoid cystic ca.	−	−	−	−	+

+, Positive; −, negative; *ca.*, carcinoma

Adenosquamous Carcinoma (Table 2)

Reactivities with Poly and KL-1 were found in adenomatous components of all cases. Reactivities with SC and PKK-1 were found in only two cases (cases 3 and 4), but not in the remaining seven cases.

Basaloid-Squamous Carcinoma and Adenoid Cystic Carcinoma (Table 3)

No reactivities with any keratin and SC were found in both basaloid-squamous and adenoid cystic carcinoma. On the other hand, reactivities with S-100 were found only in adenoid cystic carcinoma, but not in basaloid-squamous carcinoma.

So-Called Carcinosarcoma (Table 4)

Reactivities with Poly were found in carcinomatous components in three cases, but not in one case (case 4). The carcinomatous component of case 4 was composed of basaloid-squamous carcinoma, of which reactivity with keratin was

Table 4. Immunohistochemical staining in esophageal carcinoma with sarcomatous components

| | Keratin | | Vimentin | | Muscle actin | | Desmin,S-100 myoglobin | |
	Carcinoma	Spindle	Carcinoma	Spindle	Carcinoma	Spindle	Carcinoma	Spindle
Case 1	+	−	−	++	−	+	−	−
Case 2	+	−	−	++	−	+	−	−
Case 3	+	−	−	+	−	+	−	−
Case 4	−	−	−	++	−	+	−	−

++, Strongly positive; +, positive; −, negative

negative. Though reactivities with vimentin and muscle actin were found in sarcomatous component of all cases, that of desmin and myoglobin were not found.

Discussion

Esophageal carcinomas other than squamous cell carcinoma are now thought to be less rare than was previously believed. However, the histological origin of these tumors is still unclear. So we performed immunohistochemical staining about these tumors and normal esophagus, so as to compare and determine their histological origin and/or differentiation.

Adenosquamous carcinoma is the most common tumor among these groups. Previously, adenomatous component had been thought to arise from the ductal cells of esophageal glands proper [6, 7], but Takubo indicated that the incidence of intraepitherial spread in the mucosa had been about the same in carcinoma with adenomatous components and in the carcinomas without such a components, and from this result he supposed that the adenomatous components did not arise from the ductal cells, but occurred during the process of invasion by ordinary intraepitherial squamous cell carcinoma. In this study, reactivities with SC and PKK-1, which were recognized to be the specific indicators of glandular differentiation, were found only in two cases (cases 3 and 4). If the adenomatous components had been arisen in the ductal cells esophageal glands proper, reactivities of SC component and PKK-1 should be seen in most of cases. And we thought this difference in the reactivities of SC and PKK-1 among the cases of adenosquamous carcinoma had been caused by the different degree of adenomatous differentiation, but not by the difference of histological origin. So it was supposed that the adenomatous components did not originate in the esophageal glands proper, but had been formed by glandular differentiation of squamous cell carcinoma.

Basaloid-squamous carcinoma and adenoid cystic carcinoma are similar in the pathological feature [8]. Actually, the case of basaloid-squamous carcinoma often reported as adenoid cystic carcinoma [9]. In our previous report [8], we reported that both these tumors were similar in their reactivities with keratin to be the basal cells of esophageal epithelium, and suggested they were basal in origin. In this study, reactivities of S-100 was found in adenoid cystic carcinoma, but not in basaloid-squamous carcinoma. This might suggest adenoid cystic carcinoma had differentiated to the myoepithelial cells from basal cells, but this theory about the reactivities of S-100 requires further study.

Esophageal carcinoma composed of both carcinomatous and sarcomatous components have been called carcinosarcoma, pseudosarcoma, or spindle cell carcinoma, and the origin of sarcomatous component have not been clarified. On the basis of major concept, sarcomatous components were thought to arise from mesenchymal metaplasia of squamous cell carcinoma [10], but in this study, sarcomatous components of all four cases were positive for vimentin and muscle actin, but negative for desmin and keratin, and these behaviors were compatible with phenotype known as myofibroblast in the histochemical reactivities [11]. Myofibroblast was thought to be derived from fibroblast and it was also found in the stroma of invading cancers [12]. This result indicated that sarcomatous spindle cells proliferating in the stroma of the cancer are of a myofibroblast origin, probably induced under the influence of the cancer invasion.

Acknowledgments. The authors wish to thank Yoshifumi Ishii, MD for his help in this study.

References

1. Suzuki H, Nagayo T (1985) Primary tumors of esophagus other than squamous cell carcinoma. Histologic classification and statistics in the surgical and autopsied materials in Japan. Int Adv Surg Oncol 3:73–109
2. Kuwano H, Ueo H, Sugimachi K, Nokuchi K, Toyoshima S, Enjoji M (1985) Glandular or mucous-secreting components in squamous cell carcinoma of esophagus. Cancer 56:514–518
3. Takubo K, Sasajima K, Yamashita K, Tanaka Y, Fujita K, Mafune K, Wang QH (1989) Morphological heterogeneity of esophageal carcinoma. Acta Pathol Jpn 39:180–189
4. Japanese Society for Esophageal Disease (1992) Guide lines for the clinical and pathologic studies on carcinoma of esophagus, 8th edn. Kanehara, Tokyo
5. Woods GS, Warnke R (1981) Suppression of endogenous avidin-binding activity in tissue and its relevance to biotin-avidin detection system. J Histochem Cytochem 29:1196–1204
6. Kay S (1968) Mucoepidermoid carcinoma of the Esophagus, report of two cases. Cancer 22:1053–1059
7. Woodard BH, Shelburne JD, Vollmer RT, Postlethwait RW (1978) Mucoepidermoid carcinoma of the esophagus. A case report. Hum Pathol 9:352–354
8. Morisaki Y, Shima S, Yonekawa H, Yoshizumi Y, Sugiura Y, Otsuka H, Goto M, Sueyoshi S, Tsuchiya C, Tanaka S, Ogata T (1988) An Esophageal carcinoma with an adenoid cystic differentiation: An Immunohistochemical study of two cases with special reference to their histological origin-. Jpn J Cancer Clin 34:1710–1717
9. Rosai J (1989) Basaloid carcinoma. In: Rosai J (ed) Ackerman's surgical pathology, 7th edn. Mosby, St. Louis, pp 480–481
10. Battifora H (1976) Spindle cell carcinoma. Ultrastructural evidence of squamous origin and collagen production by the tumor cells. Cancer 37:2275–2282
11. Schürch W, Seemayer TA, Lagacé R, Gabbiani G (1984) The intermediate filament cytoskeleton of myofibroblasts: An immunofluorescence and ultrastructural study. Virchows Arch [A] 403:323–336
12. Seemayer TA, Lagacé R, Schürch W, Thelmo WL (1980) The myofibroblast: Biologic, pathologic, and theoretical considerations. Pathol Ann 15:443–470

Development of an Experimental Model for Spontaneous Lymph Node Metastasis of Human Esophageal Carcinoma in Nude Mice—Histopathological Analysis

Hiroshi Yoshimura, Akira Shigetomi, Tsukasa Kotoh, Kenji Suzuki, Dipok Kumar Dhar, Hiroshi Matsuura, Teruhisa Nakamura[1], Takeyuki Harada, and Shigeru Morikawa[2]

Introduction

Metastasis, a unique feature of malignant neoplasms, is the major cause of death among cancer patients. The exact mechanisms responsible for metastases are not fully understood because of the lack of proper experimental models. We established a new experimental model of spontaneous lymph node metastasis of human esophageal carcinoma in nude mice and analyzed the mode of metastasis formation histopathologically.

Materials and Methods

Animals

BALB/c nu/nu athymic mice were housed in a pathogen-free environment. All mice were 7–8 weeks old.

Tumor Cell Line

A human squamous cell carcinoma cell line (HPL-EsC-1) was established from a male patient of esophageal carcinoma. According to the morphological characteristics of the cell line, three sublines (HPL-EsC-1-K, M, S) were derived and established. Tumor cells were maintained with RPMI 1640 medium supplemented with 10% FCS and kanamycin (60 mg/ml) at 37°C in a humidified, 5% CO_2 atmosphere.

[1] Second Department of Surgery and [2] First Department of Pathology, Shimane Medical University, 89-1, Enya-cho, Izumo, Shimane, 693 Japan

Subcutaneous Inoculation in Nude Mice

Tumor cells in 0.02–0.04 ml of culture medium were inoculated in the hind foot pads.

Measurement of the Tumor Size on Inoculated Site

The thickness of tumor on the inoculated foot pad and that of the contralateral side were measured under stereoscopic microscope twice a week after inoculation. The difference in thickness was defined as tumor size. The time period during which the tumor achieved its original size of implantation was defined as the latent period.

Identification of Metastasis

At designated intervals, the mice were sacrificed. Popliteal lymph nodes were excised and fixed with 10% formalin for histological examination. Fixed tissues were embedded in paraffin, cut into 5-mm sections, and stained with hematoxylin and eosin.

Stage of Lymph Node Metastasis

According to the histopathological findings of the serial sections of the lymph nodes, the extent of cancer cell invasion into the lymph node was classified into 4 stages (Fig. 1).

Tumorigenecity and Metastatic Potential of Three Sublines of EsC-1

Four million cells of each subline were injected into the hind foot pad. All mice were sacrificed at the 3rd week after inoculation.

Effect of Inoculated Tumor Cell Number on Tumor Growth and Lymph Node Metastasis

The experiment was conducted in three groups of animals, and each group received 2, 4, or 8 million EsC-1-K cells. All mice were sacrificed when tumor size reached 3 mm, and popliteal lymph nodes were examined histologically.

Effect of Removal of Primary Tumor on Lymph Node Metastasis

Animals were devided into four groups. The distal half of the leg with tumor of all mice in each group were amputated at the 1st, 2nd, 3rd, and 4th week after EsC-1-K cell inoculation, respectively. Stumps of leg were closed with instant glue. All mice were sacrificed at the 5th week after inoculation and lymph nodes were examined histopathologically.

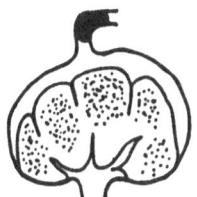

Stage 0.

Tumor cells locate in afferent lymphatic.

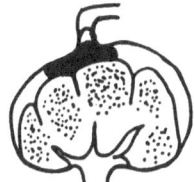

Stage I.

Tumor cells proliferate in marginal sinus.

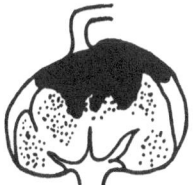

Stage II.

Tumor cells proliferate as far as intermediary sinus and invade into parenchyma.

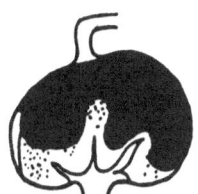

Stage III.

Tumor cells occupy more than half of the lymph node.

Fig. 1. Stages of lymph node metastasis

Treatment With Anti-Asialo GM1 Antibody

Anti-asialo GM1 antibody was purchased from Wako Pure Chemical Industries, Ltd, Osaka. After tumor cell (1 or 2 million EsC-1-K cells) inoculation, each mouse was administered 500 mg of anti-asialo GM1 antibody in 0.1 ml phosphate-buffered saline (PBS) intravenously twice a week. In the control group, mice were administered 0.1 ml saline instead of anti-asialo GM1 antibody.

Effect of Sex Difference on the Tumor Growth and Lymph Node Metastasis

To evaluate the effect of sex differences on lymph node metastasis, another two groups of mice were prepared. Mice of both sexes were injected with 4 million EsC-1-K cells into the foot pad. All mice were sacrificed in the middle of the 3rd week after inoculation and lymph node metastases were examined.

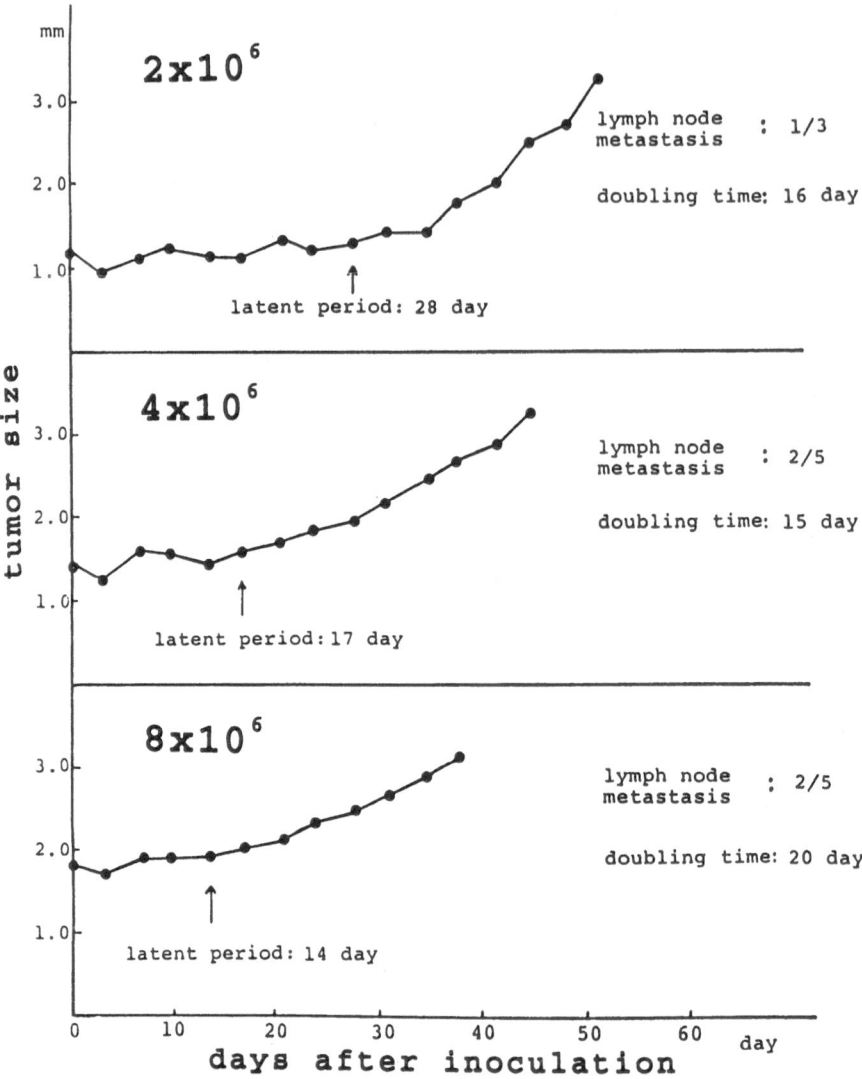

Fig. 2. Growth curves of EsC-1-K cell tumors in nude mice and incidences of popliteal lymph node metastases. Mice of each group received 2, 4, or 8 million tumor cells

Results

Tumorigenecity and Metastatic Potential of Three Sublines of EsC-1

All mice inoculated EsC-1-K and -S had tumor at the inoculated site, and the number and stage of lymph node metastasis were similar between two groups. On the other hand, EsC-1-M showed less tumorigenic and metastatic potential than the other two lines.

Effect of Inoculated Tumor Cell Number on Tumor Growth and Lymph Node Metastasis

The latent period in each group were 28, 17, and 14 days. The latent period was shown to be inversely proportional to the number of inoculated tumor cells. Lymph node metastasis was found in one out of three mice when the inoculated cell number was 2 million and two out of five were involved when the cell number was 4 and 8 million. The doubling time of each group was 16, 15, and 20 days (Fig. 2).

Estimation of the Necessary Time for Occurrence of Lymph Node Metastasis

Four out of five mice of group 4 had a relatively advanced stage of popliteal lymph node metastasis compared to mice in other groups (Table 1).

Table 1. Estimation of the time necessary for lymph node metastasis

Group of mice (amputation)	Tumor taken up/ inoculated	Tumor size (mm) mean ± SD	Lymph node metastasis	
			number	stage
1	5/5	1.8 ± 0.2	0	—
2	5/5	3.0 ± 0.3	1	I
3	5/5	4.0 ± 0.2	0	0
4	5/5	5.4 ± 0.3	4	I
				II
				II
				III

Table 2. Effect of anti-asialo GM1 antibody on tumor growth and lymph node metastasis of EsC-1-K cells in nude mice

Number of cells	Treatment	Tumor taken up/inoculated	Tumor size (mm)	Lymph node metastasis	
				number	stage
1×10^6	PBS	1/5	4.1	0	
	Anti-asialo GM1	4/5	2.3	0	
2×10^6	PBS	5/5	4.6 ± 0.3	4	I
					I
					II
					III
	Anti-asialo GM1	5/5	4.4 ± 0.2	4	I
					II
					II
					II

PBS, phosphate-buffered saline

Effect of Anti-Asialo GM1 Antibody Treatment on the Tumor Growth and Lymph Node Metastasis

Anti-asialo GM1 antibody treatment enhanced tumor formation at the inoculated site even when the number of cells was 1 million. The incidence of lymph node metastasis was not affected by anti-asialo GM1 treatment regardless of the number of inoculated cells (Table 2).

Effect of Sex Difference on Tumor Growth and Lymph Node Metastasis

Sex difference did not influence the tumor growth and lymph node metastasis.

Discussion

There are few experimental models for studies on spontaneous lymph node metastasis of human carcinomas. The experimental model in this study has clearly revealed the mode of lymphatic metastasis from the primary tumor to the popliteal lymph node. Also, histopathological findings correlated well with lymph node metastasis found clinically.

In a previous report, Kurokawa et al. [1] classified lymph node metastasis into 3 stages according to the extent of cancer cell invasion in lymph node. In the current study, we added stage 0 as a preliminary step which a pre-cancerous stage that may develop into metastasis subsequently. However, we have no evidence to confirm whether stage 0 does, in fact, progress to stage 1, 2, or 3.

Although three sublines of cancer cells (EsC-1-K, -S, -M) were derived from the same patient and had similar tumorigenecity in nude mice, the frequency of lymph node metastasis of each subline was different. The occurrence of lymph node metastasis was related to the duration of tumor growth on the primary site. At least 4 weeks were required for popliteal lymph node metastasis to develop. These results indicate that not only biological characteristics of the tumor cells but also the length of tumor growth on the primary site is an important factor for metastasis.

Nude mice have a high level of natural killer (NK) cell activity and it has been suggested that the infrequency of metastasis is attributable to the efficacy of the NK cell system [2]. In the present study, suppression of NK cell activity by anti-asialo GM1 antibody treatment enhanced tumorigenecity but not metastasis. Further study is needed to clarify the role of NK cells in this experimental model.

The growth of some esophageal cancer cell lines which have estrogen receptors are inhibited by application of estrogen [3–5]. The growth of EsC-1-K cell in nude mice was not affected by sex differences and therefore might not be regulated by sex hormones.

Clinically, patients with esophageal cancer usually have a poor prognosis when extensive lymph node metastasis occurrs. Further study regarding metastatic characteristics is an important step in the understanding of esophageal cancer. This experimental model will provide a useful research tool for studies on the biology and therapy for lymph node metastasis of esophageal cancer.

References

1. Kurokawa Y (1970) Experiments on lymph node metastasis by intralymphatic inoculation of rat ascite tumor cells, with special reference to lodgement, passage and growth of tumor cells in lymph nodes. Jpn J Cancer Res (Gann) 11:461–471
2. Kozlowski JM, Fidler IJ, Cambell D, Zuo-Liang X, Kaighn ME, Hart IR (1984) Metastatic behavior of human tumor cell lines grown in the nude mouse. Cancer Res 44:3522–3529
3. Matsuoka H, Sugumachi K, Ueo H, Kuwano H, Nakano S, Nakayama M (1987) Sex hormone response of a newly established squamous cell line derived from clinical esophageal carcinoma. Cancer Res 47:4134–4140
4. Utsumi Y, Nakamura T, Nagasue N, Kubota H, Morikawa S (1989) Role of estrogen receptors in the growth of human esophageal carcinoma. Cancer 64:88–93
5. Utsumi Y, Nakamura T, Nagasue N, Kubota H, Harada T, Morikawa S (1991) Effect of 17 b-estradiol on the growth of an estrogen receptor-positive human esophageal carcinoma cell line. Cancer 67:2284–2289

Correlation Between Expression of E-Cadherin and Metastasis and Invasion in Human Esophageal Cancer

H. Shiozaki[1], M. Miyata[1], K. Kobayashi[1], M. Inoue[1], S. Tamura[1],
H. Tahara[1], H. Oka[1], Y. Doki[1], K. Iihara[1], T. Kadowaki[1], M. Takeichi[2],
and T. Mori[1]

Introduction

Cadherins are Ca^{2+}-dependent cell-cell adhesion molecules which are possibly involved in the process of metastasis in cancer cells. We have investigated the expression of E-cadherin (E-CD), which is a subclass of cadherin expressed on cell membranes in normal esophageal epithelium. Sixty-two human esophageal cancers were studied with immunoblotting (5 cases) and immunohistochemical staining (62 cases) using monoclonal antibody for human E-CD (HECD-1) on frozen surgical specimens, and the correlation between E-CD expression and incidence of clinical lymph node metastasis and cancer invasion was investigated.

Materials and Methods

Sixty-two patients with squamous cell carcinoma of the esophagus were included in this study. They recieved no anticancerous chemo-therapy or irradiation before the operation. Tumor tissues were all obtained from surgically resected fresh specimens.

Immunohistochemical Staining Procedures

The avidin-biotin peroxidase complex (ABC) method was performed for immunostaining using HECD-1 [1].

---

[1] Department of Surgery II, Osaka University Medical School. Fukushima 1-1-50. Fukushima-ku, Osaka, 553 Japan
[2] Department of Biophysics, Faculty of Science, Kyoto University, Kyoto, 606 Japan

Evaluation of E-CD Staining

The intensity of E-CD staining for cancer cells was compared with that of the cells in normal esophagel epitelium in the same sample and were classified into the following two categories: When the intensity of E-CD staining was the same as normal epithelial cells, the cancer cells were defined as Preserved Type (P-type); if the cancer cells show very weak homogeneous or heterogeneous staining, these were defined as Reduced Type (R-type).

The clinicopathological terminology used in this report is derived from the general rules proposed by the Japanese Research Society for Esophageal Cancer [2]. All data were statistically evaluated by the chi-square test.

Results

Immunohistochemical Staining

All the normal esophageal epithelial cells, except in the most superficial keratinizing layer, strongly expressed E-CD molecules at the cell-cell boundaries (Fig. 1A,B). Reduced E-CD expression (R-type) was observed in 53 tumors (85%) of 62 primary squamous cell carcinomas. In these 53 tumors, 11 tumors showed homogeneously reduced E-CD expression (Ho-R), but the rest of them

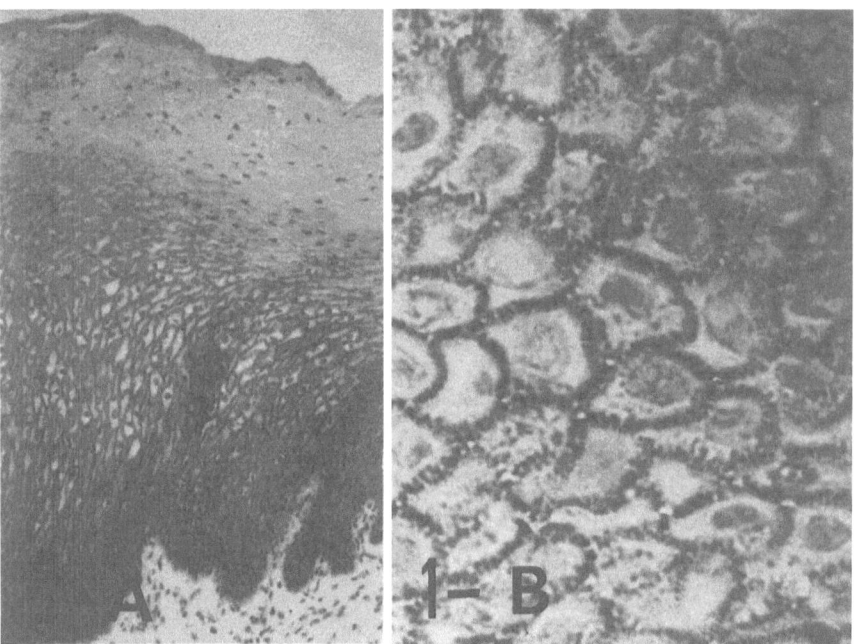

Fig. 1A,B. Normal squamous epithelial cells, except in the most superficial keratinizing layer, strongly expressed E-cadherin molecules on cell-cell boundaries. All of the specimens from 62 patients showed the same E-cadherin expression. (**A**, ×50, **B**, ×200).

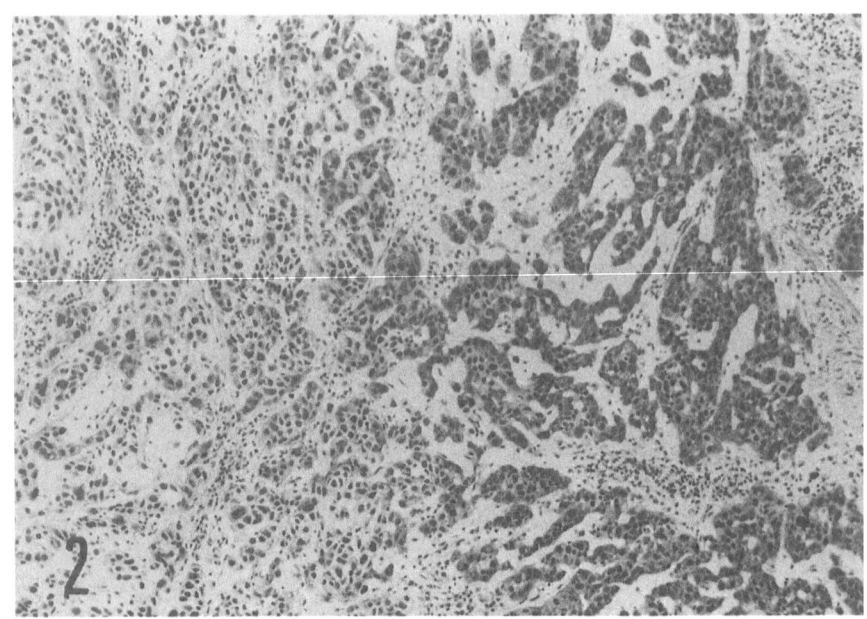

Fig. 2. Heterogeneous R-type squamous cell carcinoma. The mixture of cancer cells evaluated as E-cadherin preserved, reduced, and negative expression (×50)

Table 1. Relationship between E-CD expression and depth of invasion

Depth	No.	P-type	R-type		
			He-R	Ho-R	Total
ep	1	1 (100%)	0	0	0 (0%)
mm	2	2 (100%)	0	0	0 (0%)
sm	10	2 (20%)	6	2	8 (80%)
mp	14	0 (0%)	12	2	14 (100%)
a	35	4 (11%)	24	7	31 (89%)

* $P < 0.05$

ep, limited to intraepithelium; *mm*, invasion to muscularis mucosae; *sm*, invasion to submucosa; *mp*, invasion to muscularis propria; *a*, invasion to adventitia; *He-R*, heterogeneously reduced expression; *Ho-R*, homogeneously reduced expression; *E-CD*, E-cadherin

showed heterogeneously reduced E-CD expression (He-R) in considerable tumor subsets (Fig. 2).

Depth in Invasion

In 13 superficial carcinomas of intraepithelial (ep), muscularis mucosal (mm), and submucosal (sm) invasion, 5 patients (38%) were evaluated as P-Type. Moreover, 3 cases of ep and mm were all classified as P-Type. In 14 tumors of

Table 2. Relationship between E-CD expression and lymph node metastasis

	No.	P-type	R-type		
			He-R	Ho-R	Total
Metastatic group	47	2 (4%)	36	9	45 (96%) ⎤
Non-metastatic group	15	7 (47%)	6	2	8 (53%) ⎦ *
Total	62	9 (15%)	42	11	53 (85%)

* $P < 0.01$

proper muscle (mp) invasion, all were classified as R-Type. In 35 tumors invading the adventitia (a), 31 (89%) were evaluated as R-Type. Thus, R-Type was significantly more common in tumors invading beyond mp than in superficial carcinomas ($P < 0.05$) (Table 1).

Lymph Node Metastasis

Forty-five cases (96%) of 47 with lymph node metastasis cases were evaluated as R-Type in primary lesions. Conversely, 8 (53%) of 15 patients with no lymph node metastasis were evaluated as R-Type in the primary lesion. The frequency of reduced E-CD expression in tumors with lymph node metastasis was significantly higher than that in tumors with no lymph node metastasis ($P < 0.01$) (Table 2).

Discussion

In the presence of Ca^{2+}, cadherins play a central role in establishing and maintaining strong intercellular connections. As one subtype of cadherins, E-CD contributes to the formation and maintenance of normal and cancerous epithelial tissues [3, 4]. In order to confirm our evaluation on immunohistochemical staining, we performed immunoblot analysis (Western blotting) for four primary tumors. The E-CD expression on the immunohistochemical staining and the immunoblot analysis was correlated very exactly (data not shown) [5]. Concerning the depth of tumor invasion, the frequency of reduced E-CD expression in tumors invading proper muscle and the adventitia was higher than that in superficial carcinoma. Moreover, the frequency of reduced E-CD expression in tumors with lymph node metastasis was significantly higher than that in tumors without lymph node metastasis.

These results indicate that heterogeneous reduction of E-CD content may affect the potency of lymph node metastasis and invasion of human esophageal cancer.

References

1. Shiozaki H, Tahara H, Miyata M, Kobayashi K, Tamura S, Iihara K, Doki Y, Hirano S, Takeichi M, Mori T (1991) Expression of immunoreactive E-cadherin adhesion molecules in human cancers. Am J Pathol 139:17–23
2. Japanese Society for Esophageal Diseases: Guideline for the clinical and pathologic studies on carcinoma of the esophagus. Jpn J Surg 1976; 6:69–78
3. Takeichi M (1991) Cadherin cell adhesion receptors as a morphogenic regulator. Science 251:1451–1455
4. Nagafuchi A, Shirayoshi Y, Okazaki K, Yasuda K, Takeichi M (1987) Transformation of cell adhesion properties by exogenously introduced E-cadherin cDNA. Nature 329:341–343
5. Oka H, Shiozaki H, Kobayashi K, Tahara H, Tamura S, Miyata M, Doki Y, Iihara K, Matsuyoshi N, Hirano S, Takeichi M, Mori T (1992) Immunohistochemical evaluation of E-cadherin adhesion molecule expression in human gasric cancer. Virchows Arch [A] 421:149–156

Immunohistochemical Study of the Expression of HLA-DR Antigen and Lymphocyte Infiltration in Human Esophageal Carcinoma

Kanji Tanaka, Mika Morita, Takayuki Motohiro, Hideharu Yamanaka, Yasushi Nakane, and Koshirou Hioki[1]

Introduction

The major histocompatibility complex (MHC) class II antigen HLA-DR is known to be present on many types of immunocompetent cells, involved in a variety of immune functions, and can be found in various kinds of cancer cells of the gastrointestinal tract. It is also reported that HLA-DR is associated with tumor invasion, tumor metastasis, and patient survival [1].

The infiltration of lymphocytes surrounding tumor cells is commonly observed in solid tumors. It has been postulated that this plays an important role in an immunologic reaction against tumors and the degree of infiltration also correlates with the length of survival.

In this study, we evaluated the expression of HLA-DR antigen in relation to lymphoid infiltration in human esophageal carcinoma.

Materials and Methods

Fifty cases of primary esophageal squamous cell carcinoma were studied. Histological classification of esophageal cancer was made according to the criteria described in the Guidelines for the Clinical and Pathologic Studies on Carcinoma of the Esophagus [2]. All patients examined preoperatively showed no abnormalities on laboratory testing of liver function, serum immunoglobulin concentrations, and cellular immunity, and had received no chemotherapy or radiation prior to operation.

All specimens were fixed in 10% formalin, embedded in paraffin, cut into serial sections, and were stained using the indirect immunoperoxidase method.

[1] Second Department of Surgery, Kansai Medical University, 1 Fumizono-cho, Moriguchi, Osaka, 570 Japan

519

Mouse monoclonal antibody to HLA-DR (LN-3) was obtained from Histoclone (Seikagaku Kogyo Co., Tokyo, Japan) and human T-cell (UCHL-1) was purchased from Dakopatts (Kyowa Medics Japan, Tokyo, Japan). Fragments of horseradish peroxidase (HRP)-labeled goat F(ab')$_2$ to mouse IgG used as the second antibody were obtained from Tago Inc. (Cosmo Bio Co., Tokyo, Japan).

The grade of immunostaining of HLA-DR in cancer tissues (HLA-DR positivity) was divided into three classes as follows: 3+, more than 30% of cancer cells were positively stained; 2+, 10%–30% stained; and 1+, less than 10% stained.

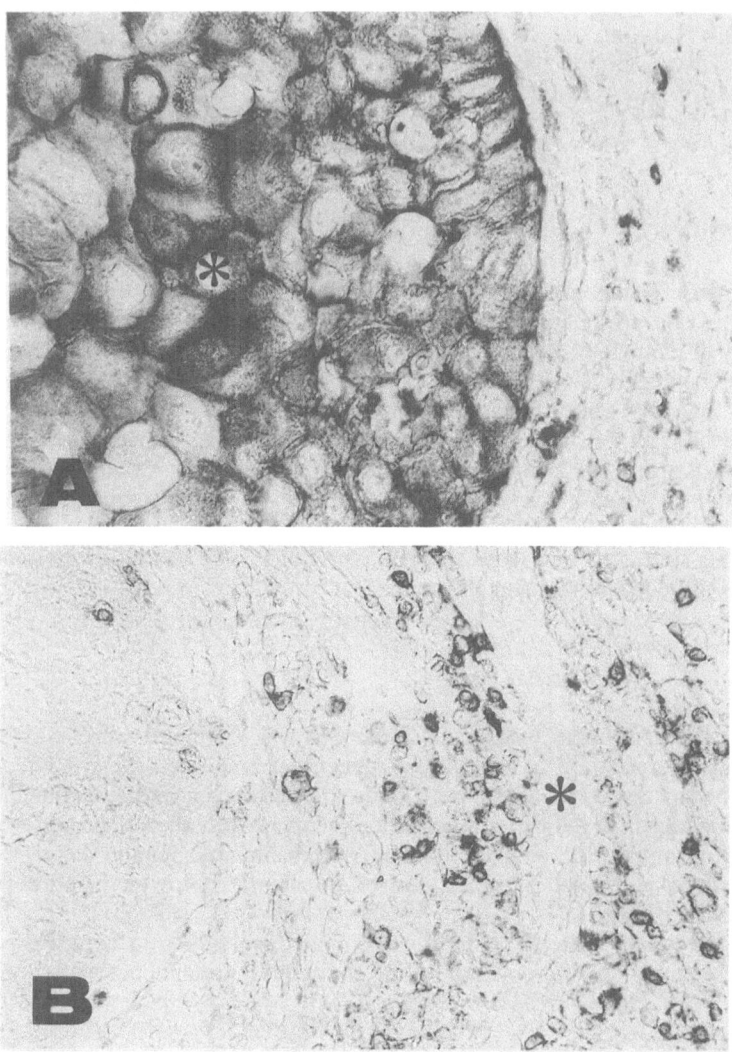

Fig. 1A,B. HLA-DR staining and the infiltration of T-cells in esophageal squamous cell carcinoma. **A** HLA-DR is stained positively in cancer cells (*). **B** T lymphocytes (UCHL-1-positive cells) infiltrate in tumor tissue (*)

The number of UCHL-1$^+$ cells were expressed as the mean number of cells per 0.16 mm^2 of tissue from the following three sites: (1) the infiltrating front of carcinoma (IF), (2) the intracarcinomatous stroma (IS), and (3) normal tissue (NR).

The data were analyzed by the Student's t-test.

Results

Various numbers of HLA-DR positive cancer cells were observed in all 50 cases of carcinoma (Fig. 1). However, more than 70% of all cases showed 1+ and 2+, and HLA-DR positivity in esophageal squamous tumor cells was rather low: 1 + ($n = 19$), 2 + ($n = 17$), and 3 + ($n = 14$).

The number of HLA-DR-positive cancer cells in the tissue increased with the degree of infiltration of UCHL 1-positive lymphocytes, not only the IF, but also the IS (Figs. 1, 2).

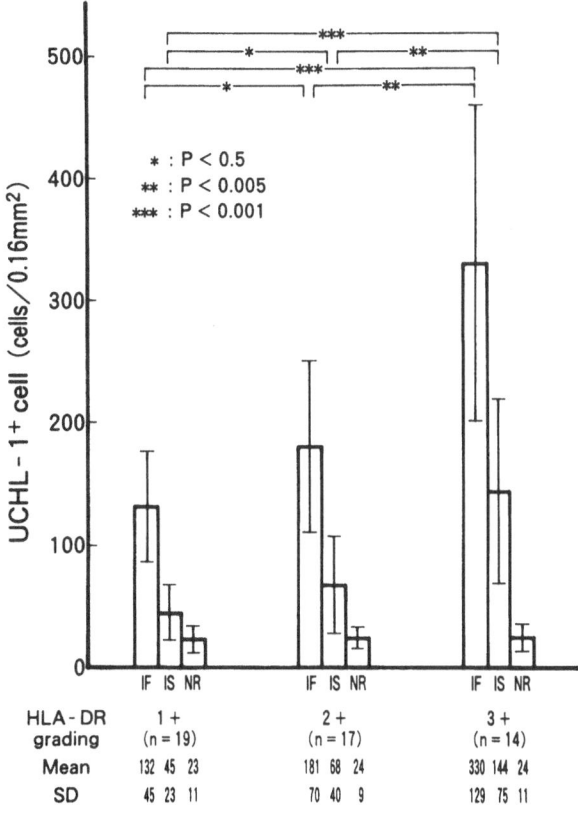

Fig. 2. The number of UCHL-1-positive cells and HLA-DR staining grades. *IF*, infiltrating front; *IS*, intra-carcinomatous stroma; *NR*, normal tissue

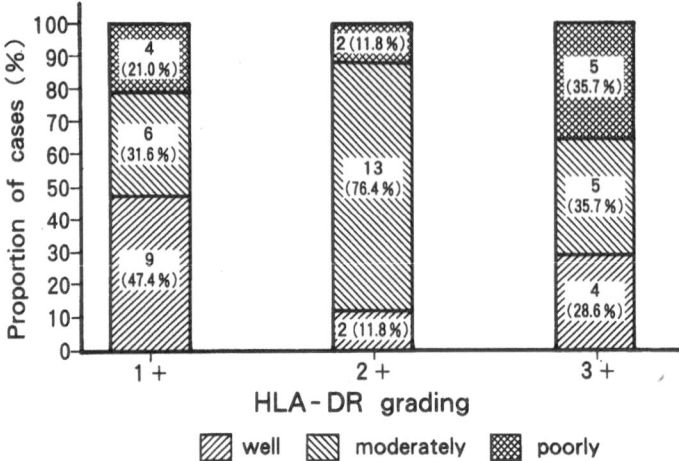

Fig. 3. The number of cases with HLA-DR staining grades and histopathological classification

Well-differentiated squamous cell carcinoma was most predominant in 1+ cases, moderately differentiated in 2+, and moderately and poorly differentiated in 3+. Conventional histopathological type of differentiation seemed to correlate with the HLA-DR staining grade (Fig. 3).

Discussion

We already hypothesized that the expression of HLA-DR in the cells appeared to be influenced by two factors relating to the microenvironment surrounding the cells: the presence of infiltrating lymphocytes, and the genotype of the cells [3].

The present study in esophageal carcinoma demonstrated that the presence of HLA-DR-positive cells was closely related to the degree of lymphocyte infiltration, which was in agreement with our previous findings in both colorectal and gastric cancers [3, 4]. Such a lymphoid infiltration seems to be one of the most important microenvironmental elements acting to induce the expression of this antigen in esophageal tumor, as with colorectal and gastric cancers.

The mechanism for the expression of HLA-DR is reported to be influenced by IFN-γ which is produced by T lymphocytes, especially if they are IL-2 receptor-positive, through the transcription of HLA-DR mRNA. On the other hand, HLA-DR is known to be involved in immune reactions including presentation of foreign antigen and induction and regulation of T cell activation. In other words, the production of HLA-DR is influenced by lymphocytes and the induction of lymphocytes infiltration is affected by HLA-DR. From this evidence, both of them are closely related to each other.

The HLA-DR staining grade in each esophageal carcinoma case was rather low and its positivity was less than 30% in 70% of all examined cases. We have already reported that it was more than 50% in 40% of colorectal cancer cases and more than 50% in 50% of gastric tumor cases [1, 5]. The HLA-DR reactivity in esophageal squamous cell cancer was lower than that in colorectal and gastric adenocarcinoma. Several human cell types naturally possess HLA-DR antigen which in the absence of obvious inflammation, and others show no reactivity with HLA-DR, which means the presence or absence of HLA-DR antigen may be phenotypically expressed in these cells defined by their own genotype. It is speculated that the expression of HLA-DR in esophageal tumors might be more likely to be affected by the genotype than by the microenvironment such as lymphoid infiltration. However, the real reason for these three cancer tissues indicating different HLA-DR positivity remains unclear.

HLA-DR antigen is reported to be a pleiocharacteristic antigen. It is involved in a variety of immune functions acting as an immunological antigen and is also detected on malignant cells as a tumor-associated antigen. It has been suggested that HLA-DR appeared to be a sort of cancer-related antigen which reflects the degree of differentiation of tumor cells especially in colorectal carcinoma [6], as with carcinoembryonic antigen (CEA) and secretory component (SC), which were shown to exhibit different patterns of distribution according to the degree of differentiation of cancer cells. This study showed that the number of HLA-DR positive carcinoma cells increased with the degree of tumor differentiation, and HLA-DR also might be related with the differentiation of cancer cells in esophageal carcinoma.

References

1. Tanaka K, Morita M, Kawanishi H, Takai S, Tsuji M, Yamamura M, Hioki K, Nagura H (1992) Malignant features of colorectal carcinoma: Correlation with HLA-DR expression. Dig Organ Immunol 26:137–142
2. Japanese Society for Esophageal Diseases (1984) Guidelines for the clinical and pathologic studies on carcinoma of the esophagus, 6th edn. Kanehara, Tokyo
3. Hirozane N, Tanaka K, Nakane Y, Yamamura M, Hioki K, Nagura H, Yamamoto M (1991) Expression of HLA-DR and secretory component antigens and lymphocyte infiltration in human gastric nonmalignant and malignant tissues: An immunohistochemical study. J Surg Oncol 46:77–86
4. Tanaka K, Nagura H, Morita M, Kawanishi H, Tsuji M, Takai S, Hirozane N, Nakane Y, Yamamura M, Hioki K, Yamamoto M (1990) Comparative study on the expression of HLA-DR antigen, tumor cell kinetics and lymphocyte infiltration in human gastric and colorectal carcinoma. Front Mucosal Immunol 1:197–198
5. Tanaka K, Yamamura M, Kawanishi H, Takai S, Tsuji M, Kwon AH, Hioki K, Nagura H, Yamamoto M (1989) Immunohistochemical study of human colorectal carcinoma for expression of CEA and HLA-DR antigens, tumor cell Kinetics, and lymphocyte infiltration. Biotherapy 3:1199–1204
6. Tanaka K, Nagura H, Hamada H, Yamamura M, Hioki K, Yamamoto M (1988) Immunohistochemical evaluation of human colorectal neoplasms for CEA, HLA class II antigen and DNA polymerase α. Dig Organ Immunol 21:209–213

Unusual Manifestation of Malignant Lymphoma of the Esophagus

Kazuhiko Inoue, Ken Haruma, Kenji Tokumo, Masaharu Yoshihara, Claudio Rolim Teixeira, Takehiro Shimamoto, Koji Sumii, Goro Kajiyama[1], and Koji Nanba[2]

Summary. Primary malignant lymphoma of the esophagus is very rare. We encountered three cases of esophageal malignant lymphoma, showing unusual manifestations radiologically and endoscopically. In all cases, the upper gastrointestinal series showed smooth swelling of folds resembling varices. Esophagoscopy showed smooth and soft longitudinal protruding lesions. A computed tomographic scan showed marked thickening of the esophageal wall. These cases were diagnosed by endoscopic giant forceps biopsy specimens as small-cell, diffuse type malignant lymphoma. We report the unusual manifestation of malignant lymphoma characterized by marked thickening of the esophageal wall.

Introduction

The commonest primary malignancy of the esophagus is squamous cell carcinoma, accounting for approximately 90% of all cases. Primary malignant lymphoma of the esophagus is very rare, representing less than 1% of all cases of lymphoma with gastrointestinal involvement [1]. In this study, we report three cases of malignant lymphoma of the esophagus, showing unusual manifestation radiologically and endoscopically.

Case Reports

Case 1

A 69-year-old woman was admitted with mild dysphagia for solid food and weight loss of 2 kg. She did not have fever, nausea, or heartburn. Physical

[1] First Department of Internal Medicine, Hiroshima University School of Medicine, 1-2-3, Kasumi, Minami-ku, Hiroshima, 734 Japan
[2] Faculty of Integrated Arts and Sciences, Hiroshima University, 1-1-89, Higashisenda-cho, Naka-ku, Hiroshima, 730 Japan

examination findings were unremarkable. The complete blood cell count was normal. An upper gastrointestinal series showed dilatation of the lower esophagus and smooth swelling of folds resembling varices (Fig. 1). Esophagoscopy showed longitudinal nodularity of the lower esophagus. The nodularity was soft and smooth, and there were no ulcers or erosions on the esophageal mucosa (Fig. 2). A computed tomographic scan indicated marked thickening of the wall of the entire esophagus. Magnetic resonance imaging showed a uniform high density in the area of the esophagus. Endoscopic biopsy was done, but a conventional biopsy specimen did not yield sufficient tissue for pathological diagnosis, so that large forceps had to be used. A large biopsy specimen revealed a small-cell, diffuse type lymphoma (Fig. 3). Chemotherapy was conducted with VEPA (vincristine, cyclophosphamide, prednisolone, and adriamycin). The thickness of the esophageal wall was subsequently reduced from 28 mm to 5 mm after two cycles of VEPA. Endoscopically, the longitudinal nodularity disappeared (Fig. 4). Biopsy specimens collected later were all negative for lymphoma. She is free of disease 63 months after therapy.

Case 2

A 65-year-old woman was admitted with dysphagia of 5 months' duration. She did not have fever, night sweats, or weight loss. Physical examination findings were unremarkable. The complete blood cell count was normal. An upper gastrointestinal series showed several large longitudinal nodularities in the middle and lower esophagus (Fig. 5). Esophagoscopy showed soft longitudinal protruding lesions whose surfaces were smooth and no ulcers or erosions were present on the esophageal mucosa. A computed tomographic scan showed marked thickening of the entire esophagus (Fig. 6). Magnetic resonance imaging showed high density in the area of the esophagus (Fig. 7). For pathological diagnosis, large biopsy forceps had to be used. A large biopsy specimen revealed a small-cell, diffuse type lymphoma. Repeated chemotherapy (three cycles of VEPA) and radiation therapy (6420 cGy) were conducted, but the thickness of the esophageal wall was not reduced. However, she is still alive 59 months after therapy.

Case 3

A 70-year-old man was admitted with epigastric discomfort. He did not have dysphagia, heartburn, or body weight loss. Physical examination results were unremarkable. The complete blood cell count was normal. An upper gastro-intestinal series showed large longitudinal nodularities throughout the entire esophagus (Fig. 8). Esophagoscopy showed soft longitudinal protruding lesions through the entire esophagus. The surfaces of the protruding lesions were smooth and their color was normal. There were no ulcers or erosions on the esophageal mucosa. A computed tomographic scan indicated marked thickening of the wall of the entire esophagus. Magnetic resonance imaging showed a uniform high density in the area of the esophagus. Examination of a large biopsy specimen revealed a small-cell, diffuse type lymphoma. Chemotherapy was conducted with VEPA. After one cycle of chemotherapy, the thickness of the esophagus improved partially, although esophagoscopic findings did not change. Another cycle of chemotherapy was carried out; however, respiratory failure of

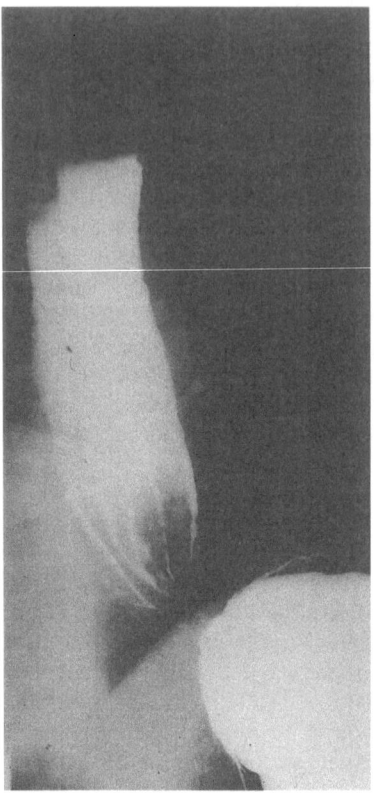

Fig. 1. An upper gastrointestinal series showed smooth swelling of folds resembling varices (case 1)

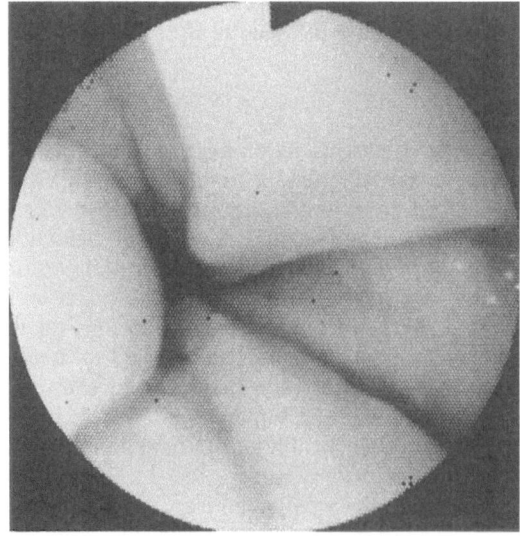

Fig. 2. Esophagoscopy showed smooth and soft longitudinal protruding lesions (case 1)

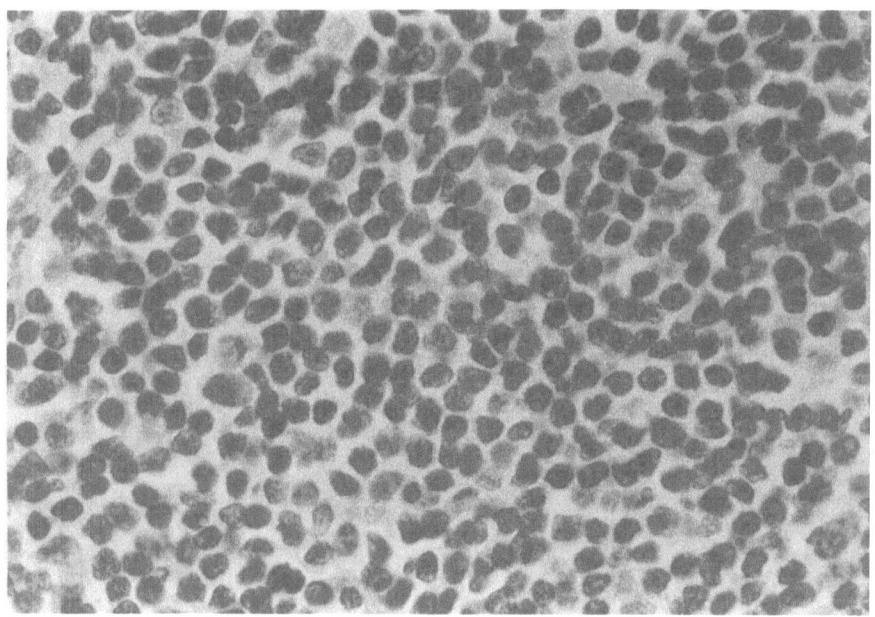

Fig. 3. A biopsy specimen revealed a small-cell, diffuse type lymphoma (case 1)

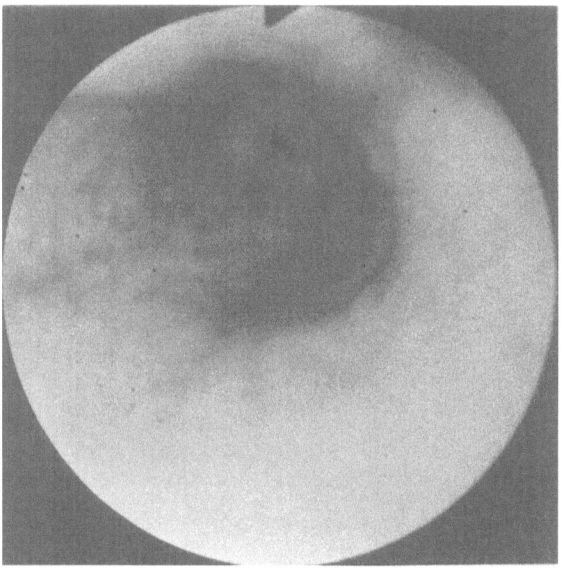

Fig. 4. Protruding lesions disappeared after therapy (case 1)

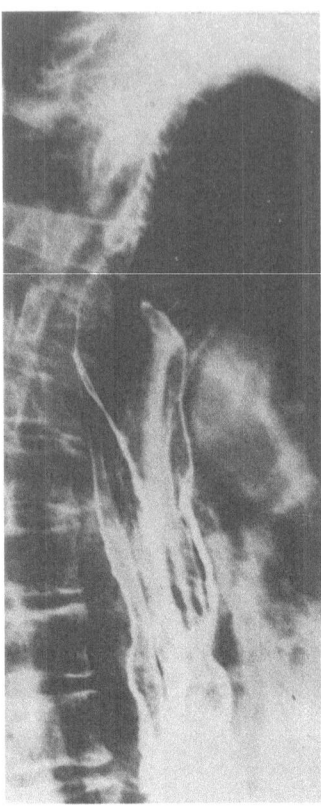

Fig. 5. An upper gastrointestinal series showed several large longitudinal nodularities (case 2)

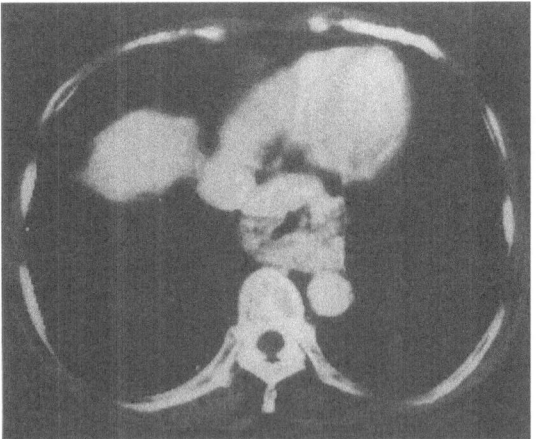

Fig. 6. A computed tomographic scan showed marked thickening of the esophageal wall (case 2)

Fig. 7. Magnetic resonance imaging showed high density in the area of the esophagus (case 2)

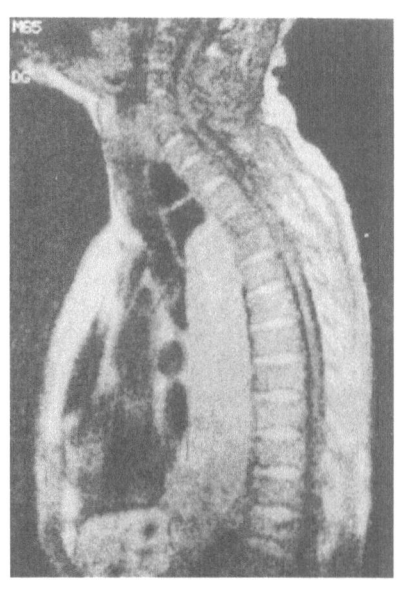

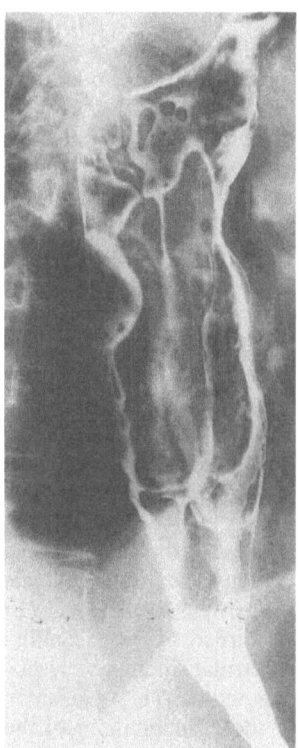

Fig. 8. An upper gastrointestinal series showed large longitudinal nodularities (case 3)

the patient prevented further therapy. However, he is free of symptoms and still alive 53 months after therapy.

Discussion

The gastrointestinal tract is the site of initial manifestations of non-Hodgkin's lymphomas in 5%–20% of all patients with the disease [1–3]. The most commonly affected site is the stomach, followed by the small intestine and ileocecal region. The esophagus is the least commonly involved hollow organ representing less than 1% of cases [1]. In 1269 cases of lymphosarcoma, only 19 patients had disease in the esophagus, with none having primary esophageal lymphoma [2]. Esophageal involvement is almost always secondary to extension of the lymphoma from the stomach or mediastinal nodes [3]. Dawson et al. [4] suggested criteria for primary malignant lymphoid tumors of the intestinal tract as follows: predominance of gastrointestinal tract lesions, with only regional lymph node involvement; absence of peripheral or mediastinal lymph node involvement; normal white blood cell count; and the absence of splenic or hepatic involvement. Based on these criteria, our three cases were all primary malignant lymphomas of the esophagus.

Malignant lymphoma of the gastrointestinal tract usually originates in the submucosa and shows various features radiologically and endoscopically. Radiologic findings previously reported in malignant lymphoma of the esophagus include polypoid masses with or without ulceration, ulcerated stenosis, a large intramural mass, a narrowed distal segment mimicking achalasia, the varicoid pattern, and multiple submucosal nodules [5–8]. Although the radiological varicoid pattern has only been reported in a few cases, smooth longitudinal swelling of folds resembling varices were found in the upper gastrointestinal series of our three patients. They had no ulcers or erosions on the esophageal mucosa. Computed tomographic scans showed marked thickening of the wall of the entire esophagus. Magnetic resonance imaging showed a uniform high density mass in the area of the esophagus. The malignant lymphomas of our three cases were characterized by marked thickening of the esophageal wall morphologically, probably as a result of the thickening of the submucosa.

Although Hricak et al. [9] demonstrated false-negative results for over one-third of cases of gastrointestinal lymphomas, our three cases were all diagnosed by endoscopic biopsy. Since conventional biopsy specimens did not yield sufficient tissue for pathological diagnosis, we had to use large forceps to obtain appropriate specimens. As malignant lymphomas originate in the submucosal layer, it is necessary to collect large specimens for pathological diagnosis. By using large forceps, we obtained specimens containing mucosal and submucosal tissue. According to the LSG (Lymphoma-Leukemia Study Group) classification [10], all three cases were small-cell, diffuse type lymphomas and all B-cell. In gastrointestinal malignant lymphomas, there are more B-cell lymphomas than T-cell lymphomas [11]. Considering the involvement of the entire esophagus, the low grade of malignancy of the lymphoma, and the age of the patients, we preferred to treat them by chemotherapy using VEPA. In one patient (case 1), the tumor improved radiologically and endoscopically, and biopsy specimens were negative for lymphoma cells after two cycles of chemotherapy. In another patient (case

3), the tumor improved partially. However, in case 2, combined chemotherapy was not effective, and the size of the tumor did not change despite additional radiation therapy. All three patients are still alive after 63, 59, and 53 months respectively. Patient 1 has not relapsed to malignant lymphoma, and the tumors of the other two patients have not increased in size. It is of considerable interest that our cases of lymphoma have all progressed slowly, and that the prognosis seems to be favorable.

Herein are reported three cases of primary malignant lymphoma of the esophagus, characterized by slow progression and marked thickening of the esophageal wall.

References

1. Brady L, Asbell SO (1980) Malignant lymphoma of the gastrointestinal tract. Radiology 137:291–298
2. Rosenberg SA, Diamond HD, Jaslowitz B, Craver LF (1961) Lymphosarcoma: A review of 1269 cases. Medicine 40:31–84
3. Herrmann R, Panahon AM, Barcos M, Walsh D, Stutzman L (1980) Gastrointestinal involvement in non-Hodgkin's lymphomas. Cancer 46:215–222
4. Dawson IMP, Cornes JS, Morson BC (1961) Primary malignant lymphoid tumors of the intestinal tract. Br J Surg 49:80–89
5. Wang CC, Peterson JA (1956) Malignant lymphoma of the gastrointestinal tract: roentgenographic considerations. Acta Radiol (Diag) (Stockh) 46:523–532
6. Caruso RD, Berk RN (1970) Lymphoma of the esophagus. Radiology 95:381–382
7. Davis JA, Kantrowitz PA, Chandler HL, Schatzki SC (1975) Reversible achalasia due to reticulum-cell sarcoma. N Engl J Med 293:130–132
8. Carnovale RL, Goldstein HM, Zornoza J, Dodd GD (1977) Radiologic manifestations of esophageal lymphoma. Am J Roentgenol 128:751–754
9. Hricak H, Thoeni RF, Margulis AR, Eyler WR, Francis IR (1980) Extension of gastric lymphoma into the esophagus and duodenum. Radiology 135:309–312
10. Suchi T, Tajima K, Nanba K, Wakasa H, Mitaka A, Kikuchi M, Mori S, Watanabe S, Mohri N, Shamoto M, Harigaya K, Itagaki T, Matsuda M, Kirino Y, Takagi K, Fukunaga S (1979) Some problems in the histopathological diagnosis of non-Hodgkin's malignant lymphoma: A proposal of a new type. Acta Pathol Jpn 29:755–776
11. Mohri N (1983) B-cell lymphomas of extranodal origin. Jpn J Clin Oncol 13:591–606

Diagnosis and Cancer Staging

Endosonography and Computerized Tomography in the Evaluation of Tumor Invasion in Esophageal Cancer After Preoperative Chemo- and Radiotherapy

G. De Manzoni, E. Laterza, S.U. Urso, G. Borzellino, L. Rodella, and C. Cordiano[1]

Introduction

Esophageal carcinoma presents a poor prognosis with 5-year survival rates not exceeding 5%, but rising to 18% for resected patients [1, 2]. Surgery is currently the most valid form of therapy for the disease, though the morbidity and mortality rates are still high [3–5].

Therefore, the selection of candidates for surgery needs to be very thorough, excluding cases which stand no chance of being cured [6].

Preoperative staging is therefore an important aid in the treatment of esophageal cancer, computerized tomography (CT) and endoscopic ultrasonography (EUS) unquestionably being the most accurate staging techniques currently available [7, 8].

From the 1980s on, in an attempt to improve the prognosis of the disease, a number of physicians began to adopt protocols involving multimodal treatment with a combination of chemo- and radiotherapy, administered preoperatively, and surgery [9, 10].

The aim of the present study was to assess the effect of multimodal neoadjuvant treatment on the accuracy of CT and EUS in the preoperative staging of depth of tumor invasion in esophageal carcinoma.

Materials and Methods

From June 1987 to June 1992, a group of 53 patients with squamous cell carcinoma of the thoracic esophagus underwent preoperative adjuvant chemo- and radiotherapy and then surgery in the 1st Division of General Surgery of the

---

[1] First Department of General Surgery, University of Verona, Borgo Trento Hospital, Piazza Stefani 1, 37126 Verona, Italy

University of Verona. The series comprised 48 males and 5 females (ratio = 10:1) with a mean age of 58.2 years (range: 41–70).

The preoperative therapeutic protocol provided for administration of Cisplatin (100 mg/m^2 on day 1) and fluorouracil (1000 mg/m^2 by continuous infusion for 96 h). High-energy radiotherapy was started at the same time and continued for a period of 3 weeks with administration of a total of 3000 Gy. At the end of this period, a second identical course of chemotherapy was given. The surgical operation was performed on average 25 days after the end of neoadjuvant therapy.

Prior to neoadjuvant treatment, all patients underwent initial tumor staging by chest x-rays, upper digestive tract x-rays, esophagogastroduodenoscopy (EGDS), thoracoabdominal CT, EUS and magnetic resonance imaging (MRI), the latter being performed only in the last 24 cases.

A second staging was done at the end of the first course of chemo- and radiotherapy with repetition of the same examinations used in the first staging.

EUS was performed using a Machida-Toshiba front-view endoscope with a 7.5 MHz linear probe at the distal end. All ultrasonographic appearances were interpreted by the same ultrasonographist, who was unaware of the CT diagnosis.

At EUS, the normal esophageal wall presents five distinct bands of different echogenicity. The first band is echo-dense and represents the acoustic interface between probe and esophageal wall; the second is relatively echo-free and corresponds to the mucosa, the third is echo-dense and corresponds to the submucosa; the fourth is relatively echo-free, corresponding to the muscularis propria; the fifth and last band is echo-dense and corresponds to the adventitia plus the acoustic interface. Depth of tumor invasion is judged on the basis of the degree of alteration or destruction of these five bands [11] (Fig. 1a,b).

CT was performed using a Siemens DR-H appliance. More than 5 mm of wall thickening was regarded as pathological: tumors with 5–10 mm wall thickening were staged as T1/T2 and those with >10 mm thickening as T3, while tumors with invasion of adjacent structures were graded as T4. Infiltration of the aorta was based on absence of the esophago-aortic fat plane and on presence of a contact angle of more than 90° between the tumor and the aortic wall [12]. In the case of the airways, compression, dislocation, and/or deformation of the tracheal or bronchial lumen was regarded as highly predictive of neoplastic invasion (Fig. 2) [13].

As regards diagnosis of lymph node involvement, CT relies entirely on volumetric criteria: lymph nodes with diameters measuring more than 10 mm were regarded as pathological [12, 14].

All 53 patients underwent surgery, and it was therefore possible to compare the results of the second preoperative staging as regards depth of tumor invasion of the esophageal wall (T staging) with the data obtained in the course of surgery and at definitive histological examination of the surgical specimens removed. The staging model adopted was the 1987 TNM-UICC model.

The CT and EUS results in this group of patients submitted to neoadjuvant treatment (group A) were compared with those of a group of 54 patients (group B) with carcinoma of the thoracic esophagus operated on in our division from 1983 to 1992, but not assigned to the multimodal neoadjuvant therapy protocol.

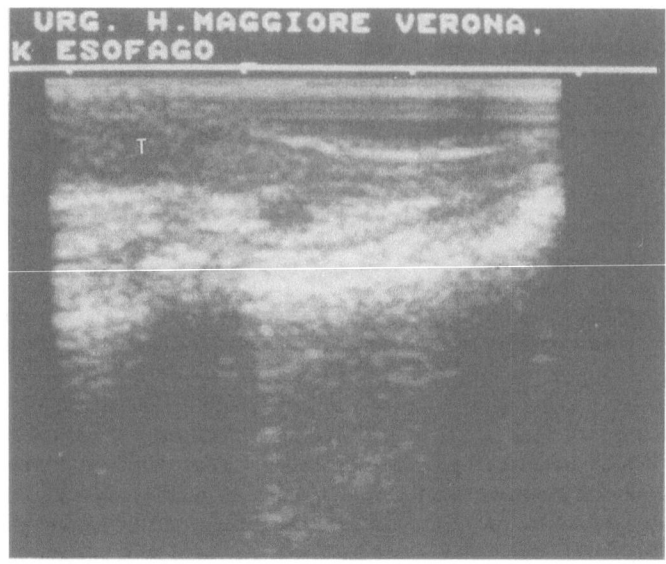

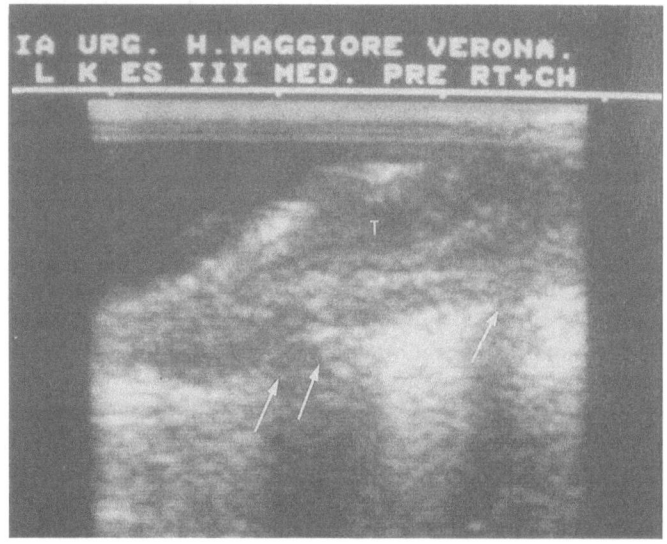

Fig. 1. a Endosonography shows T3 tumor (*T*) after chemo- and radiotherapy; malignant node (*arrow*) near the tumor. **b** The same tumor before the neoadjuvant treatment that shows airways invasion (*arrows*)

The tumors of the group B patients were also staged preoperatively by means of chest x-rays, digestive tract x-rays, EGDS, tracheobronchoscopy (TBS), CT, and EUS. EUS was performed only in 40 patients, as the technique became part of the clinical routine in our Institute only in 1987.

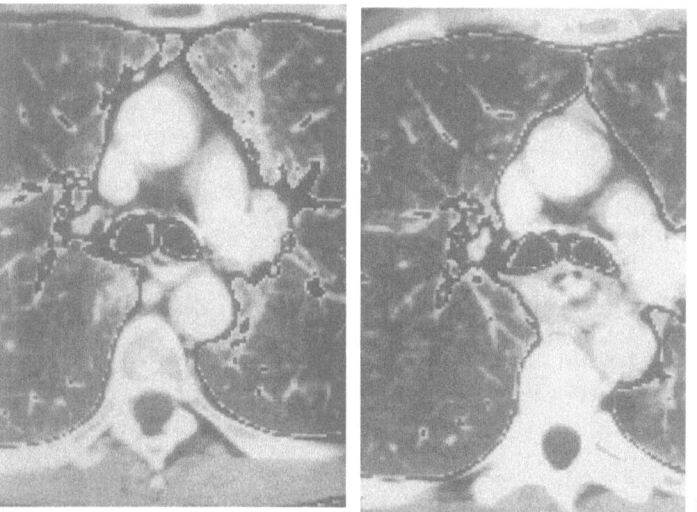

Fig. 2. a Computerized tomography (*CT*) scan of T1/T2 esophageal cancer after neoadjuvant treatment. **b** The same tumor before preoperative chemo- and radiotherapy. CT scan shows extension beyond adventitia, but tumor does not invade surrounding structures

To produce a well-matched comparison between CT and EUS findings, we grouped T1 and T2 tumors together in a single subgroup, since CT, unlike EUS, is unable to differentiate between such tumors.

In the group of patients receiving preoperative chemo- and radiotherapy, a new category emerges in terms of T staging, namely T0 tumors presenting no evidence of malignancy at histology of the surgical specimen.

Results

Endoscopic Ultrasonography

The results are presented in Table 1. It proved possible to perform the examination in 42/53 cases in group A (feasibility: 79.2%) and in 24/40 cases in group B (feasibility: 60%).

EUS yielded an accurate diagnosis in 21/42 cases in group A with an overall accuracy of 50%. The tumors were over-staged in 13 cases (31%) and under-staged in 8 (19%).

In the T0 subgroup, the diagnosis was accurate in four of ten cases (40%). In the other cases in this group, the tumors were over-staged as T1/T2 in two cases and as T3 in four cases; in all four T3 cases histology revealed the presence of abundant parietal fibrosis.

In the T1/T2 subgroup, the EUS staging coincided with the histological staging in 5/12 cases (41.6%), with tumors being over-staged in 5 cases (3 T3 and 2 T4) and under-staged as T0 in 2 cases. Within the T1/T2 group, a further subgroup of 6 cases was discernible, in which histology of surgical specimens revealed only

Table 1. Determination of wall invasion by EUS in the two groups of patients compared with pathology of the resected specimen (pT)

Pathology	Endosonography						
	CH + RT + surgery				surgery alone		
	T0	T1/T2	T3	T4	T1/T2	T3	T4
pT0	4[a]	2	4				
pT1/pT2	2	5[a]	3	2	7[b]	2	
pT3		2	8[a]	2		6[b]	1
pT4			4	4[a]		1	7[b]

EUS, endoscopic ultrasonography; *CH*, chemotherapy; *RT*, radiotherapy
[a] Overall accuracy: 21/42 (50%)
[b] Overall accuracy: 20/24 (83.3%)

microscopic neoplastic foci localized in 4 cases in the submucosa and in 2 cases in the muscularis propria and therefore regarded as T1/T2. In these 6 cases, EUS yielded the correct diagnosis in 3 cases, while 2 were over-staged as T3, and 1 under-staged as T0.

In the T3 tumors, EUS yielded a correct diagnosis in 8/12 cases (66.6%) with 2 cases over-staged as T4 and 2 under-staged as T1/T2.

Lastly, in the T4 group, the EUS diagnosis was accurate in 4/8 cases (50%), the other 4 cases being under-staged as T3.

In group B, despite the low feasibility, the results are distinctly better with an overall accuracy of 83.3% (20/24 cases), over-staging errors being made in 3 cases (12.5%) and under-staging in 1 case (4.1%).

The diagnosis was correct in 7/9 cases (77.7%) in the T1/T2 subgroup, in 6/7 cases (85.7%) in the T3 subgroup and in 7/8 cases (87.5%) in the T4 subgroup.

Computerized Tomography

The results are presented in Table 2. In group A, the overall T staging accuracy of CT was 43.3% (23/53) with over-staging in 15/53 cases (28.3%) and under-staging again in 15/53 cases (28.3%).

In the T0 tumors, CT yielded an accurate diagnosis in 3/11 cases (27.2%); tumors were over-staged as T1/T2 in 5 cases and as T3 in 3 cases.

In the T1/T2 tumors, the CT diagnosis was correct in 7/12 cases (58.3%), while in the remaining 5 cases tumors were over-staged as T3 in 2 cases and as T4 in 3. As mentioned above in the context of analysis of EUS findings, the T1/T2 subgroup contained six tumors in which histology revealed only microscopic foci of carcinoma in the submucosa or muscularis propria; in these cases, CT correctly staged four tumors, whereas the other two were over-staged as T3.

In the T3 subgroup, CT yielded an accurate diagnosis in 7/14 cases (50%) with 5 cases under-staged as T1/T2 and 2 cases over-staged as T4 with suspected invasion of the airways.

Lastly, in the T4 tumor subgroup, the diagnostic accuracy of CT was poor with only 6/16 (37.5%) correct diagnoses and as many as ten tumors under-

Table 2. Determination of wall invasion by dynamic CT in the two groups of patients compared with pathology of the resected specimen (pT)

Pathology	Dynamic CT						
	CH + RT + surgery				surgery alone		
	T0	T1/T2	T3	T4	T1/T2	T3	T4
pT0	3[a]	5	3				
pT1/pT2		7[a]	2	3	20[b]	5	
pT3		5	7[a]	2	4	7[b]	4
pT4			10	6[a]		5	9[b]

CT, computerized tomography
[a] Overall accuracy: 23/53 (43.3%)
[b] Overall accuracy: 36/54 (66%)

staged as T3, despite presenting infiltration of adjacent organs (six airways, one pericardium, three aorta).

The results obtained in group B were distinctly better than those in group A. Here, the overall diagnostic accuracy was 66% (36/54 cases) with over-staging in 9/54 cases (16.6%) and under-staging again in 9/54 cases (16.6%). The CT diagnosis coincided with the histological diagnosis in 20/25 cases (80%) in the T1/T2 subgroup, in 7/15 cases (46.6%) in the T3 subgroup and in 9/14 cases (64%) in the T4 subgroup.

Discussion

Up until only a few years ago, CT was the procedure of choice for preoperative tumor staging in patients with esophageal carcinoma, though very discordant data were reported as to its reliability. The most recent results indicate poor accuracy in T staging with values of 51%–68% [6, 8, 15–17].

A substantial improvement in esophageal cancer staging has been made in recent years as a result of the introduction of EUS in clinical practice. The accuracy of EUS is distinctly superior to that of CT, particularly in T staging, with values ranging from 77% to 94% [7, 11, 17–19].

Multimodal neoadjuvant treatment had an appreciable effect on preoperative tumor staging in our study. On comparing the CT and EUS results in patients receiving preoperative adjuvant chemo- and radiotherapy with those obtained in patients undergoing surgery alone, a distinct worsening of diagnostic accuracy is noted. This inferior diagnostic performance is not observable in the assessment of lymph node involvement (N staging) where the results of CT (56.6% versus 53.7%) and EUS (66.6% versus 70.8%) in the two groups are practically identical. It is on the T staging that preoperative adjuvant treatment has a substantial effect with a reduction of accuracy from 66% to 43.3% in the case of CT and, even more so, from 83.3% to 50% in the case of EUS.

The reduced reliability of the procedures affects all T staging grades and is caused by a number of different factors.

As regards the staging of early tumors (T1 and T2), in the group of patients receiving neoadjuvant therapy a new subgroup emerged in which the preoperative chemo- and radiotherapy produced a complete response with disappearance of the malignancy at histology of the surgical specimen. In these patients, defined as T0, it proved extremely difficult for CT (accuracy: 27.2%) and EUS (accuracy: 40%) to demonstrate the absence of cancer.

In addition to the T0 problem, we must also consider the T1 and T2 cases in which histology revealed only the presence of microscopic foci of tumor cells in the tunica submucosa and/or muscularis propria; the diagnoses formulated in these cases both by CT and by EUS are to be regarded as purely casual, in that neither procedure is capable of detecting lesions which are visible only under the microscope.

Furthermore, the gross over-staging errors committed in the early esophageal cancer subgroup by both CT (three T0 cases over-staged as T3 and three T1/T2 cases over-staged as T4) and by EUS (four T0 cases over-staged as T3 and two T1/T2 cases over-staged as T4) must be regarded as serious. In some of these patients, on the basis of these preoperative staging results, the surgeon should have declined to operate. As could be seen at subsequent postoperative histology, these gross staging errors are due to the presence of abundant post-radiation fibrosis of the esophageal wall. It is, in fact, very difficult for CT and EUS to differentiate between tumor tissue and recent post-inflammatory fibrosis [20–22].

Poor staging results were also obtained in group A for advanced cancers infiltrating neighbouring organs (T4) with numerous under-staging errors (CT accuracy: 37.5%; EUS accuracy: 40%) and patients selected for exploratory thoracotomy and/or non-radical resection.

In conclusion, multimodal neoadjuvant treatment constitutes a major obstacle to accurate preoperative staging of esophageal cancer and appreciably reduces the reliability of CT and, even more so, of EUS in estimating the depth of invasion of the esophageal wall by the malignancy. In view of these results, the surgical approach in patients receiving preoperative adjuvant therapy should be aggressive with execution of an exploratory thoracotomy in the majority of cases, excluding only those with systemic metastases or unmistakeable signs of infiltration of adjacent organs. It will only be through development of new staging techniques, allowing detection of T0 tumors and T1/T2 tumors with microscopic foci, that this approach can be modified, revolutionizing the surgical indications.

References

1. Earlman R, Cunha-Melo JR (1980) Oesophageal squamous cell carcinoma: I. A critical review of surgery. Br J Surg 67:381–390
2. Bancewicz J (1990) Cancer of the oesophagus. BMJ 300:3–4
3. Skinner DB, Ferguson MK, Soriano A, Little AG, Staszak VM (1986) Selection of operation for esophageal cancer based on staging. Ann Surg 204:391–401
4. Feketé F, Gayet B, Favas A, Langonnet F (1990) Surgical treatment of thoracic esophagus carcinoma. Dig Surg 7:86–92
5. Weiser HF, Lange R, Feussner H (1986) How can we diagnose the early stage of esophageal cancer? Diagnosis of the early esophageal cancer. Endoscopy 18 [Suppl 3]:2–10

 6. Siewert JR, Holscher AH, Dittler HJ (1990) Preoperative staging and risk analysis in esophageal carcinoma. Hepatogastroenterol 37:382–387
 7. Shorvon PJ (1990) Endoscopic ultrasound in oesophageal cancer: The way forward? Clin Radiol 42:149–151
 8. Rankin S (1990) The role of computerized tomography in the staging of oesophageal cancer. Clin Radiol 42:152–153
 9. Bains M, Kelsen DP, Beattle EJ, Martini N (1982) Treatment of esophageal carcinoma by combined preoperative chemotherapy. Ann Thorac Surg 34:521–528
10. Steiger Z, Franklin R, Wilson R, Leichman L, Seydel H, Loh JJK, Vaishamapayan G, Knechtges T, Asfaw I, Dindogru A, Rosenberg JC, Buroker T, Torres A, Hoschner D, Miller P, Pietruk T, Vaitkevicius V (1981) Eradication and palliation of squamous cell carcinoma of the esophagus with chemotherapy, radiotherapy, and surgical therapy. J Thorac Cardiovasc Surg 82:713–719
11. Tio TL, Cohen P, Coene PP. Udding J, Den Hartog Jager FCA, Tytgat GNJ (1989) Endosonography and computed tomography of esophageal cancer. Gastroenterology 96:1478–86
12. Picus D, Balfe MD, Koehler RE, Roper CL, Owen JW (1983) Computed tomography in the staging of esophageal carcinoma. Radiology 146:433–438
13. Thompson WM, Halvorsen LA, Foster WL, Williford ME, Postelthwait RW, Korobkin M (1983) Computed tomography for staging esophageal and gastroesophageal cancer. AJR 141:951–958
14. Halvorsen LA, Thompson WM (1987) Computed tomographic staging of gastrointestinal tract malignancies. Part one: Esophagus and stomach. Invest Radiol 22:1–16
15. Quint LE, Glazer GM, Orringer MB, Gross BH (1985) Esophageal carcinoma: CT findings. Radiology 155:171–175
16. Lehr L, Rupp N, Siewert JR (1988) Assessment of resectability of esophageal cancer by computed tomography and magnetic resonance imaging. Surgery 103:344–350
17. Botet JF, Lightdale CJ, Zauber AG, Gerdes H, Urmacher C, Brennan MF (1991) Preoperative staging of esophageal cancer: Comparison of endoscopic US and dynamic CT. Radiology 181:419–425
18. Date H, Miyashita M, Sasajima K, Toba M, Yamashita K, Takubo K, Onda M (1990) Assessment of adventitial involvement of esophageal carcinoma by endoscopic ultrasonography. Surg Endosc 4:195–197
19. Heintz A, Hohne U, Schweden F, Junginger T (1991) Preoperative detection of intrathoracic tumor spread of esophageal cancer: Endosonography versus computed tomography. Surg Endosc 5:75–78
20. Yoshida S, Miyamato K, Hijikata A (1990) Endosonography: Its diagnostic utilities for gastric cancer. In: Reed PI, Carboni M, Johnston BJ, Guadagni S (eds) New trends in gastric cancer. Kluwer, London, pp 78–86
21. Napoleon B, Pujol B, Berger F, Valette PJ, Gerard JP, Souquet JC (1991) Accuracy of endosonography in the staging of rectal cancer treated by radiotherapy. Br J Surg 78:785–788
22. Thoeni RF (1991) Colorectal cancer: Cross sectional imaging for staging of primary tumor and detection of local recurrence. AJR 156:909–915

Clinical Evaluation of Mucosal Cancer of the Esophagus: Analysis of 1584 Cases of Superficial Esophageal Cancer Resected in Japan

M. Endo, K. Yoshino, T. Kawano, and K. Yano[1]

Superficial Cancer and 5-Year Survival Rate

Cases of superficial cancer (pTis and pT_1 cancer) of the esophagus resected at 208 hospitals in Japan from 1984 to 1989, were collected and analyzed. A total of 1584 cases were as follows: epithelial cancer (ep cancer), 188; intramucosal cancer as far as the lamina, muscularis mucosa (mm cancer), 312; submucosal cancer (sm cancer), 996; and unknown, 88. Mucosal cancer (ep + mm cancer) totalled 500 cases (32%). Considering the long-term results related to the depth of cancer invasion, excluding death clearly due to other diseases, the 5-year survival rate of ep cancer was 97%, mm cancer was 92%, and sm cancer was 67%. This shows a significant difference between mucosal (ep, mm) cancers and sm cancer (Fig. 1).

Cancer Depth and Lymph Node Metastasis

As for the relationship between the cancer depth and lymph node metastasis in superficial esophageal cancer, no lymph node metastasis was noted in ep cancer. Lymph node metastasis was observed in 7% of mm cancer and in 4% of total mucosal cancer cases. While lymph node metastasis was noted in 35% of submucosal cancer cases (Table 1).

The long-term results related to lymph node metastasis revealed a significant difference between the 5-year survival rate of superficial cancer with (86%) and without (49%), metastasis [1].

---

[1] First Department of Surgery, Tokyo Medical and Dental University, 5-45, Yushima 1-chome, Bunkyo-ku, Tokyo, 113 Japan

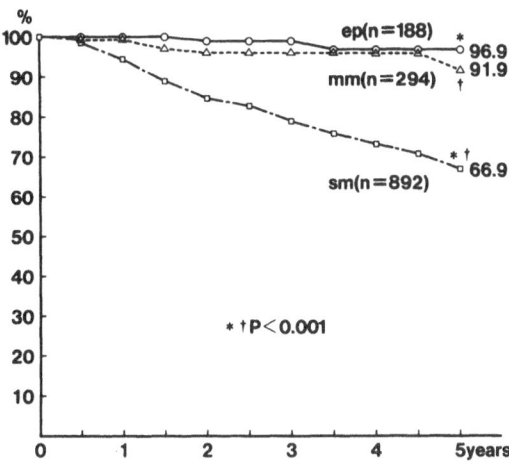

Fig. 1. Five-year survival rate of superficial esophageal cancer related to degree of depth of invasion

Table 1. Degree of depth of invasion and lymph node metastasis in superficial esophageal cancer (1498 cases)

Depth of invasion	No. of patients	No. of positive nodal involvement (%)
ep ⎫ m mm ⎭	188 ⎫ 500 312 ⎭	0 ⎫ 21 (4.2) 21 (6.7) ⎭
sm	996	351 (35.2)
Unknown	2	1

ep, epithelium; *mm*, muscularis mucosa; *m*, mucosa; *sm*, submucosa

Cancer Depth and Vascular Invasion

Lymphatic invasion was seen in 8% of mucosal cancer, and in 46% of submucosal cancer. Blood vessel invasion was observed in 2% of mucosal cancer cases and in 19% of submucosal cancer cases.

With respect to vascular invasion, the 5-year survival rate of superficial cancer cases without vascular invasion was 84% and those showing vascular invasion was 61%. The difference between these two groups was significant.

Recurrence was mostly found in submucosal cancer cases with lymphatic invasion, even if lymph node metastasis was negative.

At present, mucosal cancer and submucosal cancer of the esophagus without lymph node metastasis are included in the same category of early cancer of the esophagus according to the guidelines of the Japanese Society for Esophageal Diseases (JSDE) [2]. Considering the data provided above, however, only mucosal cancer of the esophagus can be defined as curable or clinically proper early cancer of the esophagus.

Table 2. Symptoms in mucosal cancer of the esophagus

Subjective symptoms	No. of patients (%)		
	ep ($n = 188$)	mm ($n = 312$)	Total ($n = 500$)
No symptoms	120	162	282 (56.4)
Retrosternal pain	13	21	34 (6.8)
Feeling of stenosis	12	33	45 (9.0)
Foreign body sensation	14	23	37 (7.4)
Dysphagia	4	3	7 (1.4)
Nausea	3	8	11 (2.2)
Others	24	66	90 (18.0)
Unknown	1		1

(Including double symptoms in one patient)

Table 3. Endoscopic classification of esophageal cancer (JSDE)

0. Superficial type (T_1)
   0-I   Superficial and protruding type
   0-II Superficial and flat type
     0-IIa Slightly elevated type
     0-IIb Flat type
     0-IIc Slightly depressed type
   0-III Superficial and distinctly depressed type
1. Protruding type
2. Ulcerative and localized type
3. Ulcerative and infiltrative type   (T_2–T_4)
4. Diffusely infiltrative type
5. Unclassifiable type

JSDE, Japanese Society for Diseases of the Esophagus [2]

Chief Complaints of Mucosal Cancer

Retrosternal pain and a tingling sensation in the esophagus caused by food were the most common symptoms, followed by a feeling of stenosis and generalized discomfort. No symptoms or some unrelated abdominal complaints were seen in 68% of the cases, and diagnosis of esophageal cancer was occasional (Table 2).

Endoscopic Diagnosis of Mucosal Cancer

Mucosal cancer cases were detected based on symptoms (37%), during routine health screening (33%), and during examination for other GI diseases (28%), and so on.

Endoscopy has come to play a large role in the diagnosis of mucosal cancer. Endoscopic findings of esophageal cancer are shown in Table 3 [2]. Superficial type (0-type) is defined as esophageal lesions which are considered superficial cancer at the examination.

0-type is further categorized into five basic types as follows: 0-1, 0-IIa, 0-IIb, 0-IIc, and 0-III. Of these, 0-I type indicates a superficial and protruded lesion, 0-II type a superficial and flat lesion, and 0-III type a superficial and distinctly depressed lesion. In 0-II type, 0-IIa type shows a slightly elevated lesion, 0-IIb type a flat lesion and 0-IIc type a slightly depressed lesion. When a mixture of more than two basic types is found within one lesion, a mixed type is indicated.

In this classification, mucosal cancer was commonly observed in 0-IIb flat type lesions and 0-IIc slightly depressed type lesions. Less commonly, a few small 0-IIa slightly elevated type lesions were observed.

The endoscopic staining technique with Lugol's solution can provide more precise information in the diagnosis of 0-IIb type and 0-IIc type of lesions [3].

Modalities for Detection of Mucosal Cancer

Some findings that are useful in the detection of mucosal cancer are summarized below.

When patients present with slight esophageal complaints, a tingling after a meal, or retrosternal abnormal sensation, esophagoscopy should be performed.

A periodic examination may be appropriate for high risk population, males more than 50 year of age.

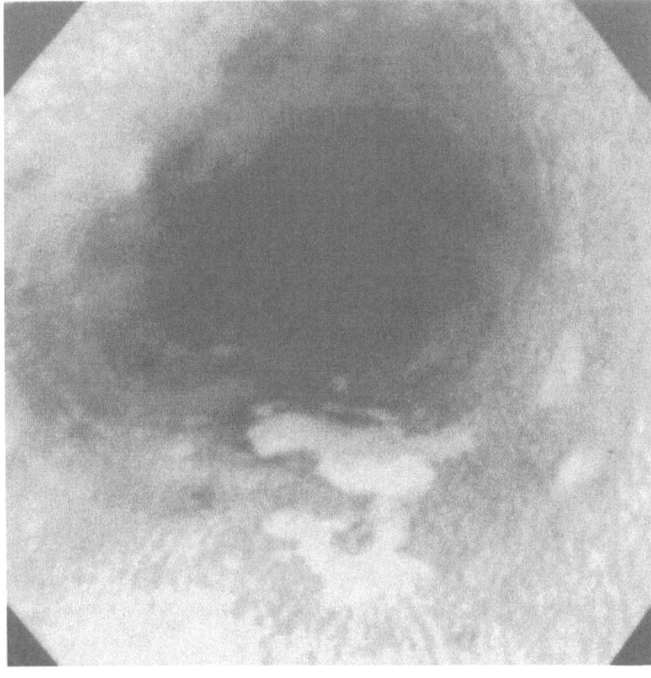

Fig. 2. An 0-IIc type of lesion 2 cm in size is demonstrated with Lugol's staining

Recently, double esophageal and gastric, colonic or head and neck cancer cases have been noted.

When abnormal findings in the esophageal mucosa are demonstrated by conventional esophagoscopy, endoscopic staining with Lugol's solution must be performed. We have experienced that some 0-IIb type of lesions could only be recognized after staining with Lugol's solution. Endoscopic staining techniques can be actively applied in periodic examination or in mass screening.

To confirm pathological diagnosis, a biopsy specimen should be taken from the unstained area.

Surgical Treatment of Superficial Cancer

As for the operative modalities, when the lesion is suspected to be mucosal cancer, less invasive operations may be indicated. Esophagectomy without thoracotomy and endoscopic resection are common. Esophagectomy and lymph node dissection under thoracotomy is usually performed for submucosal cancer cases and for positive nodal involvement cases.

Endoscopic resection is usually indicated for mucosal cancer less than 2 × 2 cm and for negative nodal involvement. However, lesion in which massive to the musculars mucosa is suspected are excluded.

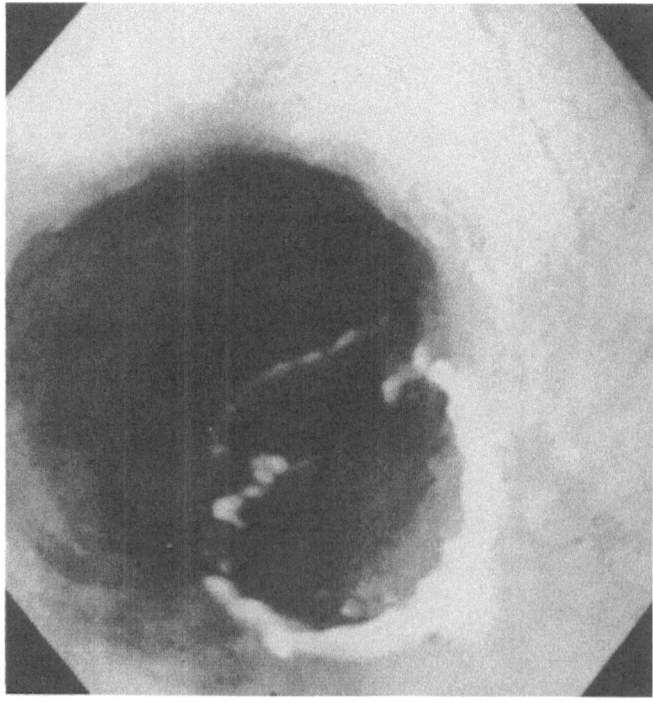

Fig. 3. A mechanically induced ulcer after endoscopic resection

In one case, a 0-IIc type of lesion was found about 2 cm in size, as shown in Fig. 2.

Figure 3 shows a picture immediately after endoscopic resection. A mechanically induced ulcer is seen.

Ulcer was cured 40 days after endoscopic resection.

Summary

All cases of superficial esophageal cancer resected between 1984 and 1989 in Japan (n = 1584) were analyzed. The frequency of mucosal cancer was 32%. Five-year survival rates of ep and mm cancer were 97% and 92%, respectively. Lymph node metastasis was observed in 4% of mucosal cancer cases, and lymphatic invasion was observed in 8%. Endoscopy and endoscopic staining with Lugol's solution is recommended for detection of mucosal cancer. As for the operative modality, minimally invasive surgery is indicated for mucosal cancer of the esophagus.

Reference

1. Endo M, Yoshino K, Takeshita K, Kawano T (1991) Analysis of 1125 cases of early esophageal carcinoma in Japan. Dis Esoph 4:71–76
2. Japanese Society for Esophageal Diseases (JSDE) (1992) Guidelines for the clinical and pathologic studies on carcinoma of the esophagus, 8th edn. Kanehara, Tokyo, pp 8–9
3. Endo M, Takeshita K, Yoshino K (1988) Oesophagoscopy for the diagnosis of superficial oesophageal cancer. Surg Endosc 2:205–208

Staging of Esophageal Cancer—Preoperative Prediction of LN-Metastases

E. BOLLSCHWEILER, A.H. HÖLSCHER, and J.R. SIEWERT[1]

Introduction

The therapeutic decision in esophageal cancer is decisively influenced by the preoperative staging especially the depth of wall infiltration of the primary tumor, lymph node metastases, and localization. Recent reports have clearly pointed out that radical lymphadenectomy is able to contribute to an improvement of prognosis especially in patients with early stages of lymph node metastases. In patients with an advanced stage of metastases, however, no improvement of survival can be effected by lymphadenectomy [1]. In addition, the radicality of lymphadenectomy also influences postoperative mortality and especially morbidity [2–4].

Whereas the staging of the depth of wall infiltration of the primary tumor in endoscopic ultrasonography (EUS) has an accuracy of 80%–90%, the results for the preoperative evaluation of an existing lymph node metastasis is much lower with an accuracy of 60%–80% for EUS. In computed tomography (CT), the accuracy ranges between 50% and 70% [5–7].

As these results are not satisfying, we turned our attention to improving the accuracy of the prediction by using a computer program. A similar program for the prediction of lymph node metastases in gastric carcinoma invented by Maruyama, showed an accuracy of more than 90% in a series of studies [5–7].

Aims of the Study

The aim of the present investigation was to establish a computer-based prediction of lymph node metastases in esophageal cancer on the basis of preoperative staging parameters together with the prediction of survival probability.

[1] Department of Surgery, Technische Universität München, Klinikum rechts der Isar, Ismaninger Str. 22, D-8000 München 80, Germany

Materials and Methods

Patients and Therapeutic Procedures

For the establishment of the program the data of 432 patients with esophageal cancer operated between 1/7/82 and 31/12/91 in the Department of Surgery of the Technical University of Munich were collected. The median age of the patients was 61.7 years with a preponderance of males to females in a ratio of 7:1. Histologically, 59% were squamous cell carcinomas and 41% adenocarcinomas of the esophagus. The squamous cell carcinomas were localized in 30% above the bifurcation, in 20% in the area of the bifurcation, and in 50% below the bifurcation, whereas adenocarcinomas were mostly localized directly above the cardia. In Table 1, further important tumor characteristics are mentioned.

In 59% of the cases, a so-called en bloc esophagectomy was performed (squamous cell cancer) and in 41% a transmediastinal esophagectomy with a standard lymphadenectomy (adenocarcinoma) was done, as has been described elsewhere [1]. The reconstruction was performed in 376 patients (87%) by gastric interposition and in 56 (23%) by colon interposition. In 69% of the

Table 1. Prognostic factors of 432 patients

	Squamous cell ca		Adeno ca	
	n	%	n	%
Number of patients	256	59.3	176	40.7
pT-category				
pT1	37	14.5	22	12.5
pT2	51	19.9	54	30.7
pT3	132	51.6	53	30.1
pT4	36	14.0	47	26.7
pN-category				
pN0	97	37.9	48	27.3
pN1	109	42.6	60	34.1
pN2 (M1 Lymph)	50	15.5	68	38.6
Metastases				
M0	245	95.7	151	85.8
M1	11	4.3	25	14.2
Grading				
G1	27	10.6	15	8.5
G2	114	44.5	73	41.5
G3	81	31.6	72	41.0
G4	34	13.3	16	9.0
R-Category				
R0	176	68.8	138	78.4
R1	53	20.7	26	14.8
R2	27	10.5	12	6.8

ca, Cancer

cases, the reconstruction was done in the anterior and in 31% in the posterior mediastinum. Seventy-two percent of the operations could be finished as an RO-resection (UICC, 1987). A preoperative radiochemotherapy (RTx/CTx) was added in 22% of the patients.

Knowledge-Based System

As a problem solution method, the heuristic classification was used [8]. The basis of science for the expert system is represented by the most important discriminating factors for the prediction of the metastatic infiltration of lymph nodes which had been detected by the multivariate procedure of logistic regression (BMDP LR). A stepwise selection of variables with the maximum likelihood ratio was performed. Variables having a calculated coefficient divided by their standard error of more than 1.8 were defined as independent.

To predict whether lymph nodes are free of metastases, a probability was calculated of which the value was between 1 (= free of LN-metastases) and 0 (= definite LN-metastases). The choice of the best cut-off point for the definition of the optimal sensitivity and specificity was performed with a receiver-operator-characteristic (ROC) curve [9]. The resulting accuracy was expressed together with a 95% confidence interval.

Probability of Survival

The data were analyzed by applying the Cox proportional hazard regression model to evaluate the most relevant prognostic factors for survival [10]. The log-linear risk function with a stepwise addition of factors with high influence on the model and elimination of the factors with a lower influence was established (BMDP 2L). The graphic display of the survival curves was done according to the Kaplan-Meier method [11].

Computer Program

For the calculations, modules of the statistics program BMDP-PC-90 (BMDP Statistical Software Inc., Cork, Ireland) were used. The programming was performed object-oriented using the software "object vision" (Borland GmbH, Starnberg, Germany).

Results

Logistic Regression Analysis

For the calculation of "prior probability" (P.P.)- the preoperative defined factors such as age and sex of the patients, preoperative radiochemotherapy, depth of tumor infiltration in EUS, histologic classification, and grading from the endoscopic biopsy, as well as localization and extent of the tumor from endoscopy, were used. If lymph node metastases had been diagnosed pre- or intraoperatively, the P.P. was given directly the value 0.

The result of the analysis shows that depth of tumor infiltration, localization and grading are independent factors for the presence of lymph node metastases

Table 2. Design matrix of the factors used in the logistic regression (patients without distant metastases)

Term	[]	Coefficient	Coefficient/SE
pT	a1	−2.382	−5.14
	a2	−2.819	−6.51
	a3	−3.019	−6.01
Local	b1	−0.887	−2.73
	b2	−0.967	−2.84
Grading	c1	−0.514	−1.98
constant		2.440	5.39

Table 3. Results of logistic regression

Term	Index	Freq.	Design 1	2
pT	1	58	0	0
	2	99	1	0
	3	169	0	1
	4	70	0	0
Local	1	113	0	0
	2	132	1	0
	3	151	0	1
Grading	1−2	197	1	
	3−4	199	1	

Freq, Frequency

in esophageal cancer. The significance of the individual factors is displayed in Table 2. The calculation of the probability that no lymph nodes are infiltrated is performed according to the equation:

$$\text{P.P. (NO)} = \frac{e^{(2.44 + ai \times pT + bi \times local + ci \times grading)}}{1 + e^{(2.44 + ai \times pT + bi \times local + ci \times grading)}}$$

where pT = depth of infiltration of the tumor [5, 6, 11, 12], local = localization of the tumor (1 = cervical − ad bifurcationem, 2 = infrabifurcal and 3 = cardia Type I), and grading = degree of differentiation of the tumor. The corresponding design matrix is shown in Table 3.

Receiver-Operator-Characteristic

Using the ROC-display, a cut-off point of 0.44 was choosen with an optimal accuracy (sensitivity of 78%, specificity of 79%). This led to an accurate prediction in 94% of the cases with lymph node metastases compared to only 55% otherwise.

Second Step of Heuristic Classification

In the second step of the analysis, a logistic regression was performed for each T-category. According to the results, factors were extracted which had an additional influence and their value was added to the prior probability.

By this classification the accuracy of the prediction, especially in T1-tumors, can be improved from 87.5% to 95.1% and in T4-tumors from 79.5% to 93.2%. The accuracy for all T-categories together is improved from 79.5% to 85.6% with a 95% confidence-interval of 82.0%−89.2%.

Discussion

The significance of an exact pretherapeutic staging is of importance because of the evaluation of the different therapeutic principles according to chance of

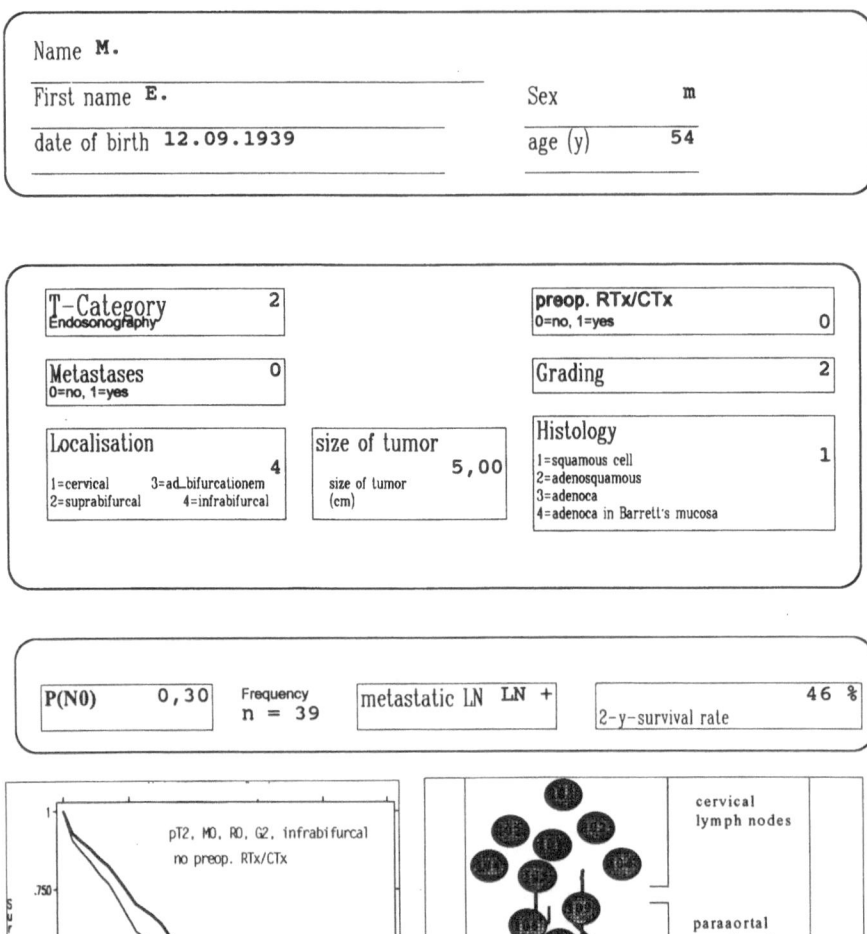

Fig. 1. Check list: Carcinoma of the esophagus—computerized pretherapeutic staging, Department of Surgery, Technical University Munich. *Pre op. RTx/CTx*, Preoperative, radio/chemotherapy

success and side effects. For example, a radical lymph node dissection is able to improve the prognosis of a tumor especially in the early stages when lymph node metastases is limited, whereas in advanced metastases the influence of lymph node dissection is limited [1]. Such an extensive resection however, has serious side effects which have to be considered for the choice of therapy together with the probability of expected survival. Whereas the T-category as one of the most important prognostic factors can be predicted with a high degree of accuracy due to the introduction of endoluminal ultrasound, results for the N-category in preoperative EUS as well as in CT scan are not satisfying [5, 6].

In the present investigation, we tried to improve the accuracy of the prediction by a computer-based decision-making program. The idea of this program was conceived by Maruyama, who has established a similar program for the prediction of lymph node metastases in gastric cancer. In this program, the evaluation showed a good accuracy [5, 13]. In Maruyama's computer program however, the data of 4000 patients with gastric cancer from one department were available so that the application of the case-comparing classification was possible. In tumors, however, which appear with a lower frequency, other classifications have to be used [8]. Therefore, a heuristic classification and in accordance with the problem the multivariate analysis of logistic regression was used as a statistical tool.

According to the results of other authors, the depth of tumor infiltration was formed to be the factors with highest influence on the frequency of lymph node metastases. However, as 43% of the patients had T3-tumors, this category in particular influences the results of the analysis to a high degree. Conversely, information of groups with a lower frequency, such as early cancers with lymph node metastases, does not change the calculation. However, especially for these groups, determining whether or not lymph nodes have infiltrated is of special importance. Therefore, separate regression analyses were performed for the different T-categories. The calculated factors were extrapolated in a way so that the addition with the prior probability led to a meaningful result.

Another important factor for lymph node metastases was the localization of the primary tumor and its histology. In agreement with other results, it was shown that the more the tumor is localized proximally, the lower the frequency of metastases [14]. In addition, it could be shown that adenocarcinomas of the esophagus have a higher frequency of lymph node metastases than sqamous cell carcinomas. It cannot be determined whether this is due to the influence of tumor localization or to different histology. It is of interest for the future if also the grading or additional classifications like DNA-ploidy may have an influence on metastases [15, 16].

By application of the statistical data, a probability for the infiltration of lymph node metastases was calculated which had an accuracy of 85.6%. This procedure leads to better or at least similar results as other methods like EUS or CT but it has the advantage of a simpler application. However, this method has to be evaluated in a prospective study.

For the results of therapy, the preoperative findings are displayed in a clear form and can be used as a check list. In addition, on this form the individual 2-year survival probability is shown numerically and graphically. The calculation is based on the most important independent prognostic factors determined by multivariate analysis: Depth of tumor infiltration, lymph node metastases, localization and histology of the tumor as well as age of the patients. The graphic display of the survival curve is done in all cases independently, whether or not lymph node metastasis is present. Another graphic shows the most frequent distribution of lymph node infiltration in the different regions according to tumor localization.

The purpose of the presented program for calculation of the probability of lymph node metastases and 2-year survival rate is to give a basis for therapeutic decisions in esophageal cancer together with the most important prognostic factors.

References

1. Siewert JR, Bartels H, Bollschweiler E, Dittler HJ, Fink U, Hölscher AH, Roder JD (1992) Plattenepithelcarcinom des Oesophagus—Behandlungskonzepte der Chirurgischen Klinik der Technischen Universität München. Chirurg 63; 693–700
2. Isono K, Ochiai T, Okuyama K, Onoda S (1990) The treatment of lymph node metastasis from esophageal cancer by extensive lymphadenectomy. Jpn J Surg 20(2):151–7
3. Kato H, Watanabe H, Tachimori Y, Iizuka T (1991) Evaluation of neck lymph node dissection for thoracic esophageal carcinoma Ann Thorac Surg. 51(6):931–524
4. Skinner DB (1991) Cervical lymph node dissection for thoracic esophageal cancer Ann Thorac Surg. 51(6):884–885
5. Bollschweiler E, Boettcher K, Hoelscher AH, Sasako M, Kinoshita T, Maruyama K, Siewert JR (1992) Preoperative assessment of lymph node metastases in patients with gastric cancer: Evaluation of Maruyama computer program. Br J Surg 79:156–160
6. Dittler HJ, Bollschweiler E, Siewert JR (1991) What is the value of endosonography in the preoperative staging of esophageal cancer? Dtsch Med Wochenschr 116(15):561–566
7. Ziegler K, Sanft C, Zeitz M, Friedrich M, Stein H, Haring R, Riecken EO (1991) Evaluation of endosonography in TN staging of esophageal cancer GUT. 32(1):16–20
8. Puppe F (1990) Problemlösungsmethoden in Expertensystemen. Springer, Berlin Heidelberg, pp 200–228
9. Fletcher RH, Fletcher SW, Wagner EH (1988) Clinical epidemiology—the essentials. Williams and Wilkins, Baltimore, pp 49–57
10. Kaplan EL, Meier P (1958) Nonparametric estimation from incomplete observations. J Amer Statist Assoc 53; 457–481
11. Cox DR (1972) Regression models and life tables. J Roy Statis Soc 34 (Series B):187–220
12. Botet JS, Kightdale CJ, Zauber AG, Gerdes H, Urmacher C, Brennan MF (1991) Preoperative staging of esophageal cancer: Comparison of endoscopic US and dynamic CT. Radiology 181:419–425
13. Kampschör GHM, Maruyama K, van der Velde CJH, Sasako M, Kinoshita T, Okabayashi K (1989) Computer analysis in making preoperative decisions: A rational approach to lymph node dissection in gastric cancer patients. Br J Surg 76; 905–908
14. Lund O, Hasenkam JM, Aagard MT, Kimose HH (1989) Time related changes in characteristics of prognostic significance in carcinomas of the oesophagus and cardia. Br J Surg 76; 1301–1307
15. Maesawa C, Tamura G, Monma N, Satodate R, Ishida K, Saito K (1991) Nuclear morphometric and DNA-content analysis of cancer cells in superficial esophageal cancer with reference to lymphynode metastases Nippon Geka Gakkai Zasshi 92(7):807–12
16. Nakamura T, Nekarda H, Becker K, Bollschweiler E, Hölscher AH, Siewert JR. Prognostic value of DNA ploidy and c-*erb* B-2 expression in adenocarcinoma of Barrett's esophagus.

Cervical Lymph Node Metastases in Thoracic Esophageal Cancer and Their Prognostic Role

Masakazu Yoshioka, Toshitada Okuma, Hirofumi Kaneko,
Yoshitsugu Torigoe, and Yoshimasa Miyauchi[1]

Introduction

It is well known that nodal metastasis of the thoracic esophageal cancer occur not only in the mediastinum and abdomen but also in the neck. Therefore, a comprehensive radical operation for the tumor should include a three-field dissection which has been discussed and performed for thoracic esophageal cancer since the 1980s [1, 2]; however, there is no general consensus about its advantages. Of note is that thoracic esophageal cancer with cervical lymph nodal involvement is defined as M1 and classified into stage IV according to the tumor, nodes, metastases (TNM) classification of the International Union Against Cancer (UICC), 1987 [3].

Cervical lymph nodes are grossly classified into two groups: the recurrent laryngeal nerve chain nodes (RLN) which consist of cervical pretracheal, paratracheal, and paraesophageal lymph nodes adjacent to cervical esophagus, and the internal jugular nodes (IJN) including supraclavicular nodes. The purpose of this study was to assess cervical lymph node metastases and to examine whether the site of the cervical lymph node metastasis impacts on patient's survival.

Materials and Methods

Patients

Three-field dissection was carried out on 68 of 142 patients who underwent transthoracic esophagectomy and reconstruction for squamous cell carcinoma of the thoracic esophagus from 1983 to 1990 in our institution. There were 57 men

[1] First Department of Surgery, Kumamoto University Medical School, 1-1-1, Honjo, Kumamoto City, Kumamoto, 860 Japan

and 11 women. The age at operation ranged from 45 to 74 years, and the average age was 62.5 years.

Operative Procedure

The esophagus is mobilized from neighboring tissues and transected at the high posterior mediastinal level with extended nodal dissection of the mediastinal lymph nodes including bilateral pulmonary hilar nodes.

After completion of this procedure, the abdominal operation and the bilateral cervical lymph node dissection with mobilization of the cervical esophagus are carried out simultaneously. Bilateral neck lymph nodes are dissected in the area from the upper levels of thyroid cartilage to the supraclavicular area and connected to the dissection of lymph nodes in the upper mediastinum.

Survival curves and rates of the patients were obtained using Kaplan-Meier distribution curves. Comparison of survival curves was carried out using the log-rank test, generalized Wilcoxon and Mantel Cox tests. Statistical calculations were also conducted using Fisher's exact test. Significant difference was accepted when P value was less than 0.05 ($P < 0.05$).

Results

Stage Distribution of the 68 Patients

Twenty-one (30.9%) of the 68 patients were Stage IV according to the histopathology (p) TNM-stage classification of the UICC, 1987, because of lymph node involvement in the neck or retroperitoneum. The 5-year survival rate of the 68 patients was 35.2%. None of the 68 patients died within 30 postoperative days and 2 patients died in the hospital.

pT of the TNM Classification and Cervical Lymph Node Metastasis

Cervical nodal disease was seen in 6 (24.0%) of the 25 patients who were classified into pT1–2 and 14 (32.6%) of the 43 patients who were classified into pT3–4. Significant difference was not seen between pT1–2 and pT3–4. Cervical lymph node metastasis was seen in 20 (29.4%) of the 68 patients.

Tumor Location and Cervical Lymph Node Metastases

Tumor location was analyzed according to the TNM classification. Cervical lymph node metastasis was seen in 1 of the 5 upper-third lesions (20.0%), 17 of the 47 middle-third lesions (36.2%) and 2 of the 16 lower-third lesions (12.5%). A significant difference was not seen in each location since the number of patients with upper- and lower-third lesions were small.

Survival Rates of the Patients With or Without Positive Cervical Lymph Nodes

The 4-year survival rates of the patients with and without positive cervical lymph nodes are 30.3% and 43.5%, respectively. However, a significant difference was not seen between the survival curves.

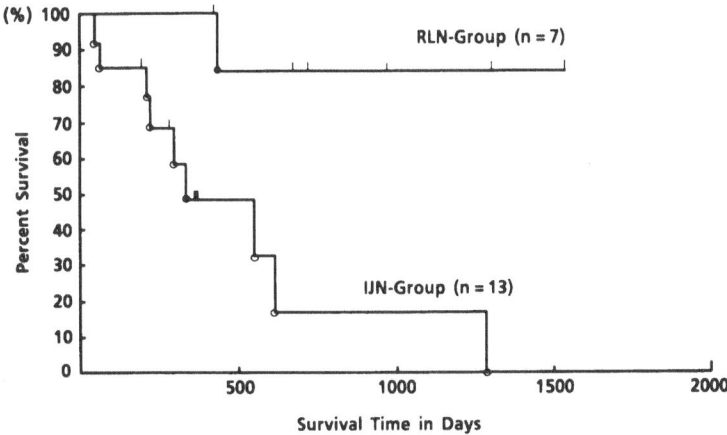

Fig. 1. Survival curves of the patients according to the site of cervical lymph node metastasis. *RLN-Group*, patients with nodal involvement limited to the recurrent laryngeal nerve chain nodes; *IJN-Group*, patients with nodal involvement of internal jugular node including supraclavicular node (*IJN*) and RLN + IJN. A significant difference was seen in each Group. Logrank test $P = 0.0057$, Generalized Wilcoxon test $P = 0.0120$, Mantel-Cox test $P = 0.0036$

Survival Rates of the Patients According to the Site of Cervical Lymph Node Metastasis

Nodal involvement limited to RLN was seen in 7 of the 20 patients (RLN Group) and nodal involvement of IJN and IJN + RLN was seen in 13 of the 20 patients (IJN Group).

Comparing the two groups revealed that the 1-, 2- and 3-year survival rates of the RLN Group were 100%, 83.3%, and 83.3%, respectively; whereas the 1-, 2-, and 3-year survival rates of the IJN Group were 48.3%, 16.1% and 16.1%. There was no survivor longer than 1277 days in the IJN Group. Survival curves were significantly different between two groups ($P = 0.010$: Generalized Wilcoxon) (Fig. 1).

Assessment of Mediastinal and Abdominal Nodal Metastasis According to the Site of Cervical Lymph Node Metastasis

Mediastinal and abdominal nodal involvements were analyzed in relation to the site of cervical lymph node metastasis. This was because a significant difference was seen in survival curves between the RLN Group and the IJN Group.

In the RLN Group, involvement of the upper mediastinal nodes was seen in three (42.9%) of the seven patients and none of them had celiac node metastases. However, in the IJN Group, positive upper mediastinal nodes were seen in 8 (61.5%), and positive celiac nodes were seen in 4 (30.8%) of the 13 patients.

Moreover, the number of patients with five or more positive nodes in the three-field areas was 2 (28.6%) in the RLN Group and 11 (84.6%) in the IJN

Table 1. Assessment of mediastinal and abdominal lymph node metastasis according to the site of cervical lymph node metastasis (1983–1990)

Lymph node	No. of RLN[a] patients Group ($n = 7$)	No. of IJN[b] patients Group ($n = 13$)
Upper mediastinum	3	8
Middle mediastinum (including hilar nodes)	3	2
Lower mediastinum	1	3
Perigastric	5	8
Celiac	0	4
No. of patients with five or more positive lymph nodes	2	11*

[a] RLN, recurrent laryngeal nerve chain nodes
[b] IJN, internal jugular nodes
* $P = 0.0223$ (vs RLN Group)

Group. A significant difference was seen between the two groups ($P = 0.0223$) (Table 1).

Discussion

Examination of the pattern of recurrence in patients having undergone esophagectomy for squamous cell carcinoma of the thoracic esophagus has revealed that there were many patients with not only distant recurrences of lung, liver and other organs, but also lymph node recurrences, especially in the cervical nodes and upper mediastinal nodes [4, 5]. Consequently, the significance of three–field dissection has been discussed for patients with squamous cell carcinoma of the thoracic esophagus in Japan since the 1980s [1, 2, 5, 6].

Several authors have reported that metastasis to cervical lymph nodes was seen in from 19% to 35% of patients who received three-field dissection for thoracic esophageal cancer [7–9]. In this study, metastasis to cervical lymph nodes was seen in 20 (29.4%) of the 68 patients. Although the cervical nodal disease was seen in more patients whose tumor penetrated the full thickness of the esophageal wall than those whose tumor invaded into the submucosal and muscle layers of the esophagus, there was no significant difference between pT1–2 and pT3–4.

Comparing the survival of the 20 patients who had positive cervical lymph node with the survival of the remaining 48 patients without positive cervical lymph node in this study, a significant difference was not seen in long-term survivals.

These data suggest that three-field dissection is useful in the surgery of patients with thoracic esophageal cancer. According to the TNM classification of the UICC, 1987, the patients with positive cervical lymph nodes are classified into Stage IV (M1). There are, however, two groups in patients with positive cervical lymph nodes as discussed above.

We demonstrated that although all patients with positive cervical lymph nodes were categorized into stage IV (M1), the patients of the RLN Group had a significantly longer survival than the patients of the IJN Group because there were many patients with five or more positive nodes in the IJN Group.

Conclusion

These results suggest that RLN should not be defined as M1 but as N1 in thoracic esophageal cancer, and that nodal disease in the neck should be classified as N1 disease, not M1.

Acknowledgments. The authors wish to thank Mr. H. Nagato for his help with statistical calculations.

References

1. Onoda S, Kouzu T, Okuyama K, et al (1989) Benefits and risks associated with dissection of three-regional lymph nodes (bilateral cervical, thoracic, and abdominal) in thoracic esophageal carcinoma. J Jpn Surg Soc 90:1619–22
2. Sasaki K, Tanaka Y, Ueki H, et al (1989) The significance of the extensive systematic lymphadenectomy for thoracic esophageal carcinoma. J Jpn Surg Soc 90:1605–08
3. Hermanek P, Sobin LH (1987) UICC international union against cancer, TNM classification of malignant tumors, 4th edn. Springer, Berlin Heidelberg New York, pp 40–42
4. Katlic MK, Wilkins EW Jr, Grillo HC (1990) Three decades of treatment of esophageal squamous cell carcinoma at the Massachusetts General Hospital. J Thorac Cardiovasc Surg 99:929–38
5. Ide H, Hanyu F, Murata Y, Kobayashi A, Yamada A, Kobayashi S (1990) Extended dissection for thoracic esophageal cancer based on preoperative staging. In: Ferguson MK, Little AG, Skinner DB (eds) Diseases of the esophagus, vol 1, malignant disease. Futura New York, pp 177–86
6. Ando N, Shinozawa Y, Kikunaga H, et al (1989) An assessment of extended lymphadenectomy including cervical node dissection for cancer of the thoracic esophagus. J Jpn Surg Soc 90:1616–18
7. Fujita H, Kakegawa T, Yamana H, et al (1989) Cervicothoracic abdominal lymph node dissection for carcinoma in the thoracic esophagus. J Jpn Surg Soc 90:1623–25
8. Tsurumaru M, Akiyama H, Udagawa H, Ono Y, Watanabe G, Suzuki M (1989) Evaluation of the collo-thoraco-abdominal dissection for the intrathoracic esophageal carcinoma. J Jpn Surg Soc 90:1612–15
9. Kato H, Watanabe H, Tachimori Y, Iizuka T (1991) Evaluation of neck lymph node dissection for thoracic esophageal carcinoma. Ann Thorac Surg 51:931–35

Scintigraphic Evaluation of Substitute Function After Esophagoplasty

Nikos Kavallieratos, Panayotis Yannopoulos[1], Michael Toubouros[2], Panayotis Tsevis[1], Angeliki Giougi[2], and Anastasia Stavraka-Kakavaki[2]

Introduction

Since no visceral tissue substitute can completely reproduce normal esophageal function, it is understandable why the criteria of life expectancy and safety predominate in choosing the viscus to be used as an esophageal replacement [1, 2]. On the other hand, in spite of the numerous reports in the literature, there are several questions that remain unanswered concerning the function of different substitutes and their influence on quality of life.

The simplicity, non-invasiveness, and quantitative properties of esophageal scintigraphy make it an attractive method to be applied in esophagoplasty evaluation. Since, as far as we know, experience in this field is still limited, we have studied different types of esophagoplasty to detect any differences in function and contribute to creating a suitable examination protocol.

Material and Methods

Twenty-five patients, 12 males and 13 females, aged at operation 12–69 years (mean age 47.5 years) were examined. They had undergone esophagectomy and substitution ($n = 20$, 80%) or bypass ($n = 5$, 20%), 1–186 months (mean 29.4 months) prior to the study ($n = 10$, 40%) or benign lesion ($n = 15$, 60%). As an esophageal substitute, stomach has been used in nine patients, isoperistaltic gastric tube in one, reverse gastric tube in three jejunum in one, isoperistaltic colon in five, and antiperistaltic colon in six. The substitute was placed in the posterior mediastinum in eight patients, substernally in eight, and subcutaneously in nine.

[1] 1st Department of Surgery, Nikea-Piraeus General Hospital, Fanarioton St. 3, 18454 Nikea, Greece
[2] Nuclear Medicin Department, Aretacion Hospital, Athens University, V. Sofias ave. 72, Athens, Greece

Table 1. Camera computer program

Delay	Total time (s)	Frame/time (s)	Frame time (s)
0	32	1/0.5	0.5
0	1280	1/10	4.0
180	240	1/10	4.0
180	240	1/10	4.0
180	160	1/10	4.0

A LFOV (large field of view) γ-camera connected with a computer has been used (Apex 409 model, Elscint). The low energy-high sensitivity collimator was placed under the supine patient since the collimator does not affect the reliability of results in this position [3]. Each patient, fasting for at least 6h, was given 10 ml of water containing 1 mCi of 99 mTc sulfur colloid and asked to take it all in a single swallow and not to swallow again for 32 s, after which time they were permitted to swallow freely. The standard program of the camera computer used for esophagus examination was modified, as shown in Table 1. During the three 180-s delay intervals, the patient was asked to sit with the help of one of the examination team, taking great care not to change their position when lying down again.

Data Acquisition

Both groups of digital scintigraphic pictures (transit-clearance) were analyzed by the computer in the same way. By means of two markers and the joystick, three regions of interest (ROI) were defined: The upper represents the proximal esophagus or pharynx in cases of pharyngolaryngectomy, the middle represents the part of the substitute at the level of the thorax, and the lower the abdominal part of it. Counts/time curves were created for the whole field examined, as well as for each ROI. The quantitative evaluation of bolus clearance at time t is given by the formula:

$$\text{transit/clearance} = \frac{E_{max} - E_t}{E_{max}} \times 100 \tag{1}$$

where E_{max} is the maximum value of the number of counts (immediately after the first swallow and E_t is the number of counts at time t.

Estimation of the ability of different viscera used as neoesophagus to propel the liquid bolus was made by comparison of clearance at examination time: a) 32 s controlling transit after a single swallowing action, b) 1312 s contolling clearance before gravity plays a role, and c) 2492 s at the end of examination. Values where roughly compared to the ones of a control group of 14 normal volunteers. A comparison of the clearance ratio due to gravity (as represented by the instant fall of the number of counts after each raising) over total clearance was made to estimate the contribution of gravity.

A more detailed assessment of transposed viscus function was made by comparison of the aforementioned values at the middle ROI. Anastomotic strictures were confirmed by low clearance of the upper ROI, while gastro- or jejuno neoesphageal reflux was diagnosed by the rise in counts above the minimal number previously recorded.

Results

Clearance values concerning all types of esophagoplasty were much lower than the transit value (32 s) in the control group (88.1%–91.5%) (Fig. 1). Among different transposed viscera, no significant tendencies were recorded, except for antiperistaltic colon which presented a much worse clearance than all other viscera (Fig. 2). Better clearance values were observed in isoperistaltic gastric tube and jejunum. These findings were more clearly presented in the study of middle ROI curves (Fig. 3). Differences in clearance values had no correlation with any symptoms, except in three patients with antiperistaltic colon: Two of them often had a feeling of fullness and vomited food even 18 h after eating, while the third had a well-tolerated feeling of contractions. Scintigraphic findings were in almost full accordance with symptomatology in patients with cervical anastomotic stricture or reflux to the transposed viscus. No differences of values were recorded in relation to substernal, subcutaneous, or posterior mediastinal position of the transplant. The role of gravity was generally highly significant in bolus propagation, with greater values in the antiperistaltic colon patients (Fig. 4). The time interval between operation and examination did not produce any differences in results. In one case involving subcutaneous transposition of about 15 cm of esophagus, upper ROI study yielded results very similar to those of normal.

Discussion

Esophageal scintigraphy is nowadays an established method of detecting abnormal esophageal motility, as well as anatomic lesions and gastroesophageal reflux; it has the advantages of speed, simplicity, quantification, and low radiation exposure [4, 5]. Experience of its use in functional evaluation of esophageal substitutes seems to be limited [6–9]. This is more true in comparing different types of esophagoplasties [10, 11].

Quantitation of this examination does present a problem. Defining some percentage of clearance (usually 50% or 25%) and measuring time as proposed by some authors [7] usually takes so much time that many other factors may affect the result. The protocol we have used has yielded values with moderate tendencies among substitutes of the same type which correlate well with our clinical impression. Use of solid or semisolid radiolabelled bolus may be advantageous when examining esophagus [12], but is not suitable, in our opinion, in examining different types of visceral substitutes as differences in gross anatomy, as well as mucosal quality, may distort the results. The combination of sitting and supine positions in this study has the advantage of factoring out the influence of gravity on bolus propagation.

Our results suggest that jejunum presents a quite good propagating activity, in accordance with manometric studies [10, 11]. It is generally accepted that the

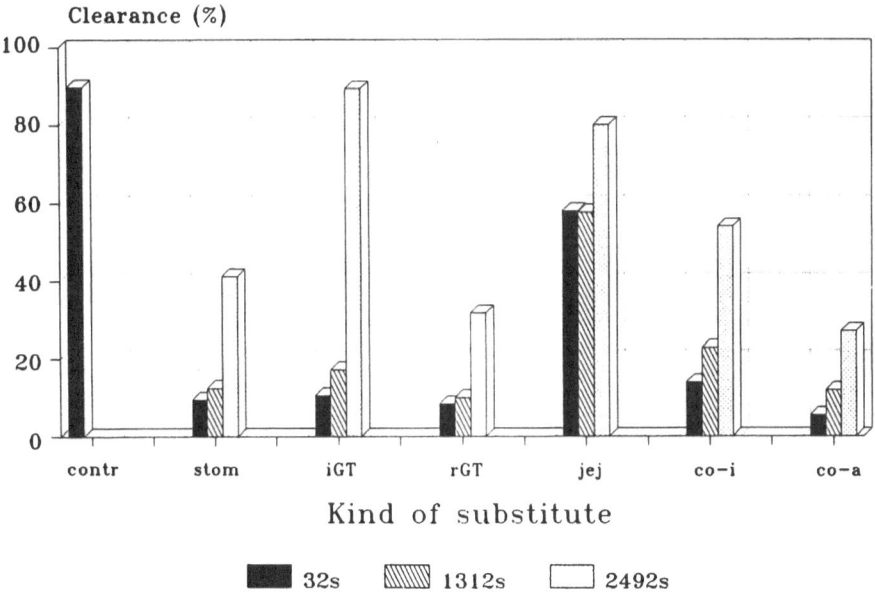

Fig. 1. Mean transit-clearance values. *contr*, control; *stom*, stomach; *iGT*, isoperistaltic gastric tube *rGT*, reverse gastric tube *jej*, jejunum; *co-i*, isoperistaltic colon; *co-a*, antiperistaltic colon

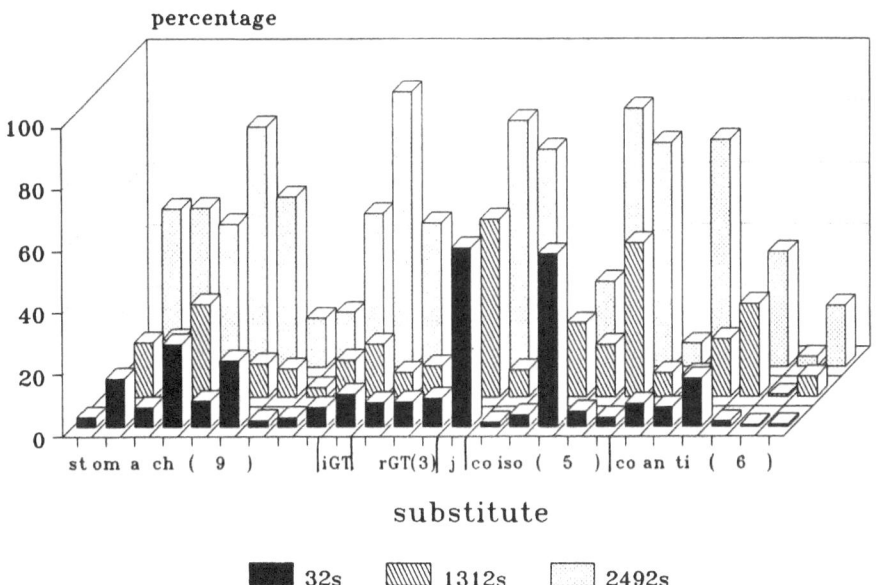

Fig. 2. Transit-clearance values of each case examined

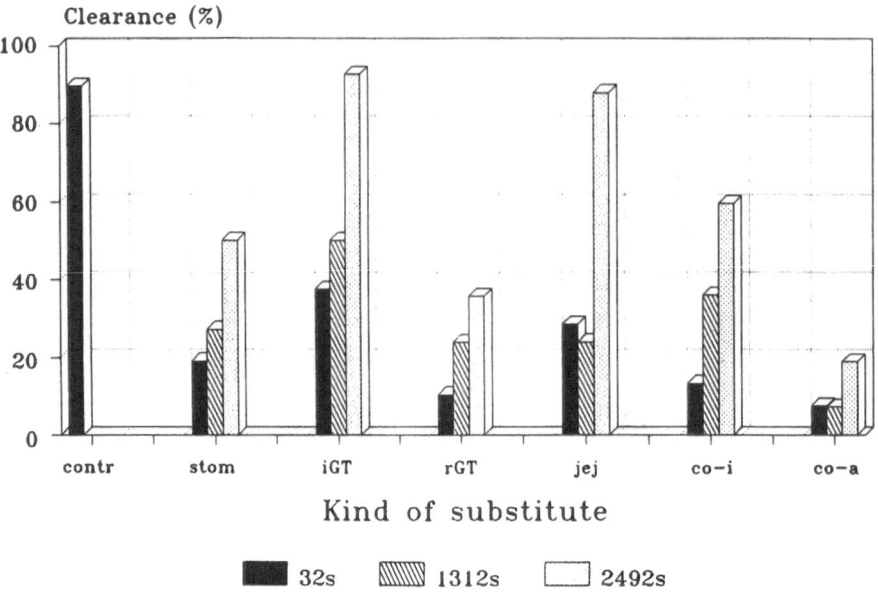

Fig. 3. Mean transit-clearance values, middle region of interest (ROI)

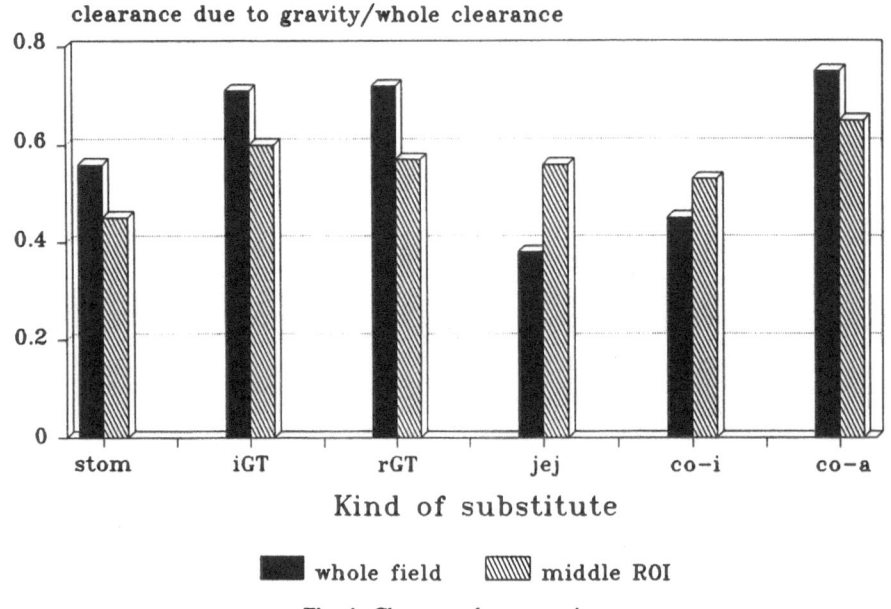

Fig. 4. Clearance due to gravity

stomach empties by means of gravity, but further attention must be paid in gastric tubes used for bypass. In our study, there is evidence of some motor activity. Worse clearance in antiperistaltic colon substitutes is evidence of sequential movement delaying bolus propagation. Further physiological evaluation of our finding of almost normal behavior of a subcutaneously transpositioned proximal esophageal stump of about 15 cm would certainly yield interesting results.

References

1. Belsey R (1983) Reconstruction of the oesophagus. Ann R Coll Surg Engl 65:360–364
2. Postlethwait RW (1983) Colonic interposition for esophageal substitution. Surg Gynecol Obstet 156:377–383
3. Klein HA (1989) The effect of projection in esophageal scanning scintigraphy. Nucl Med 15:157–162
4. Malmud LS, Fischer RS (1982) Radionuclide studies of esophageal transit and gastroesophageal reflux. Semin Nucl Med XII:104–115
5. Blackwell JN, Hannan WJ, Adam RD, Heading RC (1983) Radionuclide transit studies in the detection of esophageal dismotility. Gut; 24:421–426
6. Taillefer R, Beauchamp G, Duranceau AC, Lafontaine E (1986) Nuclear medicine and esophageal surgery. Clin Nucl Med; 11:445–460
7. Isolauri J, Koskinen MO, Markkula H (1987) Radionuclide transit in patients with colon interposition. J Thorac Cardiovasc Surg 94:521–525
8. Hinder RA (1976) The effect of posture on the emptying of the intrathoracic vagotomized stomach. Br J Surg 63:581–584
9. Bonavina L, Anselmino M, Ruol A, Borsato N, Peracchia A (1991) Valutazione funzionale del paziente operato di esofagectomia ed esofagogastroplastica intratoracica per cancro dell'esofago. Min Chir 46 [Suppl]:247–251
10. Dei Poli M, Mioli G, Gaspari G, Casalegno PA, Camandona M, Bronda M, Albertino B, Cassolino P (1991) Studio funzionale dei visceri trasposti dopo esofagectomia. Min Chir 46[Suppl]:241–245
11. Pandolfo N, Spigno L, Guiddo G, Tronfi G, Villavecchia G, Mattioli FP (1991) Valutazione funzionale dell'impianto gastrico e digiunale dopo esofagectomia. Min Chir 46 [Suppl]: 253–262.
12. Kjellen G, Svedberg JB, Tibbling L (1984) Solid bolus transit by esophageal scintigraphy in patients with dysphagia and normal manometry and radiography. Dig Dis Sci; 29:1–5

Strip Biopsy for the Diagnosis and Treatment of Superficial Esophageal Carcinoma and Esophageal Dysplasia

CLAUDIO ROLIM TEIXEIRA, KAZUHIKO INOUE, KEN HARUMA, SHINJI TANAKA, TAKEHIRO SHIMAMOTO, MASAHARU YOSHIHARA, KOJI SUMII and GORO KAJIYAMA[1]

Introduction

In order to establish a precise pathological diagnosis and to decide the correct approach for esophageal dysplasia or early esophageal cancer, it is desirable to obtain a full thickness mucosal and submucosal biopsy. Strip biopsy has proven to be effective for the treatment and for the diagnosis of flat or sessile lesions of the gastrointestinal tract [1-3]. In this study, we evaluate the efficacy of strip biopsy for the diagnosis and treatment of polypoid or flat lesions of the esophagus.

Patients and Methods

At upper endoscopy, five patients who presented with localized unstained esophageal lesions after spraying of lugol were referred for strip biopsy (Table 1).

The procedures were performed with the Olympus two-channel 2T 10 fiberscope. As this instrument is equipped with two channels, the insertion of a snare and a grasping forceps can be performed at the same time (Fig. 1). Initially, a needle forceps is used to puncture the mucosa beside the lesion, and 5-10 ml of saline solution is injected into the submucosa under the lesion. The lesion is elevated, along with its peripheral mucosa, and appears as a submucosal tumor. Then the snare device is placed around the elevated tissue held by the grasping forceps, pressed down, and tightened in preparation for resection. Resection is performed using a blended cutting and coagulation current.

[1] The First Department of Internal Medicine, Division of Gastroenterology, Hiroshima University School of Medicine, 1-2-3 Kasumi, Minami-ku, Hiroshima, 734 Japan

Table 1. Patient characteristics

Case	Age	Sex	Endoscopic diagnosis	Reason for endoscopy
1	66	M	Esophageal cancer	Pancreatic cancer
2	81	M	Esophageal cancer	Routine
3	79	M	Esophageal dysplasia	Gastric adenoma Follow-up
4	72	M	Esophageal dysplasia	Routine
5	44	M	Esophageal dysplasia	Routine

Table 2. Clinico-pathological findings

Case	Endoscopic classification	Size of resected tissue (mm)	Depth of resection	Pathology	Residual lesion
1	0-IIa	$12 \times 9 \times 4$ $4 \times 3 \times 2, 4 \times 3 \times 2$	sm	Intraepithelial carcinoma	$(-)$
2	0-I	$10 \times 7 \times 4$	sm	Submucosal carcinoma	$(+)$
3	(0-IIb)	$9 \times 8 \times 3$	sm	Severe dysplasia	$(+)$
4	(0-IIb)	$7 \times 5 \times 3$ $4 \times 4 \times 4, 4 \times 4 \times 2$	sm	Moderate dysplasia	$(+)$
5	(0-IIb)	$7 \times 3 \times 2$	sm	Mild dysplasia	$(-)$

sm, submucosa

Results

Pathology examination of the resected specimens revealed two cases of squamous cell carcinoma (one case with intraepithelial cancer and one case with submucosal cancer), one case of severe dysplasia, one case of moderate dysplasia, and one case of mild dysplasia. Two lesions, intraepithelial cancer and mild dysplasia, were completely resected and follow-up endoscopic biopsies were all negative. The patients showing submucosal cancer and severe and moderate dysplasia, had residual lesion detected at follow-up endoscopic examination. Figure 2 illustrates an esophageal cancer with submucosal invasion at the middle esophagus. Figure 3 shows the picture immediately after the strip biopsy resection. This patient with submucosal cancer was referred for radiation therapy in order to treat eventual lymph node involvement. Laser irradiation was performed in the patient with severe dysplasia and close follow-up examination was indicated in the patient with moderate dysplasia. No acute or late complications such as bleeding or perforation were encountered. Table 2 shows the endoscopic findings and the results of strip biopsy.

Discussion

By using strip biopsy, we were able to resect larger specimens of esophageal mucosa, which resulted in local cure for one case of superficial esophageal

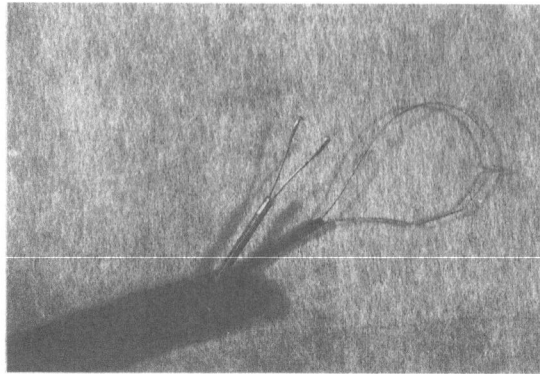

Fig. 1. The two-channel 2T 10 fiberscope

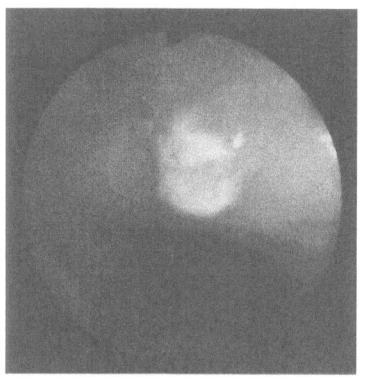
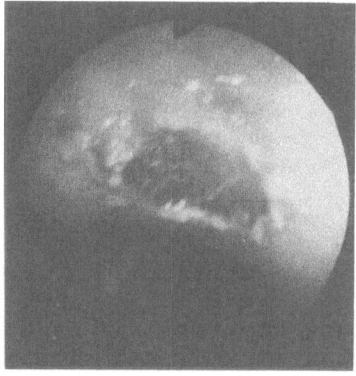

Fig. 2.   Fig. 3

Fig. 2. Esophageal cancer type 0-I, located at the middle esophagus

Fig. 3. The lesion is resected by strip biopsy. Pathology examination revealed submucosal invasion

carcinoma and one case of mild dysplasia. Moreover, a more precise pathologic diagnosis can be performed by examination of a larger specimen. As a result, we were able to diagnose submucosal invasion in one case of esophageal cancer, and the patient was referred for radiation therapy for treatment of lymph node involvement. Also, the therapeutic approach for the patients with dysplasia was influenced by the resection of larger specimens.

Recently, a new modality of esophageal mucosal resection was reported [4] which uses an external transparent tube with a central channel in which the snare is introduced. By using this tube, the need for a two-channel endoscope is eliminated and large specimens can also be resected.

In conclusion, strip biopsy proved to be an effective and a safe method for the treatment and diagnosis of sessile polypoid lesions of the esophagus.

References

1. Karita M, Tada M, Okita K (1992) The successive strip biopsy partial resection technique for large early gastric and colon cancers. Gastrointest Endosc 38:178–180
2. Karita M, Tada M, Okita K, Kodama M (1991) Endoscopic therapy for early colon cancer: The "strip biopsy" resection technique. Gastrointest Endosc 37:128–132
3. Teixeira CR, Haruma K, Teshima H, Yoshihara M, Sumii K, Kajiyama G (1991) Endoscopic therapy for gastric cancer in patients more than 80 years old. Am J Gastroenterol 86:725–728
4. Inoue H, Endo M (1990) Endoscopic esophageal mucosal resection using a transparent tube. Surg Endosc 4:198–201

Treatment of Superficial Esophageal Carcinoma with Reference to X-Ray Findings

Akiyoshi Yamada, Hiroko Ide, Reiki Eguchi, Kazuhiko Hayashi, Kazunari Yoshida, Ataru Kobayashi, and Seiichiro Kobayashi[1]

Introduction

When we treat patients with superficial esophageal carcinoma where the infiltration is limited to the mucosa or the submucosa, there are two approaches that we use. One is the extended resection of the esophagus and the other is resection of the lymph nodes around the neck, from the thoracic cavity, and from the abdominal cavity. A variety of combination therapies are then applied. However, if we expect a curative operation, we perform a minimally invasive operation such as an endoscopic mucosectomy.

A discussion of the treatment of esophageal carcinoma follows based on an analysis of the X-ray findings.

Materials

Up until 1990, 171 cases of superficial carcinoma were seen at our hospital in which no combination therapies were done before operation. These included 124 with early esophageal carcinoma without lymph node metastasis and 47 with lymph node metastasis.

The depth of carcinoma invasion was limited to the epithelium (ep) in 7 patients, the muscularis mucosae (mm) in 33 patients, and the submucosa (sm) in 131 patients (Table 1).

[1] Department of Surgery, Institute of Gastroenterology, Tokyo Women's Medical College, 8-1 Kawada-cho, Shinjuku-ku, Tokyo, 162 Japan

Table 1. Materials

Resected superficial esophageal carcinoma	171 cases[a]
Without lymph node metastasis	124
With lymph node metastasis	47

[a] Excluding preoperative combined therapy cases

Methods of Treatment and Indications

Routine treatments performed on superficial esophageal carcinoma are described below.

Endoscopic Mucosectomy and Laser Irradiation

In terms of accuracy and safety, these techniques are applied to early carcinoma cases without lymph node metastasis whose invasion is confined to the mucosa or the muscularis mucosae with a diameter of less than 2.0 cm.

Blunt Dissection

Blunt dissection can be utilized even if the carcinoma reaches the submucosal layer or if the lesions are multiple or spread over a wide area. However, blunt dissection is not applied in cases with lymph node metastasis.

Resection of the Esophagus

Esophageal resection with thoracoabdominal incision for carcinoma is generally accepted at the present time.

Due to widespread controversy, the technique and region of lymph node dissection remains unsettled.

In recent years, some doctors have recommended an extended operation in which the lymph nodes in the neck and around the bronchus as well as in the abdomen be removed. Such an invasive surgical procedure cannot be carried out in all cases.

Therefore, we must keep the depth of operation to a minimum.

Radiologic Classification of Superficial Esophageal Carcinoma

X-ray findings are defined in the guidelines of the Japanese Society for Eso-phageal Carcinoma [1], as follows:

0-I: Superficial and protruding type (Figs. 1, 2)
0-II: Superficial and flat type
  0-IIa: Slightly elevated type (Fig. 3)
  0-IIb: Flat type (Fig. 4)
  0-IIc: Slightly depressed type (Fig. 5)
0-III: Superficial and distinctly depressed type (Figs. 6, 7)

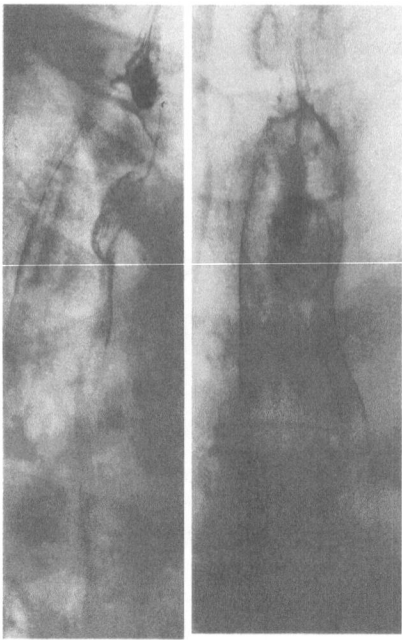

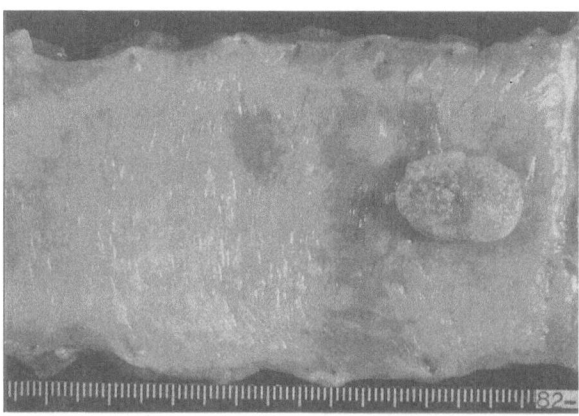

Fig. 1. 0-Iα type. A protruding lesion 2.2 cm in diameter having a well-definded border was presented in the upper thoracic esophagus. The surface is smooth although having a very fine and granular surface. This is a case of well-differentiated squamous cell carcinoma [sm, n(−), ly(−), v(−)]. Postoperative survival was 10 years. *n*, lymph node metastasis; *ly*, lymphatic invasion; *v*, vascular invasion; *sm*, submucosa

The postoperative survival curve is shown in Fig. 8. The prognosis of 0-II type is good. Only one patient with lymph node metastasis in which vessel invasion was seen, died from recurrent lymph node metastasis to the neck and the upper mediastinum (7 years postoperatively).

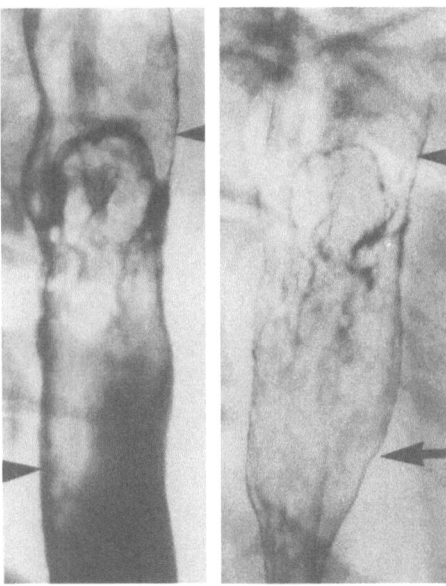

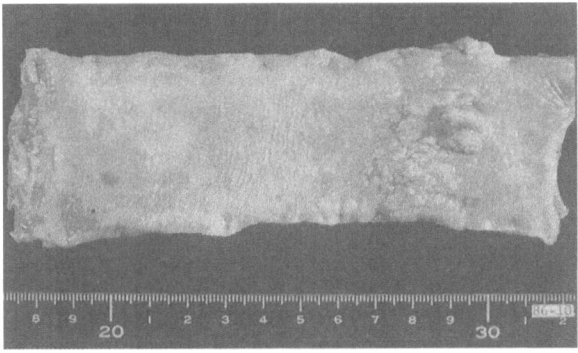

Fig. 2. 0-Iβ type. A centrally-depressed lesion 3.0 cm in diameter was present in the upper thoracic esophagus. The surface showed a nodular appearance. The analside border was undefined, with extensive erosive foci. This is a case of moderately-differentiated squamous cell carcinoma [sm, n(−), ly(−), v(−)]. Postoperative survival was 5.5 years [relapse (+)]. This patient is now receiving chemotherapy

The prognosis of 0-I as well as 0-III is very poor. So, 0-I and 0-III are each subdivided into two groups:

0-Iα: Elevation is well-defined and its surface is smooth (Fig. 1);
0-Iβ: Both contours and surface are lobulated (Fig. 2);
0-IIIα: The surrounding fold of the depressed lesion is clearly demarcated and its outline is regularly delineated (Fig. 6);
0-IIIβ: The surrounding fold is ill-defined and its outline is irregular (Fig. 7).

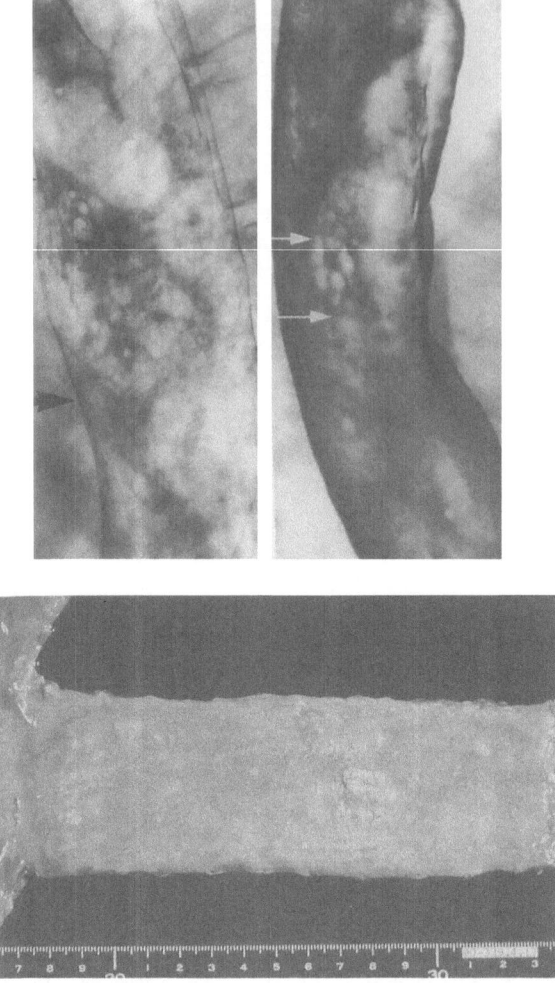

Fig. 3. 0-IIa type. An elevated lesion formed by rosette-like aggregation in nodules (1.0 cm) was found in the middle thoracic esophagus. Around this lesion, there were extensive flat foci. Moderately-differentiated squamous cell carcinoma [mm, n(−), ly(−), v(−)]. Postoperative survival was 2.5 years [relapse (−)]

The survival of 0-I type, utilizing this classification, is shown in Fig. 9. Among 0-Iα type cases, only one case died of recurrence (54 months postoperatively). In this case, blood vessel invasion was seen, but neither lymphatic vessel invasion nor lymph node metastasis was detected. Histology revealed pseudosarcoma.

The prognosis of 0-Iβ type is poor, having a 5-year survival rate of 50%.

Of the 0-III type cases (Fig. 10), no recurrence was experienced in 0-IIIα cases. Unfortunately, the 5-year survival rate of 0-III type cases is only 35%, indicating a dismal prognosis.

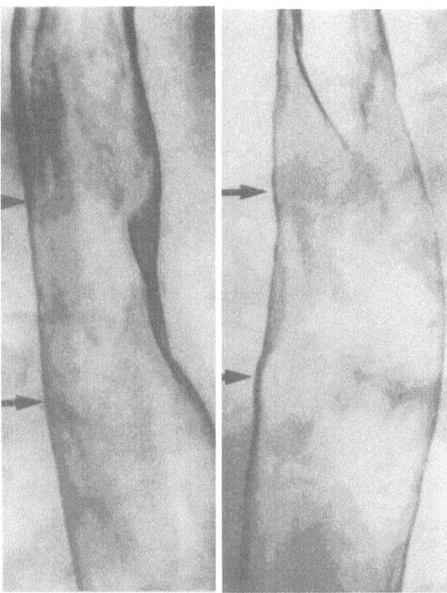

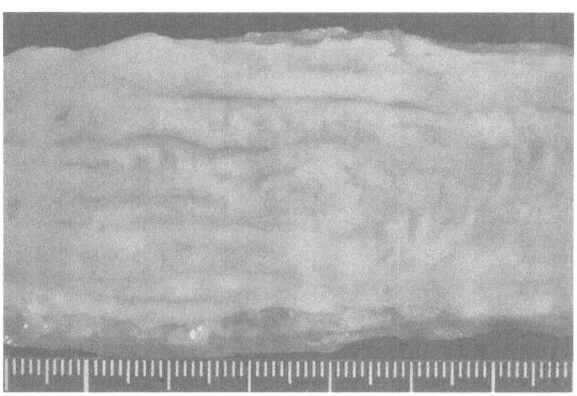

Fig. 4. 0-IIb type. An abnormal barium pattern with undefined border (3.0 cm in diameter) was found in the middle thoracic esophagus. Moderately-differentiated squamous cell carcinoma [ep, n(−), ly(−), v(−)]. Postoperative survival was 5.5 years [relapse(−)]

X-Ray Type and Depth of Invasion

The relationship between x-ray type and depth of carcinoma invasion is shown in Table 2. Almost all cases of intraepithelial carcinoma belong to 0-IIb. Most cases of 0-II type remain in the muscularis mucosae, but in some cases carcinoma penetrates into the submucosal layer. In some of these cases, a small part of the lesion invades deep into the submucosal layer, and in the remaining cases, there is only shallow invasion.

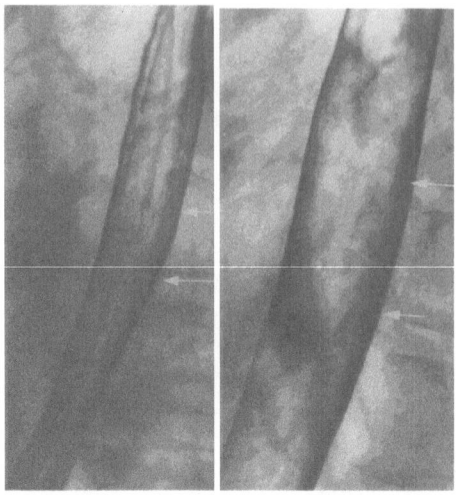

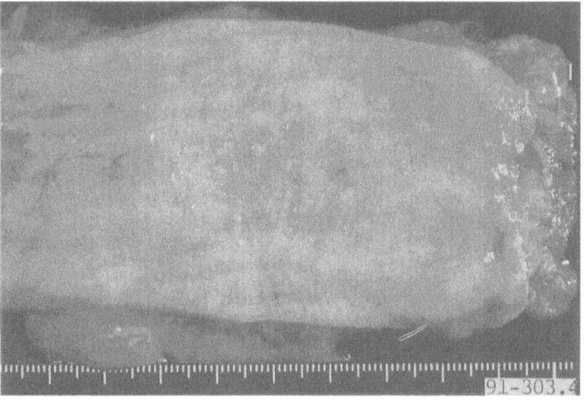

Fig. 5. 0-IIc type. An area of rough membrane (1.0 cm in diameter) was seen in the middle thoracic esophagus. A slightly depressed lesion was found in the central part of this lesion [mm (partly ep), n(−), ly(−), v(−)]. Moderately-differentiated squamous cell carcinoma. Post-operative survival was 2.5 years [relapse (−)]

Generally speaking, carcinoma of 0-I and 0-III types reaches the submucosal layer, but there is no clear relation between 0-Iα and 0-Iβ nor between 0-IIIα and 0-IIIβ as far as the prognosis is concerned.

X-Ray Type, Lymph Node Metastasis, and Vessel Invasion

The relationship of x-ray type to lymph node metastasis and vessel invasion is demonstrated in Table 3. All cases of 0-II type cases, except two, are early carcinoma with a low frequency of vessel invasion.

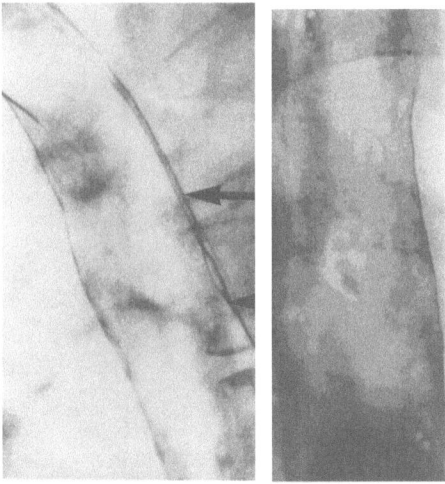

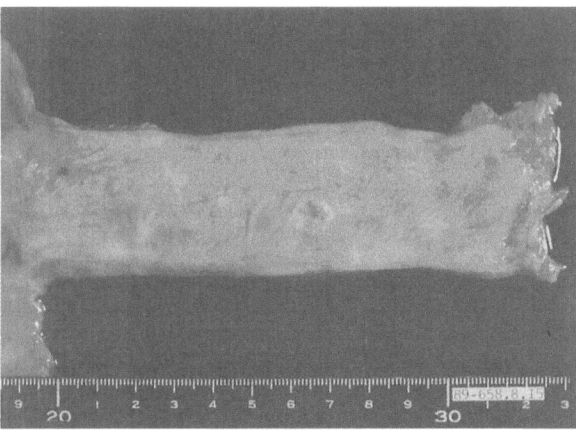

Fig. 6. 0-IIIα type. A depressed lesion with a smooth and well-defined border (1.5 cm in diameter) was present in the middle thoracic esophagus. Moderately-differentiated squamous cell carcinoma [sm, n(−), ly(−), v(−)]. Postoperative survival was 8 years [relapse (−)]

Likewise, all the cases of 0-Iα and 0-IIIα, with one exception, are early carcinoma. The one really exceptional case of 0-IIIα with lymph node metastasis is still alive and doing well. No signs of recurrence can be found even 10 years after the operation.

In 46% of 0-Iβ type and in 75% of 0-IIIβ type, carcinoma metastasizes to the lymph nodes at a high rate. Vessel invasion is noted in more than 80% of 0-Iβ and 0-IIIβ. This explains the poor recovery. Roughly 90% of 0-IIIβ types have vessel invasion. Five cases of early carcinoma of these types died due to recurrence of carcinoma. Thus, beta types show a strong tendency towards recurrence.

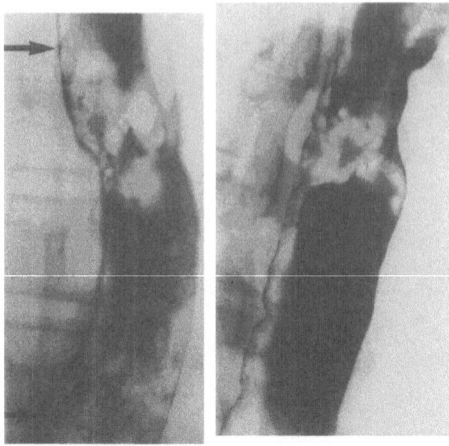

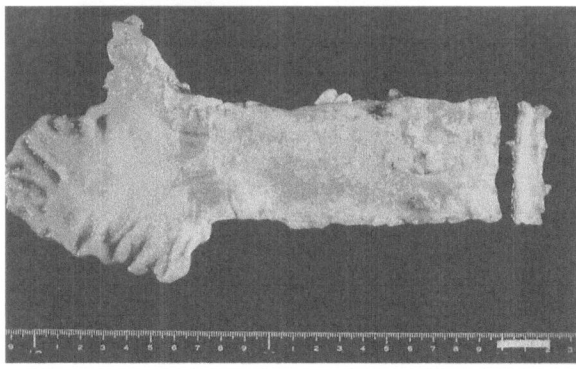

Fig. 7. 0-IIIβ type. A depressed lesion with irregular embankment and undefined border (2.0 cm in diameter) was found in the middle thoracic esophagus. There was extensive superficially sprending lesion on the anal side. Poorly-differentiated squamous cell carcinoma [sm, n2(+), ly(+), v(−)]. Postoperative survival was 8 months

Result

0-II Type

In most cases, carcinoma invades the epithelium or the muscularis mucosae. Usually, lymph node metastasis is not seen. Yet, when the surface is irregular, lymph node metastasis is sometimes found.

0-I Type

Carcinoma invasion is limited within the submucosal layer.

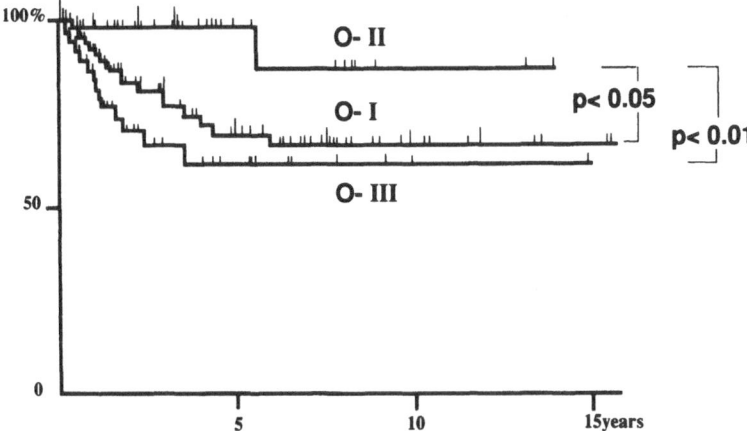

Fig. 8. Survival rates (Kaplan-Meier) in relation to x-ray types. The postoperative outcome was generally good in 0-IIα type, except for one patient with an early cancer with lymphatic invasion who died from recurrence 7 years after the operation. 0-I and 0-III types showed no significant difference in the survival curve

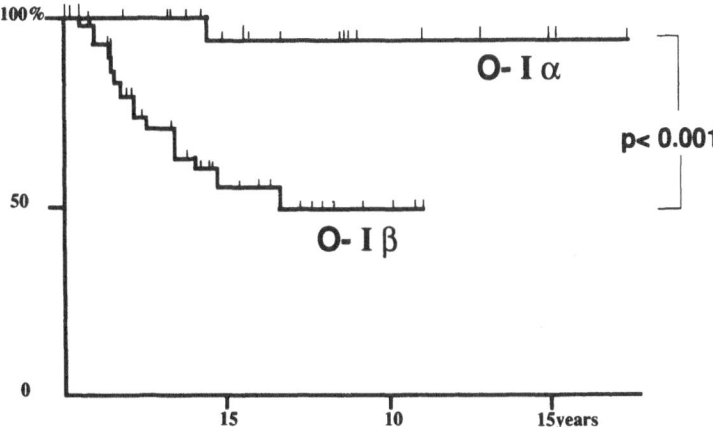

Fig. 9. Survival rates (Kaplan-Meier) in relation to x-ray type 0-I type. Only one case of death was included in 0-Iα type. In 0-Iβ type, 12 patients survived more than 5 years. However, 5 patients with early cancer relapsed and died within 5 years

0-Iα

All cases are early carcinoma without lymph node metastasis. So far, only one case died (54 months postoperatively).

0-Iβ

Lymph node metastasis and vessel invasion are detected at a high rate. The 5-year survival rate is 50%.

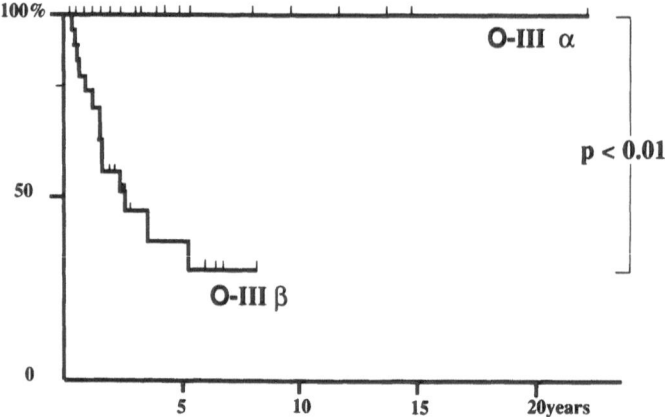

Fig. 10. Survival rates (Kaplan-meier) in relation to x-ray type 0-III. In 0-IIIα type, no patients died from relapse. In 0-IIIβ type, only 35% of these patients are still alive 5 or more years after operation. Two of the seven patients with early cancer had relapse. All patients surviving longer than 5 years were treated with postoperative chemotherapy

0-III Type

Carcinoma invades as far as the submucosal layer.

0-IIIα

All cases were early carcinoma except for one. There is no recurrence in any of these cases, and the prognosis is quite good.

0-IIIβ

Lymph node metastasis and vessel invasion are frequent. The 5-year survival rate is less than 30%. Prognosis is not always good even in early carcinoma.

Conclusion

At present there are a wide range of views regarding the method of treatment of superficial esophageal carcinoma. Therefore, we have to choose the least aggressive operation possible taking curability into consideration. To do this, we must visualize the lesion accurately before operating, utilizing diagnostic imaging.

X-ray and endoscopic examinations are ineffective when a tiny part of the lesion infiltrates deep into the esophagus. In such cases, endoscopic ultrasonography (EUS) and computed tomography (CT) are effective. We must always be alert to latent lymph node metastasis.

Before we decide the method of treatment, we have to take into account lymph node metastasis and vessel invasion, particularly in 0-Iβ and 0-IIIβ type cases.

Table 2. Correlation of x-ray type to depth of invasion

	No. of cases	Intraepithelium	Muscularis mucosa	Submucosa
0-Iα	24	0	3 (12%)	21 (88%)
0-Iβ	50	0	1 (2%)	49 (98%)
0-IIa	9	2 (22%)	5 (56%)	2 (22%)
0-IIb	9	5 (56%)	2 (22%)	2 (22%)
0-IIc	30	0	21 (70%)	9 (30%)
0-IIIα	21	0	0	21 (100%)
0-IIIβ	28	0	1 (4%)	27 (94%)

Table 3. Correlation of x-ray type to lymph node metastasis and vascular invasion

	No. of cases	Lymph node metastasis	Lymphatic invasion	Blood vessel invasion
0-Iα	24	0	5 (21%)	2 (8%)
0-Iβ	50	23 (46%)	40 (80%)	21 (42%)
0-IIa	9	0	0	0
0-IIb	9	0	1 (11%)	0
0-IIc	30	2 (7%)	8 (27%)	0
0-IIIα	21	1 (5%)	8 (38%)	3 (14%)
0-IIIβ	28	21 (75%)	20 (86%)	8 (29%)

Treatment and X-Ray Findings

0-II Type

Endoscopic mucosal excision and laser irradiation as well as operation can be indicated. When mucosal excision is adopted, an accurate diagnosis of the depth of invasion should be made before operating, utilizing EUS and CT.

0-Iα and 0-IIIα Types

Since most cases are early carcinoma, blunt dissection and radiation therapy can be performed.

0-Iβ and 0-IIIβ Types

In these types, lymph node metastasis and vessel invasion are often seen. When they occur, both resection of the esophagus with lymph node dissection and combination therapy are necessary. When the surface of the lesion is markedly irregular, extensive lymph node dissection as well as the strongest and most effective chemotherapy are mandatory.

References

1. Japanese Society for Esophageal Diseases (1992) Guidelines for the clinical and pathologic studies on carcinoma of the esophagus, 8th edn (in Japanese). Kanehara, Tokyo

The Effectiveness of Ultrasonography in Diagnosis of Cervical Lymph Node Metastasis in Preoperative Esophageal Cancer

SHIGENOBU ASAKURA, KIN-ICHI NABEYA, TATEO HANAOKA,
TETSUYA NYUMURA, YOSHITAKA NAKATA, CHOO KAKU, OSAMU KIMURA,
NOBORU SUZUKI, SHOJIROU KOIDO, MASARU ASAMI, and TAKEYUKI ASAKURA[1]

Introduction

In determining treatment procedures, it is most important to diagnose cervical lymph node metastasis of esophageal cancer preoperatively. Heretofore, the conventional criteria for ultrasonography (US) in metastatic lymph nodes, as designated in the *Guidelines for the Clinical and Pathologic Studies on Carcinoma of the Esophagus* [1] were: (1) Well defined margins, (2) irregular inner echo images, and (3) longitudinal diameter over 5 mm. Lymph nodes satisfying all three criteria were diagnosed as metastatic. Investigations were made along these lines and it was found that sensitivity was 58.3%; specificity, 97.0%; accuracy, 80.7%; false positive, 17.5%; and false negative, 1.8%. In other words, with the current diagnostic criteria, anticipated delineation ratios could not be obtained. Therefore, keeping in mind the results of occupancy ratios of cancerous lesions within metastatic lymph nodes, new criteria that would be minimally influenced by the examination apparatus or by the examinee's subjective point of view was established: (1) Ratio of longitudinal diameter to short axis over 0.5, and (2) lymph node longitudinal diameter over 0.5 cm. Lymph nodes satisfying these two criteria were considered to be metastatic. Investigations were made along these lines and it was found that sensitivity was 71.4%; specificity, 100%; accuracy, 87.7%; false positive, 10.5%; and false negative 0%. A satisfying delineation ratio was obtained.

Materials and Methods

This study was conducted on 101 patients with esophageal cancer seen in our department between July 1988 and December 1991, following preoperative cervical US. There were 86 males ranging in age between 43 and 85 years

---

[1] Second Department of Surgery, Kyorin University School of Medicine, 6-20-2, Shinkawa, Mitaka, Tokyo, 181 Japan

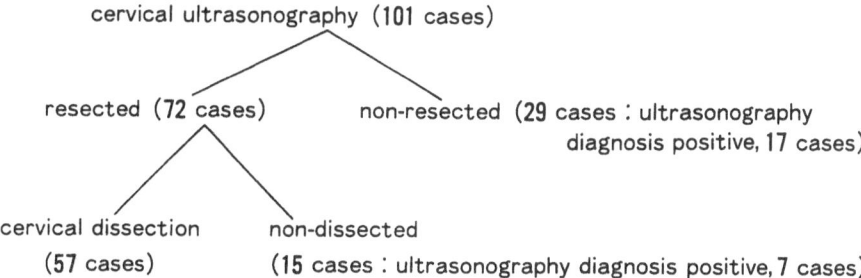

Fig. 1. Cases of cervical ultrasonography performed in preoperative esophageal cancer (July 1988 to December, 1991)

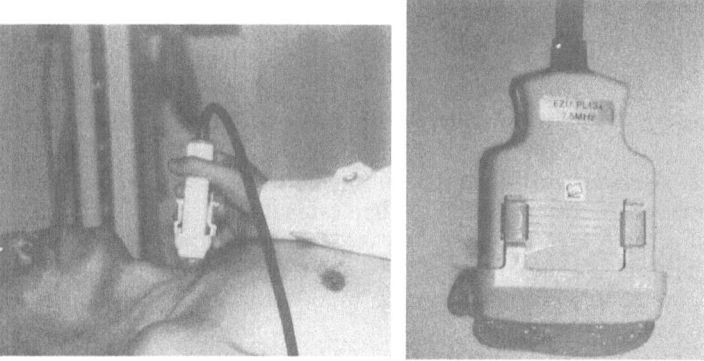

Fig. 2. Tests were made by attaching a small bag directly to the tip of the probe on Hitachi EUB 310. probe: 7.5 MHZ linear type EZU-PL 13A

(mean, 62.19 years) and 15 females ranging in age between 49 and 81 years (mean, 67.93 years). The mean age of the patients in the whole series was 64.03 years. Among the 101 patients examined by US, resection was performed in 72. Among these 72 patients, cervical lymph nodes were removed in 57. In 17 of the 29 patients who did not have a resection, and in 7 of 15 patients in whom cervical lymphadenectomy was not performed, a diagnosis of lymph node metastasis was made preoperatively by US. In these 24 patients, resection was not performed because of poor general condition or local conditions. In view of the difficulty of curative resection, a cervical lymphadenectomy was not attempted (Fig. 1).

An ultrasonic probe was used. The patient was placed supine with a pillow under the neck to maintain mild extension. Acoustic couplant gel was applied to the skin of the neck and probe was placed directly on the skin (Fig. 2). A frontal cross-section of the neck and a right and left lateral cross and longitudinal section were obtained. Lymph node nomenclature followed the guidelines for handling esophageal cancer [1]. Using conventional US diagnostic criteria for metastatic lymph nodes, (Fig. 3), the rate of cervical lymph node metastasis was evaluated.

S. Asakura et al.

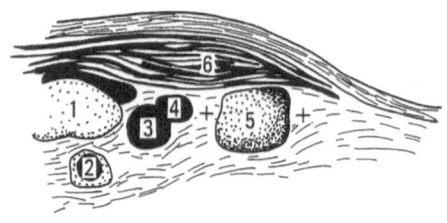 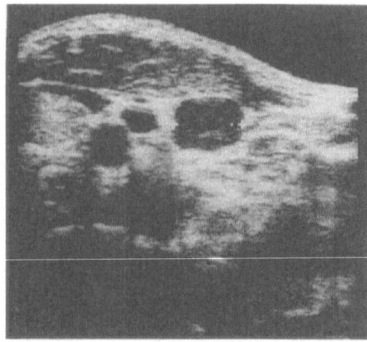

1. Thyroid gland   2. Esophagus
3. Carotid artery   4. Jugular vein
5. Lt No.104 Lymph node   6. Muscle

Fig. 3. A 60-year-old male. Im esophageal cancer ultrasonographic observations of left cervical area. Lymph nodes are indicated by a *plus*. *Im*, middle intra-thoracic esophagus

Secondly, the area of the lymph node occupied by metastatic tissue was measured in cross-sectional specimens. The ratio between the shortest and longest diameter in the lymph node (short-long diameter ratio) and the long diameter of the lymph node was then evaluated.

The relative area occupied by cancer tissue in the removed lymph node was measured on a photograph of the largest cross-section in a moderate enlargement by using a two-dimensional automatic image-analyzing system (Nikon Cosmozone 1S).

In 32 lymph nodes obtained from 14 patients in whom lymph node metastasis were correctly diagnosed by cervical US and in 1 patient in whom a false negative result was obtained, the correlation between the cross-sectional area occupied by cancer tissue the short-long diameter ratio, and the longitudinal diameter of the lymph node was evaluated.

Statistical significance between the two groups was assessed by Student's t-test, or Welch's test. The rate of occurrence was assessed by the χ^2 test (Yates).

Results

Rate of Cervical Lymph Node Metastasis

Ultrasonographic examination of the neck was performed prior to surgery for esophageal cancer in 101 patients, and 29 patients without resection and 15 patients without lymphadenectomy were excluded. The results showed that

Table 1. Preoperative cervical ultrasonography performed in 72 out of 101 cases of esophageal cancer (July 1988 to December 1991)

Cervical region dissected cases	57 cases
Metastatic cervical lymph node cases	15 cases
Metastatic cervical lymph node ratio	26.3%

15/57 patients (26.3%) in whom a cervical lymphadenectomy was performed had lymph node metastasis (Table 1).

Ultrasonographic Examination

In the 57 patients who underwent cervical lymphadenectomy, metastasis was found histologically in 14 out of 24 patients with preoperative ultrasonographic diagnosis of metastasis, a sensitivity of 58.3%.

Table 2. Results of ultrasonography diagnosis in 57 cases of cervical lymph node dissection using conventional criteria

Ultrasonography diagnosis	Histological diagnosis	Lymph node extracted cases	
		Metastasis(+)	Metastasis(−)
Metastasis(+)		14	10
Metastasis(−)		1	32
Total		15	42
Sensitivity			58.3%
Specificity			97.0%
Accuracy			80.7%
False positive			17.5%
False negative			1.8%

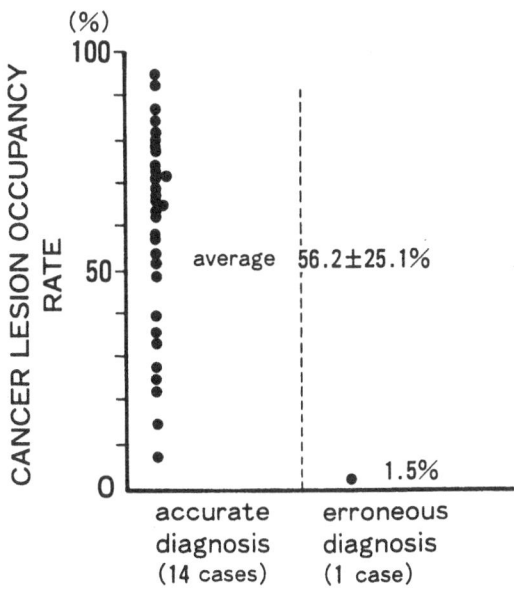

Fig. 4. Cancer lesion occupancy rate in 32 lesions of metastatic lymph nodes

Histological diagnosis was negative in 10 of these 24 patients, a false positive rate of 17.5%. In 32/33 patients with no evidence of metastasis by US, their histological diagnosis was also negative (a specificity of 97%). In one of these patients, histological examination revealed metastasis, and the false negative rate was 1.8%. The accuracy was 80.7% (Table 2).

Cancer Lesion Occupancy Rate in Metastatic Lymph Nodes

In 32 lymph nodes with metastasis, the area occupied by cancer lesion was evaluated. In 14 patients with correct preoperative diagnosis of metastatic lymphadenopathy, the cancer lesion occupancy rate ranged from 6.8%–93.1% with a mean of 56.2% ± 25.1%. In the one patient with a false negative diagnosis, the cancer lesion occupancy rate was 1.5% (Fig. 4).

The Ratio Between the Short and Longitudinal Diameters of Lymph Nodes With and Without Metastasis

The short to longitudinal diameter ratio was 0.74 ± 0.16 in 31 lymph nodes with metastasis in 15 patients. It was less than 0.5 in 5 nodes and more than 0.5 in 27. In these 15 patients, the short to longitudinal diameter ratio was 0.38 ± 0.13 in 76 nodes without metastasis from these 15 patients. ($P < 0.001$) (Fig. 5).

The Cancer Lesion Occupancy Rate and the Short to Longitudinal Diameter Ratio

The relationship between the cancer lesion occupancy rate and the short to longitudinal diameter ratio of the lymph nodes was studied. In 25 of 27 nodes

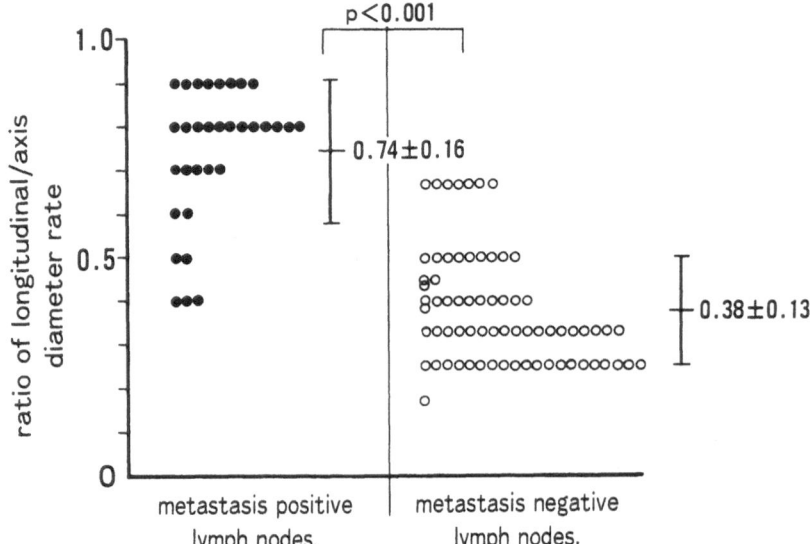

Fig. 5. Comparison of longitudinal/axis diameter of positive and negative cervical lymph nodes in 15 dissected cases

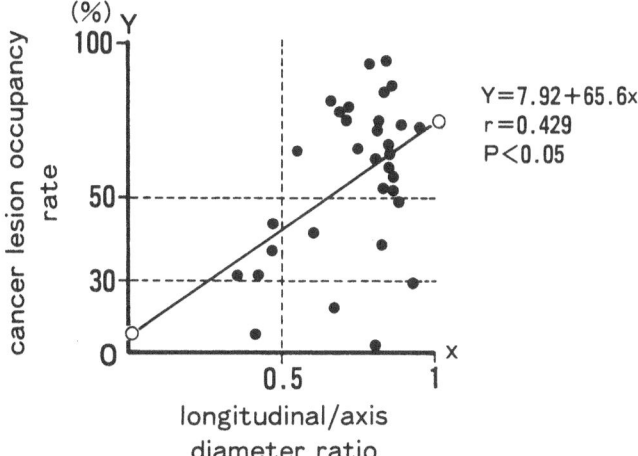

Fig. 6. Correlation of cancer lesion occupancy rate with longitudinal/axis diameter rate in 32 metastatic lymph nodes

with a short to longitudinal diameter ratio higher than 0.5, the cancer lesion occupancy rate was more than 30%. In all 22 nodes with a cancer lesion occupancy rate of more than 50%, the short to longitudinal ratio was higher than 0.5 (Fig. 6).

Comparison of Lymph Node Metastasis and Longitudinal Diameter

In 15 patients who underwent cervical lymphadenectomy, the longitudinal diameter was compared between lymph nodes with and without metastasis. The longitudinal diameter of 32 nodes with metastasis was 0.98 ± 0.32 cm, whereas that of 76 nodes without metastasis was 0.38 ± 0.15 cm ($P < 0.001$). All nodes with metastasis had diameters larger than 0.5 cm, but diameters between 0.5 and 0.9 cm were also seen in lymph nodes without metastasis (Fig. 7).

Correlation of Lymph Node Longitudinal Diameter with Cancer Lesion Occupancy Rate of Positive Lymph Node Metastasis

In 32 lymph nodes with metastasis, the cancer lesion occupancy rate was less than 30% in 5 of the 20 nodes with a longitudinal diameter between 0.5 and 1.0 cm, while it was more than 30% in the remaining 15 nodes. Among the 12 nodes with a longitudinal diameter greater than 1.0 cm, only 1 had a tumor volume less than 30%. However, one node had a cancer lesion occupancy rate of 70% with a longitudinal diameter of only 0.5 cm, and another had a longitudinal diameter larger than 1.5 cm and a cancer lesion occupancy rate of 20% (Fig. 8).

New Diagnostic Criteria

Based on the results of cancer lesion occupancy rate measurement, two factors were employed as the diagnostic criteria for evaluation of ultrasonographic

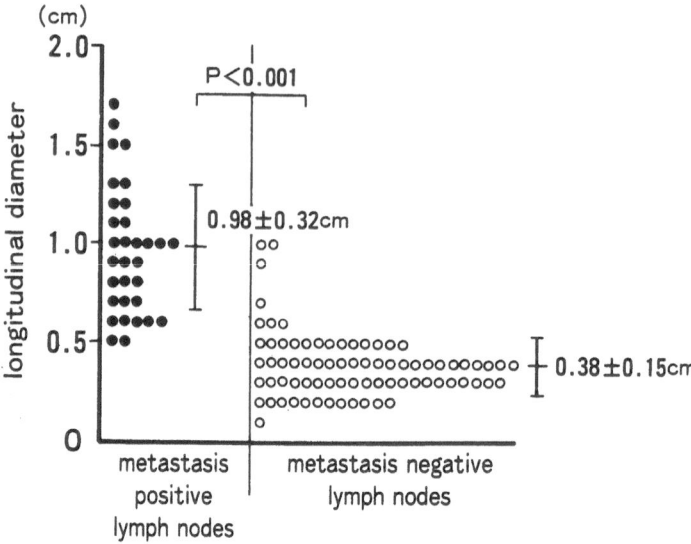

Fig. 7. Comparisons of longitudinal/axis diameter in 15 cases with metastatie cervical lymph nodes

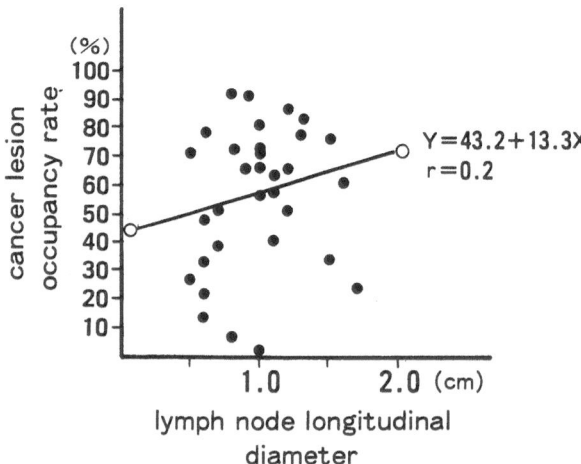

Fig. 8. Correlation of lymph node longitudinal diameter with cancer lesion occupancy rate in 32 metastatic lymph nodes

findings of the neck in 57 patients with esophageal cancer in which cervical lymphadenectomy was planned: (1) The ratio of longitudinal diameter to short axis over 0.5, and (2) lymph node longitudinal diameter over 0.5 cm. As a result, sensitivity was 71.4% (50.3% with conventional criteria), specificity was 100% (97.0%), accuracy was 87.7% (80.7%), false positive rate was 10.5% (17.5%),

Table 3. Results of ultrasonography diagnosis in 57 cases of cervical region lymph node dissection using modified criteria

Ultrasonography diagnosis	Histological diagnosis	Lymph node extracted cases	
		Metastasis(+)	Metastasis(−)
Metastasis(+)		15	6
Metastasis(−)		0	36
Total		15	42
Sensitivity			71.4%
Specificity			100.0%
Accuracy			87.7%
False positive			10.5%
False negative			0%

and the false negative rate was 0% (1.8%), indicating improvement in diagnostic capability (Table 3).

Discussion

In patients with esophageal cancer, lymph node metastasis readily occur not only in the mediastinum, but also in the neck and abdomen. For this reason, an extensive lymphadenectomy is required. In overzealous efforts for radical dissection, the recurrent nerve is often injured, leading to postoperative hoarseness and aspiration pneumonia, leading to serious complications in terms of the quality of life of the patients. For this reason, adequate removal according to the type and stage of cancer based on an accurate preoperative measurement of the lymph node metastasis is mandatory [3, 4]. One preoperative test for esophageal cancer used by us since July 1988 is preoperative US of the neck.

Since most of the cervical lymph nodes of interest are located within 3 cm of the body surface, a 7.5 MHz probe was used [5, 6]. In the initial technique, a water bath method was employed (the probe moving automatically within the waterbath), requiring marked extension of the neck, with no adjustment of apparatus position possible. Using a waterbag attachment, an attempt was made to place the bag in tight contact with the skin of the patient. This made possible fine manipulations and gave the patient more freedom of body positioning. Basically the patient must lie in a supine position and turn the neck to the right or left when necessary.

Between July 1988 and December 1991, we performed surgery for esophageal cancer with cervical lymphadenectomy in 57 patients. In 15 of these patients, cervical lymph node metastasis was positive, with a rate of metastasis of 26.3%. According to Tanabe et al. [7] and Muto et al. [8], the rate of lymph node metastasis by site was 27.2%–60% at upper intrathoracic (Iu), esophagus, 20%–22.4% at middle intrathoracic (Im), and 12.5%–23.3% at lower intrathoracic (Ei), esophagus, with higher rates tending to occur at higher sites.

Diagnosis of lymph node metastasis by cervical US has been evaluated by the diagnostic criteria of Yoshinaka et al. [9] based mainly on two elements (border echo and internal echo), by the size of lymph nodes as suggested by Ide et al. [10], Natio et al. [11], and Udagawa et al. [12], and by the short and longitudinal diameter ratio according to Tohnosu et al. [13]. At present, improved ultrasonographic apparatus has made satisfactory qualitative diagnosis of lymph nodes possible, and the available diagnostic criteria have been evaluated in detail [14]. In a clinical setting, however, it is frequently difficult to diagnose lymph node metastasis. While it is possible to diagnose metastasis based on the examiners subjective diagnostic criteria, objective figures would be more helpful. While a normal lymph node is depicted as a somewhat flattened, hypoechoic structure in the echogram [15, 16], differentiation between inflammatory and metastatic lymph nodes may be problematic. Udagawa et al. [12] and Inoue et al. [17] discussed the high probability of metastasis in the presence of notching with outward-directed convexity, in addition to the three conventional criteria for metastasis: border, internal echo, and size. The presence of an irregular granular echo within a hypoechoic area in the internal echo also suggests metastasis. However, each of these criteria is based on the subjective judgement of the examiner. In the present study, attempts were made to diagnose based on objective measured values.

We first adopted the conventional diagnostic criteria for lymph node metastasis. The high specificity and low false negative rate indicate a high degree of safety of the test. Because of the low sensitivity, the diagnostic criteria were reexamined.

The border and internal echo is readily influenced by the type of apparatus, the TV image, film, and video, and a reproducible examination under the same conditions is difficult. The two elements not readily influenced by the subjective judgment of the examiner were the short and longitudinal diameter ratio of lymph node and longitudinal diameter of the lymph node. In addition to these factors, the result of mechanical measurement of the cross-sectional area was used to determine the cancer lesion occupancy rate within the lymph node to create a new set of criteria.

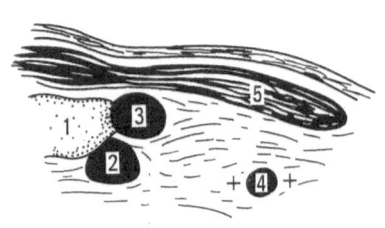
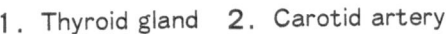
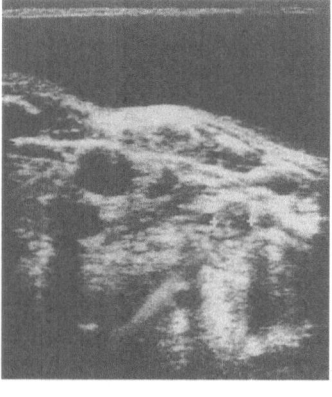

1. Thyroid gland   2. Carotid artery
3. Jugular vein   4. Lt No.104 Lymph node
5. Muscle.

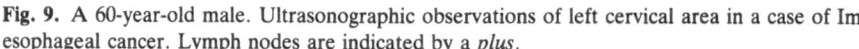

Fig. 9. A 60-year-old male. Ultrasonographic observations of left cervical area in a case of Im esophageal cancer. Lymph nodes are indicated by a *plus*.

The short to longitudinal diameter ratio in 32 removed metastatic lymph nodes was less than 0.5 in 5, and more than 0.5 in 27, with the mean of 0.74 ± 0.16. In the nodes with a short to longitudinal diameter ratio greater than 0.5, the area occupied by the cancer lesion was usually more than 30%. When more than 50% of the node was occupied by cancer, the ratio was always more than 0.5. As the area occupied by cancer increased, the short to longitudinal diameter ratio approached 1.0, creating a spheroid shape ($r = 0.429$ $P < 0.05$). In 76 lymph nodes without metastasis, the short to longitudinal diameter ratio was 0.38 ± 0.13. In 20 lymph nodes with a longitudinal diameter between 0.5 and

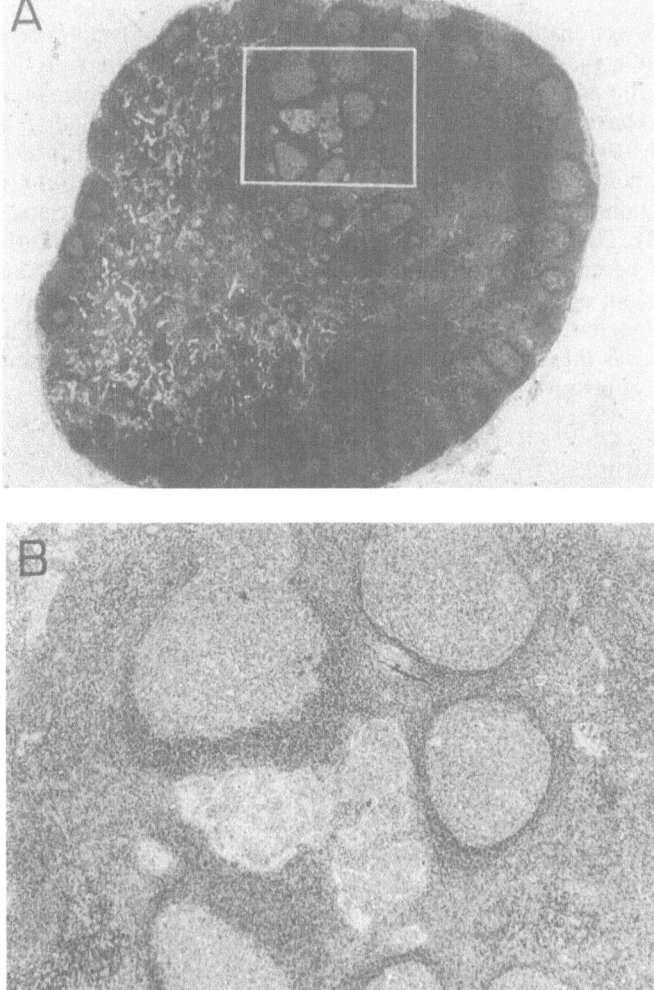

Fig. 10A,B. Left No. 104 extracted lymph node specimen. **A** Pathological examination of a false negative lymph node reveals micrometastasis in the medullary sinus (*open square*) and marginal sinus. **B** High magnification of the metastatic cancer lesion in medullary sinus

1.0 cm, metastatic disease occupied less than 30% of the cross-sectional area in 5, and more than 30% in 15. In 12 lymph nodes with diameters larger than 1.0 cm, the area occupied by cancer was less than 30% in only 1, and more than 30% in 11. As the longitudinal diameter increased, the area occupied by the tumor also increased. In one node, however, 70% of the cross-sectional area was occupied by cancer, although the longitudinal diameter was only 0.5 cm, whereas only 20% of the area was cancerous in one node with a longitudinal diameter more than 1.5 cm. In 76 removed lymph nodes without metastasis, the longitudinal diameter was 0.38 ± 0.15. Diagnosis of metastasis was more probable when the longitudinal diameter of the lymph node was more than 0.5 cm.

A cross-sectional ultrasonogram (Fig. 9) revealed one lymph node measuring 8 × 6 mm in the No104 area lateral to the left jugular vein with homogeneous internal echo and indistinct border. A diagnosis of negative metastasis was made using the conventional criteria. The fixed section of a lymph node removed from the left No104 area demonstrates a metastatic cancer lesion in the medullary sinus and marginal sinus under low power magnification (Fig. 10A). High power magnification of the metastatic cancer lesion in the medullary sinus is shown in (Fig. 10B). The homogeneous internal echo and the indistinct border probably appeared because only 1.5% of the cross-sectional area was occupied by the cancer lesion, and most of it was located in the medullary sinus. However, the short to longitudinal diameter ratio in this case was 0.75 and the longitudinal diameter was 0.8 cm. If our modified diagnostic criteria were used, a correct diagnosis of positive metastasis would be obtained.

Conclusion

The utility of ultrasonographic examination of the cervical lymph nodes prior to surgery for esophageal cancer was evaluated and compared to a new set of diagnostic criteria. By measuring the cancer lesion occupancy rate in the removed lymph nodes, a new criteria for the diagnosis of metastasis was suggested based on objective factors such as the size and shape of the nodes, rather than the subjective assessment of node quality.

A ratio of longitudinal diameter to short axis over 0.5 and a longitudinal diameter of the node larger than 0.5 cm were used as diagnostic criteria. After reevaluation of the diagnostic criteria based on these two elements, all parameters of ultrasonographic diagnosis were improved.

References

1. Japanese Society for Esophageal Diseases (1989) Guidelines for the Clinical and Pathologic Studies on Carcinoma of the Esophagus (in Japanese). Kanehara, Tokyo
3. Isono K, Onoda S, Okuyama K, Tohnosu N (1986) The significance of cervical lymph node dissection in radical operation of esophageal cancer (in Japanese) Geka Shinryo 28:529–535
4. Endo T, Ide H, Hanashi T, Murata Y, Muroi M, Saitou A, Akimoto S, Hanyuu H (1990) Use of the cervical ultrasonographic study for patients of the esophageal cancer after esophagectomy (in Japanese). Jpn J Med Ultrasonics Proceedings of the 56th Meeting, pp 463–464

5. Baatenburg de Jong RJ, Rongen RJ, Laméris JS, Harthoorn M, Verwoerd CDA, Knegt P (1989) Metastatic neck disease palpation vs ultrasound examination. Arch Otolaryngol Head Neck Surg 115:689–690

6. Hajek PC, Salomonowitz E, Turk R, Tscholakoff D, Kumpan W, Czembirek H (1986) Lymph nodes of the neck: Evaluation with US. Radiology 158:739–742

7. Tanabe G, Yoshinaka H, Baba M, Kuroshima K, Mure H, Morifuji H, Kiire A, Natsugoe S, Kawasaki Y, Suenaga H, Fukumoto T, Yotsumoto K, Matsuno M, Suenaga T, Kajisa T (1986) Cervical Lymph node Metastases in 33 Patients with Thoracic Esophageal Cancer After Modified Bilateral Neck Dissection (in Japanese). Jpn J Gastroenterol Surg 19:624–629

8. Muto T, Sasaki K, Tanaka O, Miyashita K, Katayanagi N, Hasegawa M (1988) Lymph node metastasis of thoacic esophageal cancer in the cervical region (in Japanese) Gastroenterol Surg 11:1443–1449

9. Yoshinaka H, Kajisa T, Kuroshima K, Morifuji H, Tanabe G, Baba M, Nishi M (1985) Detection of cervical lymph node metastases in esophageal cancer by ultrasound: Non-Palpable nodes localized behind the clavicle (in Japanese) Jpn J Gastroenterol Surg 18:1801–1809

10. Ide H, Murata Y, Okushima N, Muroi M, Oshibuthi H, Hanyuu H, Yamada A, Endou M (1986) Evaluation of cervical lymph node dissection for thoracic esophageal cancer (in Japanese). Geka Shinryo 28:561–566

11. Naito K, Ito K, Ito S, Naito A, Hayamizu K, Furuki T, Katsuta S, Yasutomi Y, Tomita S, Furuki Y, Fujita M, Tanimoto K, Wada T (1989) Ultrasonographic evaluation of cervical metastatic lymphadenopathy (in Japanese). Oral Radiol 29:45–50

12. Udagawa H, Tsurumaru M, Watanabe G, Ono Y, Suzuki M, Akiyama H (1986) Preoperative detection of lymph node metastasis in the neck and the superior mediastinum by neck ultrasound examination (in Japanese) Jpn J Gastroenterol Surg 19:2176–2183

13. Tohnosu N, Onoda S, Isono K (1987) Ultrasonographic evaluation of cervical lymph node metastasis in esophageal cancer with special reference to relationship between ratio of shortest and longest diameters (S/L) and cancer occupying rate (in Japanese) Jpn J Med Ultrasonics 14:501–509

14. Yoshinaka H, Kuroshima K, Morifuji H, Tanabe G, Baba M, Kajisa T, Nishi M (1985) Detection of cervical lymph node metastases in esophageal cancer by ultrasonography for non-palpable nodes behind the clavicle (in Japanese). Lymphology 8:147–150

15. Nagatomo M, Kuwajima A, Taki S, Sekiguchi R, Murakami S, Sato S, Okuyama N (1988) The size and depth/width ratio of normal lymph nodes (in Japanese). Jpn J Med Ultrasonics Proceedings of the 53rd Meeting, 11:359–360

16. Marchal G, Oyen R, Verschakelen J, Gelin J, Baert AL, Stessents RC (1985) Sonographic appearance of normal lymph nodes. J Ultrasound Med 4:417–419

17. Inoue H, Endo M, Yoshino K, Takiguchi T, Kawano T, Yamazaki S, Shimoju K, Suzuki T, Itoh K, Yamagiwa A (1990) Preoperative evaluation for cervical and upper mediastinal lymph node metastasis of esophageal cancer using conventional ultrasonography (in Japanese). Jpn J Gastroenterol Surg 23:1778–1784

Natural History of Esophageal Squamous Cell Carcinoma, with Special Reference to Evaluation of Clinical Growth Rate by Tumor Volume Doubling Time

KEN HARUMA, TADASHI TOKUTOMI, TAKEHIRO SHIMAMOTO, SHINJI TANAKA, MASAHARU YOSHIHARA, SHINYA KISHIMOTO, KOJI SUMII, and GORO KAJIYAMA[1]

Introduction

Esophageal carcinoma is a common malignancy with a poor prognosis, despite recent advances in treatment. We previously reported ten patients with rapidly growing squamous cell carcinomas of the esophagus, and showed that the rapid growth of this tumor explains both why it is seldom detected at an early stage and why prognosis is poor [1]. However, reports at variance with our findings have been published [2–4]. In particular, the selection of patients in our previous study may have presented a problem, particularly since the number was small. Moreover, to determine if tumor growth is actually rapid, it is necessary to evaluate tumor growth objectively by comparison with malignancies of other organs.

This study was conducted to evaluate the growth rate of esophageal squamous cell carcinoma in a relatively large number of patients, and to compare the doubling time with other malignancies in the gastrointestinal tract.

Patients and Methods

We reviewed the records of patients who had received upper gastrointestinal radiological and pathological studies during the 14 years between 1978 and 1991 at the Hiroshima University Hospital. For this study, we selected 22 patients based on these two criteria: (1) double-contrast esophagography had been performed more than 1 month previously, and (2) they were available for re-examination. The initial examination had been done as a part of mass screening of esophageal carcinoma in 13 patients, for gastrointestinal complaints in 6

[1] First Department of Internal Medicine, Hiroshima University School of Medicine, 1-2-3 Kasumi, Minami-ku, Hiroshima, 734 Japan

patients, for peptic ulcer in 2 patients, and as a study following radiation therapy of esophageal carcinoma in 1 patient. Of the 22 tumors found in these 22 patients, 18 had been overlooked at the initial esophagography. Four patients refused treatment.

No anticancer treatment had been administered during the observation period. Histological diagnosis of squamous cell carcinoma was confirmed by biopsy following surgical resection in 14 patients and by endoscopic biopsy in 8 who were administered radiation therapy.

Radiologic and microscopic types of esophageal carcinoma were classified according to the Guidelines for Clinical and Pathological Studies on Carcinoma of the Esophagus in Japan [5].

When tumor size was calculated, a correction was made for differences in magnification as judged from the size of the vertebrae. Tumor volume doubling time was calculated according to the method of Collins et al. [6], as modified by Schwartz [7]:

$$\text{Doubling time} = \frac{t}{10 \ (\log D_2 - \log D_1)}$$

D_1 is the tumor diameter at first measurement, D_2 is that at final measurement, and t is the interval between measurements.

Results

Data in the 22 patients with esophageal carcinoma appear in Table 1. The age, sex ratio, and location of the tumor were consistent with other reports.

The tumor diameter initially ranged from 7 to 80 mm (mean 27.9 mm). At the end of observation, it ranged from 21 to 150 mm (mean 60.6 mm). Doubling time could be determined in all but 1 of the 22 cases (patient 11), in whom the longitudinal diameter of the tumor did not change between the initial and final examination. The doubling time calculated in 21 cases ranged from 0.6 to 6.9 months (mean 3.4 months).

These cases were classified morphologically at the time of esophagography as the elevated (13 cases) or depressed type (8 cases). Doubling time for the elevated type ranged from 0.6 to 5.5 months (mean 2.4 months), and for the depressed type from 2.5 to 6.9 months (mean 5.0 months). The growth rate of the elevated type was thus more rapid. At the initial radiography, the mean doubling time in 15 patients diagnosed at an early stage was 3.8 months (1 to 6.9 months), while that of those in an advanced stage was 2.3 months (0.6 to 4.1 months). The growth rate in the advanced stage was more rapid. One illustrative case is presented.

Case Report

In case 22, a 75-year-old man, follow-up esophagography performed 4 months after the therapy of esophageal carcinoma indicated a lesion in the lower thoracic esophagus (Fig. 1a). The patient was then diagnosed as having a recurrent

Table 1. Data on 22 patients with esophageal carcinoma

Case no.	Age (years)	Sex	Radiographic appearance		Diameter (mm)		Observation period months	Doubling time months
			Initial	Final	Initial	Final		
1	61	M	Superficial elevated	Serrated	21	55	4	1.0
2	53	M	Superficial elevated	Spiral	29	150	11	1.5
3	63	M	Superficial elevated	Spiral	18	86	12	1.8
4	62	M	Superficial elevated	Tumorous	10	72	9	1.0
5	71	F	Superficial elevated	Tumorous	17	32	9	3.3
6	73	M	Superficial elevated	Superficial elevated	15	40	14	3.3
7	75	M	Superficial elevated	Tumorous	23	40	8	3.3
8	72	M	Superficial elevated	Tumorous	7	21	26	5.5
9	60	M	Superficial depressed	Tumorous	25	47	19	6.9
10	48	M	Superficial depressed	Tumorous	27	62	16	4.4
11	54	M	Superficial depressed	Funneled	100	100	15	—
12	49	M	Superficial depressed	Spiral	15	70	17	2.5
13	77	M	Superficial depressed	Funneled	25	97	19	3.2
14	76	M	Superficial depressed	Serrated	30	58	20	7.0
15	62	F	Superficial depressed	Superficial elevated	15	28	17	6.3
16	73	M	Superficial depressed	Tumorous	35	45	7	6.4
17	51	M	Superficial depressed	Tumorous	15	46	15	3.1
18	76	M	Tumorous	Tumorous	24	45	4	1.5
19	68	M	Tumorous	Tumorous	35	45	4	3.6
20	74	M	Tumorous	Tumorous	43	75	10	4.1
21	83	F	Tumorous	Tumorous	33	44	1	0.8
22	75	M	Tumorous	Tumorous	52	75	1	0.6

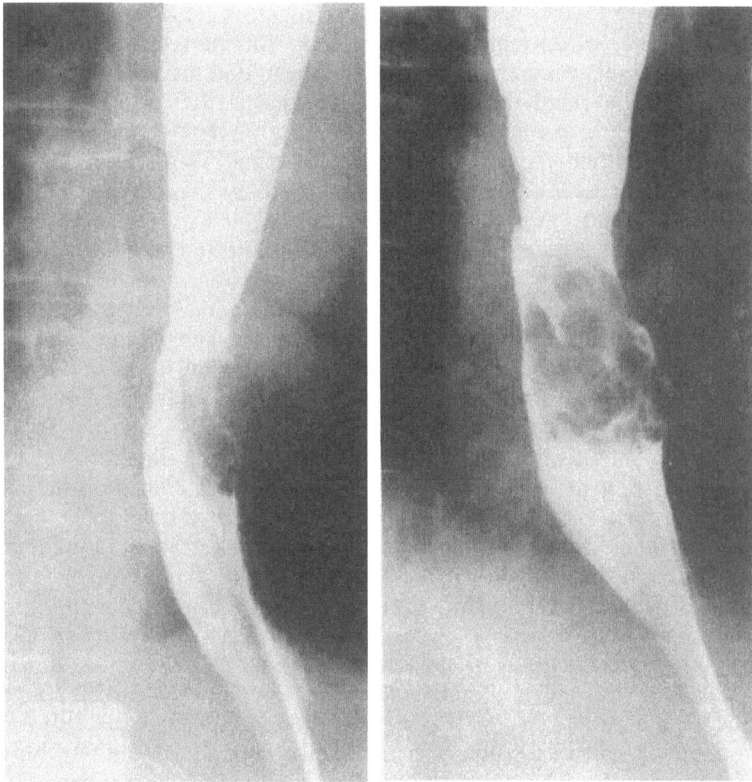

Fig. 1. A Case 22, follow-up esophagography performed 4 months after radiation therapy indicated a small filling defect. **B** One month later, it had progressed to tumorous type of advanced carcinoma

esophageal carcinoma. However, he refused further treatment. One month later, he presented with severe dysphagia, and carcinoma had progressed to an advanced stage (tumorous type) (Fig. 1b).

Discussion

Many papers have been published on the growth rate of human tumors, as this parameter is useful in evaluating survival time or therapeutic effect. In most cases, the tumors were primary or metastatic pulmonary carcinomas [8–10], breast carcinomas [11, 12], colorectal carcinoma [13–16], gastric carcinomas [17, 18], or hepatocellular carcinomas [19–21] with little study conducted on the growth rate of esophageal carcinoma. To our knowledge, the first investigation on the rapid growth of esophageal carcinoma was conducted by Takagi and Karasawa in seven cases of esophageal carcinoma studied by esophagography [22]. Several cases showing a rapid growth rate were subsequently published [23, 24]. We also reported ten cases of rapidly growing esophageal carcinomas [1];

the results agreed with those of other investigators. Guanrei et al. [4], in an endoscopic study of asymptomatic individuals for mass screening in high-risk areas of esophageal carcinoma in China demonstrated the growth of esophageal carcinomas to be relatively slow. They concluded that 3–4 years would be required for an in situ esophageal carcinoma to progress to an advanced stage. In 23 cases of untreated early esophageal carcinoma, Yanjin et al. [2] found the early stage to persist for a relatively long period. The reason for the discrepancy between our results and those of others is not clear, but may be due to differences in disease stage. Guanrei et al. [4] detected esophageal carcinoma endoscopically during mass screening. Slow growth was associated with a finding of in situ or intramucosal carcinoma. In our study, tumors were detected radiologically, meaning that they certainly involved the submucosa. Thus, tumors may grow at different rates at different stages, slowly while in situ or intramucosal, and then rapidly, even though it has been assumed that the growth of most human tumors is generally constant [6–8].

The first quantitative study of tumor doubling time in humans was made by Collins et al. [6] in 1956, and the results of this investigation were supported by numerous reports in which repeated measurements of radiographic, cutaneous, or lymph node metastases were presented. For gastrointestinal tumors, doubling time has been investigated in colorectal, gastric, or more recently, hepatocellular carcinomas. Bolin et al. [14] showed, in 27 colorectal carcinomas, that the mean doubling time was 16.5 months with a range of 2.6–78.5 months. Spratt and Spratt [15] sought the doubling time measurement data for colorectal neoplasms and calculated the mean doubling time in 98 colorectal carcinomas as 11.7 months, with a range of 1.7–333.3 months. In Japan, Tada et al. [16] found the mean doubling time of 6 colorectal carcinomas to be 13.9 months, with a range of 3.1–34.4 months. These are essentially the same. Only two reports on gastric carcinoma have been published in the English literature. Kholi et al. [17] reported the doubling time of early gastric carcinomas to be 45.2 months, with a range of 19.2–115.4 months, and that of advanced gastric carcinoma to be 5.7 months, with a range of 2.3–10.2 months. In our 12 patients with polypoid type gastric carcinoma, the mean doubling time was 10.1 months, ranging from 2.2 to 23.4 months [18]. However, the mean doubling time of esophageal squamous cell carcinoma reported here was 3.4 months, with a range of 0.6–6.9months, the values exceeding those of colorectal or gastric carcinomas, which are histologically classified as adenocarcinomas. Weiss et al. [10] demonstrated differences in the growth rates of adenocarcinomas and squamous cell carcinomas, with the latter growing more rapidly. From the results of studies on untreated primary pulmonary carcinoma, the prognosis of squamous cell carcinoma has been shown to be better than that of adenocarcinoma [25, 26]. Thus, difference in growth rates between esophageal and colorectal or gastric carcinoma may depend on histological type—whether adenocarcinoma or squamous cell carcinoma.

Recently, Sheu et al. [19] studied 28 patients with asymptomatic hepatocellular carcinomas by real-time ultrasonography, and found the doubling time to range from 1.0 to 13.3, with a mean of 4.5 months. Ebara et al. [20] reported the mean doubling time to be 6.5 months for 22 patients with cirrhosis and minute hepatocellular carcinoma <3 cm. Okazaki et al. [21], who investigated 15 patients with hepatocellular carcinomas smaller than 4.5 cm, calculated the mean doubling time to be 3.4 months, with a range of 1.4–10.2 months. The mean doubling time of hepatocellular carcinoma was similar to that of esophageal carcinoma in this study. Hepatocellular carcinoma is also generally regarded as being rapidly fatal, as with esophageal carcinoma.

In summary, our results demonstrate that most esophageal carcinomas can be diagnosed only at an advanced stage and have a poor prognosis, since the growth of esophageal carcinoma detected by esophagography is extremely rapid. Measurement of the growth rate based on doubling time may be useful for predicting the features of esophageal carcinoma and for screening and diagnostic purposes.

References

1. Haruma K, Tokutomi T, Yoshihara M, Sumii K, Kajiyama G (1991) Rapid growth of untreated esophageal squamous-cell carcinoma in 10 patients. J Clin Gastroenterol 3: 129–134
2. Yanjin M, Guangyi L, Xianzhi G, Wenheng C (1981) Detection and natural progression of early esophageal carcinoma: Preliminary communication. J R Soc Med 74:884–886
3. Rajindranath T, Nair KV, Davi RS, Devi NN (1984) Prolonged "in situ" stage in esophageal carcinoma. J Assoc Physicians India 32:445–456
4. Guanrei Y, Songliang Q, He H, Guizen F (1988) Natural history of early esophageal squamous carcinoma and early adenocarcinoma of the gastric cardia in the People's Republic of China. Endoscopy 20:95–98
5. Japanese Society for Esophageal Disease. (1976) Guidelines for the Clinical and Pathological Studies on Carcinoma of the Esophagus. Jpn J Surg 6:69–86
6. Collins VP, Loeffler RK, Tivey H (1956) Observations of growth rates of human tumors. Am J Roentgenol 76:988–1000
7. Schwartz M (1961) A biomathematical approach to clinical tumor growth. Cancer 14: 1272–1294
8. Garland LH, Coulos W, Wollin E (1963) The rate of growth and apparent duration of untreated primary bronchial carcinoma. Cancer 16:694–707
9. Spratt JS Jr, Spratt TL (1964) Rates of growth of pulmonary metastases and host survival. Ann Surg 159:161–171
10. Weiss W, Boucot KR, Cooper DA (1966) Growth rate in the detection and prognosis of bronchogenic carcinoma. JAMA 198:1246–1252
11. Kusama S, Spratt JS Jr, Donegan WL, Watson FR (1972) The gross rates of growth of human mammary carcinoma. Cancer 30:594–599
12. Heuser L, Spratt JS, Polk HC Jr (1979) Growth rates of primary breast cancers. Cancer 43:1888–1894
13. Welin S, Youker J, Spratt JS Jr, et al (1963) The rates and patterns of growth of 375 tumors of the large intestine and rectum observed serially by double-contrast enema study (Malmo technique). Am J Roentgenol 90:673–687
14. Bolin S, Nilsson E, Sjodahl R (1983) Carcinoma of the colon and rectum—growth rate. Ann surg 198:151–158
15. Spratt JS, Spratt JA (1985) Growth rates of benign and malignant neoplasms of the colon. Prog Clin Biol Res 186:103–120
16. Tada M, Misaki F, Kawai K (1984) Growth rates of colorectal carcinoma and adenoma by roentgenologic follow-up observations. Gastroenterologia Jpn 19:550–555
17. Kohli Y, Kawai K, Fujita S (1981) Analytical studies on growth of human gastric cancer. J Clin Gastroenterol 3:129–133
18. Haruma K, Suzuki T, Tsuda T, Yoshihara M, Sumii K, Kajiyama G (1991) Evaluation of tumor growth rate in patients with early gastric carcinoma of the elevated type. Gastrointestinal Radiol 16:289–292

19. Sheu JC, Sung JL, Chen DS, et al (1985) Growth rate of asymptomatic hepatocellular carcinoma and its clinical implications. Gastroenterology 89:259–266

20. Ebara M, Ohto M, Shinagawa T, et al (1986) Natural history of minute hepatocellular carcinoma smaller than three centimeters complicating cirrhosis. Gastroenterology 90: 289–298

21. Okazaki N, Yoshino M, Yoshida T, et al (1989) Evaluation of the prognosis for small hepatocellular carcinoma based on tumor volume doubling time. A preliminary report. Cancer 63:2207–2210

22. Takagi I, Karasawa K (1982) Growth of squamous cell esophageal carcinoma observed by serial esophagographies. J Surg Oncol 21:57–60

23. Sasajima K, Taniguchi Y, Morino K, et al (1988) Rapid growth of a pseudosarcoma of the esophagus. J Clin Gastroenterol 10:533–536

24. Bochna GS, Harty RF, Harned RK, Markin RS (1988) Development of squamous cell carcinoma of the esophagus after endoscopic variceal sclerotherapy. Am J Gastroenterol 83:564–568

25. Cappelen C Jr, Efskind L, Poppe E (1961) Bronchial carcinoma with special regard to prognosis. Acta Path Microbiol Scand 148 [Suppl]:23–33

26. Spratt JS Jr, Spjut HJ, Roper CL (1963) The frequency distribution of the rates of growth and the estimated duration of primary pulmonary carcinomas. Cancer 16:687–693

Resection for Esophageal Cancer

For the Debate on the Significance of Lymphadenectomy in Esophageal Cancer

Hiroshi Akiyama[1]

Introduction

Systematic lymph node dissection was proven to be effective in improving survival in patients with cancer of the thoracic esophagus, and a significant amount of discussion has been devoted to this topic. However, there are some conflicting opinions on this subject.

The frequency of lymph node metastases was assessed with respect to both tumor location and to the lymph node groups involved. Lymph node involvement due to esophageal cancer occurred extensively in the neck, mediastinum, and abdomen regardless of the tumor location in the esophagus [1]. The data suggested that the addition of a neck dissection to the conventional mediastinal and abdominal nodal dissection might improve survival.

A study was made of patients with squamous cell carcinoma of the thoracic esophagus who underwent radical lymph node dissection and were found to have no macroscopic residual tumor. However, the series excluded those with mucosal invasion. The reason for this was that nodal metastases rarely occur in patients with mucosal cancer [2]. It was concluded that cases which underwent collo-thoracoabdominal (CTA or 3-field) dissection showed a significantly better 5-year survival rate compared with that obtained by conventional thoracoabdominal (TA or 2-field) dissection.

Materials and Methods

Of 1115 cases with cancer of the esophagus, 887 cases were squamous cell carcinoma of the thoracic esophagus. Resections, including both curative and palliative, were carried out on 609 cases with a resectability rate of 68.7%.

[1]Department of Surgery, Toranomon Hospital, 2-2-2 Toranomon, Minato-ku, Tokyo, 105 Japan

Conventional thoracoabdominal (TA) dissection and collo-thoracoabdominal (CTA) dissection were carried out on 267 and 195 cases, respectively. The frequency of nodal metastases per number of cases was studied in 280 cases according to the depth of the tumor invasion. Survival rates were compared between TA and CTA dissection groups for patients, excluding those with mucosal cancers.

Results

Survival Data According to TNM Classification

Long-term results after radical resection combined with systematic lymph node dissection were studied according to the new TNM classification [3]. Figures 1 and 2 show survival curves after radical surgery with TA dissection and CTA dissection, respectively. The differences between the two groups were not clearly demonstrated by comparing the two figures. However, in pTNM stage III cases, a 5-year survival rate (58.5%) obtained after CTA dissection was significantly better than that (27.5%) obtained after TA dissection (Fig. 3). In pTNM stage IV-N (stage III due to pN-factor) cases, a 5-year survival rate (25.5%) obtained after CTA dissection was also significantly better than that (14.3%) obtained after TA dissection (Fig. 4).

Overall Survival Data

The frequency of nodal metastases varies remarkably depending on the depth of the tumor invasion. Relations between the histological depth of the tumor invasion and the frequency of lymph node metastases were studied. It is obvious

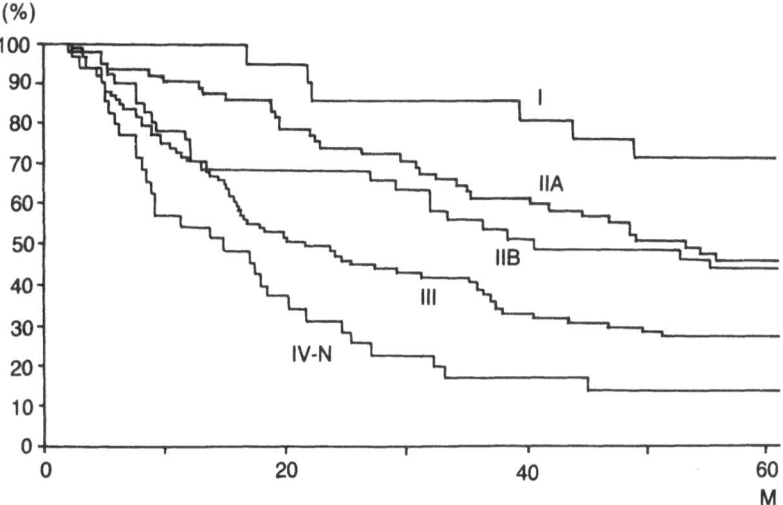

Fig. 1. Survival curves according to pTNM staging [thoracoabdominal (*TA*) dissection, *n* = 267. Stage IV due to pN-factor

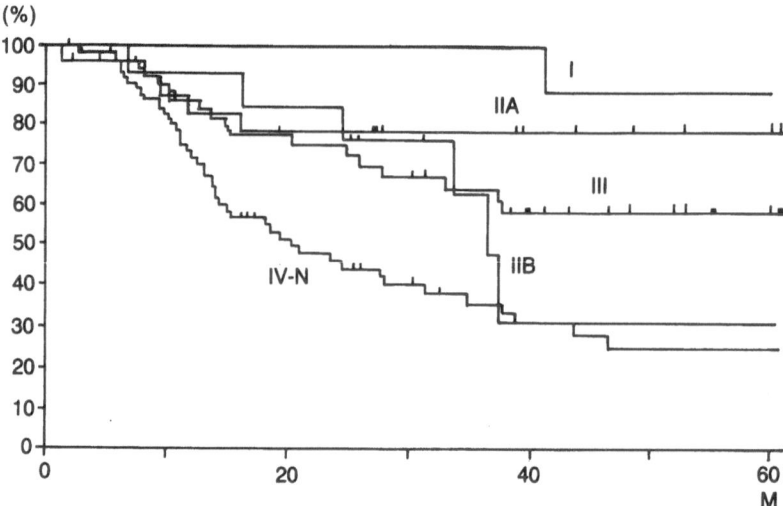

Fig. 2. Survival curves according to pTNM staging [collo-thoracoabdominal (*CTA*) dissection, *n* = 195]

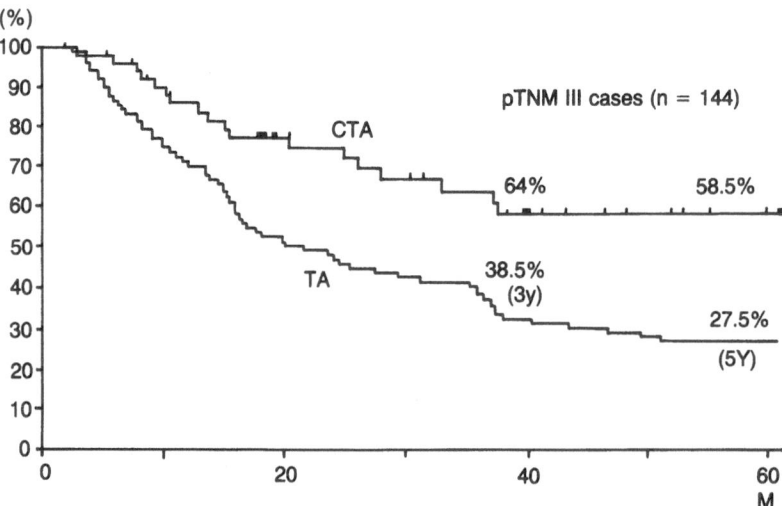

Fig. 3. Comparison of survival curves after TA (*n* = 91) and CTA (*n* = 53) dissection for pTNM stage III cases. *P* = 0.0012 for log rank test and *P* = 0.0018 for the generalized Wilcoxon test

that lymphatic spread does not occur in intraepithelial cancers. Although lymphatic spread could theoretically occur in cancers with the depth of lamina propria mucosae, no nodal metastases were found. In cancers with depth of muscularis mucosae, nodal metastases were found infrequently.

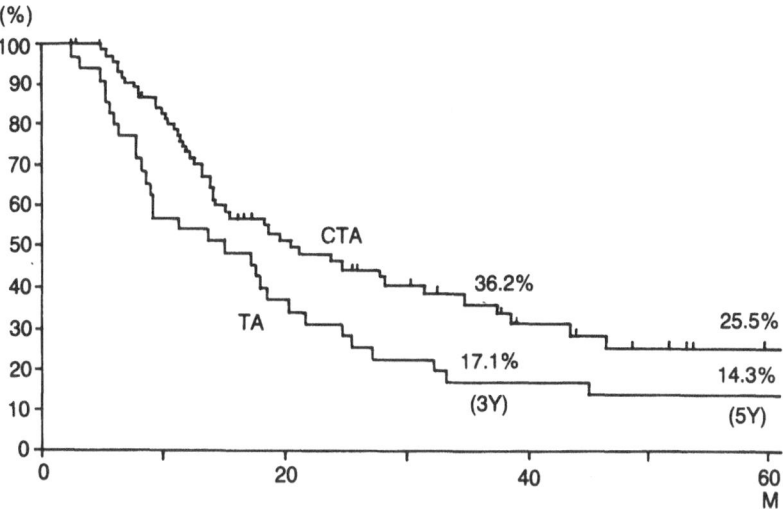

Fig. 4. Comparison of survival curves after TA ($n = 35$) and CTA ($n = 80$) dissections for pTNM stage IV (N) cases. $P = 0.0405$ for log rank test and $P = 0.0174$ for generalized Wilcoxon test

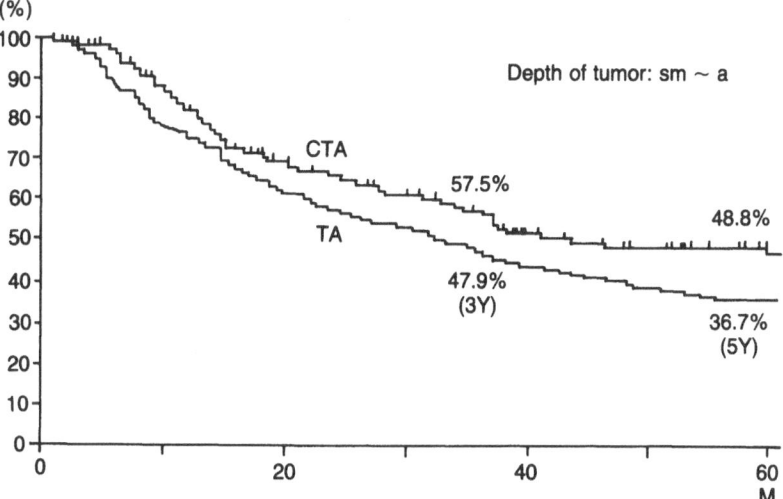

Fig. 5. Comparison of survival curves after TA ($n = 267$) and CTA ($n = 195$) dissections for patients excluding those with mucosal cancers. $P = 0.0299$ for both log rank and generalized Wilcoxon tests

In cases with submucosal tumor invasion, the frequency of lymph node metastases suddenly increased to as much as 53.5%. In cases with tumor invasion into muscularis propria and adventitia, the frequencies were 78.6% and 87.3%, respectively. Therefore, for accurate evaluation of the effect of systematic lymph node dissection, it is necessary to exclude patients with mucosal cancers.

Survival curves after radical surgery for patients, excluding those with mucosal cancers, are shown in Fig. 5. Five-year survival rates after TA and CTA dissection groups were 48.8% and 36.7% respectively. The result was significantly better in the CTA dissection group.

Discussion

The analysis and results of nodal metastases reported by the author [1] correlate well with the general concepts relating to the patterns of cancer spread. However, it should be noted that some primary cancers extend beyond a single anatomical boundary and spread into the neck, mediastinum, and abdomen. Sakata [4] described a work on the lymphatic system of the esophagus. He stated that the submucosal lymphatics mostly drain in a longitudinal fashion. The results obtained from this pioneering study coincide with our analysis of the distribution of lymph node metastases in patients with squamous cell carcinoma of the thoracic esophagus. Therefore, the spread is entirely unpredictable and for this reason, a complete eradication of the lymphatic spread is guaranteed only by a total esophagectomy with dissection of nodes in all three regions.

In recent years, it has become possible to obtain accurate information on the depth of the tumor invasion, nodal involvement, local spread, hematogenous distant metastases, and intramural tumor spread. This detailed information enables the surgeon to develop a reasonable strategy for treating esophageal cancer. Although our principle of surgical treatment for cancer of the esophagus is based on CTA dissection, the concept of type-oriented therapy [5] or malignancy-oriented strategy [1] should be kept in mind. When wide spread lymph node metastases are found in all three regions of the neck, mediastinum, and abdomen, then lymph node dissection is not indicated.

It has been shown that radical surgery combined with lymph node dissection, particularly with lymph node dissection of the three fields, has improved the cure rate of cancer of the thoracic esophagus.

Conclusion

Radical resection of cancer of the thoracic esophagus with combination of systematic lymph node dissection is recommended for improving survival. Five-year survival rates after collo-thoracoabdominal and thoracoabdominal dissections for patients, excluding those with mucosal cancer, were 48.8% and 36.7%, respectively. Thus, the long-term result was significantly better in patients treated by collo-thoracoabdominal (3-field) dissection.

References

1. Akiyama H (1990) Surgery for cancer of the esophagus. Williams & Wilkins, Baltimore
2. Akiyama H, Tsurumaru M, Odagawa H, Kajiyama Y (1993) Systematic Lymph Node Dissection for Esophageal Cancer—Effective or not?—. Dis Esoph (in press)

3. Japanese Committee for Registration of Esophageal Carcinoma. A proposal for a new TNM classification of esophageal carcinoma. Jpn J Clin Oncol 14:625–636
4. Sakata K (1903) Über die Lymphgefässe des Oesophagus und seine regionären Lymphdrüsen mit Berücksichtigung der Verbreitung des Karzinoms. Mitt Grenzgeb Med Clin 11:634–656
5. Inokuchi K (1992) Milestones along the road to improvement of results in the treatment of squamous cell carcinoma of the esophagus. In: Sato T, Iizuka T (eds) Color atlas of surgical anatomy for esophageal cancer. Springer, Berlin Heidelberg Tokyo New York, pp 1–8

Is Radical Lymphadenectomy of Value in the Surgical Treatment of Esophageal Cancer?

Bruno Zilberstein, Ivan Cecconello, Ary Nasi, and Henrique W. Pinotti[1]

Introduction

The objective of surgical management of cancer of the esophagus is twofold: To perform radical resection of the tumor and to restore effective gastric continuity. The purpose of this paper is to analyze the short- and long-term progress of patients with squamous cell carcinoma of the esophagus submitted to this procedure, regarding the importance of lymphadenectomy on long-term survival.

Subjects and Methods

This study included 121 patients with squamous cell carcinoma of the esophagus, submitted to transdiaphragmatic esophagectomy. Ages varied from 38 to 74 years with a mean of 55.2 years. Of the 121 patients, 99 (82%) were males, 70 (58%) were white, 34 (28%) negro, and 17 (14%) mulato. The esophageal region affected was cervical in 3 patients (2.5%), the upper thoracic segment in 11 (9%), the mid-thoracic seqment in 56 (46.3%), and the inferior thoracic segment in 51 (42%).

Technique

Surgery was performed by two teams working simultaneously, one in the cervical and the other in the abdominal region, according to the technique described by Pinotti et al. [1]. The surgery proceeded with dissection of the hiatal region, isolation of the abdominal esophagus, and then the fibrosed part of the

[1] Department of Surgery, São Paulo University School of Medicine, Av. Giovani Gronchi no. 4971 71, CEP 05724, São Paulo, Brazil

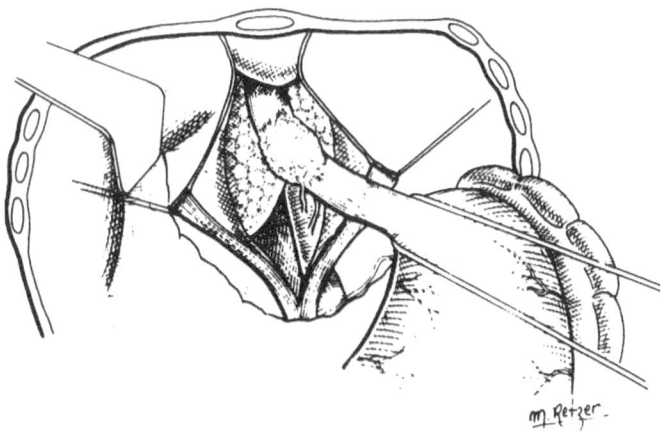

Fig. 1. Transdiaphragmatic resection. Opening of the central part of the diaphragm and dissection of the lower third of the esophagus

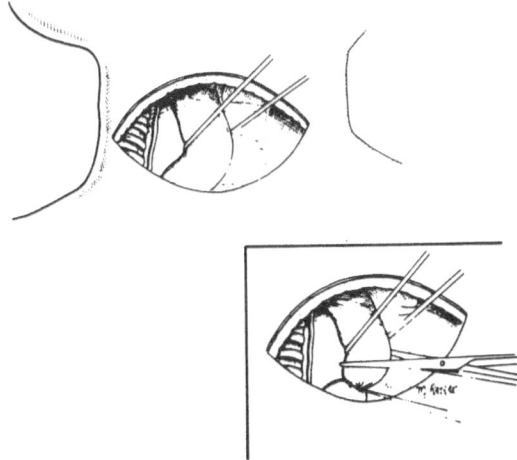

Fig. 2. Cervical esophagus section. Dissection of the esophagus at the neck, sectioning its distal segment

diaphragm was widely opened from the hiatal ring up to the xiphoid appendix. The pericardium and pleura were retracted, so ample access to the posterior mediastinum was achieved (Fig. 1). The esophagus was then dissected under direct vision and all the adjacent periesophageal tissue was removed. The mediastinal pleura was resected whenever necessary.

At the cervical level, the esophagus was resected (Fig. 2) and its distal extremity ligated and pulled toward the abdomen via the mediastinal tunnel. This caused the esophagus to assume "an inverted U" or "horseshoe" appearance (Fig. 3). This maneuver exposes the so-called "Blind Zone" which is the retrotracheal region at the level of the carina.

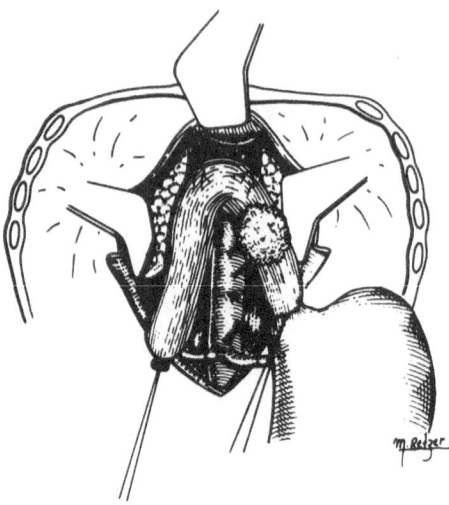

Fig. 3. "Horseshoe" maneuver. After the section of the cervical esophagus, its distal segment is pulled down to the abdomen, exposing the retrotracheal zone

Next, the final ligatures were completed and the esophagus removed from its bed. The resection was supplemented by removal of the gastric fundus and part of the lesser curvature including the branches of the left gastric artery, with the aim of promoting lymph node ressection at this level. Continuity of the food passage was achieved by gastroplasty, by passing the stomach retrosternally to the cervical region where it was anastomosed. After postoperative recovery (about 30 days), the treatment was supplemented by radiotherapy with 4500–6000 rads.

Results

In 121 cases operated on, early complications were: Traumatic injury of the recurrent nerve at the cervical level, 2 cases (1.6%); and injury to the trachea; 1 case (0.8%) which required a right thoracotomy (the patient had an uneventful postoperative course); injury to the azygous vein, 1 case (0.8%) (requiring a thoracotomy for hemostasis), and the postoperative course also was uneventful; injury to the spleen, 2 cases (1.6%) which required splenectomy; and death occurred in 12 cases (9.9%) in this series. During the early postoperative period (first 30 days), the following complications occurred:

– Fistula of the esophagogastric anastomosis at the cervical level, 27 cases (22.3%). Twenty patients showed favorable progress with spontaneous closure, only two became stenotic.
– Six cases of pleural effusion (4.9%); bronchopneumonia, 13 cases (10.7%); urinary infection, 6 cases (4.9%); evisceration, 6 cases (4.9%). Postoperative hemorrhage occurred in 3 cases (1.6%), none of which were due to bleeding of esophageal bed.

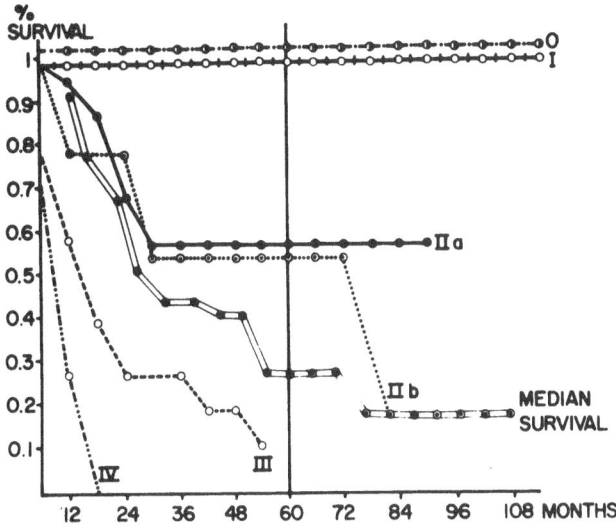

Fig. 4. Survival rate. Actuarial survival rate calculated for all patients that survived surgery (median survival). The curves are separated by stages, showing significant differences among them

This procedure enabled us to dissect 1050 lymph nodes. Involvement was noted in 165 (15.7%) of these, corresponding to 47 patients (38.8%). Lymph node involvement was negative in 60 cases (49.5%), and in 14 (11.6%) cases involvement could not be determined. Analysis of the resected specimen and the staging supplemented with the intraoperative findings showed: Stage 0, 8.3%; Stage I, 8.3%; Stage IIa, 29.7%; Stage IIb, 9.9%; Stage III, 32.2%; and Stage IV, 11.6%. Late follow-up showed a 5-year survival for the entire group of 27% and at 9 years it was 16%. According to the staging the 5-year survival was: Stages 0 and I, 100%; stage IIa 55%; stage IIb 52%; and stages III fell to 9% at 54 months and stage IV 0% (Fig. 4).

Discussion

Basic principles to be followed in the management of cancer of the esophagus should include: (1) resection of a sufficiently wide area of tumor to remove all involved tissues, if possible, (2) restitution of the digestive function to the greatest extent possible, and (3) use of the surgical technique with the lowest rate of intra- and postoperative problems. Transdiaphragmatic esophagectomy has appeared as a technical option. Initial approach by laparotomy facilitates reinforcement of staging (already defined via transdiaphragmatic approach) the possibility of resection, and the palliative or curative character of the resection, eliminating exploratory thoracotomies. The opening of the posterior mediastinum and the "inverted U" maneuver of the esophagus, expose the so called "Blind Zone" of the transmediastinal dissection so it becomes accessible, avoiding the difficulties reported by those who use this approach without opening the diaphragm. As to the type of radical surgery, with relation to lymph node dissection, with this procedure we were able to resect 1050 lymph nodes, proving that this approach enables us to dissect these structures. The rate of involvement of 15.7% is perfectly comparable to that of en bloc esophagectomy [2]. Long-term follow-up of patients demonstrated a 5-year survival of 27%. These results are as good as the results provided by those who use transpleural esophagectomy such as: Rimin et al. [3], 28%; Isono et al. [4], 12.4%; Ellis et al. [5], 21%; and Akiyama et al. [6], 34.7%. When survival was compared to staging, we verified that for stages 0 and I (early tumors), the acturial 5-year survival rate attained was identical to that reported by others [2, 7, 8]. The analysis of these results indicates that the success of surgical management in terms of survival depends more on staging than on any other criteria that might eventually be perceived [9–14]. In this series, mortality was about 10%. Akiyama [15], reported zero mortality in 41 cases and Orringer [16], reported 6.1% in 147 cases, contrasting markedly with the 20% and 30% mortality rates, reported for thoracotomy [8, 17–19]. However, most of the criticism centers around the necessity of removing all the tissue fortuitously compromised, especially the ganglionar drainage chains [20]. Therefore, authors such as Skinner [21], Akiyama [2], Ishida et al. [22], Siewert et al. [23], advocate wide dissection of the lymph node chains. Sasaki et al. [24], verified that 5-year survival with radical lymphadenectomy is 33%, decreasing to 24% without.

Radical lymphadenectomy should be based on 3 premises: (1) morbidity and mortality, (2) staging of the disease, (3) multidisciplinary management of cancer of the esophagus as a necessity. Regarding mortality, these indexes clearly increase when wide dissections are performed. Skinner [21], performing radical lymphadenectomy, reported an 11% mortality and an acturial 5-year rate of over 18% in a series of 80 patients submitted to radical lymphadenectomy. Steegmuller and Marklin [25] present a mortality rate of 36% and 5-year survival of 21%. Added to this is the fact that even those who advocate radical node dissection reported a dramatic fall in survival when the lymph nodes are involved [26]. Akiyama [2] reports an 18.5% 5-year survival rate even with radical dissection when the nodes are involved. Kasai et al. [7] reported a 38.2% 5-year survival rate when peritumoral lymph nodes are involved and 0% with distant involvement. Sorrentino et al. [27], Kodama et al. [28], and Fekete et al. [29] confirm this opinion and affirm that from a surgical point of view, resection should be considered curative when excision is complete without involvement of the margins or metastases. An analysis of the extent of lymphatic drainage of the esophagus covering the bilateral cervical region, the supraclavicular fossae, anterior and posterior mediastinum, and the abdominal, pericardial and perigastric lymph chains, shows that "sterilization" of a territory of this extent is equivalent to managing a systemic and not simply a local disease. Therefore, adjuvant treatment by radiotherapy assumes a major role and should be planned based on an overall view of the problem in an attempt to improve survival. We can conclude, therefore, that treatment of cancer of the esophagus should be multidisciplinary to improve survival, emphasizing that this will depend fundamentally on the stage of the disease [30]. The overall experience shows that this technique offers direct vision of the operative field whereas the others use blunt or blind dissection, and safe surgical procedures are possible besides removal of involved lymph node tissue which attain the goal of surgical management of esophageal cancer.

Summary. One hundred and twenty-one patients with squamous cell esophageal carcinoma were managed with cervico-abdominal esophagectomy without thoracotomy by transdiaphragmatic approach for the radical treatment of this disease. In order to assess the outcome and eventual cause of death, they were followed up for a minimum of 1 year and a maximum of 10 years or until they succumbed. The mortality for this procedure was 9.9%. The most common complication was fistula of the esophagogastric anastomosis recorded in 27 cases (22.3%). In total, 1050 lymph node were dissected and involvement was noted in 165 (15.7%), corresponding to 47 cases (38.8%). Lymph node involvement was negative in 60 cases (49.5%), and in 14 (11.6%) cases involvement could not be determined. Staging showed 10 cases (8.3%) classified as stage 0, 10 (8.3%) as stage I, 36 (29.7%) as stage IIa, 12 (9.9%) as stage IIb, 39 (32.2%) as III, and 14 (11.6%) as stage IV. The patients that survived operations underwent radiotherapy so long-term follow-up was possible. Analysis of the progress of these patients showed an actuarial survival of 5 years in 27% and of 9 years in 16%. The evaluation based on stages showed an actuarial survival rate of 5 years of 100% for stages O and I, 55% for stages IIa, and 52% for IIb. The survival rate for stage III fell to 9% at 54 months, and for stage IV it was 25% for 12 months and 0% for 18 months.

In conclusion we can state that it is possible to achieve our goal of providing a safe procedure for the surgical management of esophageal carcinoma with our technique because it is performed under direct vision and so offers a broad view of the operative field. Concerning survival, it depends fundamentally on the stage of the lesion, therefore, better results are obtained in the early stages of the disease.

References

1. Pinotti HW, Zilberstein B, Pollara W, Raia A (1981) Esophagectomy without thoracotomy. Surg Gynecol Obstet 152:344–346
2. Akiyama H (1986) Cardinals of regional lymph node dissection in surgery of thoracic esophageal cancer. In: Siewert JR, Hölscher AH (eds) Abstracts of international esophageal week, Munich, 1986. Demeter, Grafelfing, p 73
3. Rimin L, Yunkan L, Hongyi C, et al (1981) Late results of surgical treatment in esophageal carcinoma and factors influencing prognosis. Chin Med J 94:729–731
4. Isono K, Onoda S, Ishikawa T, Sato H, Nakayama K (1982) Studies on the causes of death from esophageal carcinoma. Cancer 49:2173–2179
5. Ellis Jr FH, Gibb SP, Watkins Jr E (1983) Esophagogastrectomy: A safe widely applicable and expeditious form of palliation for patients with carcinoma of the esophagus and cardia. Ann Surg 198:531–540
6. Akiyama H, Tsurumaru M, Watanabe G, Ono Y, Udagawa H, Suzuki M (1984) Development of surgery for carcinoma of the esophagusa. Am J Surg 147:9–16
7. Kasai M, Nishihira T, Kitamura K, Akaishi T, Shineka R, Sekine Y (1986) Long-term curative resection of carcinoma of thoracic esophagus. In: Siewert JR, Hölscher AH (eds) Abstracts of international esophageal week, Munich, 1986. Demeter, Grafelfing, p 103
8. Skinner DB, Soriano A, Ferguson MK, Little AG (1986) Selection of patients for en bloc esophagectomy. In: Siewert JR, Hölscher AH (eds) Abstracts of international esophageal week, Munich, 1986. Demeter, Grafelfing, p 72

9. Kurmeier A, Wehrli H, Akovbiantz A (1990) 100 consecutive cases of surgical esophagus-cardia carcinoma. Schweiz Med Wochenschr 120:502–504

10. Cederqvist C, Nielsen J, Berthelsen A, Hansen HS (1978) Cancer of the esophagus—1002 cases. Survey and survival. Acta Chir Scand 144:227–231

11. Ying-Kai W, Kuo-Chun H (1979) Chinese experience in the surgical treatment of carcinoma of the esophagus. Ann Surg 190:361–365

12. Huand GJ (1981) Early detection and surgical treatment of esophageal carcinoma. Jpn J Surg 11:399–405

13. Kinoshita Y, Endo M, Nakayama K, Sato H (1982) Clinical evaluation of 10-year survival cases after operation for upper and mid-thoracic esophageal cancer. Int Surg 67:152–161

14. Shiozaki H, Ogawa Y, Nishiyama K, Mori T (1986) Sexual difference in prognosis of esophageal cancer. In: Siewert JR, Hölscher AH (eds) Abstracts of international esophageal week, Munich, 1986. Demeter, Grafelfing, p 110

15. Akiyama H (1981) Esophagectomy without thoracotomy. In: Stipa S, Belsey RHR, Moraldi A (eds) Medical and surgical problems of the esophagus. Academic, New York, p 339 (Serono Symposium, No. 43)

16. Orringer MB (1986) Transhiatal esophagectomy for esophageal carcinoma. In: Siewert JR, Hölscher AH (eds) Abstracts of international esophageal week, Munich, 1986. Demeter, Grafelfing, p 96

17. Peracchia A, Tremolada C, Buin F, Ancona E (1982) Le traitement chirurgical du cancer de l'oesophage thoracique. Acta Chir Belg 4:355–358

18. Hankins JR, Attar S, Coughlin Jr TR, Miller JE, et al (1989) Carcinoma of the esophagus: A comparison of the transhiatal versus transthoracic resection. Ann Thorac Surg 47:700–705

19. Siewert JR, Hölscher AH, Adolf J, Bartels H, Hölscher M, Weiser HF (1986) Esophageal cancer subtotal esophagectomy with mediastinal lymphadenectomy and esophageal reconstruction with delayed urgency. In: Siewert JR, Hölscher AH (eds) Abstracts of international esophageal week, Munich, 1986. Demeter, Grafelfing, p 74

20. Chacon JP, Kobata CM (1986) Cancer of the esophagus: surgery without thoracotomy? ABCD Arq Bras Cir Dig 2:67–68

21. Skinner DB (1983) En bloc resection for neoplasms of the esophagus and cardia. J Thorac Cardiovasc Surg 85:59–71

22. Ishida K, Mori S, Okatomot K, et al (1986) Results of extended dissection of lymphnodes in operation for thoracic esophageal cancer. In: Siewert JR, Hölscher AH (eds) Abstracts of international esophageal week, Munich, 1986. Demeter, Grafelfing, p 111

23. Siewert JR, Bartels H, Lange J, Roeder JD, Hölscher AH (1990) En bloc esophagectomy—when should the digestive tract be reconstructed? Langenbecks Arch Chir 375:166–170

24. Sasaki K, Muto T, Tanka O, Soga J (1986) The significance of systemic lymphadenectomy for thoracic esophageal carcinoma. In: Siewert JR, Hölscher AH (eds) Abstracts of international esophageal week, Munich, 1986. Demeter, Grafelfing, p 112

25. Steegmuller KW, Marklin HM (1982) Resektion und Magenersatz beim thorakalen Oesophaguskarzimon. Langenbecks Arch Chir 336:43–49

26. Snnohe Y, Hiratsuka R, Dorki K (1981) Lymphnode metastases in cancer of the thoracic esophagus. Am J Surg 141:216–218

27. Sorrentino P, Ruol A, Castro C, Ferrini M, et al (1986) Prognostic significance of tumor stage and lymphnodal involvement in thoracic esophageal cancer: Our experience in 240 selected cases. In: Siewert JR, Hölscher AH (eds) Abstracts of international esophageal week, Munich, 1986. Demeter, Grafelfing, p 11

28. Kodama M, Shibata S, Shiogai Y, Yamagishi H, Oka T (1986) Analysis of surgical treatment of esophageal cancer for better clinical results. In: Siewert JR, Hölscher AH (eds) Abstracts of international esophageal week, Munich, 1986. Demeter, Grafelfing, p 112

29. Fekete F, Gayet B, Belghiti J, Langonnet F (1986) Survival results of thoracic esophageal carcinomas. In: Siewert JR, Hölscher AH (eds) Abstracts of international esophageal week, Munich, 1986. Demeter, Grafelfing, p 109

30. Zilberstein B, Cecconello I, Pollara WM, Pinotti HW (1986) Esophagectomy using a cervico-abdominal approach without thoracotomy for management of cancer of the esophagus. Results. In: Siewert JR, Hölscher AH (eds) Abstracts of international esophgeal week, Munich, 1986. Demeter, Grafelfing, p 70

Surgical Result of Esophageal Cancer Treated with Extended Lymph Node Dissection

Kaichi Isono, Teruo Kouzu, Kazuaki Okuyama, Akio Sakamoto, Yoshio Koide, and Takenori Ochiai[1]

Introduction

The relapse rate of esophageal cancer is high, especially at the cervical and supra-clavicular nodes [1]. This makes it difficult to hope for an improvement of long-term survival of the patient. In order to have curative operation, we initiated extensive three-field lymph node dissection, including the lymph nodes in the neck, mediastinum, and abdomen [2].

The present paper deals with the high proportion of lymph node metastasis and the clinical results of extensive lymph node dissection.

Materials and Method

A total of 542 patients with esophageal cancer received esophagectomy between 1965 and 1991. Among them, 388 patients received esophagectomy plus two-field lymph node dissection of the mediastinum and abdomen, and 154 patients received esophagectomy plus three-field lymph node dissection of the neck, mediastinum, and abdomen, The 1-month mortality rate was 6.4% for two-field and 2.6% for three-field lymph node dissection.

The survival rate curves were calculated by the generalized Wilcoxon test. The statistical difference between the groups was estimated by the X^2 test. Abbreviations and lymph node numbers are defined by the Japanese Society for Esophageal Diseases [3].

---

[1] Department of Surgery, School of Medicine, Chiba University, 1-8-1 Inohana, Chuo-ku, Chiba-shi, Chiba, Japan

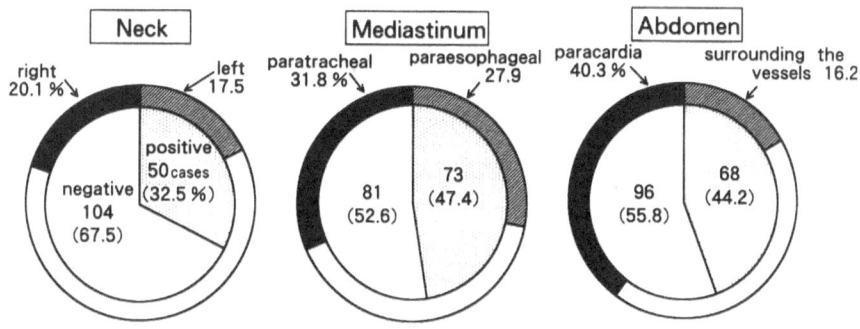

Fig. 1. Lymph node metastatic rate in relation to the field of metastasis in 154 patients receiving three-field lymph node dissection at Chiba University between 1983 and 1991

Table 1. Lymph node metastatic rate at the field of lymph node dissection in relation to cancer location (Chiba University 1983–91)

Cancer location	No. of cases	No. of metastatic cases	Field of lymph node dissection		
			neck	mediastinum	abdomen
Upper intra-thoracic	23	14	10	5	1
(*Iu*)		(60.9%)	(43.5%)	(21.7%)	(4.3%)
Middle intra-thoracic	85	63	29	41	25
(*Im*)		(71.1%)	(34.1%)	(48.2%)	(29.4%)
Lower intra-thoracic	40	27	7	13	15
(*Ei*)		(67.5%)	(17.5%)	(32.5%)	(37.5%)
abdominal (*Ea*)	6	5	2	2	5
		(83.3%)	(33.3%)	(33.3%)	(83.3%)

Results

Lymph Node Metastatic Rate in the Neck, Mediastinum, and Abdomen

Among the 154 cases receiving three-field lymph node dissection, 50 cases (32.5%), 73 cases (47.4%), and 68 cases (44.2%) showed metastatic nodes in the neck, mediastinum, and abdomen, respectively. Among the positive nodes in the neck, 17.5% were seen at the left and 20.1% were seen at the right cervical node. Paraesophageal and paratracheal nodes were metastatic in 27.9% and 31.8%, respectively. In the abdominal node, the node at the paracardia and the surrounding the vessels were metastatic in 40.3% and 16.2%, respectively (Fig. 1).

Lymph Node Metastatic Rate in Relation to Cancer Location

Table 1 shows the relationship between cancer location and lymph node metastasis in the three fields. Among the 23 cases of upper intra-thoracic (Iu)

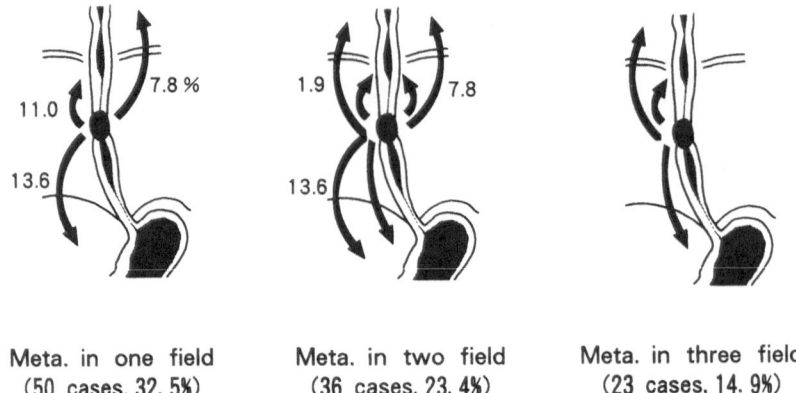

Meta. in one field (50 cases, 32. 5%)   Meta. in two field (36 cases, 23. 4%)   Meta. in three field (23 cases, 14. 9%)

Fig. 2. Lymph node metastasis to one, two, or three fields in 154 cases receiving three-field lymph node dissection. *Meta.*, metastasis

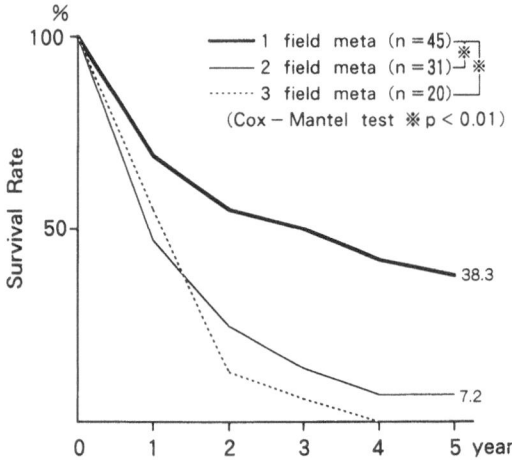

Fig. 3. Patient survival curves of patients showing one-, two-, or three-field lymph node metastasis

cancer, 14 cases (60.9%) were positive for metastasis. The fields of positive nodes were 43.5% at the neck, 21.7% at the mediastinum, and 4.3% at the abdomen.

Among the 85 middle intra-thoracic (Im) cancer, 63 cases (71.1%) were metastatic. The fields of positive nodes were 48.2% at the mediastinum, 34.1% at the neck, and 29.4% at the abdomen.

Among the 40 lower intra-thoracic (Ei) cancer, 27 cases (67.5%) were metastatic. Abdominal nodes were metastatic in 37.5%. Fifty cases (32.5%) showed metastasis to any one-field either at the neck, mediastinum, or abdomen (Fig. 2). Thirty six cases (23.4%) showed metastasis to any two fields, and 23 cases (14.9%) showed metastasis to three fields.

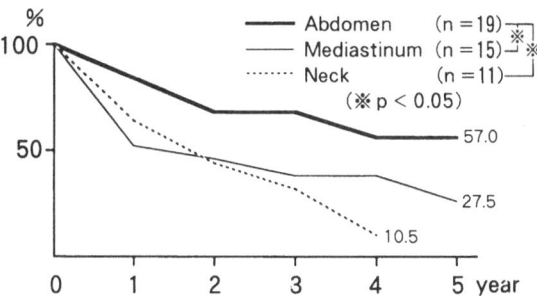

Fig. 4. Survival rate curves of patients showing metastasis to either abdominal, mediastinal, or cervical nodes

Table 2. Five-year survival rate in relation to cervical node metastasis (139 patients receiving three-field lymph node dissection—Chiba University 1983–91)

Depth of cancer Invasion	No. of cases	Meta (+)		Meta (−)		Cox-Mantel test
		(No. of 5-year survival / No. of meta cases)		(No. of 5-year survival / No. of without meta cases)		
Up to the muscularis mucosa (mm)	4	0/1		1/3	(100%)	
Involving submucosa (sm)	10	0/1		2/9	(65.8)	
Involving muscularis propria (mp)	17	0/4	(0)	4/13	(53.3)	$P < 0.001$
Invasion reaching the adventitia (a_1)	25	1/7	(16.9)	3/18	(46.8)	NS
Definite invasion (a_2)	42	0/17	(13.1)*	6/25	(34.2)	$P < 0.01$
Invasion into the neighboring structures (a_3)	30	0/9	(0)	0/21	(0)	NS
Undetermined	11	0/4	(0)*	3/7	(42.9)	NS
Total	139	1/43	(5.7)	19/96	(36.2)	$P < 0.001$

Survival Rate in Relation to Lymph Node Metastasis

Among the 154 patients receiving three-field lymph node dissection, 50 cases (32.5%) showed metastasis to one field, 36 cases (23.4%) showed metastasis to two fields, and 23 cases (14.9%) showed metastasis to all three fields (Fig. 2).

The patient survival rate curves are compared between the cases with one-field, two-field or three-field lymph node metastasis (Fig. 3). The 5-year survival rate is 38.3% in patients with one-field lymph node metastasis, 7.2% in patients with two-field lymph node metastasis, and 0% in those with three-field metastasis. The survival rate curve of patients with abdominal node metastasis were much better than patients with mediastinal or cervical node metastasis (Fig. 4).

Five-Year Survival Rate in Relation to Cervical Node Metastasis

The 5-year survival rate of 139 patients receiving three-field lymph node dissection was examined in relation to cervical node metastasis and depth of cancer invasion (Table 2). The prognosis of the patient with cervical node metastasis is poorer as compared to negative metastasis. In patients with cervical node metastasis, one patient whose cancer cells slightly invading the adventitia (a_1) survived more than 5 years.

Discussion

Surgery for thoracic and abdominal esophageal cancer includes removal of the primary lesion and lymph node dissection in the mediastinum and abdomen. In addition, radiation and chemoimmunotherapy have been performed during the pre- or postoperative periods and have improved patient survival. Nevertheless, the relapse rates at the cervical nodes have been 30%–40%, and this has been a significant obstacle to the improvement of results. Therefore, at Chiba University, we initiated extensive lymph node dissection, including the lymph nodes at neck, bilateral recurrent nerves, tracheal bifurcation, and infra-aortic arch.

The purpose of the present study was to determine the operative indications of three-field and two-field lymph node dissection by analysis of the treatment results. It was also intended to determine the area of frequent metastatic nodes and, based on that, the necessity of dissection of the node.

There are both merits and demerits to three-field lymph node dissection. One merit was improvement of the patient survival rate. The 5-year survival rate increased to 10% as compared with the results of two-field lymph node dissection. However, the demerits are: (1) the operation itself is local therapy; (2) the surgical procedure is invasive; (3) some complications such as recurrent nerve paralysis are frequent; and (4) three-field lymph node dissection is not applicable to all cases.

References

1. Isono K, Onoda S, Okuyama K, Sato H (1985) Recurrence of intrathoracic esophageal cancer. Jpn J Clin Oncol 15:49–60
2. Isono K, Sato H, Nakayama K (1991) Results of a nationwide study on the three-field lymph node dissection of esophageal cancer. Oncology 48:411–420
3. Japanese Society for Esophageal Diseases (1976) Guidelines for the Clinical and Pathologic Studies on Carcinoma of the Esophagus. Jpn J Surg 6:69–78

Pulse Oximetry for Assessment of Gastric Tube Circulation in Esophageal Replacement After Subtotal Esophagectomy

J. Salo, H. Savolainen, and L. Heikkilä[1]

Introduction

Due to its simplicity, the stomach is widely used as a substitute following an esophageal resection, particularly in malignant diseases. In cancer patients, the smaller curvature of the stomach is resected, and the left gastric, gastroepiploic and the short gastric arteries are ligated to enhance surgical radicality and to achieve added length on the esophageal conduit [1]. This technique demands extensive gastric mobilization using the Kocher manoeuver followed by an anastomosis in the neck between the esophageal remnant and the highest point of the gastric fundus. This, however, may compromise the circulation of the anastomotic area of the fundus and results in anastomotic leakage and stricture. Clinically, the fundic circulation may be difficult to assess since the fundus is vascularized only via a nonvisible submucosal plexus [2].

Pulse oximeters are widely used in the continuous assessment of arterial oxygenation in anesthetized patients. They measure the percentage of O_2 saturation of hemoglobin in the presence of a pulsating vascular bed [3, 4]. Pulse oximeters have also been used earlier in evaluating bowel perfusion in abdominal operations [5–7], but until recently, there have been no reports regarding the use of pulse oximeters in assessing the viability of the gastric tube as an esophageal replacement.

Material and Methods

Between 1990 and 1992, at the Department of Thoracic and Cardiovascular Surgery, Helsinki University Central Hospital, 32 consecutive patients, undergoing subtotal esophagectomy and cervical esophagogastric anastomosis, had

---

[1] Department of Thoracic and Cardiovascular Surgery Helsinki University Central Hospital Haartmaninkatu 4, SF-00290 Helsinki, Finland

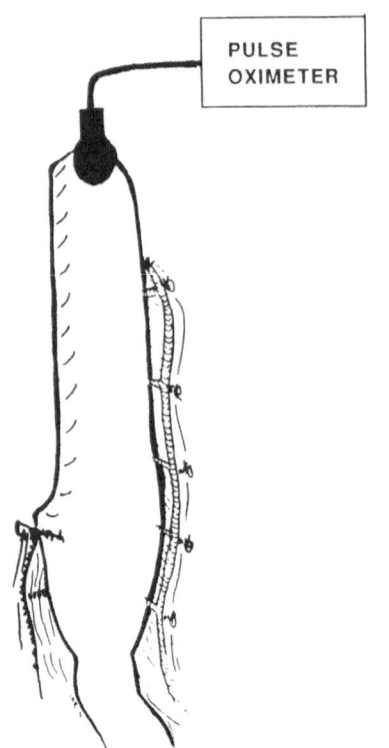

Fig. 1. Measurement of O_2-saturation in the anastomotic area of the gastric tube

PULSE
OXIMETER

the viability of the gastric tube esophageal replacement assessed, using pulse oximetry. Of these patients, 31 had cancer of the esophagus, and 1 had Barrett's esophagus with severe dysplasia. The mean age of the patients was 63 years, with a range of 43–79 years. All operations were performed under general anesthesia (isofluorane). The subtotal esophagectomy was performed using the transhiatal technique without thoracotomy [8] in 17 patients and 15 patients had transthoracic esophageal resection with mediastinal lymphadenectomy. The cervical esophagogastric anastomosis was performed to the left.

At operation, the preparation for the esophageal substitute included resecting the lesser curvature of the stomach and ligating the left gastric and gastroepiploic arteries. The short gastric vessels were also ligated. The viability of the gastric tube was detemined first clinically and thereafter with a pulse oximeter (Ohmeda, BOC Group Inc. USA). A sterile oximeter probe was applied intraoperatively and serosally to the proximal end of the gastric tube oral to the pylorus, to the middle of the gastric tube and to the intended anastomotic area of the fundus (Fig. 1). The saturation readings at each of these points were recorded approximately 20 s later. The O_2 saturation of the earlobe was used as reference in all patients. On the 7th or 8th postoperative day, the anastomosis in all patients was examined radiographically, using a water soluble contrast medium (Gastrografin) before initiating oral nutrition. A routine postoperative endoscopic follow-up-examination of the upper gastrointestinal tract (esophageal stump, anastomosis, gastric tube and proximal duodenum) was performed one to three months later in all surviving patients.

Results

In four patients, low oxygen saturation (<80%) was measured in the anastomotic area or 3–8 cm below that point. At inspection, this area appeared slightly cyanotic indicating venous engorgement. The nonperfused area was resected, and an anastomosis was performed where an oxygen saturation of 85%–90% was subsequently measured. The remaining 28 patients showed an oxygen saturation of 84%–95% in the anastomotic area of the fundus. In all patients, the oxygen saturation in the middle of the gastric tube and in the pyloric region, were slightly higher than in the fundic area. The earlobe showed O_2-saturation values of 95%–100% in all patients during the operation.

No anastomotic leaks were found on the x-ray examinations performed within 10 postoperative days. However, two patients had late anastomotic fistulas, which closed spontaneously. The oxygen saturation of the anastomotic area was 85% and 90% in these patients. All patients also underwent an endoscopic examination 1–3 months later. In three patients, a relative anastomotic stricture, one requiring dilatation, was diagnosed. These patients had oxygen saturations of 84%, 85% and 94% at the anastomotic area. The operative mortality was two patients in this study.

Discussion

Inadequate blood supply and subsequent anastomotic necrosis is probably one of the main causes of anastomotic leaks. Other factors include incomplete surgical technique, infection and perhaps, the poor general condition of the patient [9]. Clinically, assessment of the fundic blood supply may be difficult, since the fundus is vascularized only via a nonvisible submucosal plexus [2]. Slight venous engorgement, which is often present in the mobilized gastric tube, may also render the clinical evaluation of the anastomotic viability. In postmortem corrosion cast studies, Liebermann-Meffert et al. [10] found that vascularization of the uppermost 20% of the gastric tube is only through the microvascular net of the submucous vascular plexus, and is therefore very poor. Thus, they recommend resection of a 6- to 8-cm section of the cranial part of gastric tube. This procedure, however, may shorten the conduit length, so that a cervical anastomosis is no longer possible. The reliability of the pulse oximeter in the assessment of intestinal perfusion has been evaluated by Ferrara et al. [5]. They found that the pulse oximeter compared favorably with intravenous fluorescein studies, and that the pulse oximeter was superior when compared to standard clinical criteria and doppler ultrasound, in intestines compromised by arterial occlusion. The present study also shows that the circulation of the gastric tube used as an esophageal replacement, is easily assessed by pulse oximeter, which is available in almost all operating rooms. The drawback of pulse oximetry is instrument-dependent variation in the presence of hypoxemia.

References

1. Akiyama H, Tsurumaru M, Kawamura T, Oho Y (1981) Principles of surgical treatment for carcinoma of the esophagus. Ann Surg 194:438–446
2. Thomas DM, Langford RM, Russell RCG, Le Quesne (1979) The anatomical basis for gastric mobilization in total oesophagectomy. Br J Surg 66:230–233
3. Yelderman M, New Jr. W (1983) Evaluation of pulse oximetry. Anesthesiology 59:349–352
4. Kidd JF, Vickers MD (1989) Pulse oximeters: Essential monitors with limitations (editorial). Br J Anaesth 62:355–357
5. Ferrara JJ, Dyess DL, Lasecki M, Kinsey S, Donnell C, Jurkovich GJ (1988) Surface oximetry. A new method to evaluate intestinal perfusion. Am Surg 54:10–14
6. DeNobile J, Guzzetta P, Patterson K (1991) Pulse oximetry as a means of assessing bowel viability. J Surg Res 48:21–23
7. Ouriel K, Fiore WM, Geary JE (1988) Detection of occult colonic ischemia during aortic procedures: Use of an intraoperative photoplethysmographic technique. J Vasc Surg 7:5–9
8. Orringer MB (1984) Transhiatal esophagectomy without thoracotomy for carcinoma of the thoracic esophagus. Ann Surg 200:282–286
9. Peracchia A, Bardini R, Ruol A, Asolati M, Scibetta D (1988) Esophagovisceral anastomotic leak. J Thorac Cardiovasc Surg 95:685–691
10. Liebermann-Meffert D, Raschke M, Siewert JR (1989) How well vascularized is a gastric tube from the greater curvature? Fourth world congress of the International Society for Diseases of the Esophagus. Chicago, Abstract book.

Transmediastinal Esophagectomy: Comparison of Cardiopulmonary Performance After Anterior Versus Posterior Reconstruction

H. Bartels, S. Thorban, and J.R. Siewert[1]

Introduction

Cardiopulmonary complications remain one of the leading factors in post-operative morbidity and mortality following esophagectomy. To reduce these complications, new surgical methods like limited transmediastinal resection [1], endodissection of the esophagus [2] or transthoracic resection with delayed reconstruction have been evaluated [3].

Does route of reconstruction, i.e., anterior vs. posterior reconstruction, show different effects on cardiopulmonary performance following transmediastinal esophagectomy? To answer this question, we performed a controlled, prospective randomized study.

Patients

The study was performed between Oct. 1, 1986 and Dec. 31, 1988. Included were all patients with esophageal carcinoma who had a transmediastinal eso-phagectomy and reconstruction by gastric interposition. Patients who required a colon interposition, patients with preoperative radio/chemotherapy and patients with incomplete tumor resection (R1/R2-resection) were excluded. A total of 96 patients met the inclusion criteria. After informed consent, the route of recon-struction was chosen preoperatively in a random fashion. Fifty-one patients had reconstruction in the anterior mediastinum while 45 were reconstructed in the posterior mediastinum.

Concerning age, tumor type, tumor stage and preoperative risk analysis, there was no difference between the two patient groups (Table 1). All patients had Ro-resection, i.e., complete macroscopic and microscopic tumor removal.

[1] Department of Surgery, Technical University Munich, Klinikum rechts der Isar, Ismaningerstr. 22, D-8000 München 80, Germany

623

Table 1. Age, tumor type, tumor stage, and preoperative risk factors of the 96 patients in the study

	Gastric interposition		Patients (total) (*n*)
	Ant. Mediast. Group 1 (*n*)	Post. Mediast. Group 2 (*n*)	
Patients (*n*)	51	45	96
Age (x) years	61.5	59.2	60.8
Adenocarcinoma Distal esophagus	43	36	79
Squamous cell carcinoma	8	9	17
TU-stage (UICC)			
I	7	8	15
IIa	9	10	19
IIb	10	11	21
III	25	16	41
Risk			
Respiratory	14 (27.4%)	12 (26.7%)	26 (27%)
Cardiac	6 (11.8%)	4 (8.9%)	10 (10.4%)
Hepatic	6 (11.8%)	5 (11.1%)	11 (11.5%)
ASA I+II	28 (54.9%)	24 (53.3%)	52 (54.2%)
ASA >III	23 (45.1%)	21 (46.7%)	44 (45.8%)

TU, Tumor; *UICC*, Union International Cancer Classification; *ASA*, American Society of Anesthesia; *ant*, anterior; *post*, posterior; *Mediast*, mediastinal

Methods

Transmediastinal esophagectomy was performed in a standardized fashion described previously [4, 5]. After blunt dissection the gastric tube, created parallel to the major curvature [6, 7] was interposed either retrosternally (anterior mediastinum) or in the esophageal bed (posterior mediastinum). Postoperative management included positive end-expiratory pressure (PEEP) ventilation for at least 48 h in all patients [8]. Cardiopulmonary function was assessed by femoral artery catheter and balloon-tipped pulmonary artery catheter (Swan-Ganz).

Cardiac output was measured by the thermodilution technique (model 9520, American Edwards Laboratories). Arterial and pulmonary arterial (mixed venous) blood gases, pH and saturations were measured by blood gas systems (model 288, CIBA Corning Diagnostics).

The following parameters and derived values were recorded: Heart rate (HR), pulmonary artery pressure (PAP), systemic artery pressure (SAP), central venous pressure (CVP), pulmonary capillary wedge pressure (PCWP), cardiac index (CI), stroke volume index (SVI), left ventricular stroke work index (LVSWI), systemic vascular resistence index (SVRI), pulmonary vascular resistance index (PVRI), pulmonary shunt fraction (Q_S/Q_T), respiratory index (RI), oxygen delivery (DO_2), and oxygen consumption (VO_2).

Measurements were taken the day before surgery, 2 h postoperative, and then every 12 h until extubation took place [7].

All intra- and postoperative data (duration of anesthesia, blood loss, cardio-pulmonary function, days in the intensive care unit (ICU) etc.), postoperative complications and mortality were documented prospectively and evaluated in a retrospective fashion at the end of the study. Student's t-test, Wilcoxon-test and Chi^2-test were used for statistical evaluation. A P-value <0.05 was considered significant.

Results

The relevant data for hemodynamic and gas exchange values are shown in Figs. 1–3. In both groups, the intrapulmonary shunt fraction (Q_S/Q_T) was markedly increased during the immediate postoperative time as compared to preoperative values (Fig. 1). The peak in shunt volume was seen at 12 h after the procedure. Compared to reconstruction in the anterior mediastinum, respiratory function following the procedure was less compromised in patients who had reconstruction in the posterior mediastinum. This difference was significant at 24 h postoperatively.

In addition, the cardiac index was significantly decreased throughout the first 36 postoperative hours in patients who had reconstruction in the anterior mediastinum (Fig. 2). This decrease in cardiac index was primarily due to

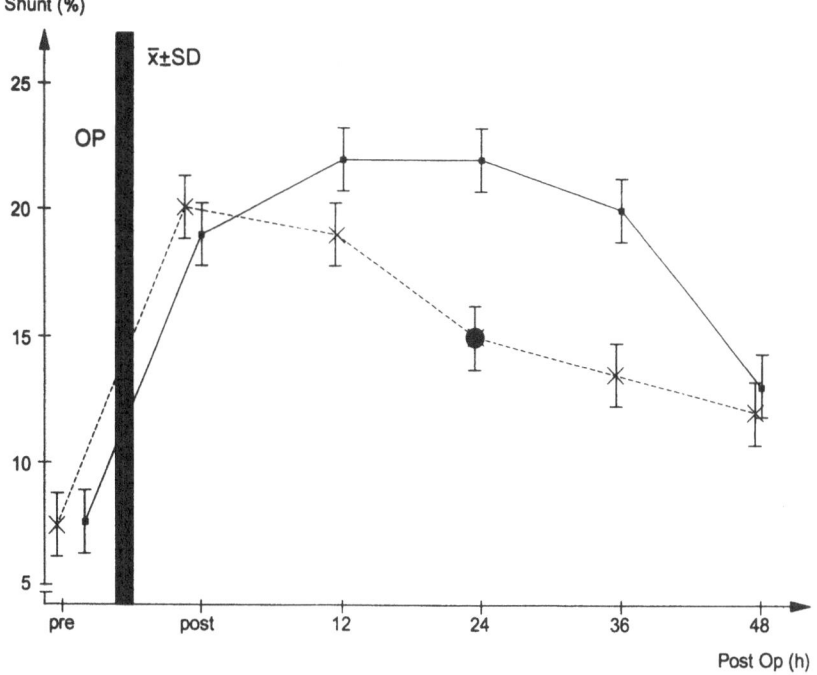

Fig. 1. Intrapulmonary right/left-shunt (Q_S/Q_T) following transmediastinal esophagectomy. *Solid squares*, anterior mediastinum (group 1, $n = 45$); X, posterior mediastinum (group 2, $n = 45$) *$P<0.05$ group 1 vs. group 2

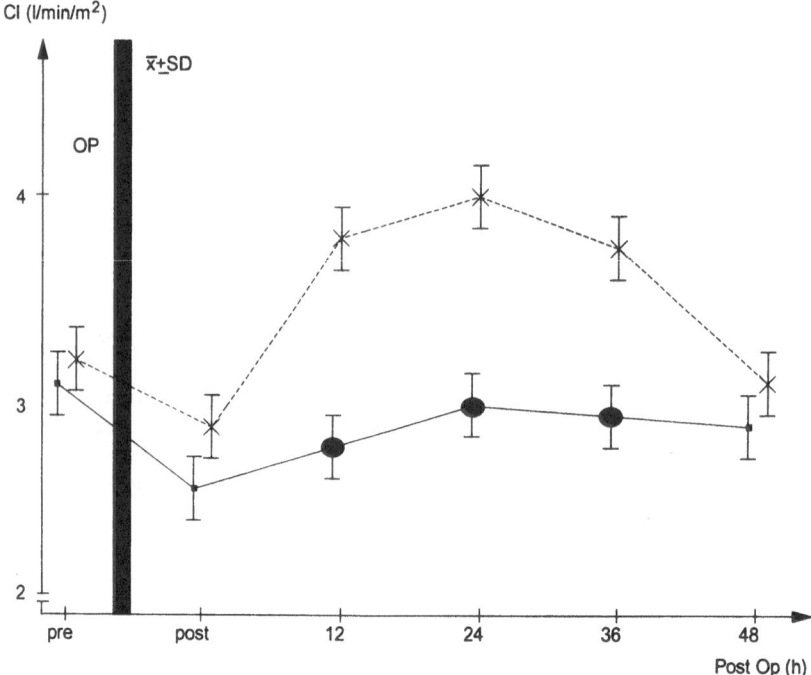

Fig. 2. Cardiac index *(CI)* following transmediastinal esophagectomy. *Solid squares*, anterior, mediastinum (group 1); *X*, posterior mediastinum (group 2) *$P < 0.05$ group 1 vs. group 2

reduction in stroke volume index, which was compromised throughout the postoperative monitoring period in these patients (Fig. 3). All hemodynamic and respiratory parameters returned to preoperative values after 48 h.

The clinical data are shown in Table 2. Duration of anesthesia, intraoperative blood loss and postoperative ventilation were similar in both groups; but compared to patients who had reconstruction in the anterior mediastinum, reconstruction in the posterior mediastinum was associated with fewer days in the ICU (9.3 days vs. 13.7 days), a decresed frequency of general complications (13.3% vs. 25%), and a lower mortality rate (2.2% vs. 5.9%).

Discussion

Following transmediastinal esophagectomy, reconstruction in the anterior mediastinum was considered superior because it allows postoperative radiation of the esophageal bed in case of local recurrence of the tumor [5]. However, tumor recurrence was found to rarely cause obstruction of the interposed organ. Furthermore, according to improvement in patients selection and resection techniques, the rate of complete tumor resection has increased to more than 90%. In these patients, the rate of local recurrence has decreased to below 10% [2].

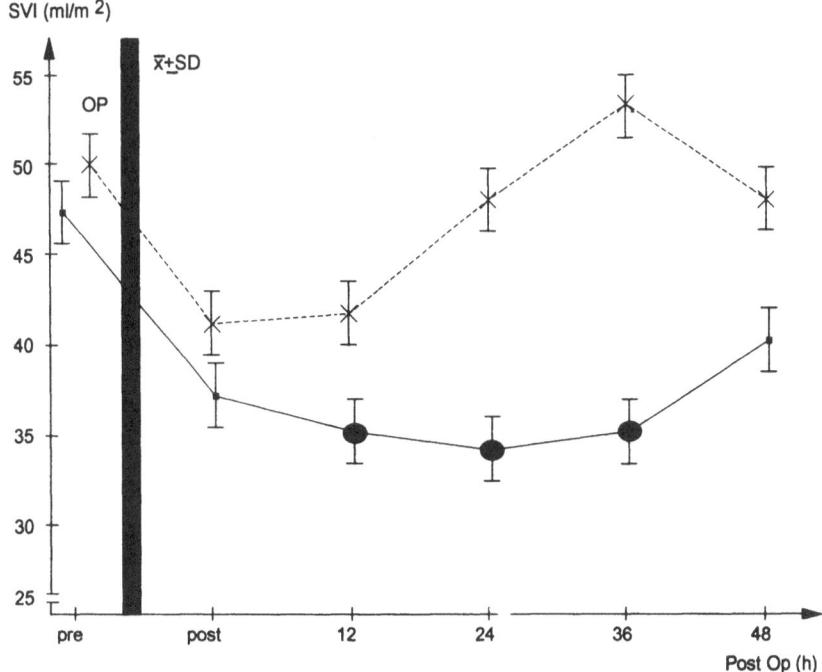

Fig. 3. Stroke volume index (*SVI*) following transmediastinal esophagectomy. *Solid squares,* anterior mediastinum (group 1); *X,* posterior mediastinum (group 2) *$P < 0.05$ group 1 vs. group 2

Due to patient selection and the higher rate of Ro-resections, local tumor recurrences were not likely in our patient population [2]. A random preoperative allocation of the route of reconstruction could therefore be justified for the present study. According to randomisation protocol, 51 patients had reconstruction in the anterior mediastinum while 45 were reconstructed in the posterior mediastinum.

Reconstruction of gastrointestinal continuity by a gastric tube in the mediastinum results in mechanical compression of the adjacent lung [8]. In the present study, this was reflected by an increase in the intrapulmonary right/left shunt (Q_S/Q_T) during the early postoperative period. This indicated more or less trauma to the lung by retrocardial manipulation during blunt dissection of the esophagus. In an experimental study, Niederle [9] has shown a significant rise in shunt fraction following transmediastinal esophagectomy compared to the transthoracic approach. Nevertheless, a lower complication rate has been repeatedly claimed for transmediastinal esophagectomy as compared to a transthoracic approach [1]. To date, a decreased risk for transhiatal esophagectomy could, however, not be confirmed in clinical trials [2, 3].

Analysis of respiratory function in our patients showed differences in respiratory function between the two routes of reconstruction (Fig. 1). The anterior reconstruction was associated with delay in normalisation of intrapulmonary

Table 2. Intra/postoperative data, complications and mortality of the 96 patients in the study

		Gastric interposition		Total ($n = 96$)
		Ant. Mediast. Group 1 ($n = 51$)	Post. Mediast. Group 2 ($n = 45$)	
Duration of anesthesia	(h)	5.1	4.9	(n.s.)
Blood loss	(U)	2.5	2.4	(n.s.)
Postop. ventilation	(h)	49.3	49.7	(n.s.)
Days in ICU	(d)	13.7	9.3	($P < 0.05$)
Hospital stay	(d)	24.3	23.8	(n.s.)
Surgical complications				
Anastom. leak		5 (9.8%)	5 (11.1%)	10 (10.4%)
Sepsis		2 (3.9%)	2 (4.4%)	4 (4.2%)
Other		4 (7.8%)	3 (6.7%)	7 (7.3%)
Total		11 (21.5%)	10 (22%)	21 (21.8%)
General complications				
Respiratory		7 (13.7%)	4 (8.9%)	11 (11.4%)
Cardiac		5 (9.8%)	1	6 (6.3%)
Hepatic		1	1	2 (2.1%)
Total		13 (25%)	6 (13.3%)	21 (21.8%)
Mortality				
30-day		3 (5.9%)	1 (2.2%)	4 (4.2%)

ICU, intensive care unit; *anastom*, anastomosis; *n.s.*, not significant

right/left shunt (Q_S/Q_T). This appears to be caused by compression of the right ventral portion of the lung.

The two routes of reconstruction in our study showed marked differences in hemodynamic function. The cardiac index, the most important cardiac parameter, dropped immediately following the surgical procedure. This drop was similar in both groups of patients and was probably secondary to hypoxia and the negative inotropic effect of anesthesia [8, 9]. Compared to reconstruction in the posterior mediastinum, reconstruction in the anterior mediastinum was, however, associated with a marked delay in normalisation of the cardiac index during the first postoperative days (Fig. 2). Obstruction of the right ventricle by the interposed gastric tube, paradox movements of the septum and the resulting compromise in the stroke volume index count for this observation [9].

Is reconstruction in the anterior mediastinum superior to posterior reconstruction after a transmediastinal esophagectomy? Our study shows no differences in blood loss, duration of postoperative ventilation, and surgical complications (Table 2). Reconstruction in the posterior mediastinum, however, had some major advantages. These are:

1. a lower rate of cardiorespiratory complications
2. a shorter stay in the ICU
3. a decreased 30-day mortality

In summary, the present study documents the superiority of reconstruction in the posterior mediastinum following transmediastinal esophagectomy. Compared to reconstruction in the anterior mediastinum, this route of reconstruction also was associated with a lower mortality and morbidity. Provided a Ro-resection has been performed, posterior reconstruction should be the procedure of choice particularly in patients with increased cardiorespiratory risk.

References

1. Orringer MB, Orringer JS (1985) Esophagectomy without thoracotomy: A dangerous operation? J.Thorac Cardiovasc Surg 85:72–80
2. Siewert JR, Bartels H, Bollschweiler E, Dittler HJ, Fink U, Hölscher AH, Roder JD (to be published) Therapiekonzepte beim Plattenepithelcarcinom der Speiseröhre. Chirurg
3. Siewert JR, Adolf J, Hölscher AH, Hölscher M, Weiser HF (1986) Oesophaguscarcinom: Transthorakale Oesophagektomie mit regionaler Lymphadenektomie und Rekonstruktion mit aufgeschobener Dringlichkeit. Dtsch Med Wschr 111:647–651
4. Akiyama H, Hiyama M, Myazazoo H (1975) Total esophageal reconstruction after extraction of the esophagus. Ann Surg 182:547–553
5. Siewert JR, Hölscher AH, Horvath ÖP (1986) Transmediastinale Oesophagektomie. Langenbecks Arch Chir 367:203–213
6. Akiyama H, Tsurumaru M, Kawamura T, Ono Y (1981) Principles of surgical treatment for carcinoma of the esophagus. Ann Surg 194:438–446
7. Liebermann-Meffert D, Siewert JR (to be published) Vascularisation of the gastric tube used for oesophageal replacement. Ann Thor Surg
8. Bartels H, Siewert JR (1988) Postoperative Intensivüberwachung nach Oesophagektomie. Z. Herz-, Thorax-, Gefäßchir 2:131–134
9. Niederle B, Burghuber OC, Roka R, Khosropour R, Lackner F (1987) Influence of transthoracic and transmediastinal esophagectomy and of various degrees of gastric filling on cardiopulmonary function. In: Siewert JR, Holscher AH (eds) Diseases of the esophagus, Springer, Berlin Heidelberg New York London Paris Tokyo, pp 237–244
10. Siewert JR, Hölscher AH, Roder J, Bartels H (1988) En-bloc Resektion der Speiseröhre beim Osophagus-Carcinom. Langenbecks Arch Chir 373:367–376.

Cancer of the Cervical Esophagus: Extent of Resection, Short- and Long-Term Results of Surgery

A. Peracchia[1], A. Ruol[2], R. Bardini[2], S. Narne[3], A. Segalin[2],
C. Castoro[2], E. Tiso[2], and S. Lazzaro[2]

Introduction

Several types of cancer can be found in the cervical esophageal region: cancer of the cervical esophagus, the hypopharynx, and recurrent or persistent ENT cancers after radiotherapy or surgery.

Tumors of the hypopharynx and cervical esophagus are often diagnosed in the late stages. These tumors can infiltrate the thyroid cartilage, recurrent laryngeal nerves, thyroid gland, or trachea, and frequently give metastases to regional lymph nodes (50%–70% of all cases). Metastases can be found bilaterally in the cervical paraesophageal, deep cervical, recurrential, paratracheal, and supraclavicular nodes. Also, the mediastinal nodes can be involved, especially in cancers of the cervical esophagus.

To date, the results of radiotherapy have been disappointing as local control and survival are low, and most patients develop significant complications or require salvage surgery [1].

Surgery is the mainstay of treatment [2]. However, postoperative complications are frequent, may be life-threatening, and often require additional surgical procedures. After surgery, local recurrence is frequent and represents the first cause of death; most local recurrences are in fact regrowth of residual disease left in situ during surgery [3, 4].

Submucosal spread along the esophagus is possible up to 3 cm in cancers of the hypopharynx, and up to 5 cm in cancers of the cervical esophagus [4]. The

[1] Department of General Surgery, Hospital Policlinico, Monteggia, University of Milan, Via Sforza, 35, 20122 Milano, Italy
[2] Department of General Surgery, University of Padua, Via Giustiniani 2, Padoua, Italy
[3] Emergency Endoscopic Service, University of Padua Ospedale Giustinianeo, Via Giustiniani 2, Padoua, Italy

treatment strategy for cancer of the hypopharynx and cervical esophagus is also conditioned by the high frequency of multiple primaries (6%–28%), most of which involve the upper aerodigestive tract [5].

Requirements of Surgical Treatment

Adequacy of resection is most important in surgery of cancers of the hypopharynx and cervical esophagus. The site and extension of cancer should dictate the size and type of pharyngo-laryngo-esophageal resection, which in turn should dictate the type of reconstruction procedure [6]. High tumors of the hypopharynx can be treated by ENT surgeons by means of partial pharyngectomy and laryngectomy. Low tumors of the hypopharynx (including tumors of the pyriform fossa apex, posterior wall, and postcricoid region) require circumferential pharyngectomy and laryngectomy. When both the hypopharynx and cervical esophagus are involved, the resection should include a circumferential pharyngectomy, laryngectomy and partial esophagectomy with at least 3 cm of resection clearance beyond the tumor. High tumors of the cervical esophagus require total pharyngo-laryngo-esophagectomy. Total esophagectomy with larynx preservation may be proposed in carefully selected patients with cancer of the distal cervical esophagus when there is a safety margin of at least 2–3 cm [4]. Another indication for larynx preservation may be a tumor treated with neoadjuvant chemotherapy or chemo-radiotherapy when adequate downstaging is obtained.

Pharyngo-laryngo-esophagectomy should include also total thyroidectomy, parathyroidectomy, and bilateral neck dissection with preservation of the jugular veins and sternocleidomastoid muscles.

Total esophagectomy is indicated [7] for the great majority of tumors of the cervical esophagus, and also for tumors of the hypopharynx when the tumor is impervious to endoscopy, has a submucosal diffusion along the thoracic esophagus, or is in the presence of a synchronous malignancy of the thoracic esophagus or cardia. Segmental cervical esophagectomy is indicated for cancers of the hypopharynx, and for selected small tumors of the proximal cervical esophagus provided that at least 3 cm of uninvolved esophagus are resected [8]. To perform partial esophagectomy, it is necessary that the tumor is pervious to endoscopy in order to rule out the presence of tumor submucosal spread or a synchronous tumor in the thoracic esophagus.

Personal Experience

Since 1967, we have observed 375 cancers involving the hypopharynx and cervical esophagus. Of these, 126 patients underwent total pharyngo-laryngo-esophagectomy. The gastric pull-up reconstruction technique was used in 109 cases, and the colon interposition technique in 17. The hospital mortality rate was 15.6% after pharyngo-gastrostomy, and 17.6% after pharyngo-colostomy. Thirty three patients underwent pharyngo-laryngo-segmental cervical esophagectomy and free jejunal or colon loop autotransplant with vascular micro-anastomoses; the hospital mortality rate was 6%. Twenty four more patients underwent miscellaneous surgical procedures.

Since 1980, clinical data have been prospectively collected and computer-stored and analyzed. Between 1980 and 1990, 291 patients with cancer of the cervical esophageal region were observed: 187 cancers of the cervical esophagus, 76 cancers of the hypopharynx, and 28 recurrent cancers of the larynx (after laryngectomy) involving the esophagus. Most tumors of the hypopharynx also involved the upper portion of the cervical esophagus.

Seventy-five of 291 (26%) of the patients had multiple synchronous or meta-chronous multiple malignancies, which were located in the upper aerodigestive tract in 63 (21.6%) of the patients. Synchronous cancers were detected in 34 (12%) of the patients. The fact that 10% of the patients (30/291) had a synchronous tumor in the upper aerodigestive tract influenced significantly the extent of resection and the cytoreductive treatment plan.

153 of 291 patients (53%) underwent surgical resection: 127 resections were curative or R0, and 26 palliative or R1–2.

106 patients underwent total pharyngo-laryngo-esophagectomy. The phar-yngoesophageal defect was reconstructed using the gastric pull-up technique in 95 cases, and a colon interposition in 11. The first choice viscus for the recon-struction after total pharyngo-laryngo-esophagectomy was the stomach since it allows long defects to be covered, is suitable also for patients with cancer spread or synchronous cancers in the thoracic esophagus, and entails lower postoperative morbidity and mortality rates than colon interposition. Colon interposition was used in patients who had previously undergone gastric operations or with concomitant gastric diseases.

To lengthen the stomach in order to easily reach the level of the hypopharynx to perform the anastomosis, at first we used a thin gastric tube. Thereafter, to preserve the intramural vascular network of the stomach and to reduce the likelihood of ischemic problems, we began using the stomach tubulized along the points where the vessels of the lesser curvature enter the stomach wall, according to Akiyama's [9] technique. At present, we prefer to use the whole stomach, as described by Collard [10]: the lesser omentum is dissected close to the lesser curvature, without using a linear stapler, according to the highly selective vagotomy technique. This technique allows the stomach to be lengthened preserving the integrity of the submucosal vascular network which provides an excellent blood supply at the top of the pulled-up stomach.

Hospital mortality rate after pharyngogastrostomy was 14.7% (14/95), and after pharyngocolostomy 18% (2/11).

The incidence of anastomotic leakage, including both clinical and asymptomatic-radiologically detected leaks, was 23% (22/95) in pharyngogastric anastomoses, and 18% (2/11) in pharyngocolic anastomoses. Most anastomotic leakages were treated conservatively by means of drainage, naso-gastric or naso-colic tube suctioning, parenteral or enteral nutrition, and broad-spectrum antibiotics. Four of the 20 patients with a leakage who were treated conservatively died. The severity of the leakage required prompt reoperation in four patients, one of whom died. The following reoperations were performed: reanastomosis in one case, T-tube drainage plus delayed skin flap repair in one case, and cervical diversion plus delayed closure of the partial stoma in two patients. This reopera-tion consists of the take-down of the anastomosis and the resuture of the posterior wall of the anastomosis, while the anterior aspect of the anastomosis is circumferentially sutured to the skin. A temporary partial stoma is thus created in the neck. After 3–4 weeks, the cervical stoma is closed by incising and rotating the adjacent skin which will form the anterior wall of the anastomosis. In the same operative session, the anastomosis is covered by direct skin suturing or using a pedicled skin flap or a myocutaneous flap.

Segmental or total necrosis of the esophageal substitute was recorded in 10.5% of the cases after gastric pull-up (10/95), and in 18% of the cases after colon interposition (2/11). Reoperation was necessary in all the cases, and consisted in the take-down of the anastomosis, resection of the necrotic segment, and temporary cervical diversion with delayed reestablishment of the continuity of the alimentary tract, according to the technique previously described.

As far as gastric pull-ups are concerned, eight patients underwent resection of the necrotic segment of the stomach, temporary cervical diversion, and delayed reestablishment of the continuity of the alimentary tract; four of these patients died. One patient underwent successful take-down of the stomach and colon interposition. One patient died of neoplastic recurrence after the establishment of two cervical stomas plus delayed free jejunal loop transplant with skin flap coverage.

As far as colon interpositions are concerned, the two patients with necrosis were treated by means of colon loop take-down and the establishment of cervical and abdominal stomas, but both died before reconstruction.

An anastomotic stricture developed in 8 pharyngogastric anastomoses: 7 were dilated successfully and one required revision of the anastomosis.

The following miscellaneous complications which required additional surgical procedures occurred in patients undergoing pharyngogastrostomy or pharyngocolostomy. A patient with the azygos vein torn during transhiatal esophagectomy required immediate transthoracic hemostasis. In a patient who had the stomach too short to reach the pharynx, two temporary cervical stomas were performed but he died of recurrence before reconstruction. In a patient undergoing gastric pull-up, the right gastroepiploic vascularization was torn so that the operation had to be shifted into a colon interposition. In a patient undergoing colon interposition, a segmentary ischemia of the colon became evident in the neck during the operation so that the necrotic segment was resected and a free jejunal loop was transplanted to cover the gap between the pharynx and the colon loop. A patient undergoing colon interposition showed defective venous drainage of the colon, which was successfully managed by means of venous microanastomoses in the neck. A patient developed chylothorax in the postoperative period and required transthoracic duct ligation.

Eighteen patients underwent laryngopharyngo-segmental cervical esophagectomy and free jejunal loop transplant. Hospital mortality was nil, and only one anastomotic leakage was recorded.

Twenty-four patients underwent total esophagectomy with larynx preservation either as primary procedure or after preoperative chemotherapy or chemoradiotherapy. To assess whether the proximal margin of section is involved by cancer, the cervical esophagus was routinely opened, checked, and stained with toluidine blue. In these cases, the anastomosis was performed at the level of the pyriform fossa. Gastric pull-up was the preferred reconstruction technique. Hospital mortality was 8.3% (2/24). Five anastomotic leakages, and 2 necroses of the esophageal substitute were recorded. Despite the fact that the larynx was preserved, a temporary or definitive tracheostomy had to be performed in several patients because of pharyngeal incoordination or intraoperative lesioning of the recurrent laryngeal nerves.

Finally, five patients underwent miscellaneous surgical procedures with one postoperative death.

Overall, 75% of the patients with cancer of the hypopharynx and 87% of the patients with cancer of the cervical esophagus underwent preoperative and/or postoperative chemotherapy or chemo-radiotherapy.

Long-Term Prognosis

The location of the tumor was the most important prognostic factor: the 5-year survival rate after curative resection for hypopharynx and cervical esophageal cancer was 37% and 18%, respectively.

The survival after curative resection was also related to the lymph node status: according to the absence or presence of lymph node metastasis, respectively, it was 43% and 25% for hypopharynx cancers, and 24% and 13% for cancers of the cervical esophagus.

While the 5-year survival rate after curative resection was 21%, the 3-year survival after palliative resection, after esophagectomy with larynx preservation, and after surgery in patients with a previous laryngectomy for cancer was 0%.

Multimodality Treatments

The therapeutic role of preoperative chemotherapy and chemo-radiotherapy has been receiving more and more attention in recent years. However, the possible advantages of these multimodality treatments in terms of improved survival should be considered with caution due to the increased risk of postoperative morbidity and mortality.

In our experience, 16 of 32 patients with an inoperable locally advanced cancer of the cervical esophagus or hypopharynx had a downstaging of the tumor and could undergo surgical resection after 2–4 cycles of chemotherapy with cisplatin ($100\,mg/m^2$ on day 1) and 5-Fluorouracil ($1000\,mg/m^2$ on days 1 through 5). Thirteen curative resections and 3 palliative resections were performed. In these patients, the postoperative mortality rate was slightly greater than after surgery alone: 3 of 16 (18.7%). The 4-year actuarial survival rate after preoperative chemotherapy and curative resection is 61%, which is promising if it is considered that these patients initially had a locally advanced, inoperable tumor.

Twenty-seven patients with a potentially resectable cancer of the hypopharynx and cervical esophagus were treated with two cycles of neoadjuvant chemo-radiotherapy (cisplatin $100\,mg/m^2$ on day 1, split course irradiation on days 1 through 5). At surgery, the tumor could be resected in 25 patients, 1 patient refused the operation, and 1 was inoperable because of progressive disease. Curative resection was performed in 21 patients, and palliative resection in 4. In seven patients, it was possible to preserve the larynx. Hospital mortality after surgery (6/25 or 24%) was almost double that of patients undergoing surgery alone, and the incidence of anastomotic leakage was very high (52% or 13/25).

After neoadjuvant chemo-radiotherapy and curative resection, the actuarial 2-and 3-year survival rates were 93% and 79%, respectively.

Conclusions

At present, cancers involving the hypopharynx and cervical esophagus can undergo surgical resection at a reasonably low operative risk and with a hope of long-term survival.

Adequate local-regional control can be achieved with pharyngolaryngo-total esophagectomy plus bilateral neck dissection. Pharyngolaryngo-segmental cervical esophagectomy and total esophagectomy with larynx preservation may be proposed in carefully selected cases. Gastric pull-up represents the first choice reconstruction technique.

While the incidence of anastomotic leakage and necrosis can be reduced using an appropriate surgical technique, most leaks can be managed conservatively. Reoperations often require familiarity with the use of free jejunal loop transplants and cutaneous or myocutaneous flaps.

The results of preoperative chemotherapy and chemo-radiotherapy are promising but the morbidity of these multimodal treatments is far from negligible. Earlier diagnosis and more effective multimodality treatments will improve the likelihood of cure.

References

1. Mendenhall WM, Pearson JT, Vogel SB, et al (1988) Carcinoma of the cervical esophagus treated with radiation therapy. Laryngoscope 98:769–71
2. Stell PM, Missotten F, Singh SD, et al (1983) Mortality after surgery for hypopharyngeal carcinoma. Br J Surg 70:713–18
3. Harrison DFN, Thompson AE (1986) Pharyngolaryngoesophagectomy with pharyngogastric anastomosis for cancer of the hypopharynx: review of 101 operations. Head Neck Surg 8:418–28
4. Gluckman JL, Weissler MC, McCafferty G, et al (1987) Partial versus total esophagectomy for advanced carcinoma of the hypopharynx. Arch Otolaryngol Head Neck Surg 113:69–72
5. Elias D, Lasser P, Eschwege F, Kac J, Zummer K (1983) Etude retrospective de 88 cas de cancers de l'oesophage cervical et definition d'une nouvelle approache therapeutique. J Chir 120:243–9
6. Lam KH, Ho CM, Lau WL, Wei WI, Wong J (1989) Immediate reconstruction of pharyngoesophageal defects. Preference or reference. Arch Otolaryngol Head Neck Surg 115:608–12
7. Kakegawa T, Yamana H, Ando N (1985) Analysis of surgical treatment for carcinoma situated in the cervical esophagus. Surgery 97:150–6
8. Germain MA, Hureau J, Trotoux J, Agossou Voyeme AK (1990) La reconstruction pharyngo-oesophagienne par transplant libre jejunal revascularise. Chirurgie 116:78–88
9. Akiyama A, Miyazono H, Tsurumaru M, Hashimoto C, Kawamura T (1978) Use of the stomach as an esophageal substitute. Ann Surg 188:606–610
10. Collard JM, Otte JB, Jamart J, Reynaert M, Kestens PJ (1989) An original technique for lengthening the stomach as an oesophageal substitute after oesophagectomy. Preliminary Results. Dis Esophagus 2:171–174

Surgical Management of Suture Insufficiency at Cervical Esophagogastrostomy After Surgery for Carcinoma of the Thoracic Esophagus

Takuo Murakami, Akira Tangoku, Hiroto Hayashi, and Takashi Suzuki[1]

Introduction

Carcinoma of the thoracic esophagus remains a surgical challenge with eso-phagectomy having an associated hospital mortality rate of about 10%–17%. One of the recommended procedures for esophageal reconstruction is to pull the stomach up into the cervical region through the posterior mediastinal and retro-sternal route.

Anastomotic leakage and stenosis after esophagogastrostomy are common complications of operative procesures for carcinoma of the thoracic esophagus.

There are a number of factors related to suture disruption. The most significant causes of suture insufficiency at the cervical esophagogastrostomy are circulatory disturbance of the reconstructed stomach and tension imposed on the suture line.

Causes of Suture Insufficiency

In the procedure to resect the thoracic esophagus and to mobilize the gastric tube, the bilateral vagus nerves are completely severed, but numerous sym-pathetic nerve fibers are preserved, such as nerves running along the right gastric and right gastroepiploic arteries. This imbalance of the autonomous nervous tone results in disturbance of blood circulation (Fig. 1).

To correct this imbalance of autonomous nervous tone and to increase arterial blood flow in the gastric tube, we perform right thoracic sympathectomy (Th5–Th10) during the thoracic procedure.

[1] Second Department of Surgery, Yamaguchi University School of Medicine, 1144 Kogushi, Ube, Yamaguchi, 755 Japan

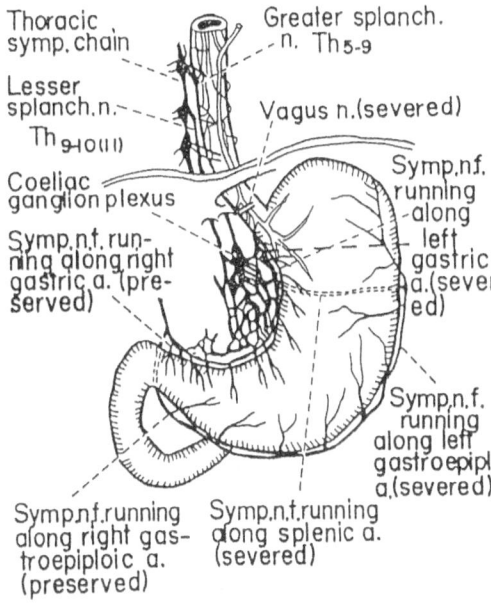

Thoracic symp.chain

Greater splanch. n. Th 5-9

Lesser splanch.n.

Th 9-10(11)

Vagus n.(severed)

Coeliac ganglion plexus

Symp.n.f. running along right gastric a. (preserved)

Symp.n.f. running along left gastric a.(severed)

Symp.n.f. running along left gastroepipl. a.(severed)

Symp.n.f. running along right gastroepiploic a. (preserved)

Symp.n.f.running along splenic a. (severed)

Fig. 1. Innervation of the gastric tube. *n.f.*, nerve fibers; *a*, artery

After construction of the gastric tube in dogs, India ink was injected into the common hepatic artery. The microcirculation in the gastric tube was observed using specimens prepared by the dry ice methanol Wintergreen method.

Results of Experimental Studies

It was demonstrated that bilateral vagotomy plays a role more significant than the division of gastric blood vessels on the left side or the loss of esophagogastric continuity, reducing blood flow in the gastric tube by 26.4% [1] (Fig. 2).

Injected India ink did not reach the mucosal surface sufficiently. Stasis and sludging in the submucosal layer were seen and opening of arteriovenous anastomoses was also observed. Fluorescence of catecholamines in the outer layer of the media and the adventitia of the right gastroepiploic artery increased markedly.

Experimentally, the construction of the gastric tube reduced the blood flow in the tip by 49.8%. Venous pressure in the splenic vein, which was elevated upwards antethoracically with the gastric tube, showed a 26% increase [2].

The disturbance of blood circulation at the tip of the gastric tube and the tension imposed on the anterior portion of the esophagogastrostomy are thought to be the main factors leading to the occurrence of anastomotic breakdown in the esophagogastrostomic region.

Right thoracic sympathectomy increased the blood flow in the tip of the gastric tube in dogs by 32.2% (Fig. 3). In the group that had undergone right thoracic sympathectomy 1–2 weeks prior to the abdominal procedure, microcirculatory disturbance was not observed. Fluorescence of catecholamines in the

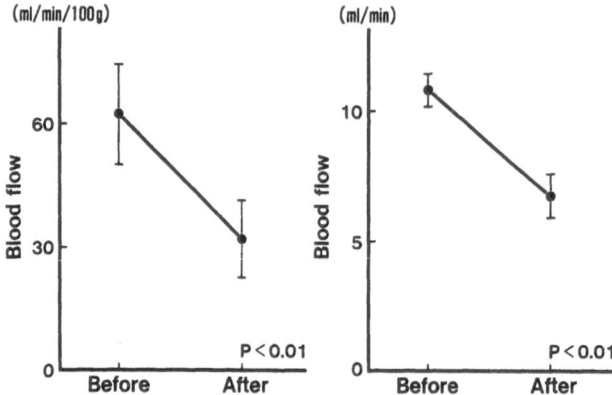

Fig. 2. Tissue blood flow in the tip of the gastric tube (*left*) and right gastroepiploic arterial flow (*right*), before and after the construction of the gastric tube

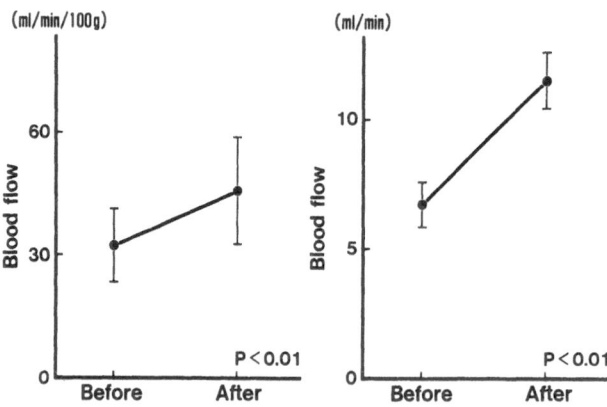

Fig. 3. Tissue blood flow in the tip of the gastric tube (*left*) and right gastroepiploic arterial flow (*right*), before and after the right (Th5–Th10) thoracic sympathectomy

outer layer of the media and the adventitia of the right gastroepiploic artery had almost disappeared [2].

Ultrasonic doppler flowmeter was used for measurement of right gastroepiploic arterial flow. A hydrogen gas clearance flowmeter was used for measurement of mucosal and submucosal blood flow of the gastric tube.

Cervical Esophagogastrostomy Using End-to-Side Anastomotic (EEA) Stapling Device

The use of a surgical stapler in esophageal operations has become popular, and many claims have been made regarding the advantages of stapling over conventional suturing techniques.

We agree that a safer anastomosis with an adequate lumen can be achieved by this means. Since 1985, we have made use of the EEA stapler (US Surgical Corp., Norwalk, Conn.) not only for intrathoracic anastomosis but also for retrosternal reconstruction.

We tried to modify the usual technique and designed a new technique in which the anvil is fixed in the lumen of the stomach for esophagogastrostomy. This procedure was performed in 64 patients at Yamaguchi University Hospital, from 1988 to May 1991. This technique is considered to be simple and easy with a satisfactory outcome.

Technique

The operation was carried out in one stage, such as total thoracic esophagectomy and lymph node dissection, through a right thoracotomy. Esophageal reconstruction with a gastric tube was performed via the retrosternal route, using a premium curved EEA instrument (CEEA; auto suture curved disposable EEA surgical stapler [US Surgical Corp.]) for the cervical esophagogastric anastomosis.

Thoracic Approach

Total thoracic esophagectomy and systemic lymph node dissection, particularly of the lymph nodes of the superior mediastinum, was performed through a right posterolateral thoracotomy.

The azygos vein was divided, preserving the deep part of the right bronchial artery to prevent pulmonary complications, and preserving the vagus nerve above the carina. Lidocaine was applied to the vagus nerve to block its action and prevent cardiac arrhythmias and arrest (by blocking the vagal reflex).

To correct the imbalance of autonomous nervous tone in the gastric tube and to increase the arterial blood flow to the gastric tube, right thoracic sympathectomy (Th5–Th10) was performed during the thoracic operation. After incision of the overlying parietal pleura, the right sympathetic trunk was resected from Th5 to Th10 together with the connecting branches.

Abdominal Approach

In the abdominal procedure, the gastrocolic ligament was severed, preserving the arcade of the right gastroepiploic vessels in the omentum. After performing en bloc dissection of the lymph nodes, including those of the lesser curvature, those around the esophageal hiatus, and those along the splenic artery, common hepatic artery and celiac axis, the gastric portion of the lesser curvature, having about one-third the width of the transverse axis, was removed using a gastrointestinal anastomotic (GIA) apparatus (auto suture multifive GIA 50 disposable surgical stapler and disposable loading unit [US Surgical Corp]).

The stomach was transected longitudinally by serial applications of the autosuture GIA instrument (five or six applications of the instrument) from the lower, lesser curvature to the paraesophageal gastric fundus without oversewing with a continuous whip stitch or interrupted suture. The duodenum and head of the pancreas were extensively mobilized to allow the gastric tube to reach the

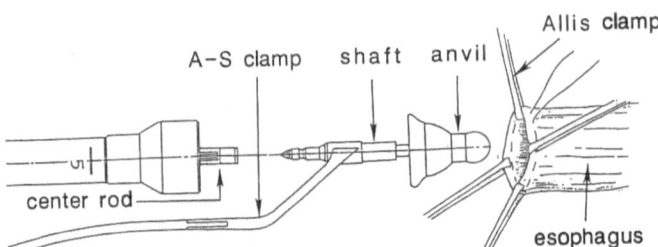

Fig. 4. The anvil with anvil shaft held with the A-S clamp (clamp created by the author) is introduced into the esophagus

desired height. A digital pyloromyotomy was routinely performed, rupturing the pylorus with gradual pressure between the externally applied thumb and forefinger.

Cervical Approach

A relatively large retrosternal tunnel was created with a wide opening at the top end of the tunnel. The gastric tube was elevated upwards retrosternally into the cervical wound after bilateral cervical lymph node dissection.

Anastomosis Using EEA Stapler in Cervical Approach [3]

The proximal cervical esophagus was prepared with a pursestring suture placed at the edge of the proximal esophagus using the pursestring instrument. The proximal esophageal edges were then grasped with four Allis clamps placed equidistantly. Next, a balloon catheter was applied intraluminally to the proximal stump of the cervical esophagus followed by gentle dilation by inflation of the balloon, and a pursestring was placed around the stump [4].

The anvil together with the anvil shaft clamped by the anvil-shaft (A-S) clamp which was produced by the author, was introduced into the lumen of the proximal esophagus, then the pursestring suture was tied into the pursestring notch on the anvil shaft (Fig. 4).

A Premium CEEA surgical stapler, 25 mm in diameter, was introduced into the stomach through the top of the gastric tube. The center rod of the EEA instrument was introduced, without the anvil and anvil shaft and with a recessed trocar tip, into the gastric tube, and the center rod was advanced proximally to the site of anastomosis. The trocar tip was advanced to perforate the posterior wall of the gastric tube, and a manual pursestring suture was placed around the instrument shaft.

After removing the trocar tip with a Babcock clamp, the anvil shaft of the esophagus was introduced from the same perforated posterior wall of the gastric tube after removal of the center rod from the posterior wall. The center rod of the gastric tube was engaged in the anvil shaft of the esophagus with the A-S clamp (Fig. 5). The manual pursestring stitches placed around the instrument shaft were tightened.

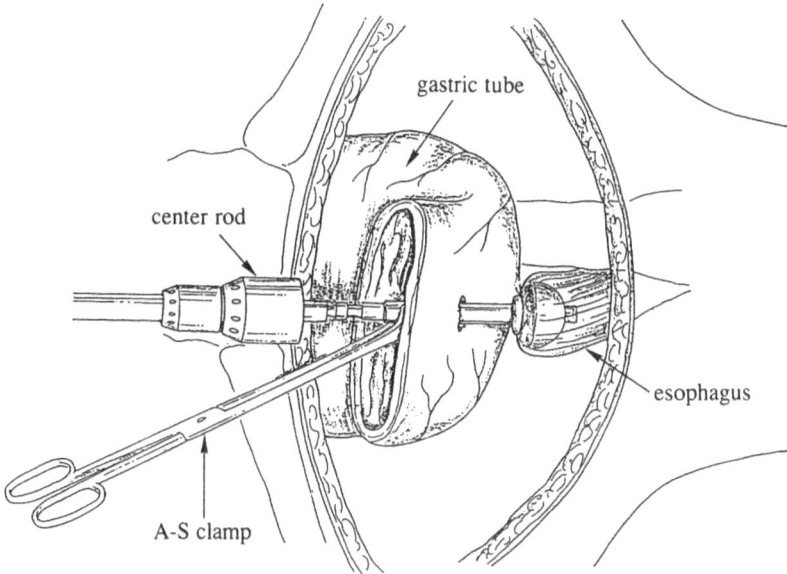

Fig. 5. The center rod of the gastric tube is engaged in the anvil shaft of the esophagus with the A-S clamp in the intraluminal portion

Table 1. Cases of right thoracic sympathectomy for carcinoma of the thoracic esophagus (1987.4–1992.12)

Reconstruction route			Leakage	Stenosis
Retrosternal route		88		
Stapled anastomosis	73		1	26
Hand-sutured anastomosis	15		1	4
Antethoracic route		2		
Hand-sutured anastomosis	2		0	0
Posterior mediastinal route		8		
Stapled anastomosis	8		0	0
Total		98	2	30

Taking care not to nip any tissue adjacent to the esophagus, the EEA stapler was tightened and fired. The anvil and the cartridge were separated, and the entire unit was removed through the incision in the stomach.

The completeness of the anastomosis was examined from the outside and inside of the stomach. The two rings were carefully inspected for their integrity and sent for pathological examination.

The remaining opening on the fundic portion of the gastric tube was resected and closed with a TA-55 stapler. The anastomotic line was oversewn in areas where the tissue was judged to be too thin.

A stomach catheter with a pH sensor was inserted into the stomach from above the pylorus, positioning the tip of the catheter to lie 5 cm below the anastomosis. A feeding tube was also inserted into the same opening. The abdomen and cervical incisions were closed.

Results of One-Stage Esophagogastrostomy in Clinical Cases

As a result of this additional procedure, the rate of primary healing of the cervical esophagogastrostomy through the retrosternal route was 98%, and the rate of successful anastomosis was 100%, showing great improvement over conventional procedures (Table 1).

References

1. Ishigami K, Murakami T, Oka M (1988) Neurovascular manipulation for safer surgery of thoracic esophageal cancer. In: Sievert JR, Holscher AH (eds) Diseases of the esophagus. Springer, Berlin Heidelberg New York, pp 437–442
2. Mii T (1981) Relationship between autonomic innervation and hemodynamics of the gastric tube for esophageal reconstruction, especially the effect of thoracic sympathectomy on the microcirculatory disturbance in the gastric tube. Arch Jpn Chir 50:747–768
3. Muehrche DD, Kaplan DK, Donnelly RJD (1989) Anastomotic narrowing after eso- phagogastrectomy with the EEA stapling device. J Thorac Cardiovasc Surg 97:434–438
4. Kumashiro R, Kamachi H, Maekawa T, Sakaida R, Inutsuka S (1990) Dilation of the stump of the esophagus and intestine with Doyen's intestinal clamp followed by application of lidocaine facilitates the stapling anastomoses. Am Surg 56:308–309

Esophageal Cancer: Surgical Treatment

Late Results of Operations on Esophagus and Cardia Tumors (1973–1990)

Attila Vörös, János Kiss, and Áron Altorjay[1]

Introduction

Tumours of the esophagus constitute 2% of all carcinomas and 4% of all the tumors of the gastrointestinal tract [1]. This type of malignant disease is one of the most problematic in oncologic surgery due to its high postoperative mortality and poor survival chances.

Subjects and Methods

Between January 1, 1973, and December 31, 1990, 1276 patients were admitted to the Department of Surgery, Postgraduate Medical University, Budapest, because of cancer of the esophagus and esophagogastric junction (Table 1). In the first 12 years, we treated esophageal tumours with standard esophagectomy and the continuity was restored by intrapleural esophagogastrostomy [2, 3]. In case of cardia tumours, we performed total gastrectomy and splenectomy, with Roux-an-Y anastomosis.

Since 1985, we have performed the resection of esophagus tumours according to Akiyama [4] by the two field dissection (mediastinal and abdominal) with resection of the minor curvature of the stomach.

Results

We analysed operative data, pathologic documentation of dissected organs, histological type, differentiation grade, gross pathology, localisation of tumour, and the TNM classification in terms of survival (life table method).

[1] Postgraduate Medical University, Department of Surgery, 1135 Budapest Szabolcs u. 35. Hungary

Table 1. Late results of operations on tumors of the esophagus and cardia

	n	%	Death	
			n	%
Total admissions	1276	100.0		
Not operated on	121	9.5		
Operated on	1155	90.5		
Operated-on patients	1155	100.0	170	14.7
Exploration	192	16.6	60	31.2
Gastrostomy	25	2.2	8	32.0
Endoprothesis	160	13.9	25	15.6
Catheter pharyngostomy	8	0.7	—	—
Bypass	48	4.1	8	16.6
Resection	722	62.5	69	9.5

Table 2. Forms of carcinoma of the esophagus and esophagogastric junction

	Well	Moderate	Poor
Esophagus	58.6%	28.6%	12.8%
Cardia	51.6%	35.4%	13.0%

Table 3. Groups according to gross pathology

	Esophagus	Cardia
Polypoid	5.0%	10.0%
Ulcerative	37.1%	32.0%
Infiltrating	52.9%	40.0%
Flat protruding	3.6%	3.0%
At mucosal level	1.4%	2.0%
Unknown		13.0%

According to histopathologic findings, esophagus tumours were classified to planocellulare keratoid carcinomas (88%), planocellulare nonkeratoid carcinomas (7%), and non-differenciated carcinoma (5%). Adenocarcinoma of the esophagogastric junction are: Tubulaire adenocarcinoma (40.4%), tubulopapillary adenocarcinoma (34.3%), sigillocellular adenocarcinoma (6.4%), muciparous adenocarcinoma (3.2%), gelatinous adenocarcinoma (1.6%), and non-differenciated carcinoma (14.1%). According to the differentiation grade, there are well, moderately, and poorly differentiated forms (Table 2).

According to gross pathology, the following groups can be identified (Table 3).

In our material, we applied the 1987 criteria of the International Union Against Cancer (UICC) [5] staging retrospectively, on the basis detailed pathological analysis to arrive at a TNM classification.

Unfortunately, in 85% of our cases, local invasion or distant metastases made curative resection impractical. Our active therapeutic attitude is illustrated by the face that one or another type of operation has been performed on 90% of patients admitted with esophageal carcinoma. These values were 97% for tumors of the lower third of the esophagus and 73% for the upper segments. In 62.5% of the patients, resection was performed. Of the resection operations, 25.5% were curative and 74.5% were palliative on the basis of surgical staging. While 71% of the tumors in the lower third of the esophagus were resected, only 50%

Table 4. Operative mortality, annual mortality rate, and chance of survival

	n	Operative mortality		Ann mort rate	Survival/month		
		n	%		Med.	Max.	Min.
Res oes curative	72	4	5.5	30	38	79	12
Res oes palliative	202	27	13.3	94	12	28	0
Res card curative	112	4	3.5	20	51	169	10
Res card palliative	336	34	10.1	65	17	41	1
Bypass	48	8	16.6	171	5	12	0
Endoprothesis	160	25	15.6	190	4	16	0
Stoma	33	8	24	173	2	12	0
Exploration	192	60	31.2	190	2	14	0
Not operated on	121	37	30.5	109	1	8	0
Total	1276						

oes, Esophagus; *card*, cardia; *Res*, resected

Table 5. Results of esophageal cancer resection

Stage	Patients		Ann mort rate	Survival/month		
	n	%		Med.	Max.	Min.
1	13	4.7	17	53	79	17
2A	59	21.5	34	36	67	12
2B	96	35.0	83	14	28	3
3	106	38.6	97	12	27	0
Total	274	100.0	58	21	79	0

of those in the upper third were resected. In the latter group, the ratio of palliative interventions increased in proportion to the decrease in resections. The absence of differences in survival and localisation in our patients proves that palliative resection is also worthwhile in cases of upper third tumors. The analysis of the survival chances reveals that the best results have been offered by curative resections, followed by palliative procedures (Table 4).

Bypass and endoprosthesis operations have not prolonged survival considerably, though they have made life more bearable by restoring the ability to swallow. Early operative death rate was also the lowest in the curative group: 3.5% for tumors located at the esophagogastric junction and 5.5% for esophageal cases. By TNM classification in our patient group, the survival was also stage-dependent (Table 5, Figs. 1, 2). Histological analysis showed that the best results may be expected in the well differentiated form of squamous cell carcinomas.

Examination of patients, according to the gross appearance of the tumor, revealed no significant differences, and no differences were discovered according to localisation as well.

Postresection studies related to age have shown the poorest survival chance for patients under 40 years of age. Staging of the tumors markedly influenced

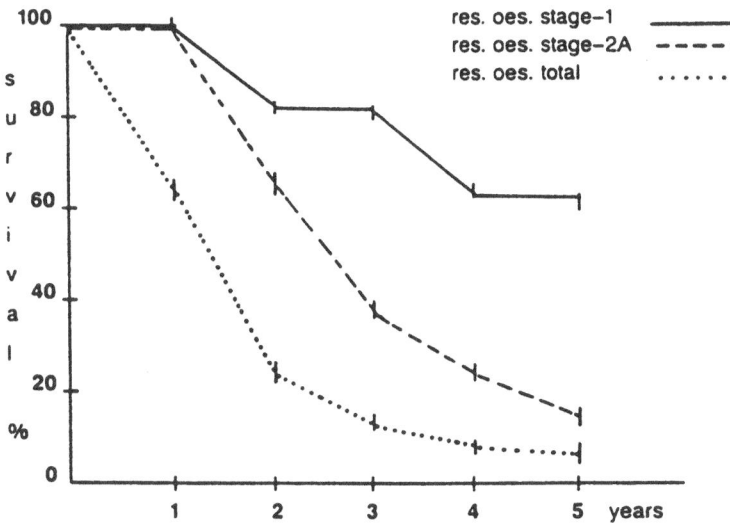

Fig. 1. Survival after esophagectomy by tumor stage-1, -2A, and overall. *res. oes.* resected esophagus

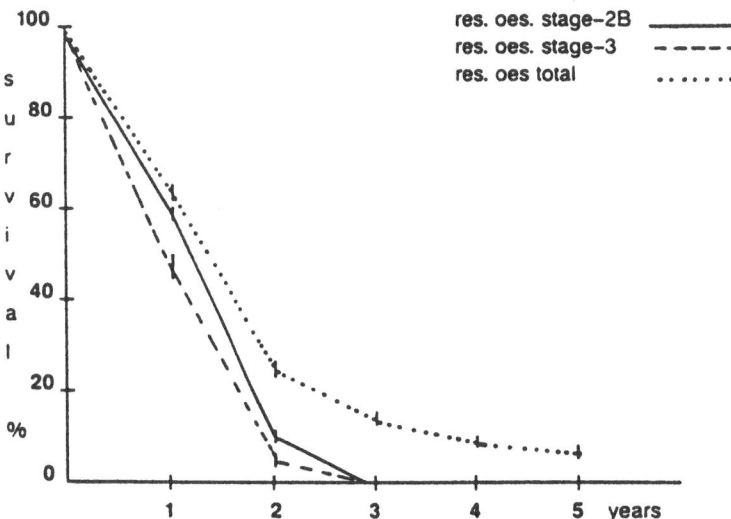

Fig. 2. Survival after esophagectomy, by tumor stage-2B, -3, and overall

the outcome of surgery for esophagogastric junction tumors as well. Significant differences in survival are demonstrated between the stages (Table 6, Figs. 3, 4).

Histological analysis has shown that the best chances of survival can be expected in patients operated on for tubulopapillary adenocarcinoma. Grade of tumor differentiation has shown significant differences in survival in favor of the

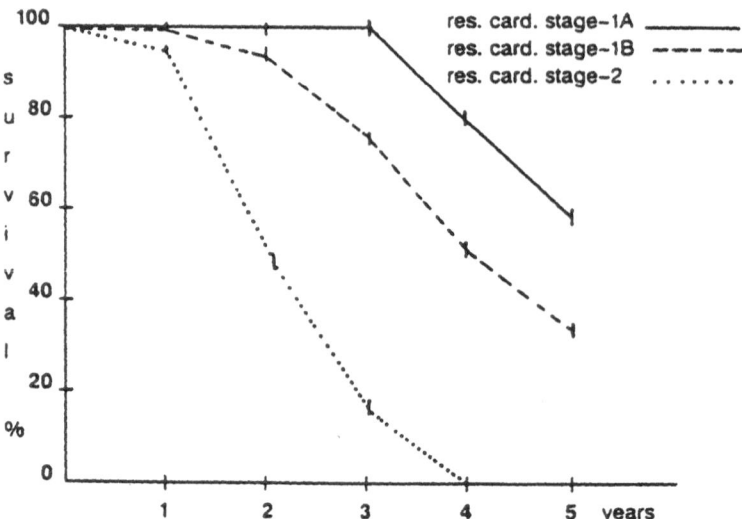

Fig. 3. Survival after total gastrectomy by stage-1A, -1B, and -2. *res. card.*, resected cardia

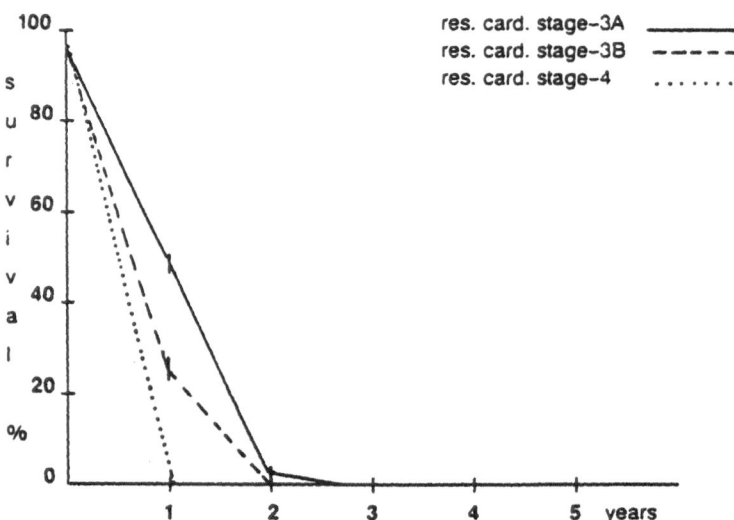

Fig. 4. Survival after total gastrectomy by stage-3A, -3B, and -4

well differentiated ones while the gross appearance of tumors had no such effect in this patient group.

In our material, the so-called bypass and endoprosthesis procedures have an average survival of 4 to 5 months in comparison to the mean of 12 to 17 months following palliative resections (Fig. 5).

Table 6. Results of cardiac cancer resection

Stage	Patients		Ann mort rate	Survival/month		
	n	%		Med.	Max.	Min.
1A	20	4.4	16	75	169	48
1B	92	20.5	19	46	147	10
2	180	40.1	46	22	42	4
3A	89	19.8	98	13	26	3
3B	36	8.0	128	9	13	2
4	31	6.9	170	5	10	1
Total	448	100.0	41	28	169	1

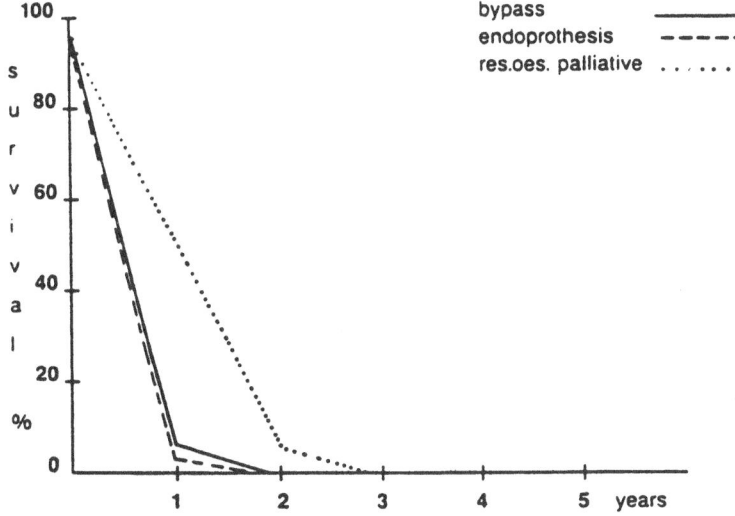

Fig. 5. Survival, palliative procedures

Discussion

Nearly 80 years ago, Franz Torek [6] proved that the tumorous esophagus could be removed successfully. Experience gained during the past decade shows that cancer of the esophagus, if recognised at an early stage, can be cured by surgical resection. Of the patients of Huang et al. [7] operated on in stage-1, 86% were still alive 5 years later. This evidence dramatically illustrates the importance of early diagnosis and disagrees with the idea that cancer of the esophagus is a basically incurable disease. In our material, we had shown that 62% of stage-1 patients had survived for 5 years after resection. In 25% of the cases, we performed curative resection, and in 75% palliative resection because of local invasion or distant metastases. In non-treated cases, survival did not exceed a few months.

In advanced cases of esophageal carcinoma, several conditions can influence the selection of treatment. Pathologic appearance of the tumour, histologic structure, expansion, grade of occlusion, possibility of complications, general condition of the patient, and the surgeon's preference.

Multiple, time demanding reconstructive operations are not recommended in palliative operations. Bypass and endoprosthesis procedures do not prolong survival chances, but they improve the quality of life by restoring the ability to swallow.

In conclusion, our goal is to prolong survival through the establishment of early diagnosis and early radical operation.

References

1. Garfinkel L, Poindexter CE, Siverberg E (1980) Cancer in black americans. Cancer 30:39
2. Ong GB, Kwong KH (1969) The Lewis-Tanner operation for cancer of the esophagus. JR Coll Surg Edinb 14:3
3. McKeown KC (1976) Total three-stage oesophagectomy for cancer of the oesophagus. Br J Surg 63:259–262
4. Akiyama H (1990) Surgery for cancer of the esophagus. Williams and Wilkins, Baltimore, pp 19–27
5. Hermanek P, Sobin LH (eds) (1987) TNM classification of malignant tumours. UICC International Union Against Cancer. Springer, Berlin Heidelberg New York London Tokyo
6. Torek F (1913) The first successful resection of the thoracic portion of the esophagus for carcinoma. Surg Gynec Obstet 16:614–617
7. Huang G, Shao L, Zhang D (1980) Diagnosis and surgical treatment of early esophageal carcinoma. Clin Med J 94:229

Adenocarcinoma of the Esophagus: Results of Surgical Treatment

A.H. Hölscher, E. Bollschweiler, M. Schüler, R. Bumm, M. Tachibana, T. Nakamura, and J.R. Siewert[1]

Introduction

Adenocarcinoma of the esophagus is of special importance because it has been showing an increasing frequency, especially in Europe and North America [1]. This tumor is mostly attributed to a malignant degeneration of the columnar cell-lined lower esophagus. The results of surgical treatment of adenocarcinoma of the esophagus were prospectively analyzed and are reported in comparison to the long-term results after resection of squamous cell cancer of the esophagus, cardia cancer, and subcardial carcinomas.

Patients

Within a 10-year period (July 1982–June 1992) 701 carcinomas of the esophagus were treated and 445 resected in our institution (resection is rate 63.5%). The series of resections with curative intention ($n = 417$) consisted of 278 squamous cell and 139 adenocarcinomas. Adenocarcinoma of the esophagus was defined by the center of the tumor being located at least 1 cm above the cardia [1–3]; 82.4% of the esophageal adenocarcinomas ($n = 113$) developed in a columnar cell-lined lower esophagus which was at least 3 cm in length. In all of these patients, specialized Barrett's mucosa was proven by histologic examination of the resected specimen, whereas in the remaining 26 adenocarcinomas, columnar metaplasia was not detected because of extensive tumor growth.

   Adenocarcinoma of the esophagus mostly occurred in men (122 males: 17 females; 8:1). The mean age of the patients was 60.1 years, with a range of 29–82 years.

---

[1] Department of Surgery, Technical University of Munich, Klinikum rechts der Isar, Ismaninger Str. 22, D-8000 Munich 80, Germany

The long-term results after the resection of esophageal adenocarcinomas in 139 patients were compared with other upper GI cancer series that were resected with curative intention during the same period, i.e., 278 squamous cell carcinomas of the esophagus, 104 so-called real cancers of the cardia, and 123 subcardial gastric cancers.

All these series had a comparable distribution of TNM stages [4]. The exact definition for adenocarcinomas of the gastroesophageal junction which is applied in our institution has been given elsewhere [1–3].

Methods

The standard type of operation for adenocarcinoma of the esophagus was trans-mediastinal abdominocervical resection with transhiatal lymphadenectomy of the lower mediastinum [5, 6]. Thirty of the transmediastinal resections were performed by endoscopic dissection from a cervical approach, using a modified mediastinoscope [7]. Reconstruction was usually performed by gastric inter-position and cervical esophagogastrostomy. In cases of an extensive Barrett's esophagus with location of the tumor in the middle third or the upper part of the lower third of the esophagus, a transthoracic en bloc resection with gastric interposition was carried out (Table 1). In a small number of patients, distal esophageal resection and total gastrectomy or total esophagogastrectomy was performed.

Squamous cell carcinomas were usually treated by transthoracic en bloc eso-phagectomy and gastric interposition. Cardia cancers and subcardial cancers infiltrating the distal esophagus were resected by abdomino-transhiatal distal esophagectomy and total gastrectomy [1, 2]. Reconstruction was performed by Roux-en-Y esophagojejunostomy.

The survival curves were calculated as actuarial survival according to Kaplan-Meyer.

Results

The median length of Barrett's esophagus in 113 patients was 5.1 cm (range 3–17.6 cm). In these patients, the median distance from the incisors to the tumor center was 36.2 cm (range 25.6–40 cm). The postoperative TNM staging of the resected carcinomas showed 46% to be T1/T2 stages, while 54% had advanced tumor stages T3/T4 (Table 2). More than two-thirds of the patients had lymph node metastases and 14% had distant metastases.

In 82% of the patients a complete microscopic and macroscopic tumor re-section was possible. Detailed results are given in Table 3. The total 30-day mortality rate was 6.5% and the 90-day mortality rate was 10.8%. Both mortality rates were lowest in patients with early esophageal cancer (Table 4).

The long-term results showed a very good prognosis for early adenocarcinoma of the esophagus, with a 5-year survival rate of 78%, whereas pT2 and pT3 cancers had a much worse prognosis, which was not significantly different between both groups (Fig. 1).

Table 1. Type of resection and reconstruction in 139 adenocarcinomas of the esophagus

Resection		
Transmediastinal subtotal esophagectomy	99	(71%)
Transthoracic en bloc esophagectomy	34	(24.5%)
Distal esophageal resection and total gastrectomy	4	(3%)
Esophagogastrectomy	2	(1.5%)
Reconstruction		
Replacement by gastric tube	129	(93%)
Colon interposition	10	(7%)

Table 2. p-TNM-staging of 139 resected adenocarcinomas of the esophagus

T-staging			N-staging			M-staging		
	n	%		n	%		n	%
pT1	28	20	No	43	31	Mo	119	86
pT2	36	26	N1	96	69	M1	15	11
pT3	42	30				Mx	5	3
pT4	33	24						

Table 3. Postoperative residual tumor (R) status in 139 patients with adenocarcinoma of the esophagus

	n	Ro	R1	R2
pT1/T2	64	61 (95.3%)	2 (3.1%)	1 (1.6%)
pT3/t4	75	53 (70.7%)	16 (21.3%)	6 (8.0%)
Total	139	114 (82.0%)	18 (13.0%)	7 (5.0%)

Table 4. Postoperative mortality of 139 patients after resection of adenocarcinoma of the esophagus

	n	30-Day mortality rate	90-Day mortality rate
pT1	28	1 (3.6%)	1 (3.6%)
pT2	36	1 (2.8%)	4 (11.1%)
pT3	42	5 (11.9%)	5 (11.9%)
pT4	33	2 (6.0%)	5 (15.0%)
Total	139	9 (6.5%)	15 (10.8%)

The survival according to pN category showed the expected favorable results for pNO status compared to pN1 (Fig. 2). Long-term survival could be achieved only by complete tumor resection, whereas none of the patients with a residual tumor status (R) of R1 or RO survived for more than 2 years (Fig. 3). Survival

Survival pT-Category

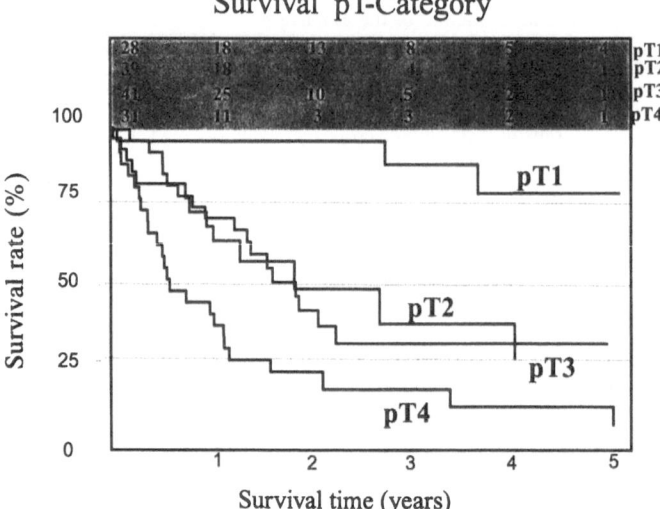

Fig. 1. Survival after resection of adenocarcinoma of the esophagus according to pT-category ($n = 139$)

Survival pN-Category

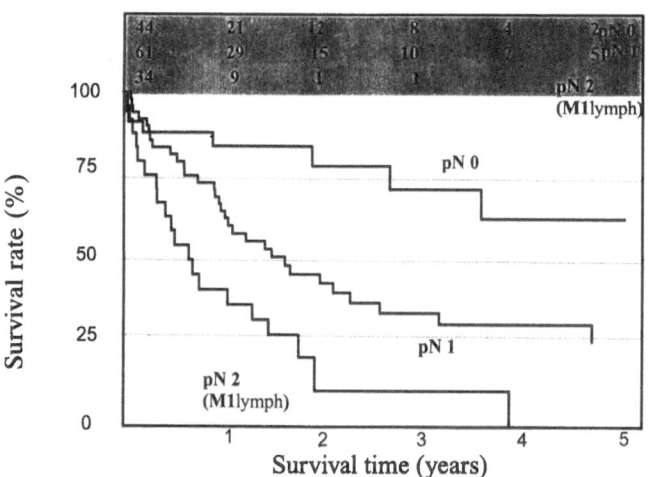

Fig. 2. Survival according to pN-category ($n = 139$)

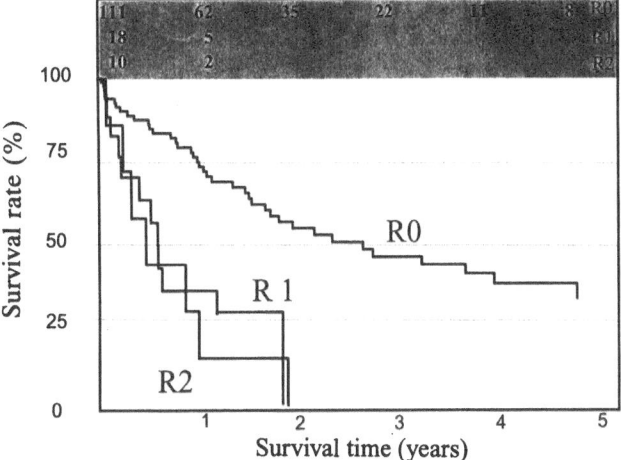

Fig. 3. Survival according to residual tumor (R)-status (n = 139); *Adenoca*, Adenocarcinoma

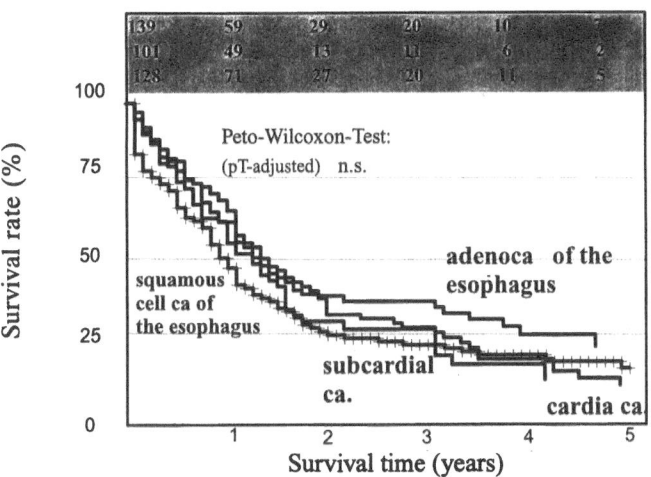

Fig. 4. Comparison of prognosis after resection of adenocarcinoma (n = 139) and squamous cell carcinoma (ca) (n = 278) of the esophagus, cardia cancer (n = 104), and subcardial gastric cancer (n = 123)

after resection of adenocarcinoma or squamous cell carcinoma of the esophagus, as well as cardia cancer and subcardial gastric cancer, did not show significant differences (Fig. 4).

Discussion and Conclusions

One-third of the resected cancers of the esophagus in our material were adenocarcinomas; 82% of these esophageal adenocarcinomas developed in a histologically-proven Barrett's esophagus. Transmediastinal esophagectomy, including endoscopic dissection from a cervical approach, is the procedure of choice for adenocarcinoma of the distal esophagus, because it allows adequate lymphadenectomy for this type of cancer [5–7]. However, more orally located adenocarcinomas, which have a tendency also to metastasize to mediastinal lymph nodes, should be removed by transthoracic en bloc esophagectomy [3]. By applying this strategy a high percentage of RO resections in advanced tumor stages can also be achieved.

Concerning the long-term results, the significant difference between the survival curves of pT1 and pT2 cancers shows again that tumor infiltration in the esophageal wall is the decisive factor. Further, the presence of lymph node metastases is of major importance for the prognosis. However, if an adequate lymphadenectomy is performed, survival is also possible in the N1 stage. The aim of surgery must be to perform a complete macroscopic and microscopic tumor resection, since long-term survival is possible only if an RO status can be achieved. The most important prognostic factors for adenocarcinoma of the esophagus are T-category, lymph node status, and postoperative residual tumor. The comparison of four series of patients with cancer of the upper GI tract with a similar distribution of tumor stages shows that the prognosis after resection does not significantly differ between squamous cell carcinoma and adenocarcinoma of the esophagus or cardia cancer and subcardial gastric cancer.

References

1. Hölscher AH, Schüler M, Siewert JR (1988) Surgical treatment of adenocarcinomas of the gastroesophageal junction. Dis Esoph 1:35–50
2. Siewert JR, Hölscher AH, Becker K, Gössner W (1988) Cardiacarcinom. Versuch einer therapeutisch relevanten Klassifikation. Chirurg 58:25–32
3. Siewert JR (ed) (1989) Breitner Chirurgische Operationslehre Band IV. Chirurgie des Abdomens 2. Oesophagus, Magen und Duodenum. Urban and Schwarzenberg, Munich
4. Hermanek P, Scheibe O, Spiessl B, Wagner G (eds) (1987) UICC:TNM-Classification of malignant tumors. Springer, Berlin Heidelberg New York
5. Orringer MB (1984) Transhiatal esophagectomy without thoracotomy for carcinoma of the thoracic esophagus. Ann Surg 200:282–288
6. Siewert JR, Hölscher AH, Horvath ÖP (1986) Transmediastinale Ösophagektomie. Langenbecks Arch Chir 367:203–213
7. Bumm R, Hölscher AH, Feussner H, Tachibana M, Bartels H, Siewert JR (1993) Endodissection of the thoracic esophagus: Technique and clinical results in transhiatal esophagectomy. Ann Surg accepted for publication

Lymph Node Dissection for Carcinoma of the Cardia—Is It Worthwhile?

Takashi Aikou[1], Nasser K. Altorki[2], David B. Skinner,[2] Masamichi Baba[1], and Hisaaki Shimazu[1]

Introduction

Adenocarcinoma arising at the cardia still remains one of the most difficult malignant neoplasms to treat. The controversial issues include the choice of the surgical approach, the extent of esophageal and gastric resection, and the need for a complete abdominal and mediastinal lymphadenectomy. The aim of this study is to clarify two specific questions. Firstly, what are the common pathways of lymphatic spread? Secondly, what is the influence of the site and number of involved nodes on survival?

Definition

Adenocarcinoma of the cardia is defined as all tumor in which the main tumor mass is centered at the esophagogastric junction (EGJ), and originates from the subdiaphragmatic esophagus, or the true EGJ, or the first 2–3 cm of the gastric cardia. For the purposes of this report, adenocarcinoma arising in the upper one-third of the body of the stomach, the gastric fundus, diffuse carcinoma (i.e., linitis plastica), squamous cell carcinoma of the distal esophagus, and adenocarcinoma arising in Barrett's epithelium are excluded.

Patients

The medical records were reviewed of 61 consecutive patients with adenocarcinoma of the cardia treated in the Departments of Surgery at the New

[1] 1st Department of Surgery, Kagoshima University Hospital, 8-35-1 Sakuragaoka, Kagoshima, 890 Japan

[2] The New York Hospital—Cornell Medical Center, 525 East 68th St., New York, NY 10021, USA

York Hospital—Cornell Medical Center and University of Chicago Medical Center over 20 years (1970–1990). There were 52 males and 9 females for a male-to-female ratio of 6:1. Patients ranged in age between 30 and 84 years with a mean and median age of 60 years. All 61 patients were surgically explored. Six patients were found to have unresectable disease, due to multiple liver disease (4), peritoneal implants (1), or direct invasion of the celiac axis by tumor (1). The remaining 55 patients underwent resection either by the en bloc resection method (34) or through a standard transthoracic esophagogastrectomy.

Pathology reports were scrutinized to determine the degree of transmural invasion, the size and location of the tumor, the total number of lymph nodes excised with the specimen, as well as the number and location of all lymph nodes involved with carcinoma. Final staging was based on the WNM system proposed by Skinner and associates [1]. Briefly, this staging system is based on wall penetration (W), lymph node involvement (N), and systemic metastases (M). W0 was assigned to neoplasms limited to the mucosa, W1 for penetration into the submucosa or into, but not through, the muscularis propria, and W2 for neoplasms penetrating through the full thickness of the wall. Lymph nodes were classified as N0 when all were negative, N1 when one to four were positive, and N2 when five or more nodes harbored metastasis. The WNM system correlates with the TNM system proposed by the UICC [2] only in the descriptions of mural invasion. W0 is equivalent to T1, W1 to T2, and W2 to T3 and T4.

Nomenclature and Statistical Method

For purposes of statistical analysis, we divided the lymph nodes according to the following nomenclature. Lower paraesophageal, middle paraesophageal, and subcarinal lymph nodes were designated as mediastinal nodes. Paracardial, lesser curvature, greater curvature, left gastric, celiac, pancreatic, and paraaortic lymph nodes were designated as abdominal nodes. Furthermore, we classified all nodal groups into three levels according to their frequency of involvement with tumor. Patients with level I disease had nodal spread in any or all of the following nodal groups: paracardial, lesser curvature, left gastric, or lower paraesophageal nodes. Level II included patients in whom nodes along the greater curvature, middle paraesophageal, or subcarinal space were the seat of metastatic disease with or without spread to glands in Level I. Level III patients had nodal metastasis to the celiac, pancreatic, or paraaortic gland.

Survival curves were computed using the Kaplan-Meier method. The general Wilcoxon test was used to quantify statistical differences. Patients were followed until either the time of death or April 31, 1991. Follow-up was complete on all operative survivors, except one.

Results

Pathways of Lymphatic Spread

An average of 35 nodes were resected per patient with the en bloc resection, versus 24 nodes for patients having a standard resection. Metastasis to the regional lymph nodes was present in 48 patients (87%) as shown in Table 1. The

Table 1. Lymph node metastasis in patients with carcinoma of the cardia

Patients	All patients $n = 55$	En bloc $n = 35$	Standard[a] $n = 20$
With lymph node metastasis	48/55 (87%)	29/35 (83%)	19/20 (95%)
Without lymph node metastasis	7/55	6/35	1/20

[a] Resections not carried out en bloc were designated "standard"

Table 2. Prevalence of nodal metastasis in abdomen and mediastinum

	Mediastinum	Abdomen	Both
All patients	1/45	15/45 (27%)	29/45 (65%)
En bloc resection	1/35	8/35 (23%)	20/35 (57%)

Table 3. Frequency of involvement of various nodal groups

	All cases (55)	En bloc (35)
Abdominal nodes		
Paracardial	39 (73%)	22 (65%)
Lesser curvature	40 (73%)	22 (65%)
Greater curvature	11 (20%)	6 (9%)
Left gastric	25 (45%)	13 (38%)
Celiac	14 (25%)	3 (8%)
Pancreatic	3 (5%)	0
Mediastinal nodes		
Lower paraesophageal	26 (45%)	17 (50%)
Middle paraesophageal	6 (11%)	4 (12%)
Subcarinal	8 (14%)	5 (15%)
Upper paraesophageal	4 (7%)	1

prevalence of nodal metastasis in the abdomen and mediastinum is shown in Table 2. Twenty-nine patients (65%) had nodal metastasis present in both the mediastinum and the abdomen. Fifteen patients (27%) had nodal metastasis limited to the intra-abdominal nodes, while in only one patient was disease restricted to the mediastinal nodes. Among 34 patients undergoing en bloc resection, the distribution of nodal metastasis was approximately the same as that for the whole group.

The frequency of involvement of the various nodal groups is shown in Table 3. The most frequently involved nodal groups were those located along the cardia and along the lesser curvature of the stomach, followed by the lower paraesophageal lymph nodes and those along the trunk of the left gastric artery. Spread occurred with nearly similar frequency to nodes along the greater curvature of the stomach, the middle paraesophageal, and the subcarinal lymph nodes.

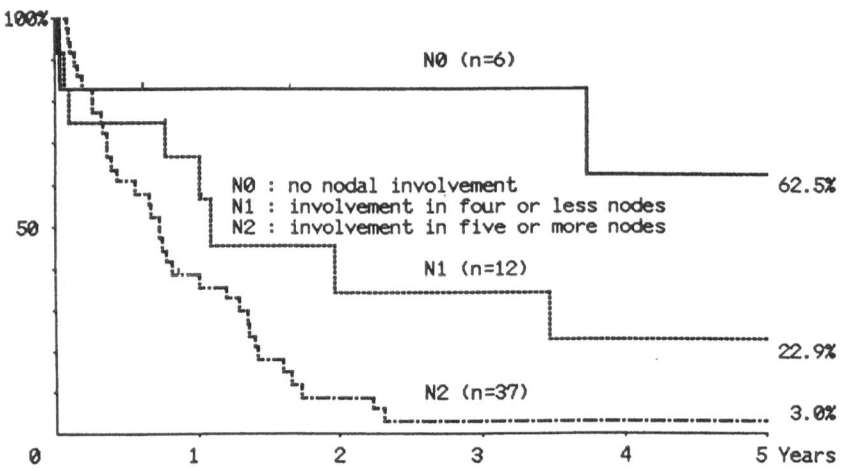

Fig. 1. Comparison of survival according to the number of positive nodes. Survival curves are determined by the Kaplan-Meier method including postoperative mortality

Influence of Site and Number of Involved Nodes on Survival

All patients surviving transhiatal and standard resections died of recurrent disease within 2 years. Among 23 patients surviving operations by the en bloc resection for more than 5 years, there were 6 (26%) long-term disease-free survivors (3/4 with negative nodes, 2/3 with one to four positive nodes, 1/16 with > four positive nodes). As for correlation between survival and the Level of nodal involvement, the median survival was 493, 278, and 239 days for patients in Levels I, II, and III respectively.

The 5-year survival rate was 62.5% in the patients with no nodal involvement, compared to 22.9% in those with one to four positive nodes. Only one patient with five or more positive lymph nodes survived 5 years after the operation, and the outcome for that group was significantly poorer than that for patients with no nodal involvement, as shown in Fig. 1.

Discussion

The prognosis of patients with adenocarcinoma of the cardia continues to be poor. Many surgical procedures for carcinoma of the cardia have been proposed [3, 4]. The evaluation of the various surgical procedures employed has been hindered by the lack of a unified surgical approach as well as the advanced stage of disease seen in the majority of patients at the time of presentation. Although the biological behavior of tumor may prove to be an important determinant of outcome, the current level of knowledge about this aspect of cancer research cannot yet be translated into therapeutic dicisions.

Clearly, the location of the cardia at the border of the thoracic and abdominal cavities presents a formidable technical challenge and requires a better under-standing of the pathways of lymphatic spread from that organ. In previous work

[5], we examined the intramural lymphatic pathways of the distal esophagus and the cardia of the stomach in 45 mongrel dogs using dye injection techniques. When dye was injected into the esophageal or gastric mucosa within 2 cm of the EGJ, an extensive network of intercommunicating lymphatics was observed advancing downward and upward across the EGJ. If the anatomic situation is similar in humans, then it is understandable that even early adenocarcinomas arising at the cardia spread quickly to lymph nodes adjacent to the gastric cardia and distal esophagus. The data shown herein as well as in previous reports [1, 3, 4] indicate that lymphatic spread of carcinoma of the gastric cardia occurs into the mediastinal and the intra-abdominal nodes in over half the cases. This pattern of nodal spread confirms the reports of DeMeester et al. [6], Akiyama and associates [7], and Castrini and Pappalardo [8].

The WNM staging system classifies nodal involvement into N1 and N2 depending on the number of nodes involved by tumor. Unlike the WNM system, staging nodal disease in the TNM system is based only on the presence or absence of nodal metastasis. Some recent reports have also suggested that long-term freedom from disease may still be possible in some patients with a limited extent of nodal involvement. The stepwise regression analysis model based on our data showed that the number of positive nodes was a significant determinant of survival. However, the difference in survival of patients with less than four positive nodes (N1) and those with five or more positive nodes (N2) was not statistically significant. This is readily explained by the small number of observations in the N1 group. Alternatively, others have suggested that two to three positive nodes may be compatible with long-term survival.

Survival was not significantly altered by the site of nodal involvement except when metastasis involved the celiac lymph nodes. In particular, long-term survival was still possible even when nodal metastasis extended into the lower mediastinum and subcarinal region. Undoubtedly, carcinoma of the cardia, like most other solid tumors, comprises a wide spectrum of disease. Patients with intramucosal tumors or those with less than transmural invasion and negative nodes are readily curable by surgical resection. On the other hand, extensive nodal spread frequently spells a dismal prognosis, especially when Level III nodes are involved. En bloc resection, in our opinion, is most suited to cases with limited nodal involvement although the critical number of nodes involved by metastatic disease is yet unclear.

In conclusion, (1) nodal metastasis in carcinoma of the cardia occurs to both mediastinal and abdominal nodes in 65% of patients; (2) the number of positive nodes is a significant determinant of survival; (3) long-term survival is possible following en bloc resection in patients with limited nodal involvement; and (4) except for celiac nodes, the location of positive nodes has no influence on survival.

References

1. Skinner DB (1983) En bloc resection for neoplasms of the esophagus and cardia. J Thorac Cardiovasc Surg 85:59–71
2. International Union Against Cancer (UICC) (1987) Hermanek P, Sobin LH (eds) TNM classification of malignant tumors, 4th edn. Springer, Berlin Heidelberg New York London Paris Tokyo

3. Moureaux J, Msika S (1988) Carcinoma of the gastric cardia, surgical treatment and long-term survival. World J Surg 12:229–235
4. Hennessy TP, Keeling P (1987) Adenocarcinoma of the esophagus and cardia. J Thorac Cardiovasc Surg 94:64–68
5. Aikou T, Shimazu H (1989) Difference in main lymphatic pathways from the lower esophagus and gastric cardia. Jpn J Surg 19:290–295
6. DeMeester TR, Zaninomotto G, Johansson KE (1988) Selective therapeutic approach to cancer of the lower esophagus and cardia. J Thorac Cardiovasc Surg 95:42–54
7. Akiyama H, Turumaru M, Kawamura T, Ono Y (1981) Principles of surgical treatment for carcinoma of the esophagus. Ann Surg 194:438–446
8. Castrini G, Pappalardo G (1981) Carcinoma of the cardia. J Thorac Cardiovasc Surg 82:190–193

Total Extended Gastrectomy Plus Transhiatal Esophagectomy for Cancer of the Cardia

E. Moreno González, I. González-Pinto, G.I. García, S.R. Gómez, S.C. Loinaz, V. Maffettone*, M.J. Bercedo, S.P. Rico, C.F. Palma, and F.M. Marcello[1]

Introduction

Cancer of the cardia has been defined as tumors which affect the esophagogastric junction, histologically being an adenocarcinoma.

Other types of malignancies have been included in the same group such as adenocarcinoma of the fundus or fornix which can affect the esophagogastric junction during its growth. Such patients should be treated by total gastrectomy extended through the hiatus to the lower segment of the esophagus to obtain sufficient free margin for a radical treatment in the upper end. Reconstruction of the digestive tract should be done by means of a long Roux-en-Y jejunal loop or an isolated jejunal loop interposed between the remaining esophagus and the duodenum. Another type of malignancy included in the same group is adenocarcinoma of the lower esophagus (probably from Barrett's esophagus) which can grow distally, infiltrating the esophagogastric junction. The approved treatment is transhiatal or transthoracic esophagectomy with more or less extensive lymphnode dissection in the upper mediastinum and the neck, but including a wider lymphadenectomy in the lower mediastinum, celiac axis, left gastric arcade, right suprapancreatic, and hepatoduodenal ligament. Esophageal replacement should be done by gastric tube ascending to the upper right thorax or to the neck through the posterior mediastinum or the substernal route.

The only point of controversy still remains in tumors located in the esophagogastric junction growing through the esophagus and the stomach almost symetrically. Several surgeons are treating such patients as gastric malignancies and others treat them as esophageal carcinoma of the lower esophagus infiltrating the esophagogastric junction. We have been proposing, since 1978, another way

[1] Hospital "12 de Octubre", "Complutense" University of Madrid, Servicio de Cirugía General, Aparato Digestivo y Trasplante de Organos Abdominales, Carretera de Andalucía Km 5,400, 28041 Madrid, Spain
* Italian CNR Fellowship

for the treatment of this less frequent type of disease, total enlarged gastrectomy extended through the mediastinum, dissecting and removal the thoracoabdominal esophagus.

Patients

During the period from January 1978 to 1990, 73 patients suffering from cancer of the cardia were treated by total extended esophagogastrectomy (Table 1). The age of the patients ranged from 34 to 74 (average 51.8) and the sex ratio (male/female) was 2.8/1.

Diagnosis was confirmed before operation by means of endoscopy and biopsy. The final diagnosis was adenocarcinoma in 71 patients, and lymphoma in 1, with liver metastasis in the left lobe. In the last patient, the diagnosis was epidermoid carcinoma. Staging of the disease was not possible although computed tomography (CT) scan was taken in 51 patients.

Methods

Operative Technique

The operation started by middle line laparotomy. Abdominal cavity was reviewed looking for lymphnode or liver metastasis. After the resectability in the abdomen was confirmed, the diaphragm was opened from the anterior border of the hiatus to the center of the diaphragm. Intramural spread through the esophagus and extension in the mediastinum was evaluated, and the feasibility of resection was confirmed.

The greater omentum was dissected free from the transverse colon; the duodenum was dissected and severed between the first and second portions. The

Table 1. Transhiatal esophagectomy

	Patients	%
Cancer of the cardia	73	25.8
Hypopharyngeal cancer	11	3.9
Esophageal cancer	171	60.4
Superior third	21	
Middle third	52	
Inferior third	44	
Distal middle third	54	
Caustic stenosis	21	7.4
Perforation	5	1.8
Reoperations	2	0.7
Total	283	100

Table 2. Cancer of the cardia

	No.	%
Esophageal replacement	73	
Right colon	55	75.3
Left colon	18	24.7
Operative mortality	6	8.2
Respiratory failure	1	
Pulmonary sepsis	2	
Abdominal sepsis	3	
Stage of the disease	68	
I	4	5.8
II	31	45.6
III	32	47.1
IV	1	1.4
Follow-up	31	45.6
Survival at 5 years	15	48.4

common bile duct, and the hepatic artery together with its branches and portal vein, were dissected and the fatty lymph tissue was removed *en bloc*. Hepatic artery on the pancreas and the celiac trunk were dissected and fatty lymph tissue around it was removed. The splenic artery was dissected at its origin, ligated, and severed. The right pillar of the hiatus was identified. The diaphragm was sectioned maintaining two centimeters around the esophagus which should be removed with the specimen *en bloc*. Through this wide diaphragmatic opening, the subcarinal segment of the esophagus was dissected under visual control removing fatty lymph tissue around the aorta and vena cava *en bloc* with the esophagus.

The middle and upper thirds of the esophagus were dissected by hand through the hiatus and the cervical incision. After the esophagus was competely mobilized, the cervical segment should be severed and pulled down by the same route. The spleen and tail of the pancreas are mobilized, the splenic vein dissected, ligated, and cut at the inferior mesenteric vein confluence, and the pancreas was cut at this point and secured by means of a stapler. The specimen, which included esophagus, stomach, spleen, tail of the pancreas, diaphragmatic border, and omentum, is completely freed and removed.

The esophagogastric substitution was done using a large segment of the left colon supplied by the left colic artery or right colon with the last 15 cm of the ileum supplied by the middle colic vessels (Table 2). Right or left colon was introduced through the mediastinum and placed in an isoperistaltic manner. Esophagus was anastomosed with the ileum in an end-to-side fashion using two layers of interrupted stitches, or one layer of interrupted stiches with absorbable material, or a running suture (monofilament, absorbable). Coloduodenal anastomosis was done in an end-to-end, one-layer, or two-layer absorbable or non-absorbable material. In only two cases, colo-duodenal anastomosis was done by circular stapler side-to-end, closing the distal end with a stapler.

Patients were transferred to the recovery room and approximately 20 h later to their wards although two patients were transferred to the ICU because they were in need of respiratory assistance.

Oral intake started between the 10th and the 13th day, reducing the total parenteral nutrition (TPN).

Results

Mortality

Six patients died during the hospital stay between the 12th and the 48th post-operative day. One due to respiratory failure (12th day), 2 pulmonary sepsis (21 and 32 days after the procedure), and 3 from abdominal sepsis and multi-organ failure between the 21st and the 48th day (Table 2). In one due to fistula of the colo-colonic anastomosis, due to subphrenic absces, pneumonia, renal failure, and sepsis with respiratory failure. The third patient had an esophago-ileal fistula which was well tolerated, and was treated by TPN; it was complicated with acute cholecystitis, cholangitis, abdominal sepsis, and liver failure after cholecystectomy.

Esophageal Leakages

Three patients suffered esophageal fistulas. One after esophago-ileal anastomosis (1.3%) and two of the esophago-colonic (2.6%) patients. All of the three were treated by conservative methods (TPN, and stop oral intake).

Survival

Sixty-seven patients survived longer than 6 months after the operation. Thirty-one patients were followed for a period longer than 5 years. Fifteen patients from this group (48.4%) survived longer than 5 years (Table 2), but 6 had symptoms of recurrent disease, and recurrence was proven in 3. According to the stage of the disease, four patients, included in stage I, were living from 1 to 5 years free of disease. Forty-five percent of stage II and 47% of stage III patients survived longer than 3 years. No patients included in stage IV survived longer than 2 years.

Lymphnode Spread

Positive lymphnodes were demonstrated in the mediastinum in 24%, in the paracardial group in 96%, and in the hilum of the spleen in 64%; the gastro-epiploic arcade was affected in 19.5% and the pyloric area in 9%.

Liver metastasis was found in one case (15 mm diatmeter). Two metastases, 10 and 20 mm were demonstrated, and one was resected.

Discussion

Cancer of the cardia has been considered almost an incurable disease, although the diagnosis due to the development of dysphagia is usually performed at an earlier stage than for gastric cancer. The cause of the worse prognosis would be the frequence of intramural spread through the submucosal lymphatic vessels in the esophagus and the involvement of mediastinal lymphnodes due to the absence of the serosa. At the same time, tumors located very close to the main lymphatic trunks in the retroperitoneum can produce a rapid spread of the disease.

Therefore, removal of the esophagus alone or the stomach would not be enough for the theoretical radical treatment of this disease.

Total gastrectomy is justified, firstly if we attend to our experience because the rate of lymphnode involvement in the greater curvature and suprapiloric area is high, and because if a partial resection is made, closure of the antral section surface, colo-gastric anastomosis, and pyloroplasty require many sutures in a very small area. On the other hand, the remnant stomach has no influence in the posprandial state of the patient.

Extension of total gastrectomy to the spleen and tail of the pancreas should be indicated if we consider the high rate of lymphnode metastasis in the hilum of the spleen and around the splenic vessels.

Total esophagectomy can be justified because the intramural spread in the esophagus produces distant metastasis in the submucosal space which can be difficult to determine due to the small diameter and covering by normal mucosa.

In any case, a free margin of 6–9 cm is always necessary. If you do so, the section of the esophagus should be almost in the upper third of the mediastinum, where the anastomosis can be made, but if complications such as leakage occur, the results could be disastrous. On the other hand, the length of the remnant cervicothoracic esophagus should not be longer than 4 cm, and its removal does not compromise swallowing ability, and it is not unusual that if we do not remove it, infiltration of the upper end of the specimen can frequently be demonstrated by the pathologists.

Tumors originating in the cardia should not be compared with those which originate in the gastric fundus (gastric cancers) or on the distal esophageal wall (esophageal cancers) mainly due to the malignant evolution of heterotopic gastric mucosal epithelium. We agreed with the standard approach treatment by means of total extended gastrectomy in the first group and total esophagectomy of the thoracoabdominal segment with the subcardial portion and lesser curvature in the second; but we consider this insufficient treatment for true cancer of the cardia.

Although the radicality of the operation appears to be very aggressive, mortality and morbidity rates do not differ from that produced by total transhiatal esophagectomy or total esophagectomy. However, survival rates are quite different from the results described with other techniques in the medical literature.

The only explanation for increased survival should be the absence of esophageal or anastomotic recurrence, and the low percentage of mediastinal or abdominal recurrence compared with other series.

We know that the group of patients is too small in consideration of the long period of time and the distribution by year reduces the number of patients too much. In the same way, the study would not be completely valid if a prospective randomized series is considered. However, the interest of our analysis is the selection of the indications and the performance of the treatment by the same group of surgeons following the results very closely for a long period of time.

The Influence of Thoracic Duct Resection on Postesophagectomy Hemodynamics: An Analysis of Changes of Atrial Natriuretic Peptide and Brain Natriuretic Peptide

Yutaka Shimada, Masayuki Imamura, Takayoshi Tobe[1],
Gotaro Shirakami[2], and Kazuwa Nakao[3]

Introduction

An en bloc resection of esophageal cancer is one of the most radical forms of esophagectomy, and includes the resection of the thoracic duct. In a previous publication [1], we examined the hemodynamic changes in 24 patients whose intrathoracic ducts were resected during esophagectomy for esophageal cancer and 3 developed severe tachycardia or postoperative shock, recovering after a massive infusion of plasma. Fluid balance analysis revealed that during surgery and for 48 h after, much more fluid was necessary for en bloc resection patients.

Recently, atrial natriuretic peptide (ANP) and brain natriuretic peptide (BNP) have been widely recognized [2, 3]. These peptides serve to discharge excess fluid from the body and recent reports [4] stated the relation between natriuretic peptides and fluid volume. This study measures changes in plasma ANP and BNP levels during and immediately after en bloc resection and standard esophagectomy and compares those results with postoperative changes in the fluid balance.

Patients and Methods

Eight patients who had en bloc resection of the esophagus for intrathoracic esophageal cancer (thoracic duct resection group; TDR group), and eight patients who had a standard esophagectomy for intrathoracic esophageal cancer without resection of the thoracic duct (Standard group) were examined. The same procedure was applied to all patients [1, 5]. In brief, a right thoracotomy

First Department of Surgery[1], Intensive Care Unit[2], and Second Department of Internal Medicine[3], Faculty of Medicine, Kyoto, University, Kawaracho-54, Shogoin Sakyo-ku, Kyoto, 606 Japan

Table 1. Patient background

	TDR group ($n = 8$) (en bloc resection)	Standard group ($n = 8$) (intact thoracic duct)
Sex (male:female)	7:1	6:2
Age years	63.3 ± 4.3	66.6 ± 15.7
Body weight (kg)	56.5 ± 4.1	52.4 ± 9.0
Duration of surgery (h)	8.63 ± 0.93	8.64 ± 0.96
Tumor extension		
T1	1	3
T2	2	3
T3	4	2
T4	1	0

TDR, thoracic duct resection

was performed through the fifth intercostal space, and the upper intrathoracic esophagus was cut after it had been freed from the posterior mediastinum. Then the posterior mediastinum lymph nodes were dissected either with or without resectioning the intrathoracic portion of the thoracic duct. After resectioning of the intrathoracic esophagus and the lymph node dissection, a retrosternal gastric tube was used as an esophageal substitute and esophagogastrostomy was performed with an end-to-end anastomotic (EEA) stapler.

Anesthesia and intraoperative fluid control were described previously [1, 6]. Briefly, all patients were intubated with a left-sided endotracheal twin-lumen tube, and the lung being operated on was ventilated during the thoracotomy using high frequency positive pressure ventilation with a Servo 900B ventilator. The rate of the intraoperative infusion of electrolyte solution was about 8 ml/kg per h.

The intraoperative fluid balance was calculated by subtracting blood loss and urinary output from the volume of electrolyte solution and blood infused during surgery. The postoperative fluid balance was calculated by subtracting the volume of urinary output and of thoracic and abdominal drainage from the volume of infused electrolytes, plasma and blood. Patients' blood samples were taken before operation, before TDR, and at 1, 3, 6, 12, 24, 48 and 72 h after TDR, and on the 7th day. TDR point was set 1 h after thoracotomy in the Standard group. The plasma contained 1000 KIU/ml of aprotinine and 1 mg/ml of ethylenediamine tetraacetic acid and was stored under −20°C until measurement. Plasma ANP and BNP levels were measured by Shiono RIA ANP and Shiono RIA BNP. Shiono RIA ANP and Shiono RIA BNP were purchased from Shionogi Co., Ltd (Osaka, Japan). Statistical analysis was performed by the students, *t*-test.

Results

There were no significant differences regarding age, sex, body weight, operation time, and tumor extension (Table 1). The fluid balance of postesophagectomy patients is demonstrated in Fig. 1. Larger amounts of fluid transfusion were

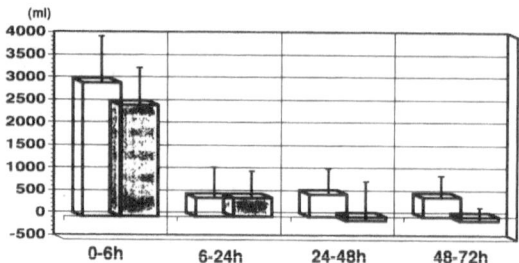

Fig. 1. Fluid balance of postesophagectomy patients. *TDR*, thoracic duct resection. *White columns*, TDR group; *dark columns*, standard group. Mean ± SD

necessary in the TDR group compared to the standard group. The fluid balance of the standard group from 24–72 h after the operation shows a minus reading.

The plasma ANP and BNP levels of esophagectomy patients are shown in Fig. 2. The plasma ANP levels increased from 48 h after the start of the operation in the standard esophagectomy group. On the other hand, the plasma ANP levels in the TDR group did not increase. The plasma BNP levels of postesophagectomy patients also increased from 24 h after the start of the operation, and the extent of these increases was larger in the standard esophagectomy group. The relation between fluid balance and plasma ANP and BNP levels is shown in Fig. 3. In spite of larger amounts of fluid transfusion, plasma ANP and BNP levels did not increase in the TDR group. Concerning the fluid balance/ANP ratio and fluid balance/BNP ratio, the fluid balance/ANP ratio of TDR group patients was higher than that of standard esophagectomy patients, and significantly higher at 72 h after the start of the operation (data not shown).

Discussion

ANP is a recently discovered hormone secreted primarily by atrial myocytes in response to local wall stretch. The combined actions of ANP on vasculature, kidneys, and adrenals serve both acutely and chronically to reduce systemic blood pressure as well as intravascular volume. The atrium releases ANP in response to atrial stretch induced by volume expansion, thus, in clinical states associated with expansion of extracellular fluid volume, plasma ANP levels rise [2]. BNP has a similar renal action. In congestive heart failure patients, the plasma BNP level rises. Contrary to ANP, BNP is secreted mainly from the ventricle and cleared from the circulation more slowly [3].

Only a few reports have previously described plasma ANP levels of esophagectomized patients [4, 7–10]. The summary of these reports is as follows: 1) Older esophagectomized patients exhibited significantly higher ANP values than those of the control group [4]; 2) plasma ANP levels were significantly higher in esophagectomized patients than in gastrectomized patients [7]; 3) plasma ANP levels of esophagectomized patients were correlated with cardiac output and pulmonary vascular resistance at 3 h after operation and on the 2nd postoperative day [8], and plasma ANP levels were also correlated with

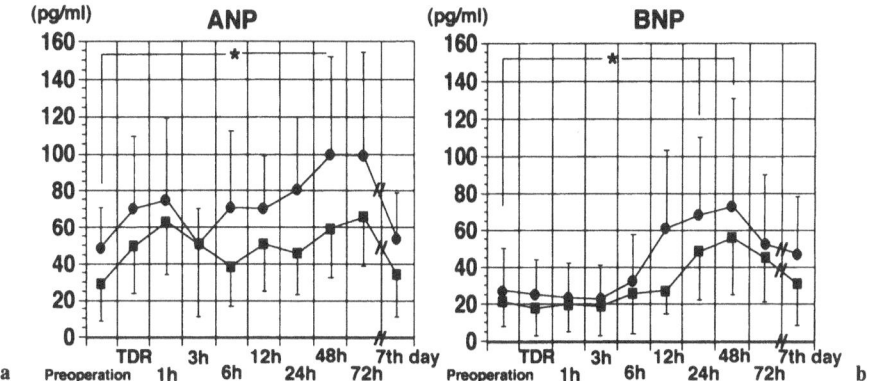

Fig. 2a,b. Changes in plasma **a** ANP and **b** BNP levels. *ANP*, atrial natriuretic peptide; *BNP*, brain natriuretic peptide. *Closed squares*, TDR group; *closed circles*, standard group. Mean ± SD. *$P < 0.05$

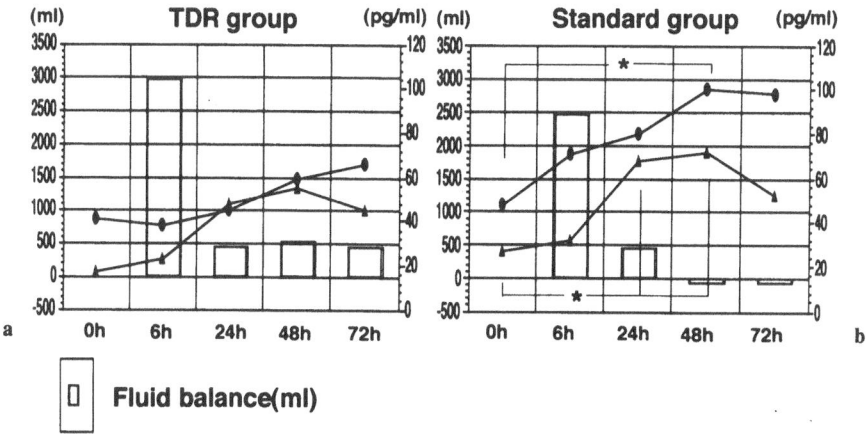

Fig. 3a,b. Relation between postoperative fluid balance and plasma ANP and BNP levels. a TDR group, **b** standard group. *Closed ellipses*, ANP (pg/ml); *closed triangles*, BNP (pg/ml). *$P < 0.05$

epinephrine and norepinephrine levels on the 1st postoperative day [9]; and 4) an inverse relationship was found between plasma ANP levels and plasma renin activity or plasma aldosterone levels [10]. Regarding plasma BNP levels and esophagectomy, no similar research exists.

In a previous publication, we described the influence of TDR on the hemodymanics of postesophagectomy patients and showed that in the TDR group larger amounts of fluid transfusion were needed compared to the Standard group. We also demonstrated that in all patients except one, following thoracic duct resection, retroperitoneal edema was observed, suggesting that in the majority of cases lymphatico-venous anastomoses are not large enough to compensate for the abrupt obstruction of the thoracic duct [1].

This study comprises the first published documentation concerning the relation between postoperative intravascular fluid volume and plasma ANP and BNP levels in TDR and standard esophagectomy patients. In order to maintain stable postoperative hemodynamics, more plasma and electrolyte solution were necessary in TDR patients compared to standard esophagectomy patients. Despite a large infusion of plasma, plasma ANP and BNP levels did not increase in TDR patients. This means that the fluid volume of the TDR group was not enough to affect the ANP and BNP levels. Obvious refilling from the third space occurred in the standard esophagectomy group on the 2nd or 3rd postoperative day. In the TDR group, however, refilling was delayed due to a decrease in plasma volume secondary to the ligation of the thoracic duct. Therefore, we conclude that en bloc resection for esophageal cancer should be performed with particular care and attention given to those hemodynamic changes caused by resection of the thoracic duct.

References

1. Imamura M, Shimada Y, Kanda T, Miyahara T, Hashimoto M, Tobe T, Arai T, Hatano Y (1992) Hemodynamic changes after resection of thoracic duct for en bloc resection of esophageal cancer. Surgery Today (Jpn J Surg) 22:226–232
2. Brenner BM, Ballermann BJ, Gunning ME, Zeidel ML (1990) Diverse biological action of atrial natriuretic peptide. Physiol Rev 70:665–699
3. Mukoyama M, Nakao N, Hosoda K, Suga S, Saito Y, Ogawa Y, Shirakami G, Jougasaki M, Obata K, Yasue H, Kambayashi Y, Inoue K, Imura H (1991) Brain natriuretic peptide as a novel cardiac hormone in humans. J Clin Invest 87:1402–1412
4. Kojima Y, Hiramatsu Y, Nakagawa A, Nishi M, Hioki K, Yamamoto M (1990) A comparative study of groups by age for the intra- and postoperative water and electrolyte management of esophageal carcinoma. Jpn J Surg 20:515–525
5. Imamura M, Ohishi K, Tobe T (1987) Retrosternal esophagogastrostomy with the EEA stapler. Surg Gynecol Obst 161:364–366
6. Imamura M, Yanagibashi K, Tobe T, Shimada Y, Naito M, Arai T, Hatano Y (1988) Transthoracic resection of esophageal cancer in patients with pulmonary dysfunction—usefulness of high frequency ventilation during thoracotomy. Ann Surg 208:601–605
7. Kojima Y (1988) Evaluation of the water-electrolyte metabolism in the patients with upper GI tract cancer—the dynamic status of secretion of a hANP levels (in Japanese with English abstract). Nippon Geka Gakkai Zasshi (J Jpn Surg Soc) 89:1603–1610
8. Kojima Y, Hiramatsu Y, Kitade H, Ogura T, Nakagawa A, Sanada T, Yamanaka H, Kawaguchi Y, Hioki K and Yamamoto M (1990) The correlation between plasma atrial natriuretic polypeptide levels (ANP) and cardiopulmonary function during the perioperative period of esophageal cancer (in Japanese with English abstract). Nihon Kyoubu Geka Gakkai Zasshi 38:1416–1423
9. Soeda K, Onoda S, Tabata Y, Hayashi H, Odaka M, Isono K (1988) Correlation of catecholamines with human atrial natriuretic polypeptides before and after surgery (in Japanese with English abstract). Igaku no Ayumi 145:133–134
10. Mitaka C, Nagura T, Sakanishi N, Tsunoda Y, Amaha K (1988) Changes in atrial natriuretic peptide after esophagectomy (in Japanese with English abstract). ICU to CCU. 12: 999–1003

Colon Interposition in the Treatment of Esophageal Carcinoma After Gastrectomy

Zhou Lun, Lin Pei-Qin, Lin Hong-Xea, and Chen Chun[1]

Introduction

The purpose of this paper is to report our experience with colon interposition (CI) in the treatment of postgastrectomy esophageal carcinoma.

Materials and Methods

During the past 16 years, 15 patients with previous gastrectomy underwent CI for esophageal squamous cell carcinoma. All 15 patients were men aged 42–71 years. The diagnosis was verified by esophagography, esophagoscopy, and histological examination. The tumor was in the middle third of the thoracic esophagus in 10 patients, in the upper third in 4, and in the lower third in 1. The length of the tumor was 3–4 cm in 6 patients and 5–8 cm in 9 patients. The period of time from gastrectomy to diagnosis of esophageal carcinoma was 3 months in one patient, 35 years in one, 6–15 years in eight, and 19–28 years in five.

The previous distal gastrectomy had been performed for benign peptic ulcer. Antecolic gastrojejunal anastomosis was then made in 12 patients and gastroduodenal anastosis in 3.

Esophagectomy and CI was performed through a right anterolateral thoracotomy and upper midline abdominal incision in 6 patients, and through above two incision with the addition of neck incision in 9 patients.

Of these 15 CI, the interposed colon and its supply artery employed are listed Table 1. CI was placed in an isoperistaltic fashion in 14 patients and an antiperistaltic fashion in 1. The route of CI was right intrathorax in 6 patients, retrosternal

[1] Department of Thoracic Surgery, Affiliated Union Hospital of Fujian Medical College, 11 Xin Quan Road, Fuzhou, Fujian, People's Republic of China 350001

Table 1. Interposed colon and its supply artery

Supply artery	Interposed colon	No. of patients
Ascending branch of left colic A.	Transverse C.	10
	Transverse C. Ascending C.	1
Ascending branch of left colic A. and middle colic A.	Transverse C.	2
	Proximal transverse C., Cecum	1
Middle colic A.	Distal transverse C., Descending C.	1

A, artery; *C*, colon

in 5, and antesternal subcutaneous in 4. The upper end of CI was anastomosed to the cervical esophagus in 9 patients and to the thoracic esophagus in 6 (anastomotic site was located on the thoracic apex in one patient and on the level of aortic arch or below aortic arch in five). The lower end of CI was anastomosed to the anterior wall of the stomach stump in ten patients, the proximal jejunal loop of gastrojejunal anastomosis in four, and the distal jejunal loop in one (the proximal jejunal loop in this patient was too short to be anastomosed).

Results

Postoperatively, one patient sustained colon graft necrosis in cervical part, a 4-cm length of necrotic colon segment was removed, and a feeding colostomy on antesternal was then performed. One patient had a cervical anastomotic leak, but the leak healed after repair. One patient with previous coronary artery disease died of acute myocardial infarction on 8 days after operation. The postoperative results of the other 12 patients were satisfactory. Follow-up observation revealed that 11 patients died within 4 months to 5 years after operation. Four patients remain alive and well 1–16 years postoperatively.

Discussion

In our experience, the pedicled colon segment can be used as an esophageal substitute for postgastrectomy esophageal carcinoma, and long-term results have been shown to be good. However, two problems concerned with CI after gastrectomy are as follows:

1. Major points of the operation include: (1) division of the adhesion among greater omentum, transverse colon, and its mesentery; between gastrojejunal anastomosis and transverse colon; (2) locate the transverse colon and gastrojejunal anastomosis; (3) identify the colic artery and its branch and select blood supply artery and colon segment to be used as a replacement; (4) the site of resection in the upper end of the esophagus depends on the exact length and adequate blood supply of the colon graft; and (5) if the ascending branch of the left colic artery is used for blood supply artery in patients with gastrojejunal anastomosis. The upper end of CI segment may be brought up directly to the

right side of the gastrojejunal anastomosis ($n = 6$) or through the opening behind the gastrojejunal anastomosis and then brought up to the left side of the gastrojejunal anastomosis ($n = 5$). The upper end of CI is then anastomosed to the esophagus. The route selected depends on increasing of blood supply and best position for extreme length of colon graft segment.

2. Effect of using colon–esophagus substitution after gastrectomy include: (1) esophageal reconstruction is sometimes difficult due to previous gastrectomy; (2) if gastrojejunal anastomosis was performed, use of the descending colon to replace the esophagus is difficult (no case in this report); and (3) adhesion in abdominal cavity and pressure of gastrojejunal anastomosis on left transverse colon may lead to shortening of the transverse colon and narrowing of the colic arteries and its branches; reduction of blood circulation of the transverse colon in some patients after gastrectomy. These lead to the inadequacy of the length and blood supply of transverse colon. Thus, the CI segment can not be brought up to the neck for cervical esophagocolic anastomosis. In comparison with the author's report [1] in 1962 (63 patients of esophageal carcinoma without previous gastrectomy), there were no instances of necrosis of CI, nor of inadequate blood supply of the transverse colon graft. The length of the transverse colon without previous gastrectomy was 31–64 cm [2]. The length from the lower margin of the throid cartilage through the anterior chest wall to the midpoint from xiphoid to umbilicus was 30–35 cm [2]. The length from the upper end of the esophagus to the cardia was 28 cm. In general, using the transverse colon only is long enough for replacement of total length of esophagus in patients without previous gastrectomy, and the esophagocolic anastomosis can be made at the neck.

In this report, the esophagocolic anastomosis was located in intrathorax in six patients; in five of them it was due to the inadequacy of the length and blood supply of the CI, and residual tumors at the upper cut edge of the esophagus were found by microscopy in three of these five patients.

The data of this series showed that shortening of transverse colon and narrowing of colic arteries and its branch after gastrectomy were related to a serious degree of adhesions in the abdominal cavity and gastrojejunal anastomosis after gastrectomy, but there was no correlation with the interval of time from previous gastrectomy to colon–esophagus substitution.

If the colon graft segment is not long enough for esophageal substitution, isolated jejunal or colon segment, residual stomach [3], or pedicled jejunal segment may be used to reconstruct the esophagus.

References

1. Li WR, Zhou L, Liang P, Lin RM (1962) Esophageal replacement by colon in the treatment of esophageal carcinoma. Chin J Surg 10:429–432
2. Liu ZZ, Zhou BJ, He XW, Zhang Z, Chai DS, Mu CZ (1988) Clinical observation on transverse colon and its application in esophageal reconstruction. Chin J Thorac Cardiovasc Surg 4:219–220
3. Lu SJ, Chen JQ, Yang JS, Chen YQ (1986) Surgical treatment of esophageal carcinoma after subtotal gastrectomy. Chin J Cancer 5:41–43

Squamous Cell Carcinoma of the Esophagus: Our Thirty Years' Experience

F. Francioni[1], R. Basile[1], P. Trentino[2], M. Trifero[2], S. Rapacchietta[2], and C. Ricci[1]

Introduction

In Italy, esophageal cancer has a mortality rate of 3.7/100000, with the majority of patients in the northern regions (Friuli-Venezia Giulia 8.1/100000, Trentino-Alto Adige 7.4/100000 Veneto 6.8/100000), probably due to alcohol consumption and smoking. In central Italy, the mortality rate is 2.1/100000 in Lazio and Abruzzi, 3.0/100000 in Umbria, 3.2/100000 in Marche, and 5.3/100000 in Toscana [1].

Since 1990, the Department of Thoracic Surgery and the Surgical Endoscopic Unit at the Second Surgical Clinic, University "La Sapienza", Rome, have started a cooperative effort to produce a correct staging for esophageal cancer patients. However, to gain insight into our undertaking, we took a look back to review the experience on esophageal cancer in a 30-year period (1960–1990), concerning 248 consecutive patients treated in our Institution.

Material and Methods

From January 1960 to December 1990, we observed 248 consecutive patients (208 men and 40 women, M/W ratio 4.6:1; age 29–83, mean 63 years) affected by squamous cell esophageal carcinoma. In our analysis, the major risk factors were alcohol consumption and smoking: 89.4% of our patients were drinking 1–21 of alcohol a day and 84.8% were smokers (more than 20 cigarettes/day). In contrast with Asian countries, diet is not a significant risk factor in esophageal cancer [2].

---

[1] Department of Thoracic Surgery, and [2] Surgical Endoscopic Unit, Second Surgical Clinic, Viale Del Policlinico, 161 University "La Sapienza", 0016 Rome Italy

Of the ten cases with idiopathic megaesophagus, eight of them were women (M/W ratio 1:4). The time delay from the beginning of the onset of megaesophagus symptomatology and cancer diagnosis was about 25 years. In three cases, the tumor was preceded by lye corrosion lesions, and the time gap between caustic ingestion and tumoral clinical onset averaged 32 years.

The neoplasia was cervical in 36 cases (14, 5%) and intrathoracic in 212 cases (85, 4%) [26 (10, 5%) to the superior, 121 (48, 8%) to the middle, and 65 (26, 1%) to the lower third].

For our retrospective analysis, the patients were divided into two groups: the first group, of 166 patients (group I), treated from 1960 to 1975 for which a precise preoperative determination of tumor staging was impossible or lacking; and the second (group II), included 82 patients treated from 1975 to 1991 and preoperatively studied, according to TNM staging [3]. The survival rates were calculated by the Kaplan-Meier method [4].

Results

In the group I, since preoperative staging was incomplete, this group was evaluated only by esophagogram and by rigid and/or flexible endoscopy. Of the 166 patients, 136 were operated on, with a resectability rate of 44% ($n = 73$). However, radical procedures (total and radical esophagectomy) were performed in only 14 of the 166 patients (8.4%), while 59 patients (35.6%) had partial esophagectomy, 8 (4.8%) had surgical bypass, 12 (7.2%) had surgical intubation, and 43 (26%) had feeding gastrostomy only. Fifteen of the 166 patients (9%) obtained a partial relief of dysphagia by dilations, and the remaining 15 had only medical therapy.

Three of the 136 operated patients (2.2%) died intraoperatively due to cardiac failure; 39 patients (28.6%) suffered early complications which caused 31 (25%) to die within 60 days postoperatively. The 5-year survival for the group I patients was 3.6% (5 of 136 operated patients).

Patients in group II, instead, were preoperatively studied, according to TNM staging, based on the results of upper endoscopy with brushing and biopsies, total body computed tomography (CT) scans, abdominal and/or cervical echography, fiberbronchoscopy, and, in the last 3 years, endoesophageal ultrasonography. Only for the last six patients was magnetic resonance (MR) imaging employed.

Overall, 19 patients (23.2%) were stage II, 48 (58.5%) were stage III, and 15 (18.3%) were stage IV (Table 1).

Of the 19 stage II patients, 18 received a total and radical esophagectomy: in 12 cases this was performed by a right thoracotomy and 6 by a transhiatal approach. The descending colon was interposed in 11 patients, the tubulized stomach in 6, and, in 1 patient who had already had a gastrectomy, a jejunal loop was used. The 19th stage II patient was endoscopically intubated due to cardiac disease.

Of the 48 stage III patients, 24 received an esophagectomy: total and radical in 11 cases, and partial in the remaining 13 patients. Total esophagectomy was performed in seven patients by thoracotomy, and in four by transhiatal approach. For reconstruction, the stomach was employed in 9 cases, and colon and jejunal

Table 1. Esophageal cancer TNM staging

Stage	Cases	%
II	19	23.2
III	48	58.5
IV	15	18.3
Total	82	100.0

Table 2. Esophageal cancer group I therapies

Therapy	Cases	%	
Refused treatment	4	2.4	
Medical therapy	11	6.6	
Intubation	12	7.2	
Dilatation	15	9.0	
Gastrostomy	43	26.0	
Surgical bypass	8	4.8	—Partial 59 (35.6%)
Esophagectomy	73	44.0 —	
			—Total 14 (8.4%)
Total	166	100.0	

Table 3. Group II therapies

Stage	Cases	Esophagectomy Total	Partial	Gastrostomy	Surgical bypass	Intub	Dilat
II	19	18	—	—	—	1	—
III	48	11	13	10	5	5	4
IV	15	—	—	8	1	2	4
Total	82	29	13	18	6	8	8

Intub, intubation; *Dilat*, dilatation

loop one time each. Among the partial esophagectomies, two were performed transhiatally only for cancer of the lower third. The tubulized stomach replaced the esophagus in 11 patients, and the colon twice. Surgical bypass by stomach was carried out in five patients. Ten patients had feeding gastrostomy. Five were intubated: only one case endoscopically, and the remaining four had dilation.

In stage IV, there were 15 patients: only one underwent a bypass with colon, one each were surgically and endoscopically intubated, eight had gastrostomy, and four dilation. Integrative radiotherapy was given in follow-up to the patients who received gastrostomy or bypass.

In group II, there was one intraoperative (1.5%) and 11 perioperative (16.6%) deaths, and the 5-year survival was 21.4% (16 of 66 operated patients). Ten of these 16 patients had a complete 5-year follow-up (Kaplan-Meier method [4]). The remaining six patients were still alive and in follow-up at the time of the study: three at 12 months from operation, one at 18 months, one at 24 months, and one at 36 months. Of the 66 operated patients, 4 dropped out, at 18, 18, 24, and 48 months, respectively (Fig. 1).

The therapeutic approaches employed in both groups are summarized, with respective percentages, in Tables 2, 3.

Discussion

The experience of our institution regarding the group I esophageal cancer patients is incomplete due to the lack of preoperative TNM staging, to the

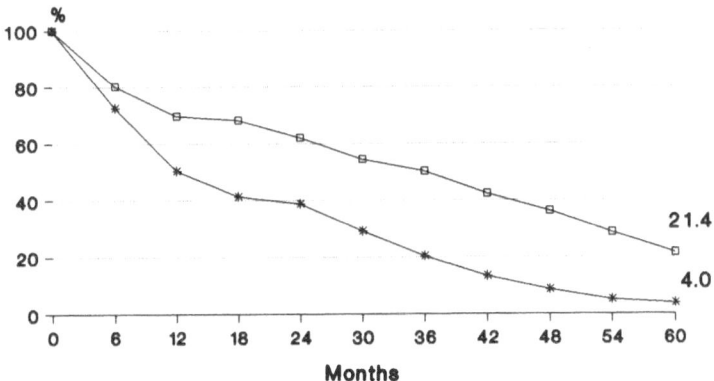

Fig. 1. Esophageal cancer 5-year survival (Kaplan-Meier method [4]). Group I, *asterisks*; group II, *open squares*

inappropriate selection of patients for surgery, and, consequentely, to the high percentage of surgical procedures which led to palliative treatment without any increase in 5-year survival. However, in group II, more accurate preoperative staging allowed us to obtain better selection of candidates for surgical treatment, with similar operability rate (82% ($n = 136$) in group I, 80.5% ($n = 66$) in group II), but with a significant decrease in the number of patients operated on in the second group; an increase in the resectability rate (from 44% to 51.2%); higher percentage of total and radical esophagectomies (from 8.4% ($n = 14$) in group I to 35.3% ($n = 29$) in group II) due to early diagnosis; decrease of intra- and perioperative deaths (respectively, 2.4% and 25% in group I, 1.5% and 16.6% in group II) and early postoperative complications (31.4% in group I, 10.6% in group II); and, above all, increase of long-term survival (from 4% ($n = 5$) in group I to 21.4% ($n = 10$) in group II) (computed by the Kaplan-Meyer statistical method).

If we compare the 5-year survivals of the two groups, 3.6% among 136 patients in the first group is a very poor percentage, such as is not found anymore in modern reports, so the 21.4% 5-year survival obtained in group II is a fair result. However, if we carefully evaluate the moderately advanced stage of the disease of our patients at the time of surgical therapy (we had no stage I patients, the majority of them being stage II and III) (Table 1), this value could be considered a good one.

Conclusions

Early diagnosis of esophageal cancer in our country is not feasible due to the lack of cancer screening programs. As the majority of patients are in an advanced stage of the disease at the time of diagnosis, preoperative evaluation is crucial to obtain acceptable 5-year survival rates of operated patients.

F. Francioni et al.

References

1. ISTAT (1982) Annuario di Statistiche Sanitarie: 1970–1978, vol 16–23. Repubblica Italiana Roma
2. Bardini R, Segalin A, Bonavina L, Anselmino M, Ruol A, Baessato M, Peracchia A (1990) Il cancro su megaesofago. Ann Ital Chir 61(3):249–52
3. AJCC (1987) Manual for staging cancer, 4th edn. JB Lippincot, Philadelphia, pp 61–6
4. Kaplan EL, Meier P (1958) Non-parametric estimation from incomplete observation, J Am Statist Assoc 53:457–481

Two-Stage Extensive Lymphadenectomy for Thoracic Esophageal Carcinoma

Takao Saito, Katsuhiro Shimoda, Yuji Shigemitsu, Tadahiko Kinoshita, Masaki Miyahara, and Michio Kobayashi[1]

Introduction

Aggressive surgery including extensive lymphadenectomy (ELA) [1, 2] is considered necessary to improve the long-term survival of patients with esophageal carcinoma. Isono et al. [1] and Kato et al. [2] reported the effectiveness of ELA on prognosis.

Surgical indication of ELA has been limited to low-risk patients because of the high surgical risks; the rate of ELA indication is around 50% (14.2%–59.8%) [3–5]. In attempts to treat the high-risk patients, we developed a two-stage ELA operation.

Patients and Method

Operative Procedures

In the two-stage operation, transthoracic subtotal esophagectomy and mediastinal lymphadenectomy were carried out as the first stage of the operation, and about 1 month later, esophageal reconstruction with the stomach or colon and abdominal and neck lymphadenectomy were done as the second stage (Fig. 1).

In one-stage operations, esophageal reconstruction as well as abdominal and neck lymphadenectomy were carried out subsequent to subtotal esophagectomy and mediastinal lymphadenectomy, on the same day and with much the same technique as the two-stage operation.

[1] The First Department of Surgery, Oita Medical University, Hasama-machi, Oita, 879-55 Japan

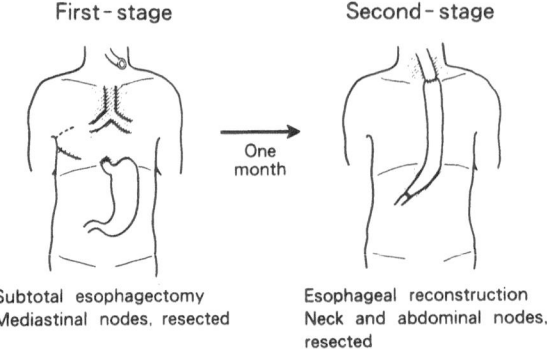

Fig. 1. Summary of two-stage operative procedures

Surgical Indication

Transthoracic subtotal esophagectomy was indicated for patients in whom impairment of the systemic state was not severe and in whom the tumor was resectable, regardless of the curability. Surgical indication of ELA was limited to patients who had curably, resectable tumors (R_{0-1} of TNM classification), excluding *in situ* cancer, and who were under 75 years of age. Selection of operative methods for ELA was determined based on impairment of the systemic state. The usual one-stage operation was selected for patients with no or mild impairment (low-risk patients) while the second-stage operation was used for those with moderate impairment (high-risk patients).

Results

Of 110 patients with thoracic esophageal cancer seen in our clinic between 1986 and 1991, 70 underwent transthoracic subtotal esophagectomy. ELA was indicated for 48 patients and completely performed in 45. Contraindications for extensive lymphadenectomy were *in situ* cancer in 1 patient, probable residual tumor (R_2) in 18 and age over 76 years in 3. Reasons why ELA was not complete were complications in two patients and other disorders in one after the first procedure of two-stage operation. The usual one-stage operation was performed in 27 low-risk patients (group A) while the two-stage operation was done for the remaining 18 high-risk patients (group B). The incidence of ELA was 94% (45/48) in patients indicated for ELA. Therefore, the use of two-stage operation contributed to increase the incidence of ELA from 56% (27/48) to 94% (45/48).

Preoperative state, surgical stress, and postoperative complications were compared between patients in group A those in group B. There were no significant differences in patient characteristics and prognostic factors including age, sex, tumor length, histologic type, TNM stage and residual tumor after treatment.

Bleeding was significantly lower in the first procedure of two-stage operation compared with the one-stage operation (765 ± 318 ml versus 1397 ± 546, respectively, $P = 0.0000$). Duration of operation was also significantly shorter in the first procedure of two-stage operation than in one-stage operation (301 ± 67 min versus 525 ± 90 min, $P = 0.0000$).

As for operative morbidity and mortality, there were no significant differences in the incidence of postoperative complications, including pneumonia (two versus two cases in groups A and B, respectively), jaundice (four versus four cases), and recurrent nerve paralysis (ten versus five cases), except that anastomotic leak (one versus three cases), and wound infections (one versus two cases) occurred more frequently in group B. There was one hospital death in each group.

The average interval time between the first and second procedures of the two-stage operation was 40 days. Effects of 40 day-delay of neck and abdominal lymph adenectomy on lymph node metastases, postoperative recurrence and 5-year survial were analyzed. The incidence of lymph node metastases was not significantly higher in group B than in group A for neck and abdominal nodes as well as for mediastinal nodes. The incidence of postoperative recurrence did not significantly differ between the two groups for all types of recurrence including lymph node. The 5-year survival rate was 35.3% for group B and 16.9% for group A, with no statistically significant difference.

Discussion

The present data are not the results of a controlled randamized study but a prospective analysis of two different groups with different systemic states. Since these two groups underwent operations during the same period and the duration of this study was relatively short, there were no changes in perioperative management and therapy. Operation was performed by the same team and the surgical technique was essentially identical in all 48 cases. Therefore, a comparison of both groups is feasible. As far as the operative risk is concerned, there was no great difference between the two groups. Thus, the two-stage operation is, in our view, an oncologically meaningful operation to extend the indication of ELA for high-risk patients with thoracic esophageal carcinoma.

References

1. Isono K, Sato H, Nakayama K (1991) Results of a nationwide study on the three field lymph node dissection of esophageal cancer. Oncology 48:411–420
2. Kato H, Watanabe H, Tachimori Y, Iizuka T (1991) Evaluation of neck lymph node dissection for thoracic esophageal carcinoma. Ann Thorac Surg 51:931–935
3. Isono K, Ochiai T, Okuyama K, Onoda S (1990) The treatment of lymph node metastasis from esophageal cancer by extensive lymphadenectomy. Jpn J Surg 20:151–157
4. Yoshida M, Iwatsuka M (1987) Extended lymph node dissection for thoracic esophageal cancer. In: Siewert JR, Hoelscher AH (eds) Diseases of the esophagus. Springer, Berlin Heidelberg, New York, pp 421–426

684 T. Saito et al.

5. Ishida K, Mori S, Okamoto K, Ohtsu T, Murakami K, Suzuki K (1987) Results of extended disection of lymph nodes in operation for thoracic esophageal cancer. In: Siewert JR, Hoelscher AH (eds) Diseases of the esophagus. Springer, Berlin, Heidelberg, New York, pp 694–696

Significance of Systematic Lymphadenectomy in Patients with Esophageal Cancer

H.D. Röher, P.R. Verreet, H. Becker, O. Horstmann, and C. Ohmann[1]

Introduction

"Surgical therapy still yields the best results in esophageal cancer!" Although the status of radio- and chemotherapy is still controversial, this quotation by Nakayama in 1979 [1] is still valid today.

However, the preferred surgical approach to esophageal resection varies and there are mainly two procedures with different demands: The transhiatal, or so called "blunt dissection", [2, 3] and the transthoracic, subtotal resection of the esophagus with systematic lymphadenectomy [4]. Proponents of the first approach suggest that abdominomediastinal esophagectomy (AM) is the safer procedure which leads to comparable 5-year survival rates [2, 5–14]. On the other hand, it is argued that the oncologic radical, transthoracic esophagectomy with systematic lymphadenectomy (TT + SLA) can be carried out with the same morbidity and mortality but with better long-term survival [4, 15–20].

We, therefore, conducted a prospective study comparing abdomino-mediastinal and transthoracic subtotal esophagectomy with systematic lymphadenectomy with regard to the following aim criteria: Perioperative complications, perioperative mortality, and long-term survival.

Patients and Methods

Between April 1986 and December 1989, we evaluated a consecutive series of esophageal cancer patients admitted to the Surgical University Clinic of Düsseldorf in a prospective clinical trial with concurrent, non-randomized groups. The only patients excluded from analysis were those with macro-

[1] Department of Surgery, Heinrich-Heine-University, Moorenstrasse 5, D-4000 Düsseldorf, Germany

scopically confirmed residual tumour, the so-called R_2 resections. It is evident that the prognosis of these patients is limited due to their residual tumor and cannot be improved by a more radical resection of the lymphatic tissue adjacent to the carcinoma. Before evaluating the aim criteria, both groups were controlled in view of structural differences in the relevant prognostic factors. These factors were: age; sex; duration of history; dysphagia; weight loss; Karnofsky scale; concurrent diseases, i.e., pulmonary risk, coronary heart disease, and liver cirrhosis; tumor type and localization; tumor length; tumor stage [21]; tumor grading; and Surgeon. The groups were compared by both univariate and multivariate analysis.

Results

Out of 136 patients with esophageal cancer, we included 87 non-R2 resections. Our overall resection rate was 68%. Approximately 50% of the patients had advanced tumor stages III and IV according to the UICC classification [21], early stage carcinoma was seen in only 12%. Even if there was no randomization, both procedures were performed in equal proportions. The overall mortality rate was 6.9% within 30 days and 10.3% before discharge (Table 1). Before evaluating the aim criteria, we compared both groups in view of stuctural differences concerning prognostic significant factors. Of the sixteen analyzed parameters, structural inequality was found in tumor localization and tumor type with more distal esophageal cancers being found in the abdominomediastinal group. Fifty percent of the transhiatal and 66% of the transthoracic resections showed lymph node metastases [22]. This imbalance however might be based on the different numbers of lymph nodes resected in both procedures (twice as many in the transthoracic group as in the abdominomediastinal group). Structural inequality in only 2 of 16 parameters is the basis for the following analysis (Table 2).

Table 1. General patient data

Number	136 unselected patients	
	92 resections (68%)	
	87 non R_2 resections	
Sex ratio	11:1	
Age	56 (40;71) years	
Histology	Squamous	81%
	Adeno	16%
Tumor stage	0, I	12%
	IIa, IIb	39%
	III, IV	49%
Approach	AM	46 (53%)
	TT + SLA	41 (47%)
Mortality	30 days	6 (6.9%)
	in clinic	9 (10.3%)

AM, abdominomediastinal; *TT + SLA*, transthoracic esophagectomy with systematic lymphadenectomy

Table 2. Multivariate analysis with stepwise logistic regression

Structural Uniformity			
Variable	Coefficient	SEM	P-value
Tumor localization	(1) −0.92	0.44	0.059
	(2) 0.52	0.44	
Tumor type	(1) 2.04	0.82	0.005
	(2) −1.92	0.92	
N-stage	−0.60	0.30	0.038

Table 3. Univariate analysis (chi-square test) revealed no significant difference between the groups

	In clinic mortality		
Approach	yes	no	total
AM	6 (13%)	40	46
TT + SLA	3 (7%)	38	41
Total	9 (10.3%)	78	87

Table 4. Multivariate analysis (multiple linear logistic regression)

Mortality before discharge			
Variable	Coefficient	SEM	P-value
Replacing organ	−1.20	0.45	0.000
Diabetes	−0.95	0.45	0.005
Pathologic ECG	−0.83	0.42	0.013
Intraoperative complications	−0.74	0.42	0.073

The first aim criteria was mortality before discharge. Looking at the mulitvariate analysis, mortality was 13% in the abdominomediastinal and 7% in the transthoracic group. The chi-square test shows no significant difference (Table 3).

Multivariate analysis of the structural imbalance shows that the choice of procedure has no influence on mortality before discharge, but there are other factors responsible for the perioperative risk. These are selection of esophageal substitute (gastric tube or colon), diabetes, pathologic ECG indicating coronary heart disease, and intraoperative complications, such as tracheal laceration and bleeding as the expression of advanced tumor stage (Table 4).

The second aim criteria was long-term survival. In the univariate analysis of the Kaplan-Meier curves and in the multivariate analysis by Cox's procedure, there is no significant difference between both curves in long-term survival (Fig. 1). Again, taking into account structural imbalances in the multivariate

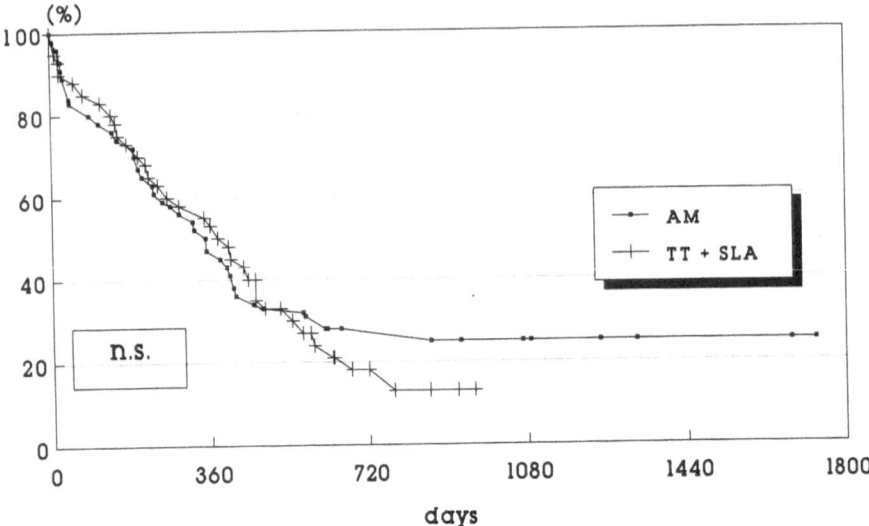

Fig. 1. Long-term survival and approach: transthoracic esophagectomy with systematic lymphadenectomy (*crosses*) versus abdominomediastinal (*closed squares*). Univariate analysis. *n.s.*, not significant

Table 5. Multivariate analysis (Cox-model)

Long-term survival			
Variable	Coefficient	SEM	P-value
Replacing-organ	1.43	0.57	0.066
Sex	1.18	0.57	0.098
Surgical radicality	0.45	0.22	0.055
Intraoperative complications	1.14	0.35	0.002
T-stage	0.67	0.27	0.028
Liver cirrhosis	2.37	0.86	0.053

analysis, there are factors other than the extent of lymphadenectomy which determine the patient's prognosis. The prognosis is usually worse for male patients with microscopically confirmed residual tumor, intraoperative complications, later T-stage, and liver cirrhosis (Table 5).

Discussion

In conclusion, we have to state that although there is a slight structural difference in tumor localization, tumor type, and probably in the N-stage in both groups, transthoracic esophagectomy with systematic lymphadenectomy and transmediastinal esophagectomy can be performed with comparable perioperative mortality.

Finally, systematic lymphadenectomy does not guarantee the expected improvements in long-term survival.

References

1. Nakayama K (1979) My experience in the management of esophageal cancer. Int Surg 64:7–11
2. Orringer MB (1988) Transhiatal esophagectomy for esophageal carcinoma. In: Siewert JR, Hölscher AH (eds) Diseases of the esophagus. Springer, Berlin Heidelberg New York, pp 697–702
3. Siewert JR, Hölscher AH, Horvath ÖP (1986) Transmediastinale Oesophagektomie. Langenbecks Arch Chir 367:203–213
4. Siewert JR, Hölscher AH, Roder J, Bartels H (1988) En-bloc Resektion der Speiseröhre beim Ösopahguskarzinom. Langenbecks Arch Chir 373:367–376
5. Barbier PA, Becker CD, Wagner HE (1988) Esophageal carcinoma: Patient selection for transhiatal esophagectomy. A prospective analysis of 50 consecutive cases. World J Surg 12:263–269
6. Finley RJ, Incluet RI (1989) The results of esophagastrectomy without thoracotomy for adenocarcinoma of the esophagogatric junction. Ann Surg 210:535–543
7. Garvin PJ, Kaminski DL (1980) Extrathoracic esophagectomy in the treatment of esophageal cancer. Am J Surg 140:772–778
8. Giuli R, Sancho-Garnuer H (1986) Diagnostic, therapeutic and prognostic features of cancers of the esophagus: Results of the international prospective study conducted by the OESO group. Surgery 99:614–622
9. Goldfaden D, Orringer M, Appelmann HD, Kalish R (1986) Adenocarcinoma of the distal esophagus and gastric cardia. J Thorac Cardiovasc Surg 91:242–247
10. Hankins JR, Attar S, Coughlin TR, McLaughlin JS (1989) Carcinoma of the esophagus: A comparison of the results of transhiatal versus transthoracic resection. Ann Thorac Surg 47:700–705
11. Peracchia A, Bardini R, Ruol A, Asolati M, Segalin A, Cavazzini F, Castoro C (1988) Blunt esophagectomy without thoracotomy for carcinoma of the esophagus: Experince with 127 patients. In: Siewert JR, Hölscher AH (eds): Diseases of the esophagus. Springer, Berlin Heidelberg New York, pp 697–702
12. Röher HD, Linn RM, Stahlknecht CD, Thon KP (1988) Zur operativen Verfahrenswahl beim Ösophaguskarzinom. Chirurg 59:582–586
13. Shahian DM, Neptune WB, Ellis FH, Watkins E (1986) Transthoracic versus extrathoracic esophagectomy: Mortality, morbidity, and long-term survival. Ann Thorac Surg 41:237–246
14. Steiger Z, Wilson RF (1981) Comparison of the results of esophagogastrectomy with and without a thoracotomy. Surg Gyn Obst 153:653–656
15. Fok M, Siu KF, Wong J (1989) A Comparison of transhiatal and transthoracic resection for carcinoma of the thoracic esophagus. Am J Surg 158:414–419
16. Ishida K, Mori S, Okamoto K, Ohtsu T, Murakami J, Suzuki K, Sato N (1986) Results of extended dissection of lymph nodes in operation for thoracic esophageal cancer. In: Siewert JR, Hölscher AH (eds) Diseases of the esophagus. Springer, Berlin Heidelberg New York, pp 697–702
17. Nishihiria T, Watanabe T, Ohmori N, Kitamura M, Toyoda K, Hirayama K, Kawachi S, Kuramato J, Kanoh T, Akashi T, Sekine Y, Kasai M (1984) Long-term evaluation of patients treated by radical operation for carcinoma of the thoracic esophagus. World J Surg 8:778–785
18. Saskai K, Muto T, Tanaka O, Soga J (1988) The significance of systematic lymphadenectomy for thoracic esophageal carcinoma. In: Siewert JR, Hölscher AH (eds): Diseases of the esophagus. Springer, Berlin Heidelberg New York, pp 697–702

19. Sugimachi K, Kitamura M, Ueo H, Tamada R, Inokuchi K (1985) Improved results of surgery for esophageal carcinoma in 148 patients. Jpn J Surg 15:190–194
20. Yoshida M, Iwatsuka M (1988) Extended lymph node dissection for thoracic esophageal cancer. In: Siewert JR, Hölscher AH (eds): Diseases of the esophagus. Springer, Berlin Heidelberg New York, pp 697–702
21. Hermanek P, Scheibe O, Spiessl B, Wagner G (eds) (1987) UICC:TNM classification of malignant tumors, 4th edn. Springer Verlag Berlin Heidelberg New York London Paris Tokyo
22. Japanese Society for Esophageal Diseases (1984) Guidelines for the clinical and pathologic studies on carcinoma of the esophagus, 6th edn. Kanetara, Tokyo

A Study on the Mode of Recurrence in Cases with Esophagectomy and Extensive Lymph Node Dissections

MASAHIKO MUROI, MISAO YOSHIDA, and NORIYUKI KUBOTA[1]

Introduction

In cases with thoracic esophageal cancer, postoperative recurrence at the posterior mediastinum and the neck are frequently observed as well as metastasis in distant organs. Extensive lymph node dissection procedures have been developed and applied in cases of thoracic esophageal cancer for these 8 years in Japan, with the expectation that a decrease in the rate of recurrence in the neck and the mediastinum would occur. In this paper, the rate and mode of recurrence among patients with thoracic esophageal cancer who underwent esophagectomy with extensive lymph node dissection at our hospital were studied. It was expected that the results would yield improved indications and postoperative care of this type of patient.

Patients and Methods

From 1985 to 1991, esophagectomy had been carried out on 176 patients with thoracic esophageal cancer at our hospital. Extensive lymph node dissection was employed in 69 cases (39%). Extensive lymph node dissection was carried out on bilateral neck, paraesophageal nodes, bilateral paratracheal nodes (including those along the anterior aspects of the trachea), infra-aortic nodes, perigastric, and celiac nodes. The 30-day operative death rate was 2.9%, and the hospital death rate was 5.6% (Table 1). In this study, 54 patients who tolerated extensive dissection were included and those who died from causes other than cancer were excluded. All patients could be classified into two groups: (1) patients who

---

[1] Department of Surgery, Metropolitan Komagome General Hospital, Honkomagome 3-18-22, Bunkyo-ku, Tokyo, 113 Japan

Table 1. Surgical results of extensive lymph
node dissection

Total no. of esophagectomies	176
No. of extensive dissections	69 (39%)
Mortality rate	2.9%
Hospital death rate	5.6%

Table 2. Characteristics of the subjects

	Recurrance	No recurrance
No. of cases	18	36
Average age (years)	57.3 ± 7.4	59.9 ± 7.5
Location		
Upper third	9%	8%
Middle third	83%	77%
Lower third	4%	8%
Multiple lesions	4%	5%

Table 3. Depth of invasion and recurrence

Parietal invasion	No. of cases (n)	No. of recurred cases (n)	Incidence of recurrence
Epithelium	1	0	0%
Mucosa	2	0	0%
Submucosa	14	1	7%
Muscularis propria	6	2	33%
Adventitia	31	15	48%
Total	54 cases	18 cases	33%

developed postoperative recurrences (18 cases) and (2) those without recurrence (36 cases). There was no significant difference between the two groups in age and location of tumor (Table 2).

Results

Depth of tumor invasion was shown to have a close relationship with the incidence of recurrence. Recurrence was found in 7% of patients with cancer invasion into the submucosa, 33% the muscularis propria and 48% in the adventitia (Table 3).

Lymph node metastasis (89%) and severe microvascular invasion (lymphatic 39% and venous 39%) were frequent in cases with recurrence, and infrequent in cases without recurrence (lymph node metastasis 42%, lymphatic permiation 8%, and veno is permiation 3%) (Table 4).

The number of positive nodes was significantly smaller ($P < 0.01$) in cases without recurrence (1.1 ± 1.9) than those with recurrence (7.9 ± 11.1) (Table 5).

Table 4. Pathological findings and recurrence

	Recurrance	No recurrance	Total
No. of cases (*n*)	18	36	54
	(100%)	(100%)	(100%)
Microvascular invasion			
Lymphatic vessel			
(−)	0%	11%	7%
(+)	61%	81%	74%
(++)	39%	8%	19%
Blood vessel			
(−)	0%	8%	7%
(+)	61%	89%	74%
(++)	39%	3%	19%
Lymph node metastasis			
(−)	11%	58%	44%
(+)	89%	42%	56%

Table 5. Number of positive lymph nodes and recurrence

	Recurrance	No recurrance
No. of cases (*n*)	18	36
Dissected nodes	95.9 ± 36.8	98.1 ± 26.8 (n.s.)
Positive nodes	7.9 ± 11.1	1.1 ± 1.9 ($P < 0.01$)

Table 6. Number of regions with metastasis and recurrence

No. of regions	Recurrance	No recurrance
	18 cases (100%)	36 cases (100%)
None	11%	58%
One	22%	25%
Two	28%	17%
Three	39%	0%
Average	2.5 ± 1.0	1.5 ± 0.7
	$P < 0.05$	

Dissecting fields were classified into three regions: The neck, the posterior mediastinum, and the upper abdomen. All patients having lymph node metastasis to all three regions developed recurrence. The average number of regions with lymph node metastasis was 2.5 ± 1.0 in cases with recurrence and 1.5 ± 0.7 without recurrence ($P < 0.05$) (Table 6).

Modes of recurrence were classified into three groups: (1) Local type— diffusely infiltrating tumor in the mediastinum, (2) distant organ type, and (3) lymph node type—local lymph node metastasis in the marginal area between the neck and the chest. The mode of recurrence was closely related to the disease-

Table 7. Mode of recurrence and disease free interval

Mode of recurrence	No. of cases (n)	Disease-free interval (days)
Local	3	182 ± 54.8
Distant	12	234 ± 94.6
Lymphatic	5	539 ± 252.2

$P < 0.05$ (Local vs Distant); $P < 0.01$

Table 8. Parietal invasion and mode of recurrence

Depth of invasion	No. of cases (n)	No. of recurrence	Mode of recurrence (Local)	(Distant)	(Mixed)
Epithelium	1	0	0	0	0
Mucosa	2	0	0	0	0
Submucosa	14	1	0	1	0
Muscularis propria	6	2	0	2	0
Adventitia	31	15	2	6	6
Total	54 (100%)	18 (33%)	2 (4%)	9 (17%)	6 (12%)

free interval. Local type recurrences developed in 185 ± 54.8 days, significantly shorter than distant organ type (234 ± 94.6 days) or lymph node type (539 ± 25.2 days) (Table 7).

Grade of parietal invasion also demonstrated a close relationship with the mode of recurrence. In cases with marked invasion into the adventitia, all three modes of recurrence were found, and local type in particular was frequently identified in this group. In cases with submucosal cancer and those with invasion into the muscularis propria, local type was not observed but distant organ metastasis was identified (Table 8).

Discussion

Lymph Node Metastasis and Parietal Invasion

Currently, extensive dissection is one way to obtain precise information on lymph node metastasis. Lymph node metastasis was found in 56% of our patients who underwent extensive dissection, and these results were similar to those reported by Akiyama et al. (59%) [1], but less than that of Kato et al. (72%) [2]. The incidence of lymph node metastasis may vary according to number of cases with each type of parietal invasion. Patients with mucosal cancer seldom demonstrated lymph node metastasis, but the frequency increases when parietal invasion reaches the submucosa or deeper [3–6], and the incidence of lymph node metastasis increases with parietal invasion. Iizuka et al. [3], who is the chairman of Japanese Committee for Registration of Esophageal Carcinoma, reviewed 5481 cases and reported that depth of invasion reflected survival. If carcinoma invasion was limited to the muscularis mucosa (mm), 10-

year survival was 50%. However, if it reached the submucosa (sm), 10-year survival dropped to 36.4%, which was not very different from the muscularis propria (25%) or the adventitia (22.5%). In our patients, incidences of recurrence were 0% in cases with mm, 7% with sm, 33% with mestasis to the muscular propria, and 40% to the adventitia. These results suggested that in cases of mucosal cancer, radical esophagectomy may not be indicated because this type of patient rarely experiences lymph node metastasis [7]. Local eradication of the mucosal lesion constitutes radical treatment for them. Extensive dissection may be indicated for cases with parietal invasion into the submucosa or deeper. On the other hand, indications of extensive dissection for cases with adventitial invasion must be evaluated in terms of the frequency of recurrence [8, 9].

Indications for Postoperative Adjuvant Therapy

The number of positive nodes is one indicator which reflected the likelihood of postoperative recurrence. Patients with two or more regions with lymph node metastasis or severe microvascular invasion are also likely to experience recurrence. Parietal invasion into the adventitia is also recurrence. Postoperative adjuvant therapies are recommended for cases with many positive nodes, metastasis in more than two regions, or tumor invasion into the adventitia.

Mode of Recurrence and Treatments

When parietal invasion was confined to the muscularis propria or less, distant organ metastasis is likely so chemotherapy should be employed following radical esophagectomy, especially for patients with many positive nodes or with severe microvascular permeation at histological studies. On the other hand, the incidence of recurrences was remarkably high in cases with adventitial invasion, and every type of recurrence was noticed. Postoperative treatment for local recurrence should be considered first because of the short disease-free interval.

Conclusions

1. Extensive lymph node dissection could be carried out at an operative death rate of 2.9% and a hospital death rate of 5.6%.
2. The number of positive nodes and the number of regions with positive nodes are reliable indicators of recurrence.
3. Distant organ metastasis may occur in cases with parietal invasion into the submucosa or the muscularis propria layer.
4. In cases with adventitial invasion, all modes of recurrence may take place. Local recurrence occurrs within a relatively shorter period of time, and this should be considered in choosing the best postoperative adjuvant therapy.
5. Extensive dissection should not be indicated for mucosal cancer of the esophagus.
6. Recurrences were frequent in cases with marked invasion into the adventitia, but indications for extensive dissection for then have not yet been clearly defined.

References

1. Akiyama H, Tsurumaru M, Kawamura T, Ono Y (1981) Principle of surgical treatment for carcinoma of the esophagus. Analysis of lymph node involvement. Ann Surg 194:438–446
2. Kato H, Tachimori Y, Watanabe H, Iizuka T, Terui S, Itabashi M, Hirota T (1991) Lymph node metastasis in thoracic esophageal carcinoma. J Surg Oncol 48:106–111
3. Iizuka T, Isono K, Kakegawa T, Watanabe (1989) Paramaters linked to 10-year survival in Japan of resected esophageal carcinoma. Chest 960:1005–1011
4. Isono K, Sato H, Nakayama K (1991) Result of a nationwide study on the three-field lymph node dissection of esophageal cancer. Oncology 48:411–420
5. Perachia A, Roul A, Baldini R, Segalin C, Castro C, Asolati M (1992) Lymph node dissection for cancer of the thoracic esophagus: How extensive should it be? Analysis of personal data and review of the literature. In: Diseases of the esophagus. Masson, Milano, pp 69–73
6. Yoshida M, Muroi M, Iwatuka M (1988) Esophagectomy with extensive lymph node sissection for esophageal carcinoma. Its availability and complications. In: Proceedings of the 4th Congress of the Japanese Section of the ISDE, Tokyo
7. Momma K, Yosida M, Sakaki H, Tajima T, Iwasaki Y, Takizawa T (1992) Endoscopic estimation of the depth of invasion in surperficial esophageal cancer. Stomach and Intestine 27(2):157–173
8. Siewert JR, Roder JD (1992) Lymphadenectomy in esophageal cancer surgery. In: Diseses of the esophagus. Masson, Milano, pp 91–98
9. Desai PB, Deshpande RK, Patil PK, Mistry RC (1992) Radical lymphadenectomy in esophageal cancer. Does it improve survival? In: Diseases of the esophagus. Masson, Milano, pp 92–99

Surgical Treatment of Intrathoracic Esophageal Carcinoma: Analysis of 481 Cases of Resected Squamous Cell Carcinoma

Masahiko Tsurumaru, Harushi Udagawa, Yoshimasa Ono, Yoshiaki Kajiyama, and Hiroshi Akiyama[1]

Introduction

Conventional surgical treatment of esophageal carcinoma does not yield a satisfactory outcome. Recurrence is frequently observed in upper mediastinal and/or cervical lymph nodes. Blood-borne metastasis is another factor contributing to the poor prognosis. Considerable effort, including extensive lymph node dissection and chemotherapy, has been directed to improving the long-term survival rate. In our department, the routine surgical treatment for thoracic esophageal carcinoma including adjuvant therapy was changed in 1984, particularly in terms of the extent of lymph node dissection. The aim of this investigation was to analyze the difference in long-term survival achieved with the surgical approaches applied before and after 1984.

Materials and Methods

We analyzed the results of treatment in 481 cases of resected squamous cell carcinoma of the intrathoracic esophagus. This analysis excluded cases of palliative resection (R2) and cases of mortality in the immediate postoperative period (within 30 days of surgery). The patients were divided into two groups. Group F (the former procedure group; F) included 276 patients who underwent esophagectomy with thoracic-abdominal lymph node dissection before 1984, when this was the routine procedure. Group L (the latter procedure group; L) comprised 205 patients who underwent esophagectomy with extensive lymph node dissection (cervical-thoracic-abdominal dissection) after 1984. In this group, adjuvant chemotherapy with cisplatin (CDDP) and 5-fluorouracil (5-FU)

[1] Department of Surgery, Toranomon Hospital, 2-2-2, Toranomon, Minato-ku, Tokyo, 105 Japan

Table 1. Background data for groups F and L

Factor	Group F	Group L	P value
Number of patients	276	205	
Sex: male/female	236/40	175/30	$P = 0.9653$
Age in years			$P = 0.0042$
Range	35–90	36–84	
Mean	61.4	59.1	
Location of tumor			$P = 0.4518$
Upper	24	25	
Middle	168	121	
Lower	84	59	

Table 2. T Categories of Groups F and L

T Categories	Group F	Group L
Tis	4	5
T1	45	45
T2	43	20
T3	155	124
T4	13	10
Tx	7	1

$P = 0.2254$ between group F and group L

Table 3. Tumor staging

TNM stage	Group F	Group L
0	4	4
1	41	30
2A	50	21
2B	41	16
3	91	53
4	36	80
(4L)	(35)	(80)

$P < 0.0001$ between group F and group L

was also administered to patients with histologically proven lymph node metastases in the cervical and/or superior mediastinal areas. The long-term survival rate was calculated by means of the Kaplan-Meier method. Differences were evaluated by the log rank test, and statistical significance was defined as $P < 0.05$.

Results

Background data for the two groups are shown in Table 1. There were 276 patients in group F and 205 in group L. There were no significant differences between the two groups in terms of sex ratio or tumor location. However, group L patients were significantly younger than those in group F.

The T categories of the two groups are presented in Table 2. Chi square analysis disclosed no significant difference between the two groups ($P = 0.2254$).

The TNM staging is shown in Table 3. A significantly higher incidence of stage 4 cancers was observed in group L. However, although group L appears to include a larger number of advanced cases than group F, we suspect this was because group F underwent less extensive lymph node dissection. If the procedure had been more extensive, it is likely that a greater number of positive distant nodes would have been detected in this group as well.

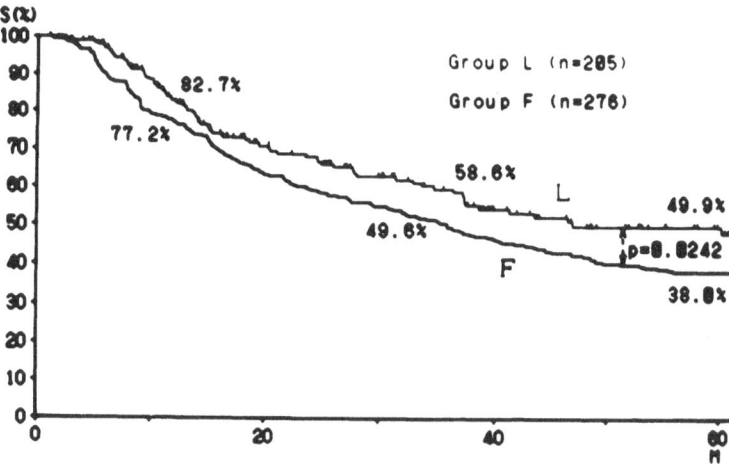

Fig. 1. Survival of thoracic esophageal carcinoma patients

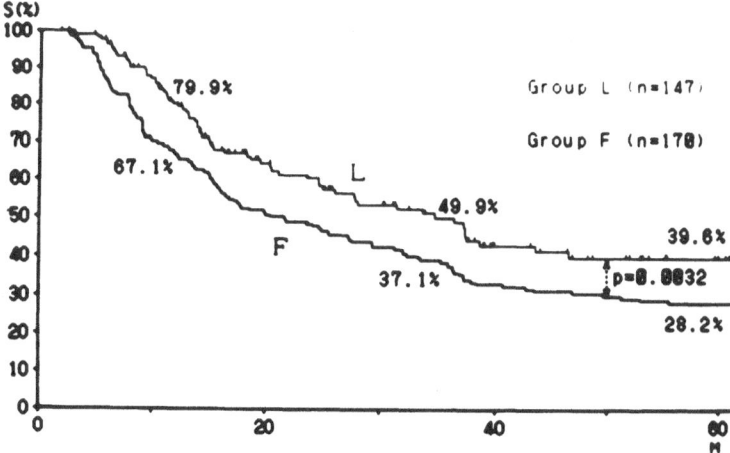

Fig. 2. Survival curves of patients with lymph node metastasis

Figure 1 shows the survival curves for the two groups. The survival rates in group L were 82.7% for 1 year, 58.6% for 3 years and 49.9% for 5 years. The survival rates were better in group L than in group F, and the difference is statistically significant ($P = 0.0242$).

Long-term survival is dependent upon many factors, the most important of which is thought to be lymph node metastasis. Figure 2 shows the survival curves of patients with lymph node involvement. The 5-year survival rates were 19.6% for group F and 28.2% for group L. This difference also is statistically significant ($P = 0.0032$).

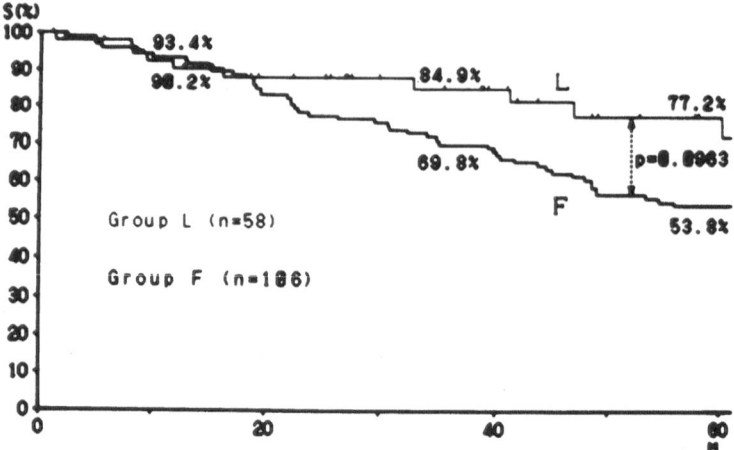

Fig. 3. Survival curves of patients without lymph node metastasis

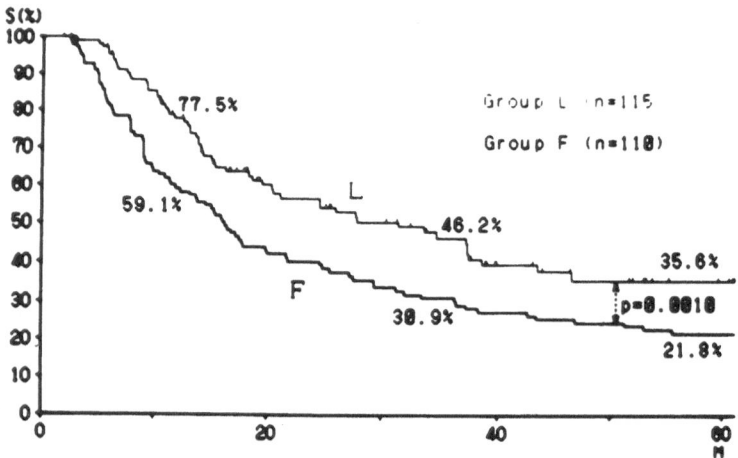

Fig. 4. Survival of patients with mediastinal lymph node metastasis

Five-year survival in patients without lymph node metastasis was longer in group L than in group F, but the difference is not statistically significant (Fig. 3). Figure 4 shows the survival curves for patients with positive nodes in the mediastinum. The 5-year survival rates were 35.6% for group L and 21.8% for group F which is a significant difference ($P = 0.0010$). Even among patients without lymph node metastasis in the mediastinum, survival was significantly longer in group L (Fig. 5).

Examination of the survival rates of patients without lymph node metastasis in the superior mediastinum, revealed a difference in outcome that is highly significant in favor of group L (Fig. 6).

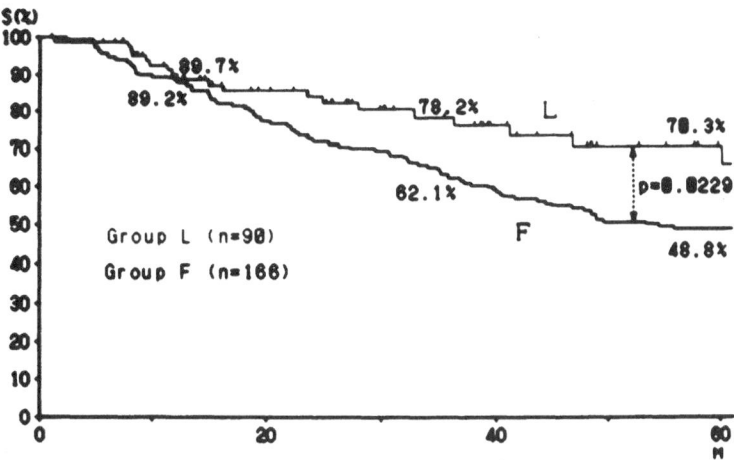

Fig. 5. Survival of patients without mediastinal lymph node metastasis

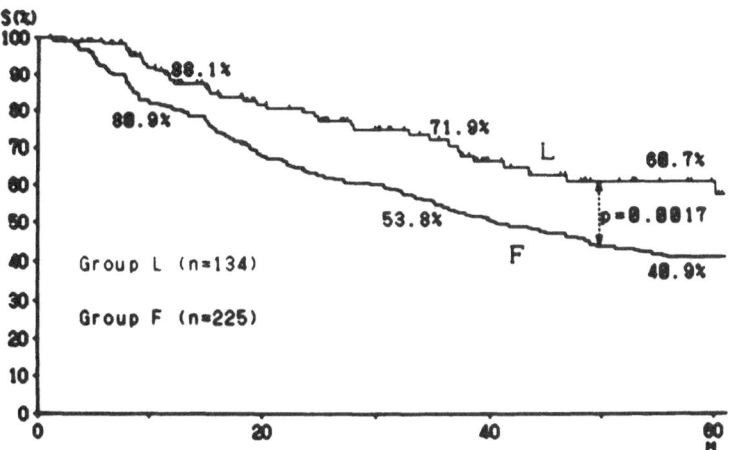

Fig. 6. Survival of patients without superior mediastinal node metastasis

Discussion

It is well known that esophageal carcinoma carries a very poor prognosis. We have frequently observed extensive lymph node metastasis in the neck, mediastinum and abdomen. Postoperative recurrence takes the form of lymph node metastasis in the cervical and/or superior mediastinal area, accompanied by symptoms of hoarseness, superior vena caval syndrome or severe cough. These facts suggest that one of the most important contributors to the poor prognosis is lymph node involvement, which was our main reason for changing our treatment protocol, including our surgical procedure and adjuvant therapy in 1984. Prior to that time, we performed two-field dissection, or thoracic-abdominal dissection. More extensive lymph node dissection especially along both sides of the recurrent laryngeal nerve in the superior mediastinum and the neck, has been applied since 1984. This procedure is termed cervical-thoracic-abdominal, or three-field, dissection. Postoperative chemotherapy is administered to patients with positive nodes in the neck and/or the superior mediastinum.

We analyzed the background data and long-term survival rates of patients treated before and after the procedures changed in 1984. TNM staging data showed a significantly higher incidence of stage 4 in group L, which suggests the possibility that metastatic lymph nodes were left behind in some patients in group F. We believe this to be the main reason for the better survival rate in group L because the survival rates of patients with no lymph node metastasis (NO and MO) were also better in group L. Patients in group F diagnosed as having no histological evidence of lymph node involvement probably included some involved nodes were missed with the less extensive lymph node dissection.

This concept proved valid for patients who were negative for lymph node metastasis in the superior mediastinum. In this subpopulation, survival was dramatically longer in group L than in group F. Since the patients in group L did not undergo postoperative chemotherapy, it can be concluded that the better outcome in this group was not a result of adjuvant therapy but rather of extensive lymph node dissection.

In summary, radical tumor excision plus cervical-thoracic-abdominal lymph node dissection combined with adjuvant chemotherapy, improved the long-term survival rate for patients with intrathoracic esophageal carcinoma.

The Results of En Bloc Esophagectomy Compared with Three-Field and Two-Field Dissection

Hiromasa Fujita, Teruo Kakegawa, Hideaki Yamana[1],
Arnulf H. Hölscher, Elfriede Bollschweiler,
and J. Rüdiger Siewert[2]

Introduction

The technique employed for radical esophagectomy performed for a carcinoma in the thoracic esophagus differs geographically in that en bloc esophagectomy is more common at hospitals in Europe and North America [1, 2], while three-field dissection is preferred in Japan [3]. The main difference between these two procedures is that cervical and upper mediastinal lymph node dissection is performed in three-field dissection and is not performed in en bloc esophagectomy. In order to evaluate the significance of such dissection, we compared the operative results for en bloc esophagectomy in the Technical University of Munich (TU Munich) with those for two or three-field dissection in Kurume University (Kurume).

Materials and Methods

In the 5 years between 1985 and 1989, 134 patients with squamous cell carcinoma in the thoracic esophagus underwent esophagectomy in TU Munich, 67 (50%) of whom underwent curative (R_0: UICC 1987) [4] en bloc esophagectomy. During the same period, 168 patients underwent esophagectomy in Kurume, 87 (52%) of whom underwent curative esophagectomy (49 patients had two-field dissection and 38 had three-field dissection). In TU Munich, en bloc esophagectomy was performed for all curatively operated patients. On the other hand, three-field dissection was performed only for patients in Kurume who were less than 70 years old, had an advanced cancer (stage II, III, and IV) and had a low risk to

[1] The First Department of Surgery, Kurume University School of Medicine, 67 Asahi-machi, Kurume, Fukuoka, 830 Japan
[2] Department of Surgery, Technical University of Munich, Ismaninger Straße 22, D-8000 München 80, Germany

703

Table 1. Clinical characteristics of patients who underwent transthoracic R$_o$ esophagectomy

		Munich	Kurume		
		En bloc	Three-field	Two-field	
No. of cases		67	38	49	
pT	pT1	9 (13%)	3 (8%)	9 (18%)	
	pT2	20 (30%)	8 (21%)	11 (22%)	
	pT3	36 (54%)	27 (71%)	27 (56%)	
	pT4	2 (3%)	0 (0%)	2 (4%)	
pN	pN0	34 (51%)[*1]	8 (21%)[*2]	18 (37%)	[*1–*2]: P < 0.01
	pN1	33 (49%)	30 (79%)	31 (63%)	
pM (LYM)	pM0	67 (100%)[*1]	33 (87%)[*2]	47 (96%)	[*1–*2]: P < 0.01
	pM1	0 (0%)	5 (13%)	2 (4%)	
Stage	stage I	8 (12%)[*1]	0 (0%)[*2]	5 (10%)	[*1–*2]: P < 0.01
	stage IIA	24 (36%)	8 (21%)	13 (27%)	
	stage IIB	10 (15%)	9 (24%)	10 (20%)	
	stage III	25 (37%)	16 (42%)	19 (39%)	
	stage IV	0 (0%)	5 (13%)	2 (4%)	

* pTNM Pathological Classification. pM(LYM): Distant lymph nodes including the cervical and coeliac nodes

postoperative complications, while the remaining patients underwent two-field dissection. The patients' characteristics according to the TNM classification are summarized in Table 1.

There was no difference in the mortality rates or in the cause of death between the patients in TU Munich and those in Kurume. The cumulative survival curves were calculated by Kaplan-Meier statistics, for all patients who died with recurrence, and also for those who died without recurrence, and these curves were compared by the generalized Wilcoxon and Log rank method.

Results

In the 67 patients from TU Munich that underwent en bloc esophagectomy, a total of 2482 lymph nodes were resected and, of these, 170 (6.8%) had positive metastasis. In 87 patients from Kurume, a total of 6035 lymph nodes were resected and 282 (4.7%) had positive metastasis. The rate of positive metastatic lymph nodes per resected lymph nodes was 2.8% (96/3392) in patients undergoing three-field dissection, and 7.3% (192/2643) in those undergoing two-field dissection.

The average number of the resected lymph nodes is summarized in Table 2. There was a significant difference in the number of resected lymph nodes among the patients who underwent en bloc esophagectomy, those who underwent three-field dissection, and those who underwent two-field dissection (each $P <$ 0.01). This difference was due to cervical and upper mediastinal lymph node dissection. During three-field dissection, an average of 26 cervical lymph nodes and 20 upper mediastinal lymph nodes were resected per patient. During two-field dissection, an average of 12 upper mediastinal lymph nodes were resected

Table 2. Average numbers of resected lymph nodes during transthoracic R_0 esophagectomy

	Munich	Kurume		
	En bloc	Three-field	Two-field	
Cervical LNs	0	$26.3 \pm 10.4^{*1}$	$3.4 \pm 9.2^{*2}$	$^{*1-*2}$ P < 0.01
Mediastinal LNs	$20.3 \pm 11.4^{*1}$	$43.8 \pm 18.6^{*2}$	$30.4 \pm 17.2^{*3}$	Each P < 0.01
upper	0	$20.2 \pm 11.0^{*1}$	$11.7 \pm 10.1^{*2}$	$^{*1-*2}$ P < 0.01
lower	20.3 ± 11.4	23.6 ± 10.1	18.7 ± 10.6	
Abdominal LNs	16.8 ± 9.3	19.1 ± 11.4	20.0 ± 11.4	
Total	$37.1 \pm 15.5^{*1}$	$89.3 \pm 28.8^{*2}$	$53.9 \pm 26.2^{*3}$	Each P < 0.01

The upper mediastinal nodes include the right recurrent nerve nodes, right paratracheal nodes, left paratracheal nodes, and infraaortic arch nodes. The lower mediastinal nodes include the periesophageal nodes, infracarinal nodes, and lower posterior mediastinal nodes. *LNs*, lymph nodes

per patient and the cervical lymph nodes were seldom resected. During en bloc esophagectomy, neither the cervical nor upper mediastinal lymph nodes were resected.

Among 38 patients undergoing three-field dissection, metastasis in the cervical lymph nodes was found in 5 patients (13%), in the upper mediastinal nodes in 19 patients (50%), in the lower mediastinal nodes in 9 patients (24%), and in the abdominal nodes in 17 patients (45%). Overall, 20 patients (53%) had metastasis in the cervical and/or upper mediastinal lymph nodes. The rate of metastasis to those nodes was lower in patients who underwent two-field dissection than in those who underwent three-field dissection ($P < 0.05$). During en bloc esophagectomy these nodes were not resected.

The 5-year survival rate was 23% in patients from TU Munich and 40% in those from Kurume. The long-term survival rates were not significantly different between the two groups, although patients from Kurume had a tendency toward better survival than those from TU Munich. Figure 1 shows the survival curves of those who underwent en bloc esophagectomy, three-field dissection, and two-field dissection. Patients who underwent three-field dissection had a better survival than either those who underwent en bloc esophagectomy ($P < 0.05$) or those who underwent two-field dissection ($P < 0.10$). There was no difference in the survival rates between those patients who underwent en bloc esophagectomy and those who underwent two-field dissection.

After the patients were divided into two groups according to whether or not they had positive lymph node metastasis, the survival curves of the three procedures were then compared again (Fig. 2). In the patients with metastasis in the lymph nodes, those who underwent three-field dissection had a better survival than those who underwent either en bloc esophagectomy or two-field dissection (both $P < 0.05$).

When the patients with metastasis in the lymph nodes were divided into two groups according to whether they had a carcinoma located in the upper/middle thoracic esophagus or in the lower thoracic esophagus, the survival curves of the three procedures were again compared (Fig. 3). In patients with a subgroup of pN1 carcinoma in the upper or middle thoracic esophagus, survival was better after three-field dissection than after either en bloc esophagectomy ($P < 0.10$)

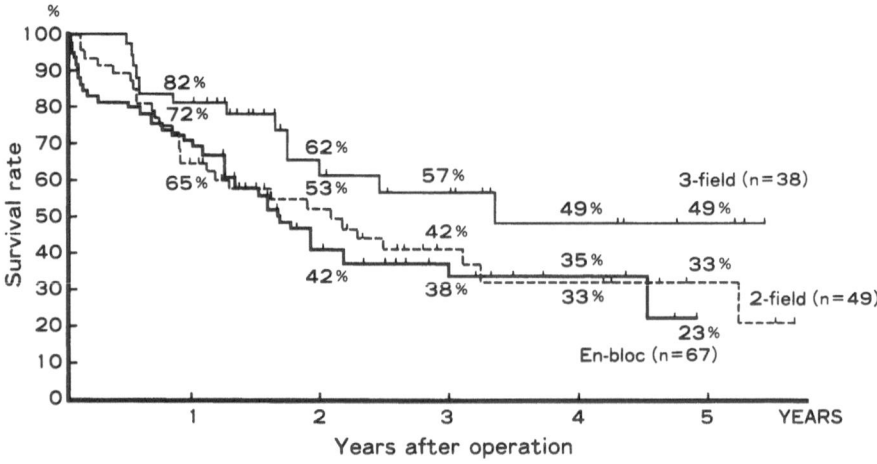

Fig. 1. Survival curves for R_0 esopagectomy: en bloc esophagectomy vs three-field dissection vs two-field dissection. Three-field vs en bloc, $P < 0.05$; three-field vs two-field, $P < 0.10$

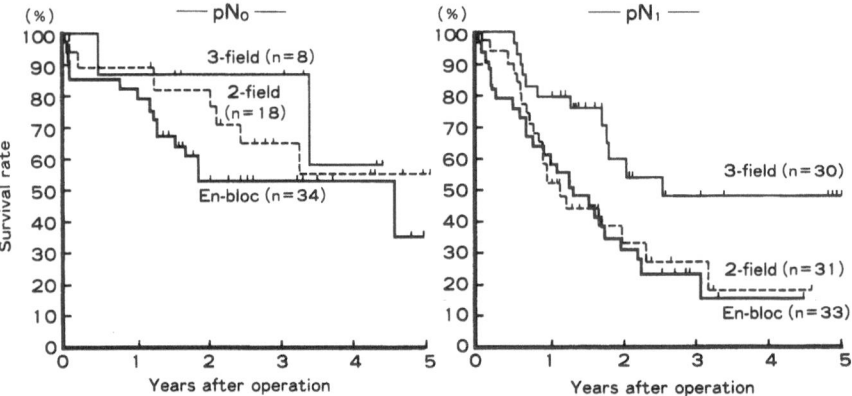

Fig. 2. Survival curves for R_0 esophagectomy in a subgroup of pN0 or pN1: En bloc esophagectomy vs three-field dissection vs two-field dissection; *pN1*, three-field vs en bloc, $P < 0.05$; three-field vs two-field, $P < 0.05$

or two-field dissection ($P < 0.05$). In patients with pN1 carcinoma in the lower thoracic esophagus, there was no difference in survival among the three procedures.

Discussion

There remains a controversy over the best surgical treatment for carcinoma in the thoracic esophagus. Orringer has performed transhiatal esophagectomy under the premise that a radical operation, including lymph node dissection

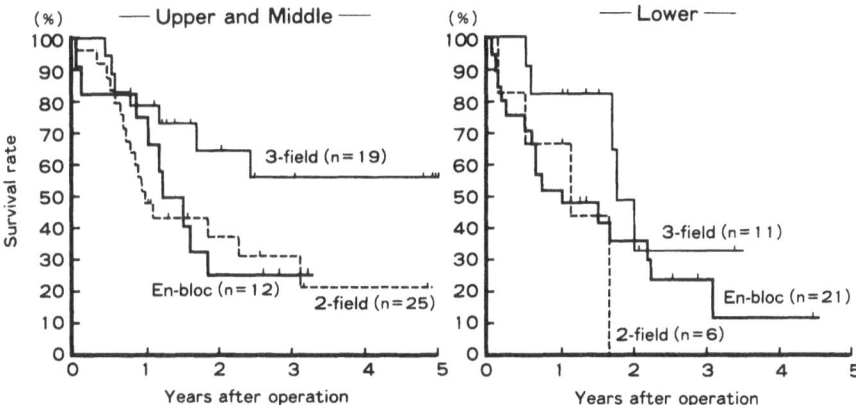

Fig. 3. Survival curves for positive lymph node metastasis and R_0 esophagectomy, in a subgroup of carcinoma in the upper and middle thoracic esophagus, and in the lower thoracic esophagus: En bloc esophagectomy vs three-field dissection vs two-field dissection; *upper and middle*, three-field vs en bloc, $P < 0.10$; three-field vs two-field, $P < 0.05$

through thoracotomy, was not necessary for esophageal carcinoma because of a preexisting high risk of systemic metastasis [5]. On the other hand, Logan had performed en bloc esophagectomy through a left thoracotomy based on the principle that the tumor should be removed with a complete covering of normal tissue [6]. Skinner followed this procedure by completely resecting the posterior mediastinal envelope together with the esophagus and regional lymph nodes, except for the aorta, vertebral bodies, and myocardium [1]. Siewert et al. performed en bloc esophagectomy through a right thoracotomy for almost every carcinoma in the thoracic esophagus and believed that resecting more lymph nodes during esophagectomy increased the survival rate [2].

In Japan, Kinoshita et al. [7] found during esophagectomy that metastasis in the right recurrent nerve nodes occurred in 31% of patients with squamous cell carcinoma in the thoracic esophagus. Sannohe et al. performed neck dissection for a carcinoma in the thoracic esophagus and found that metastases in the supraclavicular nodes were present in more than 20% of patients with carcinoma in the thoracic esophagus [8]. Sannohe reported in another study that the 4-year survival rate after three-field dissection was better than that after two-field dissection (39% vs. 21%) [9]. After this report, three-field dissection was widely adopted in Japan [3].

There is no comparative study on the efficacy between en bloc esophagectomy and three-field dissection, the two principle methods of extended radical esophagectomy for carcinoma in the thoracic esophagus. Therefore, we compared the clinical results from en bloc esophagectomy in TU Munich to those from two-field or three-field dissection in Kurume. We found that patients who underwent three-field dissection had the best survival, compared with those who underwent either en bloc esophagectomy or two-field dissection. This difference is due to the dissection of the cervical and upper mediastinal lymph nodes, in which metastasis was found in more than half the patients who underwent three-field dissection. Those metastatic nodes may be missed by en bloc esophagectomy or two-field dissection.

Based on the data presented here, we conclude that three-field dissection may offer a better chance of survival than either en bloc esophagectomy or two-field dissection for patients with a carcinoma in the upper or middle thoracic esophagus, and with metastasis in the lymph nodes, because generally these patients are likely to have metastasis in the cervical and/or upper mediastinal lymph nodes.

References

1. Skinner DB (1983) En bloc resection for neoplasms of the esophagus and cardia. J Thorac Cardiovasc Surg 85:59–69
2. Siewert JR, Liebermann-Meffert D, Fekete F, Dittler HJ, Fink U, Lukas P, Ries G (1990) Oesophaguscarcinom. In: Siewert JR, Harder F, Allgower M, Blum AL, Creutzfeldt W, Hollender LF, Peiper HJ (eds) Chirurgische gastroenterologie (in German), vol. 2. Springer, Berlin Heidelberg New York, pp 593–674
3. Isono K, Sato H, Nakayama K (1991) Results of a nationwide study on the three-field lymph node dissection of esophageal cancer. Oncology 48:411–420
4. International Union Against Cancer (1987) The general rules of the TNM system. In: Hermanek P, Sobin LH (eds) TNM classification of malignant tumours, 4th edn. Springer, Berlin Heidelberg New York, pp 5–12
5. Orringer MB (1987) Transthoracic versus transhiatal esophagectomy: What difference does it make? Ann Thorac Surg 44:116–118
6. Logan A (1963) The surgical treatment of carcinoma of the esophagus and cardia. J Thorac Cardiovasc Surg 46:150–161
7. Kinoshita I, Ohashi I, Nakagawa K, Kajitani T, Kaneda K, Tsuya A (1976) Lymph node metastasis in esophageal cancer; with special reference to upper mediastinum and measures for its treatment (in Japanese). Nippon Shyokaki Geka Gakkai Zasshi 9:424–430
8. Sannohe Y, Hiratsuka R, Doki K (1981) Lymph node metastasis in cancer of the thoracic esophagus. Am J Surg 141:216–218
9. Sannohe Y (1981) Cervical lymph node metastasis in carcinoma of the esophagus. Nippon Shyokaki Geka Gakkai Zasshi 14:1016–1022

Lymph Node Metastasis of Squamous Cell Carcinoma in the Thoracic Esophagus as a Prognostic Factor

Masamichi Baba[1], Nasser K. Altorki[2], David B. Skinner[2], Takashi Aikou[1], and Hisaaki Shimazu[1]

Introduction

In the fourth edition of the TNM classification, issued in 1987 [1], the definition of both T and N was revised and clarified: T was classified according to the depth of invasion of the primary tumor, and the perigastric nodes were added to the list of regional lymph nodes for intrathoracic esophageal cancers. It is thought that the complete removal of the tumor, including the regional lymph nodes, is necessary for the curative resection of esophageal carcinomas. The aim of this study is to clarify the anatomical spread of lymph node metastases of esophageal squamous cell carcinomas, and to determine how the number of involved nodes influences the survival of the patients.

Patients and Methods

For the 20-year period from 1969 through 1989, the medical records of 84 consecutive patients with squamous cell carcinomas of the thoracic esophagus, treated in the Departments of Surgery at the New York Hospital-Cornell Medical Center and the University of Chicago Medical Center, were reviewed retrospectively. Sixty-one (73%) of 84 patients underwent esophagectomy through a right or left thoracotomy, including 45 en bloc resections [2], and these 61 are the subject of this article.

The regional lymph nodes, as defined by the TNM for the intrathoracic esophagus, were routinely resected or sampled, but cervical and celiac nodes were sampled only when swollen lymph nodes were detected preoperatively or

[1] 1st Department of Surgery, Kagoshima University Hospital, 8-35-1 Sakuragaoka, Kagoshima, 890 Japan
[2] The New York Hospital-Cornell Medical Center 525 East 68th St., New York, NY 10021, USA

palpated intraoperatively. The actuarial method was applied to calculate survival rates and the generalized Wilcoxon test and the chi-square test were used to analyze statistical difference. Follow-up was completed to the time of death, 5 years after surgery, or April 1st, 1991.

Description of Patients and Their Tumors

There were 42 males and 19 females ranging in age from 38 to 78 years with a mean age of 61. The location of primary tumors was: the upper third of the esophagus in 8, the middle in 33, and the lower in 20. A right thoracotomy approach was performed on 40 patients and a left thoracotomy on 21, depending on their tumor sites. The extent of differentiation of the squamous cell carcinoma, as assessed histologically, was well-differentiated in 12, moderately in 28, and poorly in 18. The remaining 3 could not be assessed due to the effect of preoperative radiotherapy. Only one patient (2%) was in stage I, 18 (30%) were in stage II A, 10 (16%) in stage II B, 23 (38%) in stage III, and 9 (15%) in stage IV. Stage IV patients had no blood-borne metastases at the time of operation, but they had nodal involvement spreading beyond the regional nodes defined by the TNM.

Results

Number of Lymph Nodes

Out of 1304 lymph nodes examined histopathologically, 117 (9%) were revealed to be positive for lymph node metastases. The mean number of dissected nodes per case was 21, ranging from 3 to 60 nodes. Of 61 patients, nodal involvement was proved in 41 cases (67%), of which 30 cases had 1–3 positive nodes and the remaining 11 had more than 4 but less than 9.

Frequency of Lymph Node Metastasis

In cases where the tumor was located in the upper two-thirds of the esophagus, the percentage of cases with lymph node metastasis was 11% in the neck, 49% in the mediastinum, and 20% in the abdomen. With carcinoma of the lower esophagus, the distribution of metastases was 65% in the perigastric, 40% in the lower mediastinal, 20% in the celiac, and 10% in the middle mediastinal nodes.

Depth of Primary Tumor and Number of Positive Nodes

The incidence of involved nodes per case was 47% in cases where the tumor had invaded to muscularis propria, and was 72% in cases where the tumor had reached the adventitia. As the depth of primary tumor increased, the number of involved nodes significantly increased (Table 1).

Table 1. Depth of primary tumor and lymph node metastasis

Number of involved nodes	Depth of primary tumor				
	Submucosa	Muscularis propria	Adventitia		Adjacent structure
(−)	1 case	10	9		
1–3 nodes	1	8	18	3	$P < 0.01$
4 or more		1	5	5	
Incidence	1/2	9/19 (47%)	23/32 (72%)		8/8 (100%)

Table 2. Number/location of positive nodes and depth of tumor

Number/location of positive nodes		Submucosa	Muscularis propria	Adventitia	Adjacent structure
1–3 nodes	Cervical		1	1	1
	Regional[a]	1 case	7	17	3
	Celiac				
4 or more	Cervical				1
	Regional[a]		1	2	1
	Celiac			3	3

[a] Regional nodes, defined by the TNM classification

Table 3. Recurrence and number of involved nodes

Site of recurrence[a]	None (cases)	1–3 Nodes (cases)	4 or more nodes (cases)
Neck	3	4	1
Upper mediastinum		10	1
Middle mediastinum		1	3
Lower mediastinum, celiac axis		2	2
Anastomotic site		1	1
Bone/liver/lung	1	6	3
Skin/brain	2	3	3
Others			2
Incidence	3/20 (15%)	18/30 (60%)	9/11 (82%)

[a] Including overlapped sites of recurrence

Spread of Lymph Node Metastasis

With the patients who had one to three positive nodes, the regional lymph nodes were most frequently involved, as shown in Table 2. Cervical lymph nodes were involved in three cases in which the patients had less than three positive lymph nodes. In contrast, celiac nodes were involved only in cases with four or more positive nodes.

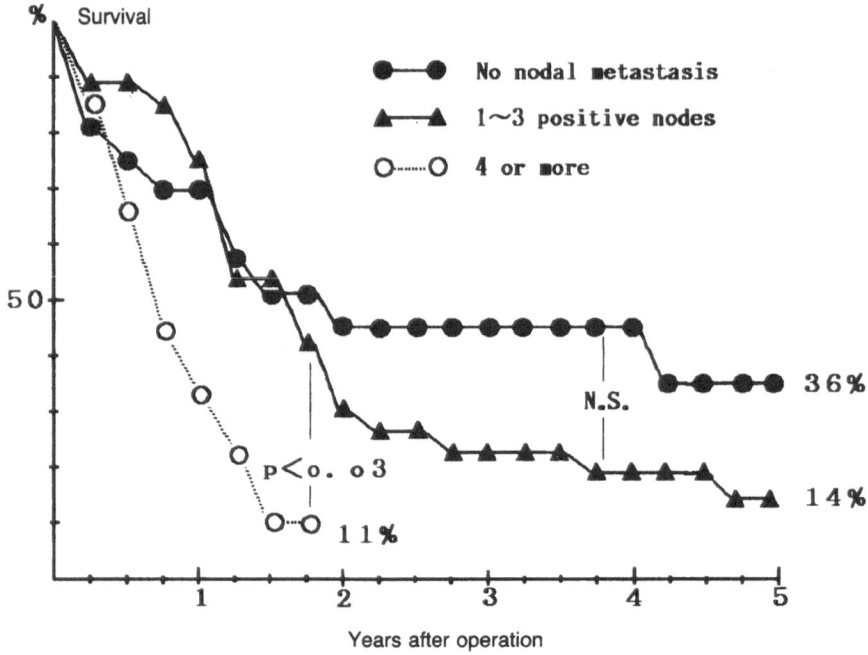

Fig. 1. Survival curves according to the number of positive nodes

Recurrence

Cervical lymph node recurrence was found in three cases even when the patients had no lymph node metastasis at the time of operation. In patients with one to three positive nodes, the most frequent site of recurrence was the upper mediastinum followed by the neck, rather than the blood (Table 3).

Outcome

The 5-year survival rate was 36% in the patients with no nodal involvement, compared to 14% in those with one to three positive nodes. Of the patients with four or more positive lymph nodes, none survived 2 years after the operation, and their outcome was significantly poorer than that of patients with one to three positive nodes (Fig. 1).

Discussion

For potential surgical cure of the patients with an esophageal carcinoma, both complete removal of the tumor and dissection of the lymph nodes is essential, taking account of the high incidence of nodal involvement. The extent of lymphatic spread mainly depends on the tumor location. In cases of tumors located in the upper two-thirds of the esophagus, upper mediastinal lymph nodes were more frequently involved than abdominal nodes. Interestingly, a single node involvement was found in the neck as the first lymph node metastasis of the tumor, although cervical lymph nodes were not routinely cleared at the time of operation. Isono et al. [3] reported that 32.5% of 117 esophagectomized patients who received three-field lymphadenectomy, i.e., dissection of the lymph nodes in the neck, mediastinum, and abdomen, were revealed to be positive for cervical lymph node metastasis. In addition, lymphatic recurrences, especially in the neck or in the upper mediastinum, were still dominant rather than blood-borne recurrences. At present, however, while the benefit of extensive lympha-denectomy remains uncertain. It is a fact that lymph node metastases in the neck and/or the upper mediastinum have a critical effect on the outcome of patients with esophageal carcinoma.

Skinner and associates [4] pointed out that metastases to lymph nodes and muscular penetration by the cancer were an important prognostic factor. As few as three or four involved nodes were critical. Abe and co-workers [5] also emphasized that with involvement of three lymph nodes or more, all patients were dead within 3 years after the operation. The presence of even a small number of lymph node metastases is deleterious to the outcome, even if the main tumor is limited to the esophageal wall. In this series, the 5-year survival rate for the patients with negative nodes was 36%. For patients with one to three positive nodes, it decreased to 14%, although there was no statistical significance in this difference, owing to the en bloc resection [2]. Conversely, the patients who had more than four positive nodes were regarded as having systemic disease even if they seemed to pass through a curative resection, because of their high relapse rate, mode of recurrences, and significantly bad prognoses.

In conclusion, the number of lymph node metastases proved to be an important prognostic factor, beneficial either in appraising potentially curable cancer or in assessing the need for postoperative chemoradiotherapy.

References

1. International Union Against Cancer (UICC) (1987) Hermanek P, Sobin LH (eds) TNM classification of malignant tumors, 4th edn. Springer, Berlin Heidelberg New York London Paris Tokyo
2. Skinner DB (1983) En bloc resection for neoplasms of the esophagus and cardia. J Thorac Cardiovasc Surg 85:59–71
3. Isono K, Ochiai T, Okuyama K, Onoda S (1990) The treatment of lymph node metastasis from esophageal cancer by extensive lymphadenectomy. Jpn J Surg 20:151–157
4. Skinner DB, Dowlatshahi KD, DeMeester TR (1982) Potentially curable cancer of the esophagus. Cancer 50:2571–2575
5. Abe S, Tachibana M, Shiraishi M, Nakamura T (1990) Lymph node metastasis in resectable esophageal cancer. J Thorac Cardiovasc Surg 100:287–291

Prognostic Factors in Patients with Squamous Cell Cancer of the Esophagus Undergoing Transthoracic En Bloc Resection

Jürgen D. Roder[1], Raymonde Busch[2], Hubert J. Stein[1], Ulrich Fink[1], and J. Rüdiger Siewert[1]

Summary. Identification of tumor characteristics which may limit survival in patients with squamous cell carcinoma of the esophagus is critical for the selection of those patients who may benefit from surgical resection and the choice of the radicality of the procedure. We evaluated the tumor characteristics which independently influenced survival in 204 consecutive patients with squamous cell carcinoma of the esophagus who had undergone en bloc resection and extensive lymphadenectomy. Multivariate analysis in the entire patient population identified the presence of residual tumor after resection, i.e., a R1 or R2 resection, and the presence and more than seven mediastinal lymph node metastases as the only independent factors influencing survival time. In a second multivariate analysis of 75 patients who survived the procedure for at least 30 days, who had a R0 resection, and who did not have preoperative neo-adjuvant therapy, only the pN category and the ratio between positive and removed mediastinal lymph nodes independently influenced survival. These data suggest that only a R0 resection, i.e., complete macroscopic and microscopic tumor removal, can increase survival in patients with squamous cell carcinoma of the esophagus. In patients with a limited number of positive mediastinal lymph nodes, the prognosis may be improved by an extensive lymphadenectomy if the number of removed mediastinal lymph nodes exceeds the number of positive nodes by a factor of at least five.

Introduction

The prognosis of a patient with squamous cell carcinoma of the esophagus undergoing resection is dependent on the general status of the patient and the characteristics of the tumor at the time of presentation. A detailed preoperative

---

[1] Department of Surgery and [2] Section of Statistics and Epidemiology, Technische Universität München, Ismaninger Str 22, D-8000 München 80, Germany

analysis of patient-dependent risk factors and subsequent improvements in patient selection for surgical resection, in combination with standardization of resection techniques and optimized perioperative management, has in recent years led to a marked reduction in operative mortality and morbidity [1, 2]. Despite these advances, resection of an esophageal carcinoma remains a major intervention associated with considerable risks and prolonged hospital and recovery time. Identification of the tumor characteristics which may limit survival following a surgical resection is therefore critical for the identification of those patients who might benefit from a surgical resection and the choice of the radicality of the procedure.

Tumor characteristics which may influence survival can currently only be reliably obtained by histologic analysis of the resected specimen. Furthermore, an accurate assessment of the tumor-node-metastasis (TNM) stage [3], which is thought to have the greatest implications for the prognosis of the patient, is dependent on complete tumor resection and adequate lymphadenectomy, to allow for an exact analysis of the tumor and nodular metastasis. Consequently, an analysis of tumor dependent prognostic factors, which may guide therapeutic decisions in the future, is useful only if it is performed in a sufficiently large patient population which has undergone a standardized resection and extensive lymphadenectomy.

In the past, the prognostic effect of tumor characteristics in patients with squamous cell carcinoma of the esophagus has been analyzed using univariate statistics [4]. However, the analyzed factors interrelate with each other. Consequently the independent influence of a single factor on the prognosis of a patient with esophageal carcinoma, can only be proven by a multivariate analysis. In the present study, we therefore assessed the independent prognostic effect of a variety of tumor characteristics in patients with squamous cell carcinoma of the esophagus who had undergone resection using multivariate analysis.

Patient Population and Methods

Between July 1982 and August 1990, a total of 454 patients with esophageal carcinoma were referred to our institution for surgical treatment. The tumor was resected in 332/454 patients accounting for a resection rate of 73.1%. These data do not include an additional 151 patients with carcinoma of cardia types II or III [5] resected during the same time interval. On histopathologic evaluation of the specimen, 128 patients had adenocarcinoma and 204 had squamous cell carcinoma. The present analysis is based on the 204 patients with squamous carcinoma. There were 179 males and 25 females with a mean age of 53.6 years (range 33–78 years)

All 204 patients with squamous cell carcinoma had a standardized en bloc esophagectomy and proximal gastrectomy via the abdominal and right thoracic route as described previously [6]. The en bloc resection comprised the proximal part of the lesser curvature of the stomach, the entire abdominal and thoracic esophagus including the azygos vein, the thoracic duct, and the surrounding lymphatic and fatty tissues. Proximal to the junction of the azygos vein with the superior vena cava an isolated lymphadenectomy was performed. All patients also had a complete lymphadenectomy of the so-called compartment II along the celiac axis. Compartment II comprises all suprapancreatic lymph nodes between the right gastric artery and the splenic hilum. The lymph nodes of the so-called compartment I, i.e., the perigastric nodes, were removed en bloc with the specimen only in the area of the proximal lesser curvature. A lymphadenectomy was not performed in the remainder of compartment I to avoid compromising the blood supply to the gastric tube. This procedure accounts for the so-called two-field lymphadenectomy as described by Akiyama [7]. Gastrointestinal continuity was restored by a gastric tube and a cervical esophagogastrostomy ($n = 178$) or colon interposition ($n = 26$).

After removal, the specimen was opened, stretched and fixed for histopathologic evaluation according to a prospective protocol. The tumor type and differentiation were classified according to the WHO criteria. In addition, the T, N, M, and R categories were assessed or reassessed according to the UICC 1987 classification [3], the presence and extent of lymphangiosis carcinomatosa was determined, and the number of removed and invaded mediastinal and abdominal lymph nodes was counted. On average, 22.9 (range 8–66) mediastinal and 19.8 (range 4–58) abdominal lymph nodes were removed with the specimen.

Patient data, the details of the operative procedure, and the histopathologic evaluation of the resected specimen were collected prospectively since July 1982. The patients were followed regularly in the tumor clinic of the Department of Surgery or by telephone contact with their primary physician. Follow-up is complete for all 204 patients with a median follow-up of 13 months (range 1–96 months). Survival rates were calculated according to the Kaplan-Meyer method [8]. For purposes of comparison, a univariate analysis of all tumor characteristics which might influence survival was performed. Significant differences were determined using a generalized Wilcoxon test [9]. Multivariate analysis (proportional hazard model of Cox [10]) was used to identify the independent prognostic effect of individual tumor characteristics. Statistical analysis was performed on a personal computer using the BMDP Statistical Software (Los Angeles, Calif.). The analyzed co-variables are shown in Table 1.

Since an accurate evaluation of the prognostic factors of a tumor can only be performed in a patient population who had standardized treatment, complete resection of the tumor, and who survived the procedure, a second multivariate analysis was performed in those patients who had no preoperative neo-adjuvant therapy, who survived the resection for at least 30 days, and who had complete tumor removal (i.e., an R0 resection). There remained 75 patients (66 male, 9 female, mean age 52.9 years, range 34–76 years) for this analysis. The distribution of factors evaluated in the multivariate analysis in these 75 patients is also shown in Table 1. Compared to the entire patient population, there were no undifferentiated tumors and a markedly higher percentage of pT1 or pT2 tumors in this population. This is primarily due to the exclusion of patients who had preoperative neo-adjuvant therapy which in our institution has been routinely performed since 1987 in patients with advanced tumors located above the tracheal bifurcation. Median follow-up in this selected population was 23 months (range 2–96 months).

Table 1. Distribution of potentially prognostic factors in patients with resected esophageal squamous cell cancer

Variables	All patients ($n = 204$)	Subgroup ($n = 75$)[a]
Age:		
30–49	82 (40.2%)	30 (40.0%)
50–59	76 (37.3%)	26 (34.7%)
60–69	38 (18.6%)	14 (18.7%)
>70	8 (3.9%)	5 (6.7%)
Sex:		
Male	25 (12.3%)	9 (12.0%)
Female	179 (87.7%)	66 (88.0)
Tumor location:		
Above tracheal bifurcation	103 (50.5%)	29 (38.7%)
Below tracheal bifurcation	101 (87.7%)	46 (61.3%)
pT Category:		
pT 1	28 (13.7%)	20 (26.7%)
pT 2	35 (17.2%)	19 (25.2%)
pT 3	105 (51.5%)	35 (46.7%)
pT 4	36 (17.6%)	1 (1.3%)
pN Category:		
pH 0	77 (37.7%)	33 (44.0%)
pH 1	127 (62.3%)	42 (56.0%)
pM Category:		
pM 0	151 (74.0%)	75 (100%)
pM 1	53 (26.0%)	0
Differenntiation:		
Well	25 (12.3%)	15 (17.3%)
Moderate	91 (44.6%)	42 (56.0%)
Poor	61 (29.9%)	20 (26.7%)
Undifferentiated	27 (13.2%)	0
R Category:		
R 0	114 (55.9%)	75 (100%)
R 1	59 (28.9%)	0
R 2	31 (15.2%)	0
Lymphangiosis carcinomatosa:		
Positive	77 (31.7%)	18 (24.0%)
Negative	127 (62.3%)	57 (76.0%)
Number of positive mediastinal lymph nodes:		
pN1 (1–3)	65 (31.9%)	18 (24.0%)
pN1 (4–8)	40 (19.6%)	13 (17.3%)
pN1 (≥8)	22 (10.8%)	11 (14.7%)
Ratio between positive and removed mediastinal lymph nodes:		
0	85 (40.7%)	33 (44.0%)
<0.2	63 (30.9%)	22 (25.3%)
>0.2	58 (28.7%)	20 (22.7%)

[a] Patients who had a R0 resection, who survived the resection for at least 30 days, and who had no preoperative neo-adjuvant radio/chemotherapy

Table 2. *P*-Values of univariate analysis

Variables	All patients ($n = 204$)	Subgroup ($n = 75$)[a]
Age	0.96	0.79
Sex	0.16	0.52
Tumor location	0.84	0.046
pT Category	<0.0001	0.04
pN Category	<0.0001	<0.0001
pM Category	<0.0001	0.26
Differentiation	0.081	0.50
R Category	<0.0001	—
Lymphangiosis carcinomatosa	<0.0001	<0.0001
Number of positive mediastinal lymph nodes	<0.0001	<0.0001
Ratio between positive and removed mediastinal lymph nodes	<0.0001	<0.0001

[a] Patients who had a R0 resection, who survived the resection for at least 30 days, and who had no preoperative neo-adjuvant radio/chemotherapy

Results

The results of the univariate analysis of prognostic factors for the entire patient population ($n = 204$) and the selected patient population ($n = 75$) who had no preoperative neo-adjuvant therapy, who survived the procedure for at least 30 days and who had complete tumor removal, i.e., and R0 resection, are summarized in Table 2.

The cumulative survival curve of the entire patient population ($n = 204$) who underwent resection of a squamous cell carcinoma of the esophagus is shown in Fig. 1. There was a rapid decline of the survival curve during the first 2 years after resection with a stabilization during the following years. Including the operative mortality, the median survival time following resection was 13 months. The cumulative survival rates after 1, 3, and 5 years were 50.4%, 21.4%, and 17.3%, respectively.

On multivariate analysis, only the presence of residual tumor (i.e., R1 or R2 resections), the presence of positive mediastinal lymph nodes (i.e. pN1 category), and more than seven positive mediastinal lymph nodes (i.e., pN1 category), and more than seven positive mediastinal lymph nodes had an independent and significant effect on survival time (Table 3). The beneficial effect of complete tumor removal on survival is illustrated in Fig. 2. The effect of mediastinal lymph node metastases is shown in Fig. 3. Survival decreased progressively with an increasing number of positive mediastinal lymph nodes and was particularly compromised in patients with more than seven positive mediastinal lymph nodes.

The survival rate for the 75 patients who had no preoperative neo-adjuvant therapy, who survived the procedure for at least 30 days, and who had complete macroscopic and microscopic tumor removal (i.e., an R0 resection), is

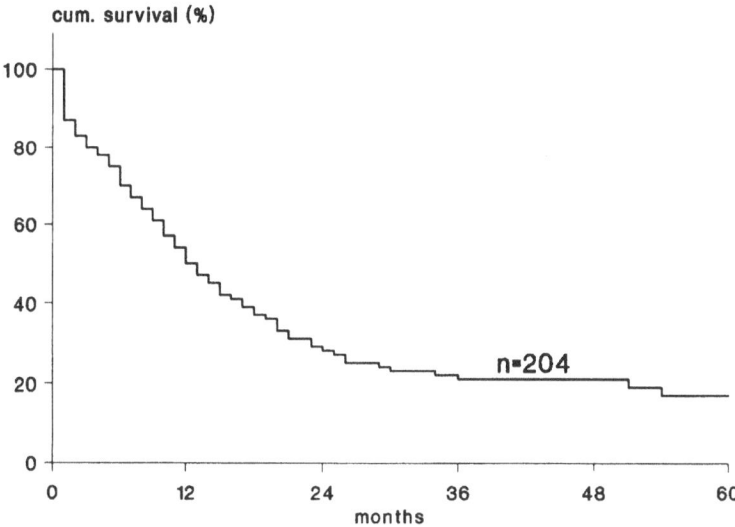

Fig. 1. Cumulative survival rate in 204 consecutive patients who underwent resection for squamous cell cancer of the esophagus

Table 3. Results of the multivariate analysis (step wise regression, enter limit 10%)

	All patients (n = 204)		Subgroup (n = 75)[a]	
	Regression coefficient	P-value	Regression coefficient	P-value
pN Category	0.43	<0.001	1.13	0.02
>7 Positive mediastinal nodes	0.87	<0.01	—	n.s.
R Category	0.55	<0.001	—	n.s.
Ratio between positive and removed mediastinal lymph nodes	—	n.s.	0.04	<0.001

n.s., not significant
[a] Patients who had a R0 resection, who survived the resection for at least 30 days, and who had no preoperative neo-adjuvant radio/chemotherapy

shown in Fig. 4. The median survival rate in this group was 21 months. The cumulative survival rates after 1, 3, and 5 years were 68.7%, 40.7%, and 31.7%, respectively.

On multivariate analysis of the prognostic factors in these 75 patients only, the presence of positive mediastinal lymph nodes (i.e., pN1 category), and the ratio between removed and positive lymph nodes had a significant and independent effect on survival time (Table 3). The effect of positive mediastinal lymph nodes on survival is shown in Fig. 5. Median survival time in patients without positive mediastinal lymph nodes (i.e., pN0 category), was 63 months compared to 13 months in patients with positive mediastinal lymph nodes (i.e., pN1 category). Cumulative 1-, 3-, and 5-year survival was 93.6%, 75.7%, and 64.9%, respec-

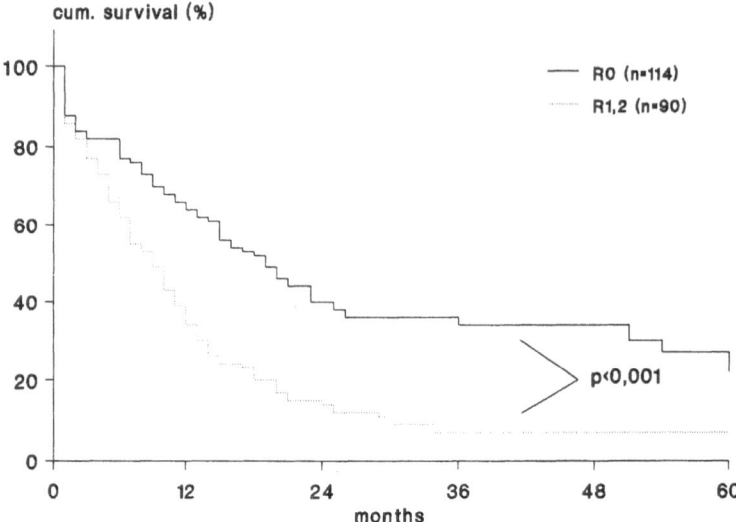

Fig. 2. Cumulative survival rates in 204 patients who underwent resection for squamous cell cancer of the esophagus and had an R0, R1 or R2 resection

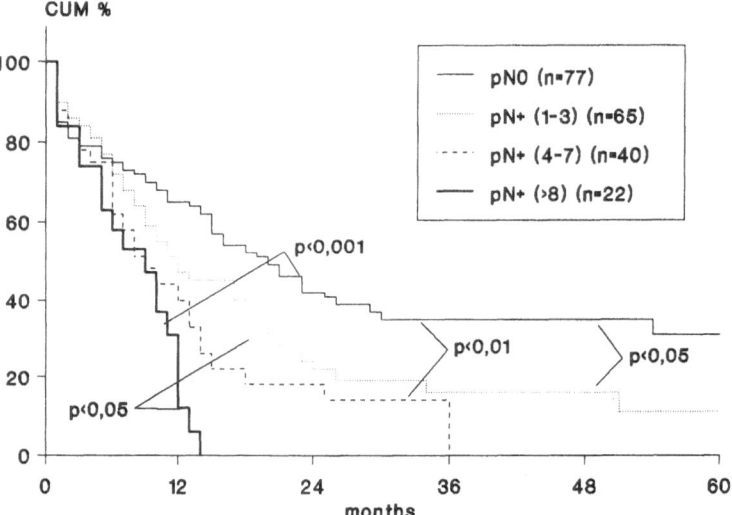

Fig. 3. Influence of the number of positive mediastinal lymph nodes (*pNt*) on the cumulative survival rate in 204 patients who underwent resection for squamous cell cancer of the esophagus

tively, in patients with pN0 disease compared to 50.4%, 14.9%. and 7.5%, respectively, in patients with pN1 disease.

Figure 6 illustrates the effect of the ratio between positive and removed mediastinal nodes on survival in patients with pN1 disease. Survival time was

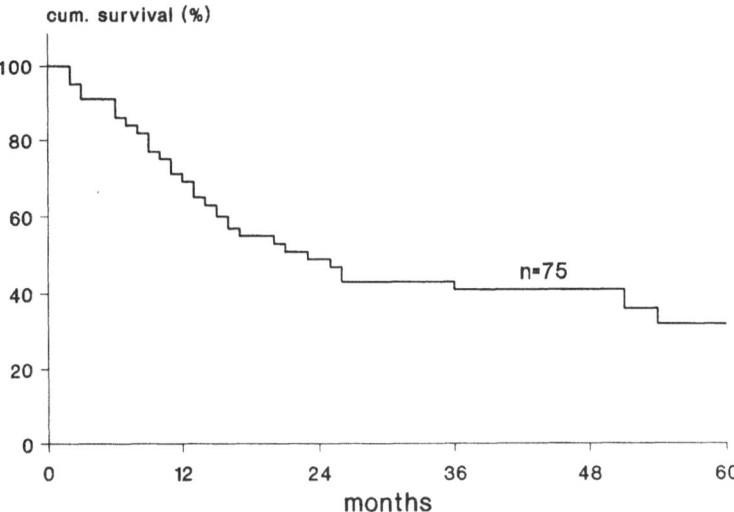

Fig. 4. Cumulative survival rate in 75 consecutive patients with squamous cell cancer of the esophagus who survived the procedure for at least 30 days, who had a R0 resection, and who did not have preoperative neo-adjuvant therapy

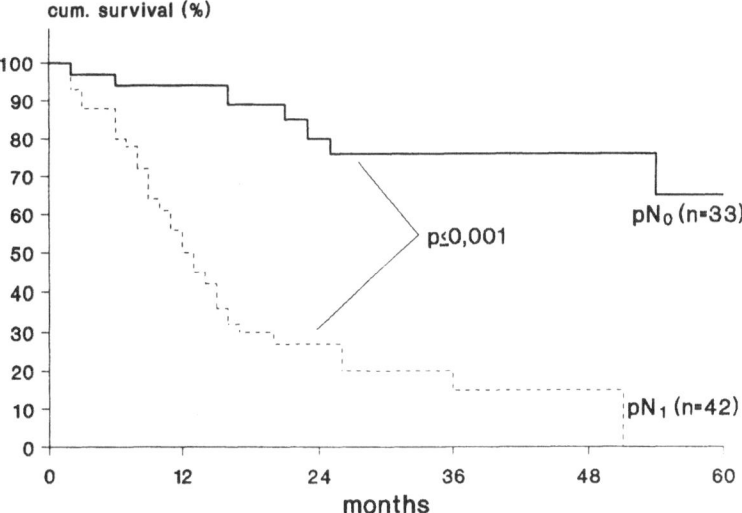

Fig. 5. Influence of the pN category on the cumulative survival rate in 75 patients with squamous cell cancer of the esophagus who survived the procedure for at least 30 days, who had a R0 resection, and who did not have preoperative neo-adjuvant therapy

significantly improved if the ratio was below 0.2, such as when the number of removed lymph nodes exceeded the number of positive lymph nodes by a factor of at least five.

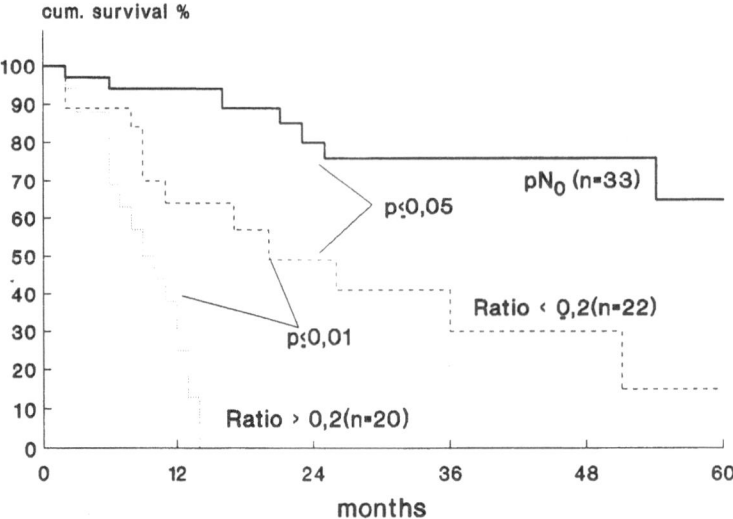

Fig. 6. Influence of the ratio between positive and removed mediastinal lymph nodes on the cumulative survival rate in the 75 patients with squamous cell cancer of the esophagus who survived the procedure for at least 30 days, who had a R0 resection, and who did not have preoperative neo-adjuvant therapy

Discussion

Following the marked reduction in operative mortality and morbidity for esophageal resections in recent years, two questions remain: Which patients benefit from surgical resection of a carcinoma of the esophagus and how extensive does the resection have to be? Currently, these questions can only be evaluated by a detailed analysis of the resected specimen and multivariate analysis of all tumor characteristics which might influence survival time. Therapeutic concepts can then be customized to the general status of the patient and the individual tumor characteristics.

A reliable multivariate analysis of prognostic factors can, however, only be performed in a sufficiently large population who: (1) has undergone extensive resection and lymphadenectomy to allow for adequate staging, and (2) has been followed for a sufficiently long period. All the prerequisites for such a multivariate analysis are given in the analyzed patient population. The data were collected prospectively using a standardized protocol in a large population ($n = 204$). All patients underwent en bloc resection of the tumor with an adequate standardized lymphadenectomy. This is reflected in the large number of mediastinal and abdominal lymph nodes available for analysis. The histopathologic analysis of the removed specimen in concert with the intraoperative evaluation also allowed a correct assessment of residual tumor (i.e., a R0, a R1, or a R2 resection). In addition, follow-up was complete for all patients.

Multivariate analysis of prognostic factors in this population identified a R0 resection and nodal status as the only independent factors influencing survival. This indicates that the goal of any resection performed for squamous cell esophageal carcinoma has to be complete removal of all microscopic or macroscopic tumor in order to improve survival time. The presence of positive mediastinal lymph nodes alone did not lead to a sudden deterioration of the survival probability. Rather, the survival probability decreased in a step-wise fashion with increasing number of positive lymph nodes indicating that, with a limited number of positive mediastinal lymph nodes, long-term survival may still be possible following a resection with adequate lymphadenectomy. Only with more than seven positive mediastinal nodes did the prognosis deteriorate. This is in accordance with data from other centers [11, 12].

In order to solely identify the influence of tumor characteristics on survival following resection, three factors which could have potentially influenced the prognosis were excluded in a second multivariate analysis. These were: (1) the operative mortality, (2) incomplete tumor resection, and (3) preoperative neoadjuvant therapy. The last-mentioned has been performed in our hospital since 1987 in patients with advanced squamous cell tumors of the esophagus located above the level of the tracheal bifurcation. This analysis confirmed again the prognostic significance of the nodal status. In addition to the pN category, the ratio between the number of positive and removed lymph nodes, however, also independently influenced survival time. A significant drop in the survival rates was noted when more than 20% of the removed lymph nodes were positive. Since this ratio can be influenced by the number of removed lymph nodes, a radical lymphadenectomy in patients with a limited number of positive mediastinal lymph nodes can decrease the ratio and may thus improve the prognosis of the patient. This is confirmed by the superior survival rates reported with radical en bloc resection and extensive lymphadenectomy as compared to a limited resection reported from other centers around the world [2, 12, 13].

Comparable published multivariate analyses in patients with esophageal carcinoma are scarce. Lund et al. [14] performed a retrospective multivariate analysis in 657 patients with squamous or adenocarcinoma of the esophagus. In this unselected population, the pT, pN, and pM stage, the tumor grading, and the age of the patient were shown to independently influence survival. Since patients in this study underwent a variety of resective or bypass procedures, these results can not be compared to the present study. In another multivariate analysis of 128 patients with squamous cell carcinoma of the esophagus who survived resection for more than 30 days, Sugimachi et al. [15] reported the presence of residual tumor as the only independent factor influencing survival. The distribution of the pT and pN categories in this study is comparable to our patient population. The rate of R0 resections in our study (55.9%) was, however, markedly higher as compared to the study by Sugimachi et al. (46.1%). In a follow-up study, Sugimachi et al. [16] evaluated the prognosis of 123 patients with squamous cell carcinoma of the esophagus who had pre-operative radio/chemotherapy. The 1-, 3-, and 5-year cumulative survival rates in this study were 55%, 27%, and 23%, respectively, and are comparable to the results achieved by an en bloc resection and lymphadenectomy alone in our population. Multivariate analysis in this study identified the DNA distribution pattern and postoperative complications in addition to the presence of residual tumor as independent prognostic factors. In a recent multivariate analysis, Theunissen et al. [17] also showed an independent effect of the pN category on survival time. In addition, they identified the presence of venous invasion as another factor independently influencing survival. However, their patient population consisted of both squamous and adenocarcinoma of the esophagus.

Common to these multivariate analyses by Lund, Sugimachi, and Theunissen is that no details about the extent of the resection and lymphadenectomy are given. A limited resection and lymphadenectomy does, however, not allow adequate staging of the nodal status. In this situation, the pN category can not be used to reliably assess the prognosis of the patient. Only an en bloc resection with extensive lymphadenectomy as performed in the present study allows correct staging of the lymph node status and an accurate assessment of its effect on prognosis.

The present multivariate analysis shows that only an R0 resection can increase survival in patients with squamous cell carcinoma of the esophagus. The independent effect of mediastinal lymph node metastasis and the ratio between positive and removed mediastinal lymph nodes can be interpreted similarly. In patients with a limited number of positive mediastinal lymph nodes, the prognosis may be improved by an extensive lymphadenectomy if the number of removed lymph nodes exceeds the number of positive nodes by a factor of at least five. On multivariate analysis, the remaining factors had no independent influence on survival time. This is in contrast to the results of several published studies using univariate statistics [4] and the univariate statistic performed in our patient population (Table 2). The contradictory results of univariate and multivariate analysis of prognostic factors reflects the shortcoming of univariate analysis which does not take into account the interrelations between the analyzed factors.

Acknowledgment. We gratefully acknowledge Professor H. Höfler, Director of the Institute of Pathology, for providing the histopathologic evaluation of the resected specimens and his expert assistance in the preparation of the manuscript.

References

1. Siewert JR, Roder JD, Fink U (1990) Fortschritte in der chirurgischen Behandlung des Plattenepithelkarzinoms der Speiseröhre. Internist 31:131–142
2. Müller JM, Erasmi H, Stelzner M, Zieren U, Pichlmaier H (1990) Surgical therapy of oesophageal carcinoma. Br J Surg 77:845–857
3. Hermanek P, Scheibe B, Spiessl L, Wagner G (eds) (1987) TNM-Klassifikation maligner Tumoren (UICC), 4th edn. Springer, Berlin Heidelberg New York, pp 42–44
4. Japanese Committee for Registration of Esophageal Carcinoma Cases. Iizuka K et al. (1989) Parameters linked to 10-year survival in Japan of resected esophageal carcinoma. Chest 96:1005–1011
5. Siewert JR, Hölscher AH, Becker K, Gössner W (1987) Kardiacarcinom: Versuch einer therapeutisch relevanten Klassifikation. Chirurg 58:25–32
6. Siewert JR, Hölscher AH, Roder JD, Bartels H (1988) En bloc Resektion der Speiseröhre beim Oesophaguscarcinom. Langenbecks Arch Chir 373:367–376
7. Japanese Research Society for Gastric Cancer. (1981) Jpn J Surg 11:127
8. Akiyama H (1980) Surgery for carcinoma of the esophagus. Curr Probl Surg XVII(2), 55–120

9. Gehan EA (1965) A generalized Wilcoxon test for comparing arbitrarily single-censored samples. Biometrika 52:203–224
10. Kaplan EL, Meier P (1958) Nonparametric estimation from incomplete observations. J Am Stat Assoc 53:457–481
11. Cox DR (1972) Regression models and life-tables (with discussion). J R Statist Soc B 34:187–220
12. Sugimachi K, Shinji O, Hiroyuki M, Massaki M, Hideo M, Hiroyuki K (1989) Clinicopathologic study of early stage esophageal carcinoma. Br J Surg 76:759–763
13. Bardini R, Castoro C, Sorrentino P, Borelli P, Ruffatto A, Ruol A, Tremolada C, ü Peracchia A (1989) Prognostic factors for squamous cell carcinoma of the thoracic esophagus after curative resection. Proceedings 4th World Congress of the International Society for Diseases of the Esophagus, Chicago, 1989, p 47
14. Lund O, Kimose HH, Aagaard MT, Hasenkam JM, Erlandsen M (1990) Risk stratification and long-term results after surgical treatment of carcinomas of the thoracic esophagus and cardia. J Thorac Cardiovasc Surg 99:200–209
15. Sugimachi K, Matsuura H, Kai H, Kanmatsu T, Inokuchi K, Jingu K (1986) Prognostic factors of esophageal carcinoma: Univariate and multivariate analyses. J Surg Oncol 31:108–112
16. Sugimachi K, Matsuoka H, Ohno S, Mori M, Kuwano H (1988) Multivariate approach for assessing the prognosis of clinical oesophageal carcinoma. Br J Surg 75:1115–1118
17. Theunissen PHMH, Borchard F, Poortvliet DCJ (1991) Histopathological evaluation of oesophageal carcinoma: The significance of venous invasion. Br J Surg 78:930–932

Esophagectomy Without Thoracotomy and Transthoracic Esophagectomy for Cancer of the Thoracic Esophagus: Analysis of 811 Patients

R. Bardini, A. Ruol, A. Segalin, M. Asolati, E. Tiso[1], and
A. Peracchia[2]

Introduction

Esophagectomy without thoracotomy was originally proposed by Denk in 1913 [1], and successfully performed in a patient with cancer of the thoracic esophagus by Gray-Turner in 1933 [2]. This procedure was virtually forgotten until the 1980s when Orringer reintroduced and popularized the transhiatal approach in patients with cancer of the thoracic esophagus [3, 4].

In our opinion, the treatment of choice for cancer of the thoracic esophagus consists of transthoracic esophagectomy through a right thoracotomy. Transhiatal esophagectomy is performed only in patients in whom thoracotomy is contraindicated due to severe respiratory failure, poor general condition, concomitant disease, and/or advanced age [5].

From 1980 to 1990, 671 and 140 patients with cancer of the thoracic esophagus underwent trans-thoracic esophagectomy and esophagectomy without thoracotomy, respectively. Short- and long-term results of the two techniques are analysed herein.

Patients and Surgical Techniques

Between 1980 and 1990, 811 patients underwent esophagectomy for cancer of the thoracic esophagus: 671 patients underwent transthoracic esophagectomy and 140 selected patients with a tumor confined to the esophageal wall who were unfit for thoracotomy underwent transhiatal esophagectomy without thoracotomy.

---

[1] Department of Surgery, Cl. Chirurgica 1 Policlinico Universitario, University of Paclua, Via Giustinini, 2 35100, Padova Italy
[2] Department of Surgery, Hospital Policlinico, Monteggia, University of Milano, Italy

Patient selection was made on the basis of accurate clinical staging including chest X-ray, barium swallow, esophagoscopy with vital staining, CT scan of the chest and upper abdomen, and panendoscopy of the upper respiratory tract and the ENT region. Laparoscopy and sonography of the liver were performed in tumors of the lower thoracic esophagus to detect small metastasis in the liver, peritoneum, and omentum. Endoscopic ultrasonography was performed in tumors pervious to endoscopy. General condition of the patient and his/her cardiac, respiratory, hepatic, and renal functions were systematically evaluated.

Bronchoscopic evidence of tracheobronchial compression or invasion by the tumor, or a suspected invasion of the aorta, pericardium, or prevertebral fascia documented by endoscopic ultrasonography, computed tomography (CT) scan, or magnetic nuclear resonance (MNR) were absolute contraindications to esophagectomy without thoracotomy. In these patients, a transthoracic approach was used when adequate downstaging of the tumor was documented after preoperative chemotherapy. Patients with distant metastatic disease were not considered candidates for surgery.

Transhiatal esophagectomy without thoracotomy is performed through a left cervicotomy and a median laparotomy. The abdominal esophagus is isolated and retracted downwards. According to Pinotti [6], the diaphragm is opened to allow an adequate exposure of the hiatal region and lower mediastinum: the thoracic esophagus can be visualized up to the carina, and the esophageal arteries and veins are identified and divided under visual control using hemoclips. Also, the tumor-containing portion of the esophagus is carefully dissected by means of digital dissection and hemostasis is obtained with hemoclips. Digital dissection is used through the cervical incision to isolate the upper thoracic esophagus, identifying the esophageal arteries and veins under visual control, and obtaining hemostasis with hemoclips. The stripping technique was never used in patients with cancer of the thoracic esophagus.

Transthoracic esophagectomy is performed through a posterolateral right thoracotomy in the fifth intercostal space. Standard lymphadenectomy includes the resection of periesophageal, subcarinal, paratracheal, and perigastric nodes located along the lesser curvature. In selected patients, enlarged three-field lymphadenectomy is performed.

Results

The mean age of patients undergoing transhiatal esophagectomy without thoracotomy and transthoracic esophagectomy was 65 and 57 years, respectively. Forty-four of 140 (31%) patients undergoing esophagectomy without thoracotomy and 29 of 671 (4%) patients undergoing transthoracic esophagectomy were older than 70 years. Severe pulmonary dysfunction or a pathologic EKG were present in 30 (21%) and 55 (39%) patients undergoing esophagectomy without thoracotomy, and in 47 (7%) and 164 (24%) patients undergoing transthoracic esophagectomy. The tumor was located in the upper, middle, and lower thoracic esophagus in 42 (30%), 46 (33%), and 52 (37%) patients, respectively, undergoing esophagectomy without thoracotomy, and in 127 (19%), 352 (67%), and 192 (29%) patients undergoing transthoracic esophagectomy.

Table 1. Tumor, pathologic TNM stage of patients undergoing curative resection

	EWT		TE	
Tis-1	36	33.9%	52	11.0%
T2	27	25.5%	130	27.5%
T3	41	38.7%	254	53.7%
T4	2	1.9%	37	7.8%
N −	67	63.2%	212	44.8%
N +	39	36.8%	261	55.2%
Stage I	34	32.0%	43	9.1%
II	36	34.0%	185	39.1%
III	24	22.6%	146	30.9%
IV (M1 Lym)	12	11.4%	99	20.9%

EWT, esophagectomy without thoracotomy; *TE*, transthoracic esophagectomy

Table 2. Postoperative complications and mortality

	EWT		TE	
Recurr. L. Nerve lesion	14	(10.0%)	32	(4.8%)
Chylothorax	1	(0.7%)	3	(0.4%)
Pulmonary complications	16	(11.4%)	71	(10.5%)
Hospital deaths	10/140	7.1%	59/671	8.8%

EWT, esophagectomy without thoracotomy; *TE*, transthoracic esophagectomy

Curative and palliative resection was performed in 106 (76%) and 34 (24%) patients undergoing esophagectomy without thoracotomy, and in 475 (71%) and 196 (29%) patients undergoing transthoracic esophagectomy. The mean duration of operation was 4.30 and 5.30 h, respectively. Mean intraoperative blood loss was 370 and 400 cc.

Stage 0-1-2 cases were more frequent in patients undergoing esophagectomy without thoracotomy (66%) than in patients undergoing transthoracic esophagectomy (48%) (Table 1). Mean tumor length was 4.6 and 6 cm, respectively. Lymph node metastases were less common in patients undergoing esophagectomy without thoracotomy (37%) than in patients undergoing transthoracic esophagectomy (55%) (Table 1).

There were 10 (7.1%) hospital deaths in patients undergoing esophagectomy without thoracotomy, and 59 (8.8%) in patients undergoing transthoracic esophagectomy. The incidence of postoperative complications, including anastomotic leak and pulmonary complications, was comparable in the two groups. Recurrent laryngeal nerve lesions were more common in patients undergoing esophagectomy without thoracotomy (10%) than in patients undergoing transthoracic esophagectomy (4.8%) (Table 2).

The overall 5-year survival was 16% and 19% after esophagectomy without thoracotomy and transthoracic esophagectomy, respectively; after curative resection it was 20% and 23%. The 3-year survival rate after palliative resection was 0% and 7%. After curative resection, 5-year survival was 29% and 41% when lymph nodes were negative, and 0% and 9% in the presence of lymph node metastasis. The site of recurrence after curative resection was documented in 35 patients undergoing esophagectomy without thoracotomy and 193 patients undergoing transthoracic esophagectomy: it was local in 50% and 39%, distant in 46% and 58%, and both local and distant in 4% and 5%, respectively.

Discussion

In the last decade, esophagectomy without thoracotomy has been performed by several surgeons in patients with cancer of the thoracic esophagus [7, 8]. The risk of severe intraoperative complications such as mediastinal bleeding or lesions of the tracheobronchial tree has been minimized thanks to increasing experience with the transhiatal approach. At present, esophagectomy without thoracotomy is considered a safe and well standardized technique with a low risk of procedure-related morbidity and mortality [4, 5]. On the other hand, the indications for this technique in patients with carcinoma of the thoracic esophagus are still controversial. Some authors believe that a curative intent is always unrealistic when dealing with esophageal cancer, and that the most realistic goal even in resectable cases is palliation of dysphagia: esophagectomy without thoracotomy is advocated as the procedure which can minimize the morbidity and the mortality rates related to esophagectomy, and prevent the potential septic complication of a thoracic anastomotic leak [3, 4].

Conversely, others authors believe that curative surgery is possible in selected patients with a localized esophageal tumor. In their opinion [9], to make cure possible, the resection should follow sound oncological principles and include the dissection of regional lymph nodes, which can be achieved only using a transthoracic approach.

At present, the problem regarding the surgical procedure of choice for cancer of the thoracic esophagus is still open. To our knowledge, there is only one controlled prospective randomized study comparing the transthoracic and the transhiatal approach; this includes 32 patients undergoing transthoracic esophagectomy and 35 patients undergoing esophagectomy without thoracotomy. Although the number of patients in each arm of the study was small and the follow-up relatively short, no difference in the morbidity and mortality rates, nor in the long-term survival was observed between the two groups of patients.

On the basis of our experience, we agree with Orringer that, from a technical point of view, esophagectomy without thoracotomy is a safe procedure both for benign and malignant esophageal diseases. However, according to the oncologic criteria, we think that use of this procedure on every patient with cancer of the thoracic esophagus is not justified. The main issue is that it is impossible to carry out a complete mediastinal lymphadenectomy which leads to possible tumor understaging. For this reason, our standard surgical approach for carcinoma of the intrathoracic esophagus consists of transthoracic esophagectomy through a right thoracotomy whenever there are no contraindications such as severe respiratory failure, poor general condition, concomitant disease, and/or advanced age. In high-risk patients in whom thoracotomy is contraindicated, transhiatal esophagectomy is performed.

The present report is not a prospective controlled study and therefore it cannot provide a significant conclusion on the advantages of transhiatal esophagectomy without thoracotomy or transthoracic esophagectomy. However, it is to be emphasized that, although the patients undergoing esophagectomy without thoracotomy were older, in worse general condition, and with an higher prevalence of severe pulmonary disfunction than patients undergoing transthoracic esophagectomy, the morbidity and mortality rates were comparable after the two surgical procedures. Moreover, the long-term results were comparable.

Conclusions

In our opinion, esophagectomy without thoracotomy is an excellent technique entailing low morbidity and mortality rates, but with oncologic limitations. It represents the ideal approach in patients with a tumor of the hypopharynx and the cervical esophagus or in patients with benign esophageal diseases requiring esophageal resection.

Transthoracic esophagectomy should be the surgical approach of choice for cancer of the thoracic esophagus. Esophagectomy without thoracotomy allows patients who are unfit for transthoracic esophagectomy to be operated on at a reasonable operative risk; however, accurate lymphadenectomy is impossible and, therefore, lymph node understaging is likely.

References

1. Denk W (1913) Zur radicaloperation des esophagus karzinoms. Zentral Chir 40:1065–1068
2. Gray-Turner G (1933) Excision of thoracic esophagus for carcinomas with reconstruction of extrathoracic gullet. Lancet II:1315–1318
3. Orringer MB (1984) Technical aids in performing transhiatal esophagectomy without thoracotomy. Ann Thor Surg 38:128–135
4. Orringer MB (1984) Transhiatal esophagectomy without thoracotomy for carcinoma of thoracic esophagus. Ann Surg 3:282–287
5. Peracchia A (1988) In: Delarue NC, Wilkins Jr. EW, Wong J (eds) CV Mosby, St. Louis, pp 210–212
6. Pinotti HW (1984) In: Via de acceso transdiafragmatico al esofago toracico y al mediastino anterior. Salvat Editores, pp 90–98
7. Peracchia A, Bardini R, Asolati M, De Vido L, Ruol A (1988) Indications et resultats de l'oesophagectomie sans thoracotomie. Actualites Digestives 6:238–240
8. Sugimachi K, Matsuzaki K, Matsuura H, Kuwano H, Ueo H, Inokuchi K (1985) Evaluation of surgical treatment of carcinoma of the esophagus in the elderly: 20 years' experience. Br J Surg 72:28–30
9. Skinner DB (1983) En bloc resection for neoplasms of the esophagus and cardia. J Thor Cardiovasc Surg 85:89

Esophageal and Gastric Cardia Carcinoma: Patient Selection for Transhiatal Esophagectomy

Chih-Yi Chen, Pei-Yen Wang, and Chun-Lieh Chen[1]

Introduction

Patients with esophageal carcinoma are often elderly and have poor nutritional and pulmonary status. Blunt transhiatal esophagectomy is an alternative surgical procedure for patients with carcinoma of the extremes of the esophagus. For the past 10 years, transhiatal esophagectomy and reconstruction with the stomach has been a choice for some patients with carcinoma of the upper or lower esophagus and gastric cardia. This report is a review of our experience with 73 patients in terms of indication and selection for this surgical procedure.

Patients and Methods

From 1983 to 1992, a total of 73 patients underwent transhiatal esophagectomy for either palliative or curative treatment of esophageal and gastric cardia carcinoma (Table 1). This series included 67 males and 6 females between 44 and 80 years of age (mean, 62 years). All patients were evaluated systemically using several clinical, radiologic, and endoscopic examinations. On the basis of these examinations, the selection of treatment was made by tumor location, chest condition, staging, aim of treatment, and patient's overall condition (Table 2).

Indications

The indications of transhiatal esophagectomy included: (1) The location of the tumor; most surgeons agree to perform transhiatal esophagectomy for the

---

[1] Division of Thoracic Surgery, Department of Surgery, Taichung Veterans General Hospital, Taiwan, ROC

Table 1. Clinical experience of transhiatal esophagectomy (Taichung Veterans General Hospital (*VGH*), 1983–1992)

Acute corrrosive injury	24
Carcinoma	73
(17% in 430 resection patients)	

Table 2. Selection of approach

Aim of surgery: Curative or palliative
General condition
Chest condition Pulmonary function
COPD, TB
previous operation
adhesion
Resection margin
Organ subsititute: Stomach—1 anastomosis
Colon—3 anastomoses
Surgeon: Surgical planning
specialities and preference

COPD, chronic obstructive pulmonary disease, *TB*, tuberculosis

normal thoracic esophagus in patients with carcinoma of the hypopharynx [1], cervical esophagus, and gastric cardia [2–5]. For carcinoma of the middle thoracic esophagus, most surgeons are against transhiatal esophagectomy as a standard procedure due to the difficulty associated with dissection between tumor and main bronchus. (2) The condition of dense adhesion in the pleural cavities, where transthoracic esophagectomy is difficult. (3) Elderly patients with respiratory insufficiency, in whom transthoracic esophagectomy may increase postoperative complications. (4) Pallative resection procedures, because mediastinal node dissection is difficult in transhiatal esophagectomy [6, 7] and (5) superficial esophageal carcinoma.

Surgical Procedures

Bronchoscopy was performed for cervical and upper esophageal lesions to exclude tumor invasion into the trachea or bronchus. On the day prior to surgery, bowel preperation was performed routinely. The patient is placed supine on the operating table with the head inclined to the right. The neck and abdomen are prepared, and an arterial line and CVP line set. When the lesion is location in the cervical esophagus, the neck is explored first to determine operability. Otherwise, the abdomen is opened through an upper midline incision. Metastastic deposits in the liver or celiac node involvement do not contraindicate resection. Before the stomach is freed, operability of the lesion is determined by palpation through the hiatus. The stomach is freed by dividing the short gastric vessels, and by preserving the right gastric and right gastroepiploic vessels. The left gastric artery is ligated at its origin and a pyloromyotomy is made.

The cervical esophagus is approached through an incision in the anterior border of left sternocleidomastoid muscle. The carotid sheath, thyroid gland, and trachea are then retracted bilaterally. The omohyoid muscle is divided, and the esophagus is separated from the trachea.

The distal esophagus is exposed by freeing it from its hiatal attachments; the hiatus is widened, and a light retracter inserted to retract the crural sling anteriorly. Wide exposure of the distal esophagus in the mediastinum is provided, then sharp dissection is carried out after visually evaluating some of the esophageal attachments and vasular components.

After the lower esophageal dissection has been completed, further mobilization of the intrathoracic esophagus is carried out by bimanual blunt dissection from the neck and abdomen, with precise separation of the surrounding tissues from the esophagus.

The esophagus is transected at the neck level if the tumor is located in the gastric cardia, and the esophagus pulled through into the abdomen. It is then transected at the mid-stomach level. Then, using the ileocolon as a reconstruction substitute through the retrosternal route, cervical anastomosis is done.

The esophagus is divided at the cardia and pulled through the neck if the tumor is located at the neck or hypopharynx. The stomach was used as a substitute through the retrosternal route and anastomosis was done at the neck or oral base level.

In some cases, transhiatal esophagectomy was performed by inversion extraction, with downward or upward stripping using the vein stripper.

Results

In 73 patients, 13 had hypopharyngeal cancer, 46 esophageal cancer (upper 9, middle 2, lower 35) and 14 had cancer of the gastric cardia. The esophageal substitute included 52 patients undergoing placement of the stomach, and 21 patients with the ileocolon. Routes for reconstruction included 64 patients in the retrosternal position, and 9 patients in the posterior mediastinum.

Twenty-three patients had postoperative pneumothorax which was treated with chest tube placement. Morbidity was 30.2%, and three patients died due to respiratory failure. The operative time ranged from 2.5 to 4.5 h (average, 3.3 h), the average blood loss was 594 ml, and the average hospital stay was 25 days. Postoperative complications are listed in Table 3.

In comparison with transthoracic esophagectomy done in the same period, a significant decrease in operative time and blood loss was noted (Table 4), but the cumulative survival time was not significantly different between these two groups.

Discussion

Transhiatal esophagectomy without thoracotomy has been shown to be associated with less morbidity and mortality than transthoracic esophagectomy [3, 7–13]. In our hospital, transhiatal esophagectomy has been performed increasingly in patients with esophageal and gastric cardia carcinoma because the associated with surgical risk palliative treatment of advanced tumor is acceptable. There is still some controversy, however, about patient selection for this operation [8, 14–16]. If the palliative nature of any currently available therapy for the treatment of carcinoma of the esophagus is accepted [3], esophagectomy without thoracotomy should be viewed with this goal in mind. The success of a palliative operation is judged by its safety and the speed with which the patient can be relieved of symptoms and returned to a normal life [3, 17]. Palliation with immediate relief of dysphagia is usually achieved by using transhiatal esophagectomy. We believe that the ideal candidate is one with

Table 3. Postoperative complications

	No.	%
Anastomotic leak	8	11.0
Hoarseness	8	11.0
Pneumonia	6	8.2
Wound infection	3	4.1
Hemothorax	2	2.7
Empyema	2	2.7

Table 4. Esophagectomy (Taichung VGH 1983–1992)

	Transhiatal ($n = 73$)	Transthoracic ($n = 292$)
Morbidity (%)	30.2	38.0
Mortality (%)	4.1	7.5
Blood loss (ml)	594 ± 34	692 ± 28
Days in hospital	25 ± 1.3	36 ± 1.6
Operative time (h)	3.3 ± 1.0	4.9 ± 0.7

a localized lesion as defined roentgenographically and endoscopically, and preferably in the cervical or upper and lower thoracic esophagus, or gastric cardia. Hemorrhage from the mediastinum can be minimized by limiting the extent of blind mobilization of the esophagus, by retraction of the hiatus to permit esophageal mobilization under direct vision. In our series, the average blood loss was less in the transhiatal esophagectomy group. The chances of complication of pneumothorax are greater in this procedure, but they are easy to treat and are generally without any sequelae.

In our series, the shortening of operative time and decrease of physiologic insult in the patient without thoracotomy may contribute to a decrease in respiratory complications, morbidity, and mortality. The most frequent cause of death following esophagectomy is mediastinitis from leakage in the intrathoracic anastomosis, and this is effectively eliminated by the esophagectomy without thoracotomy. The anastomosis in the neck ensures that an anastomotic leak will not occur in the chest and, consequently, the risk is much smaller.

Conclusions

The aim of transhiatal esophagectomy is to relieve the patient of dysphagia, pain, and bleeding associated with cancer of the upper and lower esophagus. The technique of transhiatal esophagectomy of the unaffected esophagus through the posterior mediastinum is a quick and safe method with less morbidity and mortality. The transhiatal esophagectomy can be an alternative technique in patients who have tumor in the extremes of the esophagus and are at high surgical risk due to old age or poor lung condition.

References

1. Goldberg M, Freeman J, Gullane PJ, Patterson GA, Todd TRJ, McShane D (1989) Transhiatal esophagectomy with gastric transpostion for pharyngolaryngeal malignant disease. Thorac Cardiovasc Surg 97:327–333
2. Akiyama H, Hiyama M, Miyazono K (1975) Total esophageal reconstruction after extraction of the esophagus. Ann Surg 182:547–553
3. Tryzelaar JF, Neptune WB Ellis FH, Jr (1982) 143:486–489
4. Finley RJ, Grace M, Duff JH (1985) Esophagogastrectomy without thoracotomy for carcinoma of the cardia and lower part of the esophagus. Surg Gynecol Obstet 160:49–56

5. Finley RJ, Inculet RI (1989) The results of esophagogastrectomy without thoracotomy for adenocarcinoma of the esophagogastric junction. Ann Surg 210:535–543
6. McInnes JE, Johnson WR (1987) Oesophagectomy without thoracotomy in the treatment of oesophageal carcinoma. NZ J Surg 57:819–822
7. Gotley J, Beard MJ, Cooper DC, Britton, Williamson RCN (1990) Abdominocervical (transhiatal) oesophagectomy in the management of oesophageal carcinoma. Br J Surg 77:815–819
8. Orringer MB, Orringer JS (1983) Esophagectomy without thoracotomy: A dangerous operation? J Thorac Cardiovasc Surg 85:72–80
9. Orringer MB (1984) Transhiatal esophagectomy without thoractomy for carcinoma of the thoracic esophagus. Ann Surg 200:282–288
10. Baker JW, Schechter GL (1986) Management of panesophageal cancer by blunt resection without thoracotomy and reconstruction with stomach. Ann Surg 203:491–499
11. Shahian DM, Neptune WB, Ellis FH, Watkins E (1986) Transthoracic versus extrathoracic esophagectomy: Mortality, morbidity, and long-term survival. Ann Thorac Surg 41:237–246
12. Barbier PA, Becker CD, Wagner HE (1988) Esophageal carcinoma: Patient selection for transhiatal esophagectomy. A prospective analysis of 50 consecutive cases. World J Surg 12:263–269
13. Gurkan T, Terzioglu S, Tezelman, Sasmaz O (1991) Transhiatal oesophagectomy for oesophageal carcinoma. Br J Surg 78:1348–1351
14. Mitchell RL (1987) Abdominal and right thoracotomy approach as standard procedure for esophagogastrectomy with low morbidity. J Thorac Carciovasc Surg 93:205–211
15. Mathisen DJ, Grillo HC, Wilkins EW, Moncure AC, Hilgenberg AD (1988) Transthoracic esophagectomy: A safe approach to carcinoma of the esophagus. Ann Thorac Surg 45:137–143
16. Fok M, Siu KF, Wong J (1989) A comparison of transhiatal and transthoracic resection for carcinoma of the thoracic esophagus. Am J Surg 158:41:419
17. Barbier PA, Luder PJ, Schupfer G, Becker CD, Wanger HE (1988) Quality of life and patterns of recurrence following transhiatal esophagectomy for cancer: Results of a prospective follow-up in 50 patients. World J Surg 12:270–276

Blunt Dissection for Thoracic Esophageal Cancer

Y. Karaki, M. Fujimaki, M. Saito, A. Yamada, T. Sakamoto, Y. Kuroki,
T. Sakakibara, T. Shimizu, K. Higashiyama, Y. Yamashita,
and K. Tazawa[1]

Introduction

The conventional surgical technique in treating thoracic esophageal cancer is esophagectomy using a transthoracic approach. We often use a right thoracotomy approach for transthoracic esophagectomy with posterior mediastinal lymphadenectomy. However, in patients with various complications such as cardiac, pulmonary or renal failure or with debilitated or extremely aged patients, we often conduct intrathoracic esophagectomy without thoracotomy. Although the operation has limitations in terms of curability, this method is said to be useful and safe for reducing the more serious postoperative complications. The purpose of this report is to confirm the safety and usefulness of this method based on our experience.

Patients and Methods

Since 1980, we have performed esophagectomy for thoracic esophageal cancers in 93 patients. The approaches in these cases were right transthoracic in 62 and blunt dissection in 31.

The 31 patients who underwent blunt dissection ranged in age from 51 to 85 years, with a mean of 71.2 years. The mean age of patients in the blunt dissection group was approximately 11 years greater than that of those in the thoracotomy group. The female to male ratio in the blunt dissection group was approximately 1:9 and for the thoracotomy group approximately 1:20. The location of cancer was upper (Iu) in 7 patients, middle (Im) in 42, and lower (Ei) in 13 for the thoracotomy group; and Iu in 3 patients, Im in 15, and Ei in 13 for the blunt dissection group [1].

[1] Second Department of Surgery, Toyama Medical and Pharmaceutical University, 2630 Sugitani, Toyama, 930-01 Japan

Table 1. Preoperative condition	
Diabetes mellitus	4
Double cancer	3
Pulmonary dysfunction	8
Heart failure	3
Renal failure	1

Table 2. Patient history	
Lung tuberculosis	5
Cerebral infarction	4
Myocardial infarction	4
Double cancer	2
Chronic renal failure	1
Gastrectomy (ulcer)	2

Blunt dissection is indicated for patients with complications likely to evoke serious morbidity. Table 1 shows the preoperative complications of patients who underwent blunt dissection. Among them, pulmonary failure is a frequent complication. The medical history of the patients who underwent blunt dissection is also taken into consideration and is listed in Table 2. Among them was the frequent obstacle of pulmonary tuberculosis, which makes it difficult to conduct thoracotomy.

Surgical Technique

We usually perform surgery with 2 teams (cervical and abdominal), with both starting surgery at the same time. The cervical skin incision follows the anterior border of the left sternocleidomastoid muscle exposing the cervical esophagus, followed by mobilization of the intrathoracic proximal portion of the esophagus down to the bronchus using the surgeon's index finger through the upper thoracic aperture. While the cervical procedure is under way, the other surgical team conducts the upper median laparotomy. After mobilizing the stomach, the abdominal esophagus is also mobilized and a truncal vagotomy is performed. The hiatus muscle is often transected to enlarge the hiatus. Mobilization of the distal thoracic esophagus is performed by insertion of the surgeon's hand and half the forearm into the posterior mediastinum. We do not conduct intrathoracic paraesophageal or mediastinal lymph node dissection as this procedure is basically palliative. After the complete mobilization of the esophagus, the cervical site of the esophagus is transected and pulled downward through and into the abdomen.

Results

Substitute Esophagus

In the blunt dissection group, we reconstructed the esophagus by a thin gastric tube in 23 patients (74.2%), by left colon in 3, and by right colon in 5. However, in the thoracotomy group, we used a thin gastric tube in 53 (85.5%), left colon in 7 and right colon in 1.

Route of the Substitute Esophagus

In the blunt dissection group, the routes of these substitute esophagi were posterior mediastinum in 27 patients, retrosternal in 3 and subcutaneous in 1. In

Table 3. Postoperative complications (blunt)

Pneumothorax	10
Pleural effusion	3
Atelectasis	1
Pneumonia	2
Arrythmia	2
Postoperative bleeding	2 (reoperation 1)
Tracheal injury	1 (thoracotomy, repair)
Anastomotic leakage	7
Cerebral infarction	1
Recurrent nerve paralysis	1
Pulmonary infarction	1

the thoracotomy group, most of the patients underwent reconstruction through the retrosternal route.

Surgical Time

The surgical time of blunt dissection ranged from 1 h and 50 min to 4 h and 50 min, with a mean of 2 h and 46 min.

Blood Loss

Blood loss during surgery ranged from 230 ml to 2500 ml, with an average of 793 ml.

Depth of Cancer Invasion in Resected Specimens

All the resected specimens were histologically examined and the depth of cancer invasion was classified according to the guide-lines for clinical and pathological studies on carcinoma of the esophagus presented by the Japanese Society for Esophageal Diseases [2]. Among the 31 patients who underwent blunt dissection, 2 patients had intraepithelial cancer (ep), 1 had invasion of the muscularis mucosa (mm), and 7 showed invasion of the submucosa (sm). Among the remaining 21 patients, cancer had invaded the muscularis propria (mp) in 8 patients, and the adventitia (a) in 13. These were subclassified into three types by the degree of invasion: 9 cases were a_1, 1 was a_2, and 3 were a_3.

Postoperative Complications (Table 3)

In the blunt dissection patients, pneumothorax frequently occurred, but the patient recovered within the early postoperative period after intraoperative or postoperative intrathoracic intubation in all cases. In two patients, there was an episode of postoperative bleeding from the posterior mediastinum. One of the two patients was treated conservatively and hemostasis was achieved, and the other underwent right thoracotomy for hemostasis. A tracheal tear at the point just above the carina occurred in one case with cancer in the upper thoracic esophagus, followed by repair through a right thoracotomy.

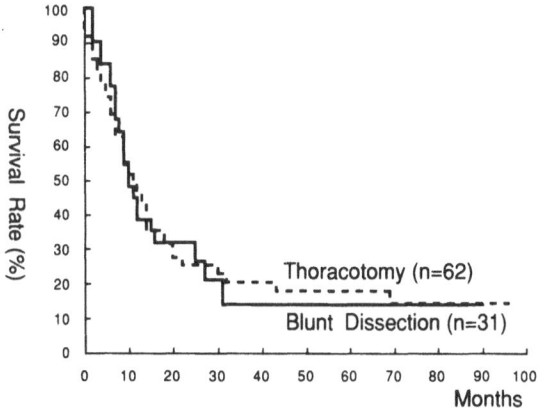

Fig. 1. Cumulative survival rate (1) (Kaplan-Meier method): Thoracotomy vs blunt dissection

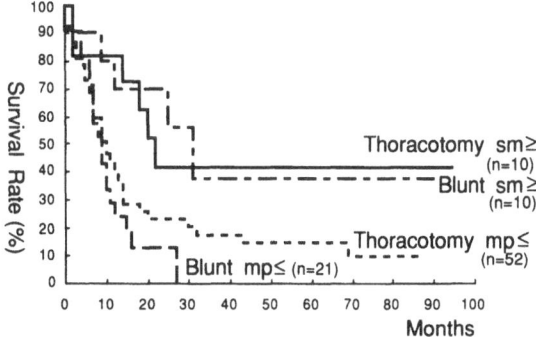

Fig. 2. Cumulative survival rate (2) (Kaplan-Meier method)

Although anastomotic leakage from the cervical anastomotic site developed in seven patients (22.6%), all leakages were minor and healed within early postoperative periods. No obvious anastomotic stenosis was observed, and there was no operative death in this series.

Prognosis

Figure 1 shows the prognoses of both the right thoracotomy group and the blunt group. These data include all the resected cases, including both the non-curative and curative ones. The 5-year survival rate was 17.9% in the former and 14.2% in the latter group. There was no significant difference between the two groups.

Figure 2 shows the prognoses of both the blunt dissection and thoracotomy groups. Patients were divided by the degree of intramural invasion. The 5-year survival rate among those with less invasive cancers (ep to sm) was 41.6% in the thoracotomy group and 37.3% in the blunt dissection group, showing no significant difference between the two groups. In the group with cancer invasion beyond the submucosa (mp to a), the 5-year survival rates were 14.4% in thoracotomy group and 0% in the blunt dissection group, with there being no significant difference between them.

Discussion

There is extensive nomenclature about the procedure for thoracic esophagectomy without thoracotomy such as: transhiatal esophagectomy without thoracotomy [3], blunt esophagectomy without thoracotomy [4], pull-through esophagectomy without thoracotomy [5], and others. These various procedures are similar in the sense that they are all non-thoracotomy techniques. However these techniques need to be classified from the viewpoint of the inclusion or exclusion of mediastinal lymphadenectomy.

According to these criteria, our procedure is defined as blunt thoracic esophagectomy without thoracotomy and without mediastinal lymphadenectomy. When discussing the prognosis of this kind of procedure, we must take this point into consideration. In the present study, there was no significant difference in prognoses between the transthoracic esophagectomy (TTE) and the blunt dissection (BE) groups. However, we can not hastily conclude that there is an advantage of BE over TTE, because the TTE group included many non-curative resection cases. To obtain a more accurate information as to whether or not these two types of procedures show the same prognoses, we must carefully conduct a comparative study such as that performed by Fok et al. [6].

As for complications, although most of the patients who underwent blunt dissection were shown to be in poor preoperative condition, there were only three serious complications and they all recovered with or without reoperation through a right thoracotomy. After our experience with a tracheal tear in one of our cases, the patients with a_2 or a_3 cancer located in the Iu were excluded from blunt (blind) dissection. Our results in terms of postoperative morbidity and mortality were not inferior to those of other investigators [3–6]. We conclude that blunt dissection for thoracic esophageal cancer as a palliative technique is safe and useful even for the patient with high risk factors for surgery.

References

1. Japanese Society for Esophageal Diseases (1976) Guidelines for the clinical and pathologic studies on carcinoma of the esophagus. Part I. Clinical classification. Jpn J Surg 6:69–78
2. Japanese Society for Esophageal Diseases (1976) Guidelines for the clinical and pathologic studies on carcinoma of the esophagus. Part II. Pathologic classification. Jpn J Surg 6:79–86
3. Orringer MB (1984) Transhiatal esophagectomy without thoracotomy for carcinoma of the thoracic esophagus. Ann Surg 200:282–288
4. Baker JW, Schechter GL (1986) Management of panesophageal cancer by blunt resection without thoracotomy and reconstruction with stomach Ann Surg 203:491–499
5. Szentpetery S, Wolfgang T, Lower RR (1979) Pull-through esophagectomy without thoracotomy for esophageal carcinoma. Ann Thorac Surg 27:399–403
6. Fok M, Siu KF, Wong J (1989) A comparison of transhiatal and transthoracic resection for carcinoma of the thoracic esophagus. Am J Surg 158:414–419

Esophageal Stripping—Experience in 82 Cases

J. López Gibert, X. Rius, and A. Sánchez Marin[1]

Introduction

There are two well known procedures to perform an esophagectomy without thoracotomy: blunt dissection and esophageal stripping. Another technique consisting of a combination of both is an initial esophagectomy with transhiatal disection followed by esophageal stripping.

The stripping procedure is a progressive and controlled esophageal pulling out of the posterior mediastinum with the aid of a venous stripper or a nasogastric tube of Wagensteen fixed in one of the sections of the esophagus. From the other section, we pull slowly causing the progressive invagination of the esophagus and its pulling out of the mediastinum (Figs. 1–3).

There are two stripping procedures depending on which way we want to extract the dissection: through the abdominal cavity or through the neck. The first one is stripping from up to down for tumours in the cardias, the other one is stripping from down to up for cervical esophageal cancer.

The stripping procedure has very precise indications. They are listed in Table 1. In the cervical esophageal cancers, total esophagectomy prevents multicentric locations. In the carcinomas of the cardias involving the esophagus, we prefer total esophagectomy with esophageal stripping and, if necessary, with transhiatal dissection compared to left thoracolaparotomy.

Material and Methods

Between January 1979 and December 1990, we performed 82 total esophagectomies with esophageal stripping. Of these, 52 involved stripping alone and the other 30 were in combination with transhiatal blunt tumor dissection.

[1] General and Digestive Surgery Department, Hospital de la Santa Creu i Sant Pau, Avda. S. Antonio María Claret no. 167, Barcelona, Spain

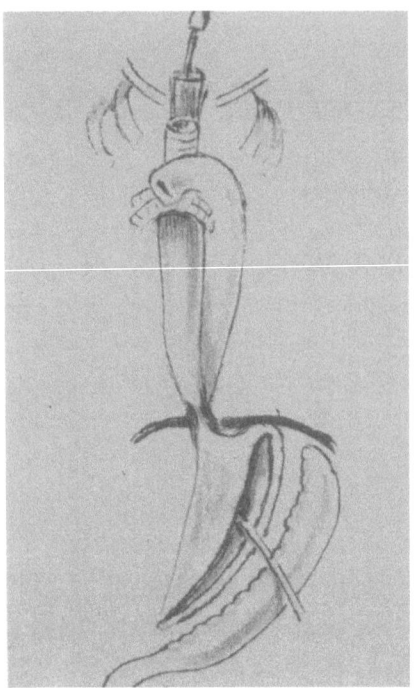
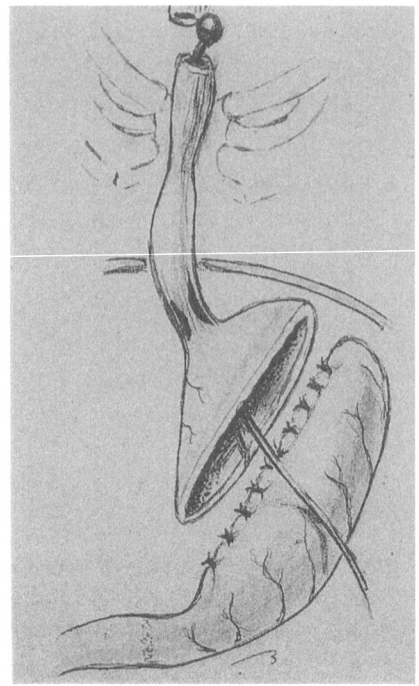

1

Fig. 1. Anatomical details of the esophageal stripping

Fig. 2. Section of cervical esophagus and vertical gastrectomy including great gastric tuberosity and lesser curvature up to incisura angularis

Except for eight patients admitted for severe caustic esophagitis and other non-tumoral pathology of the esophagus, all the resections ($n = 73$) were performed for esophageal cancers (23 epidermoid carcinomas and 50 adeno-carcinomas). They were located in the cervical esophagus in 5 patients, in the distal third of the esophagus in 31, and 37 cases were cancer of the cardias with esophageal involvement. The relation between location and pathology is shown in Fig. 4. All 37 cardial cancers were adenocarcinomas. Thirteen cancers of the distal third of the esophagus were adenocarcinomas too, probably Barret's esophagus. The histology of the other distal lesions and of all the cervival lesions was epidermoid carcinoma.

Dysphagia was the most frequent symptom and it was presented with an average of two and a half months preoperatively. Six patients had undergone gastric surgery for ulcer previously (5 gastrectomies and 1 gastroenterostomy). One patient had undergone total gastrectomy for gastric cancer and 2 years later presented relapse in esophagojejunal anastomosis.

Except for five cases of cervical location with total esophagectomy and direct anastomosis with the pharynx, in all the cases resection was nearly total esopha-

Fig. 3. Stripping procedure

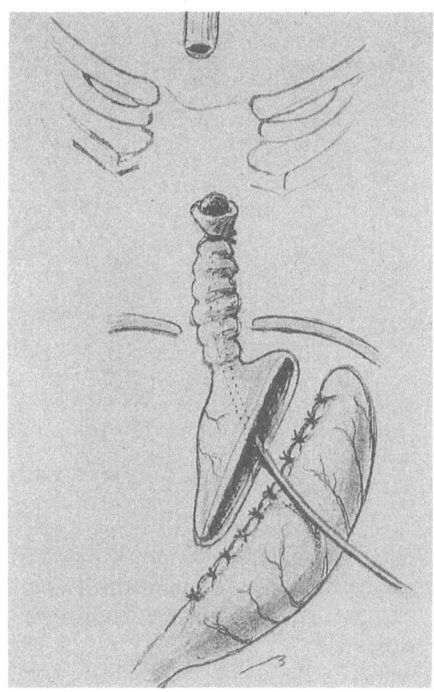

Table 1. Indications for esophageal stripping

Cervical esophageal cancer
Cardias and inferior esophageal cancer
Lymphadenectomy not needed:
  Palliative surgery
  "Cancer in situ" surgery
Contraindicated thoracotomy
Non-malignant lesions

gectomy leaving 2 cm of the cervical esophagus, near the pharynx, for the anastomosis.

The extension of the resection joined to the stripping procedures was lesser gastric curvature resection in 65 patients, esophagectomy and total gastrectomy in 14, esophagectomy with lesser curvature gastrectomy and laryngectomy in 2, and esophagectomy with jejunal resection in 1 (previous total gastrectomy).

In esophageal tumours, we performed esophagectomy with vertical gastrectomy including great gastric tuberosity and lesser curvature up to incisura angularis. We extirpate paracardial and lesser curvature ganglionar groups.

In the adenocarcinomas of the cardias with esophageal involvment, we performed total gastrectomy with splenectomy, distal pancreatectomy and omentectomy, when the procedure was curative. In palliative surgery, we performed

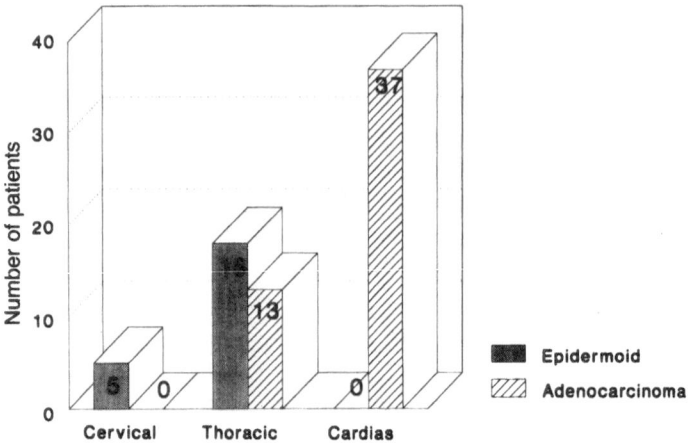

Fig. 4. Relation between location and histology

vertical gastrectomy in order to avoid coloplasty. In the patient with previous total gastrectomy, we performed esophagectomy and jejunal resection.

In the transit reconstruction, we used 57 vertical gastroplasties and 15 coloplasties.

Results

Morbidity

There were no major intraoperative complications. We had no complications associated with mediastinal bleeding. The small loss of blood observed from the posterior mediastinum stopped spontaneously or by dabbing it with gauze for a few minutes.

Cervical anastomotic leakage, confirmed radiologically, occurred in 15 patients. Only 8 patients had clinical manifestations. All the cervical fistulas closed spontaneously in 6–30 days except one which drained to the mediastinum.

Six pleural injuries occurred in transhiatal dissections in mixed stripping procedures.

Complete section of the recurrent nerve was not presented in this series. In 6 patients, there was a temporal injury probably related to fistulas of the cervical anastomosis.

One of the patients developed a coloplasty necrosis. Another case presented with tracheal injury.

Mortality

Hospital mortality was 4 of the 82 operated patients (4.8%). All the cases occurred in the esophagectomy with total gastrectomy group.

One patient developed sepsis and respiratory distress caused by anastomotic leakage which drained at the posterior mediastinum.

In the patient with previous total gastrectomy, bleeding of the jejuno-jejunal anastomosis was the cause of death.

The colic necrosis and the tracheal injury were the other causes of death.

Survival

Forty patients were operated on for cancer more than 5 years ago. Ten of them are still alive. Fourteen patients survived for more than 4 years and 23 survived for 1–4 years. Twenty-two patients died 1–4 years after the surgery.

Conclusion

In conclusion, stripping is an excellent technique when it is well indicated. There is a low morbidity rate and also low hospital mortality (4.8%) keeping in mind that all the cases were total esophagectomies, 14 combined with total gastrectomy and 6 with laryngectomy. We believe that stripping is one of the esophagectomy procedures with less complications and mortality.

Swallowing Function Before and After Esophagectomy for Treatment of Esophageal Cancer

M.A. Oliveira[1], A.H. Hölscher[2], H. Feussner[2], C. Daschner[3], C. Hannig[3], J.R. Siewert[2], and H.W. Pinotti[1]

Introduction

A total or subtotal esophagectomy represents the main therapeutical step in esophageal cancer when cure is desired or also as a palliative measure. Surgeon's goals are not only tumor radical resection, but also to allow survival under acceptable conditions.

While the morphological and functional behavior of viscera employed in digestive tube reconstruction after esophagectomies has received considerable attention in the literature [1], the same is not true with the remaining pharyngoesophageal segment.

Few authors specifically investigated the swallowing behavior in patients with esophageal carcinoma. Hambraeus et al. [2] report at least one type of pharyngeal functional abnormality in eight of nine patients which underwent esophagectomy and visceral interposition. Just five patients had been preoperatively examined, two being considered normal and two having slight functional abnormalities.

Analysis of the upper esophageal segment (UES) with conventional pull-through manometry did not disclose any major abnormality [3–5]. Feussner et al. [6] studying prospectively six patients before and after esophagectomies with gastric interposition, with manometry and cineradiography, reported minimal motility disturbances in the preoperative period which kept constant or incrased after the operation, although the findings were not correlated with clinical symptoms.

[1] Department of Gastroenterology, São Paulo University Medical School, Av. Doutor Enéas de Carvalho Aguiar, 255–900 andan São Paulo-SP-Brasil CEP: 05403-900
Departments of [2]Surgery and, [3]Radiology, Technical University of Munich (TUM), Ismaningerstraß 22, D-8000, Munich 80, Germany

With these facts in mind, a study which investigated how swallowing function is affected by an esophageal cancer, as well as its behavior in esophagectomy was carried out.

Subjects and Methods

Sixty-two asymptomatic patients served as controls (group A). Forty-four cases of esophageal carcinoma were examined: 25 (group B) just preoperatively; 14 pre- (group C1) and early posteperatively (group C2); and 5 in the late postoperative period (group D).

Clinical Evaluation

Clinical evaluation was made employing a scale which classified quality of swallowing in four degrees: degree I, asymptomatic patient—able to swallow any type of food; degree II, slightly symptomatic with occasional slowing and/or pain during swallowing—must take care with consistancy of food; degree III, moderately symptomatic—accepts semi-solids or liquids without problems—usually has problems with solids, requiring careful food preparation; degree IV, severely symptomatic—Swallows just liquids or carefully prepared semi-solid food—Regurgitation and/or vomiting during meals—Symptoms of aspiration and loss of weight.

Functional Analysis

Cineradiography

Cineradiological exams were made in the Department of Radiology, Klinikum rechts der Isar (TUM), with an Arriflex camera. Cineradiograms obtained with a rate of 50 frames/s, and reviewed after on a Tagarno film projector allowed frame-by-frame evaluation. Patients were required to swallow a standard bolus of 15 ml of barium on each sequence. Two sequences in anteroposterior (AP) projection and three in lateral projection were examined. In cases when aspiration was demonstrated, the exam was repeated 1–2 weeks later.
The following variables were selected for analysis:

A) pharyngeal wave transit time; B) vallecular retention; C) hypopharyngeal stasis; D) epiglottic closure time; and E) penetration (aspiration) of contrast medium into laryngeal vestibule and trachea.

Laryngeal Examination

Static and dynamic evaluation of vocal fold mobility (employing conventional mirror examination and flexible fiberscope) findings were classified as: A) normal; B) uni- or bilateral paresis of vocal folds; and C) uni- or bilateral paralysis of vocal folds. When some abnormality was found, a new exam was performed 1–2 weeks later.

Statistical Analysis

Comparison of values obtained pre- (group C1) and postoperatively (group C2) was made employing the Wilcoxon test for non-paired samples in the following variables:

– Pharyngeal wave transit time
– Epiglottic closure time

The NcNemar homogeneity test was used for the other cineradiological variables, in which pre- and postoperative results were classified as absent or present. In all statistical tests, probability values under 5% ($P < 0.05$) were considered significant.

Results

The results are explained in Table 1.

Discussion

Logemann [7], in an elegant review, proposes criteria for studies of treatment effects on any stage of dysphagia. The first criterion involves qualification of the disorder and the outcomes of treatment. Selection and evaluation of results from selected therapeutic methods should be based upon objective studies of the anatomy and physiology of the swallowing process in all its phases. Many methods can be used, among are included: bedside or direct clinical evaluation, videofluoroscopy, ultrasound, manometry, electromyography, and others. A reasonable consensus in medical literature indicates videofluorography or cine-fluorography as the most efficient current method for evaluating deglutition [8, 9].

In this investigation, after cineradiographic analysis, five variables were selected which were considered relevant from a clinical point of view. Pharyngeal wave transit time was registered, since current literature considers pharyngeal walls to be the main propulsive element of alimentary bolus [10], although other factors contribute to this movement, e.g., the tongue piston action [11], laryngeal movement, and pharyngoesophageal segment negative pressure [12], Epiglottic closure time was also registered. According to Curtis [13], airways

Table 1. Results of study

Variable (group)	A	B	C1	C2	D
Vallecular retention time (s/100)	61.6	64.17	56.0	60.7*	68.6
Hypopharyngeal stasis	absent	25%	21.4%	64.2%***	45%
Vallecular retention	absent	22.5%	21.4%	72.4%**	40%
Epiglottic closure time (s/100)	18.0	16.0	15.7	19.5*	20.43
Aspiration	absent	absent	absent	35.7%	absent
Dysphagia	absent	77.5%	92.8%	14.2%	absent

* Not significant; ** $P < 0.008$; *** $P < 0.003$

are protected during swallowing by three different mechanisms: Obturation of glottic fissure, through vocal folds opposition; at the vestibular level, the lumen being obliterated by ventricular folds; and at the laryngeal additus level, through epiglottic movement. Thus, any epiglottic functional disturbance, reflecting a defective closure of the laryngeal vestibule, can have potentially serious clinical consequences.

Integrated action of epiglottis and vocal folds, as protective mechanisms of the laryngotracheal block, emphazises the importance of simultaneous analysis of vocal fold mobility. Recurrent laryngeal nerve lesion, reflected by uni- or bilateral vocal fold paralysis, has been consistently registered after esophagectomies, with its incidence reaching 36% [14]. Even temporary malfunction of one of the main airway protective mechanisms can potentialize or cause aspiration of refluxed material to the respiratory tree. This event can be clearly detected in major anatomic or functional laryngeal disturbances [15, 16]. On the other hand, correlation between subtle alterations in vocal fold function and aspiration has been suggested by indirect data.

Hambraeus et al. [2] reported that pharyngeal dysfunction was more important in the first 3 weeks after esophageal operations.

Dysphagia represents the final result of a great range of clinical situations and has deserved review articles [17, 18], which propose long questionaires or algorithms, not always feasible in clinical practice. Alternatively, the status of oral ingestion in esophagectomized patients is frequently mentioned summarily after hospital dismissal [19, 20]. The analysis of the swallowing pattern made postoperatively showed a high number of asymptomatic patients. Even considering the fact that this evaluation was made in a short and relatively early period after surgical intervention, which does not exclude late stenoses at the anastomotic level, obtained data confirm that esophagogas-troplasty has as one of its main goals abolition of dysphagia. The evaluation scale used here represents a compromise between extreme simplification (good, bad, regular) and the complexity of algorithms or long questionaires, allowing also a better correlation between real clinical status and registered results after laryngeal and cineradiological exams.

Ekberg et al. [16] investigated pharyngeal function during swallowing in 22 patients with laryngeal recurrent nerve paresis: unilateral in 19 cases and bilateral in 3. Cineradiography was considered normal in three patients. The remaining patients exhibited a combination of functional abnormalities, such as abnormal epiglottic mobility (59%), defective closure of laryngeal vestibule (64%), and cricopharyngeal incoordination (28%).

Ekberg and Nylander [8] reviewing cineradiographic findings in 150 asymptomatic patients, reported variations from the normal swallowing pattern in 26 cases (27%). In seven cases, epiglottis remained in a transverse position during swallowing; in seven, cricopharyngeal dysfunction was observed; in eight, contrast penetrated the laryngeal vestibule; and one patient had a web in the upper third of the us esophagus, so a population of dysphagics without any detectable alteration and asymptomatics with multiple morphofunctional alterations.

The analysis of papers discussed above shows how difficult it is to establish a clear cause-and-effect relation between objective findings in the swallowing phase and clinical phenomena. The comparison of clinical results with those obtained at cineradiography confirm this impression. In what is essentially temporal data, decreases and increases were registered in asymptomatic individuals from which we conclude that functional abnormalities of this scale, in such a fast and dynamic phenomenon as swallowing, approaches the threshold of detectability in most cases.

Commenting morphological findings, valleculae and/or piriform synuses retention of contrast medium was visualized in ten patients (group C2) without swallowing complaints, in the postoperative period. Nevertheless, it must be remembered that pharyngeal retention of any fluid after bolus increases the possibility of aspiration of particles in the respiratory tree, a fact which can happen before, during, or after deglutition [21].

Selecting a population of patients with intrathoracic esophageal carcinoma has some intrinsic advantages when the above factors are considered. Most cases are previously asymptomatic, without neurological disease and with presumptive anatomical and functional integrity in the oropharyngeal stage of swallowing. The close temporal relationship between tumor growth and appearance of dysphagia, as well as the sudden appearances of obstructive factors eases the task of investigation, in the establishment of cause-and-effect correlations between morphofunctional alterations and clinical consequences. On the other hand, the period in which this population can be examined suffers some restrictions. Longterm survival in esophageal carcinoma is strictly related to its detection and removal in early stages, when disease in preferentially restricted to the esophagus without involvement of lymph nodes or regional ganglionary chains. Swallowing studies in the preoperative period must be based, then, in exams which are technically easy and minimally invasive, not interfering with timing of operation and incorporating, if possible, tests which already make part of preoperative routine.

Under the general title "respiratory pulmonay complications" are grouped all respiratory problems occurring after esophagectomies. This group constitutes clearly one of the main causes of morbidity and mortality after this operation.

Kawasaki [22], adopting radiological criteria and strict measures to avoid aspiration, such as keeping endotracheal tube more than 24 h after the operation and systematically draining the transposed stomach, registered a decrease in morbidity and mortality secondary to respiratory complications. Aspiration of gastric fluids to the airways was postulated as the main event in the genesis and maintenance of bronchopneumoniae in this particular group.

Therefore, the identification of patients with high risk of aspiration after esophagectomy can represent an important step in reducing morbitidy and mortality secondary to respiratory complications.

Conclusion

Minor morphological and motor pharyngoesophageal disturbances can be detected before and after esophagectomy without clinical expression. Furthermore, aymptomatic aspiration, temporary in most cases, could be a predisposing factor for respiratory complications in the early postopertive period.

References

1. Müller JM, Erasmi H, Stelzner M, Zieren U, Pichlmaier H (1990) Surgical therapy of esophageal carcinoma. Br. Heart J 77:845–847

2. Hambraeus GM, Ekberg O, Fletcher R (1987) Pharyngeal dysfunction after total and subtotal oesophagectomy. Acta Radiol 28:409–413

3. Dreuw B, Braun J, Winkeltau G, Schumpelick V (1988) Die Schluckfunktion nach Spei-serohrenersatz: Klinische und manometrische Untersuchungsergebnisse. In: SCHRIEFERS KH (ed) Chirurgisches Forum' 88 f. Experim. u. Klinische Forschung. Springer, Belin Heidelberg New York, pp 393–395

4. Catrambone GN, Iurilli L, Parodi A, Lupi P, Barra M, Devoto E (1989) A morphologic and functional study of the gastric tube as an esophageal substitute after esophagectomy for cancer. Res Surg 1:136–141

5. Bouchoucha M, Cugnenc PH, Drevillon C, Faye A, Boboc B, Arhan P, Barbier JP (1989) Functional evaluation of gastric transplants used in esophageal reconstruction. Dysphagia 4:53–57

6. Feussner H, Oliveira MA de, Daschner H (1991) Functional evaluation of the esophageal substitute. In: Fuchs KH, Hamelman H (eds) Funktions, diagnostik des obever Gastroin-testinaltraktes, in der Chirurgie. Blackwell Wissenschafts, Berlin, pp 215–221

7. Logemann JA (1987) Criteria for studies of treatment for oral-pharyngeal dysphagia. Dysphagia 1:193–199

8. Ekberg O, Nylander G (1981) Cineradiography of the pharyngeal stage of deglutition in 150 individual without dysphagia. Br J Raiol 50:253–257

9. Curtis DD, Cruess D, Dachaman A, Maso E (1984) Timing in the normal pharyngeal swallow: Prospective selection and evaluation of 16 normal asymptomatic patients. Invest Radiol 19:523–529

10. Donner MW, Bosma JF, Robertson DL (1985) Anatomy and physiology of the pharynx. Gastrointest. Radiol 10:196–212

11. Sokol EM, Heitmann P, Wolf BS, Cohen BR (1966) Simultaneous ciheradiographies and manometric study of the pharynx, hypopharynx, and cervical esophagus. Gastroenterology 51:960–974

12. McConnel FMS (1988) Analysis of pressure generation and bolus transit during pharyngeal swallowing. Laryngoscope 98:71–78

13. Curtis DJ, Hudson T (1983) Laryngotracheal aspiration: Analysis of specific neuromuscular factors. Radiology 149:517–522

14. Hugier M, Gordin F, Maillard JN, Lortat-Jacob JL (1970) Results of 117 esophageal replacements. Surg Gynecol Obstet 130:1054–1058

15. Henderson RD, Boszko A, Van Nostrand AWP (1974) Pharyngoesophageal dysphagia and recurrent laryngeal nerve palsy. J Thorac Cardiovasc Surg 68:507–512

16. Ekberg O, Lindgren S, Schultze T (1986) Pharyngeal swallowing in patients with paresis of the recurrent nerve. Acta Radio [Diagn] (Stockh), 27:697–700

17. Hendrix T, Ravich W, Buchholz D, Kashima H, Marsh B, Donner M, Jones B, Kramer S, Bosman J, Siebens A, Linden P, Robertson D (1985) The multidisciplinary approach to dysphagia. Gastrointest Radiol 10:193–261

18. Castell DO, Donner MW (1987) Evaluation of dysphagia: A careful history is crucial. Dysphagia 2:65–71

19. Matthews HR, Powell DJ, McConkey CC (1986) Effect of surgical experience of the results of resection for oesophageal carcinoma. Br J Surg 73:621–623

20. Lu YK (1987) Cancer of esophagus and esophagogastric junction: Analysis of results of 1025 resections after 5 to 20 years. Ann. Thorac Surg 43:176–181

21. Logemann J (1985) Aspiration in head and neck surgical patients. Ann Otol Rhinol Laryngol 94:373–376

22. Kawasaki K, Ogama Y, Kido Y, Mori T (1987) An important role of silent aspiration of gastric contents as a cause of pulmonary complications following surgery for esophageal cancer. Jpn J Surg 17:455–460

Dilatation in 1002 Cases of Postoperative Anastomotic Stenosis of Esophagocardial Carcinoma

Yin Niantai, Liu Fangyuan[1], and Liu Wei[2]

Introduction

During the years from 1986 to 1990, 1002 patients with postoperative anastomotic stenosis of esophacardial carcinoma were treated in our hospital by applying our self-made dilator No. 1 combined with the Japanese savary dilator and two powders called open-diaphragm-pulvis-fluid and pass-switch-pulvis-fluid. The high effective rate (98%) allows nearly all patients who have undergone resection of esophagocardial carcinoma to avoid undergoing a second operation and, therefore, the danger of operative death is reduced, especially for invalids and the aged.

The incidence of postoperative anastomotic stenosis of esophagocardial carcinoma has been reported to be 0.5%–4% [1, 2], or even as high as 5.9% according to one report [3]. The incidence is liable to go up on account of the increased popularity of this type of resection and the poor techniques used to date (the rate reached 6%–7% according to our investigation among 1002 cases).

Our dilator proves to be more convenient and more effective than those reported elsewhere [4]. It opens up a new approach to the treatment of postoperative anastomotic stenosis of esophagocardial carcinoma.

Clinical Data

Sex and Age

Among the 1002 patients, 790 (78%) were male, 212 (21.2%) were female, and the ages ranged from 19 to 82 years.

[1] Department of Thoracic Surgery, Second Teaching Hospital of Henan Medical University, Po 450003, Peoples' Republic of China
[2] Zhengzhow Third Hospital, Zhengzhou, Po 450003, Peoples' Republic of China

Diagnostic Criteria

Mild stenosis: The width of the anastomotic stoma shown on the contrast film is about 0.7 cm, and the patient is able to have a semi-liquid diet.

Moderate stenosis: The width is more or less than 0.4 cm, and the patient can only have a liquid diet.

Severe stenosis: The width is less than 0.3 cm, and the patient had difficulty taking a liquid diet or water.

Stages of Occurrence

Of the 1002 patients, 450 began to suffer from anastomotic stenosis 3 months after the resection of the tumor; 320 in 4–6 months; 11 in 6 months to 1 year; 85 in more than 1 but less than 2 years; 30 in 2 years; and 7 in over 6 years.

Classification of Stenoses and Numbers of Patients in Each Category

Circle-like irregular stenosis, 490; fish-mouth like stenosis, 310; angulation deformity, 150; obstruction with pieces of food or foreign bodies, 16; valve-like stenosis, 8 (residual of a fleshy valve in the anastomotic stoma, which connected the anterior and the posterior wall); triangular projection of the anastomat into the lateral wall of the anastomotic stoma, 7; refusal of dilatation procedure, 2; and recurrence, 19.

Effects of the Treatment

Eight hundred and ten patients were dilatated one to three times with a dilatating club 17–18 mm in diameter; 70 patients, three to five times with a club 12–16 mm in diameter; and 2 patients, six times, and the club was 15 mm in diameter. All 882 patients were relieved from obstructive dysphagia and able to have full diet. Ninety-nine patients could have a semi-liquid diet after having been dilatated seven times with a club of 14–15 mm in diameter. The patients above add up to 981; hence the effective rate of the treatment is 98%. Of the other patients, 2 refused dilatation and 19 had relapses of carcinoma. The treatment, of course, produced no harmful effects on them.

Complications and Mortality

Only one patient bled through the mouth (60 ml) as a result of dilation, but spontaneous cure took only 4 h. Obstructive exacerbation was found in eight patients, but after two days of transfusion of antibiotics, the hydrops of the anastomotic stoma disappeared, and the obstruction cleared and the patients could have a semi-liquid diet. None of the patients died from the treatment.

Manipulation of the Treatment

First, each patient fasted 4 h before dilatation and was given intramuscular injection of atropine and dolantin, and was sprayed three times into the throat with dicain (1%). Then, a metal esophagoscope was inserted into the stricture.

Next, a bougie was immediately inserted 45–50 cm. Then an appropriately-sized dilatating club was applied to the dilatation as soon as the esophagoscope was taken out. The residual of the anastomat can be brought out with a foreign body forceps. The fleshy valve is removed with a biopsy forceps or treated with laser therapy. It is desirable to treat tunnel-shaped or λ-shaped stenosis with our self-made dilator No. 1.

Spherical hard foreign bodies must not be forced out, or the esophagus will become lacerated. These foreign bodies will pass through naturally when the patients have been given 15 ml of open-diaphragm-fluid and treated with a large-sized dilatator. Patients with severe stenosis and hydrops should be given 15 ml of pass-switch-pulvis-fluid 10 min before dilatation. If half an hour of observation reveals no complications, the patient is allowed to take food 2 h later. The patient is also advised to take pass-switch-pulvis-fluid for an entire day (three times a day and 10 ml each time) so as to soften the scar and strengthen the effect.

Discussion

Earlier dilatation yields better results. Abrupt esophageal obstructions are, in most cases, brought about by foreign bodies. Some of these foreign bodies are likely to be passed through after the patients' taking open-diaphragm-pulvis-fluid.

Carcinomatous invasion is especially powerful in young patients and proper treatment should be carried out as soon as possible. A 19-year-old patient who had suffered stenosis 1 year post operatively received our treatment 3 years ago and now he is in good health, studying at high middle school.

Vital signs must be monitored while dilatation is being carried out so that emergency measures can be taken if necessary.

By combining the dilator of our own making with the Japanese one and with open-diaphragm-pulvis-fluid and pass-switch-pulvis-fluid as adjuvants, 1002 patients were able to avoid undergoing a second resection and its associated risks. The effective rate was as high as 98% with no severe complications or mortality.

Acknowledgment. This manuscript was read and revised by Associate Professor Shi Yuda.

References

1. Shao Lingfang, et al (1982) Results of the surgical treatment of 3155 cases of esophageal and cardiac carcinoma. Chin J Surg 20(1):19
2. Kang Liyuan, et al (1984) Clinical application of the circular staple device: Report on 290 cases. Chin J Surg 22(9):552
3. Lu Ping, et al (1985) Surgical treatment of stricture of esophagogastric anastomosis. Chin J Surg 23(2):93
4. Royston CMS, et al (1976) Esophageal dilation using the Eder Puestow dilators. Am J Surg 131:697

Endodissection in Transhiatal Esophagectomy: Technique and Clinical Results

R. Bumm and J.R. Siewert[1]

Introduction

Recent advances in technology enabled the construction of a mediastinoscope which enabled microsurgical dissection of structures in the posterior mediastinum [1]. We adopted this technique and constructed an advanced mediastinoscope for the endoscopic dissection of the thoracic esophagus in transhiatal esophagectomy (THE).

This article describes the intruments as well as the surgical technique, and reports the clinical results of endodissection in 30 patients operated between April 1991 and October 1992.

Methods

Endodissection

A novel mediastinoscope and suitable instruments were developed (Fa. H. Plank, Munich and Fa. K. Storz, Tuttlingen, Germany). Details on the instrument as well as on the technical equipment have been described [2]. The instrument is depicted in Fig. 1; the tissue dilatator is used in order to create a hollow space in the mediastinum because the tissues cannot be inflated by gas insufflation.

The operation requires two teams working synchronously. One team (one surgeon, one assistant) performs the endodissection while the other (one surgeon, two assistants) dissects the terminal esophagus from the hiatus and prepares the interponate. The endodissection is carried out via a left cervical

[1] Department of Surgery, Technical University of Munich, Ismaningerstr. 22, D-8000 München 80, Germany

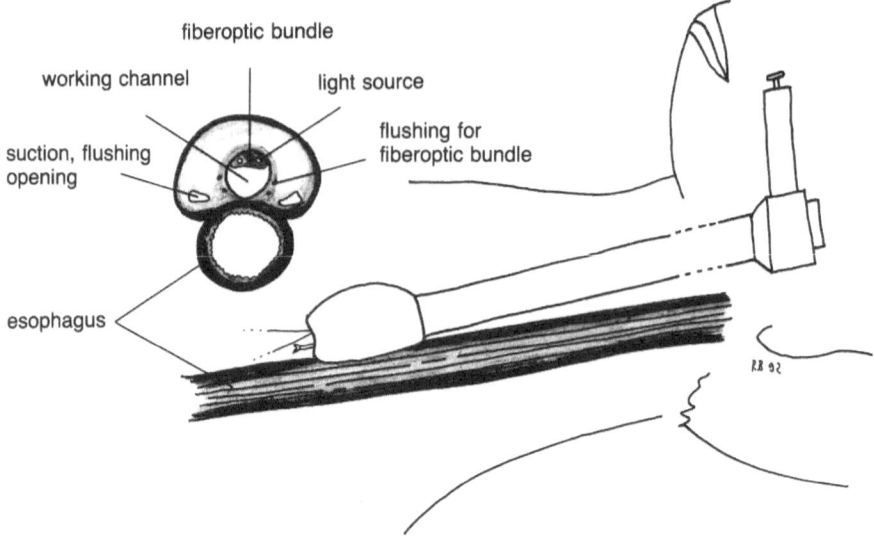

Fig. 1. Schematic depiction of the mediastinoscope used for endodissection

approach. The method was established in February 1991, tested in animal experiments between February and April 1991, and applied clinically in April 1991.

Patients

Between April 1991 and October 1992, all patients who were scheduled for a transhiatal esophagectomy underwent endodissection. All patients had undergone preoperative endoscopy, endosonography, and computed tomography (CT) scans to determine the exact tumor stage. Thirty patients (24 men, 6 women; median age was 60 years, range 35–80 years) underwent THE with endodissection. Adenocarcinoma of the esophagus was most frequent in these patients ($n = 21$, 70%), followed by squamous cell carcinoma ($n = 8$, 26.6%), and other tumors ($n = 1$, 3%). Early tumor stages dominated (T1 stage $n = 12$ [40%], T2 stage $n = 9$ [30%]) and tumors were mostly located below the tracheal bifurcation.

Results

In the 30 patients operated upon, mortality (30 days) was 6.6% ($n = 2$). One patient died from septic organ failure which was caused by a interponate necrosis; the other developed acute cardiorespiratory failure 14 days after the operation. No fatality was related to the endodissection. The perioperative complications are summarized in Table 1; the most significant complication was a lesion of the right main bronchus during lymph node dissection which was

Table 1. Perioperative complications during endodissection of the thoracic esophagus in 30 patients undergoing transhiatal esophagectomy

Peri- and postoperative complications	Patients (n)
Significant intraoperative bleeding (ligation of an intercostal vein by transhiatal approach)	$n = 1$
Postoperative bleeding (external jugular vein; cervical wound revision required)	$n = 1$
Lesion of the right main bronchus (see text)	$n = 1$
Change to transhiatally extended gastrectomy	$n = 2$

managed by thoracotomy, esophagectomy, and bronchial suture which was followed by an uneventful clinical course.

Two patients bled peri- or postoperatively (6.6%). In one case, a cervical wound revision was required (side branch of the jugular vein). Six patients (20%) had clinical evidence for a cervical insufficiency of the anastomosis. In four patients (13.3%), significant pulmonary problems such as pneumonia or pulmonary infiltrates were noted. Two patients (6.6%) developed postoperative dysphonia and showed palsy of the left vocal cord upon laryngoscopy. In one of these patients, the recurrent nerve was injured during manual suture of the cervical anastomosis; in the other case, the cause of recurrent nerve palsy remained undefined and could be attributed to the endoscopic dissection.

Discussion

Generally, we believe that THE is indicated in patients with adenocarcinoma of the distal esophagus, in which metastatic tumor spread follows a retroperitoneal route and in which mediastinal metastases are infrequent [3]. Due to the fact that these tumors are becoming more common in Europe and worldwide [4], the frequencies with which THE has to be performed in surgical units may rise. Blunt dissection of the esophagus, as it was performed during conventional THE, has some serious shortcomings: First, only the lower mediastinum is visible during this maneuver; second, the esophagus is mobilized bluntly by tearing mediastinal tissues with the risk of damage to mediastinal vessels and nerves; and third, there is only limited access to mediastinal lymph nodes. All these factors contribute to the fact that conventional THE is not very radical and, in some cases, even a dangerous procedure. After a mediastino-scope for esophageal dissection was previously described [1], we intended to develop an advanced instrument, define a surgical procedure, and evaluate the clinical results of endodissection. The preliminary results are described in this paper.

Endodissection of the esophagus is technically feasible and safe. In our study, only one major intraoperative complication (right bronchial leak) occurred, and this incidence was immediately recognized and managed by thoracotomy and bronchial suture without further morbidity. Intraoperative control of mediastinal bleeding was, except in one case, performed through the mediastinoscope. Mediastinal structures such as the back wall of the trachea, the right and left main bronchi, the vagus nerves, and the mediastinal lymph nodes can be regularily identified. In case of technical problems, the THE can be finished without major problems by conventional, transhiatal blunt dissection of the esophagus, which does not require an additional surgical access. The mobilization of the thoracic esophagus is usually complete both at and above the tracheal bifurcation; as it is sometimes difficult to inspect the lower mediastinum; this area can be dissected preferably by the transhiatal route. Due to the fact that endodissection is performed simultaneously with the abdominal approach, the total procedure of THE takes less time.

We also identified some shortcomings of endodissection. At the beginning of the procedure, anterior vision from the tip of the instrument is only centimeters. Anatomical orientation can be difficult, especially in the early stages of endo-dissection. There is continuous accumulation of fluids and blood at the tip of the instrument, which makes continuous suction and rinsing of the optical parts of the instruments indispensable. Sharp dissection of mediastinal structures is critical, and blunt division of tissue with the preparation-suction instrument in combination with monopolar thermocautery is preferred.

A systematic lymphadenectomy is not possible with this technique, but lymph node biopsies can be easily taken.

Is endodissection a benefit for the patient undergoing transmediastinal esophagectomy?

The results of this study show that the rate of postoperative complications and mortality was low. Only a few severe postoperative pulmonary complications and a low rate of recurrent nerve palsy (6.6%) were noted compared to previous studies (12%–36%) [4–11]. The latter finding may be the most important because preservation of the recurrent laryngeal nerve contributes to the pre-vention of postoperative 'silent aspiration' and pulmonary distress. The reason why endodissection reduces recurrent nerve damage is not yet identified; we speculate the main factor is that endodissection allows for anatomical pre-paration in the periesophageal tissues, which leaves the vagal nerves intact and lateralizes the recurrent nerves without tear of mediastinal structures.

These factors indicate that the use of endodissection is beneficial for patients in whom THE is indicated; however, we do not believe that these results justify extending the indication for transhiatal esophagectomy. One has to keep in mind that these results were obtained in a small series of patients with rather early stages of distal esophageal carcinoma. Maybe advanced instruments or the combination of mediastinoscopy and thoracoscopy will, in the future, allow for a complete lymphadenectomy; this would enable us to define a 'less invasive' resection procedure for patients with esophageal squamous cell carcinoma who present in a reduced clinical state or who are at risk before surgery.

References

1. Buess G, Becker HD, Mentges R, Teichmann R, Lenz G (1990) Die endoskopisch-mikrochirurgische Dissektion der Speiseröhre. Chirurg 61:308–311
2. Bumm R, Hölscher AH, Feussner H, Tachibana M, Bartels H, Siewert JR (to be published) Endodissection of the thoracic esophagus: Technique and clinical results in transhiatal esophagectomy. Ann Surg: in press

3. Akiyama H (1986) Cardinals of regional lymph node dissection in surgery of thoracic esophageal cancer. In: Siewert JR, Hölscher AH (eds) Diseases of the esophagus. Springer, Berlin Heidelberg New York, pp 416–420
4. Siewert JR (1989) Esophageal cancer from the German point of view. Jpn J Surg 19 1:11–20
5. Steiger Z, Wilson RF (1981) Comparison of the results of esophagectomy with and without thoracotomy. Surg Gynecol Obstet 153:653–656
6. Finley RJ, Inculet RI (1989) The results of esophagogastrectomy without thoracotomy for adenocarcinoma of the esophagogastric junction. Ann Surg 210 4:535–543
7. Hankins JR, Attar S, Coughlin TR, Miller JE, Hebel JR, Suter CM, McLaughlin CM (1989) Carcinoma of the esophagus: A comparison of the results of transhiatal versus transthoracic resection. Ann Thorac Surg 47:700–5
8. Barbier PA, Becker CD, Wagner HE (1988) Esophageal carcinoma: Patient selection for transhiatal esophagectomy. A prospective analysis of 50 consecutive cases. World J Surg 12:263–269
9. Finely RJ, Grace M, Duff JH (1985) Esophagogastrectomy without thoracotomy for carcinoma of the cardia and lower part of the esophagus. Surg Gynecol Obstret 160:49–56
10. Larrieu H, Millat B, Gayral F (1985) Oesophagectomies transhiatales. Chirurgie 111: 835–836
11. Orringer MB (1987) Transhiatal esophagectomy for esophageal carcinoma. In: Siewert JR, Hölscher AH (eds) Disease of the esophagus. Springer, Berlin Heidelberg New York, pp 390–393

The Impact of Close Surveillance of Barrett's Esophagus Patients on the Results of Esophagogastrectomy for Carcinoma

John M. Streitz Jr.[1], F. Henry Ellis Jr.[2], and Charles Andrews Jr.[2]

Introduction

The risk of malignant degeneration in patients with Barrett's esophagus (BE) is well known. However, the potential benefits of close surveillance of such patients in terms of the early detection of cancer and the results of esophagogastrectomy following its early detection remain poorly documented. This study was undertaken to determine whether or not there are clearly identifiable benefits from close surveillance of patients with benign BE.

Materials and Methods

Between January 1973 and July 1992, 88 patients with adenocarcinoma of the esophagus in BE were seen by us, some of whom have been previously reported [1, 2]. Twenty-one of these had been under endoscopic surveillance and were designated as the surveillance group. The remaining 67 patients were categorized as the non-surveillance group in that BE was diagnosed at the time the carcinoma was discovered. The groups were similar with respect to age and the predominance of white males (Table 1). Five patients in the surveillance group had undergone prior antireflux surgery. Four had undergone resection of an adenocarcinoma arising in BE at intervals ranging from 8 months to 10 years before the discovery of a second carcinoma while under surveillance, presumably arising from residual Barrett's mucosa remaining after the original operation.

The patients in the surveillance group were known to have had BE for varying intervals prior to the discovery of carcinoma, ranging from 6 to 120 months with a median of 22 months. Endoscopic surveillance in these patients was performed

[1] Lahey Clinic, 44 Mall Road, Burlington, MA 01805, USA
[2] The New England Deaconess Hospital—Harvard Medical School, 110 Francis Street, Boston, MA 02215, USA

Table 1. Endoscopic surveillance of Barrett's esophagus
January 1973–July 1992

	Surveillance group	Non-surveillance group
Number of patients	21	67
Age (years)		
Range	41–84	44–87
Median	62	64
Sex (M:F)	20:1	63:4
Caucasian	20	67

at intervals ranging from 1 month to 4 years with a median surveillance interval of 6 months. Four to six endoscopic biopsies were obtained from areas of mucosal adnormality and from at least two quadrants of every 2–3 cm of metaplastic epithelium.

Histology and Staging

Barrett's epithelium was classified as benign, dysplastic, or malignant based on established criteria [3]. Dysplasia was classified as low grade or high grade based on the degree of nuclear stratification, pleomorphism, enlargement, and hyperechromatism. Since there is now wide agreement among pathologists that high grade dysplasia and carcinoma in situ are synonymous [4], for purposes of staging both were considered to be T_{is} carcinomas. Staging of the resected specimens was determined according to the Manual for Staging of Cancer 1988 [5].

Statistical Methods

Survival curves were calculated by the Kaplan-Meier [6] product limit method with BMDP1L statistical software. Comparisons between the two groups were made with the Tarone-Ware [7] test. Contingency tables were analyzed using a chi square test or Fischer exact test as appropriate. Probabilities are two tailed with $P < 0.05$ regarded as statistically significant.

Surgery

Of the 21 patients in the surveillance group, all tumors were considered to be operable and 20 (95.2%) underwent resection. The one unresectable carcinoma occurred in a patient who refused operation when the diagnosis of high grade dysplasia was made. He consented to operation a year later when he began to bleed from an unresectable invasive carcinoma. Resections in these 20 patients were performed by a left thoracotomy in 2 patients, combined abdominal and right thoracic incisions (Ivor-Lewis) in 6 patients, and by a transhiatal approach in 12 patients. There were no postoperative deaths. Of the 67 patients in the non-surveillance group, 63 (94%) were considered to be operable and all but 1

Table 2. Endoscopic surveillance of Barrett's esophagus January 1973–July 1992

Stage	Surveillance group		Non-surveillance group	
	No. of patients	%	No. of patients	%
0	7		0	
I	5	75	10	26
IIA	3		6	
IIB	1		9	
III	4	25	32	74
IV	0		4	
Total	20		61	

* P = <0.001

patient were resected (98.4%). One patient operated on elsewhere is not included in the surgical statistics. The resections were performed by a left thoracotomy in 19 patients, by an Ivor-Lewis approach in 26 patients, and by a transhiatal approach in 16 patients. Two patients (3.3%) died after resection, one of a pulmonary embolism and one of a myocardial infarct.

Results

Of the ten patients in the surveillance group diagnosed as having high grade dysplasia/carcinoma in situ preoperatively, three exhibited invasive carcinoma in the resected specimen (30%). Eight of the 13 patients in the surveillance group whose resected specimen showed invasive carcinoma also revealed high grade dysplasia (62%).

The pathologic stages of the resected specimens differed significantly between the two groups (Table 2). Fifteen (75%) of those in the surveillance group were in stages 0, I, and IIA whereas 16 (26%) of those in the non-surveillance group were so staged. The findings were reversed for stages IIB, II, and IV being 25% versus 74% for the surveillance group and the non-surveillance group, respectively. These differences were significant at the $P < 0.001$ level.

Survival

Adjusted actuarial survival data was calculated for those patients operated on prior to October 1991 and differed significantly between the two groups. The rates for patients in the surveillance and non-surveillance groups, respectively, were 84.2% vs. 65.5% at 1 year, 66.2% vs. 31.8% at 3 years, and 52.9% vs. 20% at 5 years (P = 0.048) (Fig. 1). Excluding the two patients with surveillance intervals of 3 and 4 years who had Stage IIA and III tumors and the patient with resectable disease who refused operation for high grade dysplasia, the survival rate in the surveillance group increased to 93.8% at 1 year, 85.2% at 3 years, and 62.2% at 5 years (P = 0.007) (Fig. 2).

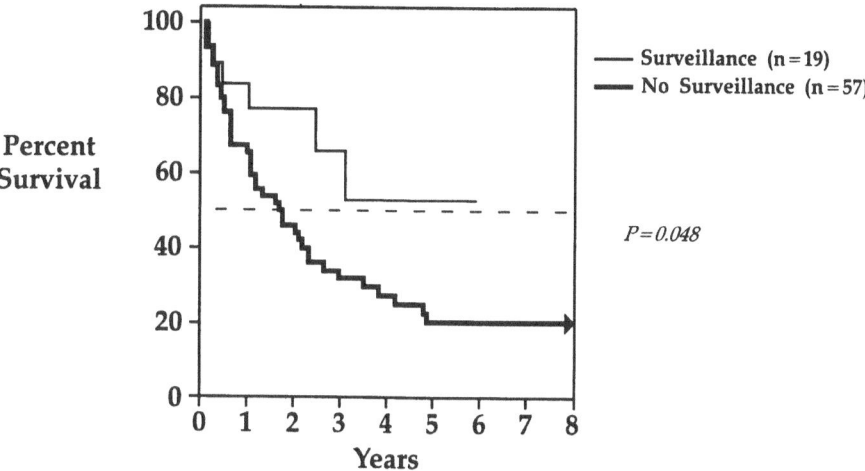

Fig. 1. Adjusted actuarial survival following esophagectomy (reproduced with permission of the Lahey Clinic)

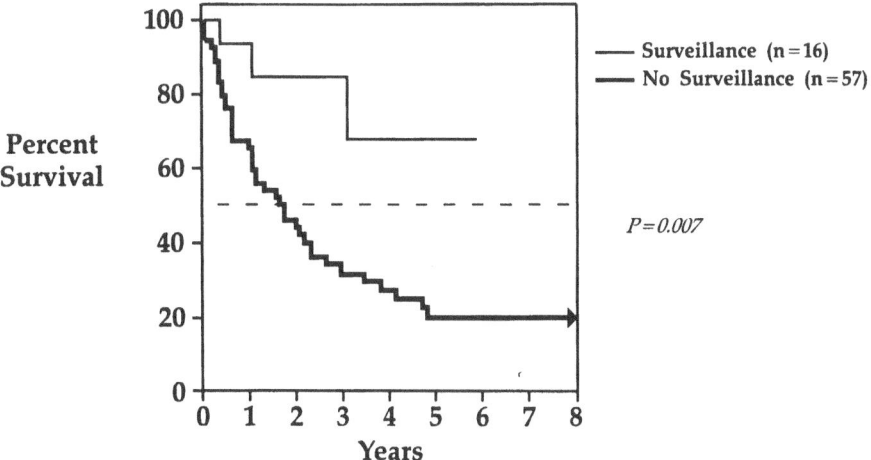

Fig. 2. Adjusted actuarial survival exclusive of one patient under surveillance who refused surgery and two whose surveillance intervals were greater than 1 year (reproduced with permission of the Lahey Clinic)

Comment

These data strongly suggest that routine endoscopic surveillance of patients with benign Barrett's esophagus permits early detection of malignant change at a curable stage, a view supported by others. Altorki et al. [8] reported their experience with nine patients with high grade dysplasia who underwent esophagogastrectomy, eight of whom had total esophagectomy with colon inter-position. Three of the nine were found to have invasive carcinoma in the resected specimen. At the time of the report, four of the nine patients were alive from 4 to 17 years after operation. More recently, Pera et al. [9] from the Mayo Clinic reported their experience with resection in patients with high grade dysplasia disclosed by esophagoscopic biopsy. Eighteen of these patients underwent esophagectomy and in 9 (50%) there was histologic evidence in the resected specimen of invasive carcinoma. The actuarial 5-year survival rate was 66.7%. Their conclusion, with which we agree, is that high grade dysplasia/carci-noma in situ is an indication for esophageal resection which can be done safely with the expectation of excellent long-term survival. There have been other ancedotal reports without detailed long-term survival evaluation reaching similar conclusions [10–13].

It is currently our practice to recommend yearly endoscopic surveillance of patients with benign Barrett's mucosa. The frequency of surveillance is increased to every 3–6 months when low grade dysplasia is identified although the benefits of increased surveillance in such patients has not been documented. Resection is advised when high-grade dysplasia/carcinoma in situ is diagnosed. The cost effectiveness of such a strategy depends on further clarification of the natural history of early dysplastic changes in the epithelium of patients with benign Barrett's esophagus.

Conclusions

1. Endoscopic surveillance allows early detection of malignant change in benign BE.
2. Early detection improves long-term post-resection survival.
3. Yearly endoscopic biopsy is an effective surveillance technique.

Acknowledgments. The assistance of Gerald J. Heatley, M.S. of the Sias Surgical Research Unit of the Lahey Clinic Medical Center in the statistical analysis of the data is gratefully acknowledged.

References

1. Streitz JM, Jr, Ellis FH Jr, Gibb SP (1991) Adenocarcioma in Barrett's esophagus: A clinicopathologic study of 65 cases. Ann Surg 213:122–125
2. Streitz JM Jr, Andrews CW Jr, Ellis FH Jr (to be published) Endoscopic surveillance of Barrett's esophagus. Does it help? J Thorac Cardiovasc Surg
3. Schmidt HG, Riddell RH, Walther B, et al (1985) Dysplasia in Barrett's esophagus. J Cancer Res Clin Oncol 110:145–152
4. Reid BJ, Haggitt RC, Rubin CE, et al (1988) Observer variation in the diagnosis of dysplasia in Barrett's esophagus. Hum Pathol 19:166–178
5. Beahrs OH, Henson DE, Hutter RVP, Myers MH (1988) Manual for staging of cancer, 3rd Edn. JB Lippincott, Philadelphia, pp 63–67
6. Kaplan EL, Meier P (1958) Nonparametric estimation from incomplete observations. J Am Statist Assoc 53:457–481
7. Tarone RE, Ware J (1977) On distribution-free tests for equality of survival distributions. Biometrika 64:156–160

8. Altkori NK, Sunagawa M, Little AG, Skinner DB (1991) High-grade dysplasia in the columnar-lined esophagus. Am J Surg 161:97–100
9. Pera M, Trastek VF, Carpenter HA, Allen MS, et al (1992) Barrett's esophagus with high-grade dysplasia: An indication for esophagectomy? Ann Thorac Surg 54:199–204
10. Reid BJ, Lewin R, VanDeventer G, et al (1986) Barrett's esophagus: High-grade dysplasia and intramucosal carcinoma detected by endoscopic biopsy surveillance (abstract). Gastroenterology 90:1601
11. Provenzale D, Wong JB, Kemp JA, Arora S (1990) Endoscopic surveillance for Barrett's esophagus: Can we afford the cost (abstract)? Am J Gastroenterol 85:1224
12. Hameeteman W, den Hartog Jager FCA, Tio TL, Tytgat GNS (1988) Early adenocarcinoma of the esophagus. In: Siewert JR, Hölscher AH (eds) Diseases of the esophagus. Springer, Berlin Heidelberg New York, pp 554–558
13. DeMeester TR, Attwood SEA, Smyrk TC, Therkildsen DH, et al: Surgical therapy in Barrett's esophagus. Ann Surg 212:528–540

Contribution of Obesity and Intra-Abdominal Fat Accumulation to Postoperative Respiratory Disorders in Patients with Esophageal Carcinoma

Yuko Kitagawa, Nobutoshi Ando, Soji Ozawa, and Masaki Kitajima[1]

Introduction

Recently, the number of obese patients has been increasing in the field of gastrointestinal surgery because of progress in early diagnosis of gastrointestinal cancer and changes in dietary habits among Japanese. There are many difficulties in postoperative respiratory management in obese patients, especially in thoracic and upper abdominal surgery such as radical esophagectomy with thoracotomy and laparotomy. Previously, the fact that massive obesity is often associated with abnormalities in respiratory function has been demonstrated [1]. Modifications in thoracic compliance, diaphragmatic function, gas exchange, and extrathoracic airway patency have been reported [2].

Recently, respiratory inductive plethysmography (RIP) has been developed which enables us to evaluate the breathing pattern quantitatively [3]. Several previous reports which measured the change in breathing pattern during trial weaning from mechanical ventilation suggest that the abnormalities in the breathing pattern represent the overall respiratory function of the patients who developed respiratory insufficiency [4].

On the other hand, the casual relationship between intra-abdominal visceral fat accumulation and several metabolic disorders has been reported [5]. The distribution of body fat can be determined by computed tomography (CT) scanning [6]. By means of these methods, we have investigated the contribution of obesity and intra-abdominal fat accumulation to the postoperative respiratory disorders in patients with esophageal carcinoma who had undergone radical surgery.

---

[1] Department of Surgery, Keio University School of Medicine, 35 Shinano-machi, Shinjuku-ku, Tokyo, 160 Japan

Methods

A total of 61 patients with esophageal carcinoma who had undergone radical surgery at Keio University Hospital (Tokyo, Japan) during the period from 1989 to 1990 were examined. These patients were divided into 3 groups according to the percentage of ideal body weight calculated by the Broca index {ideal body weight = [height (cm) − 100] × 0.9}: group A, < 90%; group B, 90%—110%; and group C, >110%. The 20 obese patients in group C were divided into two subgroups according to the intra-abdominal visceral fat area to subcutaneous fat area ratio (V/S ratio) determined by CT at the umblical level (visceral type; V/S ⩾ 0.4, subcutaneous type; V/S <0.4). In these four sub groups (A, B, C_1 and C_2), preoperative respiratory function measured by conventional spirometry (%VC, %$FEV_{1.0}$) and flow-volume curve (V_{25}, V_{50}), and by postoperative breathing patterns measured quantitatively by means of RIP were analyzed. Gas exchange conditions were evaluated by arterial blood gas analysis. Perioperative cardiovascular status was managed according to the data monitored by a Swan-Ganz catheter.

The patients were mechanically ventilated more than 24 h postoperatively, and were being weaned from mechanical ventilation when they met the weaning criteria. Weaning criteria include: stable general condition, clear consciousness, $PO_2 > 100$ mmHg and $PCO_2 < 45$ mmHg at 3 cmH O of CPAP ($FiO_2 < 0.4$), vital capacity > 10 ml/kg, tidal volume > 5 ml/kg, and respiratory frequency < 20 bpm. When the patients who were ready to be extubated were on continuous positive airway pressure (CPAP; $FiO_2 < 0.4$, and positive end-expiratory pressure (PEEP) of 3 cmH$_2$O), ribcage and abdominal movement were measured by means of RIP (Respigraph, Nims, Inc., Fla.). The %RC, which is the percentage contribution of rib cage movement to tidal volume, the Vt-RC, which is the product of Vt and %RC, and the TCD/Vt, which is the ratio of total compartmental displacement and Vt, were calculated by RIP for more than 30 min. Statistical analysis was performed by using the chi-square test.

Results

The background factors of the three groups divided according to the percentage of ideal body weight calculated by Broca index are summarized in Table 1. Although 11 of 13 visceral type obesity patients were male, all 5 subcutaneous

Table 1. Categorization by obesity

	<−10%	−10%−+10%	+10%
Broca Index % (mean)	(−20.1%)	(−2.4%)	(+24.3%)
Number	16	25	20
Age	58.4	62.4	64.8
Sex (M:F)	15:1	21:4	13:7
Operation			
Thoracotomy (+)	13	20	15
Thoracotomy (−)	3	5	5

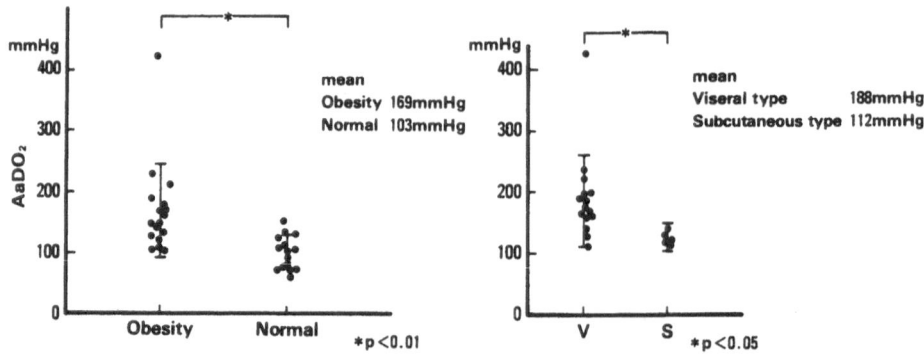

Fig. 1. Postoperative $AaDO_2$ (FiO_2 0.4)

type obese patients were female. There was no singificant difference in degree of obesity calculated by Broca index in these two groups. Although there was no significant difference between the four groups, in the preoperative resiratory parameters (%VC, %FEV$_{1.0}$, $\mathring{V}_{25}$, $\mathring{V}_{50}$, PO_2/FiO_2) and perioperative hemodynamics [cardiac index (CI), certral venous pressure (CVP), pulmonary arterial pressure (PAP), and pulmonary capillary wedge pressure (PCWP)] monitored by Swan-Ganz catheter of these four groups, mean mechanical ventilation time was prolonged in visceral type obese patients (9.8 days) than in other groups (2.6 days).

In visceral type obese patients, a significant decline of PO_2/FiO_2 with increase of $AaDO_2$ was recognized during the operation period, and such decline continued for several days after surgery compared with other groups ($P < 0.05$, Fig. 1).

In the period of weaning from mechanical ventilation, %RC, which is the percentage contribution of rib cage movement to the tidal volume measured by RIP, was significantly greater in visceral type obese patients than in group B (normal body weight) ($P < 0.01$, Table 2). Also in group A (lean patients), %RC was significantly increased compared with group B ($P < 0.01$, Table 2).

Discussion

In the field of gastrointestinal surgery, particularly in esophageal surgery, respiratory disturbance is one of the most important postoperative complications. Although the incidence of pulmonary complications has been gradually decreased by means of mechanical ventilatory support, it is still a serious problem for patients at high risk for complications, such as chronic obstructive pulmonary disease. In our experience, massive obesity is one of the risk factors of postoperative respiratory insufficiency. Obese patients who have undergone radical esophagectomy often need reinitiation of mechanical ventilatory support after weaning. On chest X-ray, higher incidence of atelectasis has been found during mechanical ventilation in the early postoperative days in obese patients. However, the pathophysiological mechanisms of postoperative respiratory insufficiency in obese patients has not been revealed.

Table 2. Respiratory inductive plethysmography

	Broca Index (%)			
	$<-10\%$	$-10\%-+10\%$	$+10\%$	
			V	S
%RC	52.5	42.1	58.5	43.4
V_T (ml/kg)	9.28	10.09	9.05	9.12
VT/T_1 (ml/kg pers)	8.17	8.51	8.47	8.20
f (/min)	14.6	14.5	15.5	14.3
T_1/T_{TOT}	0.31	0.28	0.28	0.30
TCD/V_T	1.03	1.01	1.01	1.00

$*P < 0.01$
%RC, Percentage rib cage movement; V_T, tidal volume VT/T_1, mean inspiratory flow; f, respiratory frequency; T_1/T_{TOT}, inspiratory time/total time of breath ratio; TCD/V_T, total compartmental displacement/tidal volume

In this study, these mechanisms were analyzed from a viewpoint of breathing pattern measured by RIP. On the other hand, fat distribution must be considered in analysis of pathophysiology in obese patients. A method of evaluating fat distribution by CT scanning previously developed was used in this study [6].

Perioperative hypoxemia showed a close correlation with intra-abdominal fat accumulation. In our obsevation, atelectasis on chest X-ray disappeared at weaning, and the high density area was still found in dependent area of the lung on chest CT in visceral obese patients. The reduction of functional residual capacity due to undetected atelectasis caused by the pressure of intra-abdominal accumulated fat would be one of the factors of significant decline of PO_2/FiO_2 with increased $AaDO_2$.

In the supine position, mismatch of perfusion and ventilation is more likely to increase in visceral type obese patients than in subcutaneous type obese patients. Although the other ventilatory parameters at weaning showed no difference in the four groups, diaphragmatic dysfunction indicated by significantly increased %RC measured by RIP was recognized in visceral type obese patients and lean patients. In visceral type obese patients, this disturbance of diaphragmatic ventilatory function is attributed to the pressure of intra-abdominal accumulated fat. On the other hand, increased %RC in lean patients depends on the fatigue of diaphragmatic muscle due to poor nutritional condition.

Furthermore it has been demonstrated that intra-abdominal visceral fat accumulation is associated with metabolic disorders, such as impairment of glucose and lipid metabolism, and with cardiovascular complications [7]. These results suggest that the visceral type obese patients with esophageal carcinoma have several risk factors for radical esophagectomy. Therefore, careful perioperative respiratory management for these patients in consideration of breathing pattern measured by RIP is necessary.

Acknowledgments. The authors would like to thank Dr. Junzo Takeda and Dr. Ryoichi Ochiai for their valuable advice and expert technical assistance in the analysis of the RIP data.

References

1. Barrera F, Reindeberg NN, Winters WL (1967) Pulmonary function in the obese patients. Am J Med Sci 35:785–795
2. Ray CS, Sue DY, Bray G, Hansen JE, Wasserman K (1983) Effects of obesity on respiratory function. Am Rev Respir Dis 128:501–506
3. Sackner MA (1980) Monitoring of ventilation without physical connection to the airway. In: Sackner MA (ed) Diagnostic technique in pulmonary disease. Marcel Dekker, New Yourk, pp 503–537
4. Kriege BP, Chediak A, Gazeroglu HB, Bizousky FP, Feinerman D (1988) Variability of the breathing pattern before and after extubation. Chest 93:767–771
5. Seidell JC, Bjorntorp P, Sjostrom L, Kvist H, Sannerstedt R (1990) Visceral fat accumulation in men is positively associated with insulin, glucose, and C-peptide levels, but negatively with testosterone levels. Metabolism 39:897–901
6. Tokunaga K, Matsuzawa Y, Ishikawa K, Tarui S (1983) A novel technique for the determination of body fat by computed tomography. Int J Obesity 7:437–445
7. Peiris AN, Sothmann MS, Hoffmann RG, Hennes MI, Wilson CR, Gustafson AB, Kissebah AH (1989) Adiposity, fat distribution, and cardiovascular risk. Ann Intern Med 110:867–872

A Clinical Study of Esophageal Cancer with Invasion of Contiguous Structures

Katsunobu Kawahara, Shinji Akamine, Noriyuki Itoyanagi,
Hiroharu Tsuji, Shinsuke Hara, Yutaka Tagawa, Hiroyoshi Ayabe,
and Masao Tomita[1]

Introduction

Esophageal cancer invading contiguous structures is associated with a poor prognosis. Lymph node metastases are present in the majority of cases. When the lesion extends to the diaphragm, lung, or pericardium, combined resection is relatively easy. However, when the lesion invades the aorta or tracheobronchial tree, combined resection may be technically demanding. Herein, we evaluate the indications for surgery, patient selection, and outcome after surgery in a group of patients with esophageal cancer invading contiguous intrathoracic structures.

Material and Methods

From January 1968 through December 1991, 149 patients with esophageal cancer underwent esophagectomy at our institution. In 46 of 149 patients (30.8%), the esophageal cancer was invading a contiguous structure. Forty patients were male and 6 were female. In this group, the age ranged from 46 to 78 years (mean 61 years). The tumor was located in the upper intrathoracic esophagus in 6 patients, the middle esophagus in 35 patients, and the lower intrathoracic esophagus in 5 patients. The regional lymph nodes were involved in 43 patients (93.5%) and negative in only 3 patients. The aorta was invaded by cancer in 27 patients (58.7%), the tracheobronchial tree in 19 (41.3%), the lung in 7 (15.2%), the pericardium in 5 (10.9%), the diaphragm in 2 (4.3%), and the thoracic vertebrae in 1 (2.2%). In 14 patients (30.4%), two or more structures were involved.

Combined resection of the esophagus and involved contiguous structures was performed in 22 patients. The contiguous structures were the aorta in 7 patients

---

[1] First Department of Surgery, Nagasaki University School of Medicine, Sakamoto 1-chome 7-1, 852, Nagasaki, Japan

(31.8%), the trachea or bronchus in 9 (40.9%), the lung in 4 (18.2%), the pericardium in 3 (13.6%), the diaphragm in 2 (9.1%), and the thoracic vertebrae in 1 (4.5%). Two patients underwent combined resection of the aorta and bronchus, and the aorta and the vertebrae, respectively.

Combined resection of the tracheobronchial tree was performed through a right thoracotomy in 8 patients. One patient underwent combined resection of the aorta, left main bronchus, and esophagus via a left thoracotomy. Ventilation was supported by high frequency ventilation or conventional ventilation. Sleeve resection of the main stem bronchus was performed in 2 patients and the anastomotic line wrapped with a pleural free flap. A lesion of the membranous portion of the trachea was resected in 3 patients. In 2 of these patients, a pericardial patch was placed on the membranous defect with omentopexy in one. In one patient, the membranous defect extended beyond the carina to the right main stem bronchus. The defect was repaired with Marex mesh, and covered with pleura.

Combined resection of the aorta was performed through a left thoracotomy in five patients and bilateral thoracotomy in two. In three patients, the aorta was temporarily bypassed and the invasive lesion was resected with the intrathoracic esophagus followed by prosthetic reconstruction. In four patients, permanent bypass was established above and below the aortic lesion with a dacron graft measuring 16–20 mm in diameter. Six to 11 cm of aorta was resected. The aorta was temporarily bypassed from the left subclavian artery to the aorta below the lesion. A sleeve bronchiectomy was performed and 11 cm of aorta was replaced with a 22-cm (diameter) graft. Retrosternal gastric pull-up and cervical esophagogastrostomy completed the procedure.

Adjuvant therapy, administered to 17 patients (36.9%), consisted of pre- or postoperative irradiation (35–45 Gy) and postoperative chemotherapy with bleomycin, pepleomycin, 5-fluorouracil (5-FU), or cisplatin (CDDP).

Results

Operative morbidity was 58.7% (27/46). Early postoperative complications included anastomotic leak in four patients, intrathoracic or intra-abdominal bleeding in three, respiratory failure in three, recurrent nerve paresis in two, phrenic nerve paresis in one, tracheobronchial bleeding in one, and in one patient perforation of the gastric pull-up. Late complications included aspiration pneumonia in five patients, hepatic failure in two, bile peritonitis in one, and a bronchopulmonary vascular fistula in one patient. The 30-day postoperative mortality rate was 23.9% (11/46).

The overall 5-year survival rate in the patients with esophagectomy was 12.0%; 24.8% in patients with a0 disease, 15.0% with a1 disease, and 4.5% with a2 disease (Fig. 1) [1]. No patient with a3 disease survived 3 years, and the median survival time was 174 days. Twenty-five patients (54.3%) died within 3 months. No difference in median survival was seen between patients with or without combined resection [139 and 138 days, respectively (Fig. 1)]. The median survival time of the patients who received adjuvant therapy was 152 days, which did not differ significantly from patients who received no adjuvant therapy (196 days).

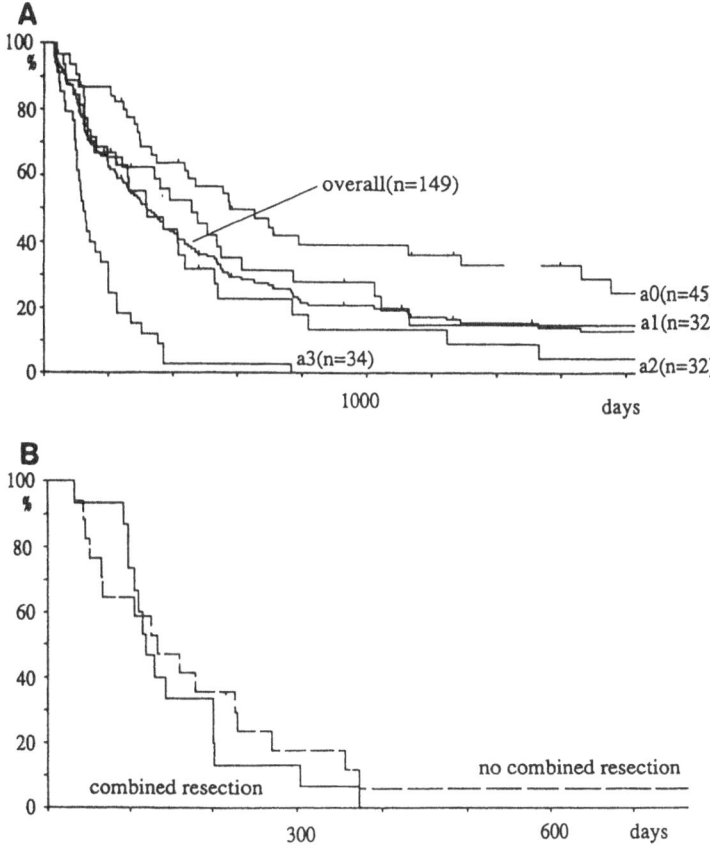

Fig. 1A,B. A Cumulative survival by the degree of esophageal wall invasion in patients with esophageal cancer. **B** Cumulative survival with and without combined resection of contiguous structures. *a0*, tumor invades muscularis propria; *a1*, tumor invades adventitia (mild invasion); *a2*, tumor invades adventitia (definite invasion); *a3*, tumor invades adjacent structures

Five of the 6 patients with combined resection of the aorta died of recurrent disease 2–6 months after surgery. One patient died of tracheal bleeding on the 6th postoperative day. One patient is alive 3 months after surgery. Four of eight patients with combined resection of the trachea or main stem bronchus died of recurrent disease 3, 7, 8, or 11 months after surgery. Other causes of death were bronchopulmonary arterial fistula 1 month postoperatively, respiratory failure due to tracheal leak, and bile peritonitis between 12 days and 32 days postoperatively.

Discussion

The prognosis of patients with a3 disease is poor with or without combined resection of contiguous structures, because the regional lymph nodes are frequently involved. Therefore, neoadjuvant therapy is required pre- or post-operatively. Recently, combined preoperative chemotherapy (5-FU, CDDP) plus perioperative radiotherapy for esophageal cancer has been found to be well tolerated, provides excellent palliation of symptoms, and allows for a high rate of resectability [2, 3]. Combined resection of the aorta or tracheobronchial tree and esophagus is more difficult than combined resection of the pericardium, diaphragm, or lungs. Palliative intubation for dysphagia in patients with advanced carcinoma of the esophagus [4] or combined endoscopic laser therapy and brachytherapy in those patients with cervical and upper thoracic tumors, in whom intubation may be unsatisfactory [5], is effective palliation for esophageal carcinoma. However, in those patients, radiation therapy, chemotherapy, or palliative intubation may predispose to aortic rupture or esophagotracheobronchial fistula. Therefore, we advocate combined resection of the aorta or tracheo-bronchial tree in patients less than 70 years old with no serious concomitant disease and other potential node involvement. These results show that aggressive surgical resection in these patients results in good long-term palliation of esophageal cancers invading contiguous structures.

References

1. Japanese Society For Esophageal Diseases (1992) Guidelines For the Clinical and Pathologic Studies on Carcinoma of the Esophagus, 8th edn. Kanehara, Tokyo, p 13
2. Naunheim KS, Petruska PJ, Roy TS, Andrust CH, Johnson FE, Schlueter JM, Baue AE (1992) Preoperative chemotherapy and radiotherapy for esophageal cancer. J Thorac Cardiovasc Surg 103:887–895
3. Carey RW, Hilgenberg AD, Choi NC, Mathisen DJ, Grillo HC, Wain JC, Logan DL, Bromberg C (1991) A pilot study of neoadjuvant chemotherapy with 5-fluorouracil and cisplatin with surgical resection and postoperative radiation therapy and/or chemotherapy in adenocarcinoma of the esophagus. Cancer 68:489–492
4. Loakakos TK, Ohri SK, Townsend ER, Fountain SW (1992) Palliative intubation for dysphagia in patients with carcinoma of the esophagus. Ann Thorac Surg 53:460–463
5. Renwick P, Whitton V, Moghissi K (1992) Combined endoscopic laser therapy and brachytherapy for palliation of esophageal carcinoma. Gut 33:435–438

Blunt Dissection for Carcinoma of the Esophagus, with Particular Reference to the Lower Thoracic and Abdominal Esophagus

Y. Yamashita, T. Hirai, H. Mukaida, T. Iwata, S. Saeki, and T. Toge[1]

Introduction

The transthoracic esophagectomy with mediastinal lymph node cleaning has been a standard surgical method for patients with esophageal carcinoma recently. However, at present in Japan, the operative indication for blunt esophageal dissection (i.e., transhiatal esophagectomy: THE) is for cases with poor prognoses or mucosal cancer. We think that, in cases of carcinoma of the lower thoracic and abdominal esophagus, even when the prognosis is good, THE can reduce the operative stress compared with the conventional right thoracotomy.

Methods

From 1982 to 1991, 49 patients with esophageal carcinoma underwent THE in our hospital. In this procedure, the lymph nodes around the lower esophagus were able to be dissected. The esophagus was reconstructed using whole stomach, through the posterior mediastinal route. Then, it was anastomosed with the cervical esophagus in layer-to-layer fashion. Of these patients, 46 had squamous cell carcinoma, two had adenosquamous cell carcinoma, and one had adenocarcinoma. The primary tumor was located in the lower intrathoracic esophagus (Ei) and abdominal esophagus (Ea) in 33 cases (67.3%), in the middle thoracic esophagus (Im) in 14 cases (28.6%), and in the upper intrathoracic esophagus (Iu) in one case (2.0%). Table 1 shows basic clinical characteristics of the patients who underwent THE, in relation to tumor location. In the patients with carcinomas in Ei and Ea, histologic stages were O in 4 cases (12.1%), I in 2 cases (6.0%), II in 3 cases (9.1%), III in 12 cases (36.4%), and IV in 12 cases

[1] Department of Surgery, Research Institute for Nuclear Medicine and Biology, Hiroshima University, 1-2-3 Kasumi, Higashi-ku, Hiroshima, 734 Japan

Table 1. Basic clinical characteristics of the patients who underwent transhiatal esophagectomy (*THE*) in terms of tumor location

	Iu	Im	Ei,Ea	Total
Stage[a]				
0	0	8 (53)	4 (12)	12 (24)
I	0	0	2 (6)	2 (4)
II	0	1 (7)	3 (9)	4 (8)
III	0	2 (13)	12 (36)	14 (29)
IV	1 (100)	4 (27)	12 (36)	17 (35)
Curability				
Curative	0	12 (80)	21 (64)	33 (69)
Non-curative	1 (100)	3 (20)	12 (36)	16 (33)
Histologic depth of invasion[a]				
ep, mm	0	5 (33)	4 (12)	16 (33)
sm	0	3 (20)	1 (3)	4 (8)
mp	0	0	3 (9)	3 (6)
a1	0	1 (7)	9 (27)	10 (20)
a2	0	4 (27)	11 (33)	15 (31)
a3	1 (100)	2 (13)	5 (15)	8 (16)
Lymph node metastasis[a]				
n0	1 (100)	11 (73)	12 (36)	24 (49)
n1	0	1 (7)	2 (6)	3 (6)
n2	0	2 (13)	10 (30)	12 (12)
n3	0	0	3 (9)	3 (6)
n4	0	1 (7)	6 (18)	7 (14)
Total	1	15	33	49

[a] According to [7] Figures in parentheses, % of total in category; *Iu*, upper intrathoracic esophagus; *Im*, middle thoracic esophagus; *Ei,Ea*, lower intrathoracic and abdominal esophagus; *ep*, epithelium; *mm*, muscularis mucosae; *sm*, submucosal; *mp*, muscularis propria; *a1*, invasion reaching the adventitia; *a2*, definite invasion to the adventitia; *a3*, invasion into the neighboring structures; *n0*, no metastasis; *n1–4*, degree expands with increasing number

(36.4%), respectively. Postoperatively, some patients, not including those at an early stage, received irradiation therapy over a T-shaped field for neck and upper mediastinum and/or etoposide, 5-fluorouracil, cis-platinum (EFP) therapy, in which *cis*-platinum (CDDP), etoposide (VP-16), and 5-fluorouracil were administered. Their postoperative complications, prognosis, and patterns of first recurrence were investigated. The survival curves after THE were analyzed by the Kaplan-Meier method.

Results

Postoperative complications are shown in Table 2. Laceration of parietal pleura happened during the operation in 12 cases (24%). However, it was easily recovered by chest tube drainage or suction via a puncture just after the surgery. A pulmonary complication was observed in eight patients (16%). Anastomotic leakage was experienced in eight patients (16%) including two with major leakage. Operative mortality was experienced in two patients. One had massive

Table 2. Postoperative complications in 49 patients who underwent THE

Site of postoperative complication	Number (percentage) of postoperative complications	
Pneumothorax	12 (24)	
Pneumonia	3 (6)	
Empyema	2 (4)	
Hemothorax	2 (4)	
Pulmonary filbrosis	1 (2)	
Hepatic dysfunction	2 (4)	
Mediastinitis	1 (2)	
Atrial fibrillation	1 (2)	
Subphrenic infection	1 (2)	
Massive bleeding	1 (2)	
Anastomotic leak	8 (16)	
Major		2 (4)
Minor		6 (12)

Table 3. Patterns of first recurrence of tumor in 31 patients who underwent THE for carcinoma in the lower third (Ei,Ea) of the esophagus, in terms of depth of tumor invasion

	Up to mp[a]	a1 or a2[a]	a3[a]	Total
Parenchyma	0	7	2	9 (29)
Lung		3	1	4
Liver		3	1	4
Bone		3		1
Lymph node	0	4	0	4 (13)
Posterior mediastinum		1		1
Pulmonary hilar		1		1
Bifurcation		1		1
Abdominal paraaortic		1		1
Dissemination	1	0	1	2 (6)
Pleural	1			1
Peritoneal			1	1
Local (remnant cervical esophagus)	0	1	0	1 (3)
Total	2	11	3	16 (51)

[a] Depth of tumor invasion, according to [7]

bleeding due to the tearing of the azygos vein during dissection of the thoracic esophagus by hand. The other was due to septic shock following acute mediastinitis.

Focusing on 33 cases with carcinomas in the Ei and Ea regions, the 5-year survival rate was 22.6% overall. The acturial survival rate in terms of curability is shown in Fig. 1. Of 30 patients in which a curative operation was performed, the pattern of first recurrence was investigated in 14 (47%) after the operation. Parenchymal recurrence (eight cases; 27%) was more frequent than that in lymph nodes (four cases; 13%), as shown in Table 3.

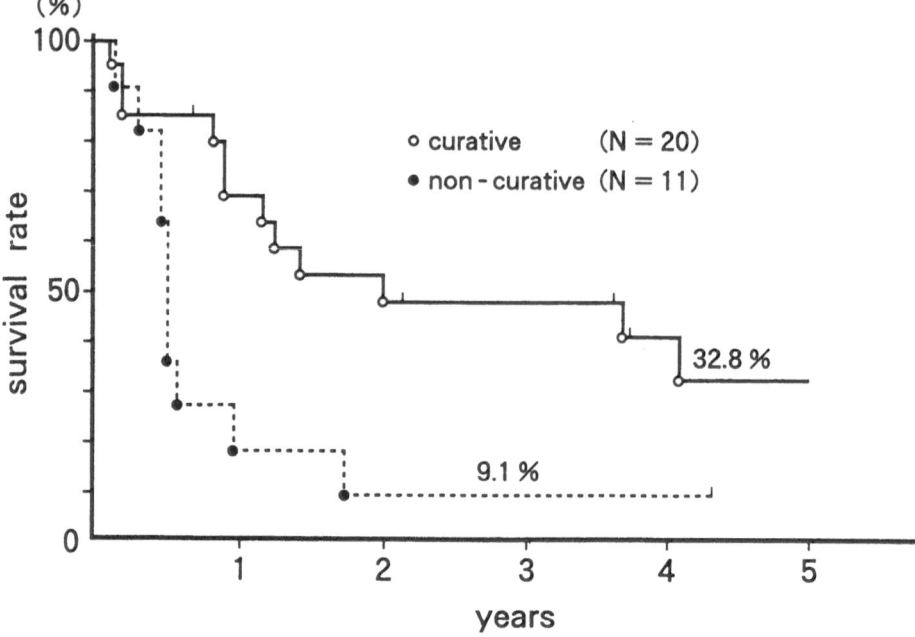

Fig. 1. Actuarial survival curves for the patients with carcinoma in the lower third (Ei,Ea) of the esophagus after transhiatal esophagectomy (*THE*), showing curative versus noncurative cases

Discussion

The postoperative course after THE was remarkably uneventful compared with that after conventional esophagectomy through right thoracotomy. The THE procedure can result in less postoperative morbidity and earlier recovery from operative stress. We have already reported the superiority of THE assessed by the recovery of immunological and nutritional indicators [1, 2]. The prognosis after THE is similar to that after the conventional transthoracic esophagectomy [3–5].

In addition, recurrence in lymph nodes after THE was less frequent than recurrence in parenchyma, although dissection of neck and upper mediastinal lymph nodes could not be carried out in THE.

In conclusion, we emphasize that carcinoma of the lower part of the esophagus should also be a suitable indication for THE [6]. A new regimen of chemotherapy seems to be necessary to improve the prognosis of patients with esophageal carcinoma with a view to preventing systemic disease.

References

1. Toge T, Kegoya Y, Yamaguchi Y, Baba N, Kuninobu H, Takayama T, Yanagawa E, Hattori T (1989) Surgical stress and immunosuppression in cancer patients. Gan to Kagaku Ryoho (Jpn J Cancer Chemother) 16:1115–1121

2. Yamashita Y, Hirai H, Mukaida H, Iwata T, Saeki S, Toge T (1991) Clinical evaluation on nutritional assessment for esophageal cancer patients in view of operative methods: Comparison between thoracolaparotomy and blunt dissection. Jpn J Metabol Nutr 25: 412–417
3. Orringer MB (1984) Transhiatal esophagectomy without thoracotomy for carcinoma of the thoracic esophagus. Ann Surg 200:282–288
4. Shahian DM, Neptune WB, Ellis FH Jr, Watkins E Jr (1986) Transthoracic versus extrathoracic esophagectomy: Mortality, morbidity, and long-term survival. Ann Thorac Surg 41:237–246
5. Hankins JR, Attar S, Coughlin TR Jr, Miller JE, Hebel JR, Suter CM, McLaughlin JS (1989) Carcinoma of the esophagus: A comparison of the results of transhiatal versus transthoracic resection. Ann Thorac Surg 47:700–705
6. Finley RJ, Grace M, Duff JH (1985) Esophagogastrectomy without thoracotomy for carcinoma of the cardia and lower part of the esophagus. Surg Gynecol Obstet 160:49–56
7. Japanese Society for Esophageal Diseases (1992) Guide lines for the clinical and pathologic studies on carcinoma of the esophagus. Kanehara, Tokyo

How Should Therapies for Superficial Cancer of the Esophagus Be Performed?

Koh Sugawara, Junzo Sayama, Tetsuro Nishihira, Katsu Hirayama, Takashi Akaishi, Ryuzaburo Shineha, and Shozo Mori[1]

Introduction

In Japan, superficial cancer of the esophagus is defined as cancer limited to the submucosa. Recently, detection of such cancer has improved due to the development of a slender fiberscope and techniques of chromo-endoscopy [1].

In this study, 59 patients with superficial cancer of the thoracic esophagus were classified according to depth of invasion and the extent of lymph node metastasis, and the prognosis in these patients was analyzed.

Methods

From 1975 through 1991, 480 patients with thoracic esophageal cancer underwent resection in our department. In 366 of these patients, curative operations with sufficient lymph node dissection were performed without preoperative irradiation or chemotherapy.

Fifty-nine of these 366 patients had superficial cancer. These 59 patients were the subjects of this study. After surgery, these 59 cases were classified into three groups according to depth of invasion: ep, intraepithelial cancer; mm, mucosal cancer (cancer invading the lamina propria mucosae or muscularis mucosae); and sm, submucosal cancer (cancer invading the submucosa).

Dissected mediastinal and abdominal lymph nodes were examined for metastasis microscopically.

The patients were treated with postoperative irradiation and/or chemotherapy according to the respective degree of lymph node metastasis and depth of invasion.

---

[1] Second Department of Surgery, Tohoku University School of Medicine, 1-1 Seiryou-machi, Aoba-ku, Sendai, 980 Japan

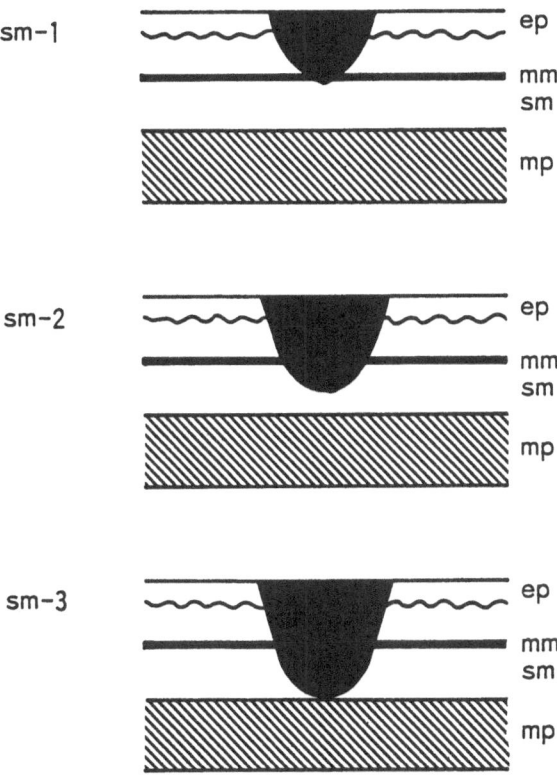

Fig. 1. Classification of submucosal invasion. The sm group was classified into three subgroups according to depth of invasion. *sm-1*, slight invasion of the submucosa; *sm-2*, invasion intermediate between sm-1 and sm-3; *sm-3*, invasion nearly to the muscularis propria

Table 1. The distribution of depth of invasion

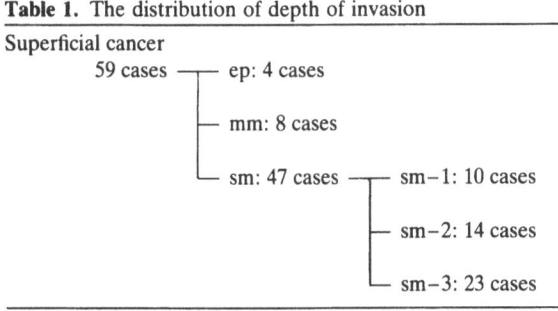

ep, epithelial cancer; *mm*, mucosal cancer; *sm*, submucosal cancer

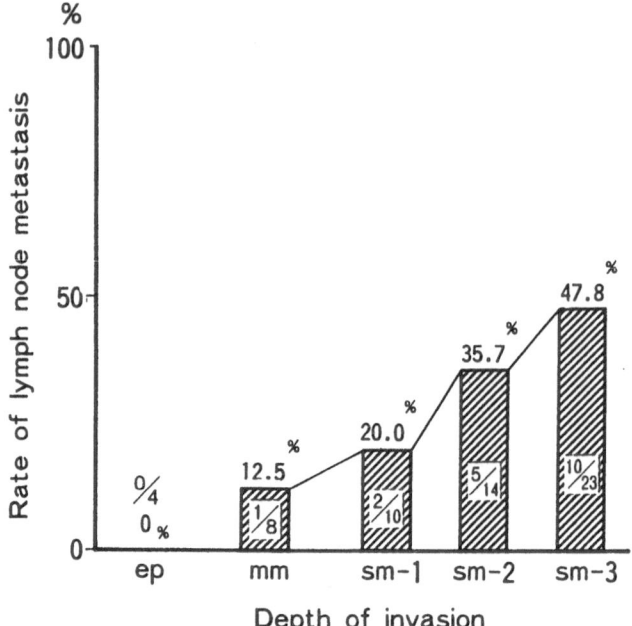

Fig. 2. Rate of lymph node metastasis according to depth of invasion

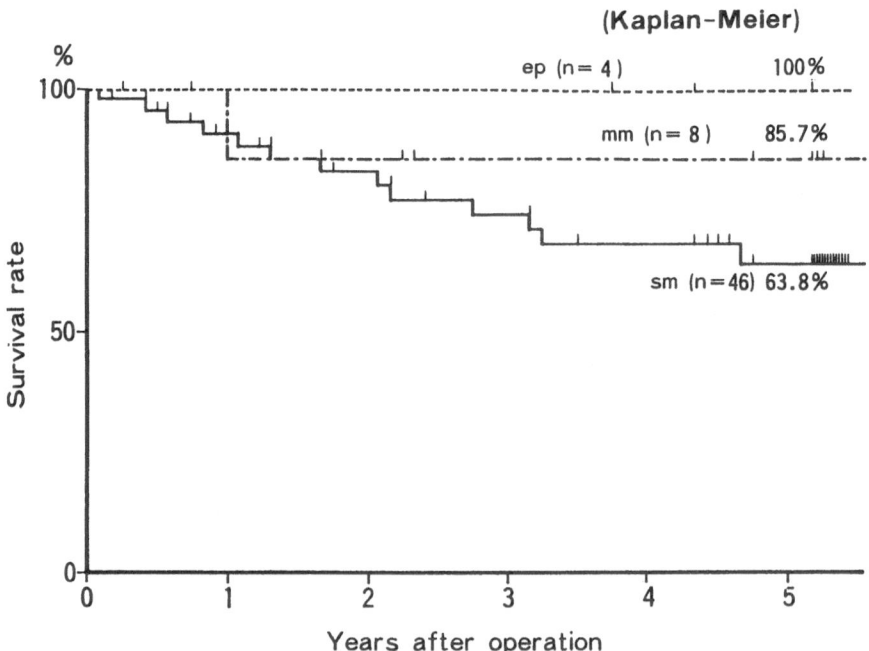

Fig. 3. Survival curve of superficial cancer according to depth of invasion

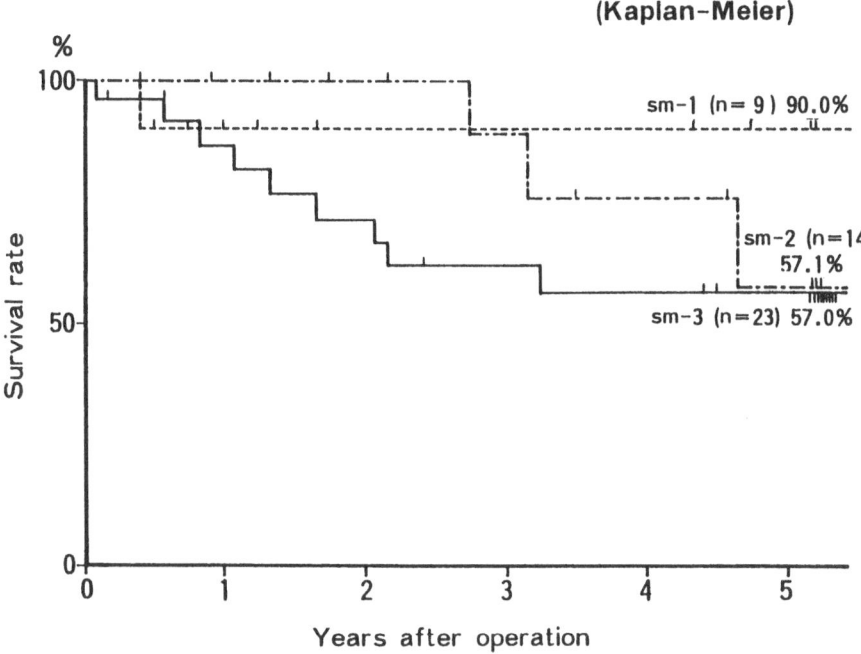

Fig. 4. Survival curve of sm cancer according to depth of invasion

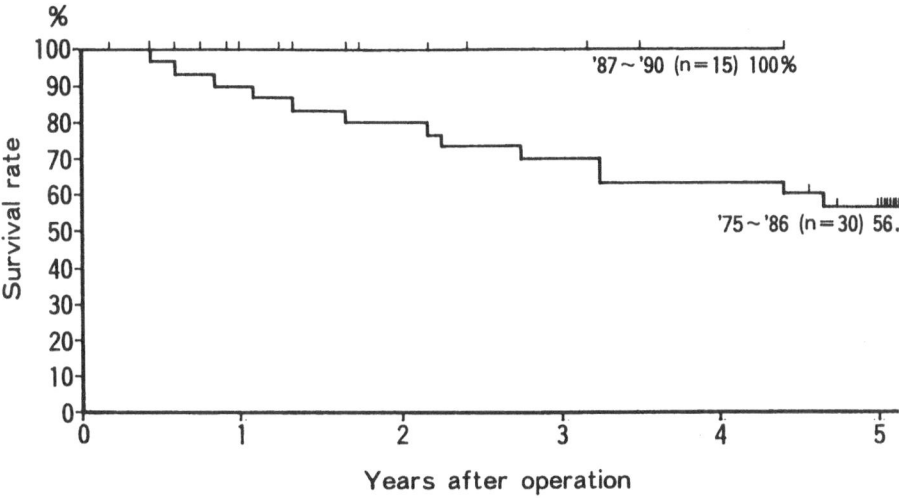

Fig. 5. Survival curves of sm cancer. Comparing the cases of sm cancer operated on from 1975 to 1986 with those from 1987 to 1990

The survival rate was calculated using Kaplan-Meier's method.

Furthermore, the sm group was classified into three subgroups according to depth of invasion for the purposes of more detailed analysis as presented in Fig. 1.

Results

The distribution of depth of invasion is shown in Table 1.

Lymph node metastasis was proven in 19 cases (32%), and 18 of these cases had invasion to the sm layer. Lymph node metastasis was strongly correlated with the depth of invasion (Fig. 2).

The 5-year survival rate of these 59 patients with superficial cancer was 69.1%. According to the depth of invasion, it was as follows: ep, 100%; mm, 85.7%; sm-1, 90.0%; sm-2, 57.1%; and sm-3, 57.0% (Figs. 3, 4).

Comparison of the cases of sm cancer operated on from 1975 to 1986 with those from 1987 to 1990 shows the survival curve of cases in the latter period to be excellent (Fig. 5).

Discussion

In this paper, 59 patients with superficial cancer were analyzed according to the depth of invasion. With the progress of carcinoma invasion, the rates of lymph node metastasis showed tendencies to increase, and 5-year survival rates showed poor tendencies. Especially, the prognosis of sm-2 and sm-3 groups were poorer. These poor prognoses were almost equal to that of advanced cases [2].

The prognosis of the sm group operated on after 1987 was excellent. One of the reasons was that the regimen of postoperative adjuvant therapy for the sm group was changed and a stronger regimen was adopted in 1986 [3]. This excellent prognosis was due not only to improvement in adjuvant therapy, but also to other factors such as postoperative management of patients, the method of lymph node dissection, etc.

Table 2. The treatment for superficial cancer

Preoperative diagnosis	Operation	Postoperative histological diagnosis	Adjuvant therapy
ep	Endoscopic resection of esophageal mucosa	ep	No treatment
		mm n($-$)	
	Blunt dissection of esophagus	mm n($+$)	Conventional therapy
		sm$-$1	(irradiation and chemotherapy)
mm	Resection of esophagus with lymphadenectomy		Aggressive therapy in the same
sm$-$1		sm$-$2	way in advancer cases
sm$-$2		sm$-$3	(irradiation, chemotherapy,
sm$-$3			immunotherapy, etc.)

ep, epithelial cancer; *mm*, mucosal cancer; *sm*, submucosal cancer

Therefore, on the basis of the results of this study, we propose the treatment of superficial cancer as outlined in Table 2.

References

1. Makuuchi H, Mitani T, Tajima T, Matimura T, Sasaki T, Sugihara T, Oomori Y, Kikunaga H, Kumagai Y (1990) Endoscopic characterization for differentiation of mucosal and sub-mucosal carcinomas in esophagus. I to Cho (Stomach and Intestine). 9:1051–1058
2. Hirayama K, Mori S (1990) Prognostic factor of early esophageal cancer. Jpn J Cancer Chemother 17(1):37–45
3. Nishihira T, Hirayama K, Shineha R, Sanekata K, Shiga K, Takano R, Mori S (1988) Improvement of treatment for carcinoma of the esophagus especially in reference to the transition of postoperative combined therapies. J Jpn Surg Soc 89(9):1479–1482

Transhiatal Esophagectomy for Intrathoracic Esophageal Cancer

Hiroyoshi Ayabe, Hiroharu Tsuji, Shinsuke Hara, Yutaka Tagawa, Katsunobu Kawahara, and Masao Tomita[1]

Introduction

Surgical treatment is the best management for the patients with dysphagia and resection should be performed unless there are any contraindications. It is generally accepted that the standard radical operation for thoracic esophageal cancer is a subtotal or total thoracic esophagectomy with intrathoracic and intra-abdominal lymph node dissection through right thoracotomy and laparotomy [1]. However, transthoracic esophagectomy has high morbidity and mortality rates [2, 3]. Therefore, for the patients with poor nutritional condition and low cardiopulmonary reserve, transhiatal esophagectomy without thoracotomy for esophageal cancer may have lower morbidity and mortality [4, 5].

The objective of this paper is to report the experience of transhiatal eso-phagectomy for thoracic esophgeal cancer in our institution.

Patients and Methods

Between 1969 and December, 1991, 172 patients underwent esophagectomy for carcinoma of the thoracic esophagus at the First Department of Surgery, Nagasaki University Hospital. Of these, 160 patients underwent transthoracic eso-phagectomy (TTE) and 12 (7.0%) had transhiatal esophagectomy (THE). All underwent immediate cervical esophagogastrostomy or esophagoileostomy with colon interposition. Of the 12 patients having THE, 9 were men and 3 were women and their ages ranged from 57 to 80 years (mean 69.3). The location of the tumor was the upper thoracic esophagus in three patients, the middle esophagus in four and the lower esophagus in five. Nine patients had dysphagia

[1]First Department of Surgery, Nagasaki University School of Medicine, 1-7-1, Sakamoto, Nagasaki, 852 Japan

Table 1. Patient characteristics

No	Age	Sex	Symptoms	Esophagogram			Associated diseases
				Type	Length	Location	
1	74	M	Dysphagia	Tumorous	7 cm	Middle	LVH
2	70	F	Dysphagia	Funnell	3.6 cm	Lower	Hypertension, heart murmur
3	62	M	Dysphagia	Serrated	5 cm	Upper	Hypertension, SSS, DM
4	60	F	Odontophagia	Tumorous	3 cm	Lower	Angina pectoris, AR
5	76	M	Dysphagia	Spiral	4.5 cm	Lower	Arrhythmia (Af), FEV 1.0, 55%
6	72	M	None	Superficial	4.5 cm	Middle	Arrhythmia (Af), Gastric cancer
7	75	F	Heartburn	Superficial	3 cm	Middle	Renal dysfunction, FEV 1.0, 50%
8	57	M	Dysphagia	Serrated	8 cm	Lower	Arrhythmia (WPW, Af)
9	80	M	Dysphagia	Spiral	8 cm	Upper	
10	76	M	Dysphagia	Serrated	4.5 cm	Upper	FEV 1.0, 59.3%
11	64	M	None	Superficial	1 cm	Middle	VC, 32.4%
12	65	M	Dysphagia	Serrated	2 cm	Lower	FEV 1.0, 33%

LVH, left ventricular hypertrophy; *SSS*, sick sinus syndrome; *DM*, diabetes mellitus; *AR*, aortic regurgitation; *Af*, atrial fibrillation; *WPW*, Wolff—Parkinson—White syndrome; *FEV* 1.0, forced expiratory volume in 1 s; *VC*, vital capaity

Table 2. Pathological findings and curability

No	Cell type	Depth of invasion	Node	Stage (UICC)	Curability
1	Squamous cell ca	ad	Negative	II A	Curative
2	Squamous cell ca	ad	Negative	II A	Curative
3	Squamous cell ca	mp	Positive (cervical)	II B	Curative
4	Squamous cell ca	mp	Negative	II A	Curative
5	Squamous cell ca	ad	Positive (paraesoph)	II B	Curative
6	Squamous cell ca	sm	Negative	I	Curative
7	Squamous cell ca	sm	Negative	I	Curative
8	Squamous cell ca	mp	Positive (cervical) (paragastric)	II B	Non-curative
9	Squamous cell ca	adj (trachea)	Negative	III	Non-curative
10	Squamous cell ca	ad	Negative	II A	Non-curative
11	Squamous cell ca	sm	Negative	I	Curative
12	Squamous cell ca	ad	Positive (paraesoph) (left gastric)	II B	Curative

sm, submucosa; *mp*, muscularis propria; *ad*, adventitia; *adj*, adjacent structure; *ca*, cancer

and one had heartburn with epigastralgia. Two patients showed no symptoms, but esophageal abnormality was observed during upper gastrointestinal examination. The length of the lesions, defined by esophagography was under 3 cm in four patients, 3–5 cm in five, and 5–8 cm in three (Table 1). All tumors were squamous cell carcinoma. According to the criteria established by the UICC in 1987 [6], three patients had Stage I, four had Stage II A, four had Stage II B, and one had Stage III on the basis of pathology findings (Table 2). The reasons for selection of THE were over 74 years of age in five cases, cardiovascular problems in five, and severe respiratory dysfunction in two.

The curative operation was performed in nine patients. However, the other three patients underwent non-curative resection because of bloody ascites (no. 8), residual cancer in the membranous portion of the trachea (no. 9), and positive margin of the esophageal stump (no. 10). Two patients were given preoperative adjuvant therepy and four had postoperative chemo and/or radiotherapy. The remaining six recieved no pre- or postoperative adjuvant therapy. An actuarial survival curve was produced according to the Kaplan-Meier method [7].

The operation was also attempted in two additional cases, but because of massive bleeding from the esophageal varices in one, and fracture of the tumor in the other, left thoracotomy was performed for completion of the procedure.

Results

The average duration of the surgical procedure including esophageal reconstruction was 4 h and 30 min (range 2 h and 55 min–5 h and 25 min). Estimated blood loss was 300 g (range 140–1085 g).

One patient had a pneumothorax due to rupture of the pleura during transhiatal blunt resection of the esophagus. This complication was treated by introducing a chest tube and establishing a continuous drainage. A tracheal tear was not observed in our series.

Table 3. Results of transhiatal esophagectomy for esophageal cancer

No	Postoperative complications	Adjuvant therapy	Outcome (years, months)			Cause of death
1	Stenosis (late)	Ra (preop) BLM (preop)	1 y	6 m	Died	unknown
2	None		8 y		Alive	
3	None	Ra Tegafur	2 y	2 m	Died	Recurrence (brain)
4	Arrhythmia (VPC)	Ra (pre and postop) CDDP, PEP	6 y	6 m	Alive	
5	None		1 y	1 m	Died	Pneumonia
6	Sputum retention Hoarseness Hemothorax		4 y	9 m	Died	Pneumonia
7	Arrhythmia (APC)		5 y	2 m	Alive	
8	Arrhythmia Leakage (minor)	CDDP, PEP		2 m	Died	Recurrence (skin)
9	Wound infection Stenosis			5 m	Died	Recurrence (neck)
10	None	Ra CDDP		8 m	Died	Toxicity of chemotherapy
11	Leakage (minor)		2 y		Alive	
12	None		1 y	9 m	Alive	

VPC, ventricular premature contraction; *APC*, atrial premature contraction; *Ra*, radiation; *BLM*, bleomycin; *CDDP*, cisplatin; *PEP*, pepleomycin

Postoperative complications occurred in six patients (50%). There was arrhythmia in three, minor anastomotic leakage in two, late anastomotic stenosis in two, sputum retention in one, recurrent nerve palsy in one, hemothorax in one, and wound infection in one (Table 3). However, these complications were improved by conservative therapy and no patients died within 30 days after operation or during the same hospitalization.

Seven patients have died, at 2, 5, 8, 13, 18, 26, and 57 months after operation. Causes of death were cancer recurrence in three patients, pneumonia in two, complications due to anti-cancer chemotherapy in one, and unknown in one. No patients had evidence of local recurrence. The remaining five patients are alive and well at 21, 24, 62, 78, and 96 months after esophageal resection (Table 3). The 1-year survival rate was 75.0%, the 2-year survival rate was 57.1%, and the 3-year survival rate was 30.5%. Four patients survived more than 4 years. None of them had any cancerous involvement of the dissected lymph nodes.

Discussion

Turner first performed esophagectomy without thoracotomy for thoracic esophageal cancer in 1933 [8]. Ong and Lee [9] in 1960 demonstrated the potential benefit of transhiatal esophagectomy without thoracotomy in the management of lesions requiring removal of the thoracic esophagus. The benefits of transhiatal esophagectomy are: (1) a short operative time, (2) ease of performance, and (3) low morbidity and mortality rates. On the other hand, the disadvantages are a lower cure rate because of incompleteness of lymph node dissection and residual tumor at the adjacent structures [10]. Therefore, the categories of patient for this procedure are: (1) those with early esophageal cancer without nodal metastasis which is diagnosed by endoscopy, radiogram, or endoscopic ultrasonography, (2) high risk patients with poor cardiopulmonary reserve, and (3) patients with previous thoracotomy with dense pleural adhesion [11]. The contraindications for this procedure are: (1) esophageal cancer which invades the adjacent structures such as the aorta and tracheobronchial tree, and (2) esophageal cancer with esophageal varices due to liver cirrhosis [10, 11]. For the former cases, radical operation through thoracotomy, simple bypass operation, or a non-operative approach such as radiotherapy should be chosen, depending on the patient's condition. For the latter cases, the risk of uncontrollable massive bleeding may require that transthoracic esophagectomy be performed.

In esophagectomy through the esophageal hiatus and upper thoracic inlet, special complications such as a tracheal tear [11, 12], bleeding from avulsion of the azygos vein or esophageal artery [13], or rupture of the esophageal tumor [14] are possible, and careful dissection is important. If these intraoperative complications occur, prompt thoracotomy is necessary to repair the condition. Left recurrent nerve paralysis occurred in 1 of the 12 patients (8.3%) in our series. This complication occurred from 3.6% to 31% of the time in reported series [13]. The cause of this complication is a transection of the left recurrent nerve at the aortic arch or an extensive traction during dissection of the cervical esophagus. The latter complication is more frequent, and careful manipulation during cervical esophageal dissection is important to prevent it.

Postoperative respiratory complications in patients with transhiatal esophagectomy have been approximately 6% (range 2%–20%) [11, 15]. In our experience, postoperative respiratory complications occurred in only one patient (8.3%), in whom there was sputum retention. The reasons for the low incidence of pulmonary complications are thought to be less surgical trauma to the lung, shorter operative time, and less pain in the chest wall after operation. The hospital mortality observed with transhiatal esophagectomy ranged between 0% and 13.3% (average 8%) in the series reported to date.

In reports which compared transthoracic esophagectomy and transhiatal esophagectomy, Shahian et al. [13] and Hankins et al. [11] stated that there was no difference in median survival between the two procedures. In our series, 4 of 12 patients survived more than 4 years and the 3-year survival rate was 30.5%, which was identical with the results of Terz et al. [10].

In conclusion, transhiatal esophagectomy should be considered for patients with early esophageal cancer without nodal metastasis, in patients with Stage I and II with poor cardiopulmonary reserve, or in patients of advanced age.

References

1. Kakegawa T, Yamana H, Fujita H, Maki J (1986) Radical operation for thoracic esophageal carcinoma. Excerpta Medica 40:122–125
2. Postlewait RW (1983) Complications and deaths after operations for esophageal carcinoma. J Thorac Cardiovasc Surg 85:827–834
3. Mattheus HR, Powell DJ, McConkey CC (1983) Effect of surgical experience on the results of resection for esophageal carcinoma. Br J Surg 73:621–623
4. Hankins JR, Miller JE, Attar S, McLaughlin JS (1987) Transhiatal esophagectomy for carcinoma of the esophagus: Experience with 26 patients. Ann Thorac Surg 44:123–127
5. Orringer MB (1988) Transhiatal esophagectomy without thoracotomy for esophageal carcinoma. In: Delarue NC, Wilkins EW, Wong L (eds) International trends in general thoracic surgery, vol 4. CV Mosby, St. Louis, pp 200–220
6. International Union Against Cancer (1987) TNM: Classification of malignant tumors, 4th edn. Springer, Berlin
7. Kaplan EL, Meier P (1985) Non-parametric estimation from incomplete observation. J Am Stat Assoc 53:457–481
8. Turner GG (1933) Excision of the thoracic esophagus for carcinoma with construction of an extra-thoracic gullet. Lancet II:1315–1316
9. Ong GB, Lee TC (1960) Pharingogastric anastomosis after esophagopharyngectomy for carcinoma of the hypopharynx and cervical esophagus. Br J Surg 48:193–196
10. Terz JJ, Beatty D, Kokai WA, Wagman LD (1987) Transhiatal esophagectomy. Ann Surg 154:42–48
11. Hankins JR, Attar S, Coughlin TR, Miller JE, Hebel JR, Suter CM, McLaughlin JS (1989) Carcinoma of the esophagus: A comparison of the results of transhiatal versus transthoracic resection. Ann Thorac Surg 47:700–705
12. Orringer MB (1984) Transhiatal esophagectomy without thoracotomy for carcinoma of the esophagus. Ann Surg 200:282–288
13. Shahian DM, Neptune WB, Ellis IH Jr, Watkins F Jr (1986) Transthoracic versus extrathoracic esophagectomy: Mortality, morbidity and long-term survival. Ann Thorac Surg 41:237–246
14. Fok JM, Siu KF, Wong J (1989) A comparison of transhiatal and transthoracic resection for carcinoma of the thoracic esophagus. Am J Surg 158:414–419
15. Garvin PJ, Kaminski DL (1980) Extrathoracic esophagectomy in the treatment of esophageal cancer. Am J Surg 140:772–778

Operative Procedure and Clinical Outcome of Carcinoma of the Thoracic Esophagus

Hiroto Hayashi, Takuo Murakami, Akira Tangoku, Hiroyuki Uchisako, Hiroshi Kusanagi, and Takashi Suzuki[1]

Introduction

One of the greatest concerns among surgeons has been to improve the operative mortality rate after radical operation for carcinoma of the esophagus. In our department, we have performed aggressive lymph node dissection of the upper mediastinum since 1980. In the present study, we evaluated this dissection and also report the results of EFP (etoposide, 5-FU, and cisplatin) therapy in the prevention of hematogenous recurrence.

Patients and Methods

From 1970 to 1992, we examined 335 patients with squamous cell carcinoma of the thoracic esophagus, for which we performed resection of the main lesion and lymphadenectomy on 286 patients (rate of resectability, 86%). The locations where the cancer was found in the resected cases were the upper intrathoracic esophagus in 41 patients, the middle intrathoracic esophagus in 186 patients, and the lower intrathoracic esophagus in 59 patients.

Results

Results of Clinicopathological Examination and Surgical Therapy

The pattern of metastases to the lymphatic system according to the location of the tumor was investigated histologically. Of the resected cases, 66% showed lymph node metastases, and there was no correlation according to location:

[1] Department of Surgery II, Yamaguchi University School of Medicine, 1144 Kogushi, Ube, Yamaguchi, 755 Japan

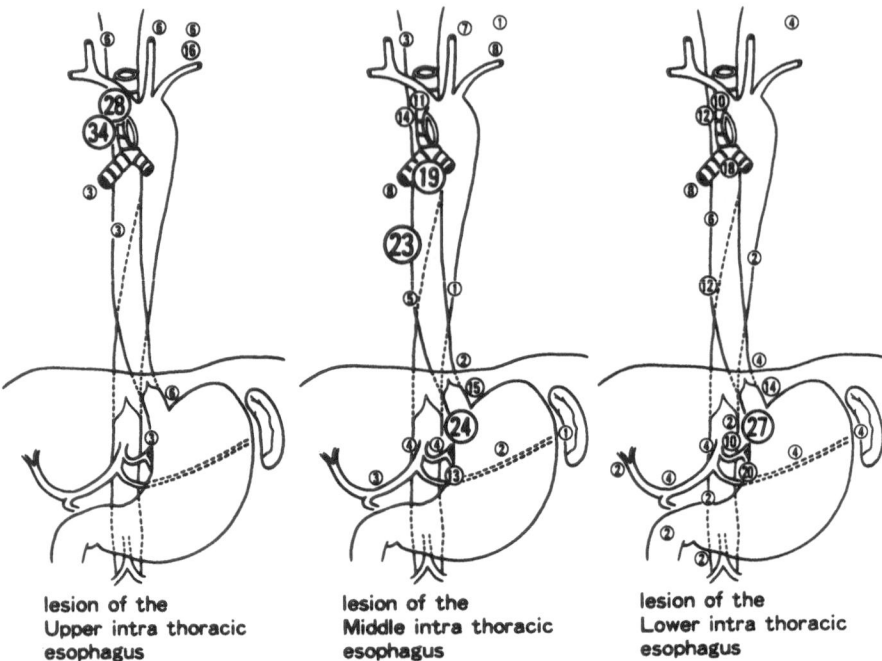

lesion of the
Upper intra thoracic
esophagus

lesion of the
Middle intra thoracic
esophagus

lesion of the
Lower intra thoracic
esophagus

Fig. 1. Lymph node metastatic rate according to tumor location. Lymph node metastasis was observed in 66% of the patients

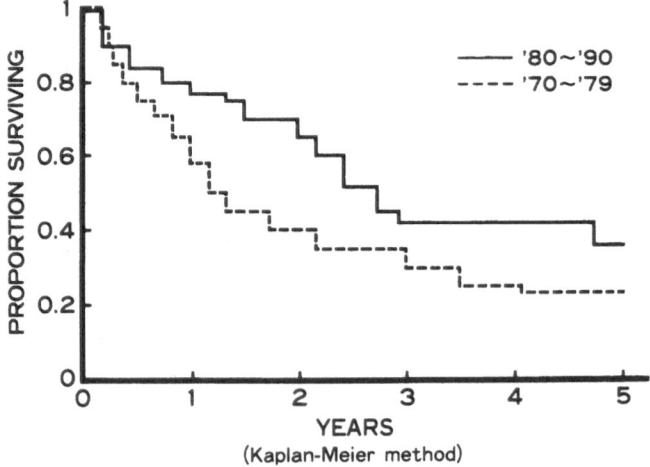

Fig. 2. The 5-year survival rate of patients who had undergone curative resection during the last 10 years was 37%, but only 24% previously

Metastasis to the upper thoracic esophagus was found in 69% of the resected cases, the middle in 67%, and the lower in 63% (Fig. 1). Skip metastasis to the cervical or abdominal lymph nodes without intrathoracic involvement was observed in 24%. In the patients examined before 1980, early recurrence within 1 year, particularly in the upper mediastinum, was observed in about a half of the patients regardless of whether or not they underwent curative resection. Lymphadenectomy with emphasis on the upper mediastinum has been performed in our department since 1980, and the prognosis improved from 32% to 42% in 3-year survival and from 24% to 37% in 5-year survival (Fig. 2).

On the basis of clinicopathological studies, lymph node dissection of the upper mediastinum was effective in improving prognosis. On the other hand, the more extensive the dissection, the higher the potential risk of postoperative pulmonary complications. During the operative procedure, we attempted to avoid injury to the right bronchial artery, the posterior pulmonary plexus, and vagal nerves by visualizing them with neurostain dye adjacent to the carina. By these preserving procedures, the incidence of postoperative pulmonary complications decreased from 22.1% to 15.6% despite extensive upper mediastinal lymph node dissection.

EFP Therapy

A total of 82 patients with a known mode of recurrence underwent curative resection since 1983. The incidence of recurrence in cervical lymph nodes has shown a decreasing trend; 17.0% with lymph node dissection in two fields (mediastinal and abdominal lymphadenectomy), 12.0% with lymph node dissection in the left cervical region only, and 10.0% with three fields (mediastinal, abdominal, and cervical lymphadenectomy). On the other hand, the frequency of hematogenous recurrence increased from 16.7% in lymph-adenectomy in two fields to 30.0% in three fields. Therefore, we consider postoperative supplemental therapy to be the most effective means of preventing hematogenous recurrence. Since 1989, we have performed EFP therapy with etoposide, 5-FU, and cisplatin on patients less than 70 years of age, on whom curative resection was the treatment of choice over chemotherapy (Table 1). Ten patients survived for more than 2 years after EFP therapy. One has died of recurrence of the upper mediastinal lymph nodes with metastasis to the lung, but the remaining nine patients are alive at the present time; the longest survival is 30 months after start of the EFP therapy.

Table 1. Regimen of EFP therapy

Drug	Dose (mg/m^2)	1	2	3	4 (day)	5	6	7	8
CDDP	30–50	↓							↓
VP-16	100–120			↓	↓	↓			
5-FU	300–500			↓	↓	↓			

CDDP, Cisplatin; *VP-16*, etoposide; *5-FU*, 5-fluorouracil; *EFP*, etoposide/5FU/cisplatin

Discussion

The prognosis of esophageal cancer, particularly of thoracic esophageal cancer, has not yet been satisfactory as compared with that of other gastrointestinal cancer. In our department, we have performed intrathoracic lymph node dissection placing emphasis on the upper mediastinum since 1980 to improve the outcome of treatment for esophageal cancer [1]. Also, analysis of the factors which affect the prognosis by multivariate analysis revealed significant correlation between the N(n)-factor (lymph node metastasis) and the prognosis of extended lymphadenectomy, and between lymph node metastasis, which is an important route of metastasis of esophageal cancer, and the effect of lymph nodes dissection with emphasis on the upper mediastinum. On the other hand, there may be a higher risk of postoperative pulmonary complications when lymphadenectomy of the cervical region and the upper mediastinum is performed. However, extended lymph node dissection is effective for prevention of postoperative pulmonary complications to identify and preserve the vagal pulmonary branch, posterior pulmonary nerve plexus, and recurrent nerve with perioperative neurostain stain, or to preserve the bronchial artery [2]. Patients are treated in ICU after operation, respiratory support is performed using Bennett 7200a, and analysis of arterial blood gas and determination of extra-vascular lung water volume are frequently performed. In thoracic upper and middle esophageal cancer, although the area of lymphadenectomy has been further extended to three fields including the cervical region, much safer operation procedures, and more careful preperi- and, postoperative management are anticipated in the future.

References

1. Hayashi H (1986) Clinico-pathological studies and the result of surgical treatment of esophageal cancer. Arch Jpn Chir 55:334–345
2. Murakami T (1978) Studies on postoperative pulmonary complications after surgery for esophageal cancer, especially the relationship between the vagus nerve and the pulmonary complication. Part 1. Clinical Observation. Arch Jpn Chir 47:413–426

Recurrence of Thoracic Esophageal Cancer After Three-Field Lymphadenectomy

Shoji Natsugoe, Hisaaki Shimazu, Heiji Yoshinaka, Masamichi Baba, Toshitaka Fukumoto, and Takashi Aikou[1]

Introduction

The prognosis for patients with carcinoma of the esophagus is poor compared with findings in the instance of malignant growths in other areas of digestive tract. The high incidence of lymph node metastasis is one of the most important factors in poor prognosis for patients with carcinoma of the esophagus. Since December 1982, we have been employing the extended lymph node dissection for thoracic esophageal carcinoma. The extended lymph node dissection signifies the type of dissection which removes the lymph nodes of three fields, namely cervical, mediastinal, and abdominal. The aims of this study are to document the patterns of recurrence after extended lymph node dissection and to evaluate the effectiveness of the 3-field lymph node dissection.

Patients and Methods

From December 1982 to May 1990, 101 patients with thoracic esophageal cancer underwent subtotal esophagectomy with 3-field lymph node dissection. All such operations were curative resections. All patients were followed up after discharge: X-ray examination was done every 1–3 months, computed tomography every 3–6 months, and ultrasonography every 6 months. Bronchoscopic and endoscopic examination was performed when necessary. All patients were observed for more than 1 year and recurrence was confirmed in 43 (42.6%). The mode of recurrence was classified into four patterns: Lymph node, visceral, both lymph node and visceral, and others.

---

[1] First Department of Surgery, Kagoshima University School of Medicine, 8-35-1, Sakuragaoka, Kagoshima, 890 Japan

795

Table 1. Incidence of recurrence by location, tumor classifications, and stage grouping

		Cases	Recurrence	Incidence (%)
Location	Upper	9	3	33.3
	Middle	65	30	46.2
	Lower	27	10	37.0
Tumor	T1	17	3	17.6
	T2	24	11	45.8
	T3	58	28	48.3
	T4	2	1	50.0
Stage	I	7	0	0.0
	II A	22	6	27.3
	II B	12	4	33.3
	III	19	11	57.9
	IV	41	22	53.7

Table 2. Relationship between recurrence and lymph node metastases

	LN-Meta(−) (%)	LN-Meta(+)
Cases	27	74
Recurrence	6(22.2)	37(50.0)
	└ $P < 0.01$ ┘	
Lymph node	5(18.5)	16(21.6)
Organ		15(20.2)
Lymph node and organ		3 (4.1)
Others	1 (3.7)	3 (4.1)

LN, lymph node

Clinical and pathological classification of carcinoma of the esophagus was based upon the TNM staging system. Statistical analysis was made using the chi square test.

Results

Incidence of Recurrence

The distribution of the location of primary tumors, tumor classification, and staging of disease are listed in Table 1. No difference was found in the incidence of recurrence by location. The frequency of T1 tumor is lower than any other T category. The incidence of advanced stages are also high.

The lymph node metastasis was histopathologically proven in 74 patients (72.3%). The incidence of recurrence was 22.2% in patients without lymph node metastasis, and 50.0% in those with metastatic lymph nodes. The difference was statistically significant ($P < 0.01$). Five patients who did not initially have lymph

Table 3. Relationship between recurrence and number of metastatic lymph nodes

LN-Meta(+)	0–5	6–
	(%)	
Cases	74	27
Recurrence	25(33.8)	18(66.7)
	└ $P < 0.01$ ┘	
Lymph node	12(16.2)	9(33.3)
Organ	9(12.2)	6(22.2)
Lymph node and organ	1 (1.4)	2 (7.4)
Others	3 (4.1)	2 (3.7)

LN, lymph node

node metastasis at operation eventually developed it. Metastasis occurred in the upper mediastinal lymph nodes in four of five patients, but no visceral occurrence was found in those patients. In other modes of recurrence, except for one case with local recurrence, lymph node metastasis was present at operation (Table 2).

The patients with recurrence were divided into two groups according to whether the number of metastatic lymph nodes was five or less or six or more positive nodes. The incidence of recurrence was 33.8% in cases with five or less, and 66.7% in those with six or more positive nodes. The difference was stastically significant ($P < 0.01$) (Table 3). No obvious difference was found in the site of recurrence between the two groups.

Patterns of Recurrence

Lymph node recurrence was found in 21 patients (48.8%), visceral recurrence in 15 patients (34.9%), lymph node and visceral recurrence in 3 patients (7.0%), and miscellaneous recurrence in 4 patients (9.3%).

The time interval from operation to recurrence in 21 lymph node recurrences was within 1 year in 12 cases, between 1 and 2 years in 9 cases, and after 2 years in 4 cases. In 15 visceral recurrences, recurrence occurred within 1 year in 11 cases and within 2 years in all other cases. Recurrences were found within 2 years in other modes of recurrence. The time interval of recurrence was longer in cases with lymph node recurrence than in those with other modes of recurrence.

The relationship between hematogenous recurrence and lymph node metastases is shown in Table 4. Visceral recurrence occurred most frequently in the lung (66.7%). Other sites in order of decreasing frequency were bone (20.0%), liver (6.7%), and skin (6.7%). All visceral recurrences occurred in patients with lymph node metastasis which extended to more than two fields in 80% of those patients.

Survival According to the Mode of Recurrence

The survival of patients with recurrence was dismal. Only seven patients are alive. Of these, six patients have had recurrent disease in lymph nodes. Four patients with lymph node recurrence have survived more than 4 years

Table 4. Relationship between hematogenous recurrence and lymph node metastases

Recurrent site	Metastatic site at operation				
	Cervix	Upper	Middle	Lower	Abdomen
Liver (n = 1)	●	●			
Skin (n = 1)		●		●	●
Bone (n = 3)	●	●●	●● ●	●●	●●
Lung (n = 10)	●● ●● ●	●● ●● ●● ●●	●● ●	●●	●● ●● ●●

Closed circles, positive nodes

Table 5. Survival according to the mode of recurrence (months)

	6M	12M	24M	36M	48M
Lymph node		●● ● ● ●	○●○ ●○ ●●● ●	● ●	○63 ○103 ○54 ●68
Organ		●● ●●● ●● ●	●● ● ● ●● ●		
Node and organ	●	○	●		
Others	●		●●●		

open circles, alive; *closed circles*, died

postoperatively. On the other hand, all the patients with visceral recurrence died within 3 years postoperatively. In particular, 12 (80%) of these patients died within 2 years. Except for one patient, all the patients with other modes of recurrence died within 2 years postoperatively (Table 5).

Discussion

To improve the treatment of patients with esophageal cancer, the current status has to be evaluated. Our analysis of recurrence after esophagectomy with 3-field lymph node dissection indicated that the incidence of recurrence was obviously high in advanced stages of disease such as stage III and stage IV. With regard to time interval from operation to recurrence, recurrence was found in 90% of patients within 2 years in spite of curative resection. Chan et al. [1] reported that evidence of residual local or metastatic esophageal malignancy was found in 81% of autopsied cases, and such universal high incidence of residual malignancy suggests that, in a fair number of cases, the disease is already in an advanced state beyond the scopy of curative treatment by the time it is detected.

Though Tam et al. [2] reported that the total local recurrence rate was 16%, in this study the incidence of local recurrence was 7% and the lymph node recurrence was most frequently found. Sugimachi et al. [3] reported that lymphatic or blood vessel invasion in instances of a malignant growth is indicative of a poor prognosis.

In this study also, the incidence of recurrence was significantly higher in patients with lymph node metastasis, especially in patients with six or more positive nodes. All visceral recurrences occurred in cases with concomitant lymph node metastasis.

The survival rate improved by the 3-field lymph node dissection as compared with the 2-field lymph node dissection. However, the outcome of patients with recurrence has remained unsatisfactory. Some patients in this study showed marked improvement on adjuvant therapy. Therefore, it is important to follow up carefully and initiate adjuvant therapy early.

References

1. Chan KW, Chan EYW, Chan CW (1986) Carcinoma of the esophagus. An autopsy study of 231 cases. Pathology 18:400–405
2. Tam PC, Cheung HC, Ma L, Siu KF, Wong J (1987) Local recurrences after subtotal esophagectomy for squamous cell carcinoma. Ann Surg 205:189–194
3. Sugimachi K, Inokuchi K, Kuwano H, Kai H, Okamura T, Okudaira Y (1983) Patients of recurrence after curative resection for carcinoma of the thoracic part of the esophagus. Surg Gynecol Obstet 157:537–540

Reduction of Operative Morbidity and Mortality in Esophageal Cancer Through Strict Prevention of Postoperative Complications

Tamotsu Kudo, Taiji Seto, Takao Hanaoka, Rikko Lee, Shinichiro Ouchi, and Yuichi Tanaka[1]

Introduction

Postoperative complications are still responsible for many deaths in esophageal cancer surgery. In the last 4 years, we achieved a great reduction of the postoperative mortality rate at 3 months after surgical treatment while also achieving satisfactory palliation of dysphagia in 100% of our patients.

The present report describes the surgical results of the patients with thoracic esophageal cancer and the essential points regarding perioperative care and management.

Materials and Methods

A total of 31 esophageal resections in the period between January 1984 and December 1987, herein referred to as the former period, and a total of 42 esophageal resections in the period between January 1988 and December 1991, herein referred to as the latter period, were performed at Nakadori General Hospital. The mean age of the patients was 63.8 years (48–78) in the former period and 59.8 (39–78) in the latter period.

In the former period, we operated relatively rapidly, as a matter of surgical policy. The stomach was commonly used as an esophageal substitute, and the colon was utilized in gastrectomized patients (Table 1). Esophageal reconstruction was done either through the posterior mediastinum or the thoracic cavity in about half of the patients, though 40% of the patients underwent surgery through the retrosternal route (Table 2). Nutritional support was provided both parenterally and enterally.

In the latter period, we switched the operative and perioperative policy. The new policy focused on preventing postoperative complications, including

[1] Department of Surgery, Nakadori General Hospital, 3-15 Minamidori, Akita, 010 Japan

Table 1. Patients and their interpositioned organs

	Number of patients	Interpositioned organ		
		Stomach	Jejunum	Colon
The former period 1984–1987	31	23	3	5ᵃ
The latter period 1988–1991	42	36	6	0

ᵃ Three of five (60%) patients died within 3 months postoperatively because of anastomotic leakage

Table 2. The reconstructive route

	Posterior mediastinum or thoracic cavity	Retrosternum	Subcutaneous
The former period 1984–1987	16	12ᵃ	3
The latter period 1988–1991	40	2	0

ᵃ Five of 12 (42%) patients died within 3 months postoperatively

the avoidance of fatal anastomotic leakage by means of strict monitoring of the blood supply and tissue viability of the reconstructive organ, especially at the suture line, which necessitated allowing sufficient operative time. The stomach was commonly used as an esophageal substitute and the jejunum instead of the colon was utilized in gastrectomized patients (Table 1). Esophageal reconstruction was done as a rule through the posterior mediastinum or the thoracic cavity (Table 2). Nutritional support was provided only parenterally in order to prevent postoperative aspiration pneumonia. Additionally, four patients in the former period and seven patients in the latter period had lymph node dissections performed in three areas: the cervical, thoracic, and abdominal regions.

Results

The majority of the patients had histologically verified advanced cancer at the time of surgery in both the former and latter periods (Table 3). Because the blood supply of the tissue and tissue viability of the reconstructive organ was strictly monitored while allowing sufficient operative time, the mean operative time required increased up to 8.3 h in the latter period from 6.5 h in the former period, though the mean blood loss during surgery was almost the same for both periods (772 ml versus 814 ml). Intraoperative re-laparotomy and/or re-thoracotomy were done in five patients in order to check the blood supply of the reconstructive organ, and the organ utilized as the esophageal substitute was switched to another organ in two patients because of insufficient blood supply in the latter period (Table 4). On the other hand, in the former period

Table 3. Patients and their histological stage

	Number of patients	Stage				
		0	I	II	III	IV
The former period 1984–1987	31	4	0	2	10	15
The latter period 1988–1991	42	7	5	3	12	15

Nakadori General Hospital, Akita, Japan

Table 4. The frequency of intraoperative re-laparotomy, re-thoracotomy and exchange of esophageal substitute

	Number of patients	Intraoperative re-laparotomy and/or re-thoracotomy[a]	Exchange of esophageal substitute[b]
The former period 1984–1987	31	0	0
The latter period 1988–1991	42	5 (12%)	2 (5%)

[a] These procedures were performed in order to check the blood supply of the reconstructive organ
[b] The exchange was done because the blood supply of the reconstructive organ had been extremely bad

three patients had repeat surgery (laparotomy and/or thoracotomy) between 5 and 30 days after the first operation because of anastomotic leakage.

Four patients (13%) within 1 month of their operation and seven patients (23%) within 3 months died in the hospital in the former period. On the other hand, none of the patients (0/42) died within 3 months of their operation in the latter period (Fig. 1). Also, satisfactory palliation of dysphagia was achieved in 100% of the procedures in the latter period from 71% (22/31) in the former period (Fig. 1).

Two patients had severe pulmonary complications that were treated successfully in the latter period: One had methicillin-resistent *Staphylococcus aureus* (MRSA) pneumonia which was treated with proper antibiotics and another patient had adult respiratory distress syndrome (ARDS) which was treated with corticosteroid administration.

Discussion

The worldwide operative mortality rate of esophageal cancer has decreased considerably in recent years. Wong and Siu [1] reported that their 30-day mortality for resection was 6% and the 3-month mortality was 13%. Kudo et al. [2] reported a 4% operative mortality rate at the Technical University of Munich between October 1986 and June 1988. Furthermore, Ellis [3] reported an

Fig. 1. The improvement in mortality rates and the satisfactory palliation of dysphagia at 3 months. In the last 4 years, we achieved great reduction of postoperative mortality at 3 months (23% → 0%), and satisfactory palliation of dysphagia (71% → 100%) in the surgical treatment of thoracic esophageal cancer

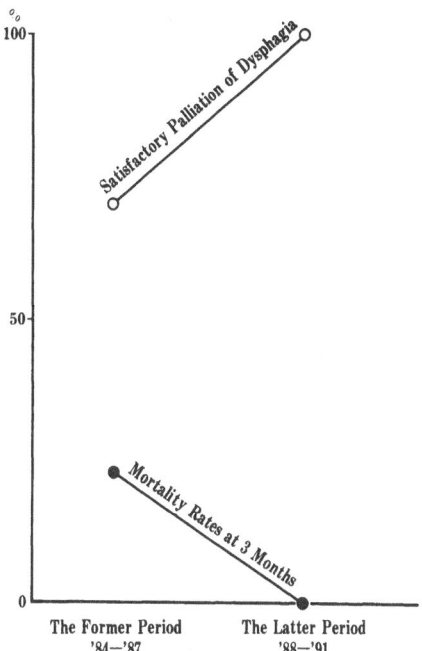

improved operative mortality rate (2.2%) at 1 month after surgery at the Lahey Clinic between 1970 and 1988. However, postoperative complications are still responsible for many deaths in the surgery of esophageal cancer, as reported by Earlam [4] who said the operative mortality rate was 33% in an analysis in the Northeast Thames region in 1981.

In our study's latter period, that is, between January 1988 and December 1991, we achieved an extreme reduction of postoperative morbidity and mortality by carrying out a strict prophylactic policy of preventing postoperative complications. Our good results might be largely due to the successful prevention of fatal anastomotic leakage. The prevention of fatal anastomotic leakage can be attributed to adequate understanding of the blood supply in the reconstructive organ [5, 6] and practical efforts at monitoring the blood supply which meant allowing longer operative time.

Although we achieved an extreme reduction of the mortality rate and also achieved up to 100% satisfactory palliation of dysphagia by performing esophageal reconstruction through the posterior mediastinum or thoracic cavity in almost all of the patients in the latter period, the posterior mediastinal (intra-thoracic) route or retrosternal route, which should be used as an esophageal reconstructive route, is still controversial. However, the posterior mediastinal route is the orthotopic and shortest route.

The question of whether the colon or the jejunum should be used as an esophageal substitute in gastrectomized patients is also controversial. However, three anastomoses are required for the use of the colon, though a Roux-en-Y configuration of the jejunal loop requires only two anastomoses. Whether to use parenteral or enteral nutritional support as postoperative nutritional support in esophageal cancer surgery is also controversial, but there is a hypothesis that total parenteral nutrition may reduce overall morbidity by reducing respiratory complications [7]. Further studies on these controversial problems are necessary before any definite conclusions can be drawn. From this study, however, we learned that sufficient care of the maintenance of an adequate blood supply and tissue viability in the reconstructive organ, especially at the suture line, should be taken during the operation, and consequently, it must be emphasized that a more carefully monitored esophageal reconstruction is superior to a rapid operation.

Conclusion

In the last 4 years, we achieved an extreme reduction in postoperative mortality at 3 months (0/42), and also achieved up to 100% satisfactory palliation of dysphagia, in esophageal cancer surgery. These good results were produced by employing a policy of preventing postoperative complications, especially fatal anastomotic leakage, which involved allowing sufficient operative time.

Acknowledgments. I wish to thank Professor S. Abo, who is a Professor at the Second Department of Surgery at the Akita University School of Medicine. Professor Abo encouraged the development of the surgery in advanced esophageal cancer.

I also wish to pay tribute to Professor J.R. Siewert, who is Professor of Surgery at the Technical University of Munich. Professor Siewert encouraged and helped, with his departmental doctor, Dr. H. Bartels, in the clinical research on the postoperative care and management following esophageal cancer surgery through three kinds of operation.

References

1. Wong J, Siu KF (1988) Squamous cell carcinoma of the esophagus. In: Delarue NC, Wilkins EW Jr, Wong J (eds) Esophageal cancer (international trends in general thoracic surgery, vol 4). Mosby St. Louis, pp 164–180
2. Kudo T, Siewert JR, Bartels H (1990) Postoperative care and management following three kinds of operation for esophageal cancer. Jpn J Surg 20:645–649
3. Ellis FH Jr (1989) Treatment of carcinoma of esophagus or cardia. Mayo Clin Proc 64:945–955
4. Earlam R (1984) Esophageal cancer treatment in north east Thames region, 1981. BMJ 288:1892–1894
5. Kudo T, Abo S, Itabashi T (1986) Prognosis of esophageal substitute in tissue viability and anastomotic leakage. In: Siewert JR, Hölscher AH (eds) Diseases of the esophagus. Springer, Berlin Heidelberg New York, pp 522–525
6. Kudo T, Abo S, Murakawa Y (1983) An experimental analysis of viability at anastomotic sites of the stomach used for esophageal reconstruction (in Japanese). Igaku no Ayumi 134:1033–1034
7. Noirot C, Bouderlique JR, Giuli R (1988) Perioperative management of carcinoma of the esophagus. In: Delarue NC, Wilkins EW Jr, Wong J (eds) Esophageal cancer (international trends in general thoracic surgery, vol 4). Mosby, St. Louis, pp 110–113

Surgical Treatment for Esophageal Cancer After Gastrectomy

Masao Yagi, Kouya Sakamoto, Wataru Fukushima, Touru Ii, Masataka Segawa, Tetsuo Hashito, Kouichi Shimizu, Ryouhei Izumi, Kouchi Miwa, and Itsuo Miyazaki[1]

Introduction

Gastroesophageal reflux is associated with a high incidence of complications such as ulcer or cancer of the esophagus [1]. Gastrectomy results in regurgitation of bile into the esophagus. However, the etiologic role of gastrectomy in esophageal cancer is still controversial [2]. Surgical treatment of postgastrectomy esophageal cancer is also investigational, because esophageal reconstruction with vascularized graft in the patient who has undergone gastrectomy is sometimes difficult due to the presence of adhesion. In this connection, we reviewed 14 cases of postgastrectomy esophageal cancer among our series.

Patients and Methods

The cause of gastrectomy was peptic ulcer in nine patients and gastric malignancy in five. Distal partial gastrectomy was performed in nine, subtotal gastrectomy with R2 lymph node dissection in four and total gastrectomy with transverse colon pancreato-splenectomy in one patient. Esophageal reconstruction using free jejunal transfer was performed in three cases (Table 1).

Results

The mean age of the 14 patients was 63.4 ± 6.4 years, and 12.6 ± 8.2 years had passed after gastrectomy. The cancer was located in the upper and middle intra-thoracic esophagus in six patients and the lower intra-thoracic and abdominal esophagus in eight patients (Table 2). Ten of the 14 patients had well or

[1] Department of Surgery II, School of Medicine, Kanazawa University, 13-1 Takara-machi, Kanazawa, 920 Japan

Table 1. Background of the patients

	Number (n)
Cause of gastrectomy	
Peptic ulcer	9
Gastric cancer	4
Gastric sarcoma	1
Procedure of gastrectomy	
Total gastrectomy (R3)	1
Subtotal gastrectomy (R2)	4
Partial gastrectomy	9
Reconstruction style (after gastrectomy)	
Roux-Y style	1
Billroth type I	7
Billroth type II	6
Postgastrectomy interval	12.6 ± 8.2 years
Treatment for esophageal cancer	
Resected: Total intrathoracic esophageal resection	8
Subtotal intrathoracic esophageal resection	4
Not resected (bypass included)	2
Reconstructed with	
Vascularized jejunum	4
Vascularized colon	5
Free jejunal transfer	3

Table 2. Clinical findings

Age and sex

	Age	Sex (F/M)
Postgastrectomy esophageal ca.	64.6 ± 6.3	1/13
Other esophageal ca.	63.4 ± 10.5	33/134

N.S.

Location of the cancer

	Iu	Im	Ei,Ea
Postgastrectomy esophageal ca.	1	5	8
Other esophageal ca.	14	97	29

$P < 0.01$

ca., cancer; *Iu*, upper intra-thoracic esophagus; *Im*, middle intra-thoracic esophagus; *Ei*, lower intra-thoracic esophagus; *Ea*, abdominal esophagus; *N.S.*, not significant

moderately differentiated squamous cell carcinoma. Curative or relative non-curative resections were performed in 12 patients. In the patients with esophageal cancer after gastrectomy, the frequencies of lower intra-thoracic and abdominal esophagus and well or moderately differentiated squamous cell carcinoma were significantly greater than other types of esophageal cancer (Table 3).

Table 3. Histological findings

Histological classification (degree of differentiation)

	Poorly	Moderately	Well
Postgastrectomy esophageal ca.	1	5	6
Other esophageal ca.	25	33	38

$P < 0.05$

Histological findings of invasion

	Invaded to mp or less,	a 1 or more
Postgastrectomy esophageal ca.	6	6
Other esophageal ca.	21	69

$P < 0.05$

Vascular invasion (ly, v)

	ly($-$)	ly($+$)	v($-$)	v($+$)
Postgastrectomy esophageal ca.	3	6	7	2
Other esophageal ca.	33	48	60	22

N.S.

Degree of lymph node metastasis

	n($-$)	n($+$)
Postgastrectomy esophageal ca.	3	9
Other esophageal ca.	33	63

N.S.

Histologic stage

	II or less	III or more
Postgastrectomy esophageal ca.	8	4
Other esophageal ca.	27	69

*$P < 0.05$

mp, involving muscularis propria; ca., cancer; ly, lymphatic invasion; v, blood vessel invasion; a1, a_1, invasion reaching the adventitia; n, lymph node metastasis

Table 4. Treatment and curability

Treatment

	Non-curative	Curative
Postgastrectomy esophageal ca.	2 (14%)	12 (86%)
Other esophageal ca.	71 (43%)	96 (57%)

$P < 0.05$

Curability

	C0	C1	C2	C3
Postgastrectomy esophageal ca.	1	4	1	6
Other esophageal ca.	28	25	5	38

N.S.

C0, absolute non-curative resection; C1, relative non-curative resection; C2, relative curative resection; C3, absolute curative resection

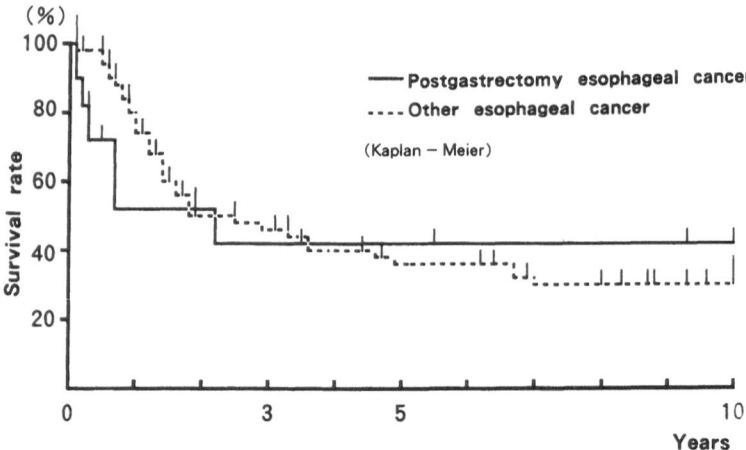

Fig. 1. Survival rate after curative or relative non-curative resction

However, the 5-year survival rate after curative or relative non-curative resection (42%) was not significantly different from that of other types of esophageal cancer (Fig. 1).

Esophageal reconstruction using free jejunal transfer was performed in three patients. The follow-up period ranged from 9 months to 4.5 years after the operation. These freely transplanted jejunums were well dilatated at the postoperative fluorostudy. Strong peristaltic waves and constriction with swallowing persisted for 3 months after the operation and disappeared within 6 months. After that, the passage of food in the transplanted jejunum was good. A positive pressure zone which moved from oral site to anal site of the transplanted jejunum was recognized on manometric study. Intermittent interdigestive electric complex and digestive irregular superimposed electric complex were observed by electromyography at 4 months and 2.5 years after the operation. Normal mucin was observed on the mucosa obtained by endoscopic biopsy.

Discussion

Gastrectomy is the main cause of regurgitation of bile into the esophagus. Bile and duodenal juice have been suggested to have carcinogenetic effects on gastrointestinal mucosa in experimental study [3]. However, the etiologic role of bile regurgitation in esophageal cancer remains controversial. Therefore, the histological background of esophageal cancer after gastrectomy was investigated. Postgastrectomy esophageal cancers are more frequently located in the lower intrathoracic and abdominal esophagus, and more frequently diagnosed histologically as either well or moderately differentiated squamous cell carcinoma compared with other esophageal cancers. Five-year survival after curative or relative non-curative resection was achieved in 42% of the patients; this rate does not significantly differ from that in patients operated on for other esophageal cancers. From these results, we suspect that the histological background of the esophageal cancer after gastrectomy may be different from that of other esophageal cancers, and that bile regurgitation to the esophagus may have a causative role in esophageal cancer.

Esophageal reconstruction with vascularized colon is most frequently used in the patient who has undergone gastrectomy. However, this is sometimes difficult because of adhesion of the mesocolon. Esophageal reconstruction using free jejunal transfer was performed in three patients in our series. The free jejunum transplanted to the anterior chest wall functioned satisfactorily as a reconstructed esophagus. We considered that the functions of the free jejunum transplanted to the anterior chest wall were satisfactory as a reconstructed esophagus, and that the reconstruction of the thoracic esophagus using free jejunal transfer is useful in patients in whom it is difficult to use vascularized graft because of previous gastrectomy or multiple abdominal surgery.

References

1. Attwood SEA, DeMeester TR, Bremner CG, Barlow AP, Hinder RA (1989) Alkaline gastroesophageal reflux: Implications in the development of complications in Barrett's columnar-lined lower esophagus. Surgery 106:764–770
2. Maeta M, Koga S, Andachi H, Yoshioka H, Wakatsuki T (1986) Esophageal cancer developed after gastrectomy. Surgery 99:87–91
3. Manson R, Filipe MR (1990) The aetiology of gastric stump carcinoma in the rat. Scand J Gastroenterol 25:961–965

Studies on Surgical Treatment for Esophageal Cancer After Gastrectomy

Mamoru Ueda, Toshiki Matsubara, Sakae Okumura, and Mitsumasa Nishi[1]

Introduction

In the surgical treatment for postgastrectomy esophageal cancer, the issues of the reconstructive method of the alimentary tract, the management of the remnant stomach, and the appoarch to the esophagus deserve special attention. We report the surgical results.

Patients and Methods

Between 1982 and 1991, 326 (283 male and 43 female) patients underwent esophagectomy for cancer of the esophagus of these, 19 (5.8%) had a history of distal gastrectomy. Clinical data on these 19 patients with postgastrectomy esophageal cancer are shown in Table 1. Of these 19 patients, 18 were male and 1 was female, ranging in age from 51 to 81 years (mean 65 years). Gastrectomy had been done due to peptic ulcer in 13 patients and due to stomach cancer in 6 patients. The reconstructive method after gastrectomy was Billroth-I in 17 patients, Billroth-II in 1 patient and Roux-en Y in 1 patient. The interval between gastrectomy and the diagnosis of esophageal cancer ranged from 2 years and 9 months to 30 years (mean 13 years and 4 months). Of the 19 patients, 1 manifested tumor in the upper thoracic esophagus, 13 tumors were in the middle thoracic esophagus, and 5 were in the lower thoracic esophagus (Table 2).

Operation for esophagectomy: (1) Approach to the esophagus. The esophagus was resected through laparotomy and right thoracotomy in 12 patients. Left

[1] Department of Surgery, Cancer Institute Hospital, Kami-Ikebukuro 1-37-1, Toshima-ku, Tokyo, 170 Japan

Table 1. Clinical data on 19 patients who developed esophageal cancer after gastrectomy

| Pt. no. | Age (years) | Sex | Previous gastrectomy | | Interval between gastrectomy and esophageal cancer | Location of esophageal cancer | Operation for esophagectomy | | | |
			cause	reconstruction			approach to esophagus	management of remnant stomach	substitute (route)	microvascular technique
1	74	M	Ulcer	Billroth-I	24 yr	Lower thoracic	Lt. thoracoabdominal	Removed	Jejunum (intra-tho.)	
2	58	M	Ulcer	Billroth-I	7 yr 6 mo	Middle thoracic	Rt. thoracotomy, laparotomy	Anastomosed	Left colon (ante-tho.)	
3	53	M	Ulcer	Billroth-I	12 yr	Upper thoracic	Rt. thoracotomy, laparotomy	Without anastomosis	Left colon (ante-tho.)	
4	73	M	Ulcer	Billroth-I	10 yr 7 mo	Middle thoracic	Rt. thoracotomy, laparotomy	Without anastomosis	Jejunum (ante-tho.)	
5	56	M	Ulcer	Billroth-II	7 yr 3 mo	Middle thoracic	Rt. thoracotomy, laparotomy	Removed	Left colon (ante-tho.)	
6	58	M	Ulcer	Billroth-I	20 yr	Middle thoracic	Rt. thoracotomy, laparotomy	Removed	Left colon (ante-tho.)	
7	52	M	Ulcer	Billroth-I	2 yr 9 mo	Lower thoracic	Lt. thoracoabdominal	Removed	Jejunum (intra-tho.)	
8	69	M	Ulcer	Billroth-I	18 yr	Middle thoracic	Rt. thoracotomy, laparotomy	Anastomosed	Right colon (ante-tho.)	+
9	74	M	Ulcer	Billroth-I	24 yr	Middle thoracic	Transhiatal without thoracotomy	Anastomosed	Right colon (post. media.)	+
10	72	M	Ulcer	Billroth-I	30 yr	Middle thoracic	Rt. thoracotomy, laparotomy	Anastomosed	Right colon (ante-tho.)	+
11	58	M	Ulcer	Billroth-I	11 yr 7 mo	Middle thoracic	Rt. thoracotomy, laparotomy	Anastomosed	Right colon (ante-tho.)	+
12	59	M	Ulcer	Billroth-I	27 yr	Middle thoracic	Rt. thoracotomy, laparotomy	Anastomosed	Ileum (ante-tho.)	
13	61	M	Ulcer	Billroth-I	5 yr	Middle thoracic	Lt. thoracoabdominal	Anastomosed	Left colon (ante-tho.)	
14	73	M	Cancer	Roux-en Y	5 yr 1 mo	Lower thoracic	Rt. thoracotomy, laparotomy	Removed	Right colon (ante-tho.)	
15	62	F	Cancer	Billroth-I	5 yr	Middle thoracic	Rt. thoracotomy, laparotomy	Anastomosed	Right colon (retro-ster.)	
16	55	M	Cancer	Billroth-I	7 yr 5 mo	Middle thoracic	Rt. thoracotomy, laparotomy	Anastomosed	Right colon (ante-tho.)	
17	81	M	Cancer	Billroth-I	19 yr 5 mo	Lower thoracic	Lt. thoracotomy	Without anastomosis	Ileum (ante-tho.)	+
18	72	M	Cancer	Billroth-I	5 yr 1 mo	Middle thoracic	Rt. thoracotomy	Without anastomosis	Ileum (ante-tho.)	
19	66	M	Cancer	Billroth-I	12 yr	Lower thoracic	Lt. thoracoabdominal	Anastomosed	Right colon (ante-tho.)	+

tho, thoracic; ster, sternal; yr, years; mo, months; Lt, left; Rt, right

Table 2. Tumor location in esophagectomy patients and gastrectomized patients (1982–1991 CIH)

Tumor location	Esophagectomy patients	Gastrectomized patients (%)
Cervical es.	5	
Upper thoracic es.	42	1 (2.4%)
Middle thoracic es.	176	13 (7.4%)
Lower thoracic es.	102	5 (4.9%)
Esophagogastric junction	1	
Total	326	19 (5.8%)

es, esophagus; *CIH*, Cancer Institute Hospital

thoracoabdominal approach was selected for limited operation in two patients who were preoperatively diagnosed as having superficial carcinoma (T1) and in two patients with far extended disease. Esophagectomy was done only through thoracotomy in two elder patients to avoid upper abdominal manipulation of a severe adhesion which developed after gastrectomy for stomach cancer, and lymphadenectomy was done through the hiatus and the diaphragma. The transhiatal approach without thoracotomy was selected in one patient who was diagnosed with mucosal cancer preoperatively. (2) Management of the remnant stomach. The remnant stomach was removed in five patients, anastomosed with a substitute in ten patients, and left without anastomosis in four patients. Involvement of perigastric nodes was present in five patients, and all had been operated on due to peptic ulcer. In all of these patients save one, the remnant stomach was removed. (3) Reconstruction of the alimentary tract. The esophagus was substituted with the right colon in seven patients, the left colon in six, the jejunum in three, and the ileum in three patiens. Routes of substitution were through ante-thoracic in 15 patients, retrosternal in 1, intra-thoracic in 2, and posterior mediastinal in 1. Microscopic vascular anastomosis was applied in 6 patients (Table 1).

Results

Treatment Morbidity

Operation mortality was 1 of 19 (5%): a 74-year-old man with lower thoracic esophageal cancer, operated through the left thoracoabdominal approach. The remnant stomach was removed and jejunum was brought up through the intra-thoracic route. Postoperative acute cardiac and renal failure resulted in death on the 7th day after surgery (case 1). Two of the 19 patients died in the 4th month due to pneumonia and liver metastasis, respectively (cases 15 and 5). The hospital mortality was 3/19 (16%).

The most common postoperative complication was anastomotic leakage or necrosis, which occured in nine patients (47%). Though one of the nine patients died of pneumonia in the 4th month, eight patients were successfully treated with minor reconstructive operations and conservative methods.

Table 3. Pathological stage-TNM classification, surgical complications and result

Patient no.	T	N	M	stage	Complications leakage	Complications others	Result alive/dead (interval)	Cause
1	3	1	1 (LYM) (OTH)	IV		cardiac failure renal failure	D (7d)	MOF
2	2	0	0	II A	+	ileus	D (1y 3m)	recur.
3	1	1	0	II B	+	pneumothorax	D (4y 6m)	recur.
4	4	X	0	III (R2)			D (3m)	recur.
5	0ª	1	1 (LYM)	IV			D (4m)	recur.
6	3	1	0	III			D (2y 9m)	recur.
7	4	1	1 (LYM)	IV			D (5m)	recur.
8	3ª	0	0	II A		pneumonia	A (3y 8m)	
9	Tis	0	0	0		pneumonia. pulmo. embolism	D (5m)	pneumonia
10	3	0	0	II A		ileus	D (2y)	malnutrition
11	3ª	0	1 (LYM)	IV	+		A (2y 4m)	
12	3	1	0	III	+		A (2y 2m)	
13	1	0	0	I			A (1y 10m)	
14	3	1	0	III	+		D (8y)	malnutrition
15	2	0	0	II a	+		D (4m)	pneumonia
16	1	0	0	I	+		A (3y 11m)	
17	3	1	0	III	+		A (2y 3m)	
18	1	1	1 (LYM)	IV			D (9m)	recur.
19	1	1	0	II b			A (8m)	

ª preoperatively irradiated

T, tumor; N, node; M, metastasis; LYM, lymph node; OTH, other; MOF, multi-organ failure; recur, recurrent; d, days; m, months; y, years

Table 4. Distribution of involved lymph nodes in esophageal cancer after gastrectomy

Patient no.	Cause of previous gastrectomy	Perigastric nodes	Middle and lower mediastinal nodes	Recurrent nerve nodes	Neck	Others
1	ulcer	+	+			
2	ulcer			+		
3	ulcer	+		+	+	
4	ulcer	+	+	+		
5	ulcer	+	+			Mesenteric nodes
6[a]	ulcer				+	
7	ulcer	+				
8	cancer		+			
9	cancer		+			
10	cancer		+	+	+	
11	cancer			+		

[a] preoperative irradiation of 70 Gy

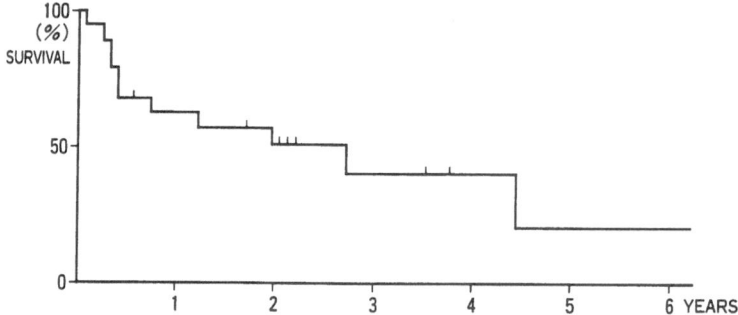

Fig. 1. Kaplan-Meier survival curves for 19 patients who underwent esophagectomy after distal gastrectomy

Pathological Staging

Histologically, all cancers were squamous cell carcinomas. The pathological stage was 0 in one patient, I in two, IIA in four, IIB in two, III in five, and IV in five (Table 3).

Except for one patient undergoing palliative operation due to cancer infiltration of the left main bronchus (case 4), lymph nodes were systematically dissected. Eleven (61%) of them had involved lymph nodes. There was no abdominal involvement in patients who had undergone gastrectomy due to gastric cancer (Table 4). This result suggests that in patients who were operated on for gastric cancer, perigastric lymphadenectomy can be omitted to reduce the degree of operative invasion.

Survival

Twelve of 19 patients died: seven died of their disease and five died of unrelated causes (one, multi-organ failure; two, pneumonia; two malnutrition). There was no cancer recurrence either in perigastric nodes or at the preserved remnant stomach. Seven patients (37%) are currently alive without disease intervals ranging from 8 to 47 months after esophagectomy. The Kaplan-Meier survival for 19 patients is depicted in Fig. 1. The 1-, 2-, 3- and 5-year survival rates were 63%, 51%, 40%, and 20%, respectively.

Discussion

Primary esophageal cancer patients who had previously undergone gastrectomy have been increasing in number recently. In particular, the number of patients who priviously underwent gastrectomy due to gastric cancer has been increasing faster than patients who underwent gastrectomy due to peptic ulcer because the treatment result of gastric cancer have been improving. Of 19 patients with previously gastrectomy esophageal cancer in our hospital, 6 (32%) had undergone gastrectomy due to gastric cancer.

The hospital mortality reported to esophageal cancer operation after gastrectomy patients were high: Nakayama et al. [1] and Konno et al. [2] reported 13% and 38%, respectively. Postoperative complications reported by Nakayama et al. [1] occured 65% of the time, and the most common postoperative complication was anastomotic leakage and necrosis. In our hospital, the hospital mortality was 16%. Postoperative complications occured 58% of the time, and postoperative anastotic troubles occured in 47%.

The distribution of involved nodes with cancer of the thoracic esophagus undergoing systematic dissection of lymph nodes, including cervical nodes, was reported by Matsubara [3] to be quite frequent along the recurrent laryngeal nerves or to the perigastric nodes. Nakayama et al. [1] reported that patients who had undergone gastrectomy due to gastric cancer had fewer involved perigastric nodes than patients who had undergone gastrectomy due to peptic ulcer. In our experiments, none of the patients who had undergone gastrectomy due to gastric cancer involved perigastric nodes which had been dissected during previous gastrectomy except for the left paracardiac nodes. In patients after gastrectomy due to gastric cancer, we think it may be necessary to dissect the left paracardiac nodes. Transthoracic dissection of that regions through hiatus and diaphragma is justified in high risk patients.

References

1. Nakayama R, Aoki A, Okazeri S, Kimura Y, Bessho T, Asagoe T, Asanuma F, Ueno S, Kuromizu J (1981) A study on surgery for carcinoma of the esophagus in the postgastrectomized patients (in Japanese). Jpn J Gastroenterol Surg 14:1267–1278
2. Konno O, Watanabe M, Abe T, Yago N, Watanabe Z, Endo Y, Inoue H, Motoki R, Teranishi Y (1989) Studies on surgical treatment of esophageal carcinoma occuring after gastrectomy (in Japanese). Jpn J Gastroenterol Surg 22:2188–2193
3. Matsubara T (1992) Pattern of lymphatic spreading in cancer of the thoracic esophagus (in Japanese). J Jpn Surg Society 93:377–387

Multimodality Treatment
for Esophageal Cancer

Leucovorin, Cisplatin, and 5-Fluorouracil for Advanced Esophageal Cancer

Toshiro Konishi, Toru Hirata, Mamoru Hiraishi, Ken-ichi Mafune, Takeshi Miyama, Kiyoshi Mori, Haruhiro Nishina, and Yasuo Idezuki[1]

Introduction

Biochemical modulation involves the use of one drug (modulating agent; modulator) to change the pharmacokinetics and/or pharmacodynamics of a cytotoxic agent (effector), in a way that the therapeutic index of the effector is enhanced [1]. The modulator is often also a cytotoxic agent, but a non-cytotoxic agent like leucovorin is sometimes used as well. The modulating agent improves selectivity or sensitivity of an effector and decreases its toxicity to normal cells via a biochemical or metabolical mechanism. Currently, several biochemical modulations such as the sequential methotrexate (MTX)/5-fluorouracil (5-FU), leucovorin (LV)/5-FU, and cisplatin (CDDP)/5-FU have been evaluated clinically in terms of their efficacy for alimentary tract malignancies.

Recently, we performed chemotherapy with a dual biochemical modulation using CDDP/LV/5-FU for treating advanced esophageal cancer. The mechanism of the dual biochemical modulation of 5-FU with CDDP and LV is such that inhibition of methionine transport into cells by CDDP increases with the concentrations of intracellular reduced folate [2] and LV [3]. Increased levels of reduced folate inhibit DNA synthesis in the tumor cells by forming a stable ternary complex conjugating with fluorodeoxyuridine monophosphate (FdUMP) and thymidylate synthetase (TS). Although several reports on CDDP/LV/5-FU in squamous cell carcinoma of the head and neck have been published [4, 5], few papers about its efficacy in esophageal cancer are published. Herein, we report our recent study on the dual biochemical modulation of 5-FU with CDDP and LV in squamous cell carcinoma of advanced esophageal cancer.

---

[1] The Second Department of Surgery, Faculty of Medicine, University of Tokyo, 7-3-1 Hongo, Bunkyo-ku, Tokyo, 113 Japan

Table 1. Grade of toxicity of CDDP/LV/5-FU according to WHO criteria

	Leukocytopenia	Thrombo-cytopenia	Anorexia	Nausea, vomiting	Diarrhea	Alopecia
1	4 (+GCSF)					
2	3	1	1	2	1	
3	3			1	1	
4			1	1		2
5	4 (+GCSF)		2			2
6	3 (+GCSF)		2		2	

GCSF, granulocyte colony stimulating factor; *CDDP*, cisplatin; *LV*, leucovorin; *5-FU*, 5-fluorouracil

Methods and Patients

Between March 1990 and May 1992, six patients were registered on this protocol. Of the six patients, three had inoperable advanced esophageal cancers with either abdominal lymph node metastases or multiple pulmonary metastases. Two patients had recurrent cancers at the lung and liver or the distant lymph nodes after esophagectomy and another patient was given this treatment as a postoperative adjuvant chemotherapy after palliative resection of the esophageal cancer. All patients had histologically proven squamous cell carcinoma.

The chemotherapy protocol consisted of cisplatin, $50\,mg/m^2$, administered intravenously during over 6 h, followed immediately by leucovorin $30\,mg/m^2$ per day and 5-FU at $500\,mg/m^2$ per day, both by bolus intravenous injection for 5 days. Customarily, sufficient hydration and antiemetic regimens were administered during the treatment and each cycle was repeated every 4 weeks.

In each lesion, the response to this treatment was analyzed from the following standard criteria. Complete response (CR) of a lesion was defined as 100% disappearance of a measurable tumor with a lack of tumor-related symptoms for a minimum of 4 weeks. A partial response (PR) was recorded as ≥50% reduction in the product of the two longest perpendicular diameters of the measurable tumor(s), persisting at least 4 weeks.

Results

Toxicity of this treatment in six patients, analyzed according to the WHO toxicity criteria, is summarized in Table 1. There was no toxic death. Grade 4 leukocytopenia was seen in two patients and grade 3 in three patients. Three patients received grenulocyte colony-stimulating factor (GCSF) administration to treat leukocytopenia. Thrombocytopenia or complaints from disturbance on alimentary tract such as anorexia, nausea, vomiting, and diarrhea were not severe in any of the patients. Two patients showed grade 2 alopecia which was the limiting factor of this treatment in both patients. Stomatitis or renal failure were not seen in our patients.

Therapeutic activities of this treatment are summarized in Table 2. Of six patients, four could be evaluated for response. In three inoperable patients who were judged unresectable due to the presence of distant metastases, all primary

Table 2. Therapeutic effect of CDDP/LV/5-FU on each lesion

	Site	Response (% reduction)	Duration (months)	Prognosis
1	Esophagus	CR (100%)	4	5 months, dead
	Liver hilus	PR		(other d.)
2	Esophagus	PR (83.7%)	6	11 months dead
	Pulmonary	NC		(pulm., liver)
3	Pulmonary	PR (86.1%)	6	11 months, dead
	Liver	CR (100%)		(pulmonary)
4	Non-evaluable	—	—	1 year alive
5	Esophagus	PR (84%)	2	6 months, dead
	Lymph node	PR		(cerebral, mediastinum)
6	Non-evaluable	—	—	2 months alive

CR, complete response; PR, partial response; pulm, pulmonary; d, disease

lesions at the esophagus showed good response to this treatment (1 CR and 2 PR). In the three patients, metastasized lymph nodes at the hepatic hilum or around the abdominal aorta showed remarkable improvement (PR) after this treatment. In one recurrent patient, liver metastasis showed complete response and pulmonary metastasis partially responded to this treatment.

Case 1 (Inoperable Case)

A 69-year-old male had a squamous cell cancer at the middle portion of thoracic esophagus (Fig. 1a), accompanied with obstructive jaundice caused from complete obstruction of the common bile duct with enlarged lymph node at the hepatic hilum. Complete disappearance of esophageal cancer was proven with both esophagogram and esophagoscopy with biopsy after 2 cycles (Fig. 1b). A percutaneous transhepatic cholangiography (PTC) drainage tube was removed successfully after recovery of patency of the bile duct.

Case 2 (Inoperable Case)

A 49-year-old male received 2 cycles of this treatment for inoperable squamous cell cancer at the middle thoracic esophagus, accompanied with multiple pulmonary metastases. Although lesions in the bilateral lung did not show any change after the treatment, the primary lesion at the esophagus showed PR (reduction rate 83.7%), which continued for 6 months.

Case 3 (Recurrent Case)

A recurrent pulmonary lesion, found 1 year after esophagectomy in a 69-year-old male, showed PR with complete disappearance of a metastatic lesion in the liver. However, after 6 cycles of this treatment, a pulmonary metastasis enlarged again and 11 months after initiation of this treatment, he died from pulmonary metastases.

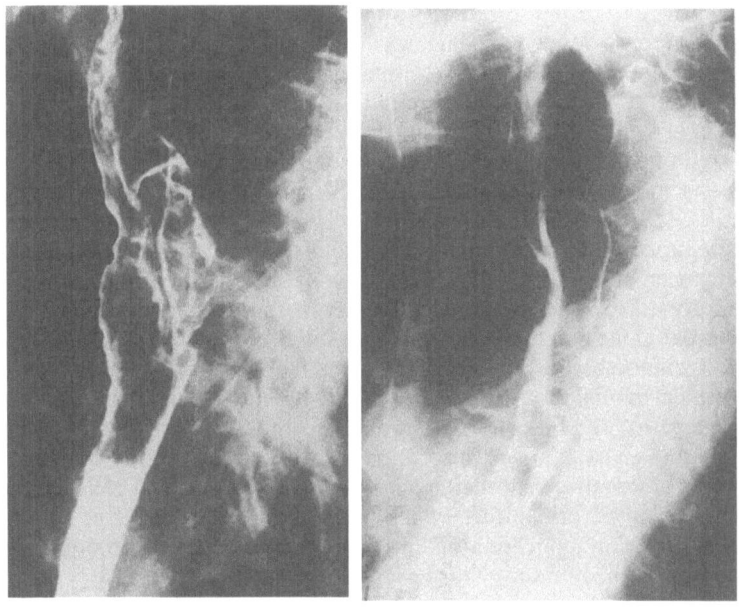

Fig. 1a,b. Complete disappearance of squamous cell cancer at the middle portion of thoracic esophagus, as seen on esophagogram (case 1)

Case 5 (Inoperable Case)

Partial response to this treatment during the period of 2 months was seen in the esophageal cancer and enlarged lymph nodes around the abdominal aorta in a 48-year-old male. His back pain caused from enlarged lymph node metastases was alleviated after this treatment.

Cases 4 and 6 could not be evaluated for response. Three inoperable patients, although the primary and metastatic lesions showed remarkable response, did not agree to receive the surgical treatment after relief of complaints from improvement of cancer lesions.

Discussion

Several biochemical modulations such as the sequential MTX/5-FU in advanced gastric cancer or LV/5-FU in colorectal cancer, have remarkably enhanced the cytotoxicity of 5-FU. However, this treatment has not yet revealed satisfactory efficacy to squamous cell cancer of esophagus [6]. Therefore, we started the newly developed dual biochemical modulation to evaluate both its efficacy and toxicity in the advanced esophageal cancer patients. Although several reports indicated superior efficacy of CDDP/LV/5-FU in treating squamous cell head and neck cancer [4, 5], no paper has reported on superiority of this treatment in esophageal cancer, except for a recent paper by Hayashi et al. [7], which reported a 72% response rate in 18 patients. From our result, a high incidence of grade 3 or 4 leukocytopenia was seen (in five of six patients). However, leukocytopenia was controllable with administration of GCSF, and symptoms of the alimentary tract, including stomatitis, were not severe. In our preliminary trial, renal failure was not seen and alopecia which occurred in 2 patients, was the limiting factor which prevented the continuation of this treatment.

This treatment may be almost tolerable in the advanced esophageal cancer patients. Although the duration of effect is not sufficiently long and the number of patients is not large enough to evaluate efficacy of this treatment in esophageal cancer, all patients who had evaluable lesions for this treatment showed good response. In this trial, a wide variety of cancerous lesions, such as primary esophageal cancer or metastatic lymph nodal, hepatic and pulmonary lesions, showed remarkable improvement after treatment. We would like to stress a dual biochemical modulation of 5-FU with combination of cisplatin and leucovorin shows superior response in treating the squamous cell carcinoma of esophagus with tolerable toxicity. We now anticipate this treatment as the pre- or postoperative adjuvant chemotherapy for advanced esophageal cancer. Decreasing occurrence of adverse effect of leukocytopenia or alopecia in this treatment may lead to safe application of this novel dual biochemical modulation on the perioperative chemotherapy for esophageal cancer.

References

1. Howell SB (1986) Biochemical modulation: Current status and considerations for the future. In: Kimura K, Yamada K, Krakoff IH, Carter SK (eds) Cancer Chemotherapy—challenges for the future. Excerpta Medica, pp 108–116
2. Scanlon KJ, Newman EM, Priest DG (1986) Biochemical basis for cisplatin and 5-fluorouracil synergism in human ovarian carcinoma cells. Proc Natl Acad Sci USA 83:8923–8925
3. O'Dwyer PJ, Cornfeld MJ, Peter R, Comis RL (1990) Phase I trial of 5-fluorouracil, leucovorin, and cisplatin in combination. Cancer Chemother Pharmacol 27:131–134
4. Vokes EE, Choi KE, Schilsky RL, Moran WJ, Guarnieri CM, Weichselbaum RR, Panje WR (1988) Cisplatin, fluorouracil, and high-dose leucovorin for recurrent or metastatic head and neck cancer. J Clin Oncol 6:618–626
5. Clark J, Dreyfuss A, Norris C, Busse P, Miller D, Lucarini J, Andersen J, Casey D, Frei E (1990) Continuous infusion cisplatin, 5-FU and high-dose leucovorin (PEL): favorable early results as induction therapy for squamous cell carcinoma of the head and neck. Proc ASCO 9:172
6. Browman GP, Archibald SD, Young JEM, Hryniuk WM, Russell R, Kiehl K, Levine MN (1983) Prospective randomized trial of one-hour sequential versus simultaneous methotrexate plus 5-fluorouracil in advanced and recurrent squamous cell head and neck cancer. J Clin Oncol 1:787–792
7. Hayashi K, Ide H, Shinoda M, Fukushima M (1992) Phase II study of cisplatin (CDDP) plus 5-fluorouracil (5-FU) and leucovorin (LCV) for squamous cell carcinoma of the esophagus. Proc ASCO 11:178

Neoadjuvant Treatment for Squamous Carcinoma of the Thoracic Esophagus

ERNESTO LATERZA, UGO S. URSO, GIOVANNI DE' MANZONI,
and CLAUDIO CORDIANO[1]

Introduction

Cancer of the esophagus has a poor prognosis. Survival rates appear to be correlated with depth of tumor invasion (T), lymph node involvement (N) and the presence of distant metastases (M). The biological behavior of the disease, characterized by early regional lymphatic spread, make it a systemic disease and explains the poor results of surgery and radiotherapy. In the last 20 years, survival rates for esophageal cancer have been less than 10% [1–2]. To obtain better results, several authors suggested many trials of different treatments including chemotherapy.

Kelsen et al. [3] and Steiger et al. [4] presented the first results of combined radiotherapy (RT), chemotherapy (ChT) and surgery, showing a complete histological response in a proportion of patients.

At our Institution, we used the Wayne State Medical University protocol of preoperative neoadjuvant radiochemotherapy [5] on 70 patients with squamous cell carcinoma (SCC) of the thoracic esophagus. Our aim was to evaluate the benefit of preoperative chemoradiotherapy on the subsequent ease of resection of locally advanced disease and assess the effect on long-term survival.

Material and Methods

From June 1987 to March 1992, 70 patients with SCC of the thoracic esophagus were entered into the study (Prot. No 01-87) (Table 1). Criteria for eligibility were as follows: age less than 70 years, no evidence of distant metastasis or tracheobronchial invasion, absence of synchronous and metachronous neoplasms,

---

[1] The First Department of General Surgery, University of Verona—Ospedale Maggiore P.le Stefani, 1 VERONA 37126, Italy

Table 1. Patient and tumor characteristics in 70 patients undergoing multimodality therapy for esophageal SCC. June 1987–March 1992

Patients	
Sex ratio (M/F); 10.6/1	
Mean age (Years); 58.4 (range 41–70)	
Tumor location	**No. of cases (%)**
Proximal third	14 (20.0)
Middle third	30 (42.8)
Distal third	26 (37.2)
Admission clinical staging (cT)	
T0	0
T1	2 (2.8)
T2	8 (11.5)
T3	34 (48.5)
T4	26 (37.3)

SCC, squamous cell carcinoma

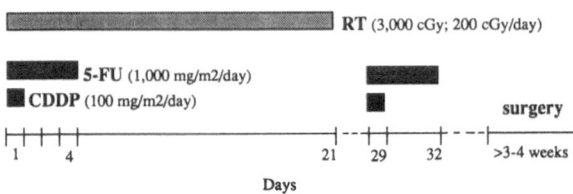

Fig. 1. Multimodality treatment plan *RT*, radiotherapy; *5-FU*, 5 fluorouracil; *CDDP*, cisplatin

absence of esophago-tracheal fistula, adequate bone marrow reserves (white blood cell count >3500/nl, platelets >100000/nl), absence of renal failure (serum creatinine <1.5 mg% and creatinine clearance >50–65 ml/min).

Patients with adenocarcinoma and hypopharyngeal and/or cervical carcinoma of the esophagus were excluded from the study. Male/female ratio was 10.6/1 (64 males and 6 females), and mean age was 58.4 years (range 41–70).

Before and 1 week after neoadjuvant treatment, patients were staged as follows: chest x-ray, barium esophagogram, esophagoscopy with biopsy, esophageal endosonography (EUS) and thoraco-abdominal computed tomographic (CT) scan. In addition, patients with upper or midesophageal cancer underwent bronchoscopy to rule out tracheal or main stem bronchus involvement.

Preoperative (cTNM), post-chemoradiotherapy (yTNM) and histopathological (pTNM) stagings were performed according to the criteria outlined by the Japanese Committee for Registration of Esophageal Disease [6]. The treatment regimen is outlined in Fig. 1.

After a variable time (mean 25 days, range 18–63 days) from the end of the last cycle of ChT, 56 patients (80%) underwent surgery. The surgical technique was chosen according to the site and the extension of the tumor, respiratory function and the general medical condition of the patient. (Table 2).

Table 2. Tumor resectability and surgical approach

	No. of cases
Resectability: 87.5% (49/56 patients)	
Operation	
Exploration	
Thoracic (endoprosthesis)	4
Abdominal (endoprosthesis)	2
Colic bypass	1
Resection	
Right thoracic and abdominal	23
Right thoracic, abdominal and cervical	19
Cervical and abdominal (transhiatal)	6
Trans-sternal (Ong procedure)	1
Total	56

The following patients received further postoperative ChT and RT (consisting of one more cycle of 5-FU and cisplatin and an additional 2000–3000 cGy of radiation): patients unsuitable for surgery, patients with unresectable disease, or those who underwent only palliative resection (residual mediastinal disease, residual disease at the proximal stump, positive non-resectable metastatic nodes). Complete follow-up (every 3 months) was obtained in all patients except one.

Results

The preoperative treatment was generally well tolerated. It was completed in 91.4% of the patients (64/70). In six patients, the treatment was interrupted because of severe complications and/or poor patient compliance (four severe cases of myelosuppression and two cases of RT-induced esophagitis). Toxicity was evaluated using standard World Health Organization (WHO) criteria. Of all the patients 35.9% presented with moderate nausea and vomiting, 31.2% had moderate myelosuppression, 9.3% moderate renal failure and 6.2% of patients a moderate esophagitis. Fourteen patients (20%) did not undergo surgery: one patient died after completion of the neoadjuvant treatment because of acute myocardial infarction, six patients were judged not suitable for surgery after restaging (three because of metastatic disease, and three because of deterioration of clinical conditions). Seven patients who had complete relief of dysphagia refused surgery.

The operability rate was 90%, (including patients who refused surgery), and 49/56 patients underwent esophagectomy (resectability rate 87.5%): 5 patients were found to be unresectable because of regional neoplastic diffusion for contiguity to mediastinal periesophageal structures, and 2 because of unresectable upper abdominal node metastasis. In all these patients, except for one who received a palliative esophageal colon bypass, an endoscopic prosthesis was placed (Table 3).

Twenty-nine patients (29/49, 59.1%) underwent operation with a curative intent (radical esophagectomy). In the remaining 20 patients (40.9%) it was impossible to entirely remove the tumor (residual disease) and metal clips were

Table 3. Surgical mortality and morbidity in resected patients

Postoperative mortality (within 30 days)	12.2% (6/49 patients)
Postoperative morbidity	No. of cases (%)
Pulmonary	12 (24.4)
Anastomotic leak	
Cervical anastomosis	8 (16.3)
Thoracic anastomosis	3 (6.1)
Chylothorax	1 (2.0)
Gastric outlet obstruction	1 (2.0)

Table 4. Postoperative histopathological tumor, node, metastasis (*pTNM*) stage in 57 patients (56 after surgery and 1 after autopsy)

Stage	TNM	No. of cases (%)
0	T0N0M0	11 (19.3)
I	T1N0M0	5 (8.7)
II a	T2N0M0	4 (7.1)
	T3N0M0	5 (8.7)
II b	T0N1M0[a]	2 (3.5)
	T1N1M0	2 (3.5)
	T2N1M0	3 (5.2)
III	T3N1M0	7 (12.3)
	T4N1M0	15 (26.5)
IV	TxNxM1	3 (5.2)
Total		57 (100)

[a] Patients with no residual esophageal tumor, but with metastasis in regional lymph nodes

positioned at the site of residual tumor as radiological markers for postoperative radiotherapy.

In the resected cases, intraoperative there was no mortality and postoperative mortality (within 30 days) was 12.2% (6/49 patients).

Intraoperative complications occurred in four cases: A rupture of the thoracic aorta during transhiatal esophagectomy that required an immediate thoracotomy and successful repair of the aorta, and three accidental spleen tears which in two cases required splenectomy. The major postoperative complications are reported in Table 3.

The average length of post-operative hospitalization was 24 days (range 13–52 days).

Histopathological assessment was performed in 57 patients (57/70, 81.4%), 56 after surgery and 1 after autopsy. Table 4 reports the pathological TNM stage grouping. No residual tumor was found in 11 cases (19.3%) and only microscopic clusters of neoplastic cells (minimal residual disease, MRD) within the esophageal wall were found in 8 cases (14%). Histopathological evaluation of the resected lymph nodes was obtained in all the 49 patients who underwent esophagectomy (an average of 12.7 nodes per patient) and it showed a neoplastic involvement in 43.9% of those cases. In 18% (2/11) of cases with no residual primary tumor (To) regional metastatic lymph nodes were found (these cases were staged as II b).

To date, 34.7% (16/42) of the resected patients have died: 14 of neoplastic progression and 2 because of unrelated causes (cerebral stroke and myocardial infarction). In the patients who underwent curative resection the incidence of locoregional recurrence was 24.1% (seven patients): five in the mediastinal region and two at an anastomotic site. The median overall survival was 23.4 months, overall 1- and 2-year actuarial survivals were 48% and 29%, respectively, and the curve was not modified at 5 years by Kaplan-Meier method. The longest survival was 55 months (a To patient). Because of the limited number of patients, we combined in the same groups nine stage II a with seven II b patients and 7 grade T1 and 7 T2 tumors. The determination of actuarial survival curves, according to the stage and the grade of infiltration of the neoplasm into the esophageal wall (T), (Figs. 2 and 3), reveals a clear superiority of survival between the patients without residual disease (grade To and stage 0) and those with residual disease ($P = 0.001$ and $P = 0.008$, respectively). All the patients with no pathological residual disease (To, N$-$/$+$) and those with only MRD in the esophageal wall are still alive (except 1 who died before surgery from an acute myocardial infarction and 1 who died on the 6th postoperative day from respiratory failure): 13 are disease-free, 3 (2 with To and 1 with MRD) showed a mediastinal recurrence after 40, 34, and 18 months, respectively, and 1 (with MRD) had an anastomotic recurrence after 16 months.

Discussion

In the last 10 years, systemic polychemotherapy has proved to be a very useful adjuvant therapy in the treatment of squamous carcinoma of the esophagus, particularly if used in conjunction with radiotherapy and/or surgery. Results obtained using these procedures together are undoubtedly promising, although not unequivocal when compared to the results of the traditional surgical treatment; however, a number of studies show an improvement of mean and long-term survival rates when compared to traditional treatments (RT and/or surgery).

Popp and et al. [7] reported a 3-year survival rate of 29% after combined treatment, as compared to that of only 4.8% in patients treated with surgery alone. Similar results were reported by Austin et al. [8], with a 3-year survival rate of 54% and 33% in patients treated with combined therapy or surgery alone, respectively. Several other experiences report 3-year survival rates between 30% and 62% [9–12]. Other authors, such as Parker and Carolyn [13] and Poplin et al. [14], although they did not obtain the same improvement in survival, support the need for further investigations on this new method of treatment.

Data obtained in our study showed a slight improvement if compared to the results of our previous experience in which 97 patients, between 1976 and 1987, were treated with surgery alone. Median survival was, respectively, 14.9 and 7.6 months in the present and previous studies and survivals at 12 and 24 months

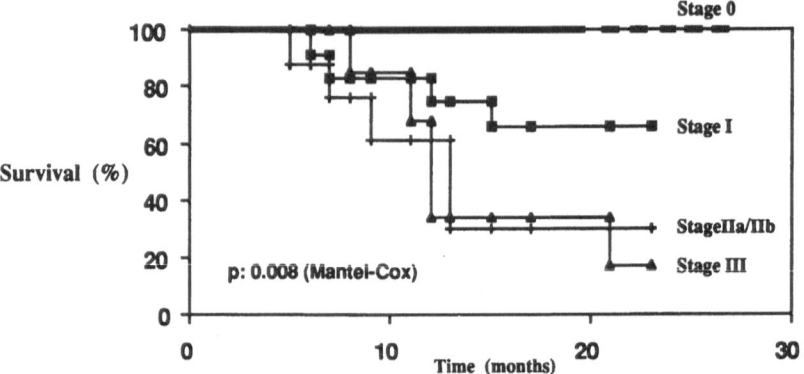

Fig. 2. Actuarial survival curves for 42 resected patients according to the histopathological stage of the disease tumor, node, metastasis (*pTNM*) Stage 0 could not be calculated because all the patients are alive

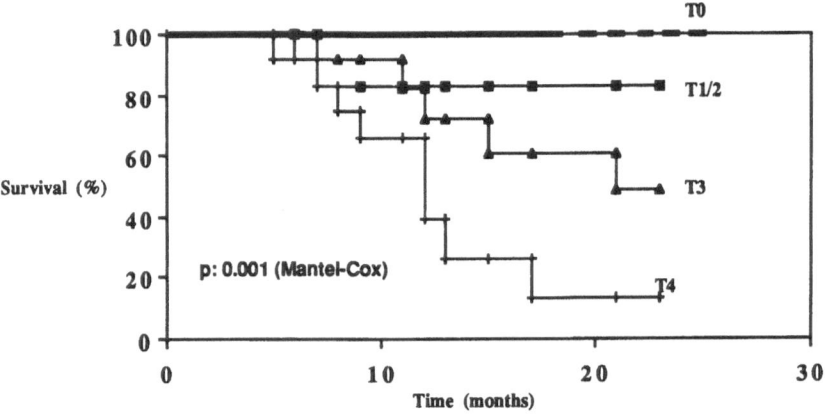

Fig. 3. Actuarial survival curves for 42 resected patients according to the grade of penetration of the tumor in the esophageal wall (*pTNM*) To could not be calculated because all the patients are alive

were 48% and 36% in this study and 29% and 19% in the previous study (the two groups are not suitable for a statistical analysis).

Another valuable aspect of the neoadjuvant preoperative treatment is the improvement of operability and resectability rates, as shown by other authors [4, 12, 15, 16]. In our study, the "down-staging" of initially unresectable tumors was 36.4% and one of these patients had no residual disease at the histological evaluation. No major side-effects were induced by chemoradiotherapy and patients showed good compliance; however, it has to be mentioned that this treatment adds to the discomfort associated with chemotherapeutic drugs, and a longer hospital stay which can deteriorate the psychological conditions of the patient (four cases of depressive syndrome).

A major interest has been raised by the cases with complete response after neoadjvant treatment. These patients account for 33% of our cases, and 17% – 56% in other studies [8–10, 12, 14, 17, 18].

Some authors, like Austin et al. [8]. McFarlane et al. [12] and Parker and Carolyn [13], do not report better results in similar groups of patients. Unexpectedly, our experience, as well as that of several others [7–11, 19], showed that the best survivals rates are obtained in these patients, with a 3-year survival rate between 70% – 100%. In our opinion, the detection of these groups of patients could influence therapeutic strategy and surgical techniques: an accurate preoperative T-staging (with a reliability similar to the histological examination), could call into question the role of surgery, as suggested by McFarlane et al. [12], or indicate other surgical options such as mediastinal lymphoadenectomy without esophagectomy, because of the possible lymphatic metastatic involvement also in To patients.

To date, the lack of such accurate staging workup, make the surgical excision of the esophagus and of the mediastinal nodes necessary so far.

References

1. Earlam R, Cunha-Melo JR (1980) Esophageal squamous cell carcinoma. A critical review of radiotherapy. Br J Surg 67:457–61
2. Launois B, Delarue D, Campion JP (1981) Preoperative radiotherapy for carcinoma of the esophagus. Surg Gynecol Obstet 153:690–2
3. Kelsen DP, Bains M, Hilaris B (1981) Cisplatin-based preoperative chemotherapy of esophageal carcinoma in adjuvant therapy of cancer. In: Salomon S, Jones (eds) Grune and Stratton, New York, pp 495–502
4. Steiger Z, Franklin R, Wilson R (1981) Eradication and palliation of squamous cell carcinoma of the esophagus with chemotherapy, radiotherapy and surgical therapy. J Thorac Cardiovasc Surg 82:713
5. Herskovic A, Leichman L, Lattin P (1988) Chemo/radiation with and without surgery in the thoracic esophagus: The Wayne State Experience. Int J Rad Oncol Biol Phis 15: 655–662
6. Japanese Committee for Registration of Esophageal Carcinoma (1985) A proposal for a new TNM classification of esophageal carcinoma. Jpn J Clin Oncol 14:655–662
7. Popp MB, Hawley D, Reiseng J (1986) Improved survival in squamous esophageal cancer. Arch Surg 121:1330–5
8. Austin JC, Postier RG, Elkins RC (1986) Treatment of esophageal cancer: The continued need for surgical resection. Am J Surg 152:592–596
9. Orringer MB, Forastiere AA, Perez-Tamayo C (1990) Chemotherapy and radiation therapy before transhiatal esophagectomy for esophageal carcinoma. Ann Thorac Surg 49:348–55
10. Lackey VL, Reagan MT, Smith RA (1989) Neoadjuvant therapy of squamous cell carcinoma: Role of resection and benefit in partial responders. Ann Thorac Surg 48:218–221
11. Hilgenberg AD, Carey RW, Wilkins EW, Choi NC, Mathinsen DJ, Grillo HC (1988) Preoperative chemotherapy, surgical resection, and selective postoperative therapy for squamous cell carcinoma of the esophagus. Ann Thorac Surg 45:357–6
12. McFarlane SD, Lucius DH, Jolly PC, Kozarek RA, Anderson RP (1988) Improved results of surgical treatment for esophageal and gastroesophageal junction carcinomas after preoperative combined chemotherapy and radiation. J Thorac Cardiovasc Surg 95:415–22
13. Parker EF, Carolyn ER (1989) Chemotherapy, radiation therapy, and resection for carcinoma of the esophagus. J Thorac Cardiovasc Surg 98:1037–44

14. Poplin E, Fleming T, Leichman L (1987) Combined therapies for squamous cell carcinoma of the esophagus: a Southwest Oncology Group Study (SWOG-8037). J Clin Oncol 5: 622–628

15. Peracchia A, Debesi B, Castoro C (1989) Results of surgery after cisplatin and 5-fluorouracil combination chemotherapy for locally advanced esophageal squamous cell carcinoma. Fourth world congress of the International Society for Diseases of the Esophagus. Chicago, September

16. Campbell WR, Taylor SA, Pierce GE, Hermrelk AS, Thomas JH (1985) Therapeutic alternative in patients with esophageal cancer. Annual meeting Southwestern Surgical Congress, Las Vegas, April

17. Leichman L, Berry BT (1991) Experience with cisplatin in treatment regimens for esophageal cancer. Semin Oncol 18:64–72

18. Stewart FM, Harkins BJ, Hahn SS (1989) Cisplatin, 5-fluorouracil, mitomycin C, and concurrent radiation therapy with and without esophagectomy for esophageal carcinoma. Cancer 64:622–628

19. Al-Sarraf M (1990) The current status of combined modality treatment containing chemotherapy in patients with esophageal cancer. Int J Radiat Oncol Biol Phys 19:813–815

Radical Radiotherapy for Inoperable Locally Advanced Esophageal Carcinoma: A Retrospective Analysis of the Treatment Results over 21-Years Experience

Tomohiko Okawa, Makiko Tanaka, Midori Kita-Okawa, Yuko Kaneyasu, Kumiko Karasawa, Ichiro Maruyama, and Kasumi Yoshikawa[1]

Introduction

Patients with inoperable advanced esophageal carcinoma are treated with radiotherapy with or without chemotherapy. In general, the 5-year survival rate is about 10% or lower for the patients curatively irradiated. This poor result is caused by the low local control rate and the high incidence of regional recurrence and distant metastasis. In contrast, in the cases of early esophageal cancer, favorable results of radical radiotherapy have been obtained which are comparable to surgery. Radiotherapy has been used for the local treatment of advanced or medically inoperable esophageal cancer for a long time.

In this report, the results of radiotherapy of our department are analyzed retrospectively, factors influencing survival are examined and the role of radiotherapy in the treatment of esophageal cancer is discussed.

Methods

During the 21 years, between 1968 and 1988, 2222 patients with esophageal carcinoma were registered by our department. Among these, the most common approach was pre- or postoperative radiotherapy with radical surgery followed by palliative radiotherapy for advanced state. The third group of 328 patients were treated by radical radiotherapy, which meant no distant lymph node or organ metastasis outside the radiation field, and these patients had no indication for radical surgery because of locally advanced tumor and/or medically inoperable tumor due to severe complications or poor performance status. These patients were given an irradiation dose of 60 Gy/6w : TDF96 or higher. Double primary cancer and multicentric cancer were used in eligible cases.

[1] Department of Radiology Tokyo Women's Medical College, 8-1 Kawada-cho, Shinjuku-ku, Tokyo, 162 Japan

Table 1. Patient and tumor characteristics of squamous cell carcinoma of the esophagus (TWMC 1968–1988, *n* 328)

Sex	Male	264
	Female	64
Age	Range 42–88 years	Mean 70.6
Location	CE	34
	UT	45
	MT	178
	LT	58
	AE	13
Length	< 5 cm	75
	5–10 cm	189
	> 10 cm	64
T (1978 UICC)	T1	59
	T2	168
	T3	101

CE, cervical esophagus; *UT*, upper thoracic esophagus; *MT*, middle thoracic esophagus; *LT*, lower thoracic esophagus; *AE*, abdominal esophagus; *TWMC*, Tokyo Women's Medical College

Patient and tumor characteristics of the 328 patients receiving radical radiotherapy are shown in Table 1. There were 264 males and 64 females, with a male:female ratio of 4.1:1. Ages ranged from 42 to 88 years with a mean of 70.6 years. Tumor length ranged from 2–18 cm with a mean of 8.0 cm. T classification by UICC (1978), 59 cases (18%) were classified for T1, 168 cases (51%) for T2, and 101 cases (31%) for T3.

The radiation field included a minimum 3-cm safety margin from the superior and inferior edge of the tumor and the width was sufficient to include the mediastinum. Since 1978, computed tomography (CT) scanning has been used to confirm the field of radiation. In principle, prophylatic irradiation of the regional lymph nodes was not performed, except in cases in which lymph node swelling was detected by CT. Radiotherapy was started with parallel-opposed anterior and posterior fields with 2 Gy fraction dose, five times a week. To avoid excessive irradiation of the spinal cord, the radiation method was changed to two posterior oblique portals, a four-field or rotation technique at 40–46 Gy. A large volume of the lung was also avoided. Total dose was 60–70 Gy/6–7 weeks (average: 66 Gy/6.5 weeks). The survival rate was calculated by the life table method (cumulative survival rate) and an evaluation of statistical significance was assessed according to the χ^2 test.

Results

Sex. Overall 5-year survival rates were 8.7%, and 5.4% in males and 21.9% in females indicating a significantly higher survival in females ($P < 0.01$) (Fig. 1).

Tumor location. Survival rate of abdominal esophagus was poor, but there was no significant difference in survival rate by tumor location.

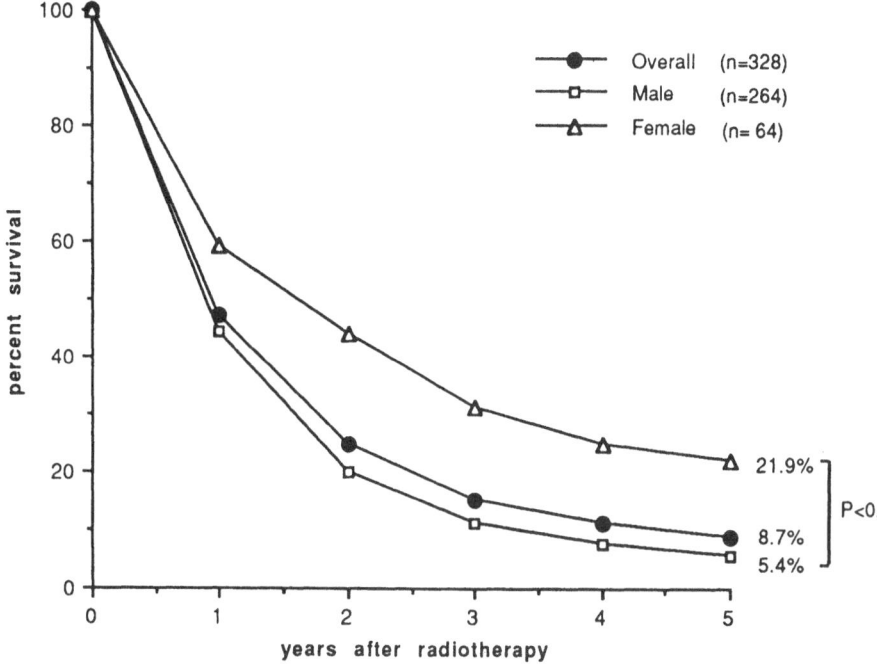

Fig. 1. Survival of esophageal cancer by sex (Tokyo Women's Medical College (*TWMC*) 1968–1988)

Tumor length. The cumulative 5-year survival rate was 15.1% in the <5 cm or less group, 8.5% in the 5–10 cm group, and 1.6% in the >10 cm group. There were no significant differences among them.

T-stage. The cumulative 5-year survival rate was 19.3% in T1, 8.4% in T2, and 3.0% in T3 (Fig. 2).

Tumor response. Initial tumor response was assessed by esophagography and endoscope within 1 month after the radiotherapy. One hundred and forty cases from 1975 to 1988 were evaluable. The cumulative 5-year survival rate was 28.2% in patients with complete response (CR), 8.1% in those with partial response (PR) and 0% in those who showed no change (NC). A significant difference between CR and PR was observed ($P < 0.05$) (Fig. 3).

Twenty-five patients have survived more than 5 years after treatment in this study (12 males and 13 females, mean age of 70 years). The locations of the tumor included the cervix (5), upper thoracic (2), middle thoracic (16), and lower thoracic (2). The mean tumor length was 6.5 cm (range 2–17 cm). Ten cases were T1, 12 were T3, and 3 were T3.

Discussion

According to the report of treatment results of esophageal carcinoma in Japan, the 5-year survival rate in 3395 resected cases from 1979 to 1982 was 26.1% [1].

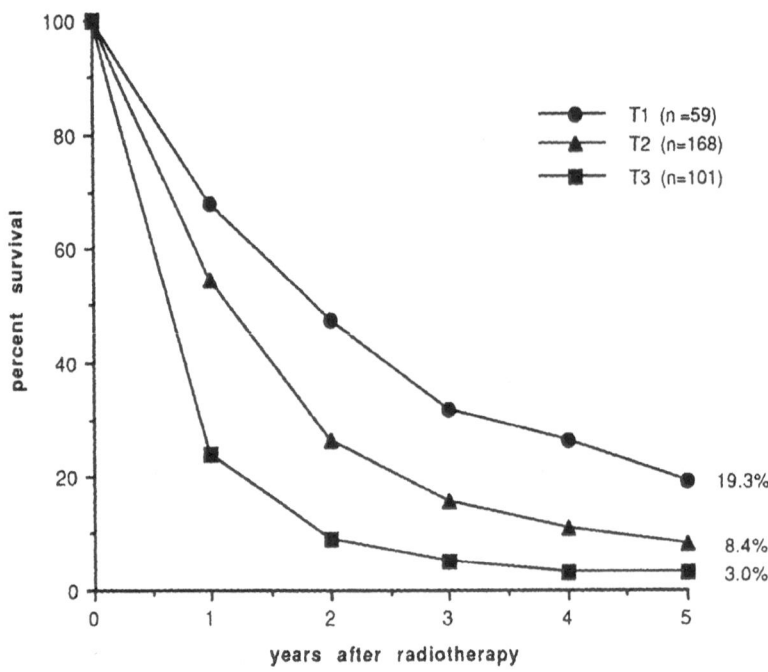

Fig. 2. Survival of esophageal cancer by T-stage (1978 UICC) (TWMC 1968–1988)

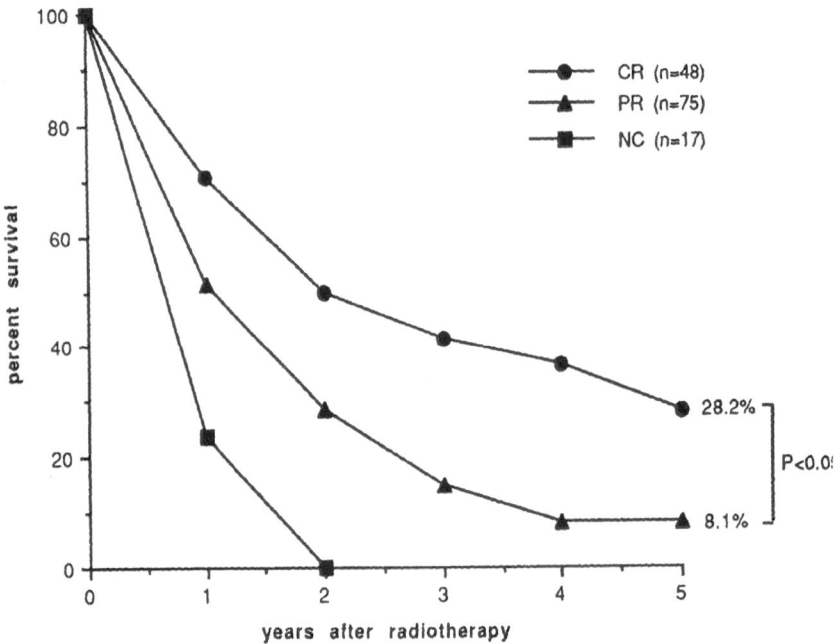

Fig. 3. Survival of esophageal cancer by tumor response (140 evaluable cases) (TWMC 1968–1988). *CR*, complete response; *PR*, partial response; *NC*, no change

Almost all of these cases were in comparatively early stages of development. Results for advanced stages were poor even if surgery was performed. In general, the majority of the patients treated by definitive radiotherapy were inoperabe locally advanced cases or were inappropriate for surgery because of severe complications. The overall 5-year survival rate of 8.7% noted in our study following radiotherapy was not satisfactory.

There have been many reports that prognosis among patients treated by either surgery or radiotherapy is more favorable for females. In our analysis, a significantly better result was obtained in females. There were no significant differences between males and females in terms of age, tumor length, and T-stage. Although the treatment results were slightly better on cervical esophagus compared with the other sites, the difference is not sufficient to explain a 5-year survival rate of over 20%.

By tumor location, the 5-year survival rate was favorable in cervical and middle thoracic carcinoma compared to abdominal esophagus, but a significant difference was not observed. As the lower esophageal tract is subject to substantial breathing movements, and the incidence of lymph node metastasis in the abdominal cavity is high, special care should be taken when determining the radiation field and dose per fraction.

By T-stage, the 5-year survival rate was better for T1 than for T2 or T3, which means that radiotherapy is generally more effective against tumors with a small volume. Recently, the proportion of definitive radiotherapy for the superficial carcinoma of the esophagus has been increasing in our hospital. Twenty-one patients with superficial carcinoma were treated by radical radiotherapy from 1975 to 1990, and the 5-year survival rate was 56.3%. This result is almost same as that of surgery.

The greatest problem in radiotherapy for esophageal cancer is the control of the primary lesion [2, 3], and in this study, primary tumor response was the most important prognostic factor. The complete response rate was 34.3% and the 5-year survival rate of that group was 28.2%. Long term survival cannot be expected in PR or NC groups, but about a half of the recurrence in CR patients was at the primary site. Elevation of the local control rate is the next most important factor to improve the cure rate of locally advanced esophageal cancer. There have been some reports that intra-luminal radiotherapy and concomitant use of chemotherapy using cisplatin (CDDP) is effective for local control [4, 5]. Optimal multimodal treatment should be studied to improve the cure rate of esophageal cancer.

References

1. Japanese Research Society for Esophageal Diseases National Cancer Center (1990). The report of treatment results of esophageal carcinoma in Japan. No. 10
2. Mantravadi RVP, Lad T, Briele H, Liebner EJ (1982) Carcinoma of the esophagus: Site of failure. Int J Radiat Oncol Biol Phys 8:1897–1901
3. Sun De-Ren (1989) Ten-year follow-up of esophageal cancer treated by radical radiation therapy: Analysis of 869 patients. Int J Radiat Oncol Biol Phys 16:329–334
4. Nishio M, Morita K, Yamada T, Hishikawa Y, Chatani M, Okawa T, Arimoto T, Kikuchi Y, Niibe H, Sugawara T, Asakawa H, Imajo Y, Hirokawa Y, Inoue T, Hirota S, Ohtake H, Dokoya T, Takegawa Y, Shibuya H, Sakai K, Watari J, Ito Y, Okazaki A, Mochizuki

S, Yamashita T, Imanaka K, Kuribayashi T, Nozue M, Masuda K, Tatsuno I, Masumoto H, Hareyama M, Ariga Y, Ogawa Y, Saito Y, Akita Y (1992) Clinical results of radiotherapy for MO esophageal cancer in Japan. J Jpn Soc Cancer Ther 27:912–924

5. Leichman L, Herskovic A, Leichman CG, Lattin PB, Steiger Z, Tapazoglou E, Rosenberg JC, Arbulu A, Asfaw I, Kinzie J (1987) Nonoperative therapy for squamous cell cancer of the esophagus. J Clin Oncol 5:365–370

High-Dose-Rate Intraluminal Brachytherapy for Advanced Esophageal Cancer: Analysis of Long Survivors

Midori Taniguchi, Yoshio Hishikawa, Koichi Kurisu, Norihiko Kamikonya, and Takashi Miura[1]

Summary. Between May 1980 and June 1987, 100 patients with thoracic esophageal cancer were treated with high-dose-rate intraluminal brachytherapy (HDRIBT) following external radiotherapy (ERT). The standard treatment protocol was 60 Gy/6 weeks of ERT and 12 Gy/1 week of HDRIBT. Follow-up time was 3–9 years (median 5 years). The 100 patients were classified into two groups according to 3-year survival after the initiation of radiotherapy. Fourteen patients survived for 3 or more years; the other 86 patients died within 3 years. The data of all patients were examined, and the following factors correlated with 3-year survival: Female sex, shorter tumor length, superficial or tumorous-type x-ray appearance before treatment, earlier stage, and better local response to treatment. In 3-year survivors, intercurrent disease was the main cause of death, while uncontrolled cancer was the main cause in the patients who died within 3 years.

Introduction

Esophageal cancer is a disease which still has a poor prognosis in spite of recent medical advances. Most patients have advanced disease at the time of presentation, which is one of the reasons for its poor prognosis. Another reason is that local tumor is not easy to control with external radiotherapy (ERT) alone [1]. However, the recent development of adjuvant radiotherapy using intraluminal brachytherapy following ERT has proven an effective treatment for localized lesions of esophageal cancer [2–4]. In our hospital, high-dose-rate intraluminal brachytherapy following ERT (ERT + HDRIBT) has been performed since May 1980. In this paper, we analyzed the data of 3-year survivors in the patients treated with ERT + HDRIBT.

[1] Department of Radiology, Hyogo College of Medicine 1-1, Mukogawa-cho, Nishinomiya, Hyogo, 663 Japan

Patients and Methods

Between May 1980 and July 1987, 100 patients with thoracic esophageal cancer were treated with ERT + HDRIBT in our department. The patients were classified into two groups according to 3-year survival from the start of radiotherapy.

For each group the following data were recorded: Age, sex, tumor site, tumor length, radiological findings of tumor, stage, other diseases present prior to treatment, presence of other primary cancer, and local response to treatment. The disease stage was classified as limited disease (LD) and extensive disease (ED): LD included disease of stages I and II according to the clinical-diagnostic classification of the AJCC classification of 1983, and ED included stages III and IV. For staging, all patients were examined by barium esophagography, endoscopy, computed tomography, and chest x-ray. Most also underwent liver scanning. Biopsy via endoscopy showed squamous cell carcinoma in all cases.

ERT was performed with either 10 MV x-rays (LMR-15, Toshiba, Tokyo) or a ^{60}Co beam (Theratron 80, Atomic Energy of Canada, Ottawa). Opposed anteroposterior/posteroanterior fields were used up to 40 Gy, followed by the rotation technique. The field was 6 cm in width, and 3 cm longer than the superior and inferior margins of the tumor. HDRIBT was performed using a high-dose-rate, remote afterloader (RAL-303, Toshiba, Tokyo). The source was ^{60}Co (2.2 Ci in May 1980 and in March 1987). The delivered dose was calculated using a computerized radiotherapy planning system (RO-7, Varian Associates, Palo Alto, Calif.). Radiation was administered to the level 5 mm below the surface of the mucosa, 1 cm from the source. Details of the technique and dosimetry of HDRIBT have been reported previously [3]. On the basis of our earlier studies of survival and local control [2, 3], complications [5–8], and autopsy results [9], the following standard treatment regimen has been developed: ERT (60 Gy in 30 fractions over 6 weeks), followed by no treatment for 1 week, followed by HDRIBT (12 Gy in 2 fractions during 1 week).

The local response was evaluated by barium esophagography and/or endoscopy 1 month after the completion of radiotherapy. The clinical efficacy was judged by the following criteria [10]: Complete response (CR), 100% regression of disease; partial response (PR), greater than 50% reduction in tumor bulk but less than 100% resolution of disease. When endoscopic biopsy showed cancer in a patient clinically CR or PR, the response was classified as neither CR nor PR. During the first 6 months of follow-up, examination was performed every month, and thereafter every 2 or 3 months. Endoscopic biopsy was performed in all patients in whom tumor recurrence was suspected.

Survival time was calculated from the beginning of radiotherapy to death, or to June 30 1990. No patients were lost to follow-up. The follow-up time was 3–9 years (median 5 years). Statistical analysis was performed using the Student's t-test or χ^2-test.

Results

Out of 100 patients, 14 patients survived for 3 years or longer. A comparison between 3-year survivors and non-survivors is shown in Table 1. Sex, tumor length, radiological appearance of tumor, stage, and local response after

Table 1. Patient and tumor characteristics: May 1980–July 1987

	Survivors		P value
	3 Years	Less than 3 years	
Age (years): range (median)	59–82 (73)	45–86 (71)	NS
Sex: male/female	8/6	74/12	0.01
Tumor site: upper/middle/lower	2/5/7	15/49/22	NS
Tumor length (cm): range (median)	1.5–8 (4.75)	1.3–22 (7.0)	0.01
Radiological findings: superficial/ tumorous/serrated and spiral/funnelled	1/7/5/1	6/13/62/5	0.05
Stage: LD/ED	14/0	34/52	0.01
Associated disease: +/−	2/12	25/61	NS
Other primary cancer: +/−	2/12	7/81	NS
Local response after treatment: CR/PR/NC	10/4/0	20/44/22	0.01

LD, limited disease; *ED*, extensive disease; *CR*, complete response; *PR*, partial response; *NC*, no change; *NS*, not significant

Table 2. Prognosis after radiotherapy

	Survivors	
	3 Years	Less than 3 years
Alive	7	0
Death from		
Cancer	2	66
Intercurrent disease	5	17
Unknown	0	1

treatment were found to be significant prognostic factors of 3-year survival. In the 3-year survivors, the female/male ratio was higher, and the mean tumor length was shorter. Superficial and tumorous-type tumor were found in 8 of the 14 3-year survivors, but in only 19 of the 86 non-survivors. All 3-year survivors had LD, but 52 of the 86 non-survivors had ED. CR rate was 71% (10/14) of the 3-year survivors and 23% (20/86) of the non-survivors.

Of the 14 3-year survivors, 7 are still alive at the time of writing. The causes of death of the 86 non-survivors are shown in Table 2. The main cause of death in patients who survived for more than 3 years was intercurrent disease.

Discussion

Several factors affect the long-term survival of patients with esophageal cancer treated by radiotherapy. Beatty et al. [11] reported that sex, tumor size, and stage correlated with patient survival, and in our series, the same results were found. Smaller tumor size and earlier disease stage are the most important factors for better prognosis after radiotherapy in patients with esophageal cancer. Thus, earlier diagnosis results in a better prognosis after radiotherapy. The clinical effect of radiation differs in patients with different types of tumor.

Radiotherapy is more effective in superficial or tumorous-type than the other types [12]. Eight of the 14 3-year survivors of our series had these types of tumor. Prior to radiotherapy, we will now be able to predict a higher likelihood of local response in patients with superficial or tumorous-type tumor than in patients with other tumor types.

Informed consent of the patient is necessary before treatment, and patients with esophageal cancer should be informed of the possibility of cure after radiotherapy. In this study, we found that factors associated with a better prognosis are female sex, smaller tumor size, earlier stage, and radio-sensitive tumor-type. In surgical candidates with these factors and a high surgical risk, we should treat with ERT + HDRIBT rather than with surgery.

References

1. Parker EF, Gregorie HB (1976) Carcinoma of the esophagus: long-term results. JAMA 235:1018–1020
2. Hishikawa Y, Tanaka S, Miura T (1985) Early esophageal carcinoma treated with intracavitary irradiation. Radiology 156:519–522
3. Hishikawa Y, Kamikonya N, Tanaka S, et al (1987) Radiotherapy of esophageal carcinoma: Role of high-dose-rate intracavitary irradiation. Radiother Oncol 9:13–20
4. Hyden EC, Langholz B, Tilden T, et al (1988) External beam and intraluminal radiotherapy in the treatment of carcinoma of the esophagus. J Thorac Cardiovasc Surg 96:237–241
5. Hishikawa Y, Tanaka S, Miura T (1984) Esophageal ulceration induced by intracavitary irradiation for esophageal carcinoma. Am J Roentgenol 143:269–273
6. Hishikawa Y, Mitsunobu M, Uematsu K, et al (1985) Histological findings of esophageal injury induced by intracavitary irradiation. Radiat Med 3:112–117
7. Hishikawa Y, Tanaka S, Miura T (1986) Esophageal fistula associated with intracavitary irradiation for esophageal carcinoma. Radiology 159:549–551
8. Hishikawa Y, Kamikonya N, Tanaka S, et al (1986) Esophageal stricture following high-dose-rate intracavitary irradiation for esophageal cancer. Radiology 159:715–716
9. Hishikawa Y, Taniguchi M, Kamikonya N, et al (1988) External beam radiotherapy alone or combined with high-dose-rate intracavitary irradiation in the treatment of cancer of the esophagus: Autopsy findings in 35 cases. Radiother Oncol 11:223–227
10. Kelsen DP, Ahuja R, Hopfan S, et al (1981) Combined modality therapy of esophageal carcinoma. Cancer 48:31–37
11. Beatty JD, BeBoer G, Rider WD (1979) Carcinoma of the esophagus: Pretreatment assessment, correlation of radiation treatment parameters with survival, and identification and management of radiation treatment failure. Cancer 43:2254–2267
12. Morita K, Takagi I, Watanabe M, et al (1985) Relationship between the radiologic features of esophageal cancer and local control by radiation therapy. Cancer 55:2668–2676

Do Postoperative Radiochemotherapy and/or Aggressive Chemotherapy for Patients with Cancer of the Esophagus Who Have Undergone Curative Surgery Contribute to Improvement of Prognosis?

Tetsuro Nishihira, Katsu Hirayama, Takashi Akaishi,
Ryuzaburo Shineha, Masabumi Katayama, Norio Higuchi,
and Shozo Mori[1]

Introduction

The most frequent sites of tumors after curative surgery of the thoracic esophagus are in the cervical region and/or mediastinum. Detailed analysis of 187 cases in our hospital showed that postoperative adjuvant therapy, namely, radiochemoimmunotherapy, improved the survival rate of patients undergoing such surgery. This indicates that such therapy prevents the recurrence of micrometastasis after curative surgery. However, the prognosis of patients with positive nodes did not improve, in spite of extensive radical surgery including lymphadenectomy. In order to improve the prognosis in such cases with positive regional nodes, a newly devised protocol of radiochemocytokine therapy including tumor necrosis factor (TNF), interleukin 2 (IL-2) and α-interferon (α-INF) has recently been performed. For patients with distant node metastasis, conventional postoperative aggressive chemotherapy under active nutritional support has been found to prolong survival. The 5-year survival rate of patients treated with aggressive chemotherapy and radiochemocytokine therapy was analyzed.

Materials and Methods

For 16 years, from 1975 to 1990, 474 out of 567 patients (83.6%) were treated with curative surgery. Of these patients, 11 operative deaths and 7 patients on whom information was unavailable were excluded. Thus, 456 patients are included in this study.

In the past 6 years, a new protocol of radiochemocytokine therapy including 40 Gy of T-shaped irradiation [1], chemotherapy with 5-FU, cisplatin and

---

[1] Second Department of Surgery, Tohoku University School of Medicine, 1-1 Seiryo-machi, Sendai, 980 Japan

Table 1. Cytokine administration and immunological studies

Cytokines
1. Kinds and doses
   r-TNF: 1×10^4 IU/day
   r-IL-2: 5×10^5 IU/day
   n-α IFN: 1×10^6 IU/day
2. Methods of administration
   a Daily 24-h continuous infusion with TPN for 30 days
   b TNF was administered first, followed by simultaneous infusion of IL-2 and IFN

Immunological studies
— Natural killer activity   — PPD skin reaction
— Analysis of lymphocyte
   surface antigens with FCM
— Peripheral lymphocytes   — Serum immunoglobulin
— Levels of serum IAP and CEA

r-TNF, recombinant tissue necrotic factor; *r-IL-2*, recombinant interleultin-2; *n-α IFN*, natural-α interferon; *PPD*, purified protein derivative; *IAP*, immunoacidic protein; *CEA*, carcinoembroyic antigen; *TPN*, total parenteral nutrition; *FCM*, flow cytometry

vindesine, and three kinds of cytokines [2] for patients who have undergone curative surgery has been adopted.

Recombinant tumor necrosis factor (1×10^4 IU per day) is administered first, followed by simultaneous infusion of interleukin-2 (5×10^5 IU per day for 30 days) and α-Interferon (1×10^6 per day for 30 days) (Table 1).

For the past 10 years, we have used postoperative aggressive chemotherapy [3, 4] for patients with positive node metastasis. This chemotherapy consists of vindesine, cisplatin, 5-FU, and adriamycin, and is called F·CAV treatment. Angiotensin II-induced hypertensive chemotherapy is always used with cisplatin and adriamycin. This therapy is performed under active enteral and parenteral nutrition of 40 Cal/kg per day.

Results

Outcome of Patients with Negative Nodes

As seen in Fig. 1, 1-, 3- and 5-year survival rates of 378 patients treated with curative surgery were 73.2%, 48.1% and 38.1%, respectively. On the other hand, in the 78 patients who underwent non-curative surgery (so-called C-O cases), 1-, 3- and 5-year survival rates were 29.5%, 8.7% and 5.2%, respectively.

Regarding the prognosis of patients without node metastasis (Fig. 2), the 5-year survival rate of the group which received radiochemoimmunotherapy including cytokines, that of the group which received only radiotherapy, and that of the group which received no postoperative combined therapy were 74.6% (68 cases), 52.7% (39 cases), and 55.3% (33 cases), respectively.

This study was done with a historical control, but the prognosis of the cytokine group (12 cases) was better than that of the group which did not receive cytokines (18 cases), although no statistical significance was noted between the two groups (Fig. 3).

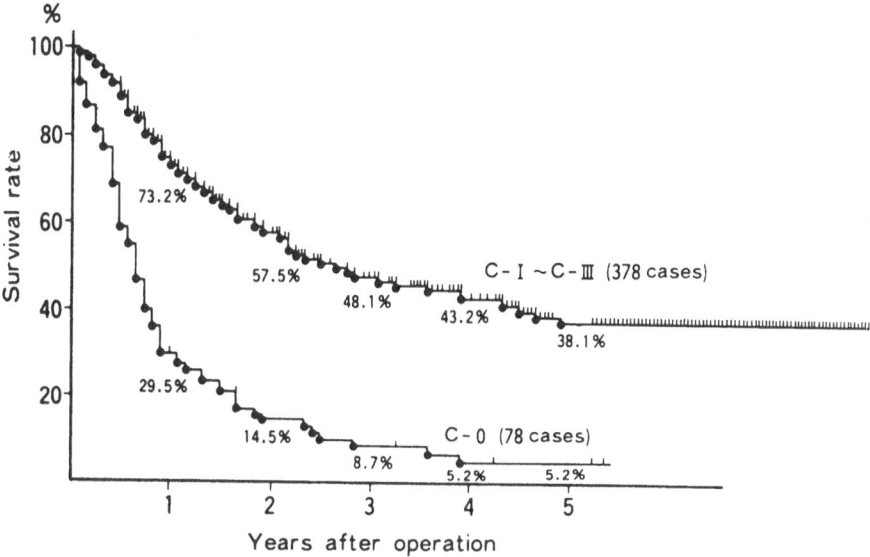

Fig. 1. Prognosis of thoracic esophageal cancer patients after surgery: Survival as related to radical (C-I~C-III) and non-radical surgery (C-O)

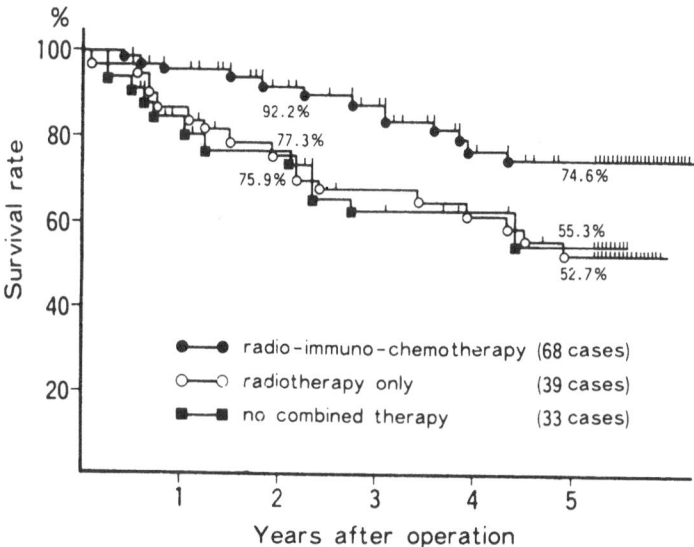

Fig. 2. Prognosis after curative surgery of thoracic esophageal cancer patients without lymph node metastasis

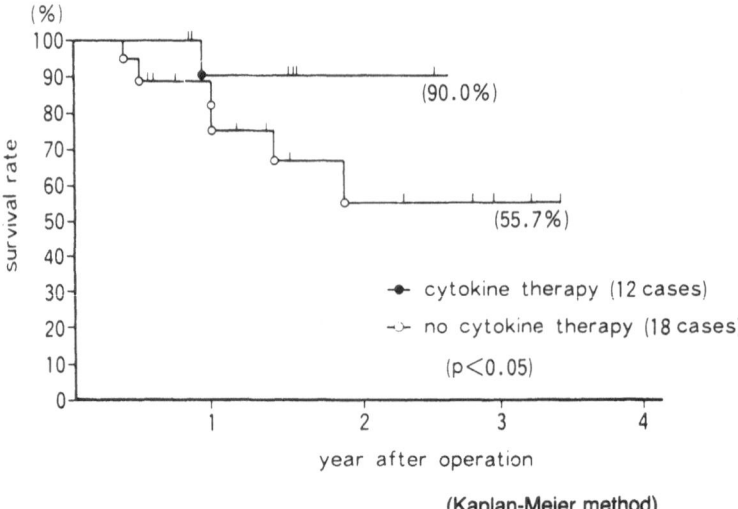

Fig. 3. Prognosis of thoracic esophageal cancer patients with regional lymph node metastasis: Comparison of therapy with and without cytokines

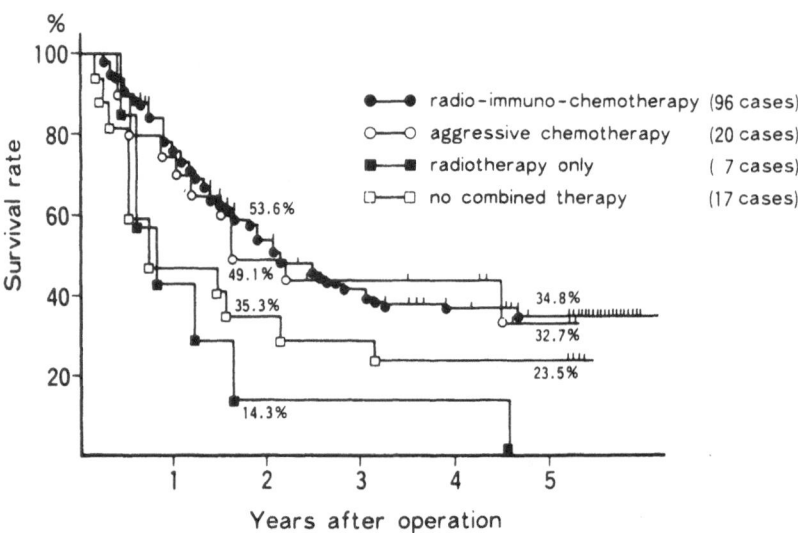

Fig. 4. Prognosis of thoracic esophageal cancer patients with positive regional nodes, $n_1(+)$ and $n_2(+)$, after curative surgery

Outcome of Patients with Regional Node Metastasis [$n_1(+)$ and $n_2(+)$]

The prognoses of patients with positive regional nodes [$n_1(+)$, $n_2(+)$] are shown in Fig. 4. Five-year survival rates of the patients who received radiochemocytokine therapy, those who were subjected to aggressive chemotherapy, and those who

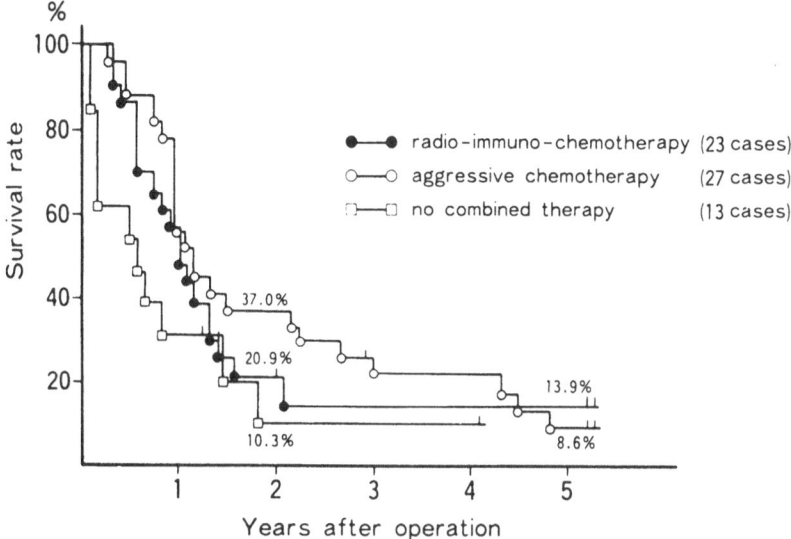

Fig. 5. Prognosis of thoracic esophageal cancer patients with distant lymph node metastasis, $n_3(+)$ and $n_4(+)$, after curative surgery

received no postoperative combined therapy were 34.8% (96 cases), 32.7% (20 cases) and 23.5% (17 cases), respectively. The prognosis of patients who received postoperative combined therapies was better than those who received no combined therapy.

Outcome of Patients with Positive Distant Nodes [$n_3(+)$, $n_4(+)$]

The outcome of 63 patients with positive distant nodes [$n_3(+)$, $n_4(+)$] is seen in Fig. 5. Two- and 5-year survival rates of the 27 patients who received aggressive chemotherapy were 37.0% and 8.6%, respectively. Two- and 5-year survival rates of the 23 patients who received radiochemocytokine therapy were 20.9% and 3.8%, respectively. There was no significant difference between the two groups. No 5-year survivors (13 cases) who did not receive combined therapies were noted.

As to the 55 cases of $n_3(+)$ and $n_4(+)$ patients with poor outcome even after radical surgery, the prognosis gradually improved and the 5-year survival rate was 14.2% in the 25 cases from 1985 to 1990. This improvement might have been due to systematic lymphadenectomy, as well as to the use of postoperative combined therapies (Fig. 6).

Strategy of Postoperative Combined Therapies for Patients with Thoracic Esophageal Cancer Who Have Undergone Curative Surgery

Epithelial cancer or muscosal cancer limited to the muscularis mucosa is not treated with combined therapy. $n(-)$ patients with cancer extending beyond the muscularis mucosa and $n_1(+)$ and $n_2(+)$ patients are treated with T-shaped

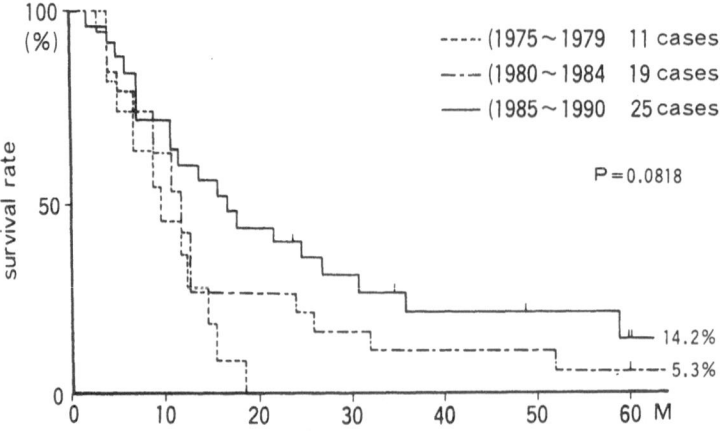

Fig. 6. Prognosis of thoracic esophageal cancer patients with distant lymph node metastasis

radiotherapy and chemoimmunotherapy including cytokines. $n_3(+)$ and $n_4(+)$ patients are usually subjected to aggressive chemotherapy with long-term active nutritional support.

Discussion

The most important prognostic factor is the degree of node metastasis. The recurrence of esophageal cancer involving regional nodes, even in patients who have undergone curative surgery, often takes place within 3 years after surgery [5]. In this paper, we report development of a new multidisciplinary treatment, including cytokines or aggressive chemotherapy with active nutritional support, to improve the prognosis in cases of cancer of the thoracic esophagus.

The prognosis of the patients who undergo non-curative surgery (C-O) is still not good, and it is unacceptable that multidisciplinary treatment including surgery has not contributed to improvement of the prognosis in such cases. In order to treat cases that have not been traditionally indicated for surgery [5] because of the extent of cancer, newly developed postoperative combined therapies for C-O cases are desired.

In light of the above stated need for improvement of prognosis, 15 years ago we started research on malignant factors of esophageal cancer [6–11]. We have put particular emphasis on cellular and molecular biological characteristics. Among over 20 kinds of gene expressions, unfortunately, no particular so-called oncogene expressions have been detected, except for epidermal growth factor, *erb-B*, *hst-1*, *int-2*, and P53 suppressor gene. The use of cellular and molecular biological characteristics for evaluating the malignancy of esophageal cancer can be expected to be applicable in the determination of treatment modalities against cancers with malignant factors.

Conclusion

Postoperative prophylactic combination therapies, namely, aggressive chemotherapy (AC) and radiochemoimmunotherapy (RCI), may help to improve the prognosis in cases of this type of cancer. It has not yet been determined which of these two therapies is adequate, but disease-oriented adjuvant therapies should be based on several markers of malignant factors, including clinicopathological findings and also cellular and molecular biological characteristics.

References

1. Kasai M, Mori S, Watanabe T (1978) Follow-up results after resection of thoracic esophageal carcinoma. World J Surg 2:543–551
2. Nishihira T, Hirayama K, Kitamura M, Shineha R, Akaishi T, Mori S (1989) Postoperative radio-cytokine therapy for patients with cancer of the esophagus involving regional node metastasis who have undergone curative surgery. In: Proceedings of the 33rd world congress of the International Society of Surgery, Toronto, October 1989, p 92
3. Nishihira T, Tan M, Kuriya Y, Ohmori N, Kitamura M, Toyoda T, Kasai M (1984) Postoperative cancer therapy for patients with carcinoma of the thoracic esophagus: an attempt of aggressive chemotherapy combined with proper nutritional support for patients with distant node metastasis. Tohoku J Exp Med 142:25–34
4. Nishihira T, Hirayama K, Shineha T, Akaishi T, Takano R, Kitamura M, Mori M (1990) Postoperative adjuvant therapies for cancer of the thoracic esophagus on the basis of the extent of node metastasis. La Chirurgia Toracica 43(1):4–12
5. Nishihira T, Watanabe T, Ohmori N, Kasai M (1984) Long-term evaluation of patients treated by radical operation for carcinoma of the thoracic esophagus. World J Surg. 8:778–785
6. Nishihira T, Hirayama K, Kitamura M, Akaishi T, Shineha R, Sekine Y, Kasai M (1989) Postoperative aggressive chemotherapy with nutritional support in case of thoracic esophageal cancer with distant lymph-node metastasis. In: Kimura K (ed) Cancer chemotherapy: Challenges for the future. Excerpta Medica, Tokyo, pp 165–173
7. Nishihira T, Akaishi T, Shineha R, Sekine Y, Sanekata K, Hirayama K, Sagawa J, Takano R, Mori S (1989) Malignant potential of esophageal carcinoma in terms of biological properties. Dis esoph II(2): 125–135
8. Hiraizumi S, Takasaki S, Nishihira T, Mori S, Kobata A (1990) Comparative study of the N-linked oligosaccharides released from normal human esophageal epithelium and esophageal squamous carcinoma. Jpn J Cancer Res 81:363–371
9. Nishihira T, Kasai M, Kitamura M, Hirayama K, Akaishi T, Sekine Y (1988) Biological characteristics of cultured cell lines of human esophageal carcinomas and tumors transplantable to nude mice originating from human esophageal carcinomas and their clinical application. In: Webber MM (ed) In vitro models for cancer research, vol 1. Carcinomas of the esophagus and colon. Florida, CRC, Boca Raton, pp 66–79
10. Tsuda T, Nakatani H, Matsumura T, Yoshida K, Tahara E, Nishihira T, Sakamoto H, Yoshida T, Terada M, Sugimura T (1988) Amplification of the hst-1 gene in human esophageal carcinomas. Jpn J Cancer Res 79:584–588
11. Takano R, Nose M, Nishihira T, Kyogoku M (1990) Increase of 1-6-branched oligosaccharides in human esophageal carcinomas invasive against surrounding tissue in vivo and in vitro. Am J Path 137(5):1007–1011

Esophageal Carcinoma Treated with Proton Beam

Shohei Koyama[1] and Hirohiko Tsujii[2]

Introduction

The prognosis of patients with esophageal carcinoma treated by external x-ray irradiation alone is poor because of local recurrence and distant metastasis [1]. To solve this problem, we have adopted a new therapeutic modality which utilizes proton beam. Proton beam has a highly defined dose distribution, resulting in no radiation exposure beyond the beam range and very little side scatter [2–4]. Thus, a study has been undertaken at the Institute of Clinical Medicine, University of Tsukuba in patients with esophageal carcinoma to receive definitive proton therapy or proton beam irradiation following external x-ray irradiation. This report describes the preliminary results from the first 15 patients who have been so treated.

Patients and Methods

Clinical characteristics of the 15 patients with esophageal carcinoma treated with proton beam are shown in Table 1. These patients had carcinoma limited to the local-regional area, which is capable of undergoing radical radiotherapy. Most of the patients were of advanced age and had associated severe concomitant diseases unrelated to the esophageal carcinoma. Six patients (case numbers 1–6) showed superficial esophageal carcinoma, and the other nine patients (case numbers 7–15) had advanced carcinoma. Histological assessnment was made according to the biopsy specimens taken from esophageal lesions. Consequently, 14 patients showed squamous cell carcinoma and 1 patient (case number 6) revealed tubular adenocarcinoma.

Department of Internal Medicine[1], Institute of Clinical Medicine, Proton Medical Research Center[2], University of Tsukuba, Tsukuba, 305 Japan

Table 1. Clinical characteristics of patients with esophageal carcinoma

	Age/sex	Location	X-ray and Endoscopic classification[a]	Vertical extension (cm)	Gross stage[a]	Associated with other diseases
(1)	68/M	Im and Ei	0-III and 0-IIc	1.5 & 1	I	Bronchiectasis Bronchial asthma
(2)	77/M	Im	0-IIc	1.5	I	Crohn's disease Renal failure
(3)	84/M	Im	0-I	2	I	Af, hypertension
(4)	69/F	Im	0-I	2	I	Epstein anomalie
(5)	64/M	Im	0-III	2	I	Respiratory failure
(6)	85/M	Ea	0-III	2	I	None
(7)	73/M	Im	2	5	III	Renal failure Hypertension
(8)	62/M	Im	1	6	III	Liver cirrhosis
(9)	84/M	Im and Ei	3	6 & 2	III	Renal failure Af, gall stone
(10)	51/M	Im–Ei	3	7	III	Liver cirrhosis Diabetes mellitus
(11)	73/M	Im	3	7	III	None
(12)	85/F	Iu	2	3	III	Diabetes mellitus Renal failure
(13)	81/F	Im	2	4	III	None
(14)	60/M	Im	2	8	III	Achalasia
(15)	95/M	Im	2	4	III	None

[a] Defined by guidelines for the clinical and pathological studies on carcinoma of the esophagus [7]. *Af*, Atrial fibrillation; *Im*, middle; *Ei*, lower; *Ea*, abdominal; *Iu*, upper

Table 2. Practical doses of x-ray and proton beams to esophageal carcinoma

	Age/sex	x-ray (Gy)	Proton (Gy)	Total dose (Gy)
(1)	68/M	16.2	52.9	69.1
(2)	77/M	50.4	30.0	80.4
(3)	84/M	50.0	36.5	86.5
(4)	69/F	40.0	45.0	85.0
(5)	64/M	40.0	40.0	80.0
(6)	85/F	0	75.0	75.0
(7)	73/M	0	86.5	86.5
(8)	62/M	0	88.5	88.5
(9)	84/M	50.4	33.0	83.4
(10)	51/M	50.4	32.4	85.4
(11)	73/M	50.4	35.0	85.4
(12)	85/M	0	75.5	75.5
		(10)[a]	(44.0)[a]	(54.0)[a]
(13)	81/F	41.4	39.0	80.4
(14)	60/M	37.8	39.0	70.8
(15)	95/M	40.0	37.0	77.0

[a] Irradiation to the mediastinal lymph nodes

Exact vertical proton irradiation control system for cancer therapy has been described previously [2–4]. The rationale of the treatment was explained to the patients, who signed a consent form before the therapy was begun. The proton beam therapy was administered to the primary lesions: single dose of 3.0–3.5 Gy was delivered five times per week. Total dose of each patient is shown in Table 2. Mean total dose was 80.4 Gy. As shown in Table 2, definitive proton therapy to the primary lesion was done in 4 of 15 patients, while the other 11 patients were treated with a combination with external x-ray (12-MeV linear accelerator) and proton beam. At the end of the radiation therapy, the x-ray and endoscopic examinations were done at regular intervals, and the clinical radiation effect was evaluated.

Results

Isodose distribution of proton beam and range compensator (bolus) design on proton computed tomography (CT) image are shown in Fig. 1. The method insured accurate localization of the proton beam with respect to tumor volume. The distributions show a rapid dose reduction from the center to the periphery of the field. Thus, the spinal cord of the patients is preferentially spared by proton technique.

Table 3 shows summary results of proton therapy to esophageal carcinoma. Tumor lesions of all 15 patients completely disappeared and a complete response (CR) was obtained. Although sufficient local control of the primary lesion was obtained, approximately 4–5 months later, most patients (9 out of 15) showed that esophageal ulcer suddenly developed at the circumference of

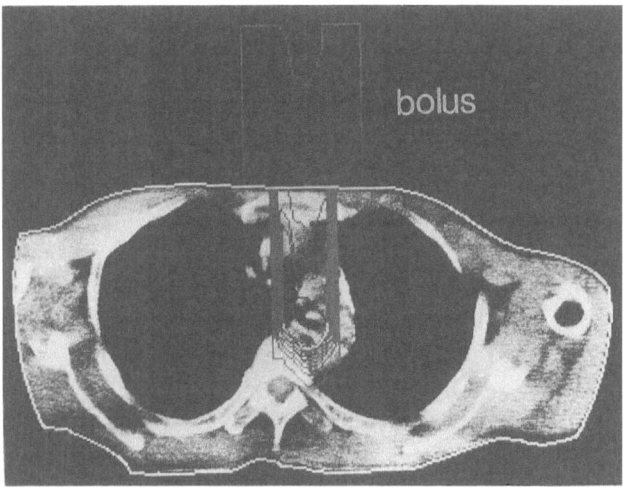

Fig. 1. Illustration of isodose curve shapes of 95%, 90%, 80%, 50%, and 10% level, and bolus shape on CT slice of an esophageal carcinoma case (single vertical field)

the primary lesion. These patients were treated with liquid diet and/or intravenous hyperalimentation (IVH), since the ulcer formation is considered to be caused by high-doses of irradiation and physical local stimuli of solid food. Then, the ulcer gradually healed without stenosis except in two patients (case numbers 2 and 15). The stenosis could be improved by endoscopic balloon dilator.

In all 6 cases of superficial esophageal carcinoma, there was no evidence of local recurrence throughout the observation. Two of the six patients died of other diseases; the period of other four patients are alive and well. In advanced squamous cell carcinoma, however, six of the nine patients showed no evidence of local recurrence of carcinoma during clinical course of observation, and three of the nine relapsed into esophageal carcinoma. Recurrence time from the end of the proton therapy was different in each case. It was observed at 44, 8, and 16 months, respectively. Five of the nine patients died; four of them died of other diseases such as hepatic failure, respiratory failure, and epiglottis carcinoma, while only one of them died of relapse of primary carcinoma. Four of these nine patients are alive and well.

Discussion

This study demonstrates that proton therapy is clinically practical, and the advantages of the irradiation for deeply seated tumor, esophageal carcinoma are now proven. Our results are based on the ability of the proton beam to provide better dose distributions than that of conventional x-ray alone. Thus, spinal cord is not dose limiting for proton therapy (Fig. 1). We could use 20%–30% higher total doses for the treatment as compared with that of conventional x-ray

Table 3. Summary results of proton therapy to esophageal carcinoma

	Age/ sex	Local response[a]	Onset of ulcer (months)	Duration of ulcer (months)	Onset of local recurrence (months)	Survival[b] (months)	Results
(1)	68/M	CR	Unknown	Unknown	No	71	Death (pneumonia)
(2)	77/M	CR	5	7	No	50	Alive
(3)	84/M	CR	5	7	No	50	Alive
(4)	69/F	CR	Unknown	Unknown	No	50	Death (acute cardiac failure)
(5)	64/M	CR	11	0.5	No	46	Alive
(6)	85/M	CR	4	0.7	No	26	Alive
(7)	73/M	CR	4	6	No	10	Death (unknown)
(8)	62/M	CR	Unknown	Unknown	No	6	Death (hepatic failure)
(9)	84/M	CR	None	None	No	32	Death (epiglottis cancer)
(10)	51/M	CR	5	6	44	48	Alive
(11)	73/M	CR	4	4	8	16	Death (recurrence)
(12)	85/M	CR	3	6	No	9	Death (respiratory failure)
(13)	81/F	CR	None	None	16	30	Alive
(14)	60/M	CR	None	None	No	17	Alive
(15)	95/M	CR	4	7	No	13	Alive

[a] Defined by guidelines for the clinical and pathological studies on carcinoma of the esophagus [7]
[b] Assessed on June 30, 1992

therapy. As a result, improved local control of primary lesion was obtained in patients, resulting in better long-term survival rate. However, at higher dose levels employed, the esophageal mucosa is dose-limiting for normal tissues. They cannot be spared because they lie within the target tumor volume. This caused the development of ulcer formation of the esophagus after the proton therapy. Similar findings have been reported by high-dose rate intracavitary irradiation following external irradiation [5]. The proton beam-induced ulcer is certainly considered to be a serious complication, but the lesions could eventually be cured by appropriate conservative treatment. Further resulting fistula or perforation did not occur. Therefore, proton therapy is still a beneficial treatment because of its efficacy in controlling local response (Table 3).

Proton therapy is indicated in esophageal carcinoma involved with intra-epithelium (ep) or muscularis mucosa (mm) of continuous malignant changes extending 20 mm or more, and in localized carcinoma that is deeper than submucosa (sm), when surgery is thought to be too dangerous to perform or the patients refuse the surgical operation. Endoscopic mucosectomy is recommended in ep and mm carcinomas less than 20 mm in size [6]. If we can choose the localized esophageal carcinoma without lymph node involvement, curative radiation therapy might be applied for these patients instead of surgical resection. Further detailed clinical evaluation of radiation effects of patients with esophageal carcinoma analyzed by repeated endoscopy and histopathological examination will be reported elsewhere.

References

1. Pearson JG (1977) The present status and future potential of radiotherapy in the management of esophageal cancer. Cancer 39:882–890
2. Inada T, Hayakawa Y, Maruhashi A, Ohara K, Kitagawa T, Akisada M, Kawachi K, Kanai T (1984) Vertical proton beam irradiation control system for cancer therapy (in Japanese). Nippon Acta Radiol 44:844–853
3. Tsujii H, Inada T, Maruhashi A, Hayakawa Y, Tsuji H, Ohara K, Akisada M, Kitagawa T (1989) Field localization and verification system for proton beam radiotherapy in deepseated tumors (in Japanese). Nippon Acta Radiol 49:622–629
4. Koyama S, Kawanishi N, Fukutomi H, Osuga T, Iijima T, Tsujii H, Kitagawa T (1990) Advanced carcinoma of the stomach treated with definitive proton therapy. Am J Gastroenterol 85:443–447
5. Hishikawa Y, Tanaka S, Miura T (1984) Esophageal ulceration induced by intracavitary irradiation for esophageal carcinoma. Am J Roentgenol 143:269–273
6. Makuuchi H, Machimura T, Soh Y, Mizutani K, Shimada H, Sugihara T, Tokuda Y, Sasaki T, Tajima T, Mitomi T, Ohmori T, Miyoshi H (1991) Endoscopic mucosectomy for mucosa carcinomas in the esophagus (in Japanese). Jpn J Gastroenterol Surg 24:2599–2603
7. Japanese Society of Esophageal Diseases (1992) Guidelines for the clinical and pathological studies on carcinoma of the esophagus (in Japanese). Kanehara, Tokyo

A New Modality of Chemotherapy in the Treatment of Esophageal Carcinoma Using Angiotensin II–Induced Hypertension and OK-432-Induced Hyperthermia

Hideyuki Kawahara*, Ken Okabayashi, Takeshi Shiraishi, Yasunori Yoshida, and Takayuki Shirakusa[1]

Introduction

In the treatment of patients with malignant tumors of the esophagus, conventional chemotherapeutic regimens have brought little improvement in long-term survival [1–3]. In view of the limited gains resulting from the therapy of these highly lethal diseases, new effective modalities are needed to improve the prognoses. The present report concerns our new method of cancer chemotherapy in combination with angiotensin II–induced hypertension and OK-432–induced hyperthermia (hypertensive-hyperthermo-chemotherapy [HHC]).

Materials and Methods

Thirty-three patients with histologically confirmed esophageal malignant tumors were entered in the study. Age ranged from 49 to 78 years with an average of 63.3. There were 25 patients with squamous cell carcinoma, 2 with undifferentiated carcinoma, and 1 patient each with adenoacanthoma, adenoid cystic carcinoma, adenocarcinoma, malignant melanoma, and others. Of these patients, 24 underwent surgery. The remaining nine were inoperable or recurrent cases. According to the staging classification of the Japanese system [4], 4 patients had stage 1 disease, 3 had stage 2, 7 had stage 3, and 17 had stage 4 (stage of the remaining 2 were unclear).

In order to elevate the blood pressure up to the "hypertensive state", Agiotensin II was administered by intravenous continuous infusion at the rate of 25 to 125 μg/hr. The mean arterial pressure was elevated to 1.5-fold but it did not exceed 150 mmHg as high as that of resting state, and was kept there for

[1] Department of Thoracic and Cardiovascular Surgery, University of Occupational and Environmental Health, 1-1 Iseigaoka Yahata-nishi-ku, Kitakyushu-shi, Fukuoka, Japan
* Current address: Kawasaki City Ida Hospital, 1272 Ida, Nakahara, Kawasaki, Kanagawa, 211 Japan

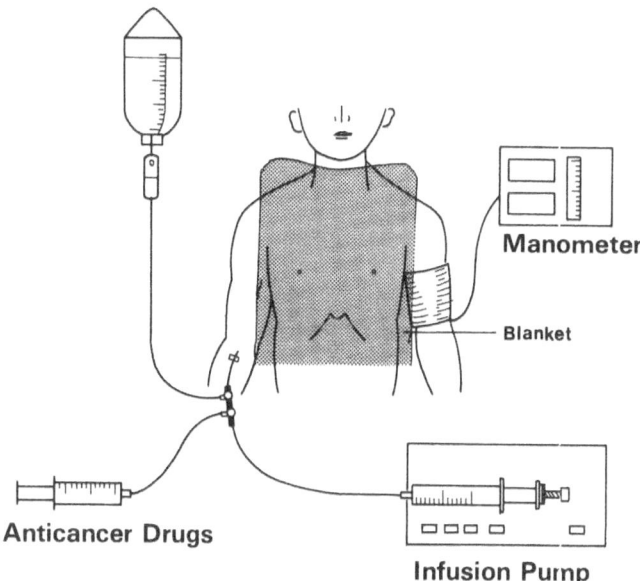

Fig. 1. Arrangement for hypertensive-hyperthermo-chemotherapy. Automatic manometer for measuring the blood pressure every minute. Heating blanket applied to the patient to diminish heat loss

Preoperative regimen

Day 1, 2. 5-FU (250~500 mg/body) c̄ HC

Day 3. ⎡5-FU (250~500 mg/body⎤
        ⎢MMC (4~8 mg/body   ⎥ c̄ HHC
        ⎣OK-432 (0.06 KE/kg) ⎦

Postoperative regimen

Day 1.   CDDP (50 mg/body) i.v.

Day 3, 5. Pep (5 mg/body) c̄ HC

Day 4, 6. Pep (5 mg/body) i.v.

Day 7.   Pep (5 mg/body)   ⎤
          OK-432 (0.06 KE/kg)⎦ c̄ HHC

Fig. 2. Treatment schedules for malignant tumors of the esophagus. *HC*, under hypertension; *HHC*, under hypertension and hyperthermia

about 20 min. During the hypertensive state, anticancer drugs were administered. Normal blood pressure was reached within several minutes after Angiotensin II was discontinued. OK-432 (0.06 KE/kg) was then given by drip infusion and was followed by the "hyperthermic state". Patients were wrapped with a heating blanket to diminish evaporative heat loss (Fig. 1).

The preoperative and postoperative chemotherapy regimens are outlined in Fig. 2. Preoperatively, 5-FU (250–500 mg/kg) was given on day 1 and 2 under hypertension, followed by a combination of 5-FU, MMC (4–8 mg/kg) and OK-432 (0.06 KE/kg) on day 3 under hypertension and hyperthermia. After a single course of this regimen, surgery was performed after an interval of 1 to 2 weeks.

Postoperative chemotherapy regimen was given starting 20 to 30 days after surgery. On day 1, CDDP (50 mg/kg) was infused with prehydration. Peplomycin (5 mg/kg) was administered by drip infusion from day 3 to 7. It was given under hypertension on days 3 and 5, and under hypertention and hyperthermia on day 7.

For unresectable patients the same chemotherapy regimen was used. Subsequent courses were given with an adequate interval.

To evaluate the clinical efficacy, survival curves of the HHC group were compared to those treated without HHC regimen (non-HHC group). Survival curves were analyzed by the Kaplan–Meier method. The Student's t-test was used for comparisons.

Results

The hypertensive state was induced in all patients during Angiotensin II infusion. Besides, the hyperthermic state over 38.5°C occurred in 91% of the patients.

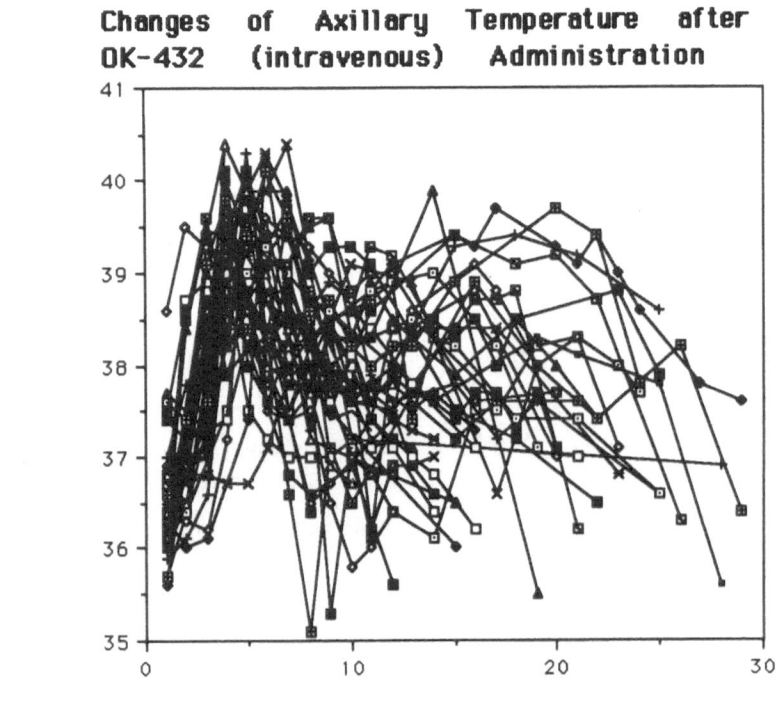

Fig. 3. Time course of temperatures recorded from the axilla

The peak temperature ranged from 38.4°C to 40.4°C with a mean of 39.6 ± 0.48°C. It was reached within 2 to 10 h with a mean of 4.7 ± 1.6 h. A mean duration of the hyperthenmic state was 7.4 ± 6.2 h (Fig. 3).

Among 24 patients who underwent surgery, 16 patients completed this regimen and the remaining 8 received the regimen only preoperatively because of their postoperative condition. Eleven patients had a single course of this regimen, 3 had two courses and 1 patient each had three or four courses. Curative resection was performed in 18 patients. Among the nine unresectable patients, three had a single course, another three had two courses, two had three courses, and one received six courses.

Survival curves are shown in Fig. 4. The 2-year survival rate was 53.4% for the HHC group and 35.8% for the non-HHC group. The 3-year survival rate was 36% and 25%, respectively. There were no significant differences between these two groups.

Of nine inoperable patients, there were two complete remissions (CR) and one partial response (PR) with a response rate of 33%. In these responding patients, remission durations ranged from 4 to 36 months.

Side effects of this regimen included shivering and chilling, high fever, and nausea and vomitting. Shivering and chilling were almost invariably seen prior to pyrexia, but no antifebrils was used against any pyrexia. Leukopenia was not prominent and there were no chemotherapy-related deaths.

Discussion

In 1977, Suzuki et al. [5] reported that the blood flow to tumor tissues selectively increases during Angiotensin II–induced hypertension without changing the flow to normal tissues. Several investigators [6, 7] have shown that tumor vessels

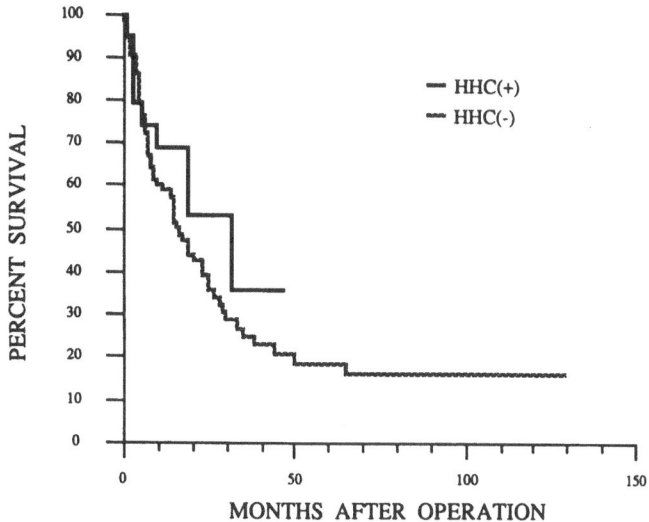

Fig. 4. Survival curve from start of therapy. *HHC*(+), patients treated with hypertensive-hyperthermo-chemotherapy, *HHC*(−), patients treated without HHC regimen

do not differentiate into arteriors or venules, thus vasoconstrictors are not effective in stimulating contraction. The absence of circulatory autoregulation in tumor vessels yields its passive dilatation secondary to Angiotensin II–induced hypertension. Under this condition, systemically administered drugs are transported concentrically both to tumors and metastatic lymph nodes. Thus, the anticancer effect of the drugs may be markedly enhanced. Most of the patients who seem to have a localized disease have micrometastasis that can not be detected by any preoperative evaluations. Systemic chemotherapy offers the only way to treat such metastatic lesions, whether it is in lymph nodes or distant organs.

On the other hand, an improved prognosis has been observed in patients with bronchogenic carcinoma exposed to pyrogenic substances by the happenstance of empyema [8]. A number of clinical and experimental investigations have suggested that fever per se may induce anticancer effects, though its basic mechanism remains obscure. Hyperthermia has been achieved by various methods, including heating blanket application, microwaves, the use of an extracorporeal circuit with heat exchanger, and the administration of pyrogens. In this series, the hyperthermic state was induced by OK-432 infusion with the aid of blanket application. OK-432 was selected because it may potentiate immunological response as well as having a pyrogenic effect, and it is a safe drug and easily available. The present study has demonstrated two CRs and one PR among nine inoperable patients. Survival curves, however, did not differ significantly between the HHC group and the non-HHC group. The failure to improve survival seemed to be a result of the insufficient dose of anticancer drugs for the adjuvant chemotherapy.

The use of Angiotensin II–induced hypertention combined with OK432–induced hyperthermia has a major theoretical advantage over conventional chemotherapy. Additional clinical experiences would be needed to evaluate this new modality.

References

1. Ravry M, Moertel CG, Schutt AJ (1973) Treatment of advanced squamous cell carcinoma of the gastrointestinal tract with bleomycin. Cancer Chemother Rep 57:493–495
2. Nabeya K (1976) The use of bleomycin in the treatment of carcinoma of the esophagus. Gan Monogr 19:177–186
3. Vogl SF, Greanwald E, Kaplan BH (1981) Effective chemotherapy for esophageal cancer with methotrexate, bleomycin and cisdiammine-dichloroplatinum II. Cancer 46:2555–2558
4. Japanese Society for Esophageal Disease (1989) Guidelines for the clinical and pathologic studies on carcinoma of the esophagus (7th edn) (in Japanese). Kanehara, Tokyo
5. Suzuki M, Hori K, Abe I, Saito S, Sato H (1977) Experimental studies on local permeation of anticancr drugs in tumor tissue. Jpn J Cancer chemother 4:97–102
6. Algire GH, Chalkloy HW (1945) Vascular reactions of normal and malignant tissues in vivo. 1. Vascular reactions of mice to wounds and to normal and neoplastic transplants. J Nat Cancer Inst 6:73–85
7. Ekelund LE, Lunderquist A (1974) Pharmacoangiography with angiotensin. Radiology 110: 533–540
8. Takita H (1970) Effect of postoperative empyema on survival of patients with bronchogenic carcinoma. J Thorac Cardiovasc Surg 59:642–668

Tumor Infiltrating Lymphocytes (TIL) and Neoadjuvant Chemotherapy in Esophageal Cancer

Toshitada Okuma, Yoshitsugu Torigoe, Keiichiro Kondo, Kenji Okamura, and Yoshimasa Miyauchi[1]

Introduction

Cisplatin (CDDP) has an antineoplastic action mechanism which directly inhibits DNA synthesis. However, another action mechanism of cytotoxic action, i.e., enhancement of spontaneous monocyte-mediated cytotoxicity (SMMC) has been reported [1].

The purpose of this study was to evaluate whether survival rate of patients with esophageal cancer could be improved as a result of inducing tumor-infiltrating lymphocytes (TIL) by administration of neoadjuvant chemotherapy (Neo-ch).

Material and Methods

Patients

Retrospective analysis of TIL was performed histologically for 149 patients with squamous cell carcinoma of thoracic esophagus resected in our hospital from 1976 to 1990. The patients were divided into three groups according to their different preoperative therapy, i.e., the surgery-alone group ($n = 22$), the pre-x-ray radiation treatment (XRT) group ($n = 41$) and the Neo-ch group ($n = 86$).

Histological Examination

TIL Grading

The microscopic paraffin sections stained by hematoxylin and eosin were taken from the center of the tumor. The intensity of TIL staining was examined in the

---

[1] First Department of Surgery, Kumamoto University School of Medicine, 1-1-1 Honjo, Kumamoto City, Kumamoto, 860 Japan

infiltrative margin of the tumor and classified into three grades. When tumor nests were thickly surrounded by TIL, it was classified as high grade. When TIL were present at moderate levels, it was classified as Medial grade, and when few TIL were noted, it was classified as Low grade.

TIL Populations

To investigate the TIL populations, paraffin sections of specimens from 84 of the 86 patients of the Neo-ch group were stained using the avidin biotinylated enzyme complex method (ABC method: Vectastain) using monoclonal mouse anti-human antigens.

Mean Number of T-Cells and Prognosis

The specimens which stained positive for T-cell antigen were examined microscopically at a magnification of 200 to quantitatively estimate the correlation between the degree of T-cell infiltration and the prognosis of the patients. The mean number of T-cells in a field of microscopic view was determined quantitatively by examining 5 fields per section for 84 of the 86 patients in the Neo-ch group. Mean numbers of T-cells were classified into 3 categories: when the mean number was less than 40, it was categorized as A; when it was between 40 and 80, it was categorized as B; and when it was more than 80, it was categorized as C.

Factors Related to TIL Grading

Factors related to TIL grading (incidence showing medial and high grade TIL) i.e., sex (male versus female), differentiation of cancer cell (poorly differentiated versus differentiated), infiltrative growth pattern (expansive versus invasive), depth of tumor invasion (T1–2 versus T3–4), lymph node involvement (positive versus negative), curability of operation (palliative versus curative), radiological response [no change (NC) versus partial response (PR)] according to the criteria of JSED [2] and histological response (Grade I versus II) according to the grading criteria of Shimozato et al. [3] were investigated for the patients in the Neo-ch group.

Administration Protocols of Neo-ch

From 1983 to 1988, the combination of CDDP, peplomycin (Pep) and Vindesine (VDS) or 5-Fluorouracil (5-FU) were used for Neo-ch. From 1989, in vitro chemosensitivity of the tumor was tested for eight antineoplastic drugs: CDDP, 5-FU, Pep, VP-16, VDS, THP-Adriamycin, mitomycin C, and methotrexate. These drugs were tested according to the method of Weisenthal using endoscopic biopsy specimens from the tumor before surgery. Three of the eight drugs showing high effectivity were selected and administered as Neo-ch.

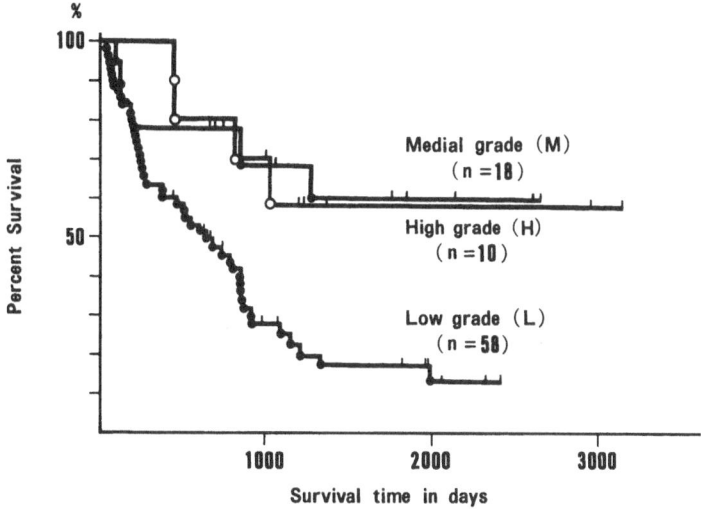

Fig. 1. Five year survival rates for Low, Medial, and High grade patients were 17.6%, 59.3%, and 58.3%, respectively. Significant differences between Low grade and Medial grade ($P <$ 0.03), and between Low grade and High grade ($P < 0.02$) were seen with generalized Wilcoxon analysis

Statistics

Survival curves and rates were obtained by the method of Kaplan-Meier. Comparison of survival curves was carried out using generalized Wilcoxon analysis. The other statistics values were calculated using the Chi-square test. Differences were considered to be significant when P was less than 0.05 ($P < 0.05$).

Results

Survival Rates According to TIL Grade

Patient survival curves according to the TIL grade are shown in Fig. 1. Survival curves of medial (n = 18) and High grade (n = 10) were significantly better than that of Low grade ($n = 58$) ($P < 0.03$, $P < 0.02$, respectively).

TIL Populations

A great number of TIL were stained positive for T-cell antigen in all specimens. Some of them stained positive for B-cell antigen and a few for macrophage antigen, but no TIL stained positive for Leu-7 antigen.

Survival Rates According to Mean Number of T-Cells

Patients survival curves based on the mean number of T-cells are illustrated in Fig. 2. A significant difference was seen in each survival curve: A vs B, $P <$ 0.02; B vs C, $P < 0.03$.

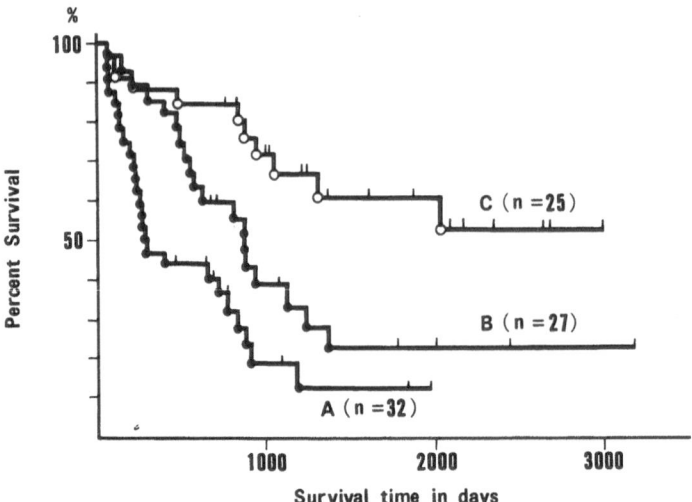

Fig. 2. Survival curves according to mean number of T-cells when the mean number of T-cells was less than 40 (*A*), between 40 and 80 (*B*), and more than 80 (*C*). Five-year survival rates of A, B, and C were 12.0%, 21.8%, and 59.9%, respectively. Significant differences were seen in each survival curve: A vs B, $P < 0.02$; B vs C, $P < 0.03$ (generalized Wilcoxon analysis)

Factors Related to TIL Grading

Significant differences were seen in the factors of depth of tumor invasion ($P = 0.0073$), curability of operation ($P = 0.014$) and histological response ($P < 0.0001$).

Preoperative Therapy and TIL

The T1 tumor specimens were excluded from this examination because there were significantly more specimens showing T1 tumor in the surgery-alone group than in the other groups, and T-factor (depth of tumor invasion) was significantly influenced by TIL grading, as mentioned above.

In the surgery-alone group, only 2 (9.1%) of the 22 specimens showed Medial grade and none showed High grade. In the Pre-XRT group, 6 (14.6%) of the 41 specimens were classified as Medial grade and only one specimen (2.4%) showed High grade.

In contrast to those findings, 13 (17.3%) of the 75 specimens in the Neo-ch group showed Medial grade and 9 (12.0%) showed High grade (Table 1).

Discussion

In an animal model of tumors, CDDP suppressed the cancer growth by inducing lymphocyte infiltration within and around the tumor [4].

Svet-Moldavsky and Hamburg reported about these findings as artificial heterogenization meaning activation of antineoplastic action by using biologic

Table 1. Preoperative therapy and TIL: Excluding PT1

TIL grade	Preoperative therapy		
	Surgery-alone group (%) (n = 22)	Pre-XRT group (%) (n = 41)	Neo-ch group (%) (n = 75)
Low grade	20 (90.9%)	34 (82.9%)	53 (70.7%)
Medial grade	2 (9.1%) $\rbrace_c$	6 (14.6%) $\rbrace_d$	13 (17.3%) $\rbrace_e$
High grade	0	1 (2.4%)[a]	9 (12.0%)[b]

TIL, tumor infiltrating lymphocytes; *XRT*, x-ray treatment; *PT1*, tumor invasion limited to submucosa
[a] vs [b] $P = 0.0650$; [c] vs [e] $P = 0.0530$; [d] vs [e] $P = 0.1449$

agents and chemical compounds [5]. It is well known that TIL were comprised of macrophages, plasma cells and T-lymphocytes, but there were very few NK-cells.

Many authors reported that TIL were pre-dominantly comprised of T-cells, of which phenotypes were CD8+ T-cells and OKT8 cells. Tahara also reported a predominance of CD8+, and CD11b- cells in TIL of esophageal cancer [6]. Rosenberg reported that these lymphocytes were cytotoxic T-cells (CTL) of which cytotoxic effectiveness against autologus tumor were shown to be from 50 to 100 times that of lymphokine-activated killer (LAK)-cells from peripheral blood lymphocytes [7].

In recent years, administering CTL derived from tumors has been studied as an adoptive immunotherapy using the method of enhancing the cytotoxic activity by generating the CTL in recombinant interleukin-2 [8].

It was unknown by what mechanism of Neo-ch TIL were induced. Considering of the findings that the most influential factor affecting TIL grading was shown to be histological response, the host immune function was activated because of regression of the tumor following the administration of Neo-ch which resulted in induction of T-cells within the tumor.

References

1. Kleinerman ES, Zwelling LA, Muchmore AV (1980) Enhancement of naturally occurring human spontaneous monocyte-mediated cytotoxicity by cis-diamminedichloroplatinum (II). Cancer Res 40:3099–3102
2. Japanese Society for Esophageal Diseases: Guidelines for the clinical and pathologic studies on carcinoma of the esophagus (8th edition), Tokyo, Kanehara (1992)
3. Shimozato Y, Oboshi S, Baba K (1971) Histological evaluation of effects of radiotherapy and chemotherapy for carcinomas. Jpn J Clin Oncol 1:19–35
4. Presnov MA, Konoalova AL, Romanova LF, et al (1978) Chemotherapy of transplantable mouse tumors with cis-dichloro-diamminplatinum (II) alone and in combination with sarcolysin. Cancer Treat Rep 62:705–712
5. Svet-Moldavsky GJ, Hamburg VP (1964) Quantitative relationships in viral oncolysis and the possibility of artificial heterogenization of tumors. Nature 202:303–304
6. Tahara H, Shiozaki H, Kobayashi K, Yano H, Tamura S, Miyata M, Wakasa K, Sakurai M, Mori T (1990) Principal lymphocyte subpopulation in local host response to human oesophageal cancer. Virchows Arch [A] 417:311–317

7. Rosenberg SA, Spiess P, Lafreniere R (1986) A new approach to the adoptive immunotherapy of cancer with tumor-infiltrating lymphocytes. Science 233:1318–1321
8. Kradin RL, Boyle LA, Preffer FI, Callahan RJ, Barlai-Kovach M, Strauss HW, Dubinett S, Kurnick JT (1987) Tumor-derived interleukin-2 dependent lymphocytes in adoptive immunotherapy of lung cancer. Cancer Immunol Immunother 24:76–85

A New Slow-Releasing Drug Delivery System for Chemically Combined Cisplatin with Chitin for Intraoperative Local Application: An Experimental Study

KENJI SUZUKI, HIROSHI YOSHIMURA, HIROSHI MATSUURA, TSUKASA KOTOH, TERUHISA NAKAMURA[1], RYOICHI TSURUTANI, and KOJI KIFUNE[2]

Introduction

In order to concentrate anticancer agents in residual cancer cells and to decrease side effects by supressing the systemic concentration of drug, we developed a new drug delivery system, Plachitin, for intraoperative local application after esophagectomy. Chitin and cisplatin were coupled by covalent bond, and in this system chitin was used as a carrier for cisplatin. Chitin is metabolized in the human body by enzymes such as lysozyme and is absorbed in 1–3 months. It is this slow breakdown of chitin that allows Plachitin to release cisplatin over a long period of time and deliver high concentrations of drug to local lesions.

In this paper, we investigated our new drug delivery system (DDS) for treatment of residual cancer cells, a system that affords long-term retention of drug in local tissues with low levels in the systemic circulation, and to show effectiveness when it was applied to solid tumors.

Materials and Methods

Preparation of Plachitin

Chitin was obtained from crab shell, which was purified by treatment with 0.1 N HCl and 1 N NaOH. The purified chitin was dissolved in amide solution and chitin fiber was obtained by wet spinning. To obtain deacetylated chitin fiber, the chitin fiber was treated with a caustic alkali solution. The deacetylated chitin fiber was reacted with cisplatin by stirring chitin fiber in 0.1% cisplatin solution.

[1] Second Department of Surgery, Shimane Medical University, Enya-cho 89-1, Izumo, 693 Japan

[2] Unitika Ltd., Research and Development Center, Ujikozakura 23, Uji, Yamaguchi, 611 Japan

The cisplatin concentration in Plachitin was varied, and in this work two different lots of Plachitin were used. One was lot no. 01003 (containing 332 mg of cisplatin in 1 g of Plachitin) and 01005 (containing 300 mg of cisplatin in 1 g of Plachitin). The content of cisplatin reacted with chitin fiber was measured by monitoring the decrease of cisplatin by high performance liquid chromotography.

Release of Platinum (Pt) from Plachitin In Vivo

The mice (ICR strain, 6-week-old, male, 30 g) were divided into two groups: Under ether anesthesia, Plachitin (lot no. 01003) at a cisplatin dose of 270 mg/kg body weight was implanted in the abdominal wall subcutaneously (group A), and 9 mg/kg body weight of cisplatin solution was injected into the peritoneal cavity (group B). Serum, kidney, and abdominal muscle were biopsied at a predetermined time and platinum (Pt) concentration was measured by flameless atomic absorption spectrophotometory (FAAS) [1]. BUN and serum creatinine was also measured.

Evaluation of Antitumor Activity and Survival Rates and Tumor Growth Rates

In this experiment, lot no. 01005 of Plachitin was used; 0.2 ml of Hanks fluid containing 2×10^6 Ehrlich cells was inoculated subucutaneously in the left inguinal region (day 0). After comfirming that subcutaneous tumors formed on day 3, tumors were treated with drugs in one of following six ways: (1) The tumors were exposed and covered with Plachitin at a cisplatin dose of 270 mg/kg body weight (group A), and at the same time, 4.5 mg/kg body weight of cisplatin solution was injected into the peritoneal cavity; (2) tumors were covered with the same dose of Plachitin (group B); (3) tumors were covered with the same weight of Plachitin used in this experiment (group C); (4) 4.5 mg/kg body weight of cisplatin solution was injected into the peritoneal cavity (group D); (5) the same dose of Plachitin was implanted in the right inguinal region contralateral to the tumor site (group E); and (6) tumor was exposed and the skin closed (group F).

After these treatments, the antitumor effect was evaluated in terms of both tumor growth rates and survival rates. Tumor size was measured with calipers twice a week, and the tumor weight was calculated by means of the following equation:

$$w = aXb^2/2$$

where a = length (mm), b = width (mm), and w = estimated weight (mg) [2]. The statistical significance between tumor weights were determined by the unpaired Student's t-test. Survival rates were obtained by confirming the life or death of mice every day. The statistical differences among the survival curves were determined by generalized Willcoxon's test.

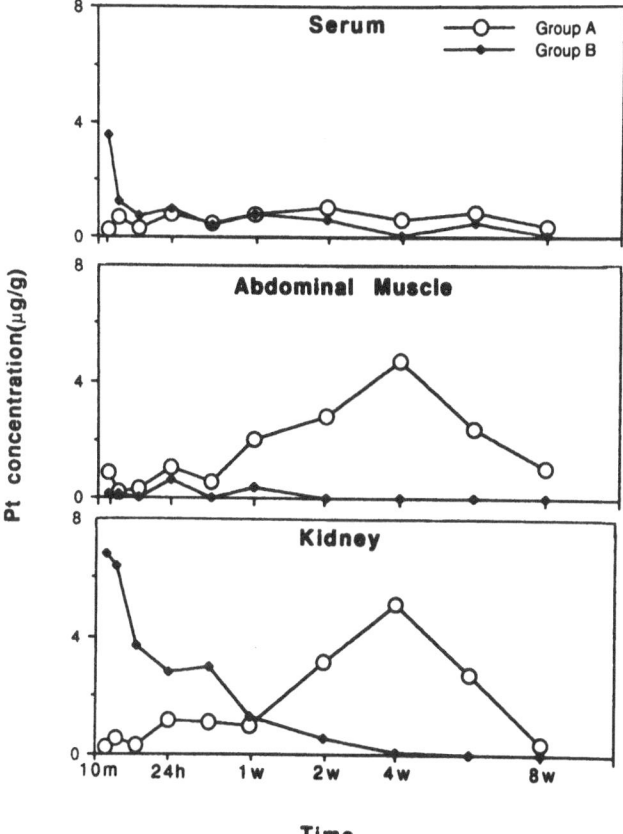

Fig. 1. Changes of platinum concentration of serum, abdominal muscle, and kidney after implanting Plachitin in abdominal wall or injecting cisplatin solution into peritoneal cavity. Five mice were used in each point, each group

Results

Release Rate of Pt from Plachitin In Vivo

In Group A, serum platinum concentration remained below $1.0\,\mu g/g$ throughout the examination period, but that in abdominal muscle increased gradually and peaked at $4.7\,\mu g/g$ at week 4. A high concentration of Pt was maintained until week 8. In group B, serum platinum was highest immediately after injection, but in the abdominal muscle it remained at a low level throughout the examination period. Kidney levels were similar to serum levels. Platinum concentrations in the kidney in both groups were almost the same as abdominal muscle (Fig. 1).

Serologic Side Effect of Plachitin and Histologic Studies

Values of BUN and serum creatinine in both groups were within normal limits throughout the examination period. Microscopic view of the kidney in group A

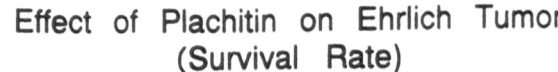

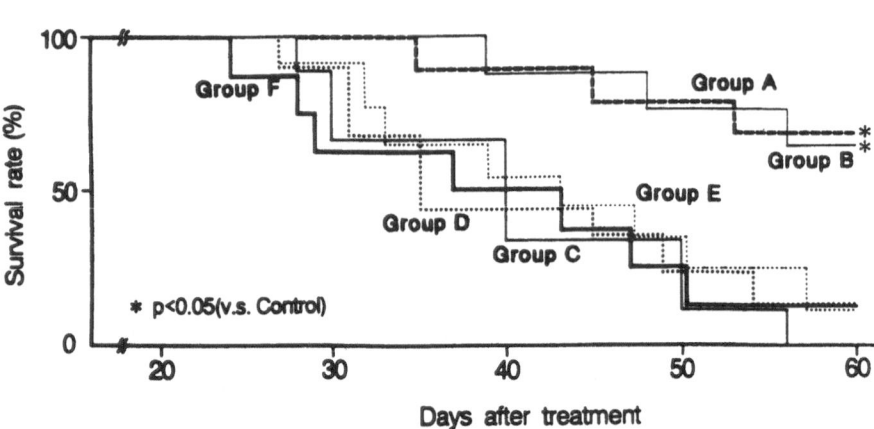

Fig. 2. Survival rates after various treatments. In group F, all mice died within 60 days. The survival curves of groups C, E, and D were similar to that of group F. On the other hand, in groups A and B, the survival rates were significantly higher than group F ($P < 0.05$), and 60-day survival rates were 77.8% and 75.0%, respectively

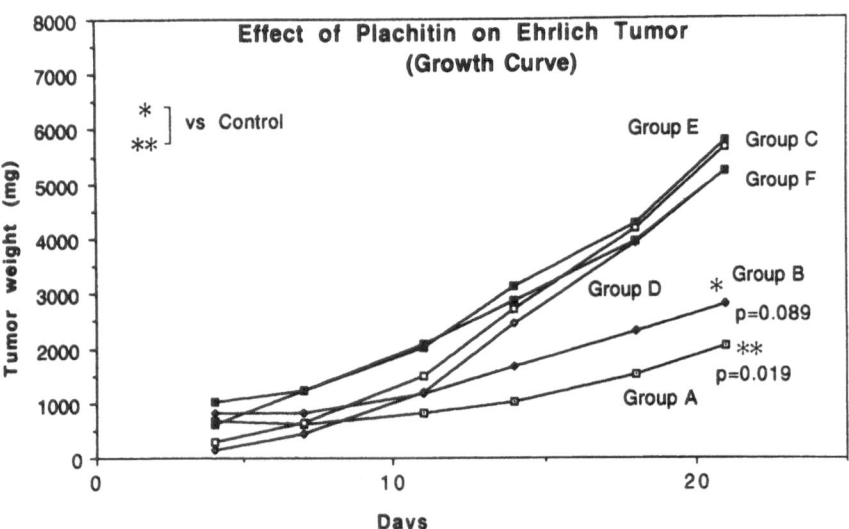

Fig. 3. Tumor growth rates after various treatments. Tumor growth of group A was supressed compared with that of the control group. That of the group B was also supressed, although it was higher than group A. Those of groups C and E were not different compared with group F. In group D, tumor growth was supressed only for first 7 days, but after that the growth curve was similar to that of group F

at week 4, when platinum concentration reached its peak level in the kidney, showed no histological abnormalities. No other specimens of kidneys showed abnormal findings.

Evaluation of Antitumor Activity

The survival rates of each group are shown in Fig. 2. Tumor growth in each group is shown in Fig. 3.

Discussion

Some investigaters reported a slow-releasing anticancer devise using cisplatin. Hecquet et al. [3] prepared cisplatin-polylactic polyglycolic acids copolymer as controlled drug delivery implants with sustained release (at least for 3 weeks), but the antitumor effect was not shown. Deurloo et al. [4] reported cisplatin release system from polyether-hydrogel formulation with a long-release period and antitumor effect by intratumoral administration.

Cancer of the esophagus is often diagnosed in an advanced stage, and it is difficult to perform the curative resection. Plachitin is intended for use in the treatment of these unresectable cancers.

It is speculated that Plachtin, chitin bounded to cisplatin, may be degraded by enzymes such as lysozyme and β-N-acetylglucosamidase [5]. The evidence that cisplatin was detected in vivo experiment supports the speculation, because cisplatin was not detected in the solution when Plachitin was left in the biological saline or in diluted hydrochloric acid (data not shown). By our analysis, it is reasonable to conclude that the amino group of deacetylated chitin reacts with cisplatin.

The dosage of Plachitin used in these experiments was decided by preliminary study which revealed that, at a cisplatin dose of 270 mg/kg body weight, Plachitin was almost equally as effective as 9 mg/kg body weight of cisplatin solution. This is the optimum dose in mice [6] and the dose of cisplatin solution administered in groups A and D was half of this dose; this dose (4.5 mg/kg of cisplatin solution) was used to evaluate the synergistic effects of cisplatin solution and Plachitin.

The result showed platinum was highly concentrated on tissue around the implanted Plachitin at least for 8 weeks, and low concentration in serum although the dose of cisplatin administrated in group A was 30-fold greater than group B. This result is certainly meets the aim of this experiment which is to increase the drug concentration at the tumor site for a long period and to decrease the concentration in systemic circulation.

The primary dose-limiting factor of cisplatin, nephrotoxity, is one of the most important problems in clinical use of Plachitin. While high concentrations of platinum were detected in the kidneys of mice in group A, serologic studies showed no renal disturbance at the dose used.

The survival rate and tumor growth rate showed apparent antitumor activity for Ehrlich tumor when Plachitin was applied locally, especially when cisplatin was injected into the peritoneal cavity at the same time. The tumor growth rate in group E was not supressed, indicating that the effectiveness of Plachitin was due to direct contact of anticancer drug with tumor cells rather than its absorption into the systemic circulation.

In conclusion, Plachitin had slow-releasing property for over 8 weeks and showed anticancer effect for solid tumors of mice by local application without any side effect in used dosage. It is expected that Plachitin may be useful in cases of unresectable cancer for palliation, and seemed to be adequate for clinical trials with the aim of evaluating the effect of local cancer treatment of human tumors.

References

1. Leroy AF, Wehling ML, Sponseller HL, Litterst CL, Gram TE, Guarino AM, Becher DA (1977) Analysis of platinum in biological materials by flameless atomic absorption spectrophotometry. Biochem Med 18:184
2. Gern RI, MacDonald MM, Schumacher AM (1972) Protocols for screening chemical agents and natural products against animal tumors and other biological systems. Cancer Chemother Reports 3:47–52
3. Hecquet B, Chabot F, Delatorre Gonzalez JC, Fournier C, Hilali S, Cambier L, Depadt G, Vert M (1986) In vitro sustained released of cisplatin from bioresorbable implants in mice. Anticancer Res 6:1251–1256
4. Deurloo MJM, Bohlken S, Kop W, Lerk CF, Hennink W, Bartelink H, Begg AC (1990) Intratumoral administration of cisplatin in slow-release devices. Cancer Chemother Pharmacol 27:135–140
5. Nakajima M, Atsumi K, Kifune K (1986) Chitin is an effective material for sutures. Jpn J Surg 16:418–424
6. Hasegawa Y, Morita M, Muto N (1980) Antitumor activity of cisplatin on experimental animal system (in Japanese). Jpn J Canc Res 7:621–630

Larynx Preserving Strategy in Patients with Squamous Cell Carcinoma of the Cervical Esophagus

M. Valente, P. Bidoli, G. Cantu, A. Santoro, V. Bedini, U. Pastorino, M. Alloisio, R. Zucali, P. Salvini, and G. Ravasi[1]

Introduction

Total laryngopharyngectomy with partial or total oesophagectomy is the standard surgical treatment for precricoid or postcricoid pharyngo-esophageal cancer [1-5].

In the reported series, the mean operative mortality was 15%, the median survival time was 16 months and the 5-year survival rate was similar to the operative mortality and not significantly greater than the poor (10%) survival obtainable with radiotherapy [6]. If incomplete resections and operative deaths are excluded (nearly 30%), the 5-year survival is 26% for pre-cricoid cancer and 17% for post-cricoid cancer in the largest reported series [1]. One-field dissection (cervical) is useful for precricoid tumours [7], but not for post-cricoid tumours, as it does not clear the upper mediastinal nodes which are to be considered regional nodes [8]. Unfortunately, cervical mediastinoscopy is not used by surgeons, traditional non-invasive staging is inaccurate in the prediction of mediastinal nodal diffusion [8], the prediction rates of endoscopic ultrasound are unknown, and two-field dissection (both cervical and mediastinal) is not performed. Lymph node status is the main prognostic factor, and the presence of lymph node metastases is the leading obstacle to complete resection and long-term survival. During the first 12 months after complete resection, most patients with post-cricoid cancer develop cervical and/or mediastinal recurrences. Nearly 20% of all patients with pre- or post-cricoid pharyngo-esophageal cancer had a previous cancer; nearly 10% have synchronous cancer and another 10% will develop metachronous cancer after treatment. The drawback of any improvement in the diagnosis and treatment of this tumour will be an increase in the metachronous cancer rate. Partial or total esophagectomy worsens the aphasia after total laryngopharyngectomy; neo-esophageal phonation is possible in only

[1] Istituto per lo Studio e la Cura dei Tumori, Via Venezian 1, 20131, Milan, Italy

30% of patients, and prosthetic or surgical tracheo-neo-esophageal phonation are not commonly performed [9–11].

With the aim to preserve the larynx in these patients, we started a phase II study on combined chemotherapy and radiotherapy with salvage total laryngopharyngectomy with total esophagectomy for squamous carcinoma of post-cricoid cervical esophageal cancer.

Methods

In order to preserve the larynx, treatment consisted of primary combined chemotherapy and radiotherapy, followed by salvage total laryngopharyngectomy with total esophagectomy in case of persistent disease or local recurrence without distant spread. Primary combined chemotherapy and radiotherapy consisted of traditional radiotherapy (30 + 20 Gy over 7 weeks) with four courses of chemotherapy (5-FU [5-fluorouracil] 1000 mg/sqm 24-h infusion, days 1–4 and cisplatin (CDDP) 100 mg/m^2, day 1).

The criteria to exclude patients from larynx preservation were contraindications to combined chemotherapy and radiotherapy, previous partial or total laryngectomy and tumor located only in the pre-cricoid pharyngo-esophageal area.

Results

From May 1985 to December 1990, 45 consecutive patients with resectable carcinoma of the cervical esophagus were treated at the National Cancer Institute of Milan. Twenty-nine patients underwent larynx-preserving treatment, whereas 16 were excluded (5 for contraindications to combined chemotherapy and radiotherapy, 4 for previous partial or total laryngectomy, and the remaining 7 for tumor located only in the pre-cricoid area) and underwent primary resection. The main features of the patients are listed in Table 1 and the main characteristics of multiple tumors in Table 2.

Four completion laryngopharyngectomies and 12 total laryngopharyngectomies, 15 with total and 1 with partial esophagectomy, were performed in the group of patients who underwent primary resection. Transhiatal gastric pull-up, the first-choice alimentary tract restoration, was performed in 13 patients, colon transposition in 2, and free jejunal transfer in the remaining patient. Hospital mortality was 0% and iatrogenic mortality (any death linked to the treatment) was 6% (1/16). One lethal pneumonia after nearly 90 days from resection and hospital discharge was linked to the treatment. Of the 29 patients who underwent larynx preservation, 4 had medical contraindications to surgery, 6 had synchronous tumors, and 2 had previous cancer. Mortality due to the toxicity of radiochemotherapy was 3% (1/29), whereas iatrogenic mortality was 7% (2/29); it could not be excluded that one myocardial infarction was linked to the treatment. The iatrogenic mortality of the adjunctive treatment for synchronous tumors was 33% (2/6), one case after surgery and the other after endoscopic dilation.

Table 1. Features of the patients

	Radiotherapy and chemotherapy	Surgery
Mean age	62	60
Female	5	6
Age >70	4	2
Previous	2	6
Synchronous	6	0
c N1	11	5
Total	29	16

c N1, involvement of the cervical nodes predicted by clinical examination

Table 2. Multiple tumors

	Previous	Synchronous	Metachronous
Larynx	5		
Esophagus		4	
Lung	3		1
Rhinopharynx	1		
Mediastinum	1		
Stomach	1	1	
Oral		1	1
Kidney			1
Total	11	6	3

A clinical complete response after chemoradiotherapy was defined as near total shrinkage of the tumor with normal mucosa at endoscopic evaluation.

With this criterion, complete responses were obtained in nearly 40% of patients. Three patients with incomplete responses underwent surgical exploration and in two of them salvage resection was possible.

By the end of January 1992, after a median follow-up of 40 months (14–79), another four patients underwent a salvage total laryngopharyngectomy for local recurrence after complete response, two with total esophagectomy and two with partial esophagectomy (jejunal transfer). The hospital mortality after salvage resection was 0% and the iatrogenic mortality was 16% (1/6); at home, after a healed pharyngo-jejunal leak, one patient had a lethal hemorrhage 120 days following resection.

Without exclusion of any patient and any cause of death, the median survival was 15 months: 22 months for larynx preservation and 11 months for primary surgery. The probability of 3-year survival was 0.30 and 0.28, respectively. Eleven of the 29 eligible patients are alive (1 with lung metastases), with a median interval from the start of treatment of 32 months (22–78). Larynx preservation was possible in 82% (9/11) of long-term survivors, and in 22% (2/9) of the long-term survivors with a preserved larynx, primary surgery for synchronous cardia carcinoma and metachronous adenocarcinoma of the lung was performed. Survival of patients is shown in Fig 1.

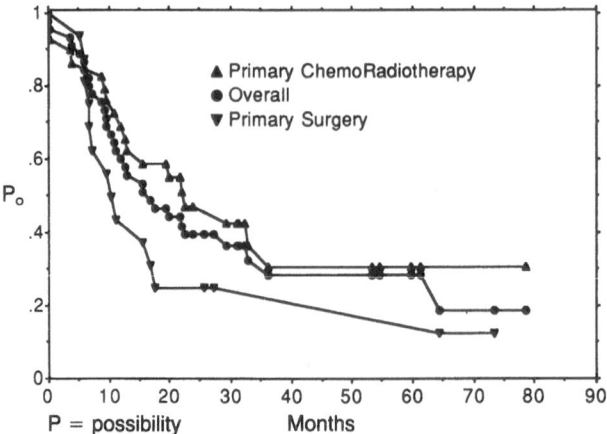

$P = possibility$

Fig. 1. Survival of the patients

Discussion

After total laryngopharyngetomy with total esophagectomy, with or without single-field cervical dissection, the prognosis for patients with post-cricoid cancer is poor. Nearly 10% of the resections are incomplete due to the presence of greater than expected nodal diffusion, nearly 15% of patients die due to causes linked with the treatment and most patients develop nodal recurrence in the upper mediastinum in the first year after resection.

In the future, accurate prediction of nodal diffusion in the upper mediastinum will be of great value to choose the adequate volume of treatment, while the use of polyvinyl prostheses could reduce the number of planned palliative total laryngopharyngectomies [12]. There are two possibilities to improve the prognosis of low cervical esophageal cancer: extended resection of the upper mediastinum or improvement of radiotherapy.

Recently, combined chemotherapy and radiotherapy has proved to be superior to radiotherapy alone [13], as measured by control of local tumors and survival; however, at the cost of increased side effects.

The data of our study shows that larynx preservation strategy with combined chemotherapy and radiotherapy is feasible and effective in patients with cancer of the cervical esophagus. It gives at least the same expected long-term results as primary surgery, preserving the larynx in nearly 80% of long-term survivors, but this approach requires selected tumors, motivated patients, interdisciplinary cooperation, and careful patient monitoring.

Summary. From May 1985 to December 1990, 45 consecutive patients with resectable pre-cricoid and post-cricoid pharyngo-esophageal cancer were treated at the National Cancer Institute of Milan. To preserve the larynx, the planned treatment was primary combined chemotherapy and radiotherapy followed by salvage resection in case of persistent disease or local recurrence without distant spread. Primary radio-chemotherapy consisted of traditional radiotherapy

(30 + 20 Gy over 7 weeks) with four courses of chemotherapy (5-fluorouracil; 5-FU, 1000 mg/m^2 24-h infusion, days 1–4 and cisplatin; CDDP, 100 mg/m^2, day 1). Sixteen patients were excluded (five for contraindications to combined chemotherapy and radiotherapy, four for previous partial or total laryngectomy, and the remaining seven for tumor located only in the pre-cricoid area) and underwent primary resection. Four completion laryngopharyngectomies and 12 total laryngopharyngectomies, 15 with total and 1 with partial esophagectomy, were performed in the group of patients who underwent primary resection. Transhiatal gastric pull-up, the first-choice alimentary tract restoration, was performed in 13 patients, colon transposition in 2, and free jejunal transfer in the remaining patient, with 0% of hospital mortality. Of 29 patients who underwent larynx preservation, 3 were medically inoperable, 2 had previous carcinoma, and 6 had 11 synchronous tumors. Iatrogenic mortality was 7% (2/29) and the iatrogenic mortality of synchronous tumor treatment was 33% (2/6). By the end of January 1992, after a median follow-up of 40 months (14–79), six patients underwent salvage total laryngopharyngectomy, four with total esophagectomy and two with partial esophagectomy with free jejunal transfer in the six patients with multiple tumors; in all these cases hospital mortality was 0%. Without exclusion of and patient and any cause of death, the median survival was 15 months: 22 months for larynx preservation and 11 months for primary surgery. The probability of 3-year survival was 0.28, 0.30 for larynx preservation and 0.25 for primary surgery. Eleven of the 29 eligible patients are alive (1 with lung metastases), with a median interval from the treatment of 32 months (22–78). Preservation of the larynx was possible in 82% (9/11) of long-term survivors, and in 22% (2/9) of the long-term survivors with a spared larynx, primary surgery for synchronous cardia carcinoma and metachronous adenocarcinoma of the lung was performed. Larynx preservation with combined chemotherapy and radiotherapy was thus shown to be effective in patients with cancer of the cerrical esophagus, giving at least the same expected long-term results as primary surgery.

References

1. Peracchia A, Bardini R, Ruol A, Castoro C, Segalin A, Asolati M, Tiso E, Bachellier C (1991) Cancer of the hypopharynx and cervical esophagus. Ann Chir 45(4):313–318
2. Mehta SA, Sarkar S, Mehta AR, Mehta MS (1990) Mortality and morbidity of primary pharyngogastric anastomosis following circumferential excision for hypopharyngeal malignancies. J Surg Oncol 43(1):24–27
3. Mehta SA, Sarkar S, Mehta AR, Mehta MS (1990) Mortality and morbidity of primary pharyngogastric anastomosis following circumferential excision for hypopharyngeal malignancies (75 cases). J Surg Oncol 43(1): 24–27
4. Moreno Gonzalez E, Hidalgo Pascual M, Landa Garcia JI, Calle Santiuste A, Seone Gonzalez J, Gomez Gutierrez M, Figueroa Andollo J, Escudero Benito F, Arias Diaz (1990) Treatment of carcinoma of the cervical esophagus and hypopharynx. J Dis Esophagus. 3(1):21–28
5. Ferguson JL, DeSanto LW (1988) Total pharyngolaryngectomy and cervical esophagectomy with jejunal autotransplant reconstruction: Complication and results. Laryngoscope. 98(9): 911–914
6. Mendenhall WM, Parsons JT, Vogel SB, Cassisi NJ, Million RR (1988) Carcinoma of the cervical esophagus treated with radiation therapy: SO. Laryngoscope 98(7):769–771

 7. Matsuura H (1988) Regional neck dissection in carcinoma of the cervical esophagus. Gan To Kagaku Ryoho. 15(4 Pt 1):574–579
 8. Peracchia A, Ruol A, Narne S, Tiso E, Segalin A, Lazzaro S, Anselmino M, Bardini R (1990) Critical analysis of the new TNM (UICC, 1987) of cancer of the cervical esophagus in relation to therapeutic decision. Acta Otorhinolaryngol Ital. 10(3):275–285
 9. Wenig BL, Keller AJ, Levy J, Mullooly V, Abramson AL (1989) Voice restoration after laryngopharyngoesophagectomy. Otolaryngol Head Neck Surg. 101(1):11–13
10. Krespi YP, Sisson GA. Wurster CF (1984) Voice preservation in postcricoid and cervical esophageal cancer. Arch Otolaryngol 110:323–326
11. Kawahara H, Shiraishi T, Yasugawa H, Okamura K, Shirakusa T (1992) A new surgical technique for voice restoration after laryngopharyngoesophagectomy with a free ileocolic graft: Preliminary report. Surgery 111:569–575
12. Goldschmid S, Boyce HW Jr, Nord HJ, Brady PG (1988) Treatment of pharyngoesophageal stenosis by polyvinyl prosthesis. Am J Gastroenterol. 83(5):513–518
13. Herskoic A, Marts K, Al-Sarraf M, Leichman L, Brindle J, Vaitkevicius V, Cooper J, Byhardt R, Davis L, Emami B (1992) Combined chemotherapy and radiotherapy compared with radiotherapy alone in patients with cancer of the esophagus. N Engl J Med 326:1593–1598

Combined Modality Treatment for Locally Advanced Squamous Cell Esophageal Carcinoma Located at or Above the Level of the Tracheal Bifurcation

U. Fink, H.J. Stein, P. Lukas, A. Gossmann, R. Schiffner, H.J. Dittler, J.D. Roder, and J.R. Siewert[1]

Introduction

Despite the advances of en bloc esophagectomy and lymph node dissection, the results of surgical resection alone in patients with advanced squamous cell esophageal cancer remain disappointing [1, 2]. Complete macroscopic and microscopic tumor removal, i.e., an R0 resection according to the UICC 1987 definition [3], provides the only chance for long-term survival in this situation [4, 5]. Due to the close anatomical relation between the esophagus, trachea, and main stem bronchi, complete macroscopic and microscopic tumor removal is particularly difficult in patients with tumors in the proximal half of the esophagus [4]. Consequently, surgical resection in patients with locally advanced squamous cell esophageal carcinoma located at or above the level of the tracheal bifurcation is usually palliative and the prognosis is dismal [4].

In recent years, a combination of chemo and/or radiation therapy with or without surgery has been investigated by several authors in an attempt to prolong survival in patients with esophageal carcinoma [5–12]. Several trials have shown that radio/chemotherapy (RTx/CTx) can induce clinical remission or complete pathologic response in a considerable number of patients [5–9]. As with other tumors of the gastrointestinal tract, multimodal therapy should increase the frequency of R0 resections and thus prolong survival in patients with locally advanced esophageal carcinoma [13]. We prospectively assessed the effect of preoperative combined RTx/CTx on resectability, frequency of R0 resections, and survival in patients with locally advanced squamous cell esophageal carcinoma located at or above the level of the tracheal bifurcation.

---

[1] Chirurgische Klinik und Poliklinik der TU München, Klinikum rechts der Isar, Ismaninger Str 22, D-8000 München 80, Germany

Material and Methods

Eligibility Criteria

Patients with histologically proven and locally advanced squamous cell esophageal cancer located at or above the level of the tracheal bifurcation who were younger than 65 years of age were eligible for combined modality treatment, i.e., RTx/CTx followed by surgical resection. The location of the tumor in relation to the tracheal bifurcation was assessed by barium esophagography and endoscopy. The carcinoma was considered as "locally advanced" when preoperative staging by computer tomography (CT) and endoscopic ultrasonography showed a T3/T4 Nx tumor, i.e., a tumor that has penetrated through the esophageal wall [3]. Systemic metastases were excluded by physical examination, CT scanning of the neck, chest, and abdomen, abdominal ultrasonography, chest radiography, and radionuclide bone scanning. Fistula or gross tumor infiltration of the trachea or mainstem bronchus were excluded by bronchoscopy.

Based on functional evaluation, the patients had to be fit for RTx/CTx and surgical resection. This required adequate pulmonary, renal, hepatic, and cardiovascular function as described in detail elsewhere [4]. Patients with a Karnofsky index below 70%, previous or second malignancies, a life expectancy shorter than 3 months, or inadequate bone marrow function were also excluded.

Patient Population and Study Protocol

Between May 1986 and December 1991, 55 patients with locally advanced squamous cell esophageal carcinoma located at or above the level of the tracheal bifurcation were included in the study. Another 95 patients with similarly advanced squamous cell esophageal carcinoma who underwent resection without preoperative RTx/CTx between 1984 and 1991 served as controls. In 17 of these 95 patients, the tumor was located at or above the level of the tracheal bifurcation. In the remaining 77 patients, the tumor was located below the level of the tracheal bifurcation.

Multimodality therapy consisted of one cycle of 5-fluorouracil (5-FU) with or without mitomycin (MMC) and 3000 cGy (rad) of radiation administered over 3 weeks followed by surgical en bloc resection. The daily fractional radiation dose was 200 cGy (rad) given 5 days per week. The radiation field included known macroscopic tumor, 5 cm of normal esophagus on either side of visible tumor, and the draining lymph nodes. During the first study period (May 1986–April 1988, 26 patients) 5-FU was administered as continuous intravenous infusion at a dose of $1000 \, mg/m^2$/day on radiation days 1–4. Mitomycin was added at a dose of $10 \, mg/m^2$ on radiation day 1. Because of frequent pulmonary complications, MMC was omitted in the second study period (October 1988–December 1991, 29 patients) and 5-FU was given as continuous infusion at a dose of $450 \, mg/m^2$/day on all radiation days. During RTx/CTx, patients had weekly physical examinations, and hematologic and biochemical studies. Toxicity of the treatment was assessed using the standard World Health Organization criteria [14].

Clinical response to RTx/CTx was assessed 1 week after completion of the RTx/CTx course using esophagoscopy, endoscopic ultrasonography, chest radiography, barium esophagography, CT of the chest and abdomen, and abdominal ultrasonography. Clinical response to RTx/CTx was classified as "complete response", "partial response", "minimal response", "no change", or "progression" according to the World Health Organization criteria [14].

Surgical resection was usually performed within 10 days after completion of RTx/CTx. Patients with a tumor of the thoracic esophagus had a standardized esophagectomy and proximal gastrectomy via the abdominal and right thoracic route as described previously [15]. The resection comprised the proximal part of the lesser curvature of the stomach, the entire abdominal and thoracic esophagus including the azygos vein, the thoracic duct, and the surrounding lymphatic and fatty tissues. Proximal to the junction of the azygos vein with the superior vena cava, an isolated lymphadenectomy was performed. This comprises the so-called 2-field lymphadenectomy. Gastrointestinal continuity was restored by a gastric tube and a cervical esophagogastrostomy. A colon interposition was used in patients with previous gastric surgery. In patients with a tumor of the cervical esophagus, a segmental cervical esophagectomy and lymph node dissection with interposition of a free jejunal transplant was performed. In all patients, the removed specimen was opened, inspected, and fixed for histopathologic evaluation. The TNM, and R (resection) categories were assessed according to the UICC criteria [3].

Data Evaluation

Patient data, side effects and response to RTx/CTx, results of the surgical procedure, and the histopathologic evaluation of the resected specimen were collected prospectively. All patients were followed regularly in our tumor clinic or by telephone contact with their primary physician. Follow-up is complete for all patients. The demographic data showed no significant differences between the various groups. Survival time was chosen as the end point of the study.

Survival was measured from the beginning of RTx/CTx or the date of resection, respectively, to the date of death or the most recent follow-up. Estimates of survival were determined by the Kaplan-Meier method for non-parametric testing [16] and compared using the log-rank test [17].

Results

Of the 55 patients with locally advanced squamous cell carcinoma enrolled in the study, 52 (94.5%) completed the full course of preoperative RTx/CTx. One patient died from severe bone marrow depression which resulted from a drug overdosage due to a protocol violation during the initial phase of the study. In another two patients, chemotherapy was stopped because of bone marrow depression. Both patients recovered.

The clinical response to preoperative RTx/CTx with or without MMC is shown in Table 1. Complete or partial clinical response was observed in 21/55 (38.2%) patients who had preoperative RTx/CTx. Eight of the 55 patients did not undergo surgical resection because of death ($n = 1$), development of systemic metastases ($n = 4$), or a deterioration of their general status ($n = 3$) during RTx/CTx resulting in a resection rate of 85.4% (47/55 patients). All eight

Table 1. Clinical response to preoperative radio/chemotherapy in patients with locally advanced squamous cell esophageal carcinoma located at or above the level of the tracheal bifurcation

	MMC/5-FU 30 Gy	5-FU 30 Gy	Total
Complete response	4/26 (15.3%)	2/29 (6.9%)	6/55 (10.9%)
Partial response	5/26 (19.2%)	10/29 (34.5%)	15/55 (27.3%)
Minimal response	6/26 (23.1%)	7/29 (24.1%)	13/55 (23.6%)
No change	7/26 (26.9%)	7/29 (24.1%)	14/55 (25.5%)
Progression	2/26 (7.7%)	2/29 (6.9%)	4/55 (7.3%)
Not evaluated	2/26 (7.7%)	1/29 (3.4%)	3/55 (5.5%)
Resection rate	23/26 (88.5%)	24/29 (82.7%)	47/55 (85.5%)

MMC/5-FU, 30 Gy, pretreatment with mitomycin, 5-fluorouracil, and 30 Gy radiation; *5-FU, 30 Gy*, pretreatment with 5-fluorouracil continuous infusion, 30 Gy radiation

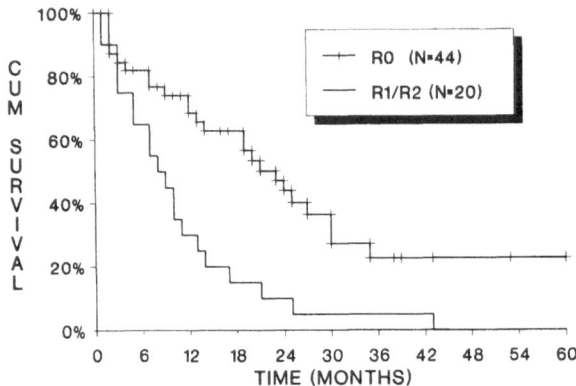

Fig. 1. Cumulative (*CUM*) survival rates in patients with locally advanced squamous cell esophageal carcinoma located at or above the level of the tracheal bifurcation according to the presence of residual tumor after surgical resection. *R0*, complete macroscopic and microscopic tumor resection (UICC 1987); *R1/2*, residual tumor after resection (UICC 1987)

patients who did not proceed to surgery had died by 8 months after the onset of RTx/CTx.

Complete pathologic response, i.e., no viable tumor in the resected specimen, was observed in 7/47 (14.9%) patients undergoing resection. An additional two patients had no viable primary tumor but positive mediastinal lymph node metastasis. In 4/47 patients who underwent resection, systemic metastases were noted on surgery. There was no significant difference in the distribution of postoperative tumor stages and median survival time between patients who had RTx/CTx with or without MMC. Independent of preoperative treatment, median survival time was, however, significantly longer in patients who had a complete macroscopic and microscopic tumor resection, i.e., an R0 resection

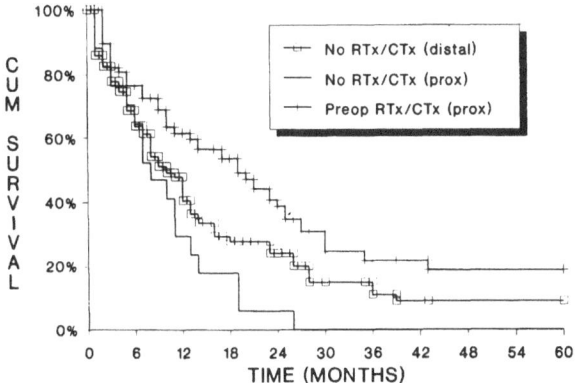

Fig. 2. Cumulative survival after surgical resection in patients with locally advanced squamous cell esophageal carcinoma according to tumor location and pretreatment. *RTx/CTx*, preoperative radio/chemotherapy; *Prox*, at or above the level of the tracheal bifurcation; *Distal*, below the level of the tracheal bifurcation

according to the UICC 1987 classification, as compared to those who had residual tumor after resection (Fig. 1).

The rate of complete macroscopic and microscopic tumor resections, i.e., R0 resections, was markedly higher in patients with locally advanced tumors of proximal esophagus who had preoperative RTx/CTx (39/47) as compared to patients with similarly advanced tumors in the proximal (5/17) or distal esophagus (36/77) who did not have preoperative RTx/CTx. This was associated with a significantly longer median survival time in patients who had preoperative RTx/CTx (Fig. 2).

Discussion

The use of chemotherapy to treat a disease with a high degree of systemic dissemination as in advanced esophageal cancer is appealing. Since some substances have cytotoxic as well as radio-sensitizing properties, a combination of preoperative chemotherapy and radiotherapy has been used by several groups to control regional tumor growth and to destroy systemic micrometastasis [5–7, 9, 12]. The present data add to the vast evidence from these studies that RTx/CTx can be used to induce substantial tumor regression including pathologic complete response in patients with squamous cell esophageal cancer. In addition, our study shows that this approach markedly increases the rate of complete macroscopic and microscopic tumor resections and thus prolongs survival in patients with locally advanced squamous cell carcinoma of the proximal esophagus.

In contrast to all other published series, preoperative RTx/CTx in the present study was performed only in patients who had advanced esophageal carcinomas at an unfavorable location, i.e., at or above the level of the tracheal bifurcation. The limited usefulness of surgical resection alone in this situation is reflected in the frequency of R0 resections performed and the dismal prognosis in the control group of patients with similarly advanced tumors in the proximal esophagus who did not have preoperative treatment. The clinical and pathologic response rates and survival time achieved with preoperative RTx/CTx in this negatively selected patient population compare to those reported in patients with earlier tumor stages at more favorable locations [6, 7, 9]. Our study suggests that this is due to the marked increase in the rate of complete macroscopic and microscopic tumor resections which even surpassed the frequency of R0 resections in patients with advanced tumors at a more favorable location, i.e., the distal esophagus.

Despite these benefits, several arguments have been raised against a more general use of preoperative therapy in patients with esophageal cancer. These include a delay in definite treatment which may result in tumor progression, a deterioration of the general condition of the patient during preoperative RTx/-CTx, and the fear of increased postoperative complications and mortality. With the preoperative RTx/CTx regimen used in the present study, esophagectomy was performed within 4 weeks of diagnosis in most patients and only 15% of the patients enrolled did not proceed to resection. The postoperative morbidity and mortality after preoperative RTx/CTx, also substantial in patients with advanced tumors, was not significantly increased compared to patients who did not have preoperative treatment.

In summary, the present study shows that with the use of preoperative RTx/CTx, complete macroscopic and microscopic tumor resection can be achieved in the vast majority of patients with locally advanced tumors in the proximal esophagus. Although this was not a randomized trial, we believe that the superior survival rates achieved with neoadjuvant therapy justifies routine use of preoperative RTx/CTx in this patient group. A randomized trial of neoadjuvant therapy in patients with locally advanced tumors located in the distal esophagus appears warranted and has been initiated at our institution.

References

1. Earlam R, Cunha-Melo JR (1980) Oesophageal squamous cell carcinoma:A critical review of surgery. Br J Surg 67:381–390
2. Müller JM, Erasmi H, Stelzner M, Zieren U, Pichlmaier H (1990) Surgical therapy of oesophageal carcinoma. Br J Surg 77:845–857
3. Hermanek P, Sobin LH (1987) UICC TNM classification of malignant tumors, 4th revised edn. Springer Berlin Heidelberg New York
4. Siewert JR, Bartels H, Bollschweiler E, Dittler HJ, Fink U, Hölscher AH, Roder JD (1992) Plattenepithelcarcinom des Ösophagus:Behandlungskonzepte der Chirurgischen Klinik der Technischen Universität Müchen. Chirurg 63:693–700
5. Steiger Z, Franklin R, Wilson RF, Leichman L, Seydel H, Loh JJK, et al (1981) Eradication and palliation of squamous cell carcinoma of the esophagus with chemotherapy, radiotherapy, and surgical therapy. J Thorac Cardiovasc Surg 82:713–719
6. Leichman L, Steiger Z, Seydel HG, Vaitkevicius VK (1984) Combined preoperative chemotherapy and radiation therapy for cancer of the esophagus:The Wayne State University, Southwest Oncology Group and Radiation Therapy Oncology Group experience. Semin Oncol 11:178–185

7. Seydel HG, Leichman, Byhardt R, et al (1988) Preoperative radiation and chemotherapy for localized squamous cell carcinoma of the esophagus. A RTOG study. Int J Radiat Oncol Biol Phys 14:33–35

8. Hilgenberg AD, Carey RW, Wilkens EW, et al (1988) Preoperative chemotherapy, surgical resection and selective postoperative therapy for squamous cell carcinoma of the esophagus. Ann Thorac Surg 45:357–363

9. Orringer MB, Forastiere AA, Perez-Tamayo C, Urba S, Takasugi BJ, Bromberg J (1990) Chemotherapy and radiation therapy before transhiatal esophagectomy for esophageal carcinoma. Ann Thor Surg 49:348–355

10. Kelsen DB, Minsky B, Smith M, et al (1990) Preoperative therapy for esophageal cancer:A randomized comparison of chemotherapy versus radiation therapy. J Clin Oncol 8: 1352–1361

11. Fink U, Pfeiffer G, Gossmann A, et al (1990) Perioperative Chemotherapie bei Plattenepithelcarcinomen des Oesophagus. Langenbecks Arch Chir [Suppl II] 107–110

12. Herskovic A, Martz K, Al-Sarraf M, et al (1992) Combined chemotherapy and radiotherapy compared with radiotherapy alone in patients with cancer of the esophagus. N Engl J Med 326:1593–1598

13. Siewert JR, Fink U (1992) Multimodale Therapiekonzepte bei Tumoren des Gastrointestinaltraktes. Chirurg 63:242–250

14. Miller AB, Hoogstraten B, Staquet M, Wonkler A (1981) Reporting results of cancer treatment. Cancer 47:207–214

15. Siewert JR, Hölscher AH, Roder JD, Bartels H (1988) En-block Resektion der Speiseröhre beim Ösophaguscarcinom. Langenbecks Arch Chir 373:367–376

16. Kaplan EL, Meier P (1958) Nonparametric estimation from incomplete observations. J Am Stat Assoc 53:457–481

17. Mantel N (1966) Evaluation of survival data and two new rank order statistics arising in its consideration. Cancer Chemother Rep 50:163–170

Evaluation of Adjuvant Therapy for Esophagectomy with Collo-Thoraco-Abdominal Lymph Node Dissection

HARUSHI UDAGAWA, MASAHIKO TSURUMARU, YOSHIMASA ONO,
YOSHIAKI KAJIYAMA, MASAMICHI MATSUDA, MASATOSHI SUZUKI,
GORO WATANABE, and HIROSHI AKIYAMA[1]

Introduction

With the introduction of cisplatin (CDDP) and new types of combination chemotherapy for the treatment of esophageal carcinoma, the use of adjuvant therapy for this disease has attracted increasing attention [1]. In this study, the effects of adjuvant chemotherapy and adjuvant radiotherapy on patients who underwent esophagectomy with collo-thoraco-abdominal lymph node dissection were investigated retrospectively.

Materials and Methods

The subjects were 234 consecutive patients with thoracic esophageal squamous cell carcinoma (Table 1). These 234 patients were divided into four groups according to the type of adjuvant therapy that they received (Table 2). Although the chemotherapy regimens varied in groups C and B, at least 50 mg of CDDP was administered in all cases. The commonest combination was two courses of CDDP and 5-fluorouracil (5-FU), in which the CDDP dose was 100 mg/m^2 and 5-FU was 1000 mg/m^2 on days 1–4 [2]. Adjuvant radiotherapy consisted of a total dose of 40 Gy of LINEAC irradiation delivered in 20 fractions over 4 weeks.

The patients in each group were staged according to the p-TNM classification. The survival of each group was calculated by the Kaplan-Meier method, and the significance of differences in survival was evaluated by the log-rank test or the generalized Wilcoxon test. The Japanese n-factor and a-factor [3] status of

[1] Department of Surgery, Toranomon Hospital, 2-2-2, Toranomon, Minato-ku, Tokyo, 10⁵ Japan

Table 1. Subjects

234 consecutive patients
   Lesions in the thoracic esophagus
   Squamous cell carcinoma
   Resected with three-field dissection
   Operated on from Feb. 1984 to Nov. 1991
   No evidence of residual tumor
   Excluding postoperative hospital deaths

Table 2. Patient groups

Group		Number
N: No adjuvant treatment		114
R: Adjuvant radiotherapy		43
Preoperative	17	
Postoperative	25	
Both	1	
C: Adjuvant chemotherapy		71
Preoperative	2	
Postoperative	66	
Both	3	
B: Both radiotherapy and chemotherapy		6
Total		234

the patients was also investigated to clarify differences of background that are not considered so meticulously by TNM staging.

Results

The survival curves of all four groups are shown in Fig. 1, and the p-TNM stage distribution is shown in Fig. 2. The longer survival of group N compared with that of groups C and R is explained by the differences in tumor stage among the three. Most of the stage 0 and I patients were in group N, and the proportion of stage IV (L) patients, i.e., patients classified as stage IV due to lymph node metastasis, was extremely high in group C. Even among the patients of the same p-TNM stage, the background data provided by the Japanese n- and a-factor classifications were not equal among the four groups (Figs. 3, and 4). However, the differences of n- and a-factor were very small among stage IV (L) patients.

   This most uniform subgroup of patients, the p-TNM stage IV (L) patients, showed the clearest differences in survival between the different types of adjuvant therapy (Fig. 5). Among the patients in p-TNM stage IV (L), those given chemotherapy survived significantly longer than those who received no adjuvant therapy. When groups N and R in Fig. 5 are combined into a *no chemotherapy* group (N + R in Fig. 6), the difference becomes even clearer.

   A similar result was obtained when the subjects were limited to those who only received *postoperative* adjuvant treatment, although the statistical significance was not so clear because of the small number of patients (Fig. 7).

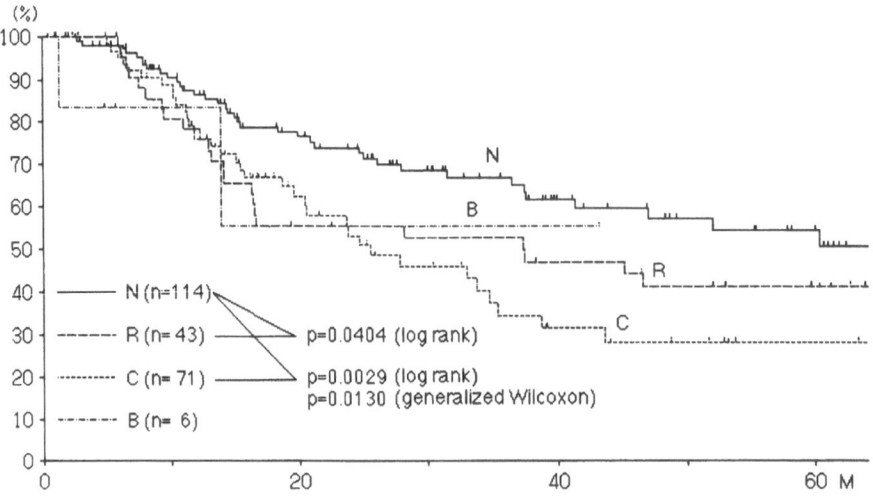

Fig. 1. Survival curves for the four groups. *M*, months

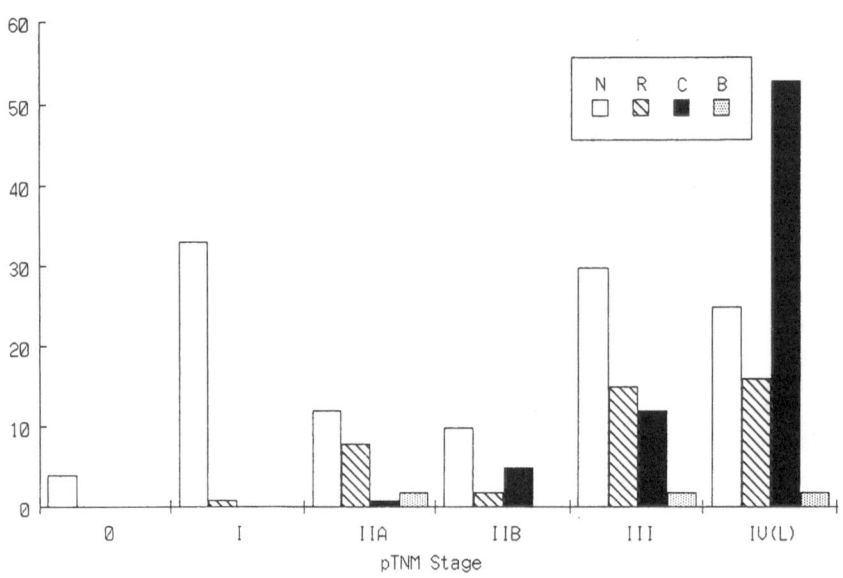

Fig. 2. p-TNM staging of the four groups

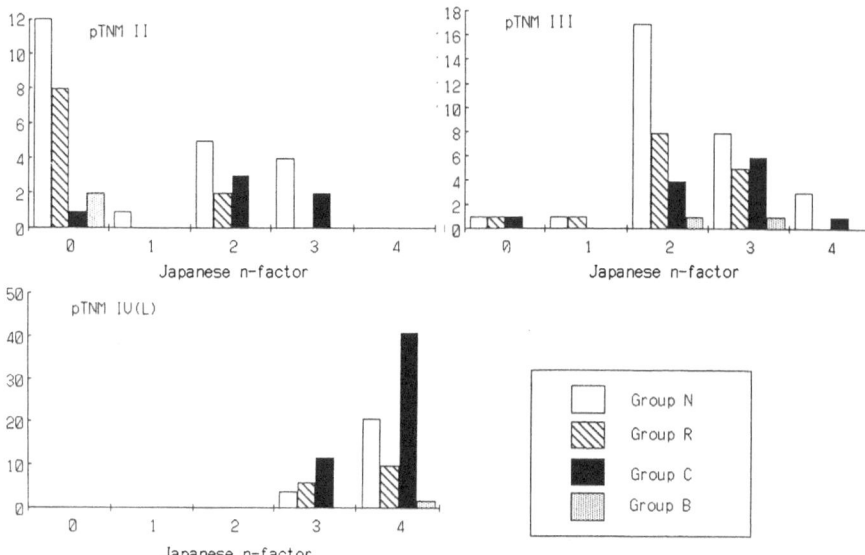

Fig. 3. Japanese n-factor distribution among p-TNM stage II, III, and IV(L) patients. IV(L), stage IV due to lymph node metastasis

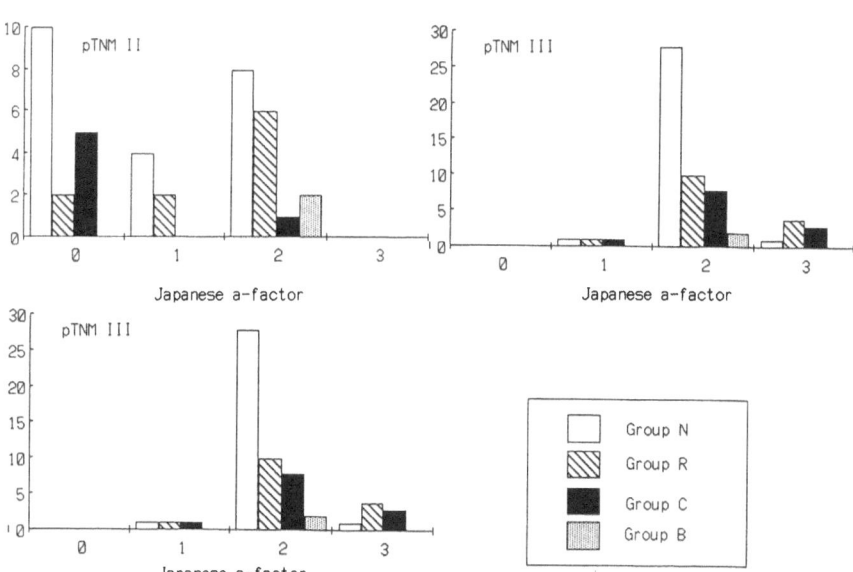

Fig. 4. Japanese a-factor distribution among p-TNM stage II, III, and IV(L) patients

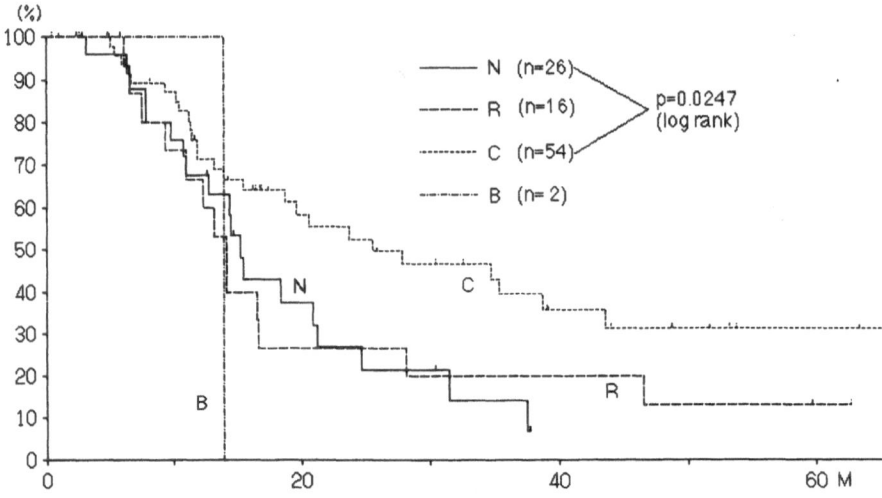

Fig. 5. Survival curves for p-TNM IV(L) patients in the four groups

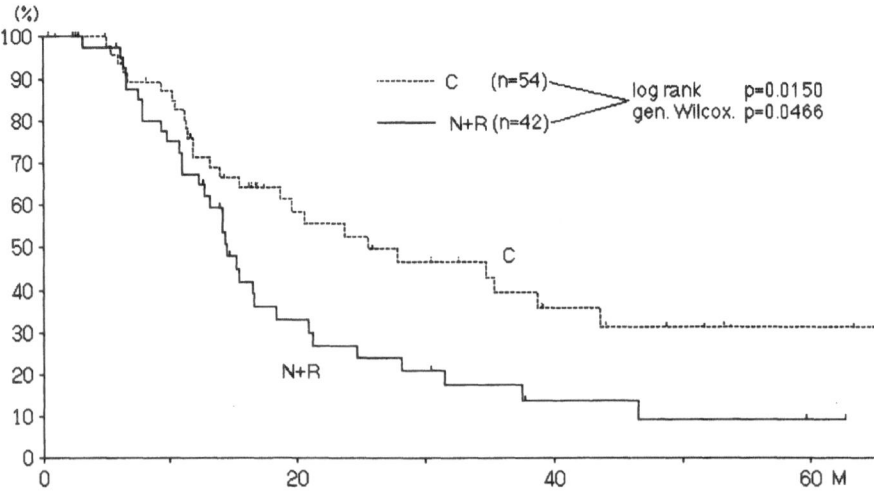

Fig. 6. Survival curves for p-TNM IV(L) patients with and without adjuvant chemotherapy

Discussion

Patients who have undergone esophagectomy with collo-thoraco-abdominal lymph node dissection (so-called 3-field dissection) are ideal subjects for the evaluation of various modes of adjuvant therapy, because they provide us with a great deal of information about lymph node metastasis [4, 5], and because such

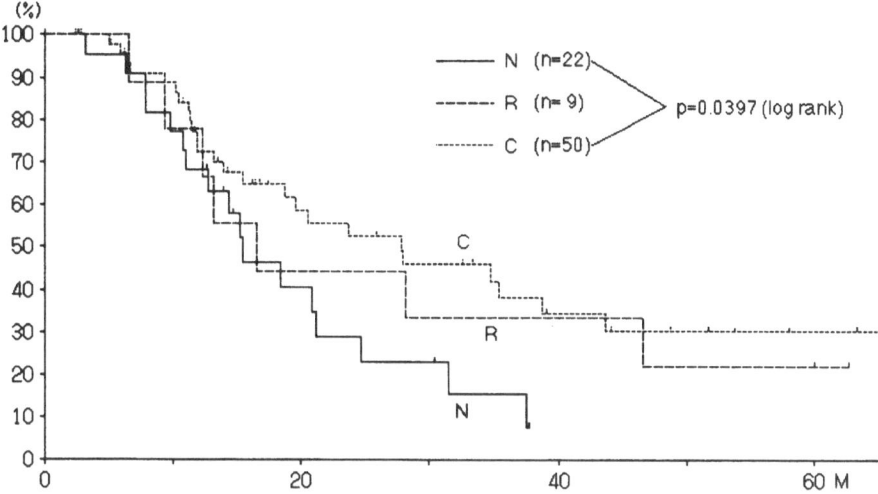

Fig. 7. Survival curves for p-TNM IV(L) patients, excluding those with preoperative adjuvant therapy

metastasis should influence the response to adjuvant therapy. It is important to determine what adjuvant treatment is effective in order to improve the prognosis of this surgical procedure, because the results are not yet entirely satisfactory.

However extensive it may be, surgery is no more than a kind of local therapy like radiotherapy, and it is not by itself a sufficient treatment for disease that has spread beyond a certain region. It seems logical that the combination of surgery and systemic adjuvant therapy should be more effective than the combination of surgery and another local treatment (e.g., radiotherapy), although the latter regimen would be more effective for the local control of disease.

Our study showed that when adjuvant chemotherapy was appropriately combined with esophagectomy and collo-thoraco-abdominal lymph node dissection, the prognosis was improved for patients with lymph node metastasis from esophageal carcinoma that is regarded as distant metastasis in the TNM system, and long-term survival could be achieved. However, in patients with less advanced disease, more precise classification and more extensive clinical data are required to reach a conclusion concerning the value of adjuvant chemotherapy.

References

1. Leichman L, Berry BT (1991) Experience with cisplatin in treatment regimens for esophageal cancer. Semin Oncol 18(1) [Suppl] 3:64–72
2. Kish J, Drelichman A, Jacobs J, Hoschner J, Kinzie J, Loh J, Weaver A, Al-Sarraf M (1982) Clinical trial of cisplatin and 5-FU infusion as initial treatment for advanced squamous cell carcinoma of the head and neck. Cancer Treat Rep 66:471–474

3. Japanese Society for Esophageal Diseases: Guidelines for the clinical and pathologic studies on carcinoma of the esophagus. Kanehara, Tokyo. 1992
4. Akiyama H (1990) Surgery for cancer of the esophagus. Williams and Wilkins, Baltimore, pp 19–42
5. Tsurumaru M, Akiyama H, Udagawa H, Ono Y, Suzuki M, Watanabe G (1990) Cervical-thoracic-abdominal lymph node dissection for intrathoracic esophageal carcinoma. Dis Esoph 1:187–196

Treatment for Recurrence of Carcinoma of the Thoracic Esophagus

MICHIHIKO KITAMURA, SHICHISABURO ABO, MASAZI HASHIMOTO, KEIICHI IZUMI, and HIROYUKI SUZUKI[1]

Introduction

Despite developments in diagnostic methods, many cases of esophageal cancer are not diagnosed until an advanced stage. Of the cases occurring during a recent period, about 70% were diagnosed at stage III or IV. Many cases of esophageal cancer have recurred after curative resection, and treatment for the recurrence is important. In order to define the important points for improving the prognosis after recurrence, we retrospectively analyzed the cases of recurrence after curative resection for thoracic esophageal cancer.

Materials and Methods

From 1972 to 1991, 64 cases of recurrence of thoracic esophageal cancer after curative resection were treated at Akita University Hospital. The primary sites of recurrence are shown in Table 1. Lymph node metastasis, especially to cervical and upper mediastinal lymph nodes, was dominant. In these 64 cases, symptoms, methods of diagnosis, tumor diameter, types of treatment, period between the onset of symptoms and the beginning of treatment, effective rates of treatment, survival curves, and survival rates were investigated.

Results

Active anticancer therapies were administered in 45 cases: irradiation in 26 cases (58%), chemotherapy in 10 cases (22%), and resection of recurrent tumor in 4

[1] Second Department of Surgery, Akita University School of Medicine, 1-1-1 Honda, Akita, 010 Japan

Table 1. Mode of recurrence

Site of recurrence	No. of cases	(%)
Lymph node	47	(73)
Neck	26	(41)
Upper mediastinum	26	(41)
Middle and lower mediastinum	7	(11)
Abdomen	6	(9)
Distant organ	23	(36)
Local (mediastinum)	11	(17)
Anastomotic site	2	(3)
Pleural and pericardial cavity	2	(3)
Others	2	(3)
Total	64	

Table 2. Method of treatment for recurrence

Method of treatment	No. of cases	(%)
Irradiation	26	(58)
Chemotherapy	10	(22)
Resection	4	(9)
Other	5	(11)
Total	45	

cases (Table 2). Mainly because of the poor condition of the patients, only palliative therapies were given in 19 cases.

The median survival period of all cases was 7 months. One-, two-, and three-year survival rates were 21%, 19%, and 5% respectively. The median survival period of patients who underwent active therapies for recurrence was 8 months and was significantly better than that of those who underwent only palliative therapies (2 months) (Fig. 1).

The mean survival period of patients who had been given irradiation was 9 months, significantly better than that of those (6 months) who had been treated with chemotherapy (Fig. 2).

Profiles of patients who had been given irradiation are summarized in Table 3. In the majority of the cases, recurrence was diagnosed based on clinical symptoms, mainly hoarseness. In four cases, recurrent tumors were detected by physical examination before the onset of symptoms, and in three cases, recurrent tumors were detected by follow-up image examination, mainly CT scan. The mean diameter of recurrent tumors was 4.4 cm. The mean diameter of recurrent tumors in patients who had been diagnosed by follow-up image examination was smaller, at 2.4 cm. The mean period between the onset of symptoms and the beginning of treatment was 2.7 months. Positive effects of the therapy were observed in 10 patients (39%). The mean survival period after treatment was 10.8 months. The results in cases which had been diagnosed by follow-up image examination were better. The rate of positive effects in patients whose tumor diameter was smaller than 4.0 cm was 55% (6/11), better than that (27%; 4/15) in patients whose tumor diameter was larger than 4.1 cm.

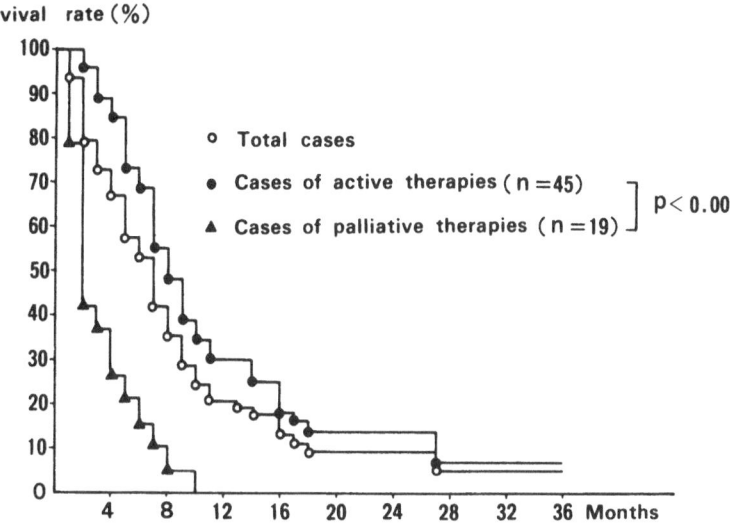

Fig. 1. Survival curves of total cases, patients who underwent active therapies, and patients who underwent palliative therapies. (Kaplan-Meier method)

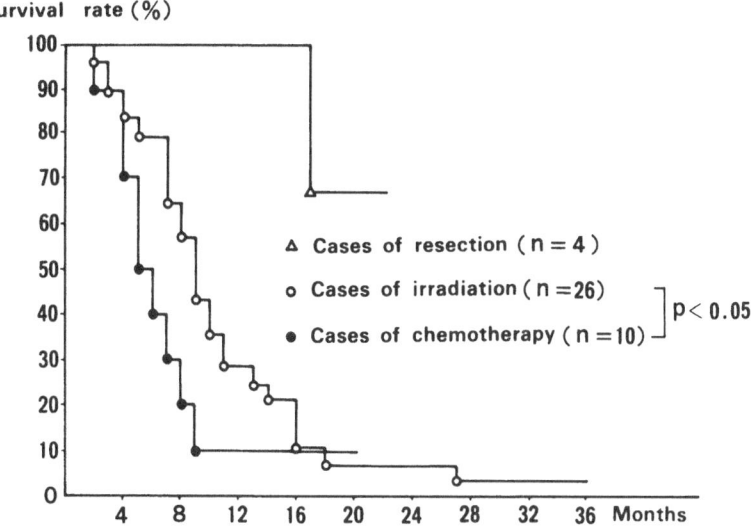

Fig. 2. Survival curves of patients who underwent resection, irradiation, or chemotherapy. (Kaplan-Meier method)

Chemotherapy was given in ten cases. *Cis*-platinum (CDDP) was mainly used (Table 4). Of these ten cases, eight cases were eligible for estimation of effects of the therapy. A positive effect was obtained in only one case and the prognosis was poor as mentioned above (Fig. 2).

Table 3. Profiles of the patients who underwent irradiation

Symptom or method of diagnosis	No. of cases	(%)	Diameter of tumor[a] (cm)	Period between the onset of symptom (diagnosis) and the beginning of treatment[a] (months)	Effective rate[b] (%)	Survival time[a] (months)
Clinical symptom	19	(73)	4.6 ± 1.6	2.8 ± 2.9	37	9.9 ± 6.2
Hoarseness	12					
Dysphagia	3					
Others	4					
Physical examination	4	(15)	4.7 ± 2.4	2.9 ± 2.8	25	8.5 ± 5.4
(Lymph node palpation)						
Follow-up image examination	3	(12)	2.4 ± 1.4	1.7 ± 1.6	67	18.8 ± 14.9
Lymph node	2		1.7 ± 0.2	2.3 ± 1.8	100	23.0 ± 18.4
Other	1					
Total	26		4.4 ± 1.8	2.7 ± 2.7	39	10.8 ± 7.6

[a] mean ± SD [b] In accordance with [5]

Table 4. Anticancer drugs for chemotherapy

Drug	No. of cases
Combination chemotherapy (CDDP used mainly)	6
CDDP	2
BLM	1
BLM + MMC	1

CDDP, *cis*-platinum; *BLM*, bleomycin; *MMC*, Mitomycin C

Table 5. Profiles of the patients who underwent resection

Case	Age	Sex	a and n[a] factor		Stage	Site of recurrence	Operation	Postoperative therapy	Prognosis
1.	63	M	a2	n3	4	Cervical lymph node	Lymph node dissection	Chemotherapy	17 months (dead)
2.	59	M	a3	n0	4	Diaphragma	Resection	Irradiation	22 months (alive)
3.	66	M	a2	n2	3	Cervical lymph node	Lymph node dissection	Irradiation	20 months (alive)
4.	60	M	a2	n2	3	Cervical lymph node	Lymph node dissection	Irradiation	6 months (alive)

[a] In accordance with [5]

Resection of recurrent tumor was performed in four cases. The sites of tumors were lymph nodes in three cases and the diaphragma in one case. The outcomes were relatively good: one patient died at 17 months after resection and the other three patients were doing well 22, 20, and 6 months after resection (Fig. 2, Table 5).

Of the other therapies, interleukin-2 (IL-2) administration [1] for pleuritis carcinomatosa or pericarditis carcinomatosa had a remarkable effect. IL-2 was administered in three patients and positive effects were observed in all three. Of these cases, one patient is still alive without recurrence 24 months after IL-2 therapy.

Discussion and Conclusion

Prognosis in cases of recurrence of esophageal cancer is poor. Nishihira [2] reported the one-year survival rate to be 13% and Shima [3] found the mean survival period to be 6.3 months. Isono [4] reported the mean survival period in cases of lymph node metastasis to be 8.4 months and that in cases of distant organ metastasis to be 4 months. Almost the same results were obtained in our study, but several factors were identified as important in improving the outcome after recurrence of esophageal cancer:

1. Maintenance of the general condition of patients to permit the administration of active therapies

2. Early detection of recurrent tumors by follow-up image examination before the onset of symptoms
3. Shortening of the period between the onset of symptoms and the beginning of treatment
4. Development of new modalities of chemotherapy
5. Application of surgical procedures, especially in cases of recurrence in cervical lymph nodes

References

1. Suzuki H (1989) Experimental and clinical studies on intrapleural instillations of Interleukin-2 (IL-2) in patients with malignant pleural effusion. Nippon Geka Gakkai Zasshi J Jpn Surg Soc 90:1922–1931
2. Nishihira T, Hirayama K, Shineha R, Sanekata K, Goukon Y, Mori S (1987) Strategies in cases of recurrent cancer of the esophagus. Saishin Igaku 42:2593–2600
3. Shima S, Yonekawa H, Yoshizumi Y, Sugiura Y, Goto M, Tanaka S (1988) The mode of recurrence after curative operation for cancer of intrathoracic esophagus. Shoukakigeka 11:2017–2022
4. Isono K (1984) The recurrence and measures after surgery for cancer of intra-thoracic esophagus. Nippon Shoukakigeka Gakkai Zasshi 17:527–536
5. Japanese Society for Esophageal Diseases (1992) Guidelines for the clinical and pathologic studies on carcinoma of the esophagus. Kanehara, Tokyo

Drug Sensitivity Tests for Human Esophageal Cancer

M. Terashima, K. Ikeda, H. Kawamura, C. Maesawa, H. Yoshinari,
K. Koeda, N. Sato, K. Ishida, and K. Saito[1]

Introduction

Recently, considerable attention has been paid to the study of systemic chemotherapy with esophageal cancer. Although relatively good response rates have been obtained compared with other gastrointestinal tumors [1], the prognosis is still worse than for other type of gastrointestinal tumors because of the poor general condition in many patients and the rapidity of tumor progression. To improve the response rate to chemotherapy and prognosis of these patients, the selection of chemotherapeutic agent is very important. The present study was designed to evaluate and compare the usefulness of in vitro human tumor clonogenic assay (HTCA), in vivo subrenal capsule assay (SRCA), SRCA with immunosuppressant (IS-SRCA) and in vitro adenosine triphosphate (ATP) assay with serum-free culture (SF-ATPA) as chemosensitivity tests in human esophageal squamous cell carcinoma.

Materials and Methods

Tumors

Fresh surgical specimens were obtained at the time of operation from patients with squamous cell carcinoma of the esophagus treated at our department: 19 for HTCA, 21 for SRCA, 33 for IS-SRCA, and 49 for SF-ATPA.

---

[1] Department of Surgery 1, Iwate Medical University, School of Medicine, 19-1 Uchimaru, Morioka, Iwate, 020 Japan

Table 1. Drug concentrations used in HTCA and SF-ATPA and the drug dosage used in SRCA and IS-SRCA

Drugs	HTCA (mcg/ml)	SF-ATPA (mcg/ml)			SRCA and IS-SRCA (mg/kg per inj.)	
Cisplatin (CDDP)	0.20	20,	2.0,	0.2	10.0	Day 1
Vindesine (VDS)	0.01	1.0,	0.1,	0.01	5.3	Day 1
5-Fluorouracil (5-FU)	1.00	500,	5.0,	5.0	150.0	Day 1
Mitomycin (MMC)		10,	1.0,	0.1	10.0	Day 1
Peplomycin (PEP)	0.40	40,	4.0,	0.4	24.0	Days 1, 3 and 5
Adriamycin (ADM)		4.0,	0.4,	0.04		
Etoposide (VP-16)		100,	10,	1.0		

HTCA, Human tumor clonogenic assay; *SF-ATPA*, ATP assay with serum free culture; *SRCA*, subrenal capsule assay; *IS-SRCA*, SRCA with immunosuppressant

Drugs

Drug concentrations used in HTCA and SF-ATPA and the drug dosage used in SRCA and IS-SRCA are shown in Table 1. The concentrations used in HTCA were one-tenth of the highest concentration pharmacologically achieved in patient's serum. Similarly, the concentration used in SF-ATPA were peak plasma concentration (PPC), 10X PPC and 1/10XPPC. In in vivo assays, the dosage was the maximum tolerated dose that did not result in toxic death (weight loss <20%).

HTCA

The method used in this study was modified from that of Hamburger and Salmon [2] and described previously [3]. Tumor specimens were cut into 1-mm pieces by scalpel and single cell suspension was obtained by enzymatic digestion. Viable cells were counted by the trypan blue exclusion method and were incubated with drugs at 37°C for 1 h. Then drugs were washed and 500,000 viable cells/ml per dish with CMRL 1066 medium, 15% horse serum (HS), several growth factors and a final concentration of 0.3% soft agar were plated onto the lower layer which consist of McCoys' 5A medium, 10% fetal calf serum, 5% HS, several growth factors, and a final concentration of 0.5% soft agar. The petri dishes were incubated at 37°C in a humidified atmosphere with 5% CO_2 for 14–21 days. Colonies were defined as aggregates of 50 or more cells, and counted by automatic colony analyzer.

SRCA

The SRCA methods followed the technique of Bogden et al. [4]. Briefly, about 1 mm^3 tumor fragments were implanted under the renal capsule of BDF_1 mice, and two diameters (length and width) of the implanted tumor were measured in situ (initial size) with a stereoscopic micrometer. The mice were divided into groups of 4–6 each, and treatment groups were administered the different drugs intravenously. At the end of the assay, each animal was killed and the tumor-bearing kidney was removed and placed under the stereoscopic microscope for measurement of the final tumor size.

IS-SRCA

As described previously [5], in order to suppress the host immunoreaction, cyclophosphamide 180 mg/kg was injected subcutaneously into mice 36 h before tumor inoculation.

SF-ATPA

Single cell suspension was obtained by enzymatic digestion in the same manner as the HTCA. Cells were plated onto 96-well microplates with serum-free medium (S-clone; SF-B) (Sanko Pure Chemical Inc., Tokyo, Japan) at a concentration of 20,000 cells/well, and cultured for 3 days with concomitant exposure to drugs as shown in Table 1. Cell viability was evaluated by measuring the intracellular ATP level using bioluminescence procedure as described by Kangas et al. [6].

Evaluation of the Assay Result

The evaluability criteria in control groups for each assay were more than 30 colonies for HTCA, more than 2×10^{-12} mol ATP level for SF-ATPA, and more than -0.05 mm tumor growth for SRCA and IS-SRCA.

The sensitivity criteria in drug treated group for each assay were more than 50% decrease of colony count from control for HTCA, more than 50% decrease of intracellular ATP level from control in SF-ATPA, and more than -0.1 mm tumor regression for SRCA and IS-SRCA.

Results

HTCA

Of 19 samples, 10 samples formed more than five colonies. In 4 of 19 tumors, more than 30 colonies were observed in the control and considered to be

Table 2. Evaluability rates and sensitivity rates of each assay

Assay	Evaluability rate (%)	Sensitivity rate (%)							
		CDDP	VDS	5-FU	PEP	MMC	ADM	VP-16	Total
HTCA	4/19	0/4	0/4	0/1	0/1				0/10
	(21)	(0)	(0)	(0)	(0)				(0)
SRCA	20/21	9/20	4/20	6/19	4/19	5/19			32/83
	(95)	(45)	(20)	(31)	(21)	(56)			(39)
IS-SRCA	30/33	8/43	3/29	4/26	2/22	12/28			30/135
	(91)	(19)	(10)	(16)	(9)	(43)			(22)
SF-ATPA	43/49	8/43	4/36	8/27	1/15	7/42	6/34	11/32	45/229
	(88)	(19)	(11)	(30)	(7)	(17)	(18)	(34)	(20)

HTCA, Human tumor clonogenic assay; *SRCA*, subrenal capsule assay; *IS-SRCA*, SRCA with immunosupressant; *SF-ATPA*, ATP assay with serum-free culture; *CDDP*, cisplatin; *VDS*, vindesine; *5-FU*, 5-fluorouracil; *PEP*, peplomycin; *MMC*, mitomycin; *ADM*, adriamycin; *VP-16*, etoposide

evaluable. Two to four drugs were tested per specimen, resulting in ten possible drug assays. In these ten drug assays, no drug showed a colony kill of more than 50% (Table 2).

SRCA and IS-SRCA

Adequate growth of the tumor in control groups was obtained from 20 of 21 tumors (95%) for SRCA and 30 of 33 (91%) in IS-SRCA. The chemosensitivity of these tumors to cisplatin (CDDP), vindesine (VDS), 5-fluorouracil (5-FU), peplomycin (PEP), and mitomycin C (MMC) were tested. In both assays, tumors showed a relatively high sensitivity rate to CDDP, MMC and 5-FU. The overall sensitivity rates were 32% for SRCA and 22% for IS-SRCA (Table 2).

Histological Analysis

Twenty-one samples for SRCA and 28 for IS-SRCA were included in a histological study focused mainly on residual tumor cells and the extent of inflammatory infiltration. In SRCA, inflammatory infiltrates were observed in 18 of 21 samples (86%). Tumor cell preservation was recognised in only nine samples (43%). In contrast, inflammatory infiltrates were observed in only 4 of 28 samples (14%), and tumor cells were persisted in 27 cases (96%) in IS-SRCA.

SF-ATPA

In 43 of 49 samples, intracellular ATP levels showed more than 2×10^{-12} mol in control wells and considered to be evaluable. In these 49 samples, a total of 229 drug assays against CDDP, VDS, 5-FU, PEP, MMC, Adriamycin (ADM), and etoposide (VP-16) were carried out. Tumor showed a relatively high sensitivity rate to CDDP, 5-FU, MMC, ADM, and VP-16 (Table 2). Clear dose-response was observed in all cytocidal drugs (data not shown).

Correlation with Clinical Results

For HTCA, one assay-clinical correlation was possible. HTCA was predictive of the clinical resistance in this patient's tumor. For SRCA, two assay-clinical correlations were possible: One was a false positive and the other was a true negative. For IS-SRCA, two correlations were possible: One was a true positive and the other was a true negative. For SF-ATPA, four correlations were possible. This assay predicted one clinical response and two clinical resistance (Table 3).

Survival Curves According to Drug Sensitivity by IS-SRCA

Of the 30 patients whose tumors were evaluable by IS-SRCA, 8 received adjuvant chemotherapy with CDDP and VDS (CDDP 70 mg/m^2 and VDS 3 mg/m^2). Of the samples from these eight patients, two were evaluated to be sensitive to CDDP or VDS, and the remaining were resistant by IS-SRCA. The survival rates were compared between these two groups (Fig. 1). All patients had stage III or IV tumor and underwent curative resection. Improvement of

Table 3. Correlations with clinical results

Assay	Tumor site	Drug sensitivity						Chemotherapy	Measurable lesion	Effect	Correlation	Overall predictive accuracy
		CDDP	VDS	5-FU	PEP	MMC	ADM	VP-16					
HTCA	Skin meta	–	–	–	–				5-FU	Skin, lung	PD	TN	1/1 (100%)
SRCA	Skin meta	+	–	+	–				5-FU	Skin, lung	PD	FP	1/2 (50%)
SRCA	Primary	+	–	+	–				VDS	Lung	PD	TN	1/2 (50%)
IS-SRCA	Primary	–	–	–	–	–			CDDP/VDS	Bone	PD	TN	2/2 (100%)
IS-SRCA	Primary	–	–	+	–	–			CDDP/VDS/5-FU	Liver	PR	TP	2/2 (100%)
SF-ATPA	Lymph node	–	–	–	–	–	–	+	CDDP/VP-16	Lymph node	MR	TP	3/4 (75%)
SF-ATPA	Lymph node	+	–	–	–	–	+	–	CDDP/5-FU	Primary	NC	FP	3/4 (75%)
SF-ATPA	Lung	–	–	–	+	–	–	–	CDDP/5-FU	Lung	NC	TN	3/4 (75%)
SF-ATPA	Primary	–	–	–	–	–	–	–	CDDP/5-FU	Primary	PD	TN	3/4 (75%)

PR, Partial response; *MR*, minor response; *NC*, no change; *PD*, progressive disease; *TP*, true positive; *TN*, true negative; *FP*, false positive

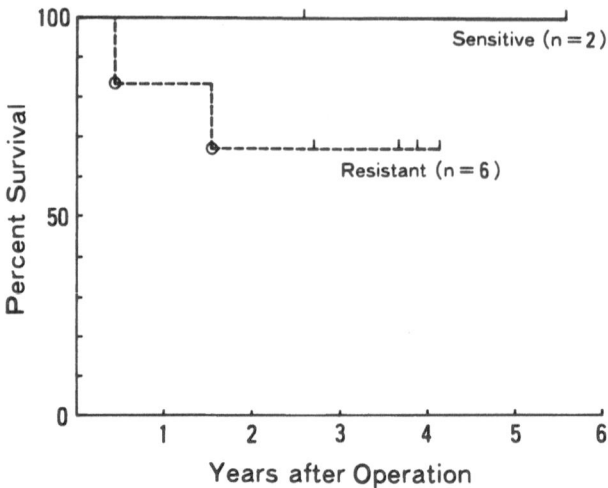

Fig. 1. Survival curves according to drug sensitivity determined by subrenal capsule assay with immunosuppressant (*IS-SRCA*)

survival time was observed when the active agents determined by IS-SRCA were administered as an adjuvant chemotherapy. However, no statistical significance was observed between these two groups by generalized Wilcoxon's test.

Discussion

Until recently, attempts to evaluate drug response against human esophageal cancer have not been made, and the usefulness of drug sensitivity tests for this type of cancer was not evaluated. Development of a two-layer semi-solid agar system by Hamburger and Salmon was a major advance which enabled the study of individual human cancer specimens in vitro [2]. A large number of studies have been performed on various types of tumor, and good clinical correlations have been reported. However, a major problem for HTCA is that not all tumors will grow and form enough colonies. Ovarian tumors, melanoma, colorectal, and breast tumors were reported to form colonies relatively well. In contrast, those from stomach, lymphoma, and leukemia showed poor colony formation [7]. In this study, esophageal tumors were also found to exhibit poor colony formation. Thus, we discontinued the use of HTCA as a drug sensitivity test for esophageal cancer.

SRCA is an in vivo test system for in situ measurement of the growth of human tumor fragments implanted under the renal capsule of mice, which is used for determining the chemosensitivity of a tumor within a 6-day period. Bogden reported that the host versus graft response would take from 7 to 12 days after implantation, and not affect the xenograft persistence until day 6 [4]. Furthermore, Bogden and Von Hoff reported on a comparative study of HTCA and SRCA that despite the large differences in these two assays, a high correlation of tumor sensitivity and resistance was obtained when the same tumors were tested against the same drugs in both SRCA and HTCA [8]. Based on these findings, we applied this system as a chemosensitivity test against human esophageal cancer.

Subsequently, several investigators have demonstrated significant host cell infiltration on day 6, and suggested that this infiltration could complicate the interpretation of the chemosensitivity results. We also demonstrated the significant host cell infiltration and poor tumor cell preservation in xenografts on day 6. From these results, we studied the effects of immunosuppressive agents, and reported the usefulness of cyclophosphamide pretreatment for SRCA against human esophageal cancer [5]. In a basic experiment, the immunosuppressive effect of cyclophosphamide pretreatment was comparable to those obtained after cyclosporine A treatment. Furthermore, cyclophosphamide was less toxic than cyclosporine A and had no influence on the activities of chemotherapeutic agents, and its excellent immunosuppressive effect was also demonstrated in clinical samples. The evaluability rate for IS-SRCA was high enough to apply this assay as a clinical chemosensitivity test, and the response rate of this assay were comparable with those of prior clinical test in each drug. This assay was considered to be a useful chemosensitivity test against human esophageal cancer.

However, the necessity of a pathogen-free environment and the complicated nature of the procedure were disadvantages of IS-SRCA, and the number of tumors and drugs that could be tested at the same time were limited. In order to develop the simple and rapid in vitro test which enables to suppress the overgrowth of the fibroblast, we studied the chemosensitivity test using serum-free culture system. In basic experiment, growth of the fibroblast was suppressed in serum-free culture and the tumor cell growth was comparable with serum supplemented culture. In addition, the measurement of intracellular ATP level was more sensitive than MTT assay. This assay could be performed with small samples such as biopsy materials and the evaluability rate was high enough. There were some problems in cut-off level or drug concentration, however the sensitivity rate of each drug was similar to those of IS-SRCA and prior clinical tests. This assay seemed to be a useful, simple, and rapid chemosensitivity test against human esophageal cancer.

Evaluation for the clinical usefulness of chemosensitivity test is very difficult. There were many discrepancies between the patients and experimental animals or in vitro conditions. However, relatively good clinical correlations were obtained in IS-SRCA and SF-ATPA. Furthermore, improvement of survival time was observed under strict clinical trials retrospectively. These data indicated the usefulness of chemosensitivity test against human esophageal cancer.

References

1. Kelsen D (1984) Chemotherapy of esophageal cancer. Semin Oncol 11:159–168
2. Hamburger AW, Salmon SE (1977) Primary bioassay of human tumor stem cells. Science 197:461–463
3. Terashima M, Ikeda K, Maesawa C, Kawamura H, Ishida K, Sato M, Saito K (1992) Drug-sensitivity testing in patients with human oesophageal squamous cell carcinoma. Eur J Cancer 28A:1347–1350

4. Bogden AE, Haskel PM, Lepage DJ, Kelton DE, Cobb WR, Eber HJ (1979) Growth of human tumor xenografts implanted under the renal capsule of normal immunocompetent mice. Exp Cell Biol 47:281–293
5. Terashima M, Ikeda K, Kawamura S, Ishida K, Satoh M, Saito K (1990) The usefulness of cyclophosphamide pretreatment for subrenal capsule assay against human esophageal cancer. Jpn J Surg 21:184–192
6. Kangas L, Gronros M, Nieminen AC (1984) Bioluminescence of cellular ATP: A new method for evaluating cytotoxic agents in vitro. Med Biol 62:338–343
7. Von Hoff DD, Casper J, Bradley E, Sandbach J, Jones D, Makuch R (1981) Association between tumor colony-forming assay results and response of an individual patient's tumor to chemotherapy. Am J Med 70:1027–1032
8. Bogden AE, Von Hoff DD (1984) Comparison of the human tumor cloning and subrenal capsule assay. Cancer Res 44:1087–1090

Local Chemotherapy of Esophageal Cancer with Bleomycin Adsorbed to Activated Carbon Particles

Mario Shimada[1], Shoji Natsugoe[1], Toru Kumanohoso[1], Takashi Aikou[1], Hisaaki Shimazu[1] and Kazuo Nakamura[2]

Introduction

Increasing interest has recently been shown in targeting cancer chemotherapy using newly designed drug delivery systems [1]. Hagiwara et al. [2] developed activated carbon particles as a drug carrier having several advantages such as selective affinity for the lymphatic system and release of a designated fixed concentration of anticancer drug over a long period.

In the present study, we prepared bleomycin (BLM) adsorbed on to activated carbon particles (BLM-CH) and BLM aqueous solution (BLM-SOL), and compared the BLM activity in the regional lymph nodes, connective tissues, liver, lung, spleen, and blood after injection of these two forms of BLM into the esophageal wall of dogs. Clinically, we measured the BLM activity in the regional lymph nodes when BLM-CH was injected into the esophageal wall.

Materials and Methods

Preparation of BLM-CH and BLM-SOL

Activated carbon particles (Activated Carbon Mitsubishi No 40, Mitsubishi Chemical Industries Co., Ltd, Tokyo), were used as an adsorbent, and BLM (Bleomycin, Nippon Kayaku Co., Ltd, Tokyo) as an anti-cancer agent. For experimental study, BLM-CH containing 15 mg of BLM was prepared by mixing 50 mg/ml of activated carbon particles with 20 mg/ml of polyvinylpyrrolidone K-30 (Nakarai Chemical Co., Ltd, Tokyo) in saline. BLM-SOL, comprised 15 mg/1.5 ml of BLM in saline. For clinical study, BLM-CH containing 30 mg of BLM was prepared as above.

[1] First Department of Surgery and [2] Department of Hospital Pharmacy, Kagoshima University School of Medicine, 8-35-1 Sakuragaoka, Kagoshima, 890 Japan

Administration Method of BLM-CH and BLM-SOL

In experimental study, 14 mongrel dogs were used. BLM-CH was administered to nine dogs and BLM-SOL to five dogs. BLM-CH or BLM-SOL (1.5 ml) was injected into the submucosa of middle esophageal wall over 1–2 min under endoscopic control. In clinical study, BLM-CH was endoscopically injected into the esophageal wall of 16 patients with esophageal cancer 1–3 days prior to operation.

Measurement of BLM Activity

In experimental study, 3 days after injection, the animals were sacrificed, and the regional lymph nodes, connective tissues, esophageal wall, liver, lung, and spleen were removed for the measurement of BLM activity. In clinical study, dissected lymph nodes were used for the measurement of BLM activity. Samples were weighed, BLM activity was calculated as micrograms of BLM per gram of tissue. Blood samples were taken at 30 min, 1 h, and 3 h after injection. BLM activity was measured by thin agar plate bioassay using Bacillus Subtilis PCL-219. The lower limit of the level detected by this assay was 0.05 µg/g.

Regional Division of Dissected Lymph Nodes and Connective Tissues

Regional lymph nodes and surrounding connective tissues were divided into the following five groups according to the classification of Aikou and Shimazu [3]: cervical lymph nodes (R-A), upper mediastinal lymph nodes (R-B), middle mediastinal lymph nodes (R-C), lower mediastinal lymph nodes (R-D), and abdominal lymph nodes (R-E). The lymph nodes of the upper mediastinal region were specially subdivided into four groups: upper thoracic paraesophageal lymph nodes (R-B1), right highest mediastinal lymph nodes (R-B2), right paratracheal lymph nodes (R-B3), and left paratracheal lymph nodes (R-B4).

Statistical Analysis

Data were statistically compared using Student's t-test, and $P < 0.05$ was considered to be significant.

Results

Distribution of BLM Activity in the Experimental Study

BLM activity was not detected in the liver, lung, or spleen. The mean ± SD (µg/g) of activity in the esophageal wall at the site of injection was 2.34 ± 0.97. Figure 1 illustrates BLM activity in both lymph nodes and connective tissues in four regions. No significant difference was found between any two values in the four regions.

Figure 2 shows the activity (µg/g) in four subdivisions of R-B. BLM activity was low in R-B2, but no significant difference was found among the other three subdivisions.

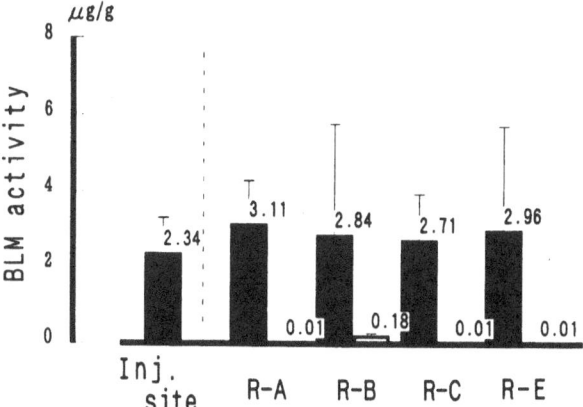

Fig. 1. Bleomycin activity in regional lymph nodes. Activity in lymph nodes (*solid bars*). Activity in connective tissues (*open bars*). *Inj. site*, injection site; *R-A*, cervical lymph nodes; *R-B*, upper mediastinal lymph nodes; *R-C*, middle mediastinal lymph nodes; *R-E*, abdominal lymph nodes

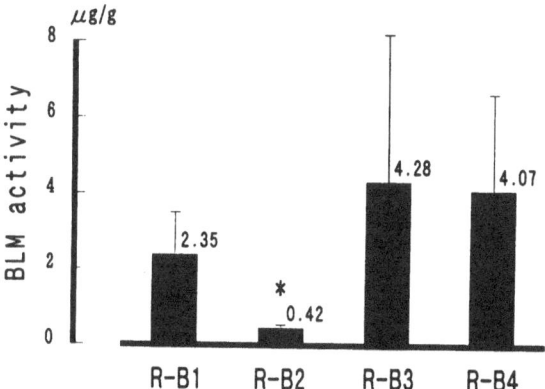

Fig. 2. Bleomycin activity in upper mediastinal lymph nodes. *$P < 0.05$ *R-B1*, upper thoracic paraesophageal lymph nodes; *R-B2*, right highest mediastinal lymph nodes; *R-B3*, right paratracheal lymph nodes; *R-B4*, left paratracheal lymph nodes

When BLM was administered in the form of BLM-SOL, BLM activity was not detected in any lymph nodes, connective tissues, or other organs examined.

Figure 3 shows the time course of changes in BLM activity in the blood, when BLM was administered in the form of BLM-CH or BLM-SOL. BLM activity at 30 min, 1 h, and 3 h after administration of BLM-CH were significantly lower than those after BLM-SOL, although levels decreased with the passage of time in both cases.

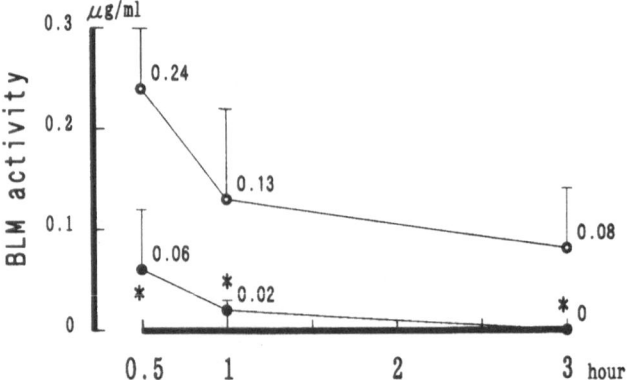

Fig. 3. Time course of changes in BLM activity in the blood. BLM-CH (*closed circles*). BLM-SOL (*open circles*) *$P < 0.05$

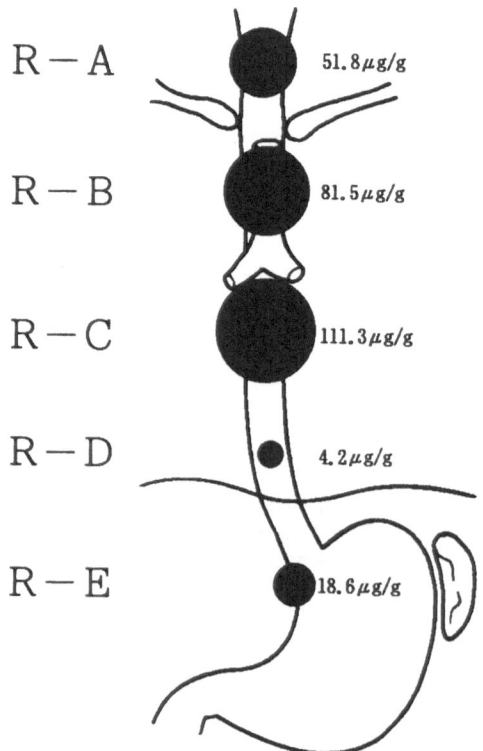

Fig. 4. Dependence of BLM activity on time in lymph nodes

Distribution of BLM Activity in the Clinical Study

The values in Fig. 4 indicate the mean activity of BLM in each of the five lymph node groups. The highest value was 111.25 µg/g observed in middle mediastinal lymph nodes (R-C). The values of cervical (R-A), upper mediastinal (R-B), and abdominal lymph nodes (R-E) were relatively high.

Discussion

Activated carbon particles have been shown to proceed easily to the lymphatic system following injection into the wall of the digestive tract [4]. The particles, when combined with an anticancer agent, gradually release the agent and keep the concentration of the cytotoxic agent in a free state at a constant level [5].

In the present study, when BLM-CH was administered into the esophageal wall, BLM activity was detected not only in the mediastinal, but also in the cervical and abdominal lymph nodes. The experimental results were in agreement with clinical findings. In the upper mediastinum also, significant BLM activity was detected both in the upper thoracic paraesophageal lymph nodes (R-B1) and in the thoracic paratracheal lymph nodes (R-B2, R-B3, and R-B4), although relatively low levels were detected in the R-B2 subdivision. The lymph nodes in the R-B2, R-B3, and R-B4 subdivisions are very difficult to dissect thoroughly by surgery. Accordingly, one might be tempted to extrapolate that BLM was also distributed to these regions clinically. However, BLM activity was not detected in any lymph nodes when BLM-SOL was administered.

When BLM-CH was injected, BLM activity in the blood was significantly lower, compared with BLM-SOL administration. The activity disappeared completely 3 h after administration. BLM activity was not detected in such organs as the liver, lung, or spleen after administration of either BLM-CH or BLM-SOL. These observations indicate that local injection of BLM-CH may not bring about serious systemic side effects.

In conclusion, we demonstrated BLM activity in a wide range of regional lymph nodes after the administration of BLM-CH into the esophageal wall. The results indicate that BLM-CH may probably become a useful tool in the targeting chemotherapy for esophageal cancer.

References

1. Tanigawa N, Satomura K, Hikasa Y, Hashida M, Muranishi S, Sezaki H (1980) Surgical chemotherapy against lymph node metastases. An experimental study. Surgery 87:147–152
2. Hagiwara A, Ahn T, Ueda T, Iwamoto A, Ueda T, Torii T, Takahashi T (1985) Anticancer agents adsorbed by activated carbon particles: A new form of dosage-enhancing efficacy on lymph nodal metastases. Anti-cancer Research 6:1005–1008
3. Aikou T, Shimazu H (1989) Difference in main lymphatic pathways from the lower esophagus and gastric cardia. Jpn J Surg 19:290–295

4. Natsugoe S, Aikou T, Shimazu H, Tabata M (1991) Lymphatic anastmoses between the distal esophagus and gastric cardia in dogs. Clinical Anatomy 4:357–365
5. Hagiwara A, Takahashi T, Ueda T, Iwamoto A, Torri T (1987) Activated carbon particles as anti-cancer drug carrier into regional lymph nodes. Anti-Cancer Drug Design 1:313–321

Advanced and Recurrent Esophageal Carcinoma: Combination Chemotherapy with Etoposide, Leucovorin, 5-Fluorouracil, and Cisplatin

Susumu Ohwada, Yuichi Iino, Seiji Nakamura,
Yoshihumi Tanahashi, Yoshiyuki Kawashima, Yukio Miyamoto, and
Yasuo Morishita[1]

Introduction

Survival of patients with esophageal carcinoma treated with surgery and/or radiation has been very poor. The clinical development of cisplatin (CDDP) based chemotherapy has changed the outcome of patients with esophageal carcinoma. The combinations of 5-fluorouracil (5-FU) and CDDP, 5-FU and leucovorin, and CDDP and etoposide are synergistic in experimental and clinical models. We have used etoposide, leucovorin, 5-FU, and CDDP in advanced or recurrent esophageal squamous cell carcinoma since January, 1991, and we evaluate herein the tumor reduction and the postoperative morbidity and mortality.

Materials and Methods

The treatment regimen was as follows: Etoposide ($50\,mg/m^2$, 3-hour infusion, days 1–5), leucovorin ($30\,mg/body$, $30\,min$, days 2–5), 5-FU ($400\,mg/m^2$, 10-hour infusion, days 2–5), and CDDP ($100\,mg/m^2$ day 1) (ELF-P). Recombinant human granulocyte colony stimulating factor ($75\,\mu g$, subcutaneous, days 8–12) was given. Saline was added to maintaining the urine volume over $2000\,ml/day$ for an additional 7 days. Granisetron was given for nausea or vomiting. Patients often required this treatment more than twice every 4 weeks.

Response criteria were as follows: Complete response (CR), the complete disappearance of all clinical evidence of existing lesions for over 4 weeks; partial response (PR), a $50\% < 100\%$ reduction in the sum of the products of two perpendicular measurements taken of all measurable lesions lasting over 4

---

[1] The Second Department of Surgery, Gunma University School of Medicine, 3-39-15 Shouwa-machi, Maebashi, Gunma, 371 Japan

Table 1. Patients and characteristics production advanced carcinoma

Patient	Age	Sex	Anatomical Size Location (cm)	Histology	T	N	M	Response	Treatment	Outcome
Advanced carcinoma										
1.	58 yrs	M	Middle 9.0	Well	3	1	1 Lym	PR	Surg	8 weeks, died
2.	69 yrs	M	Middle 6.2	Well	3	1	1 Lym	PR	Surg	17 months, alive
3.	56 yrs	M	Upper 5.3	Undiff	2	0	1 Lym	NC	Surg-ELFP	3 months, died
4.	55 yrs	M	Middle 9.0	Poor	4	1	0	NC		3 months, died
5.	65 yrs	M	Middle 7.5	Poor	4	1	0	PR		7 months, died
6.	75 yrs	F	Middle 2.7	Poor	2	1	1 Lym, H	PD		7 months, died
7.	46 yrs	M	Upper 5.0	Poor	4	1	0	CR	RT-ELFP	15 months, alive
8.	62 yrs	M	Middle 6.0	Poor	3	2	0	PD	RT	9 months, died
9.	60 yrs	M	Lower 9.0	Poor	1	1	1 Lym	PD		3 months, died
10.	61 yrs	M	Middle 10	Poor	4	0	0	PR	Surg	8 months, alive
11.	56 yrs	M	Lower 9.6	Poor	4	0	0	PR	Surg	7 months, alive
12.	66 yrs	M	Upper 8.0	Mod	4	0	0	PR	RT	6 months, alive

Patient	Age	Sex	Histology	Recurrent Sites	Response	Treat	Outcome
Production recurrent carcinoma							
13.	56 yrs	M	Poor	Cervical, Axillar, Mediastinal Lym	PR	RT	3 months, died
14.	55 yrs	M	Well	Cervical, Mediastinal Lym, Skin	PR		6 months, died
15.	59 yrs	M	Mod	Cervical, Mediastinal Lym	PR	RT	15 months, died

Well, Well differentiated; *mod*, moderately differentiated; *poor*, poorly differentiated; *undiff*, undifferentiated squamous cell carcinoma. *Lym*, lymph nodes; *H*, liver; *surg*, surgery; *RT*, radiation; *yrs*, years; *PR*, partial response; *NC*, no change; *CR*, complete response; *PD*, progressive disease; *ELF-P*, etoposide, leucovorin, 5-FU, CDDP

weeks; no change (NC), a ± 25% change in tumor size over 4 weeks; progressive disease (PD), a > 25% increase in the sum of the products of two perpendicular measurements taken of all evaluable lesions, or the appearance of new lesions. The final assessment of chemotherapy effectiveness in patients who underwent resection can be made pathologically.

Results

Fifteen patients (advanced 12, recurrent 3) with histologically confirmed esophageal squamous cell carcinoma and measurable disease were enrolled in this study. The mean age was 59.9 years (46–75 years) and WHO performance status (PS) was: grade 0 in ten patients grade 1 in three, and grade 2 in two (Table 1). One complete and nine partial responses (response rate 67%) were observed. Among the 12 patients with advanced carcinoma, 7 patients (58%) achieved a response (Table 2). Sixty-seven percent of distant lymph node metastasis obtained a partial or complete response, and 80% of regional lymph nodes achieved a partial response (Table 3). One patient had complications of broncho-esophageal fistula during chemotherapy.

Neoadjuvant ELF-P Therapy

Five (41%) patients underwent radical resection after ELF-P chemotherapy. One CR patient refused operation. Surgical resection was performed through a right thoracotomy in three-field (cervical, mediastinal, and abdominal) lymph-

Table 2. Results (median duration of response = 4.3 months)

Number of patients	CR (%)	PR (%)	NC (%)	PD (%)	Response rate
15	0	10 (67%)	2 (13%)	3 (20%)	10 (67%)
Results in advanced carcinoma					
Number of patients	CR (%)	PR (%)	NC (%)	PD (%)	Response rate
12	0	7 (58%)	2 (17%)	3 (25%)	7 (58%)
Results in recurrent carcinoma					
Number of patients	CR (%)	PR (%)	NC (%)	PD (%)	Response rate
3	0	3 (100%)	0	0	3 (100%)

CR, Complete response; *PR*, partial response; *NC*, no change; *PD*, progressive disease

Table 3. Results according to metastatic sites

Localization	Number of patients	CR (%)	PR (%)	NC (%)	PD (%)	RR
Local tumor	12	0	7 (58)	4 (33)	1 (8)	58
M1-lymph nodes	6	1 (17)	3 (50)	0	2 (33)	67
Lymph nodes	5	0	4 (80)	0	1 (20)	80

CR, Complete response; *PR*, partial response; *NC*, no change; *PD*, progressive disease; *RR*, response rate

Table 4. Toxicity according to who criteria

	WHO Grade				
Toxicity	0	1	2	3	4
Nausea, vomiting	10	3	0	2	0
Appetite	6	3	3	3	0
Alopecia	0	9	6	0	0
Diarrhea	15	0	0	0	0
Neurotoxicity	14	1	0	0	0
Nephrotoxicity	15	0	0	0	0
Thrombocytes	12	2	0	1	0
Leukocytes	6	1	1	5	2
Hemoglobin	13	1	0	1	0

adenectomy. Four patients were reconstructed by poststernal esophagogastric and one mediastinal esophagocolonic anastomosis with end-to-end stapling device. Two patients had complicated infections (thoracic wound two, intrapleural one). One of the infections was associated with lung abscess due to methicillin-resistant *Staphylococcus aureus* (MSRA) and this patient was the only postoperative death. No anastomotic leakage after resection occurred. Postoperative mortality and morbidity rates were 20% and 40%, respectively. Histological effectiveness of chemotherapy was moderate.

Toxicity

Toxicity of the ELF-P regimen, according to WHO standard criteria, is shown in Table 4. Hematologic toxicity with leukocytes grade 3 or 4 occurred in seven patients (47%), and grade 3 thrombocytes were found in one patient (7%). Loss of appetite grade 2 or 3 was present in 40% of patients. All patients showed hair loss, and grade 2 alopecia was seen in six patients (40%). These toxicities were clinically tolerable and reversible.

Discussion

Cisplatin-based combinations for esophageal squamous carcinoma are reported to show response rates from 15% to 76% [1, 2], however, patients prognosis still remain unsatisfactory. We have to establish a better regimen to improve the survival of the patients with esophageal carcinoma. There are several theoretical advantages to the use of chemotherapy prior to surgery [3, 4]. Studies of neoadjuvant chemotherapy indicate a high response rate to chemotherapy and suggest improved survival.[5] The response rate obtained in our study was higher than the studies of selected phase II trials [5]. An analysis of the pooled data for overall mortality, morbidity, and anastomotic leak rate after resection shows no difference between surgery alone or surgery with preoperative radiation therapy and/or chemotherapy [5]. In our study, infections were a major cause of mortality and morbidity after neoadjuvant chemotherapy following resection. The anastomotic leak was not increased by neoadjuvant chemotherapy. In conclusion, ELF-P induced a high response rate (67%) in advanced and recurrent esophageal carcinoma. Also, leukocyte and thrombocyte toxicities were moderate and well tolerated. We need further comparative studies of chemotherapy with surgery to surgery alone, or chemotherapy-surgery versus chemotherapy plus concurrent radiotherapy-surgery in patients with advanced esophageal squamous carcinoma.

References

1. Kelsen DP, Lichter A, Roth JA (1990) Carcinoma of the esophagus. American Society of Clinical Oncology Educational Booklet p 69
2. Leichman L, Berry BT (1991) Experience with cisplatin in treatment regimens for esophageal cancer. Semin Oncol 18:64–72
3. Fisher B, Gunduz N, Saffer EA (1983) Influence of the interval between primary tumor removal and chemotherapy on kinetics growth of metastasis. Cancer Res 43:1488–1492
4. Goldie JH, Coldman AJ (1984) The genetic origin of drug resistance in neoplasms: Implications for systemic therapy. Cancer Res 44:3643–3645
5. Kelsen DP, Bains M, Burt M (1990) Neoadjuvant chemotherapy and surgery of cancer of the esophagus. Semin Surg Oncol 6:268–273

Preoperative Chemotherapy with Cisplatin/5-FU/Leucovorin for Squamous Cell Carcinoma of the Esophagus

Kazuhiko Hayashi, Hiroko Ide, Reiki Eguchi, Kazunari Yoshida,
Ataru Kobayashi, Takeshi Endo, Tomoko Hanashi,
and Akiyoshi Yamada[1]

Introduction

The result of chemotherapy for esophageal carcinoma has been disappointing because of low response rates and little evidence of prolongation of life. In our institute also, patients with far advanced esophageal squamous cell carcinoma (SCC) had been treated with neoadjuvant chemotherapy on some protocols [1-2], and their responses and survival rates have been insufficient. However, recent in vitro studies have suggested synergy between cisplatin and 5-FU if the intracellular pools of reduced folates are increased [3-7]. Leucovorin is metabolized to the biochemically active form 5,10-CH2-FH4, and this cofactor augments- the cytotoxicity of fluorouracil (FUra) through stabilization of the ternary complex of 5-fluorodeoxyuridine monophosphatase (FdUMP), and thymidilate synthase (Fig. 1).

Additionally, this concept might be successfully applied in clinical situations to the combination chemotherapy of cisplatin, 5-FU, and leucovorin in the initial treatment of the patients with esophageal SCC.

Patient Eligibility

Patients with histologically confirmed SCC were eligible for this study. All patients had a history and physical examination, assessment of disease, chest X-ray, electrocardiogram, and blood cell counts and chemistries, and were required to have bidimensionally measurable lesions. Eligibility requirements also included a WHO performance status of 0 or 1, adequate bone marrow (WBC $> 3000/ml$, platelet count $10^4/ml$), liver (bilirubin $< 2 mg/dl$), and renal (creatinin $< 1.5 mg/dl$) functions.

[1] Department of Surgery, Institute of Gastroenterology, Tokyo Women's Medical College, 8-1, Kawada-cho Shinjuku-ku, Tokyo, 162 Japan

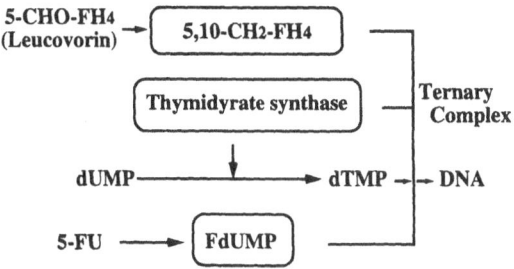

Fig. 1. Modulation of 5-FU by leucovorin

Of the 21 patients, 2 women and 19 men were included in this study between September 1990 and June 1991. The characteristics of the patients are listed in Table 1: Mean age was 62 years (range 47–73), and 17 patients were PS 0 and 4 were PS 1. According to the American Joint Committee on Cancer (AJCC) staging system [8], three patients has stage IIB, eight had stage III, and ten had stage IV. Patients were monitored with regular blood counts, renal function tests, and clinical examinations during each course, and they provided informed consent in keeping with our institutional policy.

Treatment

The treatment plan is showed in Table 2. All patients were treated with cisplatin $70\,mg/m^2$ on day 1, and 5-FU $700\,mg/m^2$ and leucovorin $20\,mg/m^2$ on days 1–5 preoperatively. After prehydration, cisplatin was given intravenously over 3 h, 5-FU 24-hours continuous iv, and leucovorin iv bolus. This cycle was repeated after 3–4 weeks in 14 cases; 7 cases had only one cycle of the chemotherapy for the evaluation of dose escalation, but this was not due to medical reasons. To reduce nausea and vomiting, it was recommended that patients receive a combination of metoclopramide iv, methylpredonisolon iv, and domperidone rectal suppository before each course of chemotherapy. Responses were assessed by endoscopy, upper GI series, endoscopic ultrasonography, and CT scan every 2 weeks after chemotherapy and were evaluated in accordance with the World Health Organization (WHO) criteria [9].

Results

All patients' characteristics are listed in Table 3. Of those, 21 patients received combination chemotherapy of CDDP, 5-FU, and leucovorin preoperatively according to the protocol, and one patient was found to have stage IIB (patient 1) achieved complete remission (CR) with negative biopsy findings, but a minute cancer nest still existed in the esophageal gland on the resected speciment. Two of three patients with stage IIB, 2/8 with stage III, and 7/10 with stage IV achieved partial remission (PR). The responses were seen within 2 weeks after the first cycle in all responders. Table 4 shows the objective response rate (CR

Table 1. Patient characteristics

Characteristics	Number of patients
Sex	
Male	19
Female	2
Age	
Median, 62 years	
Range, 47–73	
Site of disease	
Upper thoracic	3
Mid-thoracic	10
Lower thoracic	8
Stage	
IIB	3
III	8
IV	10
Histology	
Por.	4
Mod.	13
Wel.	4

por., poorly differentiated; *mod.*, moderate; *wel.*, well differentiated

Table 2. Treatment plan

Day	First Cycle					Second Cycle					40~
	1	2	3	4	5	21	22	23	24	25	
CDDP 70 mg/m^2	↓					↓					Operation
5-FU 700 mg/m^2	↓	↓	↓	↓	↓	↓	↓	↓	↓	↓	
Leucovorin 20 mg/m^2	↓	↓	↓ .	↓	↓	↓	↓	↓	↓	↓	

CDDP, cisplatin; *5-FU*, 5-fluorouracil

+ PR) was 57.1% (12/21; 95% confidence interval [CI] = 36.0 − 78.2). Every patient received curative operation within 4 weeks after the start of chemotherapy. The overall median follow-up period was 7.3 months, while their survival has not been reached.

Clinical observations and pathological findings revealed that widespread intraepithelial lesions of the four T1 carcinoma had completely or almost disappeared, and five intramural metastasis of four T3 and one T4 carcinoma decreased remarkably. One of the most interesting findings of this treatment is the excellent response of superficial lesions. This response was very likely due to the enhanced activity of 5-FU by leucovorin in the mucosal layer.

Table 3. Clinicopathological characteristics, response, and survival. Patient 5 died of mutiple organ failure 1 month after chemotherapy. Patients 3, 6, and 8 were lost of recurrent progressing tumor (mediastinal lymph nodes)

Patient sex/age	TMN-stage		Location	Histology	No. of cycles	Response to chemotherapy	Definitive treatment	Survival (months)
1. M/53	T1N1M0	IIB	Middle	por.	X2	CR	S	13
2. M/64	T3N1M1	IV	Lower	mod.	X2	NC	S + IOR	12
3. M/59	T3N1M0	III	Lower	mod.	X2	MR	S + RT	11 Dead
4. M/64	T1N1M1	IV	Middle	mod.	X2	PR	S + RT	11
5. M/69	T3N1M1	IV	Lower	mod.	X1	PR	S	1 Dead
6. M/61	T3N1M0	III	Upper	mod.	X2	MR	S + RT	4 Dead
7. M/47	T3N1M1	IV	Middle	mod.	X2	NC	S + RT	9
8. M/52	T3N1M1	IV	Lower	por.	X2	PR	S + RT	8 Dead
9. M/63	T4N1M1	IV	Middle	mod.	X2	PR	S + RT	9
10. M/66	T2N1M1	IV	Lower	wel.	X2	PR	S + IOR	3 Dead
11. M/63	T2N1M0	IIB	Upper	mod.	X1	PR	S + RT	7
12. M/61	T3N1M0	III	Lower	por.	X2	PR	S	7
13. M/60	T3N1M0	III	Middle	mod.	X1	NC	S	7
14. M/69	T3N1M0	III	Upper	mod.	X1	MR	S	6
15. F/73	T3N1M0	III	Middle	mod.	X1	MR	S	5
16. M/58	T1N0M1	IV	Middle	wel.	X2	PR	S + RT	5
17. M/53	T3N1M0	III	Middle	wel.	X2	PR	S	5
18. M/61	T1N1M0	IIB	Middle	por.	X1	PR	S	5
19. M/69	T3N1M1	IV	Lower	mod.	X1	PR	S	5
20. M/71	T3N1M1	IV	Lower	wel.	X2	MR	S	1
21. M/61	T3N1M0	III	Middle	mod.	X2	NC	S	1

S, surgery; *RT*, postoperative radiotherapy; *IOR*, intraoperative radiotherapy; *TNM*, tumor node metastasis; *CR*, complete response; *PR*, partial response; *NC*, no charge

Table 4. Clinical response

	CR	PR	MR	NC
Stage				
IIB	1/3	2/3		
III		2/8	4/8	2/8
IV		7/10	1/10	2/10

MR, minimal response

Toxicities

Overall toxicities were considered acceptable (Table 5). Almost all patients experienced oral or pharyngeal mucositis. Such toxicity was apparently enhanced by the addition of leucovorin [10] and this fact indicates that leucovorin at the dose of $20 \, \text{mg/m}^2$ employed in this trial substantially enhanced the effect of 5-FU. Allopurinol mouthwash was used to prevent oral mucositis [11] and steroid ointment was applied to the erosions and ulcers. In addition, due to the other gastrointestinal toxicities such as nausea and vomiting, most of the patients required parenteral hyperalimentation to maintain an adequate diet. WHO grade 1 and 2 leukopenia were both observed in 24%, and grade 1 and 2 renal dysfunction was seen in 20% and 24%, respectively. Grade 1 and 2 liver

Table 5. Toxicity (n = 21) according to the WHO criteria [9]

	Grade 1	Grade 2	Grade 3
Oral mucositis	8	5	5
Nausea/vomiting	8	9	2
Alopecia	8	8	
Leukopenia	5	5	
Anemia	5	3	
ECG		3	
Renal dysfunction	4	5	
Liver dysfunction	3	3	

dysfunction both occurred in 14%, and grade 2 transient arrythmia in 14%. These toxicities were reversible within 3–4 weeks after each course of chemotherapy.

Discussion

The activity of the combination of cisplatin and 5-FU on esophageal cancer are now well demonstrated with a response rate of 35%–57% [2, 12–14]. According to the results of phase I and II studies of cisplatin, 5-FU and leucovorin in patients with head and neck cancer [15], we applied this combination for the first time to the treatment of esophageal squamous cell carcinoma [16], and here we described the results in detail. In our past studies on the chemotherapy of esophageal carcinoma, no combinations could achieve CR. In this study, we could obtain excellent results (CR + PR = 57%, 95% CI = 36.0 − 78.2) and did not experience severe toxicities against the neoadjuvant chemotherapy with no dropping out before operation. Furthermore, no drug-related enhancement of surgical morbidity was observed. The considerable toxicity of this regimen was mainly manifest as oral mucositis, leukopenia, alopecia, and nephrotoxicity, but these adverse effects were well tolerated by the patients. Intraepithelial lesions and intramural metastasis of advanced cases showed responded well, thereby suggesting that this combination of chemotherapy might be recommended for the initial treatment of superficial carcinoma of the esophagus. This study provides preliminary data which might show a trend in advantage of the neoadjuvant chemotherapy of esophageal SCC. In conclusion, this therapy has shown excellent activity, and low toxicity as neoadjuvant chemotherapy for patients with esophageal cancer.

References

1. Iizuka T, Kakegawa T, Ide H, Ando N, Watanabe H, Takagi I (1991) Phase II evaluation of combined cisplatin and vindesine in advanced squamous cell carcinoma of the esophagus: Japanese esophageal oncology group trial. Jpn J Clin Oncol 21:176–179
2. Iizuka T, Kakegawa T, Ide H, Ando N, Watanabe H, Tanaka O, Takagi I, Isono K, Ishida K, Arimori M, Endo M, Fukushima M (in press) Phase II evaluation of cisplatin and 5-

fluorouracil in advanced squamous cell carcinoma of the esophagus: Japanese Esophageal Oncology Group Trial. Jpn J Clin Oncol

3. Ullman B, Lee M, Martin DW (1978) Cytotoxicity of 5-fluoro-2-deoxxuridine: Requirement for reduced folate cofactors and antagonism by methotrexate. Proc Natl Acad Sci 75:980–983

4. Waxman S, Bruckner H (1982) The enhancement of 5-fluorouracil antimetabolite activity by leucovorin, menadion and alphatocopherol. Eur J Cancer Clin Oncol 18:685–692

5. Evans RM, Laskin JD, Hakala MT (1981) Effects of excess folates and deoxyuridine on the activity and site of action of 5-fluorouracil. Cancer Res 41:3288

6. Keyomarsi K, Moran RG (1987) Folinic acid augmentation of the effects of fluoropyrimidines on murine and human leukemic cells. Cancer Res 46:5229–5235

7. Mini E, Moran BA, Bercino JR (1987) Cytotoxicity of fluoroxyuridine and 5-fluorouracil in human T-lymphoblast leukemia cells: Enhancement by leucovorin. Cancer Treat Rep 71:381–389

8. American Joint Committee on Cancer Staging and End-Results Reporting: Manual for Staging of Cancer. (1978) AJC, Chicago

9. Handbook for reporting: Manual for staging of cancer treatment. (1979) WHO-offset publication No. 48. World Health Organization

10. Figoli F, Sileni VC, Gulisano M, Maggian P, Fosser V (1989) Leucovorin calcium enhancement of mucositis after continuous infusion fluorouracil and short infusion cisplatin (letter) J Clin Oncol 7:680

11. Clark PI, Slevin ML (1985) Allopurinol mouthwashes and 5-fluorouracil-induced oral toxicity. Eur J Surg Oncol 11:267–268

12. Carey RW, Hilgenberg AD, Wilkins EW, Choi NC, Mathisen DJ, Grillo H (1986) Preoperative chemotherapy followed by surgery with possible postoperative radiotherapy in squamous cell carcinoma of the esophagus:Evaluation of the chemotherapy component. J Clin Oncol 4:697–701

13. Hilgenberg AD, Carey RW, Wilkins EW, Choi NC, Mathisen DJ, rillo HC (1988) Pre-operative chemotherapy, surgical resection, and selective postoperative therapy for squamous cell carcinoma of the esophagus. Ann Thorac Surg 45:357–363.

14. Kies Ms, Rosen ST, Tsang TK, Shetty R, Schneider PA, Wallemark CB, Shields TW (1987) Cisplatin and 5-fluorouracil in the primary management of squamous esophageal cancer. Cancer 60:2156–2160.

15. Vokes EE, Choi KE, Schilaky RL, Moran MJ, Guarnieri M, Weichselbaum RR, Panje WR (1987) Cisplatin, fluorouracil and high dose leucovorin for recurrent or metastatic head and neck cancer. J Clin Oncol 6:618–626

16. Hayashi K, Ide H, Shinoda M, Fukushima M (1992) Phase II study of cisplatin (CDDP) plus 5-fluorouracil (5-FU) and leucovorin (LCV) for squamous cell carcinoma of the esophagus. Proc Am Soc Clin Oncol 11:178

A Prospective Randomized Trial of Pre- and Postoperative Chemotherapy in Patients with Esophageal Cancer

Junsuke Shibata, Hiroyuki Naito, Akira Kawaguchi, Yoshihiro Endo, and Masashi Kodama[1]

Introduction

Most patients with esophageal cancer are at an advanced stage when they were referred to surgeons, and the prognosis is generally poor. However, operative mortality rates after radical operation for esophageal cancer have decreased with improvement of operative procedures and perioperative care.

The factors which hinder the survival rate are organ metastasis and recurrence in the lymph nodes at the neck and upper mediastinum.

To reduce the recurrence in the lymph nodes, we have employed three-field lymph node dissection of the bilateral cervical, mediastinal, and abdominal regions since 1985.

This time, we tried a prospective, randomized study of pre- and postoperative chemotherapy to the patients with esophageal cancer undergoing curative operation to determine its effectiveness in long-term survival.

Materials and Methods

Twenty-eight patients with cancer of the thoracic esophagus were randomized to receive either immediate surgery or pre- and post operative chemotherapy from January 1988 to July 1992.

Patients with non-curative operation or superficial mucosal cancer were excluded. Our operative procedure is total thoracic esophagectomy through right thoracotomy with three-field lymph node dissection.

The treatment schedule consists of a combination of cisplatin, vindesine, and pepleomycin as Kelsen [1] reported (Fig. 1).

[1] First Department of Surgery, Shiga University of Medical Science, Tsukinowa-cho Seta, Otsu Shiga, 520-21 Japan

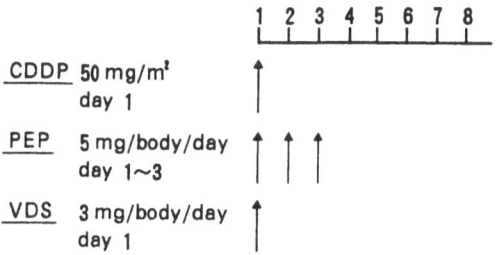

Fig. 1. Chemotherapy for esophageal cancer. *CDDP*, cisplatin; *PEP*, pepleomycin; *VDS*, vindesine

Table 1. Characteristics of patients

		Control	Chemotherapy
No. of patients		15	13
Sex (M:F)		13:2	13:0
Mean age in years (range)		64.1 (45–72)	61.8 (46–72)
Location	Upper	2	1
	Middle	9	8
	Lower	4	4
Stage	1	3	2
	2	3	2
	3	7	5
	4	2	4
Histology	Well	7	8
	Mod	5	3
	Poor	3	2

Cisplatin $50 \, \text{mg/m}^2$ and vindesine $3 \, \text{mg/day}$ were delivered on day 1 and pepleomycin on days 1–3. This chemotherapy was given once before operation and repeated starting 3–4 weeks after operation once a month if the patient's condition allowed it. Cisplatin was delivered with adequate pre- and post-hydration with antiemetics. Characteristics of the patients are shown in Table 1. Patients with stage 3 and 4 comprised 60% (9/15) of the control group and 69.2% (9/13) of the chemotherapy group. There was no difference between the two groups.

Result

All the patients received preoperative chemotherapy as scheduled and underwent curative operation 10–14 days after chemotherapy. The 30-day operative mortality rate was 0% and there was no drug-related death. The major toxicities were anorexia, nausea, vomiting, and leukocytopenia. Anorexia was seen in all patients. Nausea and vomiting were seen in 76.9% (10/13) even with the use of antiemetics. Leukocytopenia was also common, but no patients had white blood counts of <1000 cells/mm³. Thrombocytopenia was uncommon. Renal dysfunction of >2.5 mg of serum creatinine occurred in only 7.7% (1/13)

Table 2. Recurrent cases of esophageal cancer

No.	Age	Sex	Site	Invasion	Degree of lymph node metastasis	Stage	Outcome (years postop)
Chemotherapy group							
1.	72	M	Im.	a2	n3	st IV	X Paraaortic LN (3)
2.	64	M	Im.	a2	n3	st IV	O Mediastinum LN
3.	70	M	Im.	a2	n2	st III	X Bone Skin
4.	56	M	Ei.	a1	n1	st II	X Liver, Skin
5.	46	M	Ei.	mp	n3	st IV	X Liver
Control group							
1.	68	M	Im.	mp	n2	st III	O Cervical LN (3)
2.	60	M	Iu.	mp	n0	st I	O Cervical LN
3.	59	M	Im.	a1	n2	st III	X Bone
4.	69	F	Im.	sm	n0	st 0	X Mediastinum
5.	56	M	Im.	a1	n0	st II	O Liver lung
6.	45	M	Im.	a2	n3	st IV	X Lung
7.	57	M	Im.	a2	n3	st IV	X Liver
8.	69	M	Ei.	a2	n2	st III	X Liver
9.	65	M	Iu.	a2	n2	st III	X Lung

——— : disease free   ········· : recurrence

Iu, upper thoracic; *Im*, middle; *Ei*, lower; *X*, dead; *O*, alive; *sm*, submucosa; *mp*, muscularis mucosa; *a1*, adventitia (reaching); *a2*, adventitia (definite invasion); *n1*, metastasis to group 1

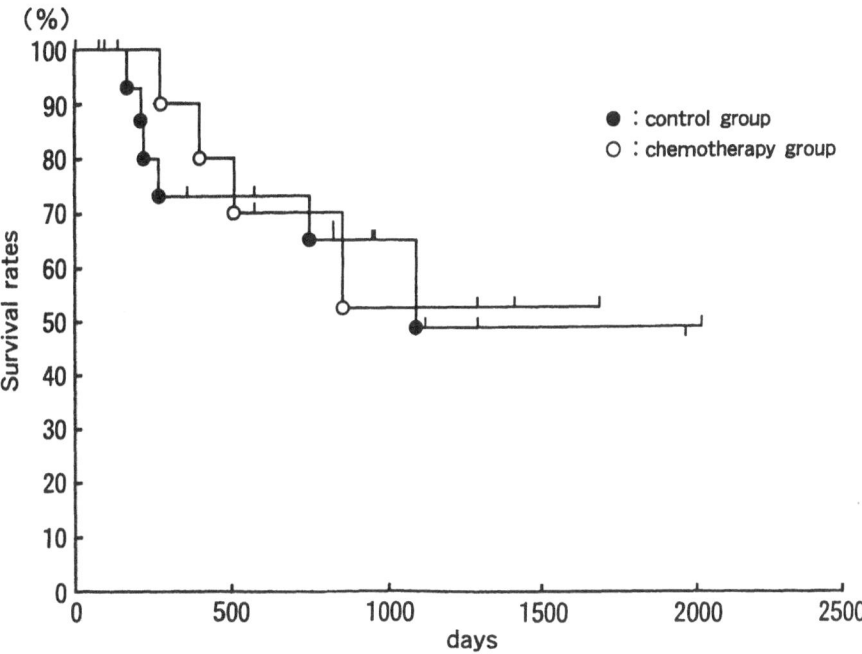

Fig. 2. Survival curves of curatively resected esophageal patients with or without pre- and postoperative chemotherapy

because of pre- and post-hydration and the use of diuretics. Toxicity of this schedule was tolerable and no patients discontinued this schedule because of toxicity. Recurrences were seen in five cases in the chemotherapy group and nine in the control group (Table 2). The mean times to recurrence were 15 and 12.3 months, respectively. One in five cases in the chemotherapy group and three in nine in the control group are alive with recurrence. Metastases to the lymph nodes were seen in five cases about 1 year after operation. Organ metastases (lung, liver, and bone) were seen in nine cases within 1 year after operation, but bone metastasis was not. Survival curves were compared between the two groups (Fig. 2). The 1- and 3-year survival rates were 88.9% and 53.3% for the chemotherapy group, and 72.5% and 66.7% for the control group respectively. They were a little better in the chemotherapy group than in the control group. Survival rates in relation to the depth of cancer invasion, the degree of lymph node metastasis, and stage were also analyzed, but there were no significant differences between the two groups.

Discussion

Most of the patients had recurrence in the lymph nodes and/or organs (liver, lung, and bone) after surgery. We used combined preoperative irradiation and surgery, but preoperative irradiation did not increase 5-year survival in spite of increasing the rate of resectability and curability. Since advanced cancer is a systemic disease, systemic treatment is expected [2, 3]. Kelsen [1] reported that a three-drug combination of cisplatin, vindesine, and pepleomycin is effective in the treatment of esophageal cancer. A prospective, randomized study is necessary to see the effects of chemotherapy, and we changed the schedule and dosages of the three drugs for our patients as mentioned before.

The results showed that the incidence of recurrence and 1- and 3-year survival rates are better in the chemotherapy group than in the control group, though the differences are not statistically significant.

Kelsen [1] and other investigators reported that the maximum degree of response was seen after two courses of chemotherapy, and also that chemotherapy will have little or no effect on the course of the disease in non-responding patients. We had 10–14 days from the end of chemotherapy to surgery, and it is rather short to evaluate the effects on tumors. When we started this trial, we thought that it is difficult to give chemotherapy twice or three times before operation because of drug toxicity and the interval required. Because of the lack of definitive differences between the two groups, we are trying to design a modified treatment schedule referring to other reports [4, 5].

References

1. Kelsen DP, Bains M, Hilaris B, Chapman R, McCormack P, Alexander J, Hopfan S, Martini N (1982) Combination chemotherapy of esophageal carcinoma using cisplatin, vindesine, and bleomycin. Cancer 49:1174–1177
2. Sasaki T, Makuuchi H, Sugiura T (1988) Evaluation of preoperative irradiation therapy for carcinoma of the esophagus. In: Siewert JR, Holscher AH (eds) Diseases of the esophagus. Springer, Berlin Heidelberg New York, pp 313–316
3. Huang J, Gu Z, Wang J, Wang M, Zhang W, Yin B, Zhang G, Liu S, Wang Y (1990) Combined preoperative irradiation and surgery versus surgery alone for squamous cell carcinoma of the midthoracic esophagus: A prospective randomized study in 360 patients. In: Ferguson M, Little A, Skinner D (eds) Diseases of the esophagus. Futura, Mt Kisko pp 275–281
4. Herskovic A, Martz K, Al-Sarraf M, Leichman L, Brindle J, Vaitkevicius V, Cooper J, Byhardt R, Davis L, Emami B (1992) Combined chemotherapy and radiotherapy compared with radiotherapy alone in patients with cancer of the esophagus. New Engl J Med 326:1593–1598
5. Forastiere A (1992) Treatment of locoregional esophageal cancer. Semin Oncol 19:57–63

Preoperative Concurrent Chemotherapy and Radiotherapy of Squamous Cell Carcinoma of the Thoracic Esophagus: A Pilot Study Report

ANDRZEJ W. SZAWLOWSKI[1], SLAWOMIR FALKOWSKI[2], TADEUSZ MORYSINSKI[3], ANNA NASIEROWSKA-GUTTMEJER[4], ANDRZEJ KARWOWSKI[5], MAREK KRAWCZYK[5], and ANDRZEJ KULAKOWSKI[1]

Introduction

In Poland, 1300 new cases of carcinoma of the esophagus are registered each year and it ranges from 1.1 in women to 4.8 in men per 100,000 population [1]. Most of the esophageal cancer patients admitted to the hospitals are in an advanced stage of the disease, and this is mainly responsible for the low operability/resecability rates and therefore poor long-term results of treatment (5-year survival is around 4%, the lowest of all gastro-intestinal cancers). Since no significant progress in early diagnosis has been observed, the attempts to improve the results concentrate on combining other modes of treatment (e.g., radio- and/or chemotherapy) before surgery (Fig. 1). Currently, surgery, whenever possible, remains the treatment of choice for carcinoma of the esophagus aimed at palliation or cure, whether or not it is associated with radiotherapy pre- and/or postoperatively. The place and the role of chemotherapy (combined or monotherapy) in the treatment program for esophageal carcinoma is still unproven, and is under evaluation for its potential benefits by ongoing prospective clinical trials.

Here, we present the first Polish experience based on the results of a pilot study of preoperative application of chemotherapy and concurrent radiotherapy for advanced squamous cell carcinoma (SCC) of the thoracic esophagus. The aim of this study was to evaluate the dose-related tolerance and response rates before the start of a multicenter prospective and randomized clinical trial in Poland. The morphological pattern of response found in our patients is presented separately elsewhere in this issue.

Departments of Surgical Oncology[1], Chemotherapy[2], Radiotherapy[3], and Tumour Pathology[4], The Maria Sklodowska-Curie Memorial Cancer Center and Institute of Oncology, 15, Wawelska Street, 00-973 Warsaw, Poland. [5] Department of General and Hepatic Surgery, Medical Academy, Warsaw, Poland

927

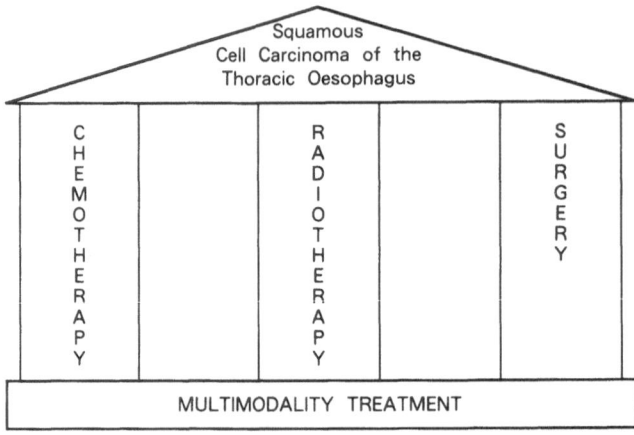

Fig. 1. Toward a new strategy in the treatment of advanced squamous cell carcinoma of the thoracic esophagus

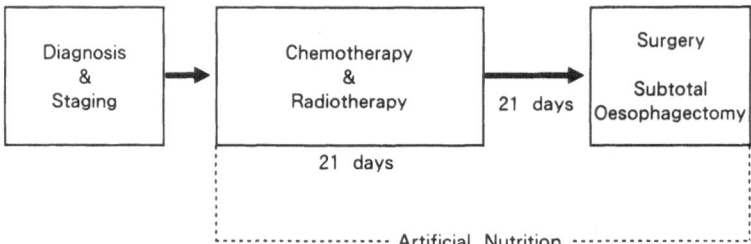

Fig. 2. Treatment program for pilot group of patients with advanced squamous cell carcinoma of the thoracic esophagus

Methods

Between June 1990 and June 1991 at the Maria Sklodowska-Curie Cancer Center and Institute of Oncology, Warsaw, Poland, 15 consecutive patients with SCC of the thoracic esophagus were treated according to the program presented in Fig. 2. All were considered as candidates for either palliative or potentially curative esophagectomy. Prior to treatment, imaging studies (chest x-ray, barium esophagogram, chest computed tomography (CT) or magnetic resonance imaging (MRI) scans, and abdominal ultrasonography were performed to evaluate the extent of the disease. The criteria of eligibility are listed in Table 1. Pretreatment data for all patients are presented in Table 2. The tumors were classified according to the UICC TNM system both before and after treatment [2].

The treatment protocol was similar to the one reported by Forastiere et al. [3] and consisted of 21 days of continuous IV infusion chemotherapy (cisplatin and 5-fluorouracil) and concurrent radiotherapy (Fig. 3), followed by a 3-week rest. Esophagectomy was performed around the 42nd day of treatment.

Table 1. Criteria of eligibility for pilot study of preoperative concurrent chemo- and radio-therapy for advanced squamous cell carcinoma off the thoracic oesophagus

1. Histologically confirmed squamous cell carcinoma of the thoracic esophagus
2. Age under 70 years
3. Distant metastates excluded (M0)
4. Karnofsky performance status above 70%
5. Normal hematologic and renal function (WBC >3500 cells/µl, platelets 100 000 cells/µl, creatinine clearance >50 ml/min)
6. Normal pulmonary function tests
7. No prior treatment for carcinoma of the gastrointestinal tract
8. Informed consent of the patient

Table 2. Pilot group of patients treated concurrently by preoperative chemo- and radiotherapy

No	Age	Sex	Tumor localization[b] (cm)	Tumor length (cm)	Radiologic type	TNM
1[a]	45	M	27	9	Serrated	T3N0M0
2	59	M	38	3	Serrated	T1N0M0
3	59	F	34	6	Spiral	T2N0M0
4[a]	64	F	25	8	Funnelled	T3N0M0
5	65	M	30	5	Serrated	T2N0M0
6	63	M	30	5	Spiral	T2N0M0
7[a]	48	M	25	11	Funnelled	T3N0M0
8	68	M	24	12	Funnelled	T2N0M0
9	63	M	30	12	Serrated	T2N0M0
10[a]	60	M	25	7	Funnelled	T3N0M0
11	53	M	22	10	Spiral	T2N0M0
12	40	M	30	10	Serrated	T2N0M0
13	53	M	25	9	Spiral	T2N0M0
14	58	M	35	8	Serrated	T2N0M0
15	62	M	26	9	Serrated	T2N0M0

[a] Preoperative death, [b] The distance from the upper incisors to the lesion
TNM, tumor node metastasis

Cisplatin (DDP) was administered on days 1–5 and 17–21 at a dose of 20 mg/m^2/day. 5-Fluorouracil (5-FU) was administered throughout the 21 days of treatment at a dose of 300 mg/m^2/day. Radiation (Co^{60} therapy) was delivered through the anterior field encompassing the tumor volume with 5 cm longitudinal margins and 2 cm lateral margins. Daily fractions of 200 cGy, 5 days a week, to a total of 3000 cGy over 15 days of irradiation were planned.

Anti-emetics (e.g., Torecan, metoclopramide, dexamethasone) were not given prophylactically during the treatment unless indicated by clinical signs (e.g., nausea, vomiting). Parenteral nutrition (Aminomel Salvia from Boehringer Laboratory as a source of nitrogen, glucose and Intralipid from KabiVitrum as a source of lipids) supplemented by electrolytes and vitamins and totalling

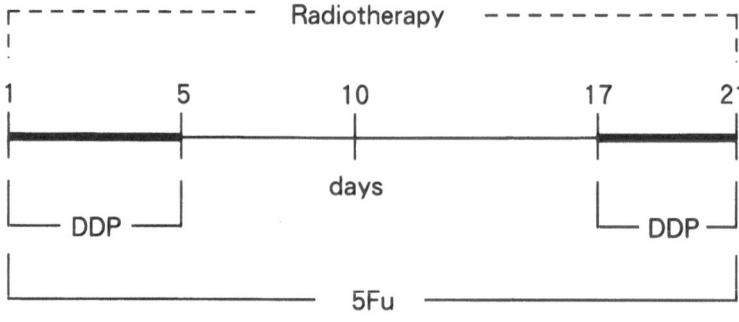

Doses :
DDP- 20mg ⁄ m² ⁄ 24hrs.
5Fu- 300mg ⁄ m² ⁄ 24hrs.
Radiotherapy (Co⁶⁰) - 3000 cGy (Fractions = 200 cGy)

Fig. 3. Preoperative treatment protocol design

1200–1600 calories (normonutrition) was infused via a jugular catheter in those patients in whom oral caloric intake was inadequate. Hematological toxicity was considered when WBC was below 3500 and/or platelet count was below 50 000. In these cases, the chemotherapy was stopped and resumed after recovery of hematological parameters.

Barium esophagograms were repeated every week during chemo- and radio-therapy to evaluate the tumor response to the treatment. Clinical tolerance was defined as good if the preoperative treatment was completed without interruptions and bad if it had to be prolonged or even discontinued as a result of uncontrolled nausea, vomiting, and/or hematological toxicity.

About 3 weeks after completion of chemo- and radiotherapy, the patients were operated upon either at the Department of Surgical Oncology, the Maria Sklodowska-Curie Memorial Cancer Center and Institute of Oncology or at the Department of General and Hepatic Surgery, Medical Academy in Warsaw. Esophagectomy associated with two-field lymph node dissection (mediastinal and abdominal) was performed using either the modified Ivor-Lewis approach [4] or Akiyama's procedure [5] with esophagoplasty using isoperistaltic stomach tube retrosternally.

All operation specimens were examined by the same pathologist to assess post-therapy tumor degeneration and necrosis. The response to treatment was categorized as either complete (CR), partial (PR), or stable disease (SD), and was based on a comparison of the initial and preoperative imaging studies, as well as on postoperative pathological findings. Thus, CR was defined as dis-appearance of all signs and symptoms of the tumor with no histopathological evidence of residual tumor in the resected specimen. PR was defined if dis-appearance of all signs of the tumor was evidenced by imaging studies, but residual tumor was found microscopically in postoperative specimens. SD patients had no appreciable change in tumor mass on imaging studies and no signs of tumor degeneration or necrosis on histopathological examination.

Table 3. Preoperative treatment (chemo- and concurrent radiotherapy) toxicity data

Toxic reaction	No. of patients
Leukopenia	9/15 (60.0%)
Thrombopenia	7/15 (46.6%)
Esophagitis	15/15 (100%)
Nausea	7/15 (46.6%)
Diarrhea	2/15 (13.3%)
Fever (>37.8°C)	6/15 (40.0%)
Cardiotoxicity	2/15 (13.3%)
Hepatotoxicity	2/15 (13.3%)

Table 4. Post-therapy results: preoperative concurrent chemo- and radiotherapy followed by surgery

No	Clinical tolerance	Surgical procedure	Postoperative complications	Tumor response	pTNM
1[a]	Bad	—	—	SD	T4N0M0
2	Good	Ivor-Lewis	Horner syndrome	PR	T1N0M0
3	Good	Ivor-Lewis	Hydrothorax	CR	T0N0M0
4[a]	Bad	—	—	SD	—
5	Good	Akiyama	—	PR	T2N0M0
6	Bad	Ivor-Lewis	—	PR	T1N0M0
7[a]	Bad	—	—	SD	T4N1M0
8	Bad	Akiyama	Abdominal wound eventration	PR	T2N1M0
9	Good	Akiyama	—	PR	T1N1M0
10[a]	Bad	—	—	SD	T4N1M0
11	Good	Laparotomy	—	PR	—
12	Good	Akiyama	Wound sepsis	PR	T1N0M0
13	Good	Laparotomy	—	PR	—
14	Good	Akiyama	—	PR	T2N1M0
15	Bad	Ivor-Lewis	—	PR	T1N0M0

[a] Preoperative death

CR, complete response; *PR*, partial response; *SD*, stable disease

Results

Full preoperative treatment protocol was completed in all patients except for one (case 6) due to severe toxicity and bad clinical tolerance. Overall preoperative treatment toxicity data are listed in Table 3.

All patients had subjective improvement in food passage but to a lesser extent in cases with radiologic funnel-type lesions as compared to serrated and spiral lesions. In general, radiologic funnel-type esophageal tumors were found to show the worst response to preoperative treatment.

Four patients died preoperatively due to post-chemo- and radiotherapy complications such as tracheobronchial fistula and septic shock resulting from aspiration pneumonia ($n = 2$) and/or bone marrow aplasia ($n = 4$). Postmortem examinations were performed in all cases except one (case 4) because her family refused to consent to such a procedure; however, previous esophagograms performed during the preoperative treatment showed signs of marked regression of the tumor mass.

Of the operated patients, 9/11 (81.8%) underwent esophagectomy with no 30-day postoperative mortality. The two remaining patients were disqualified from esophagectomy, in one case (case 11) due to inextirpable nodular mass at the celiac trunk and in the second (case 13) due to extensive liver cirrhosis and portal hypertension. In both cases, exploratory laparotomy confirmed these findings.

Discussion

DDP and 5-FU were chosen for preoperative chemotherapy because of their known activity in SCC [6-9] and because of their established role as radiation sensitizers [10, 11]. Both drugs were administered by continuous IV infusion to increase cytotoxicity and radiation enhancement. The same type of treatment was previously used by Leichman et al. [12], Poplin et al. [13], and Seydel et al. [14]. CR in patients undergoing resection was reported as 26%, 25%, and 29%, respectively. We had only one CR case (11.1%).

The basic aim of this study was to assess if the treatment plan could be effectively accomplished based on dose-related tolerance and response. As it was a pilot study, we are not allowed to make any definitive statements. However, we may conclude that preoperative chemo- and concurrent radiotherapy which we have applied to our patients may be effective as a neoadjuvant or remission-inducing modality in combined treatment of SCC of the esophagus, but the radiologic funnel-type lesions should probably be considered as bad responders. The treatment protocol is indeed burdening to the patients, causing, in some instances, fatal complications even before surgery. Therefore, individual tolerance should certainly be taken into consideration.

References

1. Zatonski W, Tarkowski W, Chmielarczyk W, Tyczynski J (1990) Cancer in Poland. National Cancer Registry, Warsaw, pp 29-56
2. Illustrated Guide to the TNM/pTNM classification of malignant tumors (1992). International Union Against Cancer (3rd edn.). Springer, Berlin Heidelberg New York, pp 62-70
3. Forastiere AA, Orringer MB, Perez-Tamayo C, Urba SG, Husted S, Takasugi BJ, Zahurak M (1990) Concurrent chemotherapy and radiation therapy followed by transhiatal esophagectomy for local regional cancer of the esophagus. J Clin Oncol 8(1):119-127
4. Lewis J (1946) The surgical treatment of carcinoma of the oesophagus with special reference to a new operation for growths of the middle third. Br J Surg 34:18-27
5. Akiyama H, Miyazono H, Tsurumaru M, Hashimoto C, Kawamura T (1978) Use of the stomach as an esophageal substitute. Ann Surg 188(5):606-610

6. Forastiere AA, Belliveau JF, Goren MP, Vogel WC, Posner MR, O'Leary GP (1988) Pharmacokinetic and toxicity evaluation of 5-day continuous infusion versus intermittent bolus cis-Diamminedichloroplatinum (II) in head and neck cancer patients. Cancer Res 48:3869–3874

7. Lokich JJ, Shea M, Chaffey J (1987) Sequential infusional 5-fluorouracil followed by concomitant radiation for tumors of the esophagus and gastrointestinal junction. Cancer 60:275–279

8. Byfield JE, Barone R, Mendelsohn J, Frankel S, Quinol L, Sharp T, Seagren S (1980) Infusional 5-FU and x-ray therapy for non-resectable esophageal cancer. Cancer 45:703–708

9. Rich TA, Lokich JJ, Chaffey JT (1985) A pilot study of protracted venous infusion of 5-fluorouracil and concomitant radiation therapy. J Clin Oncol 3:402–406

10. Dewit L (1987) Combined treatment of radiation and cis-diamminedichloroplatinum (II). A review of experimental and clinical data. Int J Oncol Biol Phys 13:403–426

11. Pinedo HM, Karim ABMF, van Vliet WH, Snow GB, Vermorken JB (1983) Daily cis-dichlorodiammineplatinum (II) as a radio-enhancer: A preliminary toxicity report. J Cancer Res Clin Oncol 105:79–82

12. Leichman L, Steiger Z, Seydel HG, Vaitkevicius VK (1984) Preoperative chemotherapy and radiation therapy for patients with cancer of the esophagus. A potentially curative approach. Semin Oncol 11:178–185

13. Poplin E, Fleming T, Leichman L (1987) Combined therapies for squamous cell carcinoma of the esophagus, a Southwest Oncology Group Study (SWOG 8037). J Clin Oncol 5:622–628

14. Seydel HG, Leichman L, Byhardt R, Cooper J, Herskovic A, Libnock J, Pazdur R, Speyer J, Tschan J and the Radiation Therapy Oncology Group (1988) Preoperative radiation and chemotherapy for localized squamous cell carcinoma of the esophagus: ARTOG study. Int J Radiat Oncol Biol Phys 14:33–35

High-Dose-Rate Intraluminal Brachytherapy for Small Superficial Esophageal Carcinoma

KOICHI KURISU, YOSHIO HISHIKAWA, MASAYUKI IZUMI, MIDORI TANIGUCHI, and NORIHIKO KAMIKONYA[1]

Introduction

Recent remarkable progress in high-dose-rate intraluminal brachytherapy (HDRIBT) has contributed to the treatment of esophageal cancer. This method is particularly effective for patients with early disease stage [1, 2]. We previously reported that a complete response was gained by HDRIBT alone in the patients with small superficial esophageal cancer and the treatment protocol of HDRIBT alone was recommended for these patients [3, 4]. However, a longer period of observation revealed different results. In this study, our purpose is to analyze local control, regional lymph node control, and survival relative to three radiotherapy protocols combined with HDRIBT for superficial esophageal carcinoma. We will describe the disadvantage of HDRIBT alone for patients with small superficial esophageal cancer; this method should be limited to patients with serious systemic disease.

Patients and Methods

Patients

Between May 1986 and March 1991, 109 patients were treated with HDRIBT with or without external radiotherapy (ERT) in the Department of Radiology at Hyogo College of Medicine. Of these, 17 (16%) had small superficial esophageal carcinoma without lymph node and distant metastases. Endoscopic biopsy proved squamous cell carcinoma in all of the tumors.

These 17 patients were divided into three groups according to the treatment method: The patients in group A were treated with HDRIBT only; the patients

[1] Department of Radiology, Hyogo College of Medicine, 1-1, Mukogawa-cho, Nishinomiya Hyogo, 663 Japan

Table 1. Characteristics of patients and tumors

	Group A (n = 8)	Group B (n = 5)	Group C (n = 4)
Sex			
Male	7	5	2
Female	1	0	2
Median age, years	63.5	81.0	80.5
(range)	(52–82)	(59–88)	(79–85)
P.S.			
0–2	7	4	4
3–4	1	1	0
Median tumor length, cm	1.0	2.5	2.8
(range)	(1.0–2.0)	(1.5–2.5)	(2.0–3.0)
Endoscopic findings			
Protruded	6	4	2
Flat	2	0	1
Excavated	0	1	1
Tumor location			
Cervical	1	0	0
Upper	3	0	0
Middle	2	3	4
Lower	2	2	0

P.S., Performance Status

in group B were treated with HDRIBT following ERT (ERT + HDRIBT); and those in group C were treated with HDRIBT followed by ERT (HDRIBT + ERT).

Pretreatment characteristics of patients and tumors according to the groups were as shown in Table 1. In group A, all patients had serious associated condition including liver cirrhosis ($n = 4$), cerebral infarction ($n = 2$), diabetes mellitus ($n = 1$), lung tumor ($n = 1$), and postoperative condition after resection of gastric cancer ($n = 2$). Additionally, one patient developed hepatoma 2 months after radiotherapy and was treated with transhepatic arterial embolization. In group B, diabetes mellitus and liver cirrhosis were recognized in each patient, and all patients in group C had no problem except esophageal cancer.

Radiotherapy

HDRIBT was performed using a high-dose-rate, remote afterloader (RAL-303, Toshiba, Tokyo). The source was Co^{60}. The delivered dose was calculated using a computerized radiotherapy planning system (RO-7; Varian Associates, Palo Alto, Calif.). Radiation was administered to the level 5 mm below the surface of the mucosa, 1 cm from the source. Details on the technique and dosimetry of HDRIBT have been previously reported [2].

ERT was performed with 10 MV x-rays (LMR-15, Toshiba, Tokyo). Opposing anterior and posterior parallel treatment fields were used up to 40 Gy, followed by the rotation technique. The field was 6 cm in width, and 3 cm longer than the superior and inferior margins of the tumor.

In group A, all patients were treated with HDRIBT alone. Seven patients received 24 Gy (4 fractions over 2–3 weeks) and the other one received 18 Gy (3 fractions over 2 weeks). In group B, all patients were treated with ERT + HDRIBT. Three patients received 60 Gy (30 fractions over 6 weeks) ERT plus 6 Gy (1 fraction) HDRIBT, the other one received 60 Gy (30 fractions over 6 weeks) ERT plus 12 Gy (2 fractions over 1 week) HDRIBT, and the last one received 56 Gy (28 fractions over 5.5 weeks) ERT plus 6 Gy (1 fraction) HDRIBT. In group C, all patients were treated with HDRIBT + ERT. Three patients received 12 Gy (2 fractions over 1 week) HDRIBT plus 60 Gy (30 fractions over 6 weeks) ERT, and the other one received 12 Gy (2 fractions over 1 week) HDRIBT plus 50 Gy (25 fractions over 5 weeks) ERT.

Follow-Up Studies

All patients underwent endoscopy within 1 month after completion of radiotherapy. Subsequently, endoscopy or esophagography was performed every month during the next 6 months; after that, the examination was done once every 2 or 3 months. Endoscopic biopsy was performed in all patients in whom tumor recurrence was suspected.

Statistics

Survival time was calculated from the beginning of radiotherapy to death, or to September 30, 1992. No patients were lost to follow-up. The median follow-up time for survivors was 23 months (range: 19–78 months). Statistical analysis was performed using the Student's t-test or the chi-square test.

Results

Tumor Response

The tumor in all 17 patients had completely disappeared when the first endoscopic study was done, within 1 month after radiotherapy.

Treatment Failure (Table 2)

Local Recurrence

Local recurrence in groups A, B, and C was 50% (4/8), 0% (0/5), and 25% (1/4), respectively. In Group A, the median time to local recurrence was 9 months (range: 7–22 months) after radiotherapy. Case 14 in group C showed local recurrence 7 months after radiotherapy. Case 4 was again treated with HDRIBT (total dose, 12 Gy) for local recurrence, 7 months after the first HDRIBT, and regrowth of the tumor was recognized 29 months after the second HDRIBT. Case 8 was treated with ERT (total dose, 50 Gy) for local recurrence, 8 months after HDRIBT, and the tumor has been well controlled until now.

Table 2. Survival and cause of death

Group/Case	Local recurrence	Lymph node metastasis	Distant metastasis	Survival (months)	
Group A					
1	No	No	No	36	dead[a]
2	No	Yes	Yes	27	dead
3	No	Yes	No	16	dead
4	Yes	No	No	41	dead
5	No	Yes	No	37	dead
6	Yes	Yes	No	27	dead
7	Yes	Yes	No	21	dead
8	Yes	No	No	27	alive
Group B					
9	No	No	No	78	alive
10	No	No	No	26	dead[a]
11	No	Yes	No	19	dead
12	No	No	No	23	alive
13	No	No	No	6	dead[a]
Group C					
14	Yes	No	No	12	dead
15	No	No	No	22	alive
16	No	No	No	2	dead[a]
17	No	No	No	19	alive

[a] intercurrent death

Lymph Node Metastasis

Lymph node metastasis was recognized after radiotherapy in 62.5% (5/8) of patients in group A, 20% (1/5) in group B, and 0% (0/4) in group C. In group A, the median time to lymph node metastasis was 8 months (range: 3–17 months) and mediastinal lymph node metastasis was found in four patients (cases 2, 3, 6, and 7), cervical lymph node metastasis in two patients (cases 2 and 7), and abdominal lymph node metastasis in one patient (case 5). Case 11 of group B had cervical lymph node metastasis 16 months after radiotherapy.

Distant Metastasis

Only one patient (case 2) of group A had lung metastasis 47 months after radiotherapy and the other 16 patients had no distant metastasis.

Survival and Cause of Death

Survival and cause of death in all patients are shown in Table 2. Intercurrent death was found in four patients (cases 1, 10, 13, and 16). The other death was caused by cancer, including local recurrence, lymph node metastasis, and distant metastasis.

Discussion

Esophageal cancer is a disease that still has a poor prognosis despite recent medical advances. The disease is advanced in most of patients at the time of initial diagnosis, which is one reason for its poor prognosis. Another reason is that the local tumor has not been easily controlled with ERT alone [5]. In contrast, for patients with an early disease stage, the prognosis of the patients treated with surgery [6] or ERT + HDRIBT [1] is good.

In our previous reports on the treatment of small superficial esophageal carcinoma [3, 4], we recommended HDRIBT alone as the treatment protocol because of the complete response after treatment; however, in this study, longer observation of these patients showed a 50% local recurrence rate (group A). This result suggested that the dosage of 24 Gy in four fractions of HDRIBT was not enough to control the small superficial esophageal carcinoma.

As for lymph node metastasis, about 30% of the patients with small superficial esophageal carcinoma had regional lymph node metastasis in clinicopathological studies [6, 7]. In this study, 62.5% of the patients had lymph node metastasis in group A; and, with one exception, all of the patients in groups B and C had no lymph node metastasis. From the dose distribution of HDRIBT, the rapid dose fall-off is found, and this is the reason for the high rate of regional lymph node metastasis observed after HDRIBT alone because of the lower dose for controlling lymph node metastasis. However, ERT was very effective for occult lymph node metastasis in groups B and C.

From the results of this study, patients with small superficial esophageal carcinoma should be treated with ERT + HDRIBT or HDRIBT + ERT. However, longer observation is necessary to determine which protocol will yield superior results; HDRIBT alone is indicated for the patients with serious systemic disease due to the increased difficulty of performing of ERT under such conditions.

References

1. Hishikawa Y, Tanaka S, Miura T (1985) Early esophageal carcinoma treate with intracavitary irradiation. Radiology 156:519–522
2. Hishikawa Y, Kamikonya N, Tanaka S, Miura T (1987) Radiotherapy of esophageal carcinoma: Role of high-dose-rate intracavitary irradiation. Radiother Oncol 9:13–20
3. Hishikawa Y, Kurisu K, Taniguchi M, Kamikonya N, Miura T (1989) Small, superficial esophageal carcinoma treated with high-dose-rate intracavitary irradiation only. Radiology 172:267–270
4. Hishikawa Y, Kurisu K, Taniguchi M, Kamikonya N, Miura T (1991) High-dose-rate intraluminal brachytherapy (HDRIBT) for esophageal cancer. Int J Radiat Oncol Biol Phys 21:1133–1135
5. Parker EF, Gregorie HB (1976) Carcinoma of the esophagus: Long-term results. JAMA 235:1018–1020
6. Sugimachi K, Ohno S, Matsuda H, Mori M, Kuwano H, Ide H (1989) Clinicopathologic study of early stage esophageal carcinoma. Surgery 105:706–710
7. Yoshinaka H, Shimazu H, Fukumoto T, Baba M (1991) Superficial esophageal carcinoma: A clinicopathological review of 59 cases. Am J Gastroenterol 86:1413–1418

High-Dose-Rate Intracavitary Irradiation in the Surgical Treatment of Cancer of the Thoracic Esophagus

SHOHEI OGOSHI, YOSUKE TANAKA, YOSHINOBU OHMORI, TAI-ICHI TOKI, TATSUO TAMIYA[1], YASUHIRO OGAWA, and TOMOHO MAEDA[2]

Introduction

Thoracic esophageal cancer upon diagnosis is frequently found to be already advanced and also to have metastasized to the lymph nodes even in the early stages. Current surgical treatment operatively excises lymph nodes in three major areas (cervical, thoracic, and abdominal). It is difficult to know whether this operative treatment always contributes to the therapeutic improvement. However, advances in surgery have led to greater understanding about the ease with which esophageal cancer metastasizes to the lymph nodes. Accordingly, extensive dissection is not very effective particularly for advanced cancer. We feel that a new approach is needed to improve therapeutic results for the treatment of advanced esophageal cancer.

In gynecology, high-dose-rate intracavitary irradiation (remote-controlled after-loading system, RALS), when used with surgery, has presented good results, particularly for cancer of the uterine cervix. This fact has led us to employ intracavitary irradiation therapy combined with surgery for the treatment of squamous cell carcinoma of the esophagus because of the histological similarities to cancer of the uterine cervix. Although the number of clinical cases receiving this treatment to date and follow-up observation period for these cases have been limited, all patients, regardless of having been resected or not (bypass), have become able to continue oral feeding while receiving long-term irradiation. There were no deaths due to the operation or during hospitalization and the patients were all eventually discharged from hospital. Based on these results, it is viewed that this combined therapy will be a new strategy to the treatment of esophageal cancer.

[1] The Second Department of Surgery and [2] Department of Radiology, Kochi Medical School, Nankoku, Kochi, 783 Japan

Patients and Methods

Patients and Operation

Twenty-three patients with thoracic esophageal cancer and confirmed with squamous cell cancer received this radiotherapy postoperatively. The patients were divided into two groups: those who underwent total resection of the thoracic esophagus (15 patients) and those who were not resected (8 patients). The nonresected (bypass) cases included patients whose lesion was not radically resectable, patients preoperatively diagnosed as having extensive metastasis to the lymph nodes in the abdomen, and patients diagnosed as unable to receive resection due to their general condition, such as cardiac or pulmonary complications.

Esophageal Reconstruction

Esophageal substitute of the patients, both for resected and bypass cases, were performed with a thin (3-cm width) gastric tube along the greater curvature of the stomach using the linear stapler (GIA or Proximate-PLC 50) by our original method [1, 2]. In both resected and bypass cases, as a rule, the anastomosis was performed by hand in end-to-end fashion through the retrosternal route. After anastomosis, a decompression tube was inserted nasogastrically and total parenteral nutrition was initiated for postoperative nutrition.

Excision of Lymph Nodes

In the thorax, paraesophageal lymph nodes alone were excised following the total resection of the thoracic esophagus, while lymph nodes around the superior mediastinum, trachea and tracheal tree were left intact. Regarding dissection of abdominal lymph nodes, the dissection of the paracardial lymph nodes associated with gastric tube construction was performed in both resected and non-resectted cases, but it was not extended beyond these lymph nodes. As for cervical region, only lymph nodes on the left side involving gastric tube construction were excised leaving those on the right side intact.

Intubation of Tube for Intracavitary Irradiation

After thoracic esophagectomy in the resected cases, the tube was inserted from a small skin incision on the left abdomen in the same manner as a drain. The tip of the tube was led from the esophageal hiatus through the esophageal bed, reaching the suprasternal notch. The tube is made of silicon having an inner diameter of 10 mm. To guarantee asepsis, the end of the tube was closed in duplicate using surgical wire. For non-resectable cases, a tube with the same inner diameter as the one used in the resected cases was also used; however, the end of the tube was kept open because asepsis is not necessary with this procedure. After the retrosternal bypass operation using isoperistaltic thin gastric tube along the greater curvature, the abdominal esophagus and the jejunum were anamotosized in loop- ρY fashion, and jejunostomy was performed on the oral jejunum loop fixed on the left abdominal wall. The tube was led from the

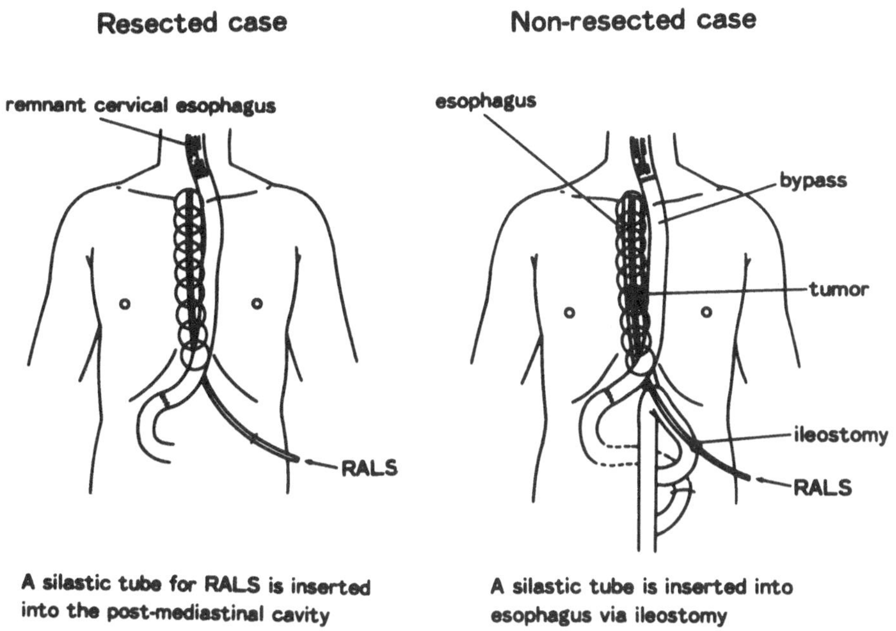

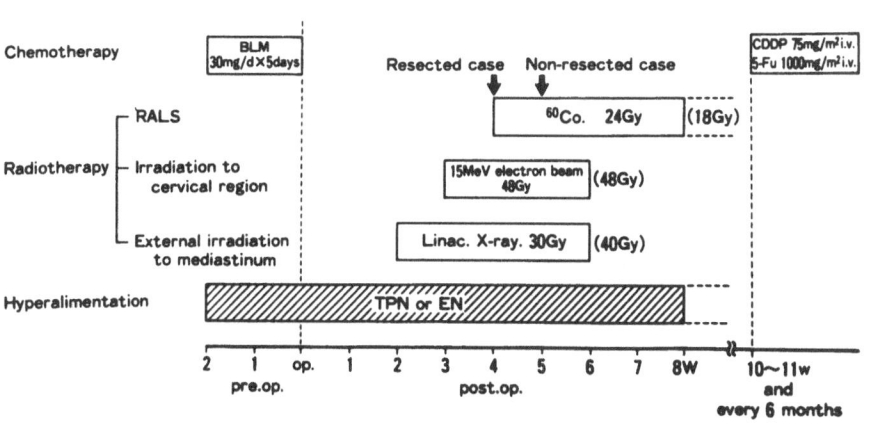

Fig. 1. Reconstruction and intubation for remote-controlled after-loading system (*RALS*)

Fig. 2. Multidisciplinary treatment by KOCHI system to esophageal cancer. *BLM*, bleomycin, *CDDP*, cisplatin; *5-Fu*, 5-fluorouracil

jejunostomy through the unresected esophageal cavity until it reached the stump of the cervical esophagus. In the event that stenosis due to a tumor prevented tube insertion, the tube should be inserted halfway first and then introduced to the upper thoracic esophagus upon intracavitary dilatation by external radiation (Fig. 1.).

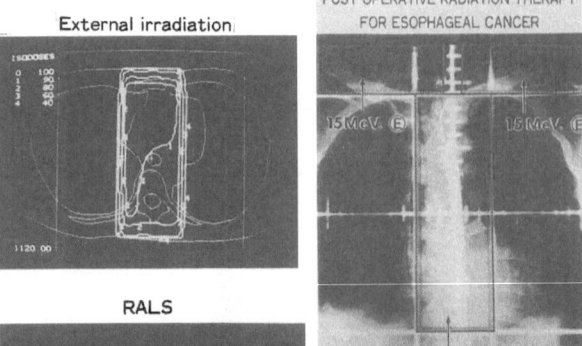

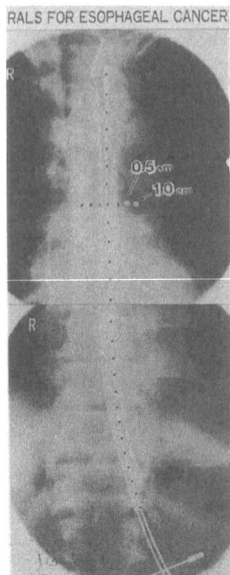

Fig. 3. Dose distribution

Pre- and Postoperative Adjuvant Therapy

Perioperative radiotherapy and chemotherapy, our standardized KOCHI system, are shown in Fig. 2. This method was rescheduled depending on the patient's condition, particularly upon change in the leucocyte count. After confirming by postoperative x-ray that there was no postoperative anastomotic leak, the external irradiation of the local area by linac x-ray and of the cervical area by linac electron ray was initiated after the patients resumed oral feeding, followed by intracavitary irradiation with ^{60}Co. Intracavitary radiation was performed from the suprasternal notch to the esophagel hiatus through the esophageal bed with a distance of 1 cm and a 3-cm width. Biological effective dose was 30–40 Gy (Fig. 3). The external irradiation dose to the cervical and local area was 48 Gy, and 30 Gy or 40 Gy, respectively (Fig. 3).

Results

This report presents the clinical results of patients who were treated at our institution during a 2-year period starting from January 1990. The results for the 15 resected patients are summarized in Table 1, while the results for the 8 non-resected patients are summarized in Table 2. When external and intracavitary irradiation were started, all the patients became capable of oral intake approximately 10 days after the operation. In non-resected patients having persistent stenosis due to carcinoma lesion, external irradiation was first chosen to clear

Table 1. Resected cases (patients who underwent esophagectomy)

Case No.	Age	Sex	Location	Length (cm)	Stage[a]	Reconstruction	Chemotherapy	Prognosis
1	60	M	Im	2	I	Gastric tube	CDDP 100 mg 5-FU 4000 mg	Alive (1 y 11 m)
2	63	M	Iu-Im	8	IIA	Gastric tube	CDDP 100 mg 5-FU 4000 mg	Alive (1 y 9 m)
3	52	F	Im	6	IIB	Gastric tube	CDDP 100 mg	Alive (1 y 7 m)
4	79	M	Im	2	0	Gastric tube	None	1 y
5	69	M	Im-Ei	4	I	Gastric tube	CDDP 75 mg 5-FU 4000 mg	Alive (1 y 5 m)
6	65	M	Im	4	I	Gastric tube	CDDP 100 mg 5-FU 4000 mg	Alive (1 y 5 m)
7	63	M	Im-Ei	7	IV	Gastric tube	CDDP 100 mg 5-FU 4000 mg	10 m
8	72	M	Im	4	IIA	Gastric tube	None	Alive (1 y 4 m)
9	54	M	Ei	3	IIA	Gastric tube	CDDP 75 mg 5-FU 4000 mg	Alive (1 y 2 m)
10	50	F	Im	7	IIA	Gastric tube	CDDP 75 mg 5-FU 4000 mg	Alive (1 y 1 m)
11	51	F	Im	3	IIA	Colon	None	Alive (9 m)
12	67	M	Im	4	IV	Gastric tube	CDDP 100 mg 5-FU 4000 mg	Alive (8 m)
13	59	M	Iu	4	I	Gastric tube	None	Alive (2 m)
14	64	M	Ei	3	I	Colon	None	Alive (2 m)
15	56	M	Ei	3	III	Gastric tube	None	Alive (1 m)

[a] Clinical stage based on TNM classification, UICC, 1987 [9]   1990.1–1991.12
CDDP, cisplatin; *5-FU*, 5-fluorouracil; *y*, years; *m*, months; *Im*, middle thoracic esophagus; *Iu*, upper intrathoracic esophagus; *Ei*, lower intrathoracic esophagus

the stenosis, and the intracavitary irradiation was initiated via the inserted tube. As a rule, postoperative chemotherapy was given with reference to leucocyte counts, and all the patients who could complete it. All resected and bypass patients were discharged from the hospital in good condition. In bypass patients, the unresected tumor can be checked by x-ray or endoscopy retrogradely via jejunum fistula inserted with the radiation tube. Other patients are presently being kept on the treatment, and all are having oral intake and anticipated to leave the hospital soon. No deaths occurred during the study while the patients were in hospital. Figure 4 shows the typical findings before and after treatment in bypass patients. Stenosis caused by the tumor mass can be observed in the middle of the esophagus before treatment. Endoscopy revealed a narrow lumen obstructed by the tumor mass. One year after treatment the esophageal wall was completely constricted but the tumor mass had disappeared. No tumor mass and obstruction were observed by endoscopy and cancer cells were not found in the biopsy specimen taken after treatment.

The 1-year survival rate of the patients undergoing radical resection and treated by RALS according to the KOCHI system was 90%, while the 2-year rate is 80% (Fig. 5). They are still receiving chemotherapy every 6 months.

Table 2. Non-resected cases (patients who underwent bypass operation)

Case No.	Age	Sex	Location	Length (cm)	Stage[a]	Operation	Chemotherapy	Prognosis
1	68	M	Im	8	III	Bypass · gastrostomy	CDDP 100 mg 5-FU 4000 mg	1 y 7 m
2	45	M	Ei	7	III	Bypass · gastrostomy	CDDP 120 mg 5-FU 6400 mg	1 y 2 m
3	54	M	Im-Ei	11	III	Bypass · ileostomy	CDDP 100 mg 5-FU 4000 mg	Alive (1 y 5 m)
4	70	F	Im	5	II	Total gastrostomy · ileostomy	None	Alive (1 y 4 m)
5	62	M	Im-Ei	9	III	Bypass · ileostomy	CDDP 100 mg 5-FU 4000 mg	11 m
6	63	M	Im-Ea	9	III	Bypass · ileostomy	CDDP 100 mg 5-FU 4000 mg	Alive (9 m)
7	72	M	Im-Ea	9	III	Bypass · ileostomy	CDDP 100 mg 5-FU 4000 mg	Alive (8 m)
8	60	M	Im	10	III	Bypass · ileostomy	CDDP 100 mg 5-FU 4000 mg	Alive (5 m)

[a] Clinical stage based on TNM classification, UICC, 1978 [9] 1990.1–1991.12
Ea, abdominal esophagus

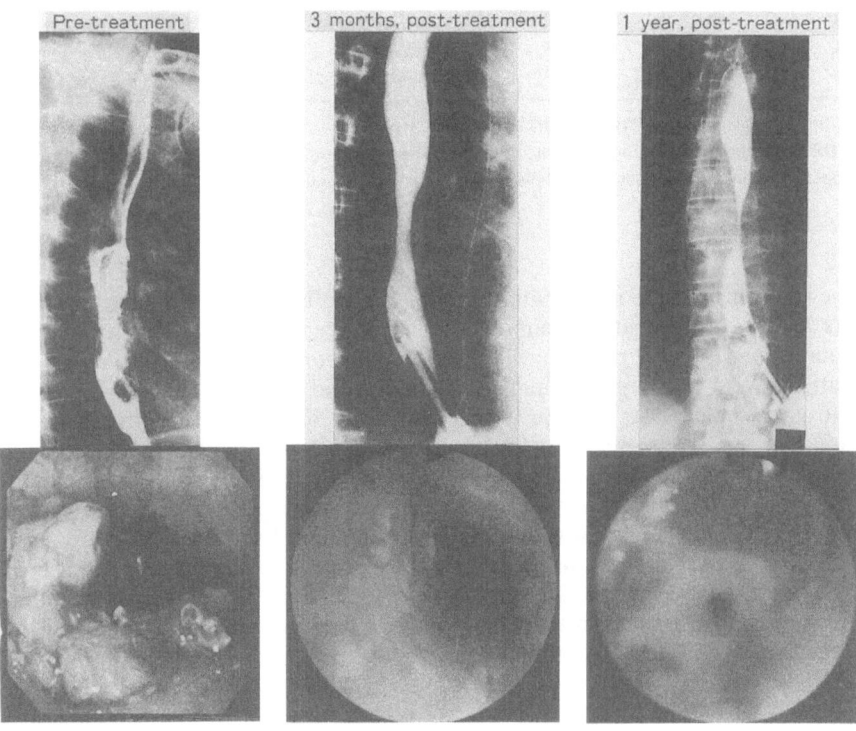

Fig. 4. Radiologic and Endoscopic Findings

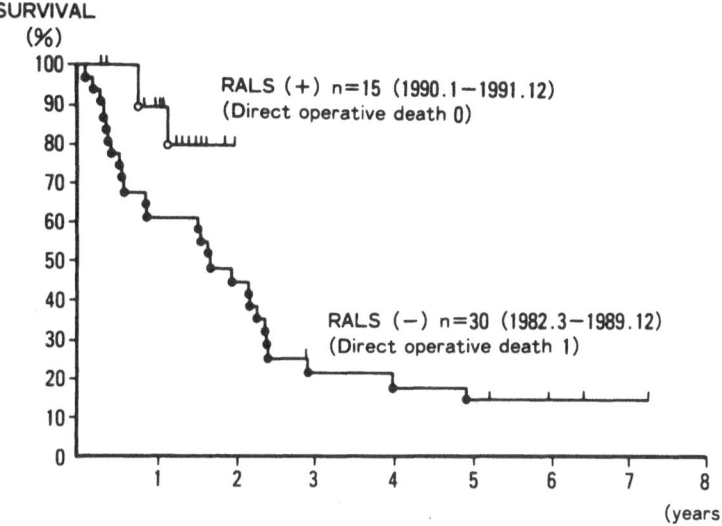

Fig. 5. Survival rates after esophagectomy with and without RALS (Kaplan-Meier method)

to adjuvant therapy, the irradiation was performed with reference to patient condition at appropriate intervals. Four patients received granulocyte colony stimulating factor (G-CSF) to keep leucocyte counts within normal range.

Discussion

Even today, most cases of esophageal cancer are first identified in the later stages of development. Furthermore, even when a local tumor is in an early stage, it tends to quickly metastasize to the lymph nodes. The metastasis rate reported in Japan is over 50% for a mm-depth tumor and over 70% for a sm-depth tumor [3]. In this regard, it is always essential to be prepared to treat the patients from the viewpoint of advanced cancer. In addition, as compared to other gastrointestinal cancers, surgical invasion becomes extensive in esophageal cancer, and the patients are generally elderly. Thus, the rate of operative or in-hospital mortality is relatively high.

High-dose-rate RALS has been long used in gynecology, in combination with surgery, to successfully treat cancer of the uterine cervix. Such irradiation therapy has led us to try intracavitary irradiation for the treatment of esophageal cancer [4, 5]. In radiology, low-dose-rate intracavitary irradiation and local irradiation on advanced cancer via the tube inserted from the mouth have been attempted with good results [6, 7]. Leichman et al. reported a 1-year survival rate of 80% when radiotherapy and chemotherapy were combined [8]. However, the combination of high-dose-rate intracavitary irradiation and esophagectomy or bypass surgery applied to the entire posterior mediastinum area for the resected case and to the entire unresected esophagus for the non-resected case has not been reported anywhere.

The practice of combining irradiation and chemotherapy (KOCHI system), was based on our clinical experience as well as on other reports. In spite of the campaign for early medical check-ups, it is still very common to see the diseases diagnosed when they are in an advanced stage upon patient admission to the hospital. In such cases of esophageal cancer, extensive excision of the lymph nodes becomes therapeutically less significant, and even in the event that an extended excision could be performed, there is a therapeutic limit. In other words, it could be that lymphatic vessels are merely destroyed. In fact, there are many cases of local recurrence probably due to surgical dissemination. It is now generally recognized that an increase of resection rate does not necessarily reflect an increase in therapeutic improvement in any type of advanced cancer.

In contrast to gastric cancer, true en bloc resection including lymph nodes is not possible because the serosa is not present in the esophagus and the lesion has proceeded to neighboring structures. Extreme excision of the opposite side of the thoracic cavity is not possible. This appears to be the reason for the poor therapeutic outcome. In our methods, external and intracavitary irradiation are to be performed on the remaining tissue of the esophagus bed, and electron irradiation is for cervical lymph nodes. Abdominal paracardial lymph nodes, which have the highest rate of metastasis, are surgically excised. However, more clinical data and longer observation periods are needed before it can be determined whether this combination therapy can replace the conventional surgically-oriented extensive excision.

References

1. Ogoshi S, Ohmori Y, Tamiya T, Yonezawa T (1985) Preparation of isoperistaltic tube along the greater curvature with GIA instrument and its esophageal reconstruction (in Japanese). Operation 39:1409–1415
2. Ogoshi S, Tamiya T (1992) Esophageal substitute with a thin gastric tube along the greater curvature (in Japanese). Gastroenterol Surg 15:1549–1559
3. Isono K (ed) (1990) Survey report of the 44th annual meeting of the Japanese Society for the Diseases of the Esophagus (in Japanese). Chiba, Japan, 6, 1990
4. Hishikawa Y, Tanaka S, Miura T (1985) Early esophageal carcinoma treated with intracavitary irradiation. Radiology 156:519–522
5. Hyden EC, Langholz B, Tilden T, Lam K, Luxton G, Astrahan M, Jepson J, Petrovic Z (1988) External beam and intraluminal radiotherapy in the treatment of carcinoma of the esophagus. J Thorac Cardiovasc Surg 96:237–241
6. Hishikawa Y, Kamikonya N, Tanaka S, Miura T (1987) Radiotherapy of esophageal carcinoma: role of high-dose-rate intracavitary irradiation. Radiother Oncol 9:13–20
7. Hishikawa Y, Kurisu K, Taniguchi M, Kamikonya N, Miura T (1991) High-dose-rate intraluminal brachytherapy (HDRIBT) for esophageal cancer. Int J Radiat Oncol Biol Phys 21:1133–1135
8. Leichman L, Herskovic A, Leichman CG, Lattin P, Steiger Z, Taparzoglou E, Rosenberg JC, Asfaw I, Kinzie J (1987) Nonoperative therapy for squamous cell cancer of the esophagus. J Clin Oncol 5:365–370
9. UICC edited by Hermanek P and Sobin LH (1978) TNM classification of malignant tumors, 4th edn. Springer-Verlag Berlin Heidelberg, 1987

Resectable Esophageal Carcinoma: Preoperative Versus Postoperative Radiochemotherapy

Hiroshi Matsuura, Kenji Suzuki, Tsukasa Kotoh, Hiroshi Yoshimura, Shunichi Abe, and Teruhisa Nakamura[1]

Introduction

It is generally accepted that chemotherapy and radiotherapy for esophageal carcinoma provide significant palliation, and multiple modality therapy has become the common trend during the past two decades [1, 2]. Surgery continues to be the cornerstone of treatment, and most protocols consist of surgical therapy combined with these adjuvant therapies. Preoperative radiation therapy was introduced in the 1960s and is still in use with promising results [3, 4]. However, there are several reports indicating that preoperative therapy neither improves the resectability nor the survival rate of patients who undergo resection [5, 6].

One concern is whether these therapies should be given preoperatively or after surgery. The aim of this study is to clarify the relative merits of "initial" management of patients suffering from esophageal carcinoma through a controlled, prospective, and randomized study. We report herein the effects on survival rate and the morbidity and mortality associated with preoperative and/or postoperative therapy for resectable esophageal carcinoma.

Patients and Methods

From 1988 to 1991, 56 patients with esophageal carcinoma were admitted to our institution, and 40 of these patients were enrolled in this study. (Criteria for enrollment are outlined below.) These patients were divided into two groups (group A and group B) in a prospective randomized fashion. In group A, the first cycle of radiochemotherapy was given 3 weeks before and the second 4–5 weeks after operation. In group B, both cycles were carried out postoperatively

[1] Department of Surgery II, Shimane Medical University, Ehya-cho 89-1 Izumo, Shimane, 693 Japan

at 4 weeks interval. Regimen of each cycle of radiochemotherapy consisted of: (1) irradiation with a total of 30.6 Gy in 17 installments, (2) cisplatin ($50 \, mg/m^2$ IV on days 1 and 15), and (3) 5-FU ($400 \, mg/m^2$/day as a continuous IV infusion on days 1 through 28).

Patients with resectable squamous cell carcinoma of the thoracic esophagus with adequate bone marrow (leukocyte count more than $4000/mm^3$, platelet count more than $100,000/mm^3$), renal (creatinine clearance more than 60 ml/min) and hepatic (serum glutamic oxaloacetic transaminase and serum glutamic pyruvic transaminase levels less than 100 IU) functions were chosen for this study. Furthermore, patients having serious cardiac, renal, or pulmonary complications were excluded. Pathologic diagnosis and classification of the cases were performed according to the rules established by the Japanese Society of Esophageal Diseases [7].

Table 1. Clinicopathologic characteristics

Variables	Group A (n = 19)	Group B (n = 20)	P Value
Sex			
Male	18	19	NS
Female	1	1	
Age (years)	64.7 ± 6.7	63.8 ± 7.5	NS
Location of tumor			
Upper	2	4	NS
Middle	14	10	
Lower	3	6	
Length of tumor	7.5 ± 2.3	6.5 ± 2.9	NS
Depth of penetration			
Submucosa	3	3	
Proper muscle	2	3	
Invasion into adventitia	7	7	
Invasion into the neighboring structures	7	8	
Lymph node metastasis			
Negative	10	4	<0.05
Positive	9	16	
Histologic stage			
0–2	6	0	NS
3	4	8	
4	9	12	
Histologic type			
Well	5	6	NS
Moderately	10	12	
Poorly	2	2	
Unknown	2	0	
Esophagectomy			
Subtotal	18	20	NS
Distal	1	0	

NS, not significant

Data were analyzed using the chi-square test and Student's t-test. Survival curves were calculated by the method of Kaplan-Meier. Comparisons were done by the generalized Wilcoxon test. A P value of less than 0.05 was considered to be statistically significant.

Results

Among the 40 patients entered into this study, 20 were in group A, and 20 in group B. Out of 20 patients in group A, 1 was excluded because of the patient's refusal to undergo the operation after preoperative therapy. Clinicopathologic details of the two groups are given in Table 1. There were no significant differences between the two groups with regard to age, sex, location of the tumor, histologic type, or depth of penetration. However, lymph node metastasis was more frequent in group A than in group B ($P < 0.05$), and relatively earlier stage of carcinomas were slightly higher in group A than group B. Except for one patient in group A, all the operations were carried out in one stage: Subtotal esophagectomy and reconstruction using gastric tube was done in all but one patient who received a distal esophagectomy with reconstruction by jejunal interposition.

Table 2. Postoperative morbidity

	Group A (n = 19)	Group B (n = 20)
Lung (%)	4 (21.1)	6 (30.0)
Pneumonia	4	5
Atelectasis	0	2
Thorax (%)	4 (21.1)	9 (45.0)
Pyothorax	1	2
Effusion	2	4
Pneumothorax	1	1
Bleeding	0	1
Mediastinal abscess	0	1
Leakage (%)	4 (21.1)	2 (10.0)
Major	1	2[a]
Minor	3	0
Recurrent nerve palsy (%)	5 (26.3)	5 (25.0)
Intercostal neuralgia	1	1
Supraventricular tachycardia	1	1
Intra-abdominal abscess	1	1
DIC	1[b]	0
Cholestasis	1	0
Herpes zoster	1	0
Delilium	0	3
Ileus	0	1

DIC, disseminated intravascular coagulation
[a] One of two died within 30 days
[b] Died within 30 days

Fourteen patients (74%) in group A completed the treatment regimen as planned, and the postoperative portion of the regimen could not be completed in 5 (26%) because of postoperative complications ($n = 2$), early stage ($n = 2$), and toxity ($n = 1$). On the other hand, in group B, 11 patients (55%) completed the planned regimen, and 7 (35%) had one cycle of radiochemotherapy because of: postoperative complications ($n = 1$), toxicity ($n = 4$), and patient's refusal ($n = 2$). In the other 2 patients in group B, no radiochemotherapy could be given due to postoperative complications.

Toxicity of radiochemotherapy occurred in five (26%) patients in group A and seven (35%) in group B. In group A, three patients had renal insufficiency (creatinine clearance less than 60 ml/min), in one leukopenia (less than 2000/mm³), and in one severe nausea and vomiting. In group B, two patients had renal insufficiency, in two leukopenia, in one nausea and vomiting, and one had abdominal pain and diarrhea.

The operating time was 388 ± 54 min in group A and 359 ± 57 min in group B, and the blood loss was 1057 ± 684 g in group A and 838 ± 715 g in group B. There was no significant difference between the two groups with regard to these operating factors.

The postoperative mortality and morbidity are listed in Table 2. One postoperative death was encountered in each group. There was no significant difference between the two groups with regard to pulmonary complications and anastomotic leakage.

The survival curves of groups A and B are shown in Figure 1. Three-year survival rates were 32.7% and 40.4% in groups A and B, respectively, and the difference between the two curves was not statistically significant. Total hospital

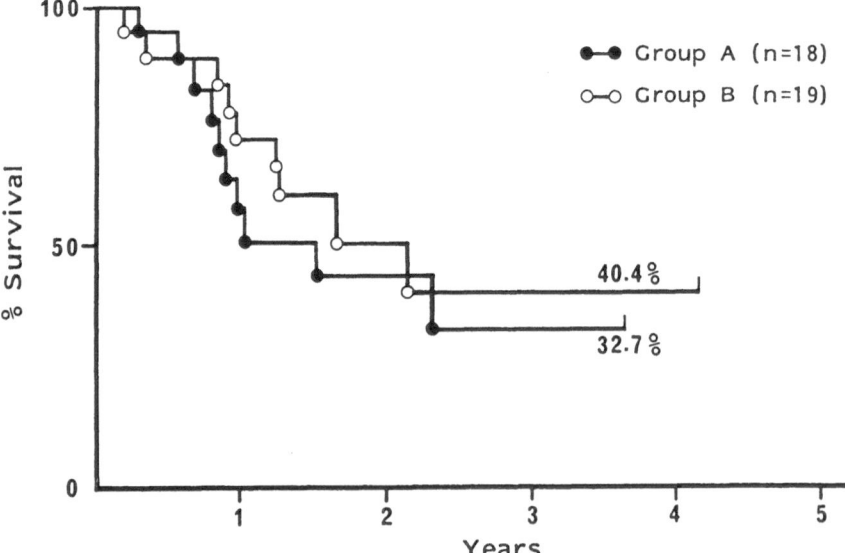

Fig. 1. Postoperative survival rates of the two groups. There were no statistically significant differences between the two groups. Operative deaths were excluded from these survival curves

stay was 152.7 ± 81.1 days in group A, and 92.5 ± 32.7 days in group B, a significant difference ($P < 0.01$). Moreover, the duration from diagnosis of the esophageal carcinoma to the operation was 62.3 ± 9.6 days in group A, which was obviously longer than that of 17.1 ± 5.9 days in group B.

Discussion and Conclusions

The use of preoperative chemoradiotherapy for the treatment of esophageal carcinoma has the theoretical advantage of improving local control. Preoperative irradiation often reduces the size of the primary tumor, local invasion, and metastatic lesions making the resection more feasible and easier. Moreover, irradiation decreases the possibility of dissemination of cancer cells by manipulation at operation [4]. It seems that the lower incidence of lymph node metastasis in the preoperative group in this study could be the therapeutic effects of the radiochemotherapy.

On the contrary, preoperative treatment has produced marked immunosuppression in patients with esophageal carcinoma [8], and this disturbed immune function prior to the operation may contribute to the increased incidence of postoperative complications and the risk of dissemination of cancer cells. However, in this study, preoperative radiochemotherapy did not adversely affect surgical morbidity and mortality.

Iizuka et al. [6] reported that preoperative radiotherapy reduced survival significantly compared to the group without it. The EORTC group [5] reported no improvement of survival rate by preoperative therapy, and our results were in accordance with this report. The other factor to be considered is the substantially prolonged hospitalization in group A, which was clearly demonstrated in this study. Although long-term follow-up data remained unavailable and the number of patients were insufficient because of the recent implementation this protocol, postoperative therapy alone seemed to be more feasible than a combination with preoperative therapy for resectable esophageal carcinoma.

Acknowledgment. We wish to thank Dr. Dhar Dipok Kumar for his comments on this manuscript.

References

1. Stewart FM, Harkins BJ, Hahn SS, Daniel TM (1989) Cisplatin, 5-Fluorouracil, Mitomycin C, and concurrent radiation therapy with and without esophagectomy for esophageal carcinoma. Cancer 64:622–628
2. Kelsen D (1982) Treatment of advanced esophageal cancer. Cancer 50:2576–2581
3. Clifton EE, Goodner JT, Bronstein EL (1960) Preoperative irradiation for cancer of the esophagus. Cancer 13:37–45
4. Sugimachi K, Matsufuji H, Kai H, Matsuda H, Ueo H, Inokuchi K (1986) Preoperative irradiation for carcinoma of the esophagus. Surg Gynecol Obstet 162:174–176
5. Eortc (1985) Preoperative radiotherapy for carcinoma of the esophagus: Results of a prospective multicenter study. In: DeMeester TR, Skinner DB (eds) Esophageal disorders: Pathophysiology and therapy. Raven, New York, pp 367–371

6. Iizuka T, Ide H, Kakegawa T, Sasaki K, Takagi I, Ando N, Mori S, Arimori M, Tsugane S (1988) Preoperative radioactive therapy for esophageal carcinoma. Randomized evaluation trial in eight institutions. Chest 93:1054–1058
7. Japanese Society of Esophageal Diseases (1976) Guidelines for the clinical and pathological studies on carcinoma of the esophagus. Jpn J Surg 6:1–39
8. Tsutsui S, Morita M, Kuwano H, Matsuda H, Mori M, Okamura S, Sugimachi K (1992) Influence of preoperative treatment and surgical operation on immune function of patients with esophageal carcinoma. J Surg Oncol 49:176–181

Postoperative Irradiation for Esophageal Carcinoma

Shogo Yamada, Yoshihiro Takai, Kenji Nemoto, Yoshihisa Kakuto, Yoshihiro Ogawa, Akihiko Hoshi, Kiyohiko Sakamoto[1], Tetsuro Nishihira, and Shozo Mori[2]

Introduction

Postoperative irradiation for curative resection of esophageal carcinoma has been used in order to eradicate micro-dissemination and micro-metastases. Generally, a long T-shaped field is employed for postoperative irradiation, and the risk of radiation myelopathy increases even at low doses when the irradiated volume of the spinal cord enlarges. Some questions arise about the postoperative irradiation: First, whether its effectiveness outweighs the risk; second, for which patients it is indispensable; third, what is the optimal dose of irradiation; fourth, whether combined chemotherapy improves the prognosis; and fifth, what the actual incidence of radiation myelopathy is. We analyzed data compiled over the last decade.

Materials and Methods

During the period from 1980 through 1989, 179 esophageal carcinomas were curatively resected and underwent postoperative irradiation of more than 30 Gy at the Department of Radiology, Tohoku University School of Medicine. There were 151 males and 28 females, and the average age of these patients was 60.3 ± 7.7 (34–84) years. Histopathologically, 168 tumors were diagnosed as squamous cell carcinoma, 7 as undifferentiated carcinoma, 3 as adenocarcinoma, and 1 as adenosquamous cell carcinoma. Twenty-four tumors were located at the cervical esophagus, 22 at the upper thoracic portion, 88 at the mid-thoracic portion and 45 at the lower thoracic portion. According to the American Joint Committee on Cancer (AJCC) classification, 21 patients were classified into stage I, 54 stage IIA, 21 stage IIB, and 83 stage III. Eighty patients had no lymph node metastasis at the time of surgical treatment, and 99 had some lymph node metastases.

[1] Department of Radiology, [2] Second Department of Surgery, Tohoku University School of Medicine, Seiryomachi 1-1, Aoba-ku, Sendai, 980 Japan

Table 1. Patients' characteristics and details of treatment by
tumor staging

	Stage				Total
	I	IIA	IIB	III	
Sex					
Male	19	42	20	70	151
Female	2	12	1	13	28
Age (years)					
30–39	0	0	1	2	3
40–49	1	3	0	5	9
50–59	6	19	10	30	65
60–69	10	26	8	38	82
70–79	4	6	2	8	20
Mean (years)	62.2	60.5	59.4	60.0	60.3
Radiation dose (Gy)					
30–39	1	6	0	7	14
40–49	12	28	19	61	120
50–59	8	20	2	12	42
60–69	0	0	0	3	3
Mean (Gy)	43.6	43.1	41.5	41.9	42.4
Chemotherapy					
None	12	27	5	24	68
FT or mild	3	11	4	11	29
BLM or PLM	3	10	9	35	57
CDDP + VDS	3	6	3	12	24
ADR + MMC	0	0	0	1	1
Total	21	54	21	83	179

FT, futraful; *BLM*, bleomycin; *PLM*, peplomycin; *CDDP +
VDS*, cisplatin + vindesine; *ADR + MMC*, adriamycin +
mitomycin C

Anterior-posterior parallel opposed field was used for postoperative irradiation with 10 MV photons. A total dose of 30–60 Gy was delivered at 2 Gy per
fraction with a T-shaped field including the bilateral supraclavicular region and
the whole mediastinum. Different chemotherapeutic agents were combined with
postoperative irradiation. Details of patients' characteristics and treatment are
shown in Table 1.

The Kaplan-Meier method was utilized for the calculation of survival rates
from the beginning of irradiation and a statistical comparison of survival rates
was performed with Log rank test and generalized Wilcoxon test. Multivariate
analysis for survival time, using Cox's proportional hazard mode [1] was carried
out to evaluate prognostic factors.

Results

Relapse

Table 2 shows relapsed sites. Relapse was observed in 30% of all patients, and
the frequency of inner field recurrence was the highest. The incidence of lung

Table 2. Relapsed sites

	Inner field	Lung	Abdomen	Others	None	Unknown
Tumor location						
Cervical	5 (24%)	0 (0%)	0 (0%)	1 (5%)	15 (71%)	3
Upper	2 (10%)	4 (20%)	0 (0%)	2 (10%)	12 (60%)	2
Middle	14 (18%)	6 (8%)	3 (4%)	0 (0%)	54 (70%)	11
Lower	4 (10%)	2 (5%)	4 (10%)	0 (0%)	30 (75%)	5
Stage						
I	1 (5%)	3 (14%)	0 (0%)	0 (0%)	17 (81%)	0
IIA	7 (14%)	1 (2%)	0 (0%)	0 (0%)	43 (84%)	3
IIB	2 (11%)	1 (6%)	2 (11%)	1 (6%)	12 (67%)	3
III	15 (22%)	7 (10%)	5 (7%)	2 (3%)	39 (57%)	15
Lymph node metastasis						
Negative	9 (12%)	4 (5%)	1 (1%)	0 (0%)	63 (82%)	3
Positive	16 (20%)	8 (10%)	6 (7%)	3 (4%)	48 (59%)	18
Radiation dose (Gy)						
30–39	3 (25%)	1 (8%)	0 (0%)	0 (0%)	8 (67%)	2
40–49	16 (15%)	7 (6%)	6 (6%)	3 (3%)	76 (70%)	12
50–59	6 (17%)	3 (8%)	1 (3%)	0 (0%)	26 (72%)	6
60–69	0 (0%)	1 (50%)	0 (0%)	0 (0%)	1 (50%)	1
Chemotherapy						
None	10 (17%)	7 (12%)	0 (0%)	0 (0%)	43 (72%)	8
FT, mild	2 (9%)	0 (0%)	1 (4%)	1 (4%)	19 (83%)	6
BLM, PLM	11 (21%)	3 (6%)	6 (11%)	1 (2%)	32 (60%)	4
CDDP + VDS	2 (10%)	1 (5%)	0 (0%)	1 (10%)	17 (81%)	3
ADR + MMC	0 (0%)	1 (100%)	0 (0%)	0 (0%)	0 (0%)	0
Total	25 (16%)	12 (8%)	7 (4%)	3 (2%)	111 (70%)	21

Upper, upper thoracic portion; *middle*, middle thoracic portion; *lower*, lower thoracic portion

metastasis was higher in patients with primary tumor at upper or middle thoracic portion, and that of abdominal metastasis was higher in patients with tumor at the middle or lower thoracic portion. The relapse rate of stage III patients was significantly worse than that of the other stages ($P < 0.01$). Although there was no significant difference, inner field recurrence was more frequent in patients with irradiation doses of 30–39 Gy. There was no difference in relapse pattern between the 40–49 Gy group and the 50–59 Gy group. Bleomycin (BLM) or Peplomycin (PLM) group had a higher relapse rate than the other chemotherapy groups, but the difference was not significant.

Survival Rate

Survival rates by various categories are shown in Table 3. There was no difference in survival rates of male and female patients. The survival of younger patients was significantly higher than that of older ones ($P < 0.05$), despite the fact that there was no relationship between age and tumor staging (Table 1). Stage IIA patients had much better survival rates than those in stage III ($P <$

Table 3. Survival rates by various categories

	No. of cases	Survival rate (%)				
		1-year	2-year	3-year	4-year	5-year
All cases	179	79.9	64.2	56.1	49.9	43.3
Sex						
Male	151	80.1	64.9	57.4	49.8	41.8
Female	28	78.6	60.7	49.5	49.5	49.5
Age (years)						
−49	12	100.0	100.0	82.5	82.5	68.7
50−59	65	80.0	64.6	60.0	58.2	54.0
60−69	82	80.5	63.4	53.2	42.3	32.8
70−	20	65.0	45.0	40.0	32.0	32.0
Stage						
I	21	85.7	81.0	81.0	74.2	64.9
IIA	54	85.2	79.6	77.7	67.2	57.8
IIB	21	76.2	66.7	56.7	50.4	28.8
III	83	75.9	49.4	35.8	32.8	32.8
Lymph node metastasis						
n0	80	86.2	81.2	79.9	69.3	60.4
n1	99	74.7	50.5	36.9	34.3	29.6
Radiation dose (Gy)						
30−39	14	92.9	71.4	57.1	57.1	57.1
40−49	120	80.0	61.7	53.7	48.0	42.0
50−59	42	78.6	71.4	66.7	56.6	46.3
60−69	3	33.3	33.3	0		
Radiation dose (Gy)						
n0						
40−49	41	85.4	82.9	82.9	72.5	62.4
50−59	32	87.5	78.1	78.1	65.1	55.3
n1						
40−49	79	77.2	50.6	38.6	35.3	31.6
50−59	10	50.0	50.0	30.0	30.0	15.0
Chemotherapy						
None or FT	97	78.4	66.0	59.5	50.4	42.3
BLM or PLM	57	82.5	59.6	49.1	45.6	40.4
CDDP + VDS	24	83.3	70.8	61.9	61.9	(−)
Chemotherapy						
n0						
None or FT	56	83.9	78.6	76.7	64.0	53.8
BLM or PLM	14	92.9	85.7	85.7	78.6	71.4
CDDP + VDS	10	90.0	90.0	90.0	90.0	(−)
n1						
None or FT	41	70.7	48.8	35.7	32.3	26.8
BLM or PLM	43	79.1	51.2	37.2	34.9	30.2
CDDP + VDS	14	78.6	57.1	41.7	41.7	(−)

n0, no lymph node metastasis; n1, lymph node metastasis

Table 4. Multivariate analysis by Cox's proportional hazard model

Variable	Scoring		Score Chi-square	Probability (P) Chi-square
Sex			0.3662	0.5451
	Male	1		
	Female	2		
Age (years)			12.87.2	0.0003
Tumor location			0.1119	0.7380
	Cervical	1		
	Upper	2		
	Middle	3		
	Lower	4		
Stage			12.7357	0.0004
	I	1		
	IIA	2		
	IIB	3		
	III	4		
Lymph node metastasis			17.3807	0.0001
	n0	1		
	n1	2		
Radiation dose (Gy)			1.1471	0.2841
Chemotherapy			0.6620	0.4157
	None or FT	1		
	BLM or PLM	2		
	CDDP + VDS	3		

0.001). Patients without lymph node metastasis at the time of operation had a significantly better prognosis than patients with metastasis ($P < 0.00001$). No advantage was found in survival when radiation dose was increased from 40 to 50 Gy, regardless of whether or not lymph node metastases were present. Although the difference was not significant, patients treated with CDDP + VDS had slightly better survival than the others; this was more notable in patients without lymph node metastases.

Prognostic Factors

Multivariate analysis by Cox's model revealed that the following variables were significantly important prognostic factors: age, stage, and the presence of lymph node metastasis. On the other hand, sex, radiation dose, and combined chemotherapy did not affect survival time (Table 4).

Cause of Death

Of 108 patients who died before this analysis, 74 died due to cancer (4 stage I, 11 stage IIA, 10 stage IIB and 49 stage III), 27 died due to intercurrent disease (6 stage I, 14 stage IIA, 2 stage IIB, 5 stage III), and 2 died due to complications (1 stage IIA, 1 stage III). Most stage IIB and stage III patients died of cancer.

Radiation Myelopathy

Radiation myelopathy was observed in seven patients (3.9%). Six of them (three in the 40–49 Gy group and three in the 50–59 Gy group) complained of sensory disturbance, and one (in the 50 Gy group) had Brown-Sequard syndrome. The incidence of radiation myelopathy was 3% in the 40–49 Gy group and 9% in the 50–59 Gy group, but the difference was not significant.

Discussion

Five-year survival rate of curatively resected and non-irradiated esophageal carcinomas is reported as 11.5%–30% [2–5]. In our data the 5-year survival rate was 43.3%; postoperative irradiation seems to improve survival.

Younger age, lower tumor staging, and the absence of lymph node metastasis were favorable prognostic factors. Younger patients had no specific characteristics regarding stage, radiation dose, and chemotherapy; their residual tumor cells are possibly radiosensitive. Stage IIB, stage III, or patients with lymph node metastasis had a higher occurrence of relapse, lower survival rate, and higher incidence of cancerous death in spite of the postoperative irradiation. The irradiation dose was probably insufficient and the tumor had already spread outside the irradiation field. Post-operative irradiation for these patients seems valueless.

There was no advantage when irradiation dose was increased from 40 Gy to 50 Gy, either in the relapse rate or in the survival rate, and the incidence of radiation myelopathy increased with the dose. We concluded that a total dose of 40 Gy is sufficient for postoperative irradiation using T-shaped large field.

References

1. Cox DR (1972) Regression models and life tables. J Royal Stat Soc Series B 34:187–220
2. Launois B, Delarue D, Campion JP, Kerbaol M (1981) Preoperative radiotherapy for carcinoma of the esophagus. Surg Gynecol Obst 153:690–692
3. Sugimachi K, Kitamura M, Inokuchi K, Ohsato K, Yoshimatsu H, Matsuura K, Inuzuka S, Ono Y, Furusawa M, Hata K, Kakegawa T, Ohtake H, Tomita M, Honbo Z, Kobayashi M, Shirabe J, Ashizawa A, Miyauchi Y, Akagi M, Takahashi M, Koga Y, Watanabe K (1986) Clinical results of esophageal cancer in Kyushu district—Analysis of 2126 cases. J Jpn Soc Cancer Ther 21:1423–1432
4. Mei W, Xian-Zhi G, Weibo Y, Guojun H, Liang-Jun W, Da-Wei Z (1989) Randomized clinical trial on the combination of preoperative irradiation and surgery in the treatment of esophageal carcinoma: Report on 206 patients. Int J Radiat Oncol Biol Phys 16:325–327
5. Arnott SJ, Duncan W, Kerr GR, Walbaum PR, Cameron E, Jack WJL, Mackillop WJ (1992) Low dose preoperative radiotherapy for carcinoma of the esophagus: Results of a randomized clinical trial. Radiother Oncol 24:108–113

Clinical Trial of Preoperative Chemotherapy, Intraoperative Radiotherapy, and Esophagectomy for Lower Esophageal Carcinoma

Reiki Eguchi, Hiroko Ide, Tutomu Nakamura, Kazuhiko Hayashi, Kazunari Yoshida, Ataru Kobayashi, Fujio Hanyuu[1], Akiyoshi Yamada, Makiko Tanaka, and Tomohiko Ookawa[2]

Introduction

The most clinically important mode of recurrence after operation for patients with esophageal cancer is paratracheal lymph node metastasis. On the other hand, abdominal lymph node metastasis after the operation is also commonly recognized in patients, especially those with lower esophageal cancer. Patients with recurrent abdominal lymph node metastasis complain of abdominal pain, anorexia, or other generalized symptom, and will be able to take nothing per os soon after the operation. To avoid abdominal lymph node metastasis after operation, we have been treating patients with advanced lower esophageal cancer with combined preoperative chemotherapy, intraoperative radiotherapy (IOR) and esophagectomy.

While IOR is commonly applied in the treatment of advanced carcinoma these days, there are few reports of IOR for esophageal carcinoma [1, 2], and none concerning intraoperative abdominal radiotherapy for esophageal carcinoma. The focus of this paper is the evaluation of IOR.

Patients and Methods

From September 1989 to June 1992, 61 patients with advanced cancer in the lower third of the esophagus underwent esophagectomy. In these patients, ten patients were treated with combined preoperative chemotherapy, IOR, and radical esophagectomy. On admission, all patients had remarkable abdominal lymph node metastasis detected by ultrasonography (US) or computed tomography (CT).

Medical College, 8-1 Kawada-cho, Shinjuku-ku, Tokyo, 162 Japan

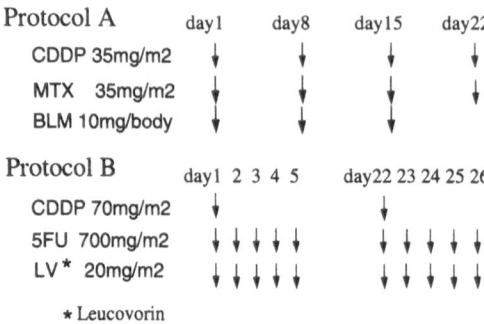

Fig. 1. Two protocols were selected for preoperative chemotherapy. *CDDP*, cisplatin; *MTX*, methotrexate; *BLM*, bleomycin; *5-FU*, 5-fluorouracil

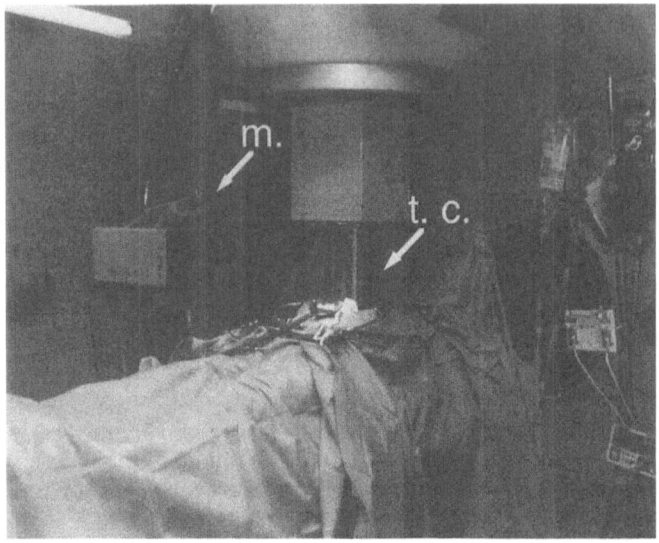

Fig. 2. The treatment cone through which an electron beam was delivered was set close to the celiac axis through laparotomy. *M*, monitor (ECG, PaO$_2$); *t.c.*, treatment cone

There were two protocols for preoperative chemotherapy: A, [cisplatin (CDDP) 35 mg/m^2 + methotrexate (MTX) 35 mg/m^2 + bleomycin (BLM) 10 mg/body iv bolus] every week (four courses); and B, [CDDP 70 mg/m^2 + Leucovorin 20 mg/m^2 iv bolus + 5-fluorouracil (5-FU) 700 mg/m^2 iv continuously] every 3 weeks (two courses) (Fig. 1).

Two or 3 weeks after chemotherapy, the patients underwent surgical treatment. Laparotomy, construction of the gastric tube, and abdominal lymph node dissection (with pancreatosplenectomy in some cases) were performed before IOR for patients who underwent esophagectomy through a right thoracotomy. While they were under general anesthesia, the patients were transported to

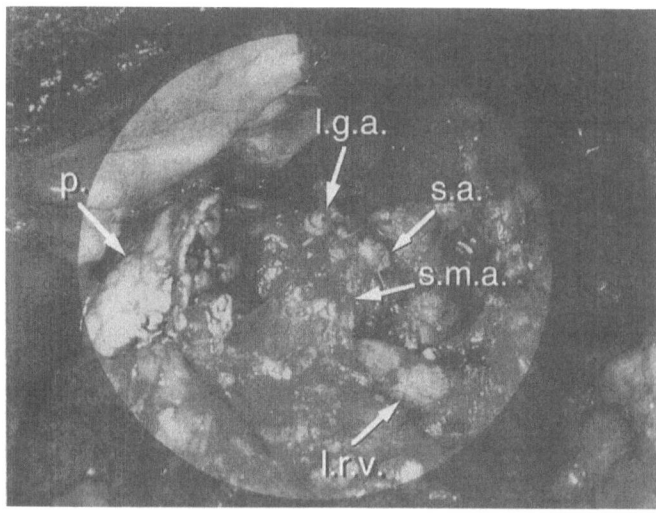

Fig. 3. The radiation field was defined around the celiac axis (*bright round area*). Irradiation was performed after lymphadenectomy and pancreatosplenectomy. *l.g.a.*, left gastric artery; *l.r.v.*, left renal vein; *s.a.*, splenic artery; *s.m.a.*, superior mesenteric artery; *p.*, pancreas

the radiation room where IOR was carried out before esophagectomy. The radiation field was defined around the celiac axis and a single dose of 25 Gy with 9–12 MeV was delivered to the field through a round treatment cone of 8–10 cm in diameter (Figs. 2, 3). After irradiation, the patient was taken back to the operation room and underwent right thoracotomy and esophagectomy with mediastinal (and cervical) lymph node dissection and reconstruction of the passage. For patients who underwent esophagectomy through left abdominothoracotomy, mediastinal lymphadenectomy and esophagectomy were often performed before IOR.

Diagnosis of the mode of recurrence was made with clinical findings, US CT scan, and autopsy.

Results

Six patients received preoperative chemotherapy according to protocol A, and in four patients with tumor localized near the esophagogastric junction, left-sided abdominothoracic esophagectomy was performed. In the other six patients, a right-sided thoracic approach was chosen. In addition, seven patients underwent pancreatosplenectomy (Table 1).

All the patients were classified as stage III or IV histologicaly. The number of resected metastatic lymph nodes of the patients was 2–14 (mean = 7.5). Partial remission was achieved in five patients, but in the other five patients response to preoperative chemotherapy was poor (Table 2).

Duodenal stenosis caused by IOR was revealed in two patients 2–3 months after treatment (Fig. 4). In five patients, recurrent tumor was recognized. While

Table 1. Summary of treatment

Case	Age	Sex	Preoperative chemotherapy protocal	Approach of esophagectomy	Pancreato-splenectomy	Intraoperative irradiation
1	66	M	A	thoracotomy	–	25 Gy–10 MeV
2	64	M	A	left	+	25 Gy–10 MeV
3	66	M	A	right	+	25 Gy– 9 MeV
4	52	M	A	right	–	25 Gy–12 MeV
5	62	M	A	right	+	25 Gy–12 MeV
6	64	M	A	right	+	25 Gy– 9 MeV
7	55	F	B	left	+	25 Gy–12 MeV
8	64	M	B	left	+	25 Gy–12 MeV
9	54	M	B	left	+	25 Gy–12 MeV
10	66	M	B	right	–	25 Gy–12 MeV

Table 2. Pathological features

Case No.	pTNM classification			Stage	No. of metastatic lymph nodes	Response to chemotherapy
	pT	pN	pM			
1	pT4	pN1	pM0	III	8	None
2	pT3	pN1	pM1	VI	12	None
3	pT3	pN1	pM1	VI	6	Partial
4	pT3	pN1	pM0	III	2	Partial
5	pT2	pN1	pM1	VI	14	Partial
6	pT3	pN1	pM1	VI	14	None
7	pT3	pN1	pM0	III	6	Partial
8	pT3	pN1	pM0	III	3	None
9	pT3	pN1	pM1	VI	6	None
10	pT4	pN1	pM1	VI	4	Partial

TNM, tumor node metastasis

no lymph node metastasis was revealed around celiac axis (i.e., within the radiation field), in two patients (cases 5 and 7), recurrent abdominal lymph node metastasis was found outside of the radiation field (Fig. 5). Four patients died of cancer less than 12 months postoperatively, but five patients are still alive, in whom the longest survival term was 28 months (Table 3). One patient died of causes unrelated to the disease (at 3 months).

Of the patients with many (12–14) metastatic lymph nodes, those who underwent esophagectomy without IOR lived less than 1 year after operation, and two of three patients who underwent esophagectomy with IOR lived over 1 year (Fig. 6).

Discussion

Intraoperative radiotherapy was reported by Pack and Livingstone [3] and Henschke et al. [4] in 1940 and 1944, and was developed in Japan by Abe et al. [5, 6]. However, the literature contains few reports which describe the details

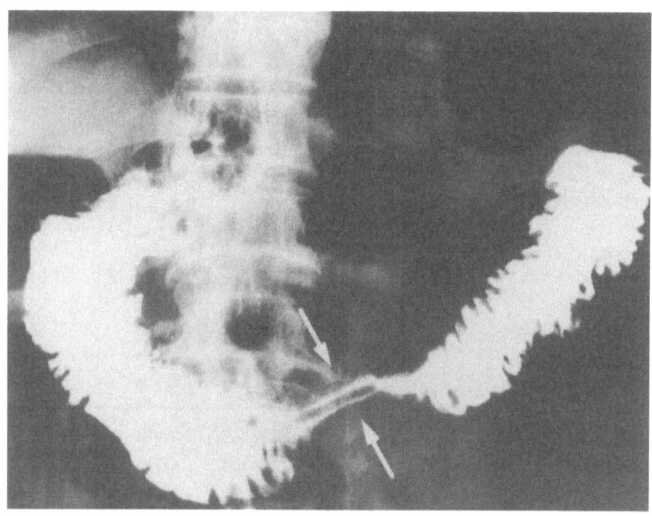

Fig. 4. Stenosis of IIIrd(-IVth) portion of the duodenum (*arrows*) was revealed 2 months after intraoperative radiotherapy (*IOR*)

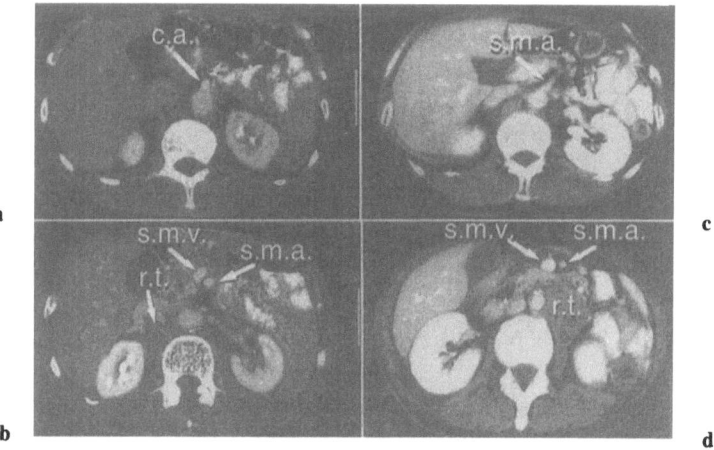

Fig. 5a–d. In patients who underwent esophagectomy with IOR, no recurrent tumor was revealed around celiac axis (**a, c**), but metastatic lymph node was recognized outside of the radiation field after the therapy (**b, d**). (**a, b**, cases; **c, d**, case) *c.a.*, celiac axis; *r.t.*, recurrent tumor; *s.m.a.*, superior mesenteric artery; *s.m.v.*, superior mesenteric vein

of IOR in esophageal carcinoma [1, 2], and all of them are related to IOR of mediastinal irradiation for esophageal carcinoma. So there are no reports of intraoperative abdominal radiotherapy for esophageal carcinoma as a means of avoiding recurrent abdominal lymph node metastasis. Intra-operative mediastinal radiotherapy is a very reasonable form of treatment considering the mode of

Table 3. Clinical results

Case	Postop. major complications	Postoperative therapy	Mode of recurrence	Survival
1	Renal failure	Chemotherapy	Vertebra	2 Months
2	Duodenal stenosis	Irradiation	Cervical LN	12 Months
3	—	Chemotherapy	—	28 Months + NED
4	Anastmotic leakage	—	—	26 Months + NED
5	—	Chemotherapy	Abdominal LN	21 Months + AWD
6	Anastomtic leakage	—	Liver and vertebra	7 Months
7	—	Chemotherapy	Brain and abdominal LN	7 Months
8	—	—	—	6 Months + NED
9	Pancreatic fistula	—	—	6 Months + NED
10	Duodenal stenosis	Irradiation	—	3 Months[a]

NED, no evidence of disease; *AWD*, alive with disease; *LN*, lymph nodes
[a] Died of causes unrelated to the disease

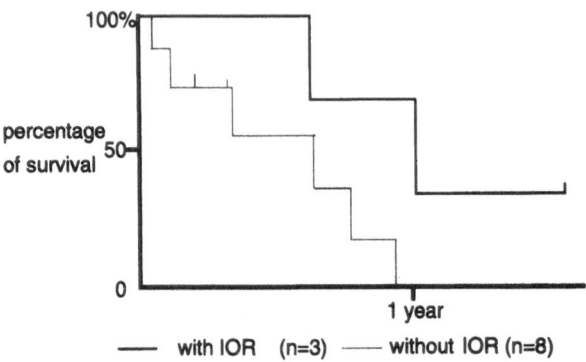

Fig. 6. Survival rate of patients with 12–14 lymph node metastases who underwent esophagectomy with IOR had a tendency to be better than that of patients without IOR

Table 4. Location of recurrent abdominal lymph node metastasis[a]

Common hepatic artery LN	26%
Celiac artery LN	74%
Mesenteric LN	37%
Para-aortic LN	53%
Other LN	5%

LN, lymph nodes;
[a] Study of 19 patients with abdominal lymph node metastasis after esophagectomy who did not receive intraoperatire radiotherapy (*IOR*)

recurrence after esophagectomy for thoracic esophageal carcinoma. Since recurrent abdominal tumor cannot be disregarded clinicaly, intraoperative abdominal radiotherapy must be applied to treatment of lower-third esophageal cartinoma.

In the authors' institute, most recurrent metastatic lymph nodes in 19 patients with recurrent abdominal tumor who had undergone esophagectomy without IOR between January 1980 and June 1992 were mainly found around celiac axis (Table 4). Owing to this result, the radiation field was defined around the celiac axis, which includes lymph nodes around the common hepatic and superior mesenteric arteries. We selected a treatment cone of 8–10 cm in diameter, but the shape and a size must be investigated further on an individual basis. One of the most favorable characteristics of an electron beam is that depth, dose, and distribution of irradiation can be regulated by adjusting the amount of energy of the beam. We thought 9–12 MeV would be required to irradiate the field after lymphadenectoy.

According to the results of combined preoperative chemotherapy, IOR, and esophagectomy, no recurrent tumor was revealed within the radiation field, while recurrent abdominal tumor was recognized outside the field in two patients. The prognosis of the patients who underwent esophagectomy with IOR was better than that of patients without IOR. These result suggests that combined therapy might be a realistic alternative in properly selected patients.

However, because duodenal stenosis caused by IOR was observed in 20% of the patients after treatment, it is necessary to keep the duodenum away from the radiation field or to protect it with a lead plate.

References

1. Ogata M, Tamura Y, Kawamura A, Hikita T, Maeda T, Ogawa Y, Inomata Y, Hirakawa K, Takeda A, Tatibana Y (1984) Intraoperative radiation therapy of esophageal cancer. J Clin Surg 39:369–375
2. Ozawa Y, Kizumi H, Minamide J, Tokunaga M, Fukano F, Osaka Y, Kitamura T, Yamashita K, Shibata T, Hayakawa J (1992) Results of intraoperative radiation therapy for upper mediastinal dissection of esophageal carcinoma. Jpn J Cancer Clin 38:11–15
3. Pack G, Livingston E (1940) Palliative irradiation of gastric cancer. In: Pack G, Livingston E (eds) Treatment of cancer and allied disease, vol 2. Paul B. Hoeber, New York, pp 1088–1109
4. Henschke U, Henschke G (1944) Zur Technik der Operationsbestraphlung. Strahlentherapie 74:228
5. Abe M, Fukuda M, Yamano K, Matsuda S, Handa H (1971) Intraoperative irradiation in abdominal and cerebral tumours. Acta Radiol 10:408–416
6. Abe M, Takahasi M, Yabumoto E, Adachi H, Yosii M, Mori K (1980) Clinical experiences with intraoperative radiotherapy of locally advanced cancers. Cancer 45:40–48

Treatment for T4 Cancer
of the Intrathoracic Esophagus

A. Yamada, M. Fujimaki, K. Higashiyama, Y. Kuroki, T. Sakakibara,
T. Shimizu, T. Sakamoto, Y. Karaki, and K. Tazawa[1]

Introduction

Cancer of the intrathoracic esophagus has a very poor prognosis. The prognosis
is particularly poor in cases accompanied by tumor invasion into other organs
(i.e., T4 cases). T4 cancer of the intrathoracic esophagus is treated by various
methods, including surgical resection, and conservative treatment, depending on
the organs invaded, the degree of invasion, lymph node metastasis, organ
metastasis, and the patient's general condition. We recently analyzed the results
and problems of various therapies for this cancer. In this study, the UICC's
TNM classification of esophageal cancer was employed.

Subjects

Between October 1979 and December 1990, we treated 192 cases of esophageal
cancer. Of these cases, 69 (35.9%) were classified as T4 by computed tomography
(CT), magnetic resonance imaging (MRI), endoscopic ultrasonography (EUS),
and bronchoscopy before a therapeutic method for individual cases was decided.
These 69 cases were selected for the present study. The stage of cancer was III
or IV in all patients. The tumor-occupying site was the upper third of the
esophagus in 11 cases, the middle third in 45, and the lower third in 13.

Our therapeutic strategy for T4 cancer of the esophagus was as follows. Cases
with metastasis to organs were treated by chemotherapy. In cases where tumor
had invaded the surgically resectable organs such as the pericardium and the
disphragm, without any extensive lymph node metastasis, or in cases where
narrow regions of the thoracic aorta, trachea, or bronchi had been invaded, we

[1] The Second Department of Surgery, Toyama Medical and Pharmaceutical University, 2630
Sugitani, Toyama-shi, Toyama, 930-01 Japan

performed surgical resection and postoperative radiochemotherapy, considering the age and general condition of patient. The other cases were first treated by a combination of hyperthermo-radio (Linac 30 Gy) -chemotherapy (bleomycin [BLM], *cis*-platinum [CDDP], 5-fluorouracil). Surgery and postoperative radiochemotherapy were considered if patients showed partial or complete responses to this combination therapy. Cases showing no change after the combination therapy were treated either by additional radiotherapy (Linac, total 50–60 Gy) and chemotherapy, or by bypass operation or esophageal prosthesis.

Therapeutic Methods and Cases

Seventeen patients first received nonoperative therapies (NO group). Of these patients, 3 later received an esophageal prosthesis (EP group), and 8 underwent a bypass operation (BO group). Surgical resection was performed in 44 patients (68.3%). Sixteen of these patients had received combination therapy before surgical resection. In 14 patients, right thoracotomy was performed for surgical resection (PRT group), while blunt dissection was performed for resection in 2 (PBD group). Radical operation was possible in 6 (37.5%) of these 16 patients. Twenty-eight patients first underwent surgical resection, via right thoracotomy in 23 patients (RT group) and blunt dissection in 5 patients (BD group) (Table 1). Radical operation was possible in only 4 (14.3%) of these 28 patients.

The organ most frequently invaded by tumor was the thoracic aorta. Invasion to this organ was observed in 34 patients. In addition, the tumor invaded the main bronchus in 9, the trachea in 5, the diaphragm in 4, and the pericardium in 1. Surgical resection was performed in 76.5% of the patients with aortic invasion, in 55.6% of those with bronchial invasion, in 40% of those with tracheal invasion, and all cases of invasion into the pericardium or the diaphragm. Invasion into two or more organs was observed in 13 patients. In all 13 of these patients, the aorta was one of the invaded organs. The surgical resection rate was 46.2% for these 13 patients (Table 2).

Table 1. Various treatments for T4 cancer

Nonoperation (NO)	17
Esophageal prosthesis (EP)	3
Bypass operation (BO)	8
Resection without POCT	28
Right thoracotomy (RT)	23
Blunt dissection (BD)	5
Resection with POCT	16
Right thoracotomy (PRT)	14
Blunt dissection (PBD)	2
Total number	69

POCT, Preoperative combination therapy (hyperthermia plus radio-chemotherapy)

Table 2. Organ of invasion by T4 cancer

Treatment	NO(EP)	BO	PRT + PBD	RT + BD	Total No.
Thoracic aorta	4	4	10	16	34
Trachea	2	1	1	1	5
Main bronchus	2(1)	2	3	2	9
Pericardium	0	0	0	1	1
Diaphragm	0	0	0	4	4
Others	2	0	0	1	3
Aorta + trachea	2	1	0	1	4
Aorta + bronchus	1(1)	0	1	1	3
Aorta + pericardium	1	0	0	0	1
Aorta + lung	0	0	0	1	1
Aorta + Pericardium + Diaphragm	3(1)	0	1	0	4

NO, nonoperative therapy; *EP*, esophageal prosthesis; *BO*, bypass operation; *PRT + PBD*, preoperative combination therapy plus right thoracotomy or blunt dissection; *RT + BD*, right thoracotomy or blunt dissection without preoperative combination therapy

Table 3. Prognosis of T4 cancer

Treatment	Number of patients	Survival (months) (mean ± SD)
NO	17	8.65 ± 9.93
EP	3	6 ± 1
BO	8	3.13 ± 1.83
PRT	14	6.64 ± 5.19
PBD	2	6 ± 5
RT	23	12.70 ± 15.56
BD	5	9.6 ± 4.41

Results

All patients died. Two deaths (one in the BO group and the other in the PRT group) were operative deaths. One patient in the PRT group and two in the RT group died of other diseases. The mean survival period was 8.65 months for the NO group, 6 months for the EP group, 3.13 months for the BO group, 6.64 months for the PRT group, 6 months for the PBD group, 12.70 months for the RT group, and 9.6 months for the BD group. Thus, the survival time was longest for the RT group and shortest for the BO group. Among radically operated patients, the mean survival period was 5.5 months for six patients undergoing PRT and 25.5 months for four undergoing RT. Thus, radical operation by RT resulted in longer survival periods (Table 3).

Conclusion

Despite various therapies, the prognosis of T4 cancer of the intrathoracic esophagus was very poor. The prognosis was best in the RT group. The percentage of patients who underwent radical operation was not high in the RT group. The relatively good prognosis in the RT group may be explained by relatively less severe invasion into organs and the effectiveness of postoperative combination therapy. The prognosis was poorest in the BO group. Although the primary purpose of bypass operation is to improve the ability to ingest food orally, this purpose was achieved only in a few patients in BO group, suggesting the necessity of reviewing the indications for bypass operation. The prognosis was poor for the NO group. Of patients in this group, those who later received an EP showed satisfactory improvement in oral food ingestion. Although the prognosis was not good in patients who received preoperative combination therapy, the results from these patients suggest that preoperative combination therapy increases the percentage of patients who can receive radical operation.

Discussion

In patients with T4 cancer (advanced cancer) of the intrathoracic esophagus, radical operation is often impossible and the prognosis is very poor. The incidence of lymph node metastasis or organ metastasis is very high for these cases. In treating this type of cancer, it is essential to select a therapeutic method, considering the prognosis and the quality of life. In patients not indicated for operation, we have recently begun to use a combination of hyperthermia and radiochemotherapy, according to the method reported by Fujimaki et al. [1]. This combination therapy resulted in a high response rate. If the systemic condition permits, we often perform surgical resection after this kind of preoperative therapy. The percentage of cases in which radical operation was possible after such preoperative therapy was high. We will continue to apply this preoperative combination therapy for the purpose of improving the prognosis. Regarding chemotherapy, Bernal et al. [2] recently reported the usefulness of combined CDDP and 5-fluorouracil therapy. If this combination chemotherapy is additionally combined with hyperthermia, the response rate may be further increased. On the other hand, if patients with very poor general condition and severe dysphagia are expected to survive for only about 3 months, it seems reasonable to consider the use of less invasive esophageal intubation which is solely aimed at enabling food ingestion.

References

1. Fujimaki M, Katoh H, Tazawa K, Yamashita I, Sakamoto T, Yamada A (1990) Adjuvant hyperthermia in nonresectable esophageal carcinoma. In: Diseases of esophagus, vol I, malignant diseases. Futura, New York, pp. 317–322
2. Bernal AG, Cruz JJ, Sanchez P, Munoz A, Nieto A, Fonseca E, Calle R, Gomez JL (1989) Four-day continuous infusion of cisplatin and 5-fluorouracil in head and neck cancer. Cancer 63:1927–1930

Efficacy of Hyperthermia for Advanced Esophageal Carcinoma

Tetsuro Shimizu, Hiroshi Kato, Shigeru Takemori, Masahiro Okamoto, Tomohiro Saito, Iwao Yamashita, Akira Yamada, Takashi Sakamoto, Yoshiaki Karaki, Kenji Tazawa, and Masao Fujimaki[1]

Introduction

The prognosis of patients with advanced cancer of the esophagus is very poor. To control advanced esophageal carcinoma nonoperatively, irradiation and chemotherapy have been applied. However, the clinical effectiveness of these treatments has not been satisfactory. Hyperthermia has recently received attention since neoplastic cells have been reported to have greater heat-sensitivity than normal cells, and because this method has been confirmed to enhance the anticancer effect of radiation and some anticancer drugs. We have employed multidisciplinary treatment consisting of radiotherapy, chemotherapy, and hyperthermia, since 1985 [1]. This treatment protocol was derived from basic experiments using cultured cells of human cancer of the esophagus. This is a report of our study on the efficacy of hyperthermia in combined treatment.

Patients and Methods

Radiochemotherapy combined with hyperthermia was administered to 35 patients (33 males and 2 females) with advanced esophageal carcinoma which either required preoperative treatment or was unresectable. The patients ranged in age from 44 to 81 years (mean 65.1 ± 9.42 years). The location of the main lesion was intrathoracic esophageal in 31 patients, hypopharyngeal in 1, cervical in 2, and abdominal in 1. The tumor diameter ranged from 3 cm to 20 cm, with an average of 8.4 ± 3.9 cm. The histological type determined by examination of biopsy or resected specimens was well-differentiated in 6 patients, moderately

[1] The Second Department of Surgery, Faculty of Medicine, Toyama Medical and Pharmaceutical University, 2630 Sugitani, Toyama City, Toyama, 930–01 Japan

Table 1. Patient characteristics

Number of Patients	35	Histologic type	
Sex Male	33	Squamous cell carcinoma	
Female	2	Well differentiated	6
		Moderately differentiated	19
Age	44–81 years	Poorly differentiated	6
	(mean: 65.1 ± 9.42)	Unknown	1
Location of lesion		Small cell carcinoma	3
Hypopharyngeal	1 (2.9%)		
Cervical	2 (5.7%)	Pretreatment clinical classification	
Intrathoracic	31 (88.6%)	TNM classification	
Upper	6 (17.1%)	T4	27 (77.1%)
Middle	22 (62.9%)	Tumor invaded aorta	12 (34.3%)
Lower	3 (8.6%)	bronchus	8 (22.9%)
Abdominal	1 (2.9%)	trachea	8 (22.9%)
		pericardium	2 (5.7%)
Length of lesion	3–20 cm	others	3 (8.6%)
	(mean: 8.4 ± 3.9)	N1	29 (82.9%)
		M1	2 (5.7%)

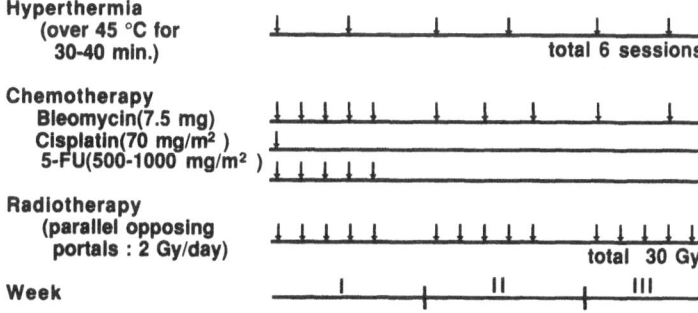

Fig. 1. The protocol of radiochemotherapy combined with hyperthermia for advanced esophageal carcinoma. *5-FU*, 5-fluorouracil

differentiated in 19 patients, and poorly differentiated squamous cell carcinoma in 6 patients. There were 3 cases of small cell carcinoma (Table 1).

Regarding pretreatment clinical classification, in 27 (77.1%) patients, invasion to contiguous structures was considered to be present: the aorta was found to have tumor invasion in 12 patients, the trachea in 8, the bronchus in 8, and the pericardium in 2. As preoperative treatment for cases showing extensive infiltration to other organs or distant metastasis, radiochemotherapy with hyperthermia under a no-operation policy was performed as follows.

As shown in Fig. 1, each patient received 2 Gy/day delivered at opposing angles for a total of 15 sessions over the course of 3 weeks. Continuous 24-h subcutaneous injection of 7.5 mg of bleomycin for a total of ten injections was administered as chemotherapy during the early period of this study. Later,

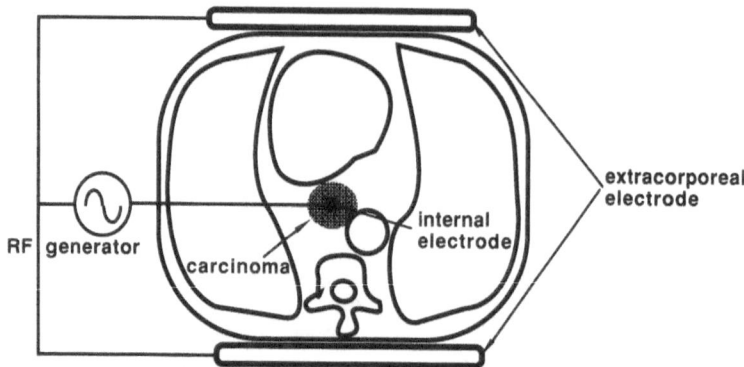

Fig. 2. Hyperthermia delivery for esophageal carcinoma. *RF*, radiofrequency

cisplatin in combination with 5-fluorouracil was employed. Hyperthermia was performed with intraluminal heating twice a week for a total of six sessions, using a Japan Crescent, (Tokyo) IH-500 T apparatus (radiofrequency [RF], 13.56 MHz). For patients with unresectable carcinoma, adjunctive treatment was used whenever possible.

Figure 2 shows the schema of hyperthermia delivery. Intraluminal heating was effected with an intraesophageal applicator (the Second Department of Surgery, Toyama Medical and Pharmaceutical University Model), inserted under pharyngeal anesthesia, and two extracorporeal applicators placed on the chest and back. The temperature, measured with a sensor placed on the tumor surface during hyperthermia, ranged from 42°C to 44°C during the early study period; however, since 1988, a temperature exceeding 45°C, sustained for more than 30 min, has been used. A temperature exceeding 45°C at the tumor surface could be obtained immediately after the beginning of the treatment using low radiofrequency at power of less than 100 W. Since heating could be obtained at lower power, no water cooling system was necessary in almost all the patients during the later study period, and no skin damage was observed.

The efficacy of treatment was determined by endoscopic or radiologic evaluation of the local and histological effects about 1 month after completion or discontinuation of treatment.

Results

The average doses of the combined therapy are shown in Table 2. The number of hyperthermia sessions ranged from 2 to 12 sessions (mean 5.2 ± 2.2 sessions).

The effectiveness rate was 80.0%. Eight (22.9%) patients showed complete response (CR), 20 (57.1%) partial response (PR), 6 (17.1%) no change (NC), and 1 (3.3%) progressive disease (PD).

After treatment, surgical operation was performed in 16 patients, in 15 of whom the tumor was resectable (resectability rate, 42.9%); the remaining patient underwent a bypass operation with a gastric tube. Of the 15 surgically treated

Table 2. Average doses of combined therapy

Hyperthermia (sessions)	5.2 ± 2.2 times
Radiation (dose)	42.3 ± 22.2 Gy
Chemotherapy	
Bleomycin ($n = 17$)	82.9 mg/body
Cisplatin ($n = 26$)	144.0 mg/body
5-Fluorouracil ($n = 10$)	3375.0 mg/body

Table 3. Effects of multidisciplinary treatment

Local response			Histologic effects of preoperative treatment		
Complete response	(CR)	8 (22.9%)	Ineffective	(Grade 0)	0 (0.0%)
Partial response	(PR)	20 (57.1%)	Slightly effective	(Grade 1)	5 (33.3%)
		6 (17.1%)	Moderately		
No change	(NC)	1 (3.3%)	effective	(Grade 2)	6 (40.0%)
Progressive disease	(PD)		Markedly effective	(Grade 3)	4 (26.7%)
Effectiveness	(CR + PR)	80.0%	Histologic effectiveness	(Grade 2 + 3)	10 (66.7%)

Based on the criteria of the Japanese Society of Esophageal Diseases [2]

patients, 10 underwent intrathoracic esophagectomy with thoracotomy, 3 blunt dissection, and 2 pharyngolaryngo-esophagectomy. The histological study of the resected specimens revealed absence of viable tumor cells in 4 (26.7%) patiens (markedly effective), and in 6 (40.0%) patients the combined therapy was assessed to be moderately effective based on the criteria of the Japanese Society of Esophageal Diseases [2] (Table 3).

During the treatment period, leukocytopenia, which was the most frequent complication and was considered to be due to myelosuppression, was seen in eight patients, pulmonary fibrosis in four patients, interstitial pneumonitis in two, hypercalcemia in three, transient renal dysfunction induced by combined cisplatin in three patients, esophagobronchial fistula in one, and fungal uveitis in one patient. Leukocytopenia and renal dysfunction improved within 1–2 weeks of discontinuation of the treatment, but pulmonary fibrosis was fatal. Complications considered to be due to hyperthermia itself were not recognized.

The survival rate at 1-year was 37.9% in all patients, 51.9% in resected cases, and 20.3% in unresectable cases. At the time of writing, the longest survivor has a postoperative survival period of 4 years and 7 months.

Discussion

Complete removal is the essential treatment for esophageal carcinoma. While the treatment results for esophageal carcinoma have improved in association with developments in surgical technique, diagnostic procedures, and anesthesia, the prognosis of patients with advanced cancer of the esophagus remains very poor, since these patients are often no longer candidates for a curative resection. The clinical effectiveness of radiotherapy and chemotherapy in advanced

esophageal carcinoma has not been satisfactory. The effectiveness of hyperthermia was demonstrated in a basic study carried out on three cell lines
established from human esophageal carcinoma in the authors' department [3],
and this method was confirmed to enhance the anticancer effect of radiation and
some anticancer drugs. In addition, with the development of a hyperthermia
applicator for use in the esophageal lumen by Sugimachi et al. in 1983 [4],
it became possible to perform hyperthermia at selected sites. We therefore
employed hyperthermia in combination with radiotherapy and chemotherapy
in patients who either required preoperative treatment or had nonresectable
tumor. The two clinical advantages of multidisciplinary treatment for patients
with advanced esophageal cancer are that it often reduces the size of the lesion
bringing about improvement in such aspects of quality of life as oral digestion,
and that the local control minimizing the number of cancer cells invading to
contiguous structures facilitates curative resection and improves patient prognosis. Radiochemotherapy combined with hyperthermia was locally effective,
yielding an overall effectiveness of 80.0% and a resectability rate of 42.9%.
Dysphagia that had been present prior to treatment disappeared in almost all
patients.

It is important to evaluate histological effectiveness, since the survival rate
of the patients in whom treatment is assessed to be "markedly effective" is
excellent compared that in those in whom it "ineffective" or "moderately
effective" [5]. In this study, treatment was "markedly effective" in 26.7% of the
patients. To increase this rate is the purpose of nonoperative multidisciplinary
treatment.

Generally, the antitumor effects of hyperthermia are considered to be greater
at higher temperature. To attain a high temperature in the deep layer of the
lesion, the temperature at the surface of an advanced tumor should be maintained at a higher level. Improvements in the hyperthermia applicator have
increased the safety and ease of maintaining the tumor surface temperature at
above 45°C at a low radiofrequency power of less than 100 W.

During the course of the combined therapy, serious complications, particularly pulmonary fibrosis, which was fatal, were noted. Thus, other chemotherapeutic drugs such as cisplatin were employed instead of bleomycin during
the later period of the study. Careful consideration of the other complications
will be required in the future.

Hyperthermia in combination with radiochemotherapy for advanced esophageal carcinoma was found to increase locally observd therapeutic effects.
However, the prognosis of the patients remains unfavorable. This is considered
to be attributable mainly to lymphatic and hematogenic metastasis, and indicates
the necessity for further study of combined chemotherapy. In addition, more
effective heating procedures and methods of preventing complications are also
important factors in increasing histological effectiveness.

Conclusion

Radiochemotherapy combined with hyperthermia for advanced cancer of the
esophagus is locally effective. In this study, an overall effectiveness of 80.0%
and temporary improvement in the quality of life of the patients, such as

resumption of oral digestion, were obtained. While a fairly good local effect was obtained, there were several serious complications during the course of the combined therapy, and the outcome was unfavorable. These indicate the necessity for further study on more effective heating and combined therapeutic procedures, and methods of preventing complications.

References

1. Fujimaki M, Katoh H, Tazawa K, Yamashita I, Sakamoto T, Yamada A (1990) Adjuvant hyperthermia in nonresectable esophageal carcinoma. In: Ferguson MK, Little AG, Skinner DB (eds) Disease of the esophagus, vol. 1: Malignant diseases. Futura, New York, pp 317–322
2. Japanese Society for Esophageal Diseases (1992) Guidelines for the clinical and pathologic studies on carcinoma of the esophagus. Kanehara, Tokyo, pp 32–58
3. Shinbo T, Katoh H, Saitoh M, Saitoh T, Shimizu T, Otagiri H, Tazawa K, Fujimaki M (1989) Effect of thermotherapy on human esophageal carcinoma in culture and clinical cases. Gan to Kagaku Ryoho (Jpn J Cancer Chemother) 16(4):1899–1904
4. Sugimachi K, Inokuchi K, Kai H, Sogawa A, Kawai Y (1983) Endotract antenna for application of hyperthermia to malignant lesions. Jpn J Cancer Res (Gann) 74:622–624
5. Sugimachi K, Kai H, Matsufuji H, Ueo H, Inokuchi K (1986) Histopathological evaluation of hyperthermo-chemo-radiotherapy for carcinoma of the esophagus. J Surg Oncol 32:82–85

Palliative Treatment
for Esophageal Cancer and Others

The Development of "Through-Bougie Esophageal Prosthesis Intubation" and Its Evolution to an "Extinctive Type"

Hiroyoshi Koizumi, Junji Minamide[1], Norio Aoyama, Yukihiro Ozawa[2], Haruo Sekino[3], and Hajime Kurabayashi[4]

Introduction

There are two basic techniques for esophageal prosthesis intubation: Pulsion and traction. The pulsion technique is superior to the traction technique in that there are fewer associated complications. Also, there is less invasion to the patient. Even so, with pulsion, general anesthesia is sometimes necessary, in cases of highly advanced stricture, to pass a prosthesis with or without the support of esophagoscopy or an introducer. With some cases of highly advanced stricture, it is necessary to use a general anesthesia, to be able to pass the prosthesis through.

We were using esophageal bougies to dilatate the stricture after esophagectomy. On extension of this technique, we developed our intubation method, namely "through-bougie esophageal prosthesis intubation". As is the case with bougienage, the whole procedure is undertaken while the patient is awake.

In 1984, we reported our first cases in cooperation with Sumitomo Bakelite Co. [1, 2]. From our experiences in 57 trial cases, we were assured of the superiority of our technique over other conventional methods. Anyone who has had experience with bougienage can perform this procedure safely, easily and without anesthesia.

[1] First Division of Surgery, Kanagawa Cancer Center, 54-2 Nakao-cho, Asahi-ku, Yokohama, 241 Japan
[2] First Department of Surgery, Yokohama City University School of Medicine, 3-9, Fukuura, Kanazawa-ku, Yokohama, 236 Japan
[3] Tokyo Medical Office, Mitsui Mutual Life Insurance Co., 2-25 Tsuruya-cho, Kanagawa-ku, Yokohama, 221 Japan
[4] Fundamental Research Laboratory, Sumitomo Bakelite Co., Ltd., 495 Akiba-cho, Tozuka-ku, Yokohama, 245 Japan

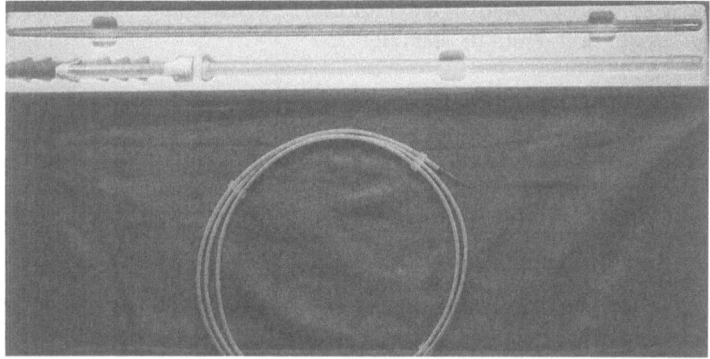

Fig. 1. An intubation set of a flexible esophageal prosthesis and a guide-wire

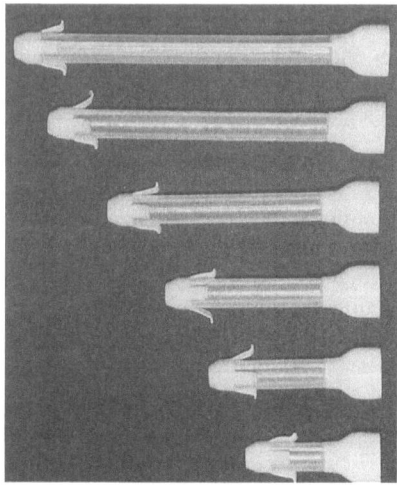

Fig. 2. A flexible prosthesis

The actual procedure of our technique, and the results from the 57 cases we experienced, are presented.

In addition, an advanced type of prosthesis, under development, will be introduced. This new prosthesis is made of "food additives," and will dissolve in a controlled period of time.

Materials

Flexible prosthesis, esophageal bougie, pusher tube, and a wire make up one set for this method (Fig. 1).

1. Esophageal bougie: Made of vinyl chloride, 70 cm in length, 10 mm in diameter with a tunnel of 1.4 mm in diameter.
2. Prosthesis: Urethane was the original material used. We found that this was too hard against the wall of the esophagus, and in some cases, led to a pressure necrosis. We devised a new flexible type of prosthesis made from silicone rubber that is strengthened with a nylon spiral in its wall. The tube is available in six lengths (portion between the funnel-shaped proximal portion and the distal portion with three winged flange)—3, 5, 7, 10, 13, and 15 cm (Fig. 2). The outer diameter of the prosthesis measures 13 mm, with an inner diameter of 10 mm.
3. Pusher tube: A polyethylene tube with an 11-mm inner diameter, and 50 cm in length.
4. Guide wire: A stainless steel wire, 0.055 inches in diameter and 200 cm in length. The distal 20 cm is flexible.

Intubation Procedure

Our intubation technique is quite simple:

1. Measure the length of a stricture from the contrast film. Select a prosthesis tube that is 2 cm to 3 cm shorter in length than the stricture so as to avoid necrosis caused by the wings against a normal esophageal wall.
2. Position the patient in an upright position. The patient is then asked to swallow contrast media, so that the passage and the stricture can be noted, by the operator.
3. The x-ray table is adjusted, so that the patient lies supine. A wire is passed through the center tunnel of the esophageal bougie.
4. Lidocaine jelly is applied to the tip of the bougie. The bougie is advanced until the tip has passed the entrance of the esophagus. Then, the wire is

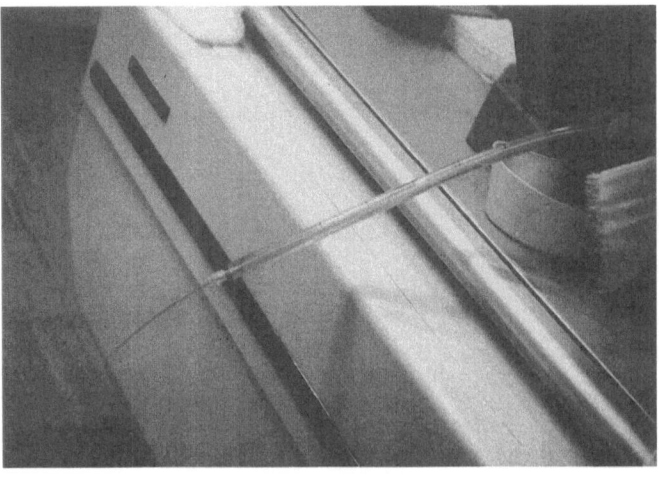

Fig. 3. Dilatation of the esophagus

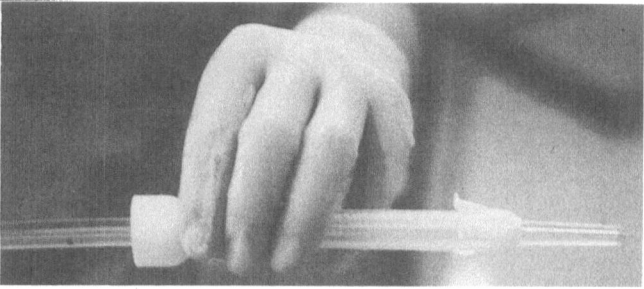

Fig. 4. A prosthesis and an esophageal bougie

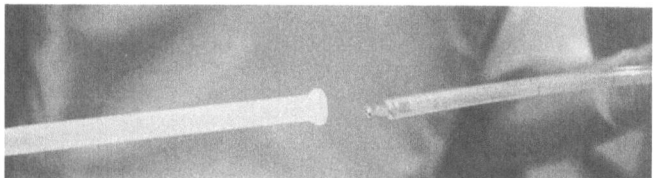

Fig. 5. A pusher tube and an esophageal bougie

inserted through the anal end of the stricture. The bougie is pushed forward, guided by the wire until it is clear that the head of the bougie has passed the anal end of the stricture.

5. The patient is then moved into the right decubitus position. The patient must wait for a few minutes, with the bougie at the stricture, for dilatation. (Fig. 3) Then the bougie is pulled out, with the wire left behind.

6. Lidocaine jelly is applied to the bougie. Then, the prosthesis is mantled over the bougie. (Fig. 4)

7. The pusher tube is guided through the bougie from the proximal end of the bougie. (Fig. 5)

8. The bougie, assembled with the prosthesis and the pusher tube, is advanced toward the oral cavity guided by the wire. Lidocaine jelly should be applied over the whole set. (Fig. 6a,b)

9. The prosthesis is then pushed down through the stricture. This process should be observed on the fluorescent monitor.

    In summary, the whole procedure consists of a repetition of the same sequence: First, bougienage; second, the sending of the prosthesis into the stricture.

10. The funnel-shaped end of the prosthesis will stop its further advancement as it reaches the oral side of the stricture.

11. The bougie is pulled out first by pushing down slightly on the prosthesis with the pusher tube.

12. The pusher tube is pulled out with a slight rotation, while under fluorescent observation, so that the prosthesis is kept in position.

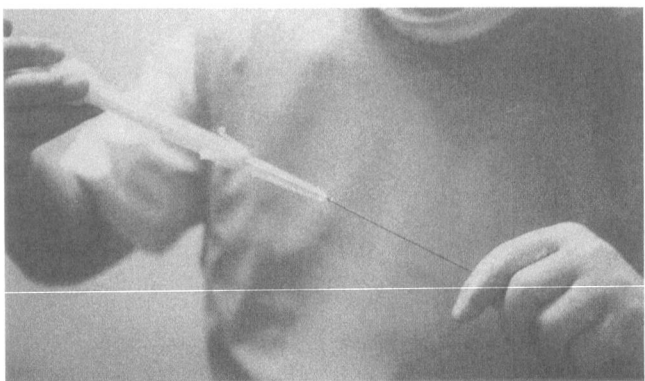

a

b

Fig. 6a,b. A bougie, assembled with a prosthesis and a pusher tube, proceed along the wire whose tip has been already passed through the stricture

13. Finally, the wire is removed and the prosthesis is left in the stricture. (Fig. 7a–d)
14. The x-ray table is adjusted, so that the patient is in an upright position. A contrast media study is performed to make certain the prosthesis is in the correct position and that the passage is smooth. This procedure will take 10–15 min.
15. The patient will be able to take meals in an hour.

An actual case is shown next:

This case involves a 64-year-old man. He had had a total gastrectomy, and because of recurrence, had not been able to take even water and had been living on total parenteral nutrition (TPN). After the intubation, he was free from any i.v. line and he was able to return home happily. (Fig. 8)

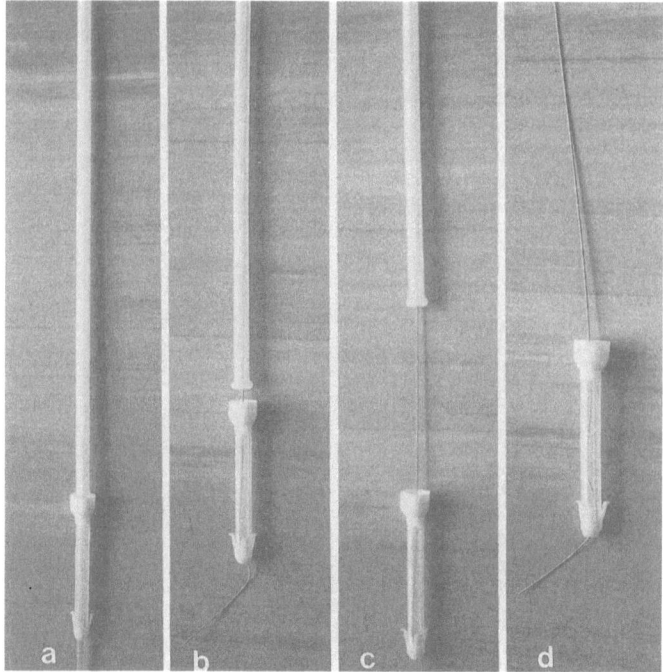

Fig. 7a–d. Procedure of the prosthesis placement

Results

We experienced 57 cases between 1983 and 1992. (Table 1) The most common cases, 21 in all, were of Esophagobronchial (E-B) fistula, due to esophageal cancer, and there were 14 cases of inoperable esophageal cancer.

The complaints after the prosthesis intubation were as shown in Table 2. Complications occurred in 5 cases (Table 3). The status of food intake, both before and after intubation is compared in Table 4.

Of all intubated patients, 94.7% (54) were on nothing by mouth (npo) or a clear liquid diet before intubation. After intubation, 94.7% (54) could start a diet of 30% or more of gruel, building towards a regular diet.

Two of the three patients that were on a more than 30% gruel diet had to go through intubation a second time, after the first prosthesis had slipped down into the stomach and spontaneous excretion occured.

The two cases on npo after intubation, were due to complications.

Discussion

We found "through-bougie prosthesis intubation" to be superior to all other methods of intubation. Through the historical efforts of trying to solve this difficult problem of esophageal stricture, bougienage has been the oldest and the

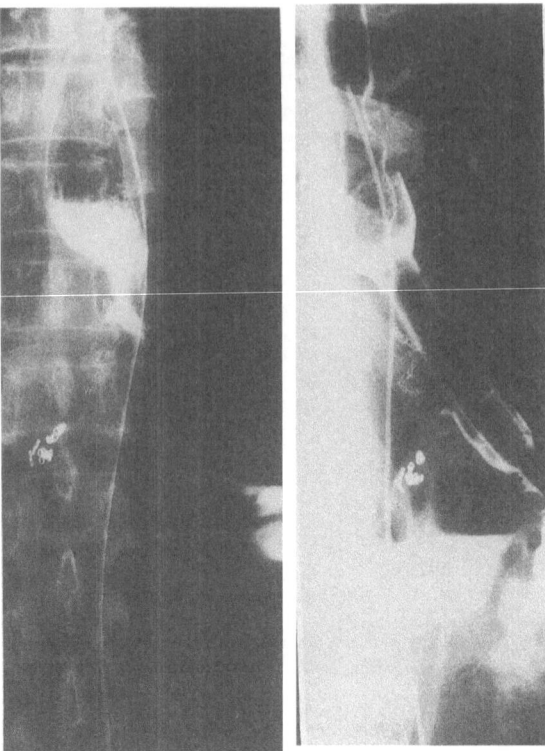

Fig. 8. Contrast film before and after the intubation. Total parenteral nutrition (*TPN*) line is also shown in the film

Table 1. Through-bougie esophageal prosthesis intubation (1983.12–1992.3)

	Reasons		Survival (average)	
Esophageal cancer	Inoperable	14	3–150	(62) days
	E-B fistula	21	3–226	(67)
Stomach cancer	Inoperable	8	11–241	(88)
	Recurrence postop	9	17–454	(190)
Extraluminal mass	Thyroid cancer	1	51	
	Lung cancer	1	15	
Cicatrix	Laryngeal ca postop	1		
	Esoph ca postop (anast)	1		
	Esoph ca postop (stomach tube)	1		
E-B, Esophagobronchial		57		

most fundamental means of making the passage. Our method is superior because of its simplicity. The procedure is similar to bougienage in that the procedure is repeated twice and that the patient is awake for both procedures. The patient can take meals soon after the procedure has been performed.

Table 2. Complaints after the intubation

		%
None	30	52.6
Feeling of foreign body	16	28.0
Pharyngeal pain	14	24.6
Feeling of oppression	12	21.0
Thoracodorsal pain	7	12.3
Substernal pain	4	7.0
Heartburn	1	2.3

None, Indicates lowest level of complaints with routine endoscopic examination of the esophagus

Table 3. Complications

		%
None	52	91.2
Slipping off	2	3.5
Perforation	1	1.8
Bleeding to transfusion	1	1.8
Mediastinitis	1	1.8

Table 4. Food intake after the prosthesis placement

Diet	Before	(%)	After	(%)
Nothing by mouth	30	(52.6)	2	(3.5)
Liquid food	24	(42.1)	1	(1.8)
30% Gruel	2	(3.5)	1	(1.8)
50% Gruel	1	(1.8)	6	(10.5)
Full gruel	0		45	(78.9)
Regular food	0		2	(3.5)

There are only a few reports on "awake intubation." In 1977, Majima et al. reported their experiences [3]. Most likely, the procedure was too complicated, so it did not become widely accepted. Our method, in contrast, is simple and has been more widely accepted than we had expected. Among the reports on the esophageal intubation, there is a radical opinion by some doctors that the esophageal bypass operation is out-of-date and no longer a good choice for treatment of esophageal stricture [4]. We do not agree with this view.

Our principle assumption is that an artificial material should only be used as a last resort. Unfortunately, deaths do occur with esophageal bypasses. However, it is doubtful that intubation should be performed in such cases if a bypass operation is possible. We believe that the indications for a bypass operation itself must be reexamined. We have performed esophageal bypass on 5 patients in the past 5 years. All of the five patients were discharged from our hospital on a more favorable diet than might have been the case after intubation.

There are many cases where a bypass operation is not indicated, and the only choice is intubation.

Our indications for intubation are:

When there is no other possible means for the patient to take meals orally.

Note 1: Those patients who are on a 50% or higher gruel diet do not fall into this category.

Note 2: After intubation, patients can return home to enjoy a better quality of life.

In Japan, our views on what the indications for intubation are, differ distinctly from the reports we see from overseas.

Angorn and Haffejee [5] give us a list of indications from his experiences in 2,785 cases by either pulsion (2446 cases by Procter-Livingstone tube—Latex products, Johannesburg, South Africa), or by traction (339 cases by Celestin tube—Latex Products; Medoc Co., England). In all of these cases, procedures were conducted with the patient under general anesthesia.

Palliative intubation was indicated for patients in the following categories:

(1) Medical contraindications to surgery or radiotherapy
(2) Irreversible physical debility
(3) Clinically detectable invasion of adjacent organs or distant dissemination
(4) Dysphagia resulting from recurrence following surgery or radiotherapy
(5) Malignant strictures of the upper thoracic esophagus longer than 6 cm
(6) Upper thoracic tumors causing complete dysphagia (if the lesion is considered curable, i.e., is less than 6 cm, intubation is followed by radiotherapy)
(7) Demonstrable tracheoesophageal or bronchoesophageal fistula
(8) Nonresectability established at laparotomy on thoracotomy

Points 5 and 6 in particular, are doubtful, since the indication is based on the length of the stricture.

Esophagectomy is the first choice of treatment in Japan. In current practice, nonresectability would be determined before laparotomy or thoracotomy; thus such examples as those in point number 8 are not likely to be true today because the degree of invasion by the tumor can now be diagnosed well beforehand due to recent advances in fiberscopic echograms.

Our efforts to develop an ideal type of esophageal prosthesis began early on. Our final goal was/is to develop a prosthesis which would not stay in the body longer than we wanted it to. We thought it best if the prosthesis were to dissolve altogether while in place. Possiblly, we have found an ideal material for a new type of prosthesis. It is polyuronide. Polyuronide is a food additive that is one of the thickening agents used in making jams and ice cream.

At present, we are carrying out experiments with polyuronide to try to find a way of controlling the time in which the prosthesis would take to dissolve.

Our patients was a 67-year-old male, who had a spiral shaped stricture, in his mid-esophagus, 10 cm in length. The prosthesis had been intubated 4 days prior to esophagectomy (Fig. 9). The esophagus was resected together with the prosthesis. Our prosthesis was found to be losing its original form (Fig. 10).

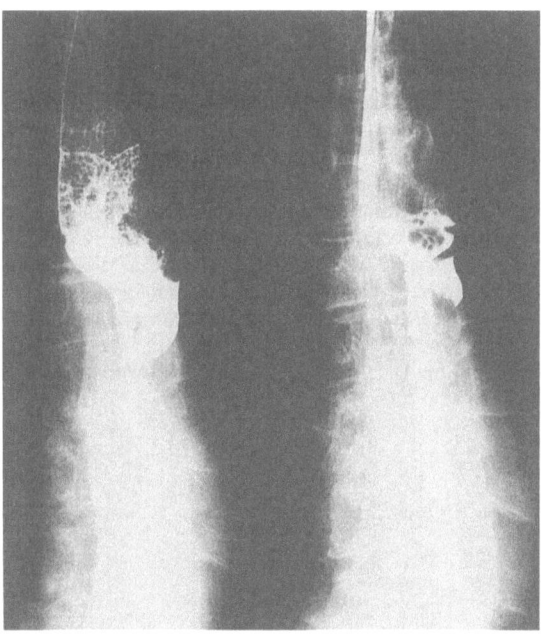

Fig. 9. An extinctive type of prosthesis. Before and after the intubation

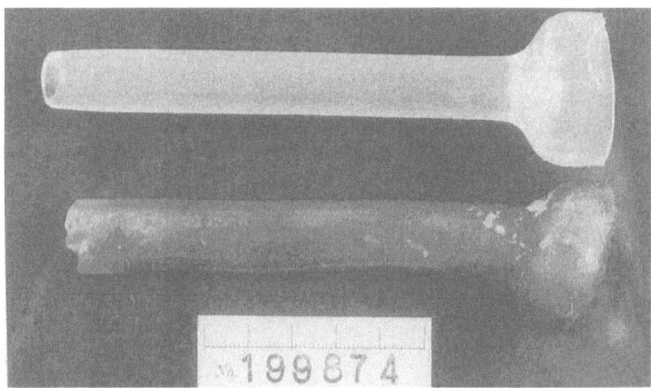

Fig. 10. Extinctive type of prostheses. Before use and 4 days after the intubation was removed from resected esophagus

Historically, esophageal intubation has been used as a last resort. However, with the successful development of our new "extinctive type prosthesis," the doctor will have many more options open to him. The range of indications will be greatly expanded to include all strictures due to esophageal carcinoma.

References

1. Aoyama N, Koizumi H, Abe S, Kurosawa T, Suzuki H, Sekino H (1984) Esophageal prosthesis intubation as a palliative treatment for esophageal stricture. Yokohama Med J 35:35–43
2. Koizumi H, Aoyama N, Akaike M, Sekino H (1986) Through-bougie esophageal prosthesis intubation. In: Kasai M (ed) Esophageal cancer. Excerpta Medica Amsterdam, pp 227–230
3. Majima M, Inoe K, Saito N, Morikawa S, Sakamoto T, Nagamine S (1977) Newly devised esophageal tube: Review of 29 cases. J Jpn Soc Cancer Ther 12:139–148
4. Konno O, Koyama S, Kogure M, Terashima S, Haga Y, Sagawa K, Sato Y, Inoue H, Motoki R (1991) Study on bypass operation and esophageal prosthesis as palliation for unresectable esophageal cancer. Jpn J Gastroenterol Surg 24:1163–1168
5. Angorn IB, Haffejee AA (1988) Endoesophageal intubation for palliation in obstructing esophageal carcinoma. In: Delarue NC, Wilkins EW, Wong J (eds) Esophageal cancer. C.V. Mosby, St. Louis, pp 410–419

Results of Two Types of Substernal Gastric Bypass for Advanced Esophageal Cancer

Toshihiro Hirai, Yoshinori Yamashita, Hidenori Mukaida, Takashi Iwata, Shuji Saeki, and Tetsuya Toge[1]

Introduction

Despite the availability of various devices and the advances which have been made in the field of surgery and radiation therapy, the prognosis of advanced esophageal cancer still remains poor. In fact, most die within 1 year under very miserable conditions.

We considered bypass surgery as a possible treatment of choice for advanced esophageal cancer involving the adjacent organs or that with distant lymph node and/or parenchymatous metastasis. The aim of bypass surgery was to carry out multidisciplinary treatment using radiation, immunochemotherapy and/or hyperthermia under better oral intake.

One hundred and two cases with advanced esophageal cancer were treated with bypass surgery and assessed from 1973 to 1991. The analysis of these cases is presented herein.

Materials and Methods

Patients

From 1973 to 1991, 306 cases of esophageal squamous cell carcinoma were treated at Hiroshima University Hospital. Of these 306 patients, 102 (33.3%) underwent bypass surgery. The indications for bypass surgery were determined as follows: (1) direct invasion to the neighboring organs, (2) distant lymph node or parenchymatous metastasis, and (3) high risk cases due to combined complications.

[1] Department of Surgery, Research Institute for Nuclear Medicine and Biology, Hiroshima University Kasumi 1-2-3, Minami-ku, Hiroshima, 734 Japan

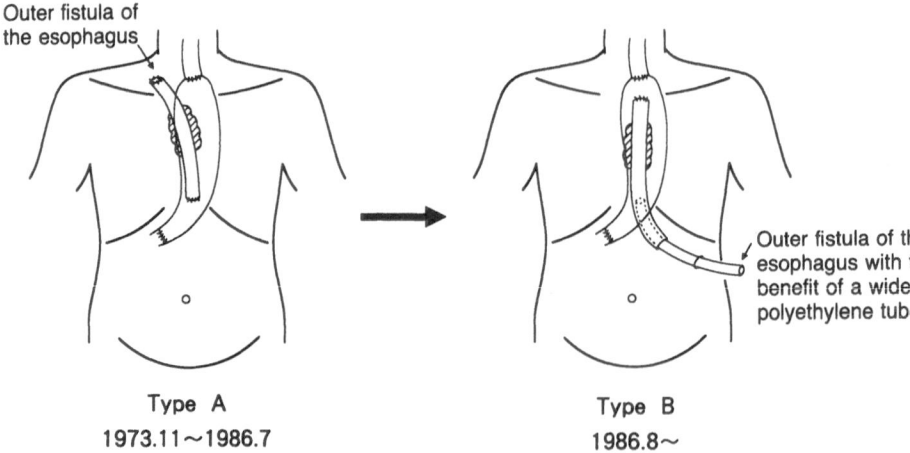

Outer fistula of the esophagus

Outer fistula of the esophagus with the benefit of a wide polyethylene tube

Type A
1973.11~1986.7

Type B
1986.8~

Fig. 1. Two types of operative procedures of substernal gastric bypass

Two types of bypass surgery (Type A and B) were introduced to these 102 cases (Type A in 79 cases and Type B in 23 cases). We will present a detailed analysis of 23 cases of Type B in this paper because that of Type A has already been reported [1].

Operative Methods

Until 1986, we had chosen Type A method as a bypass operation (Fig. 1) wherein the abdominal esophagus is divided and immediately closed by a running suture in advance. Then, the cervical esophagus was divided and the distal esophageal stump was pulled out to the right supraclavicular region for external esophagostomy. The gastric tube or full stomach tube was pulled up to the neck via the retrosternal route and anastomosed to the proximal end of the cervical esophagus after a U-shaped removal of the manubrium sterni. The aim of the esophagostomy was as a means to administer anticancer drugs. From 1981, hyperthermia was introduced as an anticancer modality because it was very easy to perform using the esophagostomy.

The Type B method differs from Type A in that the outer fistula of the esophagus had been made in a downward direction in the left hypochondrial region with the benefit of a wide polyethylene tube, 2 cm in diameter, which was inserted into the proximal end of the divided abdominal esophagus and fixed there. The distal stump of the divided cervical esophagus has been closed by a running suture.

Characteristics of 23 Cases of Type B

Table 1 shows the characteristics of 23 cases who underwent the Type B method. The average longitudinal length of the tumor in x-ray was 9.9 cm. Twenty two of 23 cases showed invasion to the adjacent organs.

Table 1. Characteristics of 23 cases with type B method

Age	51–85 years (average: 63.7 years)
Sex	Male: 19 Female: 4
Location of tumor	Upper thoracic: 5 Middle thoracic: 16 Lower thoracic: 2
X-ray type of tumor	Spiral: 21 Funnel: 2
Longitudinal length of tumor	4.7–15 cm (Average 9.9 cm)
Depth of tumor invasion[a]	22 Cases showed invasion to adjacent organs

[a] Judged by CT and/or others

Preoperative

  Lipiodol - Bleomycin 45 mg inj. into the submucosal layer of the esophagus with endoscope

Postoperative

  1. Initial therapy

     a. EFP therapy (Over 2 cycles every 4 weeks)

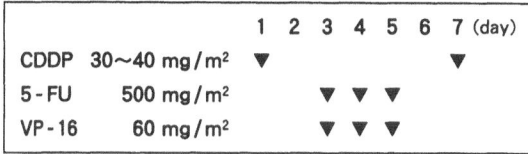

     b. Lineac 10 MV X - ray 60 Gy (long T)

     c. Hyperthermia (43~45 ℃, 60 min. 2 times / week)

     d. LAK therapy

  2. Maintenance therapy

     5 - FU 150~200 mg / day p.o.

Fig. 2. Recent multidisciplinary treatment after bypass operation. *EFP*, CDDP, 5-FU, and VP-16; *CDDP*, cisplatin; *5-FU*, 5-fluorouracil; *VP-16*, etoposide; *LAK therapy*, lymphokine activated killer cell adoptive therapy

Multidisciplinary Treatment After Type B Method

The modalities employed in the multidisciplinary treatment used in the Type B method were quite varied: chemotherapy in 22 cases, radiation therapy in 17 cases, hyperthermia in 8 cases, and lymphokine activated killer cell adoptive immunotherapy (LAK therapy) in 3 cases. Figure 2 shows the most recent schedule employed. Chemotherapy with cisplatin (CDDP), 5-fluorouracil (5-FU), and etoposide (VP-16) (EFP therapy) and radiation therapy were performed concomitantly.

Statistical Analysis

The survival rate was calculated by the method of Kaplan-Meier.

Table 2. Postoperative complications

	Type A	Type B
Anastomotic leakage	25 (31)	5 (26)
Major	9 (11)	1 (4)
Major	16 (20)	5 (22)
Necrosis of the bypass organ	2 (3)	0
Other troubles of the bypass organ	2 (3)	1 (4)
Pneumonia	14 (18)	1 (4)
Pulmonary fibrosis	2 (3)	0
Atelectasis	2 (3)	0
ARDS	1 (1)	0
Lung edema	1 (1)	1 (4)
Renal failure	1 (1)	0
Liver failure	1 (1)	0
Total cases	79	23

ARDS, acute respiratory distress syndrome

Results

Postoperative Complications

The postoperative complications of Type A and B methods are shown in Table 2. Major anastomotic leakage occurred in 11% in the Type A method, but 4% in the Type B method. In Type A, the pulmonary complications of pneumonia, pulmonary fibrosis, atelectasis, adult respiratory distress syndrome (ARDS) and lung edema occurred in 14 cases (18%), 2 cases (3%), 2 cases (3%), 1 case (1%) and 1 case (1%), respectively. In Type B, pneumonia and lung edema occurred in one case (4%) each. Ten (12.6%) of 79 cases of Type A died within 30 days of operation mainly due to pulmonary complications and anastomotic leakage, but no such mortality occurred in Type B. The postoperative complication rate of Type B was much less than that of Type A.

Survival Rate

Figure 3 shows the actuarial survival curve of the cases who underwent a Type A bypass, excluding 10 cases of postoperative death. One-year survival was 13.3% and only 2 cases survived over 5 years. Figure 4 shows the actuarial survival curves of the 23 cases who underwent a Type B bypass. One-year survival rate of the total cases was 36.6%. Furthermore, in the cases without other non-curative factors, except for invasion to the adjacent organs and those who completed postoperative therapy, 1-year survival was 53.9%. Of 23 cases, 19 were able to be discharged from the hospital and live in their homes.

Oral Intake After Type B Method

Figure 5 shows the levels of oral intake after a Type B bypass. As compared with preoperative oral intake, 13 cases (57%) showed improvement, 2 cases

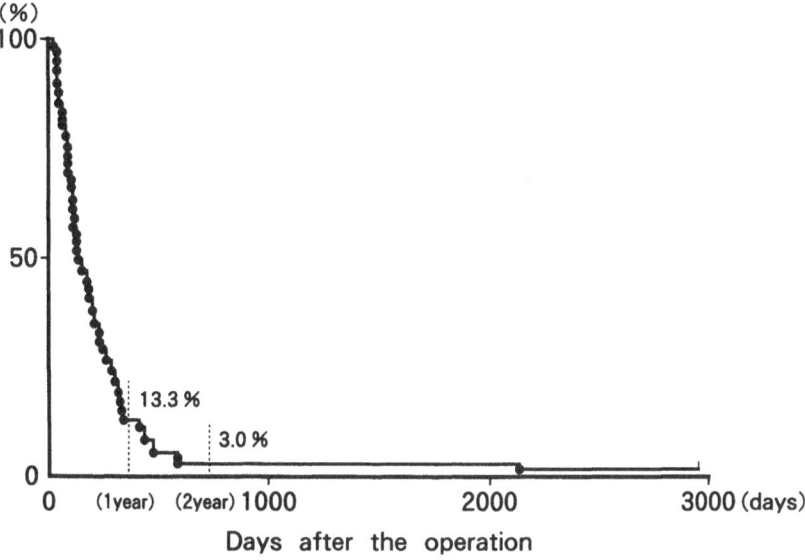

Fig. 3. Actuarial survival curve of patients with Type A method ($n = 69$)

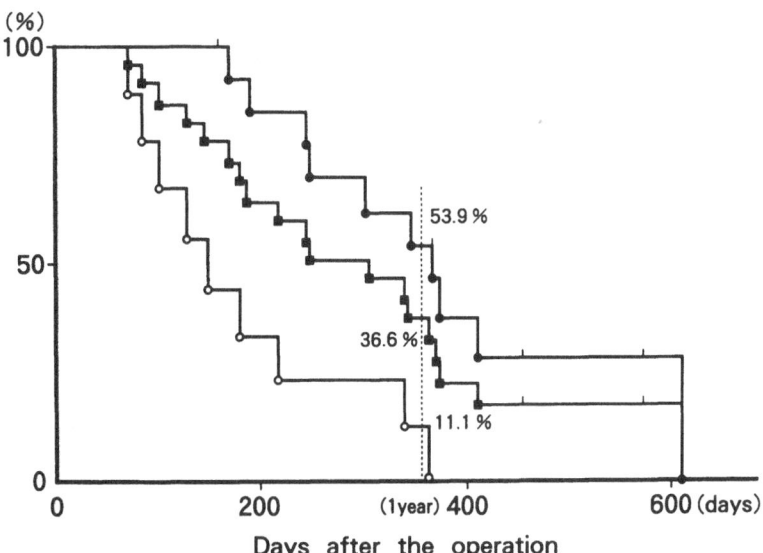

Fig. 4. Actuarial survival curves of patients with Type B method. *Closed circles*, patients without other non-curative factors, except for invasion to the neighboring organ, who have completed postoperative therapy ($n = 14$); *open circles*, other patients ($n = 9$); *closed squares*, total number of patients ($n = 23$)

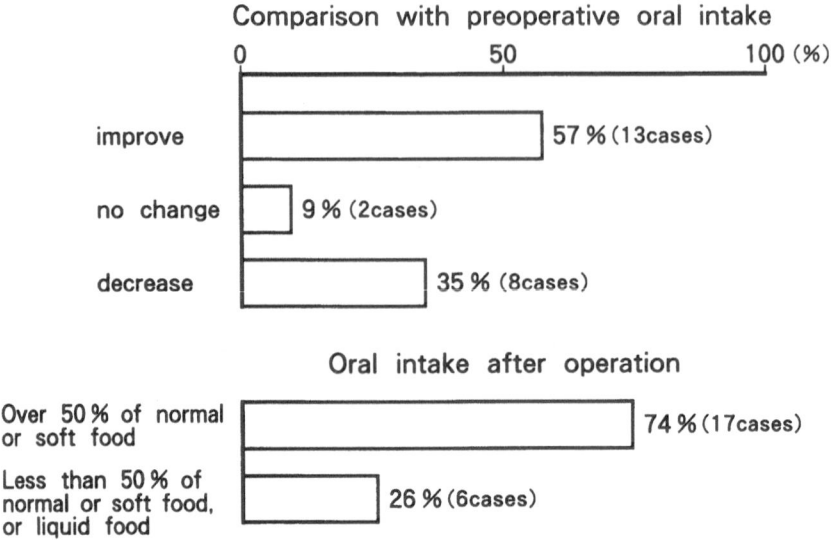

Fig. 5. Oral intake in 23 patients after Type B bypass operation

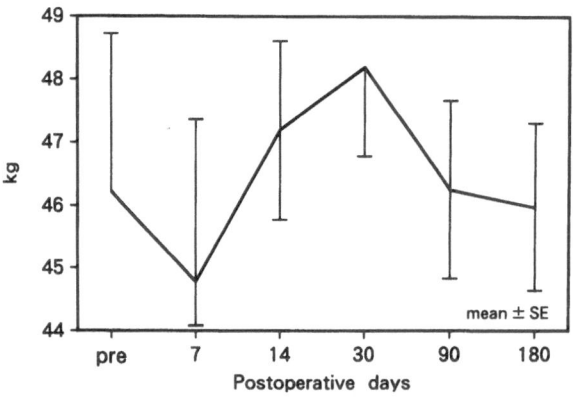

Fig. 6. Changes of the body weight of patients with Type B method

(9%) had no change, and 8 cases (35%) showed a decrease. Seventeen cases (74%) could take more than 50% of normal or soft food after recovery from the operation.

Body Weight Change After Type B Method

Figure 6 shows the changes in body weight after a Type B bypass. The curve revealed quick recovery from the loss of body weight after the operation and good maintenance until 6 months.

Discussion

The optimum method in patients with inoperable advanced esophageal cancer remains controversial. The gastric bypass to these cases is generally disagreeable because it has a high rate of postoperative complications as a palliative surgery [2]. Pulsion intubation or laser therapy are now more popular because they are safe procedure and have high success rate as there is no chance of causing dysphagia [3, 4]. Angorn and Haffejee [4] reported a randomized prospective study of pulsion intubation vs retrosternal gastric bypass for palliation of unresectable carcinoma of the upper thoracic esophagus and concluded that pulsion intubation is the preferred palliative procedure because of fewer complications and a lesser degree of postoperative catabolism. However, survival and relief from dysphagia following intubation or laser therapy are too short as reported [5, 6].

Our aim of the bypass surgery was not only to make oral intake possible but also to carry out the intensive multidisciplinary treatment using radiation, immunochemotherapy and/or hyperthermia under better oral intake and improve their survival. Until 1986, we had chosen the Type A bypass, but there was some difficulty regarding the operative procedure, such as performing esophagostomy in the supraclavicular region, and also had major postoperative complications which resulted in postoperative death in 10 cases (12.7%). These major complications disturbed the postoperative treatments and followed poor prognosis. These facts led us to change the operative procedure to Type B. The Type B method was simpler and easier to perform than Type A. In Type B, an esophagostomy was made in the left hypochondrial region through a wide polyethylene tube. The wide tube was removed 2 or 3 weeks after the operation and the wide fistula remained. The reason for using a wide polyethylene tube was to make a wide fistula to provide easy access of the inner probe used in hyperthermia treatment. Type B showed fewer postoperative complications and no case died within 30 days after operation. Moreover, the 1-year survival rate was 36.6%, and 74% of them could take more than 50% of normal or soft food. These results revealed that the bypass surgery was never a dangerous operation and the intensive multidisciplinary treatment under good conditions contributed to the improvement of the survival rate.

References

1. Hirai T, Yamashita Y, Mukaida H, Kawano K, Toge T, Niimoto M, Hattori T (1989) Bypass operation for advanced esophageal cancer—An analysis of 93 cases. Jpn J Surg 19:182–188
2. Wong J, Lam KH, Wei WI, Ong GB (1981) Results of the Kirschner operation. World J Surg 5:547–552
3. Reimann JF, Lux G, Demling L (1986) Palliative laser treatment of malignant stenosis in the upper gastrointestinal tract. Endoscopy 18:21–26
4. Angorn IB, Haffejee AA (1983) Pulsion intubation vs retrosternal gastric bypass for palliation of unresectable carcinoma of the upper thoracic esophagus. Br J Surg 70:335–338
5. Fuchs KH, Freys SM, Schaube H, Eckstein AK, Selch A, Hamelmann H (1991) Randomized comparison of endoscopic palliation of malignant esophageal stenosis. Surg Endoscop 5:63–67

6. Sander R, Hagenmueller F, Sander C, Riess G, Classen M (1991) Laser versus laser plus afterloading with iridium-[192] in the palliative treatment of malignant stenosis of the esophagus: a prospective, randomized, and controlled study. Gastrointest Endosc 37:433–440

Bypass Operation with Pedicled Jejunum for Unresectable Intrathoracic Esophageal Cancer

Masayuki Higashino, Harushi Osugi, Noriaki Maekawa, and Hiroaki Kinoshita[1]

Introduction

The number of cases of intrathoracic esophageal cancer detected early has been increasing in Japan, but most cases are still advanced when detected. Such cancer readily infiltrates the aorta, trachea, and lungs due to their anatomical proximity, and combined resection can be difficult, often preventing curative excision. The bypass operation performed for such patients is only palliative therapy, but it can make discharge from hospital possible if the patient can eat.

The surgery may prevent aspiration pneumonia when there is an accompanying esophagopulmonary fistula. We once did bypass operations using a gastric tube, but since 1986, we have used a pedicled jejunum. Here, we reviewed patients who underwent bypass operations with a pedicled jejunum, comparing them to those for whom a gastric tube was used, to evaluate the usefulness of Roux-en-Y bypass operation with a pedicled jejunum.

Subjects and Methods

Of the 156 patients with primary intrathoracic esophageal cancer admitted to our hospital from January 1986 to March 1992, resection of the lesion and reconstruction of the digestive tract were performed in 111 cases (71%). Of the 45 other patients, 30 were treated by radiotherapy and chemotherapy only, and 15 underwent a bypass operation. A pedicled jejunum was used in 11 patients and a gastric tube was used in 4 patients. These 15 patients were the subjects.

We compared the two kinds of bypass operations (Fig. 1) in terms of the reason for the operation, operating time, amount of operative bleeding; and

[1] Second Department of Surgery, Osaka City University Medical School, 1-5-7 Asahimachi, Abeno-ku, Osaka, 545 Japan

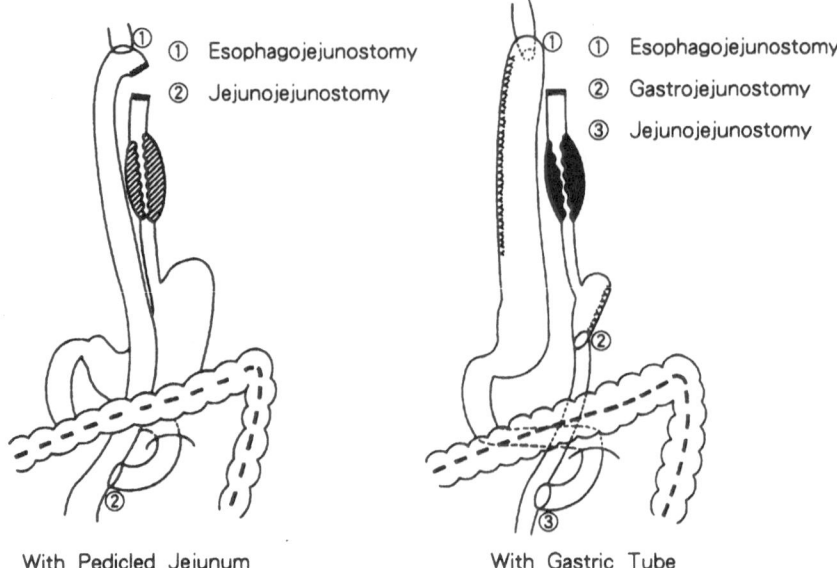

Fig. 1. Bypass operation

whether there was anastomotic leakage, whether there was postoperative pneumonia, whether oral intake was possible after surgery, and whether the patient was discharged. For more meaningful comparison of the operating time and the amount of operative bleeding, the time and amount of bleeding during thoracotomy were subtracted when there was exploratory thoracotomy.

The χ^2 test was used for evaluation of significance.

Results

Reasons for Bypass Surgery

The most common reason for bypass surgery was fistula formation with the trachea or bronchi ($n = 6$). Infiltration to the trachea or bronchi without fistula formation was detected in three patients. Thus, in 9 of the 15 patients (60%), infiltration of the trachea or bronchi was detected. Invasion of the aorta was found in five patients. Thus, except for one patient who underwent surgery because of renal failure, the bypass operation was necessary because of two factors: invasion of the trachea or bronchi, and invasion of the aorta.

Operating Time and the Amount of Bleeding

The mean time of the bypass operation with a pedicled jejunum was 2.8 h (range, 1.5–4 h). The amount of bleeding was between 50 and 435 ml, with a mean of 240 ml.

The mean time of the bypass operation with a gastric tube was 4 h (range,

3–5.5 h). The amount of bleeding was between 305 and 1030 ml, with a mean of 604 ml. The surgery with a pedicled jejunum was better in terms of operating time and amount of bleeding (both, $P < 0.05$).

Anastomotic Leakage

Anastomotic leakage (Table 1) occurred in 2 of the 11 patients undergoing surgery involving a pedicled jejunum. In one case, reoperation was needed because the jejunum had became necrotic at day 3 after surgery. At reoperation, the elevated jejunum in the subcutaneous space, oral to the outlet of the peritoneal cavity, had turned dark red. A hematoma was found in the mesentery in that region, so a returning disturbance of venous blood flow was suspected. In the other case, leakage in the cervical anastomosis was noticed at day 6 after surgery.

Conservative treatment did not lead to spontaneous closure, so reconstruction with a free jejunal graft was performed 2 months later. Anastomotic leakage occurred in one of the four patients undergoing surgery involving a gastric tube.

Postoperative Pneumonia

Before surgery, six patients had an esophagopulmonary fistula and two patients (cases 4 and 7) had aspiration pneumonia (Table 1). The pneumonia resolved after surgery in one case (case 7), but tracheostomy was needed because of postoperative pneumonia in the other. Three of the nine subjects developed postoperative pneumonia due to anastomotic leakage in two cases.

Two of the three patients had undergone bypass with a pedicled jejunum and one patient had undergone bypass with a gastric tube.

Oral Intake After Surgery and Discharge from Hospital

Two of the three patients with anastomotic leakage could not eat normally: one died of liver failure 1 month after surgery, and the other died of pneumonia 4 months after surgery (Table 1). Spontaneous healing of the anastomotic leakage did not occur. The other patient with such leakage underwent a second operation.

Three patients, including the two with untreatable leakage, died in hospital. The other 12 patients were discharged. Nine had undergone surgery with use of a pedicled jejunum and three had undergone surgery with use of a gastric tube.

Discussion

Combined resection of the lung, trachea, and aorta is now being undertaken and is sometimes used for esophageal cancer. We did resection and reconstruction in 111 (71%) of 156 cases of esophageal cancer. In one case, esophagopulmonary fistula and pulmonary abscess called for emergency combined resection of the middle and lower lobe of the right lung and intrathoracic esophagus. However, in most cases, in which the carcinoma is in an advanced stage, there are extensive lymph node and circulatory metastases, and combined resection

Table 1. Postoperative complications and course

	With pedicled jejunum					With gastric tube			
Case	Anastomotic leakage	Pneumonia	Oral intake		Postoperative course	Case	Anastomotic leakage	Pneumonia	Oral intake		Postoperative course
1.	−	−	Yes	8 pod	Discharge	12.	+	+(Tracheostomy)	No		Hospital death
2.	−	−	Yes	7 pod	Discharge	13.	−	−	Yes	8 pod	Discharge
3.	−	−	Yes	7 pod	Discharge	14.	−	−	Yes	8 pod	Discharge
4.	−	+(Tracheostomy)	Yes	15 pod	Hospital death	15.	−	−	Yes	9 pod	Discharge
5.	+(Necrosis)	+(Tracheostomy)	No		Hospital death						
6.	−	−	Yes	7 pod	Discharge						
7.	−	−	Yes	5 pod	Discharge						
8.	−	−	Yes	10 pod	Discharge						
9.	−	−	Yes	7 pod	Discharge						
10.	+	−	Yes	58 pod	Discharge						
11.	−	−	Yes	7 pod	Discharge						

pod, postoperative days

is rarely possible. For unresectable esophageal cancer, radiotherapy and chemo-therapy are used. Many such patients cannot eat normally and aspiration pneumonia occurs because of an esophagopulmonary fistula. We have adapted bypass surgery for such cases.

Generally, unresectable esophageal cancer is treated by bypass operations that use the stomach. However, the risk is high in most patients for whom such surgery is considered, and a safer method is desirable. Patients with an esophagopulmonary fistula, those with severe stenosis in which an esophageal prothesis is impossible, and those with a strong wish to eat normally should be considered for bypass surgery.

Thirteen (87%) of the 15 subjects given a bypass operation could eat normally after surgery, but with esophageal intubation, the figure is less than 10%, and reports state that 30% develop recurrent dysphagia [1] and that 44% have developed tube dysfunction [2]. According to Burt et al. [3], esophageal intubation for 14 patients with esophagopulmonary fistula did not prolong life compared with a palliative treatment. The reason given was that a prosthesis could not block reflux of saliva and gastric contents through the fistula.

When Burt et al. [3] performed bypass surgery using the stomach and colon for 28 patients with an esophagopulmonary fistula, the 30-day mortality rate (25%) was significantly lower than with combined resection and intubation. For these reasons, we prefer bypass surgery to intubation in cases of unresectable esophageal cancer in which oral intake is impossible.

The stomach and colon are often used in bypass surgery, probably because a gastric tube is familiar to surgeons, who use it in reconstruction after esophagectomy.

In 1986, we tried elevation of a pedicled jejunum in case 1, with multiple diverticular of the entire colon after gastrectomy, taking into consideration vascular anastomosis in the mesentery on the proximal side of the jejunum. Results were satisfactory.

The stomach is left intact, so the surgery has little effect on respiratory function. Anastomosis to the remaining part of the stomach and pyloroplasty can be omitted, thus controlling reflux of the gastric contents into the remaining esophagus, which becomes a problem when there is an esophagopulmonary fistula.

We found use of a gastric tube preferable in 4 (33%) of the 15 patients treated since 1986, because the jejunum could not be elevated. The marginal vascular arcades were not continuous in two patients, twisting of the intestine after elevation was predicted from the distance between the intestine and the continuous vascular arcade in one patient, and the mesentery was short and thick due to mesenteric fatty tissue in one case. Barlow [4] examined 257 postmortem cases and reported that 16% had partial disappearance or narrowing of the vascular arcade, and that there was no vascular arcade in 6%.

Of our subjects, reconstruction with a pedicled jejunum would have been possible in two of the four patients given a gastric tube because of the shape of the vascular arcade, but the jejunum was not used because its twisting after elevation was predicted. Such twisting can be prevented by anastomosis of the blood vessels at the cervix so as to divide the blood vessels supplying the marginal vessels in the mesentery into two blood supplies, but we consider this inappropriate except for radical operations.

Lorentz et al. [5] also reported cases in which elevation of the jejunum to the neck was anatomically difficult, although leakage was rare when such elevation was possible.

The main purpose of bypass surgery is to make normal eating possible. The difference in the incidence of anastomotic leakage with a pedicled jejunum and a gastric tube was insignificant, so a pedicled jejunum seemed to be fairly safe. In a recent large-series report [5], leakage occurred in 19% of patients after resection, but in 45% of patients after bypass. In our subjects, 20% (3/15) had leakage after bypass, but again this was higher than the 10% after resection. In the report of Lorentz et al. [5], the leakage rate was 26% with the jejunum and 45% with the whole stomach, and this difference was significant, but in our study, the difference depending on the organ used was not significant.

In 11 (73%) of the 15 subjects, normal eating became possible soon after the operation, and 13 patients were discharged. No significant differences were observed in these points between the two groups. The Roux-en-Y bypass operation with a pedicled jejunum took less time and caused less bleeding, so surgical risk was lower.

References

1. Diamantes T, Mannel A (1983) Oesophageal intubation for advanced oesophageal cancer: The Baragwanath experience. Br J Surg 70:555–557
2. Pfleiderer AG, Goodall P, Holmes GKT (1982) The consequences and effectiveness of intubation in the palliation of dysphagia due to benign and malignant strictures affecting the oesophagus. Br J Surg 69:356–358
3. Burt M, Diehl W, Martini N, Bains MS, Ginsberg RJ, McCormack PM, Rusch VW (1991) Malignant esophagorespiratory fistula: Management options and survival. Ann Thorac Surg 52:1222–1229
4. Barlow TE (1955) Variations in the blood supply of the upper jejunum. Br J Surg 174:473–475
5. Lorentz T, Fok M, Wong J (1989) Anastomotic leakage after resection and bypass for esophageal cancer: Lessons learned from the past. World J Surg 13:472–477

Quality of Life After Laser Therapy in Patients with Inoperable Cancer of the Esophagus and Gastric Cardia

A. Moraldi[1], P. Ginevri[1], C. Iascone[2], S. Stipa[2], and C.U. Casciani[1]

Introduction

Many patients with carcinoma of the esophagus and gastric cardia, when first seen, are inoperable either because of advanced disease or extremely poor general condition. Then the only therapeutic goal in these patients is palliation of dysphagia, to improve their quality of life until death occurs from cachexia, metastatic disease, or cardio-respiratory insufficiency. Resolution of malignant dysphagia with recanalization of the esophagus and gastric cardia by endoscopic Nd:YAG (neodymium:yttrium-aluminum-garnet) laser photocoagulation was introduced in the early 1980s; since that time many patients have been success-fully treated because the method has been accepted more and more in the last few years. In fact, laser therapy has some characteristics such as ease of performance, short or no hospitalization, low morbidity and practically no mortality, which are indispensable for a treatment that is only palliative and for patients with a life expectancy that is usually less than 6 months.

The aim of the study was to assess the real risk-benefit ratio of laser therapy in treating patients with unresectable cancer of the esophagus and esophago-gastric junction, and to evaluate recanalization, failure, and complication rates, and especially the quality of life, considering the degree of relief from dysphagia, necessity of endoscopic follow-up examination or retreatment, and the possibility of hospitalization until death.

---

[1] Clinica Chirurgica, Università degli Studi di Roma "Tor Vergata", Ospedale S. Eugenio, P. le dell'Umanesimo, 10, 00144, Rome, Italy
[2] Istituto di 1ᵃ Clinica Chirurgica, Università degli Studi di Roma "La Sapienza", Viale del Policlinico, 00161, Rome, Italy

Methods

From January 1987 to March 1992, 61 patients with cancer of the esophagus, 25 patients with cancer of the cardia, and 22 patients with anastomotic recurrence after total gastrectomy or esophagectomy, for a total of 108 patients, were referred to our gastrointestinal (GI) endoscopy service. All these patients were inoperable because of advanced stage of disease, poor general condition, cardio-respiratory problems, or because they refused to undergo surgery. There were 81 males and 27 females, with a mean age of 68 years (range 44–92). The laser source was both a contact neodymium:YAG laser (Surgical laser technology; maximal power output of 60 W) and non-contact neodymium:YAG laser (Medilas 2; maximal power output of 100 W). When necessary, patients were previously dilated by Celestin or Savary-Gillard dilators to allow a safer treatment by a retrograde technique. Usually two laser sessions were necessary to obtain a complete tumor recanalization, with a 3- to 4-day interval between sessions. Laser therapy was performed under local anesthesia (tetracaine, administered in tablets form) and, only for patients who so requested, under general sedation by propofol.

Treatments were performed without hospital stay, with the exception of a very few elderly patients, in extremely poor condition, who required hospital admission for a safer and more comfortable treatment. Patients were usually controlled 4 weeks after the first treatment and then every month until death. If a mild dysphagia was present at the time of control, the patient was only dilated; if tumor overgrowth was observed, the patient was retreated by laser. If dysphagia occurred 1–2 weeks after laser therapy, the patient was treated by endoscopic intubation.

Results

Laser therapy was considered successful if the patient could eat a free diet or a semi-solid diet with sufficient calorie intake. Fifty-one out of 61 patients (84%) with cancer of the esophagus were successfully treated and 9 (15%) were considered as failures: 1 patient developed a tracheo-esophageal fistula 3 days after laser therapy and was treated by endoscopic intubation. Eight out of the nine failures were intubated and one patient died before any treatment could be done. Twenty-one out of 25 patients (84%) with cancer of the gastric cardia were successfully recanalized, whereas 3 of the 4 failures were intubated and 1 patient died before any treatment. We had no complications in this series of patients. The dysphagia-free mean time (the time interval during which the patient is able to eat a normal diet after laser therapy), among the 72 recanalized patients with cancer of the esophagus and cardia was 2.5 months and the mean survival 6 months.

It is interesting to point out that adequate recanalization does not always correspond to a successful functional result. If we consider the 86 treated patients with cancer of the esophagus and cardia, in 72 we had an adequate recanalization, but only 60 patients could have a regular diet (that is, 70% of the overall treated patients or 83% of the recanalized patients); 9 patients could eat a semisolid diet (12%); and 3 patients could not eat at all (5%), notwithstanding the patency of the viscus.

In the group of patients with anastomotic recurrence (esophago-jejunostomy after total gastrectomy for cancer of the stomach and intrathoracic esophago-gastroplasty for cancer of the cardia or lower esophagus) 19 out of 22 (86%) were successfully treated and 3 patients must be considered as failures (2 were intubated and 1 died before any treatment). No complications were observed in this group.

Looking at the entire group of 108 patients referred to our Institutions, the reasons why, in 17 cases, we were not able to recanalize the viscus are essentially technical: our inexperience in the first cases (most of the failures), tumors where the infiltrating component was prevalent or stenosing tumors with no possibility of dilatation. In most of the patients with adequate recanalization but persisting dysphagia, the tumor was longer than 7–8 cm, involved the esophageal muscle for a long segment and, in some instances, the esophagopharyngeal junction.

A few patients underwent laser therapy only once because they died within the first 2 months of follow-up. The majority of patients were treated twice, and in fact a second laser treatment usually associated with one or more dilatations, provided a good palliation until death occurred. Only four patients were hospitalized, a few days before they died for extremely poor general condition and severe cachexia.

Discussion

In patients with carcinoma of the esopnagus and gastric cardia, at the time of presentation, the disease is very aften too advanced to be radically cured; then palliation of dysphagia is the most important therapeutic goal. The ideal palliative treatment should provide normal swallowing by a quick and safe method with a short hospital stay, low complication rate, and no mortality. Surgery is an excellent method of palliation but related morbidity and mortality rates are too high; surgical intubation has been generally abandoned in favor of the more practical endoscopic method, which involves less morbidity. The role of radical radiotherapy, intracavitary radiation, or chemotherapy must still be defined; in many patients treatment is not terminated because of worsening of dysphagia, side effects, or progressive deterioration. Laser therapy at present seems to be the most attractive method; the resolution rate of dysphagia is very high, with no complications and no hospital stay, the treatment is low cost, and if necessary, may be repetitive. A recent study on long-term results of endoscopic laser therapy tried to define parameters that could predict the long-term outcome in order to better define the indications and limitations of Nd:YAG laser therapy [1]. Improvement after initial laser treatment, a tumor length of 6 cm, and adenocarcinoma confirmed by histology, were the most significant parameters affecting long-term outcome. It is interesting to note that for patients with advanced carcinoma or squamous cell carcinoma, the cumulative probability of remaining symptomatically improved at 3 months was almost the same, but the difference became significant at 6 months. This effect of histology, according to the authors, is probably the result of differences in tumor kinetics, and the fact that adenocarcinoma has a longer doubling time than squamous cell carcinoma. On the other hand, another prospective study trying to define parameters of survival during laser treatment [2], revealed that survival was statistically independent of histology, location, and length of tumor. In contrast, this study found that the relationship between survival and the degree of stenosis and dysphagia both before and after laser treatment was significant. These data support the concept that adequate nutrition is extremely important in these debilitated patients.

In fact, there are reports in the international literature which describe an increased survival for patients treated by laser. Siegel et al. [3] demonstrated a 70% improvement in survival for patients so treated compared to the control group. The mechanisms by which laser therapy prolongs survival are not clear and the authors include these possibilities: decreased tumor bulk, improved nutrition with improvement of immune function, decreased incidence of aspiration pneumonia, an increased sense of well-being depending on the resolution of dysphagia that is extremely important also from a psychological point of view.

If we look at the more recent trials of laser therapy and endoscopic intubation for palliation of malignant dysphagia, we can state that both methods are successful in relieving dysphagia but the complication rate and mortality are much higher in the intubated group; moreover, for patients treated by laser, the long-term results in terms of recurrent dysphagia and quality of life are much better [4–6].

Laser therapy and intubation are effective in relieving dysphagia and both should be considered to be complementary to each other. For patients in poor general condition, endoscopic intubation may be the treatment of choice because it provides speedy palliation and obviates the need for repeat treatments; for all other patients, laser therapy should be attempted first.

If the result is good, further treatment sessions can be arranged to prolong palliation; if the result is mediocre, endoscopic intubation should be considered.

Laser therapy is also indicated for patients with tight, impassable stricture, if the tumor occurs high in the esophagus, if it is largely exophytic, or if it has caused significant bleeding [6].

In conclusion, laser therapy, when possible, is the best method of palliation because it is a low-risk procedure, resolution of dysphagia can be achieved in most cases, and it offers a good quality of life until death occurs.

References

1. Naveau S, Chiesa A, Poynard T, Chapt JC (1990) Endoscopic Nd:YAG laser therapy as palliative treatment for esophageal and cardial cancer. Dig Dis Sci 35:295–301
2. Stange EF, Dylla J, Fleig WE (1989) Laser treatment of upper gastrointestinal tract carcinoma: Determinants of survival. Endoscopy 21:254–257
3. Siegel HI, Laskin KJ, Dabezies MA, Fisher RS, Krevsky B (1991) The effect of endoscopic laser therapy on survival in patients with squamous cell carcinoma of the esophagus. J Clin Gastroenterol 13:142–146
4. Loizou LA, Grigg D, Atkinson M, Robertson C, Bown SG (1991) A prospective comparison of laser therapy and intubation in endoscopic palliation for malignant dysphagia. Gastroenterology 100:1303–1310
5. Hahl J, Salo J, Ovaska J, Haapiainen R, Kalima T, Schroder T (1991) Comparison of endoscopic Nd:YAG laser therapy and esophageal tube in palliation of esophagogastric malignancy. Scand J Gastroenterol 26:103–108
6. Barr H, Krasner N, Raoul A, Walker RJ (1990) Prospective randomized trial of laser therapy only and laser therapy followed by endoscopic intubation for the palliation of malignant dysphagia. Gut 31:252–258

Preoperative Total Parenteral Nutrition in Patients with Cancer of the Esophagus or Stomach

Heinz Becker, Ansgar Roehrborn, Christoph Ebener, and Hans Dietrich Roeher[1]

Introduction

Poor nutritional status is known to have a negative impact on perioperative morbidity and mortality. At the time of hospital admission, up to 80% of cancer patients present with a reduced nutritional status [1]. However, attempts to improve the nutritional situation prior to surgery even by means of preoperative total parenteral nutrition (TPN) often failed [2]. Therefore, the role of preoperative TPN in patients with cancer of the esophagus or stomach is still controversial.

Patients and Methods

Between January 1990 and June 1992, 191 patients were admitted for cancer of the esophagus or stomach to our hospital. Only patients in whom esophagectomy or gastrectomy was planned were eligible for the study. After informed consent had been obtained, 122 patients were stratified according to their nutritional risk. Patients were of high risk if two of three criteria were positive (albumin <3500 mg/dl; prealbumin <21.8 mg/dl; body weight <95% ideal body weight). High risk (HR) patients were randomized to receive preoperatively either a low caloric TPN (HR-LC) ⟨250 g of glucose, 50 g amino acids 1400 kcal⟩ or a high caloric TPN (HR-HC) ⟨250 g glucose, 100 g amino acids, 100 g fat, 2350 kcal⟩ regimen. Low risk patients (LR) received either the high caloric total parenteral nutrition (LR-HC) or volume substitution (50 g glucose). All regimens were equal in volume (2500 ml), trace elements, and vitamins. Infusion was given for 7–14 days prior to surgery. Infusion solutions used were: Aminoplasmal PO® and

---

[1] Department of Surgery, Heinrich-Heine University, Düsseldorf, Moorenstraße 4, D-1000 Düsseldorf, Germany

Table 1. Preoperative nutritional status at time of admisson

	High risk ($n = 22$)	Low risk ($n = 43$)
Age (years)	61 (53.7/66.5)6	59 (50/64)
Height (cm)	172 (165/178)	174 (169/179)
Weight (kg)	63.5 (56/75)	76 (69/83)
BW (% IBW)	96.5 (82/114)	107 (100/115)
Weight loss (kg)	6.5 (1.5/11.3)	5 (0/5)
Tot, prot (g/dl)	7.2 (7/7.8)	7.4 (6.9/7.7)
Albumin (g/dl)	3.35 (3/3.59)	3.97 (3.58/4.4)
Prealb. (mg/dl)	19.3 (815.2/20.2)	24.7 (22.8/27.1)
Transf. (mg/dl)	255 (205/284)	260 (227/291)

BW, body weight; *IBW*, ideal body weight; *Tot Prot*, total protein; *Prealb*, prealbumin

Table 2. Postoperative complications

	HR-LC ($n = 10$)	HR-HC ($n = 12$)	LR-Vol ($n = 17$)	LR-HC ($n = 26$)
Death (30 days)	1 (10%)	0	0	1 (4%)
Death (hospital)	1 (10%)	0	0	1 (4%)
Sepsis	2 (20%)	0	3 (18%)	5 (19%)
Pneumonia	2 (20%)	1 (8%)	4 (24%)	4 (15%)
Wound problems	2 (20%)	1 (8%)	5 (29%)	6 (23%)
Anastomotic Leak	2 (20%)	1 (8%)	6 (35%)	8 (30%)
Reintubation	1 (10%)	1 (8%)	3 (18%)	3 (12%)
Renal failure	0	0	0	0
Postop stay (days)	18.5 (12/31)	15 (13/18)	20 (15/34)	25.5 (15/40)

HR, high risk; *LR*, low risk; *HC*, high caloric TNP (total parenteral nutrition); *LC*, low caloric TNP; *LR-Vol*, low risk volume substitution

Lipofundin MCT® 20% (Braun Melsungen, Germany). Fifty-seven patients were excluded from the study because the planned therapy was changed or the TPN was not performed according to the protocol.

Results

Sixty-five patients remained in the study, of whom were 22 were high risk and 43 were low risk. The nutritional status of both groups is shown in Table 1. The analysis of preoperative risk factors, intraoperative management and tumor pathology was comparable between the treatment groups in each stratification arm.

The overall mortality of all patients remaining in the study was low, 3% (2/65). High risk patients seemed to improve from preoperative high caloric TPN (Table 2). The rate of severe complications (e.g., pneumonia, anastomotic leakage, sepsis, death) and the number of complications in each patient (Fig. 1)

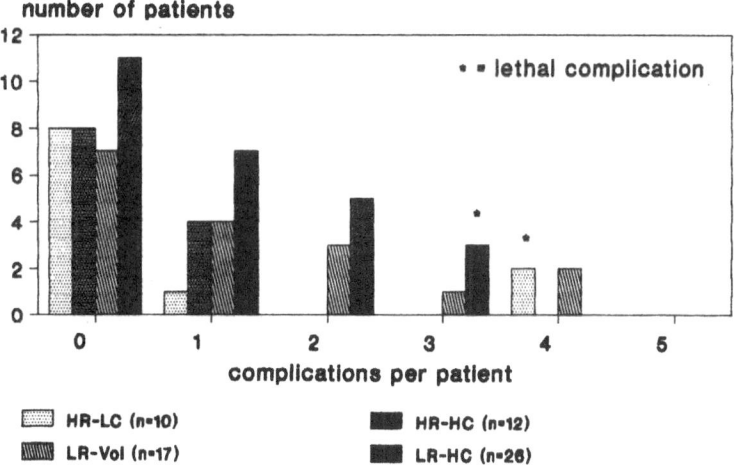

Fig. 1. Preoperative TPN: postoperative complications. Multiple complications in each patient: anastomotic leak, sepsis, pneumonia, reintubation, acute renal failure, severe infection (peritonitis, mediastinitis, phlegmonia, abscess). *TPN*, total parenteral nutrition; *HR-LC*, high risk-low caloric; *HR-HC*, high risk-high caloric; *LR-HC*, low risk-high caloric; *LR-Vol*, low risk-volume substitution

were lower in patients treated with preoperative high caloric TPN for at least 7 days. As expected, low risk patients did not show a difference in the postoperative outcome between the two preoperative treatment arms.

Conclusion

High caloric preoperative TPN seems to reduce perioperative morbidity and mortality in patients with cancer of the esophagus or stomach who had a poor nutritional status at the time of admission to the hospital. Therefore, our results confirm findings of the Veterans Affairs Total Parenteral Nutrition Cooperative Study Group that have been published recently [3].

References

1. Dewys WD, Begg GG, Lavin PT, et al (1980) Prognostic effect of weight loss prior to chemotherapy in cancer patients. Am J Med 69:491–497
2. Klein S, Simes J, Blackburn GL (1986) Total parenteral nutrition and cancer clinical trials. Cancer 58:1378–1386
3. Veterans Affairs Total Parenteral Nutrition Cooperative Study Group. (1991) Perioperative total parenteral nutrition in surgical patients. N Engl J Med 325:525–532

Pulmonary Function During Exercise Before and After Radical Esophagectomy for Esophageal Cancer

FUMIKAZU MAEDA, MASAYUKI HIGASHINO, HARUSHI OSUGI,
NORIAKI MAEKAWA, and HIROAKI KINOSHITA[1]

Introduction

For radical esophagectomy, branches of the vagus nerve, the posterior plexus, and the bronchial artery often resected to complete lymph node dissection. These injuries can be a cause of late postoperative pulmonary complications. However, spirometory shows minimal differences between patients with and without such injuries. To clarify the relationship between such injuries and late pulmonary complications, we did exercise tests before esophagectomies and again in the late postoperative stage.

Patients and Methods

Twenty patients (16 men and 4 women), who underwent radical esophagectomy, were studied by spirometory and an exercise test on two occasions, once before surgery and again at least 3 months after surgery (Table 1). The esophagus was reconstructed with the gastric roll in 17 patients and with the colon in 3. Postoperative spirometory was done 3–18 months after surgery, and the exercise test was done 4–17 months after surgery. In the exercise test, a bicycle ergometer was used, with stepwise increments in the workload, and heart rate (HR), tidal volume (TV), ratio of dead space (VD/TV), O_2 uptake ($\dot{V}O_2$), and CO_2 output ($\dot{V}CO_2$) were measured (RM-300, Minato Medical Science Company, Osaka, Japan). Partial pressure of oxygen in arterial blood (PaO_2) and partial pressure of carbon dioxide in arterial blood ($PaCO_2$) were analyzed with the patient both at rest and during maximum exercise.

[1] Second Department of Surgery, Osaka City University Medical School, 1-5-7 Asahi-machi, Abeno-ku, Osaka, 545 Japan

Table 1. Clinical features of patients

Patient	Age	Sex	Smoking history	Weight (kg)		Area of body surface (m²)		Hugh-Jones		Symptom limit		N	n	Lymph node dissection
				(Pre)	(Post)	(Pre)	(Post)	(Pre)	(Post)	(Pre)	(Post)			
1	43	M	–	61	51	1.64	1.51	1	1	FA	FA	3	0	+
2	63	F	–	53	42	1.42	1.28	1	3	FA	D	0	0	–
3	73	M	–	57	57	1.53	1.55	1	3	FA	FA	0	0	–
4	63	F	–	52	40	1.39	1.26	1	2	FA	D	0	0	–
5	66	M	+	68	54	1.75	1.58	1	–	D	D	3	3	+
6	60	M	+	59	58	1.61	1.60	1	–	FA + P	FA	3	3	+
7	66	F	–	49	40	1.38	1.27	1	2	P	D	2	2	+
8	56	M	+	60	50	1.70	1.58	1	1	P	FA	2	0	+
9	63	M	+	51	39	1.52	1.37	1	3	FA	D	2	2	+
10	64	M	+	63	53	1.69	1.59	1	1	FA	FA	2	2	+
11	50	M	+	41	38	1.36	1.33	1	2	FA	D	2	0	+
12	66	M	+	52	46	1.51	1.45	1	2	FA	D	2	0	+
13	49	M	+	40	44	1.30	1.37	1	1	P	D	3	2	+
14	59	M	+	51	47	1.49	1.40	1	3	FA	D	2	2	+
15	59	M	+	55	51	1.65	1.60	1	1	FA	D	0	0	–
16	56	M	+	42	38	1.38	1.32	1	2	D	D	3	3	+
17	77	M	–	55	45	1.61	1.47	1	2	FA	D	0	0	–
18	57	M	+	41	39	1.35	1.32	1	2	FA	D	2	2	+
19	58	F	–	39	35	1.26	1.20	1	2	FA	D	4	0	+
20	77	M	–	55	45	1.61	1.47	1	2	D	D	2	0	–

M, male; F, female; FA, fatigue; D, dyspnea; P, palpitation; N, macroscopic findings of lymph node metastasis; n, microscopic findings of lymph node metastasis

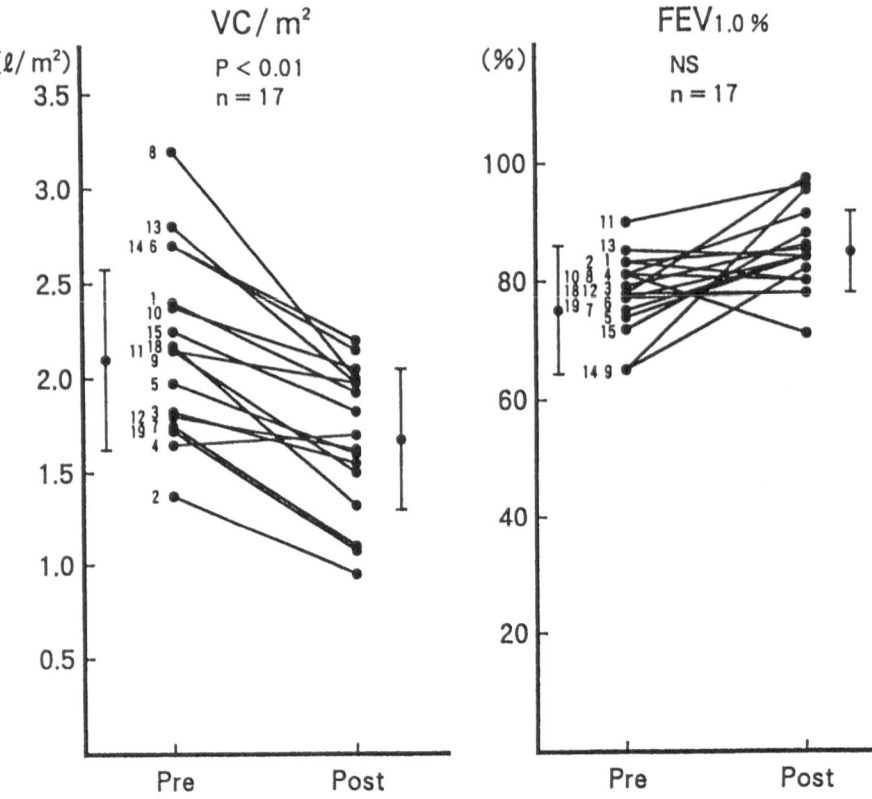

Fig. 1. The vital capacity (*VC*) was lower after surgery than before, but the forced expiratory volume (*FEV*)$_{1.0\%}$ was unchanged

Results

Before surgery, all patients were at stage 1 of the Hugh-Jones dyspnea scale. After surgery, five patients were at stage 1, nine were at stage 2, and four were at stage 3.

The vital capacity (VC) was lower after surgery than before ($P < 0.01$ for both), but the forced expiratory volume (FEV)$_{1.0\%}$ was unchanged (Fig. 1).

Before surgery, exercise was limited by fatigue in 14 patients and by dyspnea in 3 patients. After surgery, exercise was limited by fatigue in 5 patients and by dyspnea in 15 patients. In seven patients, the reasons for stopping exercise were the same before and after surgery.

The TV during maximum exercise was lower after surgery than before ($P < 0.01$).

The $\dot{V}O_2$ during maximum exercise was lower after surgery than before (23.2 vs 20.7 ml/min/kg, $P < 0.01$) (Fig. 2). The $\dot{V}CO_2$ during maximal exercise was also lower after surgery than before ($P < 0.01$).

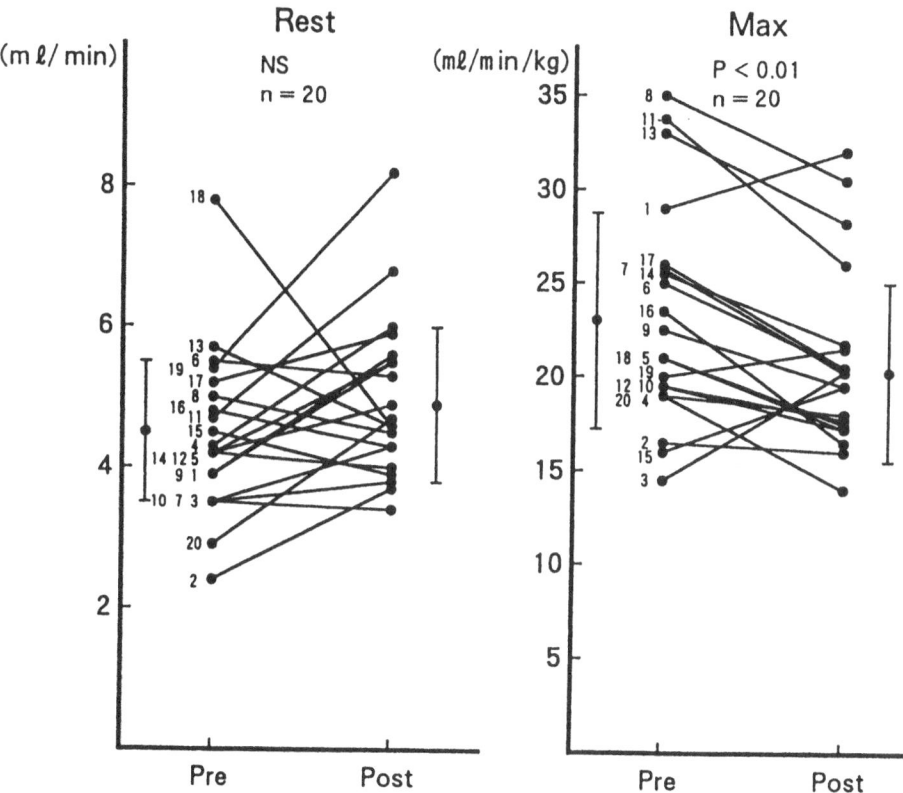

Fig. 2. The $\dot{V}O_2$ at rest was unchanged, but the $\dot{V}O_2$ during maximum exercise was lower after surgery than before (23.2 vs 20.7 ml/min/per kg)

The $\dot{V}O_2$ during maximum exercise and the VC were lower after surgery in the 14 patients who underwent radical dissection, but not in the other 6 patients. These values were also lower after surgery in patients with a history of smoking, but not in those without smoking. The patients were divided into two groups based on age (mean $\geq$ 60, mean $<$ 60), but the VC was not changed, and the $\dot{V}O_2$ was lower after surgery in the older group.

There was no difference between the mean HR at rest. The HR at maximum exercise was lower after surgery than before. (146.0 vs 139.2 beat/min). When the patients were classified by age, history of smoking, or type of operation, there were no differences in HR at maximum exercise based on the width of lymph node dissection.

The O_2 pulse ($\dot{V}O_2$/HR) at maximum exercise was lower after surgery than before (8.21 vs 6.75 ml O_2/beat, $P < 0.01$).

There were no differences in PaO_2 or in $PaCO_2$ either at rest or during maximum exercise based on the width of lymph node dissection.

Discussion

Pulmonary complications in the early postoperative stage have been examined in many cases, but little work has done to study such complications in the late stage. We evaluated the respiratory function in the late stage using the exercise test.

Williams and Brenowitz [1] reported that preoperative spirometory was useful for predicting postoperative pulmonary complications. Subsequently, VC and quadrant diagram using $FEV_{1.0\%}$ have been widely used. Recently, the differences in the effect of various factors, such as surgical procedures and operating time have been examined.

In the patients with esophageal cancer, a study on the relation between the preoperative respiratory function and postoperative pulmonary complications stated that vital capacity, forced expiratory volume 0.5 s percent ($FEV_{0.5\%}$), $FEV_{1.0\%}$, and maximum ventilatory volume (MVV) were correlated with late postoperative pulmonary complications [2, 3].

In this study, a significant decrease in VC is observed postoperatively, but there is no significant difference in the $FEV_{1.0\%}$. The respiratory pattern in exercise becomes shallow and rapid compared with the preoperative state and the influence of restrictive defect impairment becomes more clear due to exercise in the postoperative late stage (Fig. 3). The maximum $\dot{V}O_2$ and maximum $\dot{V}CO_2$ are respiratory measures in exercise and used as parameter showing the maximum capacity for locomotion. A significant decrease in the maximum $\dot{V}O_2$ and in maximum $\dot{V}CO_2$ suggest a decrease in exercise tolerance postoperatively. We think that changes in the respiratory pattern with exercise worsen the ventilatory efficiency during gas exchange and cause fatigue of the respiratory muscles, leading to suspension of exercise. Comparison of the causes of suspension at the largest movement before and after the operation seems to suggest this.

Next, we divided patients into groups to investigate related factors. The effects observed in the postoperative late stage were stronger in the patients who underwent 3-region lymph node dissection, smokers, and patients over the age of 60. Thus, we consider that various preoperative and perioperative factors affect the quality of life of patients in the postoperative late stage.

Conclusion

After surgery, all patients developed restrictive ventilatory impairment: the VC was decreased, and there was no change in $FEV_{1.0\%}$.

Radical dissection and a history of smoking can contribute to pulmonary restriction long after surgery. Esophagectomy caused no chronic change in blood gases, probably because the patients had had enough time to compensate for some of the changes in lung volume. Ventilation during exercise after surgery was faster and shallower than it had been during exercise before surgery. This pattern of ventilation can be important in exercise limitation by impairing gas exchange and by causing ventilatory muscle fatigue. Restrictive ventilatory impairment is the main long-term pulmonary complication of surgery for esophageal cancer. This complication is accentuated by exercise, particularly if it includes radical dissection.

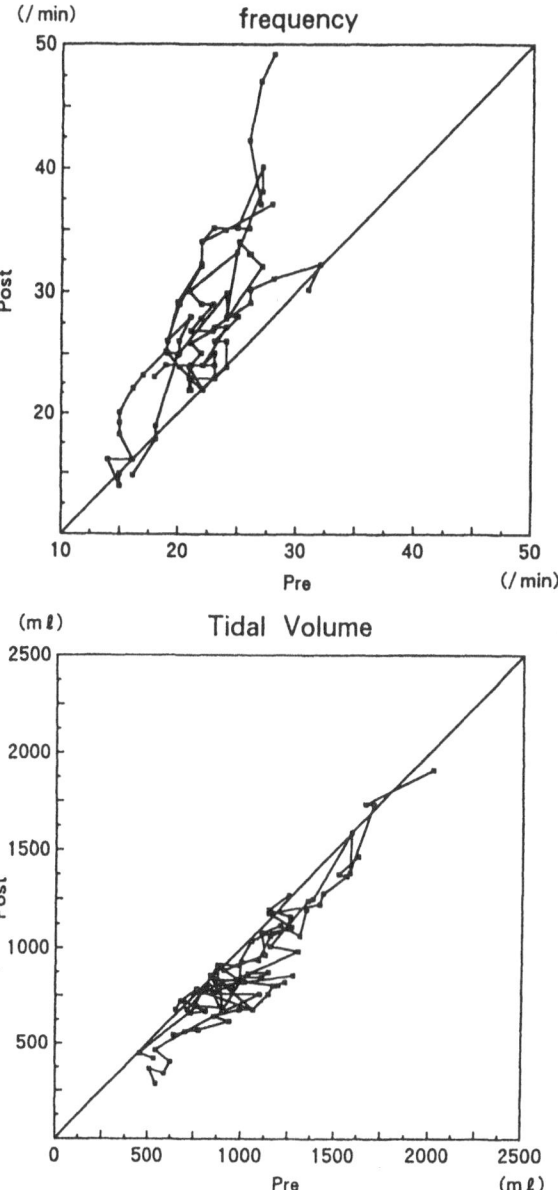

Fig. 3. The respiratory pattern in exercise becomes shallow and rapid compared with the preoperative state

References

1. Williams CD, Brenowitz JB (1976) "Prohibitive" lung function and major surgical procedures. Am J Surg 132:763–766
2. Doki K, Sannohe Y, Hiratsuka R, Shirakusa T (1980) Study on relation between the preoperative exam for the pulmonary function and the postoperative respiratory complications after surgical treatment of patients with esophageal cancer. Journal of Japanese Association for Thoracic Surgery 28:51–58
3. Oomori T (1967) Postoperative pulmonary complication following radical operation for cancer of esophagus and cardia. Journal of Japanese Association for Thoracic Surgery 15:40–52

Recombinant Human Growth Hormone Improves Postoperative Protein Retention of Patients Receiving Esophagectomy

Tsuguhiko Tashiro, Kazuya Takagi, Yoshiya Mashima, Hideo Yamamori, Masahiko Nishizawa, and Nobuyuki Nakajima[1]

Introduction

Surgical treatment for esophageal cancer, which includes thoracotomy, laparotomy, and three-field lymph node dissection [1] followed by reconstruction, is one of the most severe operative procedures resulting in an increased protein catabolism with supressed immune function. Growth hormone has a strong anabolic effect and became applicable for clinical use owing to the availability of recombinant human growth hormone (rhGH) by the development of bioengineering techniques. The effects of rhGH in the stressed state were investigated experimentally and clinically.

Materials and Methods

Experimental Study

Thirty-one Sprague-Dawley male rats (purchased from Takasugi Farm, Japan) weighing approximately 200 g were catheterized into the superior vena cava and were fed exclusively by total parenteral nutrition (TPN) [2] providing 6.2 g of amino acid/kg per day and 200 kcal/kg per day. Six days later, a 20% third degree scald burn was made on the back of the rats by dipping into 95°C water for 15 s. Recombinant human growth hormone (rhGH) of 200 mU per day was given subcutaneously to 16 rats for 3 consecutive days pre- and postburn days (GH group). The same volume of saline was given to 15 rats (Control group).

Urinary excretion of total nitrogen and 3-methylhistidine (3-MH) were measured every day before and after burns. Twenty-four hours after burn,

---

[1] The First Department of Surgery, Chiba University Medical School, 18-1 Inohana, Chuo-ku, Chiba, 260 Japan

Table 1. Effects of recombinant human growth hormone on liver, skeletal muscle, and whole body retertion of burned rats

	NB mg N/day	S g prot/day	B	Liver N mg N	Muscle N mg N	3-MH mg/day
"HGH" (n = 16)	17 ± 54*	2.8 ± 0.6**	2.7 ± 0.3**	210 ± 21**	36 + 2**	0.48 ± 0.10
"Control" (n = 15)	23 ± 42	2.3 ± 0.3	2.5 ± 0.2	176 ± 31	28 ± 3	0.47 ± 0.11

M ± SD. * $P < 0.05$, ** $P < 0.01$ vs "Control"

HGH, human growth hormone; *3-MH*, 3-methylhistidine; *prot*, protein; *N*, nitrogen

whole-body protein turnover was measured according to the method of Stein et al. [3] modified in our laboratory.

After the determination of whole-body protein turnover, all rats were sacrified. Liver and gastrocnemius muscle were taken and stored frozen. Nitrogen content of liver and skeletal muscle protein were measured by the Micro-Kjeldahl method.

Clinical Study

Thirteen patients receiving esophagectomy for thoracic esophageal cancer, the invasion depth of which were assessed as M or SM with No by the intra- and postoperative macroscopic findings, were divided into two groups (GH and Control). Six patients received 24 IU/day of rhGH for 5 consecutive post-operative days by constant intravenous infusion with TPN (GH group). Saline was infused to seven patients (Control group). All patients were fed exclusively by TPN pre- and postoperatively providing 2.0 g/kg per day of amino acid and 30 kcal/kg per day.

Urinary excretion of total nitrogen and 3-MH were measured every day. Serum GOT, GPT, creatinin, blood urea nitrogen (BUN), and total bilirubin were also measured. Whole-body protein turnover was measured preoperatively and on the 3rd postoperative day (3 POD) by the constant infusion of ^{15}N-glycine, which has been previously described [4].

The study protocol was approved by the Ethics Committee of Chiba University Medical School, Chiba, Japan. Informed consent was obtained prior to conducting these studies.

Results

Experimental Study

Nitrogen balance on the first postburn day was -22.8 ± 41.9 mg N/day in the Control group, whereas 16.6 ± 53.9 mg N/day in the GH group (Table 1). Improvement in the nitrogen balance following the administration of rhGH in burned rats was statistically significant ($P < 0.01$).

Whole-body protein turnover (Q) was 3.7 ± 0.2 g · protein/day in the Control group, whereas if was found to be 4.0 ± 0.4 g · protein/day in the GH group, which was significantly higher than control ($P < 0.01$). Whole-body protein syn-

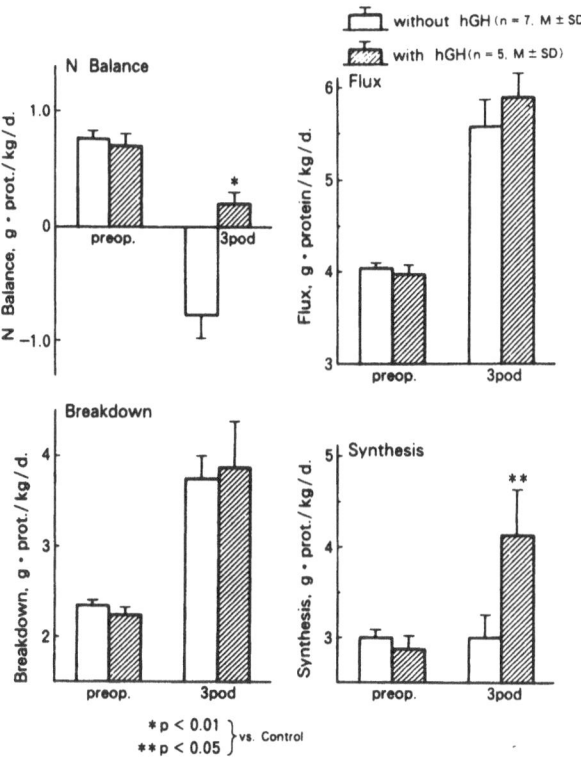

Fig. 1. Pre- and postoperative protein kinetics in patients who underwent esophagectomy with or without rhGH. *rhGH*, recombinant human growth hormone; *N*, nitrogon; *POD*, postoperative day

thesis (S) and breakdown (B) were both significantly greater in the GH group when compared with controls. The increase of synthesis was far greater than that of breakdown in the GH group. Nitrogen content of liver and gastrocnemius muscle were both significantly greater in the GH group when compared with those in the Control group ($P < 0.01$, and $P < 0.01$, respectively). Urinary excretion of 3-MH, however, was not significantly different between the groups.

Clinical Study

Positive nitrogen balance is rarely observed in patients who received esophagectomy. Cumulative nitrogen balance 2–5 POD was -273.6 ± 97.6 mg N/kg per day in control patients. In the patients who received rhGH, however, a positive nitrogen balance of 70.2 ± 55.3 mg N/kg per day was achieved. The improvement of nitrogen retention was statistically significant ($P < 0.01$).

Whole-body protein flux, synthesis, and breakdown tended to increase in the patients who received rhGH postoperatively. Above all, whole-body protein synthesis on 3 POD of 4.5 ± 0.7 g · protein/kg per day in the GH group was significantly greater than that of 3.0 ± 0.6 g · protein/kg per day observed in the

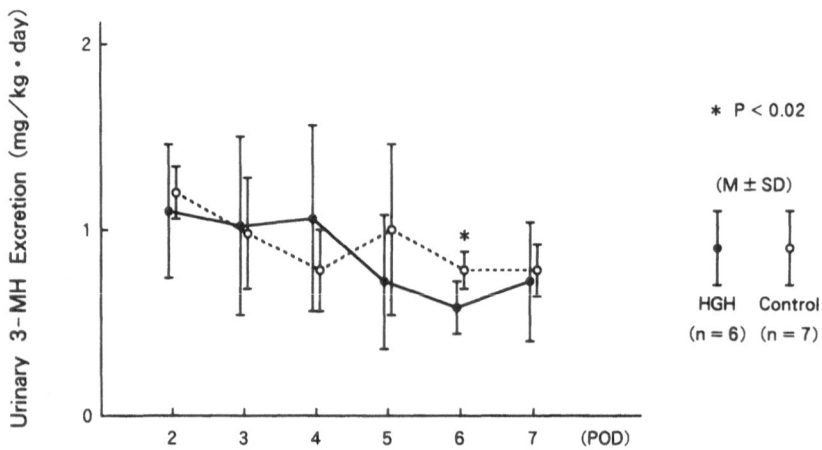

Fig. 2. Daily urinary excretion of 3-methylhistidine (*3-MH*) in patients fed by TPN with or without rhGH following esophagectomy. *TPN*, total parenteral nutrition; *rhGH*, recombinant human growth hormone

Control group ($P < 0.01$, Fig. 1). Urinary excretion of 3-MH demonstrated no significant difference between the groups with and without rhGH throughout the study (Fig. 2).

Serum GOT and GPT showed slight elevation postoperatively, but no difference was observed between the groups (Fig. 3). BUN and total bilirubin were lower in the patients with rhGH, and the differences were statistically significant on the late postoperative days (Fig. 4).

Discussion

We reported the improvement of nitrogen retention and protein kinetics by increasing the dose level of amino acid of TPN in moderately stressed states such as in the early postoperative phase following gastrectomy or colorectal operation, but not in the severely stressed patients receiving esophagectomy [5].

Growth hormone is well known to promote the increase of lean body mass. Our experimental study demonstrated that 200 mU/day of rhGH to the burned rats significantly improved nitrogen retention. In the clinical study, 24 IU/day of rhGH significantly improved postoperative nitrogen retention, and made it possible to achieve a positive nitrogen balance even in an early postoperative period of the patients receiving esophagectomy. Approximately 20 IU/day of rhGH reportedly improved the nitrogen balance of stable malnourished [7], injured or burned patients [8], and septic and/or traumatized patients [9]. Ward et al. [10] and Jiang et al. [11] reported that approximately 10 IU/day of rhGH reduced nitrogen excretion in patients receiving major gastointestinal surgery. In contrast, no improvement of protein metabolism was observed in burned patients by Belcher et al. [12], and in generalized septic patients by Gottardis et al. [13]. Appropriate dose levels of rhGH has yet to be determined.

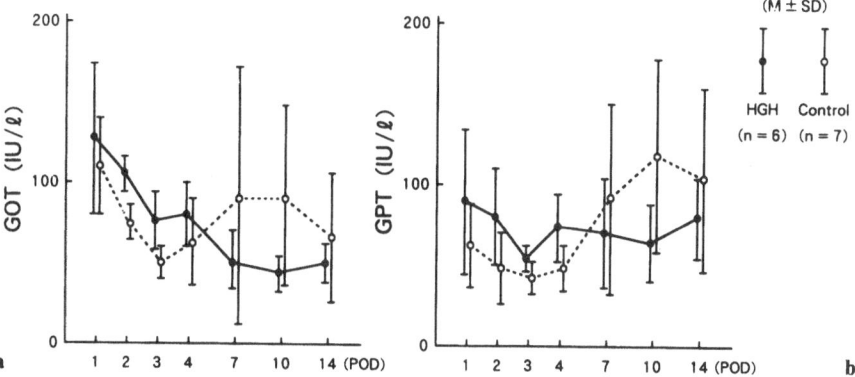

Fig. 3. a Serum GOT and **b** GPT in patients with or without rhGH following esophagectomy. *GOT*, glutamic oxaloacetic transaminase; *GPT*, glutamic pyruvic transaminase; *rhGH*, recomb inant human growth hormone

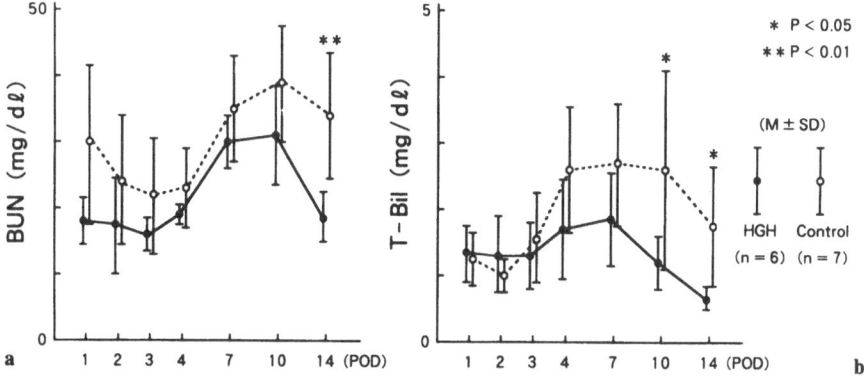

Fig. 4. a Blood urea nitrogen (*BUN*) and **b** total bilirubin (*T-Bil*) in patients with or without rhGH following esophagectomy. *rhGH*, recombinant human growth hormone; *POD*, post-operative day

The mechanisms of the improvement in protein metabolism by the administration of rhGH has been investigated from the kinetic point of view. In our experiment, protein kinetics using the constant infusion of ^{15}N-glycine demonstrated significantly increased whole-body protein turnover rates of the burned rats recieving rhGH. Greater increase of whole-body protein synthesis resulted in a significant improvement of nitrogen balance. Significantly increased nitrogen content of liver and gastrocunemius muscle and unchanged urinary excretion of 3-MH in rats receiving rhGH indicated the increase protein synthesis of liver and skeletal muscle. The results of our clinical study coincided well with those of the experiment with rats. Whole-body protein turnover, synthesis and breakdown tended to increase, and the increase of synthesis was statistically significant. Thus the improvement in nitrogen balance during administration of rhGH was becaue of an increased rate of protein synthesis rather than reduced catabolism. This finding is consistent with those of others [9–11, 14, 15].

Amelioration of protein metabolism is associated with many beneficial effects. In the early postoperative period following esophagectomy, it may be seen by increased respiratory muscle strength and ability to cough, breathe deeply, and to be weaned from the ventilator [11]. Enhanced wound healing may accelerate postoperative recovery, reduce the hospital stay [16], and shorten surgical convalescence. Increased immune function [17] may diminish susceptibility to infection and reduce morbidity and mortality of the patients who recieved esophagectomy.

Recombinant human GH did not affect hepatic or renal function. Furthermore, rhGH prevented a rise in BUN and total bilirubin which are frequently manifested following esophagectomy. Thus, it was confirmed that rhGH can be safely used with many beneficial effects includng the nutritional advantages.

References

1. Isono K, Sato H, Nakayama K (1991) Results of nationwide study on the three-field lymph node dissection of esophageal cancer. Oncology 48:411–420
2. Tashiro T, Meng HC (1981) A technique for long-term parenteral nutrition in unrestrained weaning rats. Jpn J Ped Surg 17:667–673
3. Stein TP, Leskiw JM, Buzby GP (1980) Measurement of protein synthsis rates with ^{15}N-glycine. Am J Physiol 239:E294–E300
4. Tashiro T, Yamamori H, Mashima Y (1984) The measurement of whole-body protein turnover in surgical patients recieving total parenteral nutrition (TPN). Jpn J Surg Metab Nutr 18:403–409
6. Fujisaki Y, Tashiro T, Mashima Y, Yamamori H (1992) Adequate requirement of energy and protein in postoperative total parenteral nutrition. Jpn J Surg 93:119–127
7. Ziegler TR, Young LS, Manson JM, Wilmore DW (1988) Metabolic effects of recombinant human growth hormone in patiens recieving parenteral nutrition. Ann Surg 208:6–16
8. Ziegler TR, Young LS, Ferrari-Baliviera E, Demling RH, Wilmore DW (1990) Use of human growth hormone combined with nutritional support in a critical care unit. JPEN 14:574–581
9. Douglas RG, Humberstone DA, Haystead A, Shaw JHF (1990) Metabolic effects of recombinant human growth hormone: isotopic studies in the postabsorptive state and during total parenteral nutrition. Br J Surg 7:785–790
10. Ward HC, Hailiday D, Sim AJW (1987) Protein and energy metabolism with biosynthetic human growth hormone after gastrointestinal surgery. Ann Surg 206:56–61
11. Jiang Z, He G, Wang X, Yang N, Zhu Y, Wilmore DW (1989) Low dose growth hormone and hypocaloric nutrition attenuate the proteincatabolic response after major operation. Ann Surg 210:513–525
12. Belcher HJCR, Mercer D, Judkins KC, Shalaby S, Wise S, Marks V, Tanner NSB (1989) Biosynthetic human growth hormone in burned patients: A pilot study. Burns 15:99–107
13. Gattardis M, Benzer A, Koller W, Luger TJ, Puhringer F, Hack IJ (1991) Improvement of septic syndrome after administration of recombinant growth hormone (rhGH). J Trauma 31:81–86
14. Manson JM, Smith RJ, Wilmore DW (1988) Growth hormone stimulates protein synthsis during hypocaloric parenteral nutrition. Ann Surg 208:136–142
15. Horber FF, Haymond MW (1990) Human growth hormone prevents the protein catabolic side effects of predonisone in humans. J Clin Invest 86:265–272

16. Herndon DN, Barrow RE, Kunkel KR, Broemeling L, Rutan RL (1990) Effect of recombinant human growth hormone on donor-site healing in severely burned children. Ann Surg 212:424–431
17. Crist DM, Kraner JC (1990) Supplemental growth hormone increases the tumor cytotoxic activity of natural killer cells in healthy adults with normal growth hormone secretion. Metabolism 39:1320–1324

Usefulness of Posterior Mediastinal Reconstruction After Esophagectomy in Case of Esophageal Cancer with Palsy of Recurrent Laryngeal Nerve

Harushi Osugi, Masayuki Higashino, Noriaki Maekawa, Taigo Tokuhara, Hiroaki Kinoshita[1], and Hironobu Ochi[2]

Introduction

In cases of esophageal cancer, metastasis to the lymph nodes alongside the recurrent laryngeal nerve (RLN) is found in high incidence, namely 25%. Palsy of the RLN may develop after the dissection of these nodes, even if the nerves were preserved surgically. In patients with metastasis to these nodes, the palsy of the RLN is observed before operation. Functional changes in the pharynx and cervical esophagus after the reconstruction of the intrathoracic esophagus have not yet been reported. To find an appropriate reconstructive procedure in the cases of esophageal cancer with palsy of the RLN, postoperative swallowing function was examined quantitatively by scintigraphy in the patients who had undergone a reconstruction via various routes.

Patients and Methods

Thirty-three patients and 12 healthy volunteers (controls) entered this study. All patients were subjected to resection of the intrathoracic esophagus for esophageal cancer through right thoracotomy. Thirteen patients who had a reconstruction using a gastric roll through the retrosternal route without RLN palsy were classified into the retrosternal (RS) group. Among the 20 patients who had a reconstruction using a gastric roll through the posterior mediastinal route, 12 patients without RLN palsy were classified into the posterior mediastinal (PM) group, and the other 8 patients with RLN palsy formed the PM-palsy group.

Esophageal scintigraphy was performed after a 4-h fast. After a few practices with unmarked water, patients took a bolus of 10 ml of water containing 185 MBq

[1] Second Department of Surgery and [2] Radionucleology, Osaka City University Medical School, 1-5-7, Asahimachi, Abeno-ku, Osaka, 545 Japan

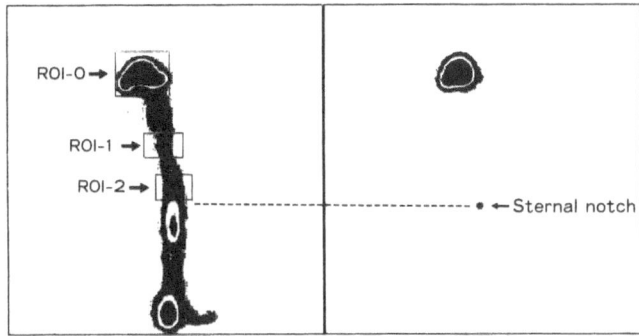

Fig. 1. Setting of regions of interest (*ROI*)

of ^{99m}Tc pertechnetate, and held it in their mouth. Then patients were instructed to swallow the radioactive liquid in a single swallow in front of a large-field scintillation camera, so that the mouth, pharynx, and esophagus were seen in the same field. Data were collected at time intervals of 0.2 s. These studies were performed twice, once sitting and once supine. Time activity curves were generated for three regions of interest (Fig. 1): the oral cavity (ROI-O); a region of 24 × 36 mm in the upper cervical esophagus (ROI-1); and the lower cervical esophagus (ROI-2). The results of calculations were expressed as mean ± one standard deviation. The Student's two-tailed independent *t*-test was used to determine the statistical significance of the differences in the results of the study groups.

Results

Radioactivity in ROI-O decreased rapidly after deglutition and reached a post-deglutition plateau. The time-activity curves in ROI-1 and 2 showed single peaks that reflected the passage of radioactive liquid following the decrease in radio-activity in ROI-O, and then reached plateaus (Fig. 2). Four objective parameters were derived from each time-activity curve (Fig. 3). Transit time to ROI-1 and 2 was obtained as the time-lag from the beginning of the deglutition to the appearance of the top of the peak. The widths of the peaks, indicating the retention time of the radioactive liquid in ROI-1 and 2, were obtained as the time from the beginning of the peak to the start of the post-passage plateau. The height of the peak in ROI-1 and 2 and the plateau level in each ROI were expressed as the ratio (%) to the original amount of radioactivity in ROI-O before deglutition, because the radioactive counts of the whole bolus in the mouth were slightly different in each study.

The results of studies in a sitting position are shown in Table 1.

In the supine position, the levels of plateau of ROI-O were higher than 50% of the original isotope in four patients of the RS group. Because more than a half of the radioactive liquid was not able to be propelled to the esophagus, these four patients were eliminated from the evaluation of the results in ROI-1 and 2. The results are shown in Table 2.

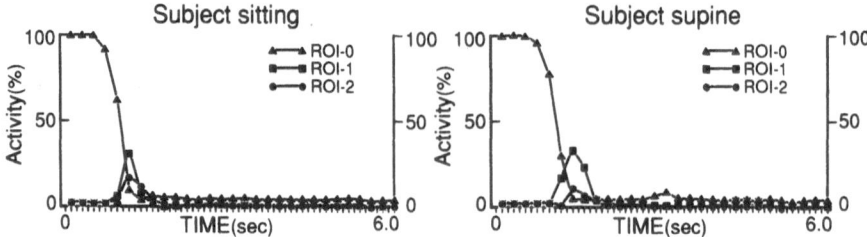

Fig. 2 Time-activity curves for controls

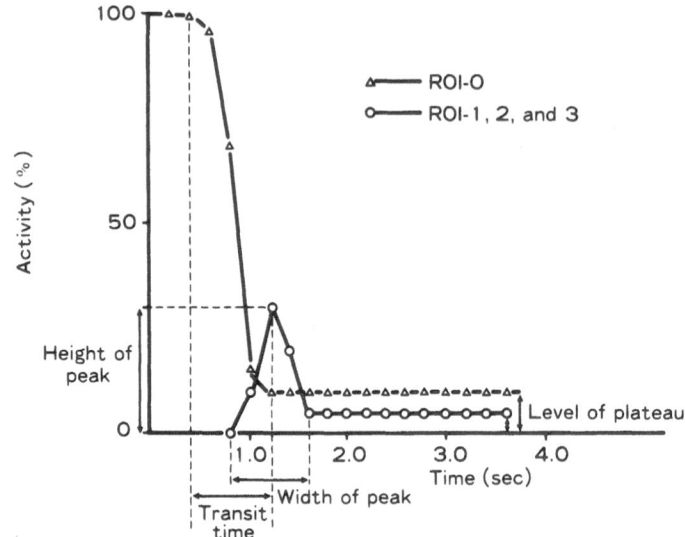

Fig. 3 Typical time-activity curve and numerical values obtained

Discussion

The assessment of esophageal function using radioactive material was first introduced by Kazem in 1972 [1]. Esophageal scintigraphy has been employed by some authors to study the function of the organs utilized for reconstruction after the intrathoracic esophagectomy [2]. However, those studies aimed at evaluating clearance of the swallowed material in the esophageal substitute such as the colon or stomach, which had been denervated. No study evaluating the functional differences according to the route of reconstruction has been reported. Recent developments of the computer facilitated more accurate analysis of esophageal function. Also, a significant change of swallowing function on alteration of position in normal volunteers was detected by scintigraphy recently [3]. The present study was designed to evaluate the clearance of swallowed material from the oral cavity and upper esophagus by the reconstructive routes,

Table 1. Numerical values with the subject sitting

	ROI-0	ROI-1			
	Level of plateau (%)	Transit time (s)	Height of peak (%)	Width of peak (s)	Level of plateau (%)
PM group	8.8 ± 2.4	0.5 ± 0.1 *	21.7 ± 6.9	0.7 ± 0.1	2.1 ± 1.9
PM-palsy group	8.3 ± 5.6	0.6 ± 0.1	25.3 ± 15.3	0.7 ± 0.1 **	1.8 ± 1.7
RS group	15.8 ± 11.2 *	0.6 ± 0.2 *	34.8 ± 15.9 *	1.0 ± 0.2 *	4.8 ± 5.5 *
Controls	6.7 ± 2.9	0.5 ± 0.1	21.9 ± 5.1	0.7 ± 0.2 *	0.6 ± 0.5

	ROI-2			
	Transit time (s)	Height of peak (%)	Width of peak (s)	Level of plateau (%)
PM group	0.6 ± 0.1	15.4 ± 9.1	0.8 ± 0.2	2.3 ± 1.4
PM-palsy group	0.7 ± 0.1 *	13.6 ± 5.0 **	0.9 ± 0.1 **	2.5 ± 1.4
RS group	0.9 ± 0.2 *	36.7 ± 28.6 *	1.4 ± 0.2 *	11.1 ± 14.8 **
Controls	0.6 ± 0.1 *	14.1 + 3.1 *	0.8 ± 0.1 *	0.9 ± 0.5

* $P < 0.05$
** $P < 0.01$
PM, posterior mediastinal; *RS*, retrosternal; *ROI*, region of interest

Table 2. Numerical values with the subject supine

	ROI-0	ROI-1			
	Level of plateau (%)	Transit time (s)	Height of peak (%)	Width of peak (s)	Level of plateau (%)
PM group	9.4 ± 3.5	0.6 ± 0.2	25.4 ± 8.1	0.9 ± 0.2	2.0 ± 1.7
PM-palsy group	10.5 ± 2.4 **	0.6 ± 0.2	27.8 ± 6.2	0.8 ± 0.2 *	1.1 ± 0.4
RS group	26.8 ± 25.1 *	0.7 ± 0.2	38.2 ± 23.2	1.0 ± 0.1	3.2 ± 4.2
Controls	8.4 ± 5.0	0.6 ± 0.1	28.6 ± 7.9	0.9 ± 0.2	0.1 ± 0.3

	ROI-2			
	Transit time (s)	Height of peak (%)	Width of peak (s)	Level of plateau (%)
PM group	0.7 ± 0.2	23.2 ± 8.1	1.2 ± 0.2	4.6 ± 2.1
PM-palsy group	0.8 ± 0.3 **	24.0 ± 9.0 **	1.2 ± 0.3 **	3.6 ± 1.8 **
RS group	1.0 ± 0.2 *	57.2 ± 23.6 *	2.2 ± 0.7 *	18.2 ± 9.7 *
Controls	0.8 ± 0.2	21.7 + 6.9 *	1.1 ± 0.2 *	2.3 ± 1.2 *

* $P < 0.05$
** $P < 0.01$
$n = 9$ in the RS group ROI-0

and the effect of RLN palsy. As the movement of the swallowed material is quick in the pharynx and upper esophagus, the accumulated radioactivity was measured every 0.2 s.

To evaluate the preferred reconstructive procedure in the patients with RLN palsy, the swallowing function in such patients whose esophagi were reconstructed through the retrosternal space should be compared with those who had posterior mediastinal reconstruction. The patients with RLN palsy whose esophagi were reconstructed retrosternally were studied in the preliminary stages, but they were not able to keep their positions in front of a scinti camera after a swallow, because of a cough as a result of aspiration. Therefore, quantitative evaluation was not possible in those patients.

The patients of the RS group showed significantly more radioactivity remaining in the oral cavity after the swallow than the patients of the PM group, PM-palsy group, and controls in sitting position. In the supine position, this tendency became more remarkable; four patients in the RS group were not able to make an efficient swallow. This suggests that the patients who had a retrosternal reconstruction may develop an aspiration following regurgitation.

Prolonged transit time in the RS group suggested that, in the patients who had retrosternal reconstruction, the swallowed material moved significantly slower in the cervical esophagus. The widening of the peak in the time-activity curve can be caused by prolonged retention of radioactive liquid in each ROI, or longitudinal spitting of the bolus of the liquid swallowed into the esophagus. Despite the observation that in the RS group, significantly more radioactivity remained in the oral cavity after a swallow than in the other three groups, the peaks in ROI-1 and 2 were significantly higher and wider in the RS group. This implied that in the RS group, a larger bolus of water remained in the cervical esophagus significantly longer than in the PM group, PM-palsy group, or controls. This tendency became clearer in the supine position than in the sitting position. In swallowing in the supine position, the bolus of water is progressed purely by pharyngoesophageal functions such as pharyngeal projection and esophageal peristalsis, without the effect of gravity. The results of this study corresponded well to the fact that the patients who had retrosternal reconstruction have a high incidence of cervical dysphagia. This study proves that the patient who had posterior mediastinal reconstruction, even if RLN palsy occurs, can swallow more physiologically than those who had retrosternal reconstruction. Therefore, in patients likely to experience RLN palsy, posterior mediastinal reconstruction is useful to prevent pulmonary soilage after an operation.

Esophageal scintigraphy was a sensitive and objective method of studying esophageal function. Esophageal transit can be evaluated more physiologically and quantitatively by scintigraphy than cineradiography, which necessitates the swallowing of barium of high specific gravity, and also involves a large dose of radioexposure.

References

1. Kazem I (1972) A new scintigraphic technique for the study of the esophagus. Am J Roentgenol 115:681–688
2. Isolauri J, Koskinen MO, Markkula H (1987) Radionuclide transit in patients with colon interposition. J Thorac Cardiovasc Surg 94:521–525
3. Osugi H, Higashino M, Kinoshita H, Shimonishi Y, Omura M, Ikeda H, Oda J, Ochi H (1992) Quantitative evaluation of deglutition in the upper esophagus by scintigraphy. Jpn J Nucl Med 29:1237–1243

Small Cell Carcinoma of the Esophagus: Report of Three Cases and Review of Literature

KEN-ICHI MAFUNE[1], YOICHI TANAKA[1], KAIYO TAKUBO[2], NOBUYUKI UCHIDA[3], SHUGO AKAZAWA[3], and KICHISHIRO FUJITA[1]

Introduction

Undifferentiated small cell carcinoma is a highly malignant tumor arising usually from the lung. This lung tumor is distinct from the other types of tumors in terms of biological and clinical behavior. Responses to multi-drug combinations are seen in over 80% of lung small cell carcinomas, whereas they are frequently disseminated and the outcome after surgery as primary therapy is terrible [1–3]. Therefore, small cell carcinomas of the lung are mostly treated with radiation and chemotherapy even in early stages of disease.

Small cell carcinoma of the esophagus is a rare tumor, showing extremely aggressive behavior. Several reports indicate that chemotherapy for small cell carcinoma of the lung was effective in the treatment of small cell carcinoma of the esophagus [4–6]. We have already reported a case with this type of lesion who survived more than 1 year with chemotherapy alone [7]. We herein describe three patients with small cell carcinoma of the esophagus who were treated differently at Saitama Cancer Center over the past 3 years, including the former reported case. For these small cell carcinomas of the esophagus, we have performed a chemotherapy using cisplatin [cis-dichlorodiammine-platinum (II), (CDDP)], etoposide (VP-16), and vindesine sulfate (VDS) (Table 1).

Furthermore, we reviewed English and Japanese literature. About 150 cases of esophageal small cell carcinoma have been reported so far, and 79 of them are Japanese cases including our series of 3 patients. We discuss here especially about these reported cases in Japan.

[1] Abdominal Surgery Clinic, Saitama Cancer Center Hospital, 818 Komuro, Ina, Saitama, 362 Japan
[2] Division of Clinical Pathology, Tokyo Metropolitan Geriatric Hospital, 35-2 Sakae-cho, Itabashi-ku, Tokyo, 173 Japan
[3] Gastroenterology Clinic, Saitama Cancer Center Hospital, 818 Komuro, Ina, Saitama, 362 Japan

Table 1. Chemotherapy for small cell carcinoma of the esophagus at Saitama Cancer Center

Agent	Dosage	Schedule
CDDP	100 mg/body i.v. infusion	: Day 1
VP-16	120 mg/body i.v. infusion	: Day 2, 3, 4
VDS	3 mg/body i.v.	: Day 5

For one course
CDDP, cisplatinum; *VP-16*, etoposide; *VDS*, vindesine sulfate

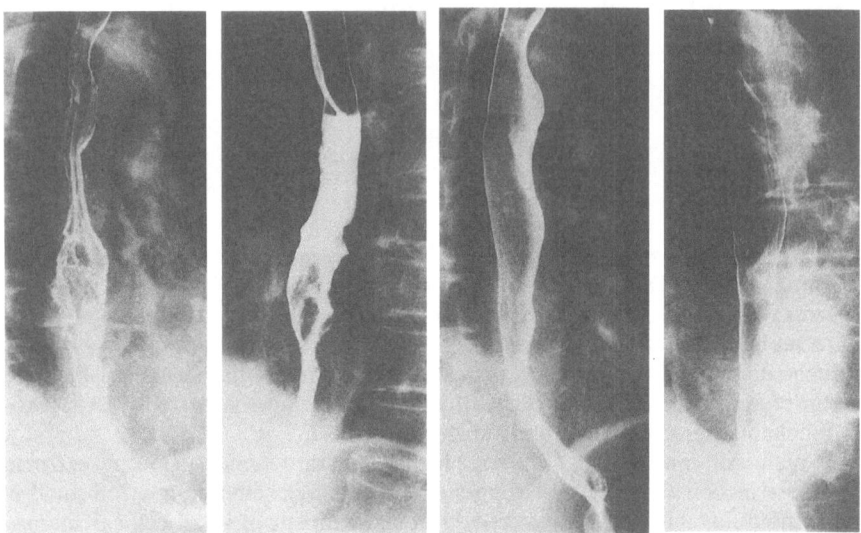

a

Fig. 1a,b. a Esophagram showing an ulcerative lesion in the middle to lower third of the esophagus (before chemotherapy). **b** Repeat esophagram after two courses of chemotherapy demonstrating resolution of primary lesion (case 1)

Case Reports

Case 1

A 72-year-old man, who had complained of slight dysphagia for 2 months, was referred to Saitama Cancer Center on September 20, 1989. Barium study and endoscopic examination revealed an ulcerated tumor in the middle third of the esophagus (Fig. 1a). Biopsy specimen taken during endoscopy showed small cell carcinoma of the esophagus (Fig. 2). Immunohistochemically, tumor cells were stained positively for neuron-specific enolase (NSE) and epithelial membrane antigen (EMA). Serum NSE was 11 ng/ml (normal range, <10 ng/ml).

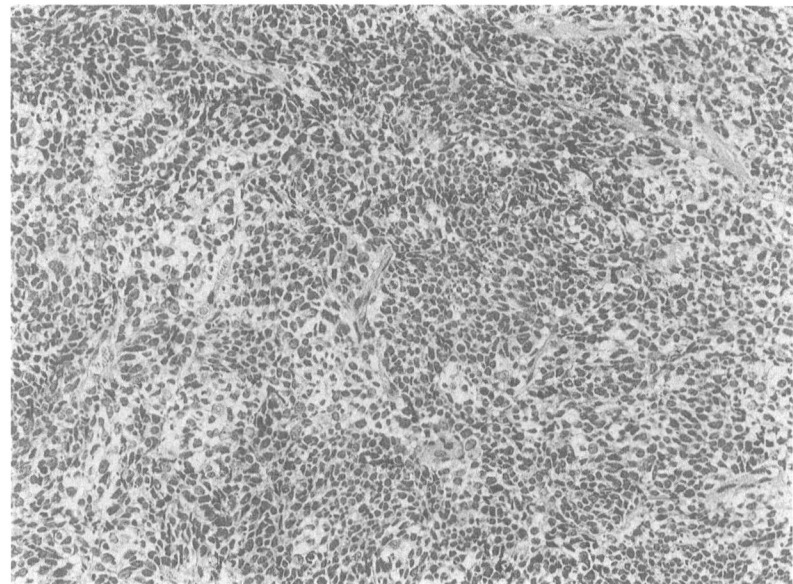

Fig. 2. Biopsy specimen showing undifferentiated small cell carcinoma (case 1)

This patient was admitted to Saitama Cancer Center on September 26. On admission to the hospital, there was evidence of recent hoarseness, and a hard supraclavicular mass was palpable. The remainder of the physical examination was unremarkable. Chest x-ray and bronchoscopy were almost normal. Ultrasonography (US), endoscopic ultrasonography (EUS) and computed tomography (CT) showed large lymph node metastases in the neck, the upper mediastinum, and the abdominal cavity. Because of widespread lymph node metastases, he underwent two courses of the chemotherapy, instead of surgery, using CDDP, VP-16, and VDS from October 6 and from November 22. Endoscopic examination after one course of chemotherapy showed a smaller and flatter tumor with a shallower ulceration compared with the finding before the chemotherapy. After the second course of this chemotherapy, the tumor could not be detected by a barium swallow (Fig. 1b). This patient was discharged with no complaint on December 22, 1989.

The patient was readmitted on February 13, 1990 for a repeat course of the chemotherapy and discharged on February 18. Endoscopic examination showed a small protruded lesion covered with normal epithelium. Furthermore, the patient underwent a chemotherapy using VP16 (150 mg/day p.o.) at the outpatient clinic from March 12, however this chemotherapy was stopped because of his appetite loss and fever on April 16. He was readmitted on June 12, 1990 for another course of chemotherapy using CDDP, VP-16, and VDS, and was discharged on July 7. Even after this treatment, the patient complained of cough, and his general condition was becoming worse. He was admitted to our hospital on September 3, 1990. Chest x-ray showed hydrothorax, and cytological examintion revealed cancer cells in the pleural effusion. The patient underwent a different chemotherapy using CDDP and 5-fluorouracil (5-FU) (CDDP 120 mg/body iv infusion, day 1; 5-FU 1000 mg/body iv infusion, days 1, 2). However, the condition of the patient was not improved, and he died of pleuritis carcinomatosa on October 25, 1990, 13 months after the first visit and 12 months after the first chemotherapy.

Case 2

A 65-year-old woman who had complained of epigastral discomfort for 2 months was referred to Saitama Cancer Center on November 7, 1990. Barium study and endoscopic examination showed an ulcerative tumor in the middle to lower esophagus (Fig. 3a). Biopsy revealed anaplastic small cell carcinoma of the esophagus. CT, US, and EUS revealed large lymph node metastases in the upper mediastinum and the abdominal cavity. The serum NSE level was 7.3 ng/ml.

This patient was admitted for surgery on December 4, 1990. However, because invasion to the trachea and widespread metastases to lymph nodes were suspected, the patient underwent the chemotherapy using CDDP, VP-16, and VDS starting from December 12, 1990. After one course of chemotherapy, the primary tumor and large metastases were reduced in size, but the esophageal cavity became stenotic (Fig. 3b).

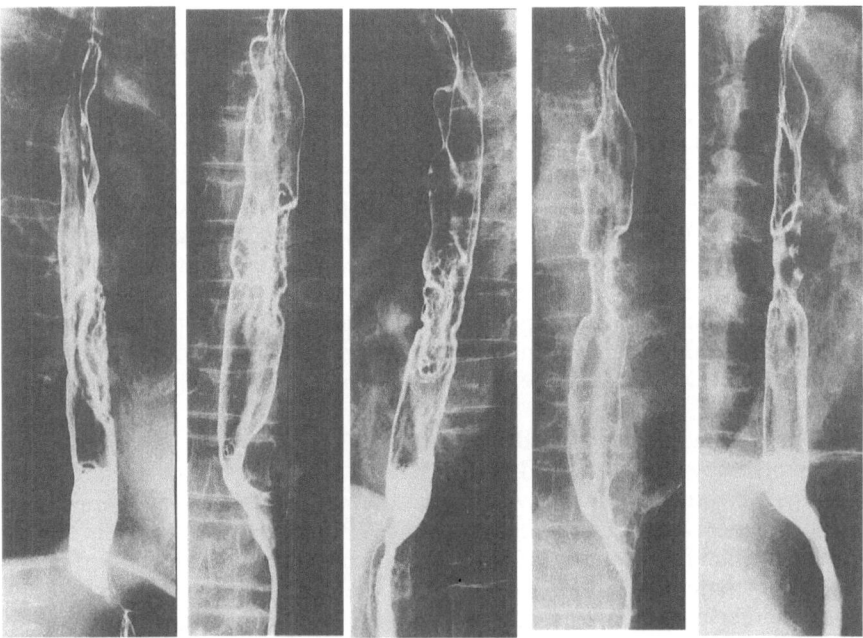

a

Fig. 3a,b. a Pretreatment esophagram showing an ulcerative lesion in the middle to lower third of the esophagus. **b** Repeat esophagram after one course of the chemotherapy showing a smaller but more stenotic primary lesion (case 2)

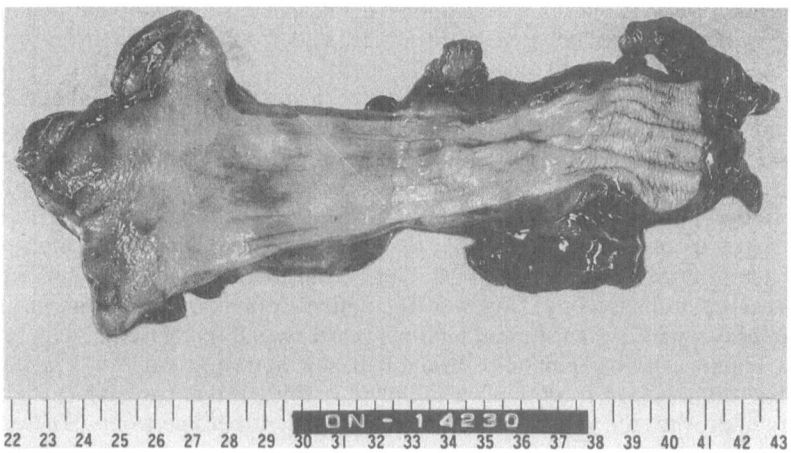

Fig. 4. Resected specimen showing an ulcerative tumor invading adventitia of the esophageal wall (case 2)

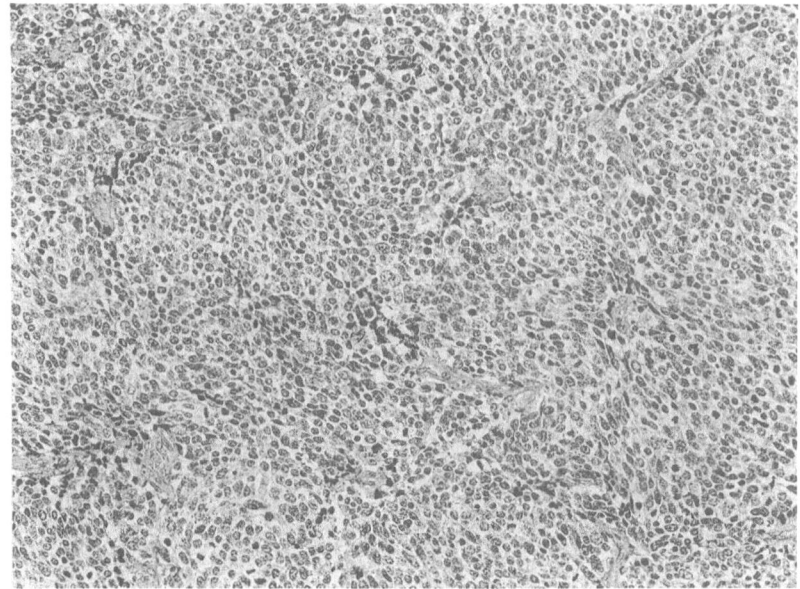

Fig. 5. Microscopic examination indicating small cell carcinoma of the esophagus (case 2)

Esophagectomy and reconstruction with stomach tube was performed on January 12, 1991. The tumor was not resected completely because of direct invasion to the trachea. Histologically, the resected specimen showed that a 4.3 × 2.5 cm-sized small cell carcinoma in the middle to lower esophagus (Figs. 4, 5). It had invaded the adventitia of the esophageal wall and metastasized to the lymph nodes from the mediastinum (paratrachea, subcarina, and pulmonary hilar nodes) to the abdomen (paracardiac, and the left gastric artery nodes). Marked lymph vessel and blood vessel infiltrations were also observed. Histologic effect of the chemotherapy could not be seen in this specimen. Immunohisto-chemically, the tumor cells were stained positively for NSE.

This patient underwent the chemotherapy using CDDP, VP-16, and VDS from February 27, 1991, however bronchoscopic examination showed three protruded tumors at the membrane part of the trachea and carina. She under-went irradiation (Linac total 50 Gy) for the residual and recurrent tumors at the trachea from March 25 to April 24, 1991. After this treatment, no tumor could be seen by bronchoscopy. However, the patient complained of severe headache from May, and CT scan showed multiple (more than 80) metastatic brain tumors and meningeal dissemination. Brain metastases were treated by irradiation (Linac total 40 Gy) from June 6 to July 13, 1991. Although brain metastases were improved, the general condition of the patient became worse. The patient died of large mediastinal lymph node metastases on August 12, 1991, 9 months after the first visit and the first chemotherapy, and 7 months after surgery.

Case 3

A 49-year-old man whose chief complaint was back pain for 2 months was referred to Saitama Cancer Center on March 1, 1991. Esophagogastrography and endoscopy showed a large ulcerative tumor in the lower esophagus, extended into the cardia (Fig. 6). A biopsy revealed this tumor to be undifferentiated small cell carcinoma. CT and US revealed a large lymph node metastases near the cardia and widespread lymph node metastases in the abdominal cavity. The serum NSE level was 5.6 ng/ml.

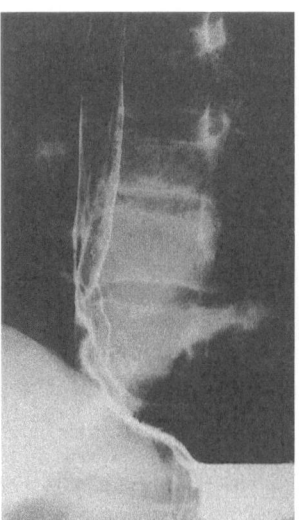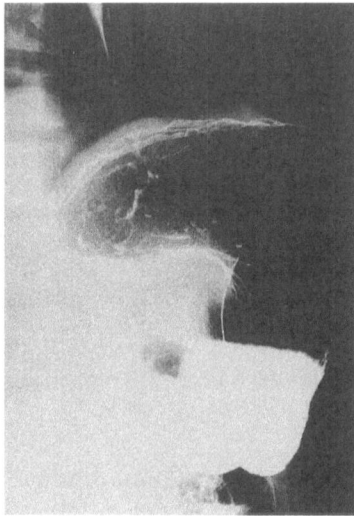

Fig. 6. Barium esophagogastrogram revealing an infiltrative tumor in the lower esophagus to cardia (case 3)

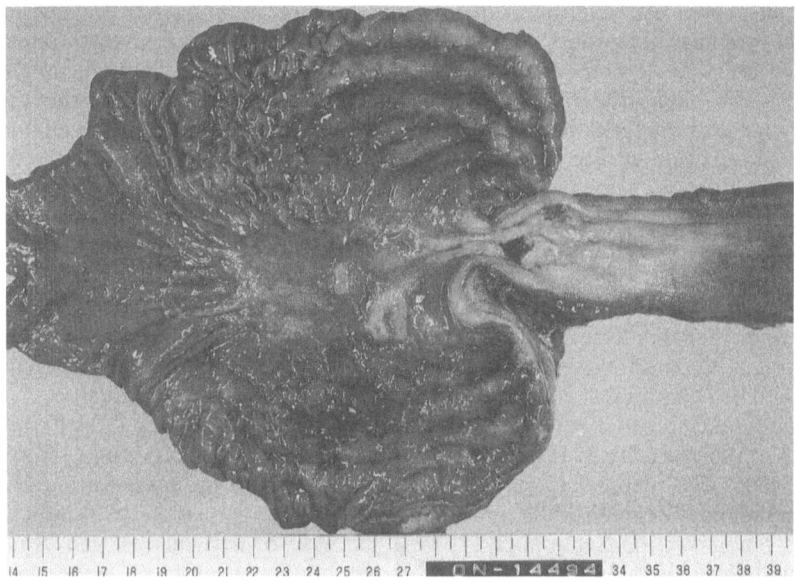

Fig. 7. Resected specimen showing an ulcerative tumor in the lower third of the esophagus infiltrating into the stomach (case 3)

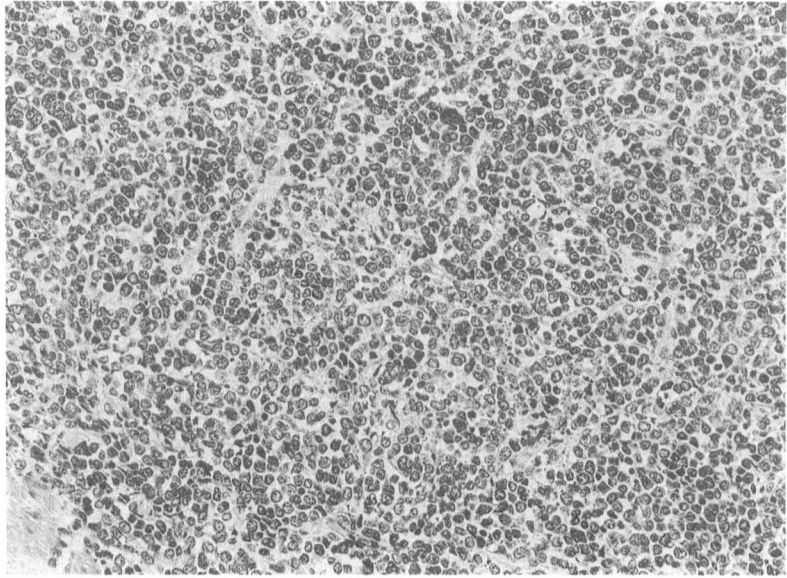

Fig. 8. Histological examination indicating undifferentiated carcinoma, small cell type (case 3)

The patient was admitted our hospital for surgery on March 27, 1991. Subtotal esophagectomy and total gastrectomy, and reconstruction with transverse colon were performed on April 2, 1991. As there was a large lymph node metastasis along the left gastric artery, invading the pancreas, the tail of the pancreas, spleen, and left adrenal gland were co-resected. Lymph node metastases were spread throughout the abdominal cavity but not in the upper mediastinum. Resected specimen showed a large 22.0 × 17.0 cm tumor which had three ulcers: two shallow ones in the cardia and one deep one in the lower esophagus (Fig. 7). Histological cell type of this tumor was undifferentiated carcinoma, small cell type (Fig. 8). Microscopically, this tumor widely metastasized to the abdominal lymph nodes such as perigastric, left gastic artery, common hepatic artery, splenic artery, celiac, and para-aortic nodes. Marked lymph and blood vessel infiltration were observed. Immunohistochemically, NSE, EMA, and cytokeratin staining were positive in the cancer tissue.

This patient underwent two courses of chemotherapy using CDDP, VP-16, and VDS from May 8, 1991 and from June 5, 1991. He was discharged on July 13, 1991. The general condition of the patient was becoming worse, and he complained of appetite loss and edema of the face and upper extremities. He was readmitted on September 11, 1991, because of hypotension and cyanosis. This patient died of large mediastinal lymph node metastases on September 12, 1991, 6 months after the first visit and 5 months after surgery.

Discussion

Small cell carcinoma of the esophagus was first reported by McKeown [8] in 1952. In Japan, Taniguchi et al. [9] reported the first two cases in 1973. About 150 cases of this lesion have been reported so far in English and Japanese literature, and 79 cases have been reported in Japan alone, including our 3 patients in this report.

These Japanese cases consisted of 64 men and 15 women, and the mean age was 69 years (range, 42–78 years). These patients usually complained of dysphagia, chest pain, almost the same as patients with typical esophageal cancer. Only one patient complained of spasms due to brain metastases. The distribution of esophageal tumors was as follows: upper third, 3; middle third, 30; lower third, 17; middle to lower, 11; upper to lower, 2; and lower to stomach, 1. Most tumors arise from the middle and/or lower third of the esophagus. This is thought to be because Kulchitsky's cells, which may be the orgin of this tumor, exist more in the middle-lower esophagus [10]. When this lesion was diagnosed, 84% (31/37) of these cases had metastases to lymph node, liver, and brain. Furthermore, the follow-up of 49 patients was described in these reports. Only 9 cases were alive (range, 2–24 months) at last follow-up. The mean survival period of the 40 expired cases was 8.1 months (range, 22 days–29 months). These data indicate that this small cell carcinoma is extremely aggressive.

Treatments selected for this esophageal lesion were described in 45 cases. The mean survival months of these cases according to treatments were as follows: surgery, 9.1 ($n = 26$) [surgery alone, 4.5 ($n = 8$); surgery + chemotherapy, 8.1 ($n = 6$); surgery + radiation, 2 ($n = 2$); surgery + chemotherapy + radiation,

12.8 ($n = 10$)]; chemotherapy alone, 10 ($n = 8$); radiation alone, 11 ($n = 1$); and chemotherapy + radiation, 9.1 ($n = 10$). Furthermore, we also selected 10 cases who survived more than 1 year after diagnosis or after treatment. Treatments selected for them were as follows: surgery alone, 1; surgery + chemotherapy, 1; surgery + chemotherapy + radiation, 3; radiation + chemotherapy, 3; and chemotherapy alone, 2. These reports in Japan showed that the outcome after surgery as the only therapy for small cell carcinoma is terrible and most cases had already metastasized when the disease was diagnosed. There was a case of early cancer (superficial cancer without metastasis) which recurred after surgery in 9 months [11]. Furthermore, there have been several reports that chemotherapy alone was effective in the treatment of small cell carcinoma of the esophagus [4–7].

We describe herein three cases of small cell carcinoma of the esophagus treated differently, and the patient who did not undergo surgery survived longer than other two cases. Our experience suggests that chemotherapy should be selected as primary therapy for small cell carcinoma of the esophagus instead of surgery. Therefore, the treatment program should emphasize the use of poly-drug regimens active in small cell carcinoma of the lung. In addition, prophylactic whole-brain irradiation could be one therapeutic option for small cell carcinoma of the esophagus because this tumor sometimes metastasizes to the brain.

However, the outcome after surgery combined with both chemotherapy and irradiation was not bad. There are still times when surgical therapy may be appropriate. For example, resection of primary tumor could be selected for advanced tumors which had responded effectively to chemotherapy and irradiation. Resection of primary tumor with lymph node dissection could be selected for tumors in early stage followed by intensive chemotherapy with or without irradiation. For complete cure of this esophageal lesion, the latter may be a hopeful treatment program. In any case, it is true that results of current therapies for esopahgeal small cell carcinoma are not satisfactory. Further clinical trials will be required to establish more effective treatment programs.

References

1. Bunn PA Jr, Cohen MH, Ihde DC, Fossieck BE, Matthews MJ, Minna, JD (1977) Advances in small cell bronchogenic carcinoma. Cancer Treat Rep 61:333–342
2. Brader LE, Cohen MH, Selawry OS (1977) Treatment of bronchogenic carcinoma. II. Small cell cancer. Cancer Treat Rev 4:219–260
3. Greco FA, Einhorn LH, Richardson RL, Oldham RK (1978) Small cell lung cancer: Progress and perspective. Semin Oncol 5:323–335
4. Kelsen DP, Weston E, Kurts R, Cvitokovic E, Lieberman P, Golby RB (1980) Small cell carcinoma of the esophagus. Treat by chemotherapy alone. Cancer 45:1558–1561
5. Levenson RM Jr, Ihde DC, Matthews MJ, Cohen MH, Gazdar AF, Bunn PA Jr, Minna JD (1981) Small cell carcinoma presenting as an extrapulmonary neoplasm: Sites of origin and responses to chemotherapy. J Natl Canc Inst 67:607–612
6. Tanabe G, Kajisa T, Shimizu H, Yoshida A (1987) Effective chemotherapy for small cell carcinoma of the esophagus. Cancer 60:2613–2616
7. Uchida N, Akazawa S, Tanaka Y, Takubo K (1991) A case report of small cell carcinoma of the esophagus treated by chemotherapy alone (in Japanese). JJCDO 1:105–110
8. McKeown F (1952) Oat cell carcinoma of the esophagus. J Pathol Bacteriol 64:889–891

9. Taniguchi K, Iwanaga T, Kosaki G, Horai T, Sano M, Tateichi R, Taniguchi H (1973) Two cases of ACTH-producing esophageal cancer (in Japanese). Saishin Igaku 28:1834–1837
10. Ho K-J, Herrera GA, Jones JM, Alexander B (1984) Small cell carcinoma of the esophagus: Evidence for a unified histogenesis. Hum Pathol 15:460–468
11. Kuwano H, Ikeda M, Tatsuda Y, Okamura K, Sugimachi K, Inokuchi K, Iwashita A, Enjoji M (1981) Early esophageal cancer of oat cell carcinoma-like appearance: Report of a case (in Japanese). Rinsho Geka 36:1651–1654

The Clinicopathological and Prognostic Evaluation of 12 Primary Undifferentiated Small Cell Carcinomas

Ataru Kobayashi, Hiroko Ide, Reiki Eguchi, Kazuhiko Hayashi,
Kazunari Yoshida, Yoko Murata, Takeshi Endo, Tomoko Hanashi,
Tutomu Nakamura, Akiyoshi Yamada, Fujio Hanyu,
and Seiichiro Kobayashi[1]

Introduction

Undifferentiated small cell carcinoma is a rare disease and, since the first case was reported by McKeown [1] in 1952, no more than 100 cases have been reported [2]. The prognosis is usually extremely poor, and the best treatment has not yet been established, though several cases that obtained fair prognosis by the multidisciplinary treatment were seen.

In the present study, we report on 12 cases of undifferentiated small cell carcinoma plus clinicopathological and prognostic evaluation.

Patients and Methods

From 1965 to 1991, we experienced 12 cases of undifferentiated small cell carcinoma, and its incidence was 0.7% of the 1812 resected esophageal cancers during the 27-year period in our institution.

Results

In 26 years, we had 12 cases of undifferentiated small cell carcinoma. Table 1 shows the clinical features of those cases.

Sex and Age Distribution

Ten patients were males and two were females, and the mean age was 63 (range 55–80)

[1] Department of Surgery, The Institute of Gastroenterology, Tokyo Women's Medical College, 8-1 Kawada-cho, Shinjuku-ku, Tokyo, 162 Japan

Table 1, Clinical features of 12 cases of undifferentiated small cell carcinoma

Case no.	Age/ sex	Symptoms/duration	Tumor site	Size (T)	N	M	Stage
1.	57 M	Dysphagia 5 months	Middle	9 cm (T1)	N1	M1LYM	IV
2.	57 M	Swallowing discomfort 4 months	Middle	2 cm (T1)	N1	M0	I
3.	55 M	Swallowing discomfort 6 months	Middle	3 cm (T1)	N1	M0	I
4.	59 M	Swallowing discomfort 6 months	Middle	1 cm (T1)	N0	M0	I
5.	59 M	Dysphagia 6 months	Middle	14 cm (T4)	N1	M1LYM	VI
6.	65 F	Dysphagia 2 months	Middle	9 cm (T3)	N1	M0	III
7.	72 M	Dysphagia 2 months	Middle	5 cm (T2)	N1	M0	II B
8.	81 M	Dysphagia 2 months	Middle	9 cm (T4)	N1	M1LYM	IV
9.	55 M	Dysphagia 4 months	Lower	9 cm (T3)	N1	M1LYM	IV
10.	77 F	Dysphagia 1 month	Middle	8 cm (T4)	N1	M1LYM	IV
11.	69 M	No complaints	Middle	5 cm (T2)	N1	M1LYM	IV
12.	61 M	Dysphagia 5 months	Middle	9 cm (T3)	N1	M0	III

TNM, tumor node metastasis

Chief Complaints and Duration

Eight patients were seen as dysphagic, swallowing discomfort was present in three, and no complaint in one. These duration ranged from 2 to 6 months.

Tumor Site

Eleven cases were located in the middle thoracic esophagus, and the remaining cancer was in the lower thoracic esophagus.

TNM Staging

In T-categories, the tumor size ranged from 1 to 9 cm (four T_1, two T_2, three T_3, three T_4 cases). In N-categories, there were 11 N_1, cases, and 1 N_0 cases. In M-categories, half of the cases were M_0 and the rest were 6 M_1. Their stages were stage I in three, II B in one, III in two, and IV in six cases.

Next is shown as the pathological features of the 12 cases (Table 2).

Table 2. The pathological features of 12 cases of undifferentiated small cell carcinoma of the esophagus

Case no.	Gross type	Microscopic	ly	v	Special Staining	
					Grimelius	s-100
1.	Superficial (plateau)	Undiff.SCC	+	+		
2.	Superficial (plateau)	Oat cell	+	+		+
3.	Superficial (plateau + ulcerative)	Oat cell	+	+		+
4.	Superficial (subepithelial)	Oat cell	−	−		+
5.	Advanced (ulcerative)	Undiff.SCC	+	+	+	−
6.	Advanced (ulcerative)	Oat cell	+	+	−	−
7.	Advanced (ulcerative)	Undiff.SCC	+	+	−	−
8.	Advanced (ulcerative)	Undiff.SCC	+	+	+	+
9.	Advanced (ulcerative)	Oat cell	+	+	+	+
10.	Advanced (ulcerative)	Oat cell	+	+		+
11.	Advanced (ulcerative)	Oat cell	+	+		+
12.	Advanced (ulcerative)	Undiff.SCC	+	+		+

ly, Lymphatic *v*, vascular; *SCC*, small cell carcinoma

Gross Type

Four cases were superficial and eight were advanced cases. Among the superficial cases, two were plateau-like, one was plateau + ulcerative, and one subepithelial type. An advanced cases were ulcerative type.

Microscopic Type

Seven cases were oat cell type, and five were undifferentiated squamous cell type. Concerning lymphatic and vascular invasion, 11 cases were positive in both lymphatic and vascular invasion. In special staining, we did Grimelius in 5 (3/5 were positive) and s-100 staining in 11 cases, of which 10 were positive.

Next, we will discuss one superficial (case 4) and 1 advanced (case 11) case.

Case 4

Example of superficial type (Fig. 1). An esophagogram revealed a flat plateau lesion in the middle thoracic esophagus. Endoscopically, the 0-I lesion was seen in the right wall of the esophagus. A tumor mucosectomy first, followed by two courses of chemotherapy (cisplatin [CDDP] $80\,mg/m^2$ + VP − 16 $70\,mg/m^2$), subtotal esophagectomy, and lymph node dissection by right thoracotomy. Pathologically, the cancer had invaded the submucosal layer in the cut surface of mucosected specimen, and there was no remnant cancer tissue in resected specimen.

Case 11

Example of advanced type (Fig. 2). An esophagogram revealed an ulcerative lesion in the middle thoracic esophagus. Pathologically, the cancer had invaded

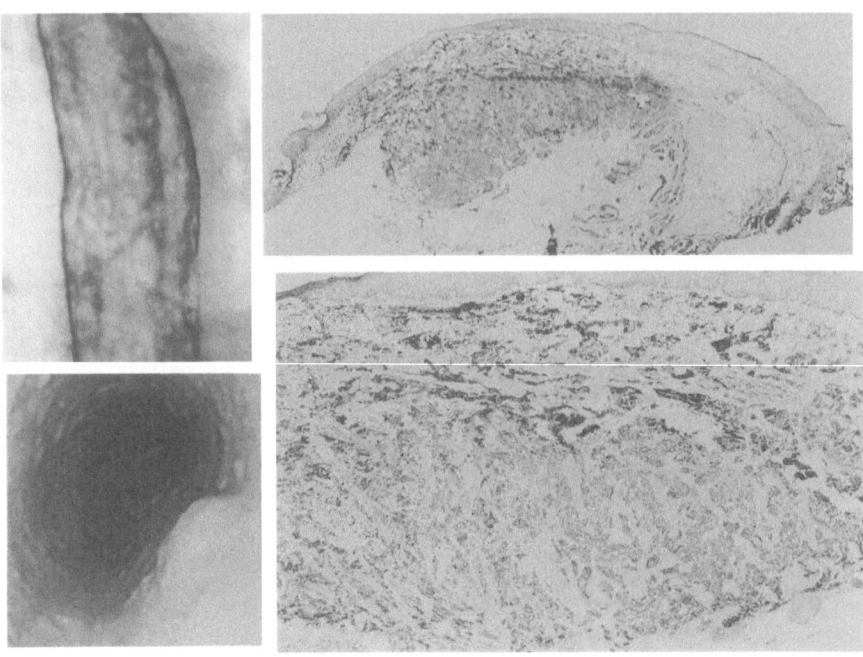

Fig. 1. Example of superficial type. *Left upper* is esophagographic findings (flat plateau lesion), *left lower* is endoscopical findings (0-I type). *Right upper* is cut surface of mucosectomized specimen and *right lower* is high magnification of this tissue. The cancer invaded the submucosal layer

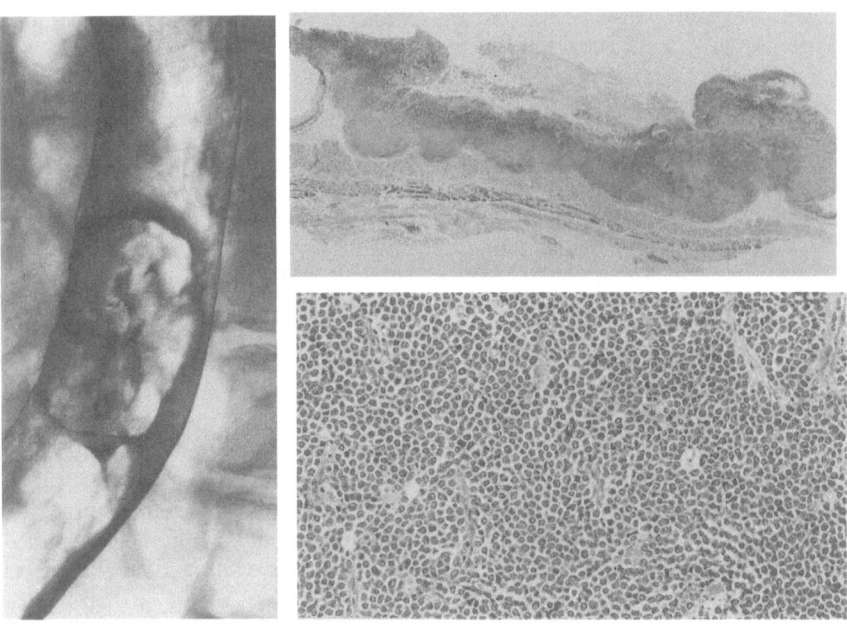

Fig. 2. Example of advanced type. *Left* are the esophagographic findings (ulcerative type), *right upper* is cut surface of resected specimen of cancer which invaded the muscular layer. *Right lower* is pathological findings of this cancer, characterized as typical small cell type

Table 3. Treatment and prognosis

Case no.	Treatment	Outcome	Cause of death
1.	Preop.RT(20 Gy) + Ope(R1)	Dead (6 months)	Liver meta.
2.	Ope(R1) + postop.RT(50 Gy)	Dead (18 months)	Unknown
3.	Ope(R1) + postop.CHT(CDDP + VDS)	Dead (19 months)	Liver meta.
4.	Mucosectomy + preop.CHT(CDDP + VP-16) + Ope(R0)	Alive (13 months)	
5.	Ope(R2)	Dead (2 months)	LN meta.
6.	Ope(R1) + postop.RT(60 Gy)	Dead (4 months)	Unknown
7.	Ope(R1) + postop.RT(50 Gy)	Dead (7 months)	LN meta.
8.	Ope(R2)	Dead (5 months)	Local recurrence
9.	Ope(R1)	Dead (4 months)	Liver, bone meta.
10.	Ope(R2)	Dead (3 months)	Bone meta.
11.	Ope(R1) + postop.CHT(CDDP + VDS)	Dead (4 months)	Pleuritis carcinomatosa
12.	Ope(R1) + postop.CHT(CDDP + VP-16)	Dead (6 months)	Lung meta.

RT, Irradiation; CHT, chemotherapy; Ope, operation; L.N., lymph node; meta., metastasis; CDDP, cisplatin; VP-16, etoposide; VDS, vindesine

the muscular layer in the cut surface. Microscopically, uniform small round cells with scanty or copious cytoplasm and hyperchromatic or vesicular nuclei, and tumors were arranged in sheets.

Table 3 shows each patient's treatment and prognosis.

Treatment

Four patients were treated by surgery alone, four by resection and irradiation, and four by resection and chemotherapy.

Prognosis

Eleven patients have since died (2–19 months postoperatively). Only one patient has lived more than 1 year. The cause of death was metastases to the liver in two patients, lymph node in two; and liver and bone, bone, lung metastasis; local recurrence, and pleuritis carcinomatosa in one each; and unknown in two.

Discussion

Small cell carcinoma is common in the lung, but in other organs the incidence is rare. Undifferentiated small cell carcinoma was reported in approximately 100 cases over the last 40 years.

The incidence was reported to be 0.05% by Kelsen et al. [4], 2.4% by Briggs and Ibrahim [5]; and 7.6% by Horai et al. [3]. In our institute, the rate was 0.7% (12/1812). The sex ratio male:female was 10:2, i.e. the condition was much more common among males than females, and the age distribution was 55–80 years.

The most common complaint was dysphagia and the duration was within 6 months, an extremely short period. In the tumor location, almost cases were located in middle thoracic esophagus.

Concerning TNM-staging, the sizes varied and even though tumor size was small, lymph node metastasis was almost always positive. Therefore, in the M-categories, M1LYM was the most common factor (6/6 cases); the staging was 6 T_4 cases in 12 (50%). That meant undifferentiated small cell carcinoma was generally advanced by the time of diagnosis.

Macroscopic findings revealed that the plateau or subepithelial shape is common in superficial cancer. In contrast, the ulcerative shape in advanced cancer first appeared to chiefly occupy the subepithelial layer, then the epithelial layer was destroyed with tumor invasion. Lastly, the ulceration was appeared.

Microscopic findings revealed that seven cases were oat cell type and the remaining five were undifferentiated small cell type. According to lymphatic and vascular invasion, there was a high tendency (11/12) of the cancer to invade. Also, in special staining, 3/5 were positive for Grimelius, and 8/11 for S-100 stain. Horai et al. [3] defined the histological criteria of small cell carcinoma of the esophagus as solid sheets without a centripetal gradient of maturity to the epidermoid carcinoma, ribbon like, and/or streaming patterns consisting of small, spindle–shaped cells. While the presence of argyrophilic cells under Grimelius stain is considered to be a confirmative evidence for the diagnosis of small cell carcinoma; the failure to demonstrate argyrophil tumor cells may be attributed to the paucity of their neurosecretory granules.

Then, the efficacy of the multidisciplinary treatment seen in the results was not satisfactory. Regarding the prognosis, 11 patients died (8 within 6 months) and only 1 is alive. The longest-term survival was only 19 months. Severe vascular invasion and hematogenous (liver, bone, lung) and lymphatic metastasis were the main causes of death seen even in the short-term.

In conclusion, primary undifferentiated small cell carcinoma of the esophagus is a rare tumor with extremely bad prognosis like small cell carcinoma of the lung. Our goal is to identify undifferentiated small cell carcinoma in the early phase to increase the effectiveness of multidisciplinary treatment. It is hoped that the prognosis will be improved each year.

References

1. McKeown F (1952) Oat-cell carcinoma of the esophagus. J Pathol Bacteriol 64:889–891
2. Shimizu T, Kato H, Yamashita I, Saito T, Takemori S, Nakamura K, Horai I, Yamada A, Shimazaki K, Otagiri H, Sakamoto T, Karaki Y, Tazawa K, Fujimaki M (1990) A case report of small cell carcinoma of the esophagus. J Gastroenterol Surg 23(3):753–757
3. Horai T, Kobayashi A, Tateishi R, Wada A, Taniguchi H, Taniguchi K, Sano M, Tamura H (1978) A cytologic study on small cell carcinoma of the esophagus: Cancer 41:1890–1896
4. Kelsen DP, Weston E, Kurtz R (1980) Small cell carcinoma of the esophagus: Treatment by chemotherapy alone. Cancer 45:1558–1561
5. Briggs JC, Ibrahim NB (1983) Oat cell carcinoma of the esophagus. A clinocopathological study of 23 cases. Histopathology 7:261–277

Relationship Between the Esophagus, Trachea, and Pleura

D. Liebermann-Meffert[1], W. Huber[1], B. Häberle[2], L.J. Wurzinger[2], and J.R. Siewert[1]

Introduction

The location in a loose areolar connective tissue bed permits esophageal mobility within the mediastinum during swallows and respiration [1]. In general, it also allows the esophagus to be bluntly stripped from the mediastinum without any hazard during blunt transdiaphragmatic esophagectomy [2–6]. However, tracheal and pleural tears or tracheoesophageal fistula formation have repeatedly complicated blunt dissection, adjuvant chemotherapy, and irradiation [7]. This event may be due to pathological adhesions, on the other hand it also may be based on normal anatomical structures attaching the esophagus to its neighboring tissue.

Can the complications be explained on a morphological basis? Our knowledge of the tissue relationships of the upper human mediastinal organs is poor and textbook descriptions inadequate. To meet optimal surgical requirements, the purpose of this study was to investigate firstly in normal human specimens the proximity of esophagus, trachea, and pleura; and secondly the upper mediastinum in regard to potential esophageal attachments, if there are any, which may be located between its cranial anchorage at the cricoid cartilage and the tracheal bifurcation.

Material and Methods

Twelve human autopsy specimens, 8 male and 4 female, aged 21 to 80 years were studied. Five were cadavers from the anatomical dissecting theater (TU München) and six *en bloc* specimens of thoracic organs were obtained from fresh corpses of a forensic Medical Institute (LMU München).

Departments of Surgery[1] and Anatomy[2], Technical University of Munich, Technische Universität Klinikum rechts der Isar, Ismaningerstr.22 D-8000 München 80, Germany

After inspection of the topographical relationships of esophagus, trachea, vessels and nerves, pleura, and spine, large specimens containing the mediastinum and its organs were removed *en bloc*. These were fixed in formaldehyde solution for 3 weeks. Beginning with the cricoid cartilage down 5 cm caudal to the tracheal bifurcation, macroscopical transverse consecutive tissue blocks were cut equidistantly at intervals of 1 cm. Serial histological plane sections 15 μm thick were made from each block and stained using different techniques. The positional relationships between tissues, organs, and connecting structures were evaluated, measured, and documented both in the transverse and craniocaudal extension.

Results

Originating from the posterior margin of the cricoid cartilage, the esophagus accompanied the trachea presenting a slight left side deviation. Located in the ventral portion of the posterior mediastinum and along its trajectory through the chest it was embedded in loose areolar tissue, except for its anterior surface. There, the distance to the posterior aspect of the trachea remained less than 0.5 mm in our specimens for 7 to 8 cm down to the tracheal bifurcation. With the division into principal bronchi, the distance to the left bronchus progressively enlarged to 3 mm, and areolar connective tissue became interspersed. The pleura, after appearing 3 to 5 cm caudal to the cricoid cartilage, was 0.5 to 5 mm distant from the esophagus.

The bundles of the lamina muscularis were wrapped in delicate connective tissue sheaths (perimysium, epimysium) that were continuous with the sur-

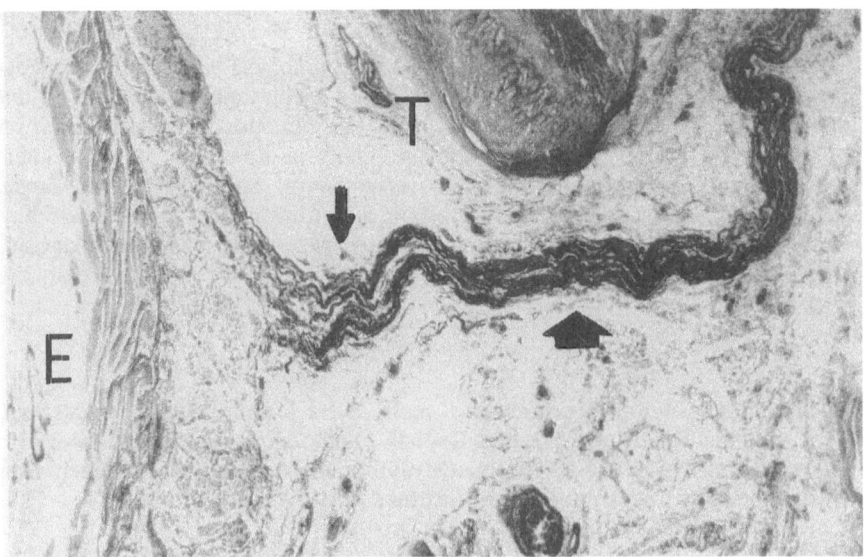

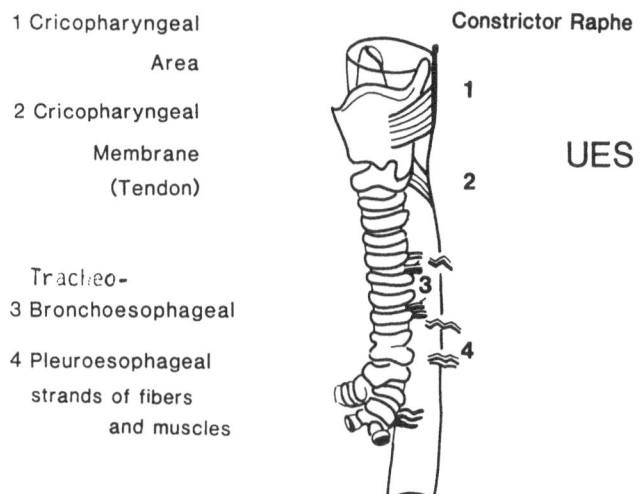

1 Cricopharyngeal
Area

2 Cricopharyngeal
Membrane
(Tendon)

Tracheo-
3 Bronchoesophageal

4 Pleuroesophageal
strands of fibers
and muscles

Constrictor Raphe

UES

Fig. 2. The anchoring structures of the upper half of the esophagus. The esophagus, which lies mobile in the posterior mediastinum in a bed of loose areolar connective tissue, is anchored at the cranial end (*1*) to the cricoid cartilage by the cricopharyngeal tendon (*2*). Delicate membranes (*3* and *4*) stabilize the area more distal down to the tracheal bifurcation. *UES*, upper esophageal sphincter

rounding tissues; this included parts of the fibrous membrane of the trachea extending between the adjacent hoops where the cartilages were incomplete.

The transverse histological section showed distict fiber strands between esophagus and trachea, at varying number and size, but in all the specimens (Figs. 1 and 2). They inserted most often in lateral position in the irregular dense connective tissue that formed the tracheal membrane or in the perichondrium of the cartilages, travelled towards the lateral aspect of the esophageal wall to radiate close to the esophageal muscle and became continuous with the perimysium (Fig. 1). Coiled in the histological cross section they presented "stretched" lengths between 1 and 7 mm, and thicknesses of 30 to 300 μm (1000 μm in one case). When analysed in the consecutive serial sections, the "cords" were found to represent laminary membranes of 1.5 mm to 3 cm craniocaudal extension. The membranes consisted of mainly elastic and collagen fibers and, occasionally, contained striped or smooth muscle bundles.

A larger number of similar fiber strands originated in all our specimens dorsal and lateral from the esophagus, radiating into the meshes of the periesophageal connective tissue space or inserting into the tissue of the pleura.

Discussion

The esophagus, the vessels for its blood supply and the vagal nerves including their recurrent laryngeal branches are contained in the posterior mediastinum that occupies the space between the trachea and pericard and the spine and that extends from the neck to the diaphragm [6].

The stabilization of the esophagus is mainly provided at its proximal end by the tendinous insertion of its musculature to the cricoid cartilage in the neck. Unlike the common construction of the digestive tube, the esophagus possesses neither mesentery nor serosal envelope. The location within the loose areolar connective tissue at the mediastinum permits not only the appropriate movements of the esophagus [1] but also offers as a rule no resistance to a blunt pull through stripping of the esophagus in surgery [2–6] as long as the tumor is confined to the esophageal wall and no inflammatory adhesions are present.

The intimate proximity of the trachea, esophagus, and pleura and the lack of any essential partition sheaths paves the way for easy spread of malignancy and fistula formation. The close local relationship that continues all the way down to the tracheal bifurcation, is on the other side, characterized by the presence of joint structures. These are tiny, delicate laminary membranes, individually varying in number and size, which insert predominantly at the lateral aspects of both the trachea and esophagus. The membranes are by far smaller and shorter than the long gross fibroelastic cords which Laimer in 1883 referred to in his picture [8] later adopted by Netter [9]. Their orientation longitudinal with the esophagotracheal axis, was wrongly pictured [8, 9] because it was found to be regularly transverse. Another factor for the stabilization of the esophagus that has not been appreciated hitherto are the numerous fine membranes that anchor it laterally in the connective tissue network of the mediastinum, dorsally (presumably) to the prevertebral fascia, and connect the esophagus with the pleura. One may admit that these short anchoring membranes restrict the mobility of the esophagus. Yet, the extensibility of collagen membranes and the elastic component with the ability to recoil will yield adequate mobility when stretched under normal tension. When the tiny membranes are torn, they may easily break without damage of either tracheal or pleural wall; however, the unpredictable presence of individually broader membranes may cause damage when the esophagus is stripped during esophagectomy. Therefore, mediastinoscopic dissection during transdiaphragmatic esophagectomy may be a benefit to reduce the incidence of tears in case unusually strong membranes are present.

References

1. Dodds WJ, Stewart ET, Hodges D, Steff JJ, Arndorfer RC (1983) Movement of the feline esophagus associated with respiration and peristalsis. J Clin Invest 52:1–13
2. Akiyama H, Miyazono H, Tsurumaru M, Hashimoto C, Kawamura T (1978) Use of the stomach as an esophageal substitute. Ann Surg 88:606–620
3. Orringer MB, Orringer JS (1983) Esophagectomy without thoracotomy: A dangerous operation? J Thorac Cardiovasc Surg 85:72–80
4. Liebermann-Meffert D, Lüscher U, Neff U, Rüedi ThP, Allgöwer M (1987) Esophagectomy without thoracotomy: Is there a risk of intramediastinal bleeding? A study on blood supply of the esophagus. Ann Surg 206:184–192
5. Siewert JR, Bartels H, Lange J, Roder JD, Hölscher AH (1990) En bloc esophagectomy—when to reconstruct the food passage? In: Ferguson MK, Little AG, Skinner DB (eds) Diseases of the esophagus, vol I. Malignant Diseases. NY, Mt. Kisco, Futura, pp 253–260
6. Duranceau A, Liebermann-Meffert D (1991) Embryology, anatomy, and physiology of the esophagus. In: Orringer MB, Zuidema GD (eds) Shackelford's surgery of the alimentary tract, vol I, The esophagus, 3rd edn. Saunders, Philadelphia, pp 3–49

7. Orringer MB: Complications of esophageal surgery. (1991) In: Orringer MB, Zuidema GD (eds) Shackelford's surgery of the alimentary tract, vol I, The esophagus, 3rd edn. Saunders, Philadelphia, pp 434–459
8. Laimer E (1883) Beitrag zur Anatomie des Oesophagus. Med.Jb (Wien) 333–388
9. Netter FH (1971) The Ciba collection of medical illustrations, vol 3, Digestive system. Part I: Upper digestive tract. Ciba Pharmaceutical Company, New York, pp 44–45

Percutaneous Endoscopic Gastrostomy (PEG) For Treatment of Dysphagia

U. Goebel, H. Kolvenbach, S. Arens, and A. Hirner[1]

Introduction

Dysphagia may occur in different diseases of the upper gastrointestinal tract. Even if a patient is not able to swallow, enteral nutrition is preferable to parenteral nutrition. Since nasogastric tubes cause severe psychological and nursing problems, we perform the percutaneous endoscopic gastrostomy (PEG) as an alternative method.

Methods

The data of our patients treated by PEG gastrostomy was analyzed retrospectively with regard to demographic parameters, indication, mode of anaesthesia and complications.

Via PEG, a gastric feeding tube was placed either using the "pull method", described by Gauderer et al. [1], or the "push method", according to Russel et al. [2].

The "Pull Method"

With the patient in supine position, gastroscopy was performed and the stomach was insufflated until positive diaphanoscopy showed direct contact of gastric and abdominal wall (Fig. 1) [3]. After percutaneous puncture, a guiding cord was passed into the stomach under endoscopic control, grasped with a biopsy forceps and pulled out of the patients mouth (Fig. 2).

---
[1] Chirurgische Universitätsklinik, Sigmund-Freud-Str. 25, W-5300 Bonn 1, Germany

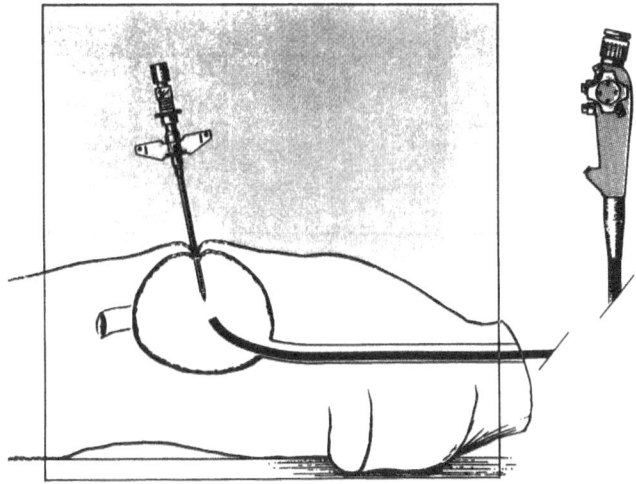

Fig. 1. Gastroscopy performed in the supine position (from [3])

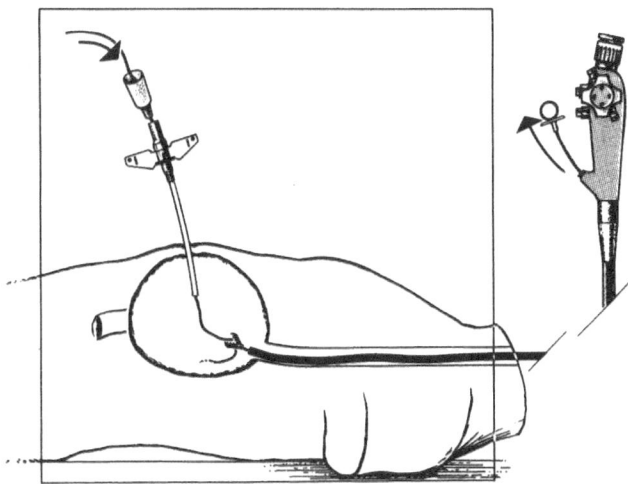

Fig. 2. A guiding cord is passed into the stomach and grasped with forceps (from [3])

This cord was tied to the distal end of a specally prepared tube, which was then pulled retrograde, down to the esophagus and stomach and through the abdominal wall, Leaving only the reserve head of the tube inside the stomach (Figs. 3, 4).

The correct position of the PEG tube was finally verified endoscopically and radiologically. Feedings were begun 24 h postoperatively.

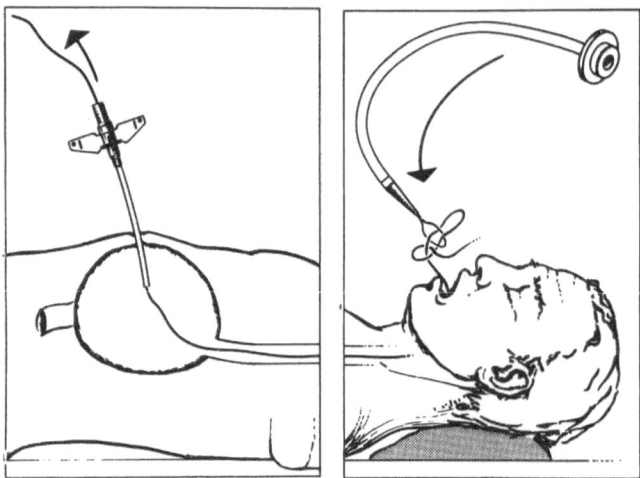

Fig. 3. A tube is pulled through the esophagus and abdominal wall leaving only the reserve head of the tube inside the stomach (from [3])

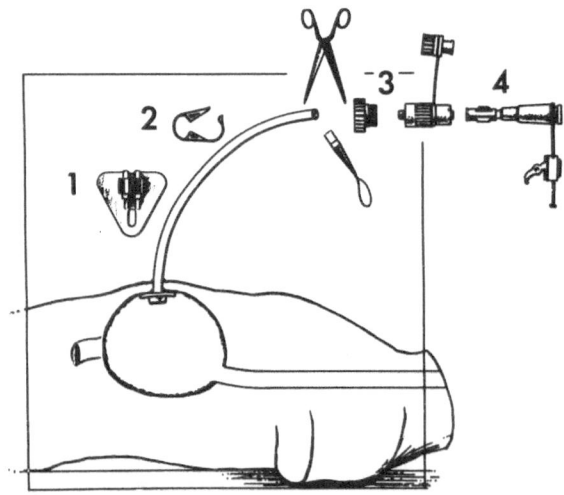

Fig. 4. Tube apparatus (from [3])

Results

General Parameters

From April 1985 to November 1991, PEG was performed in 78 patients (45 male, 33 female). Mean age was 57.7 years, ranging from 24 to 87 years. The "pull method" was applied in 71 patients, while 7 patients underwent the "push

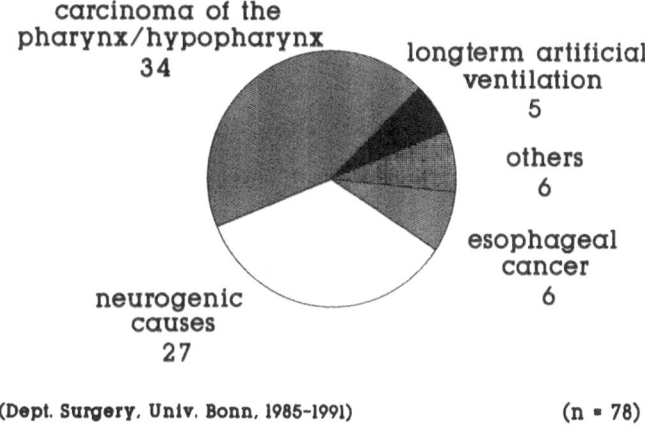

carcinoma of the
pharynx/hypopharynx
34

longterm artificial
ventilation
5

others
6

esophageal
cancer
6

neurogenic
causes
27

(Dept. Surgery, Univ. Bonn, 1985-1991)   (n = 78)

Fig. 5. PEG indications

method". In more than 65% ($n = 51$) of the patients, treatment could be performed using local anaesthesia, but 27 patients needed general anesthesia. The mean operative time was 23.5 min.

During the observation period, the PEG tube was carried for an average time of 227 days. Three patients have been feeding enterally via PEG for more than 3 years now.

Indications

The indications for PEG are shown in Fig. 5. The majority of patients ($n = 40$) suffered from malignant diseases of the oral cavity and the esophagus. Also, severe neurological impairment, especially pseudobulbar paralysis, frequently ($n = 27$) was an indication for PEG.

Five patients showed profound respiratory failure and needed long-term artificial ventilation.

Miscellaneous indications ($n = 6$) included central bronchial carcinoma with bronchoesophagial fistula and severe facial trauma. In cases of advanced malignant occlusion of the common bile duct (pancreatic cancer, proximal cholangicarcinoma), PEG was performed to allow an external/internal drainage of the bile fluid after percutaneous transhepatic cholangiostomy.

Complications

Complications associated with PEG are shown in Figs. 6 and 7. Complications were relatively frequent after PEG, but could easily be managed in most cases. It was always possible to treat local infections of the abdominal wall ($n = 7$) conservatively without removal of the PEG tube. In 14 cases, an exchange of the feeding tube was necessary because of tube-associated complications. In 12 cases, this could be performed on an outpatient basis. Diarrhea was, in all cases, treated successfully by feeding with products of lower osmolarity.

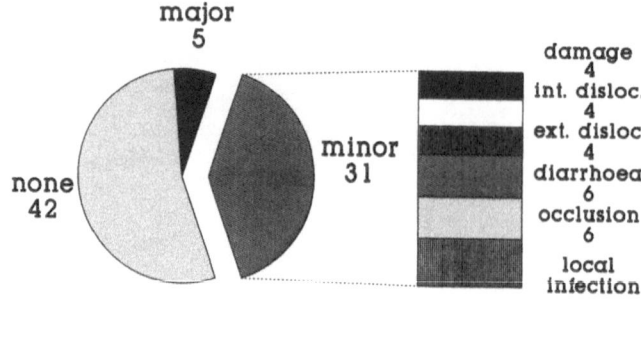

(Dept. Surgery, Univ. Bonn, 1985-1991)   (n = 78)

Fig. 6. Minor PEG complications

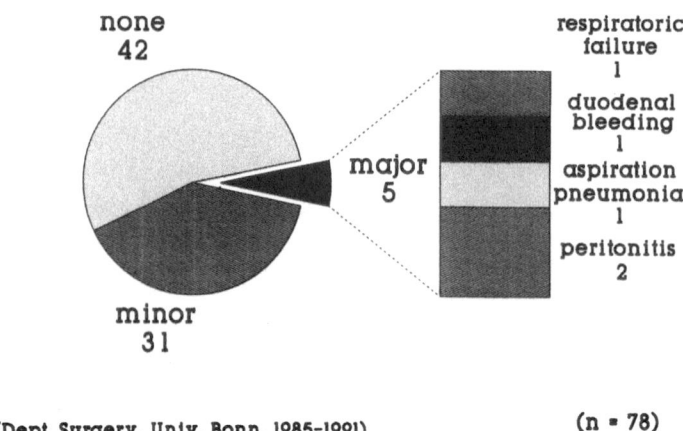

(Dept. Surgery, Univ. Bonn, 1985-1991)   (n = 78)

Fig. 7. Major PEG complications

There was one gastrointestinal bleeding from the duodenal bulb due to internal dislocation of the PEG tube. In another patient, the PEG caused peritonitis. Both patients survived after surgical treatment and intensive care management. We observed an aspiration pneumonia in one patient, which was treated successfully by artficial respiration and antibiotics. Two fatal complications observed in our group were not due to PEG, but were related to the patients' underlying diseases:

- Peritonitis after perforated appendicitis under the condition of long-term artificial ventilation
- prolonged respiratory failure in a patient with pseudobulbar paralysis

Discussion

According to the literature [4–8], we found the percutaneous, endocopically controlled gastrostomy to be a safe, handy, and cheap procedure to maintain enteral nutrition in dysphagia of various origins. Performed under local anaeshesia, it is suitable for in patient as well as outpatient use.

PEG should be performed for the following indications:

- Impossible or insufficient oral nutrition for longer then 4 weeks, due to:
  - Tumor-associated dysphagia
  - Neurogenic dysphagia
  - Long-term respiratory therapy
- Supportive nutrition (e.g., during oncologic therapy)

Contraindications for PEG are:

Absolute	Relative
Negative diaphanoscopy	Previous gastric resection
Coagulation disorders	Massive ascites
Ileus	Immunosuppression
Peritonitis	Unfitness for anesthesia
Peritoneal dialysis	

References

1. Gauderer MWL, Ponsky JL, Izant RJ (1980) Gastrostomy without laparotomy. A percutaneous endoscopic technique. J pediat Surg 15:872–875
2. Russel TR, Brotman M, Norris F (1984) Percutaneous endoscopic gastrostomy: A new simplified and cost-effective technique. Am J Surg 148:132
3. Kolvenbach H (1992) Kuenstliche Ernaehrung durch Sonden (to be published) In: Dengler HJ, Zierz S, Jerusalem F (eds) Amyotrophe Lateralsklerose. Georg Thieme, Stuttgart
4. Keymling M, Schroeder M, Woerner W (1985) Erfahrungen mit der perkutan endoskopisch kontrollierten Gastrostomie (PEG). Med Welt 36:1297–1301
5. Jung M, Harz C, Pimentel F (1991) Perkutane endoskopische Gastrostomie. Dtsch med Wschr 116:1063–1068
6. Stellato THA, Gauderer MWL, Ponsky JL (1984) Percutaneous endoscopic gastrostomy following previous abdominal surgery. Ann Surg 200/1:46–50
7. Ponsky JL, Gauderer MWL, Stellato THA (1983) Percutaneous endoscopic gastrostomy, review of 150 cases. Arch Surg 118:913–914
8. Ponsky JL, Gauderer MWL (1989) Percutaneous endoscopic gastrostomy: Indications, limitations, techniques, and results. World J Surg 13:165–170

Disturbance of the Coagulatory System Before and After Surgery for Esophageal Cancer—Clinical Significance and Therapy

Akira Usuba, Osamu Konno, Yukio Endoh, Hitoshi Inoue, and Ryoichi Motoki[1]

Introduction

Invasion, of the body results in activation of proteinases that regulate various functions to maintain homeostasis. Depending on the degree of the invasion, the body may activate proteinases to the point where even the normal tissue may be destroyed. Multiple organ failure and mortality may occur.

The blood coagulation factors consist of 12 factors, I–XIII (no VI factor). Excluding fibrinogen (I), tissue thromboplastin (III), Ca^{2+} (IV), V, VIII, and XII, the remaining 6 factors are proteinases, which are activated if the body is invaded [1]. Radical resection of esophageal cancer is one of the most high risk operation. We clarified that hypercoagulability develops after surgery for esophageal cancer, and it is related closely to postoperative complications [2]. The purpose of this study was to determine hypercoagulability in patients surgically treated for esophageal cancer, and to evaluate the effects of the synthetic proteinase inhibitors (PI) on hypercoagulability.

Material and Methods

Thirty-eight patients with esophageal cancer who underwent radical resection were studied. Of these, 4 patients received nafamostat mesilate 150 mg/day (FUT [3] group), 8 patients received gabexate mesilate 2000 mg/day (FOY [4] group), and 3 patients received urinastatin 300 000 U/day (MRC group) for 3 days after surgery, and 23 patients (control group) did not receive proteinase inhibitor. (Nafamostat mesilate [Futhan®] was obtained from Torii and Co

[1] First Department of Surgery, Fukushima Medical College, 1 Hikarigaoka, Fukushima, 960-12 Japan

[Tokyo, Japan] and Banyu Pharmaceutical Co [Tokyo, Japan]. FOY® was obtained from Ono Pharmaceutical Co [Osaka, Japan] and urinastatin [Milaclid®]
was obtained from Mochida Pharmaceutical Co [Tokyo, Japan].) No significant
differences were observed in each group for following factors: age, body weight,
the time needed for surgery, the volume of intraoperative bleeding, and the
volume of intraoperative blood transfusion. Blood samples were collected at
the before the operation and at 1, 3, 5, and 7 postperative days (POD). We
measured the following 16 parameters: 3 parameters of platelet system [platelet
count (PLT), β-thromboglobulin (β-TG), and platelet factor 4 (PF$_4$)], 6 parameters of the coagulation system [prothrombin time activity (PT), activated partial
thromboplastin time (APTT), fibrinogen (FBG), antithrombin III (AT III),
fibrinopeptide A (FPA), and thormbin–AT III complex [TAT]], and 7 parameters the fibrinolytic system [fibrinopeptide B β$_{15-42}$ (B β), plasminogen (PLG),
antiplasmin (α$_2$PI), tissue plasminogen activator (t-PA), euglobulin lysis time
(ELT), D-dimer (DD), and plasmin-α$_2$PI complex (PIC)].

TAT, PIC, and DD were compared among the FUT, MRC and control
groups, and euglobulin lysis time (ELT) among the FUT, FOY, and control
groups.

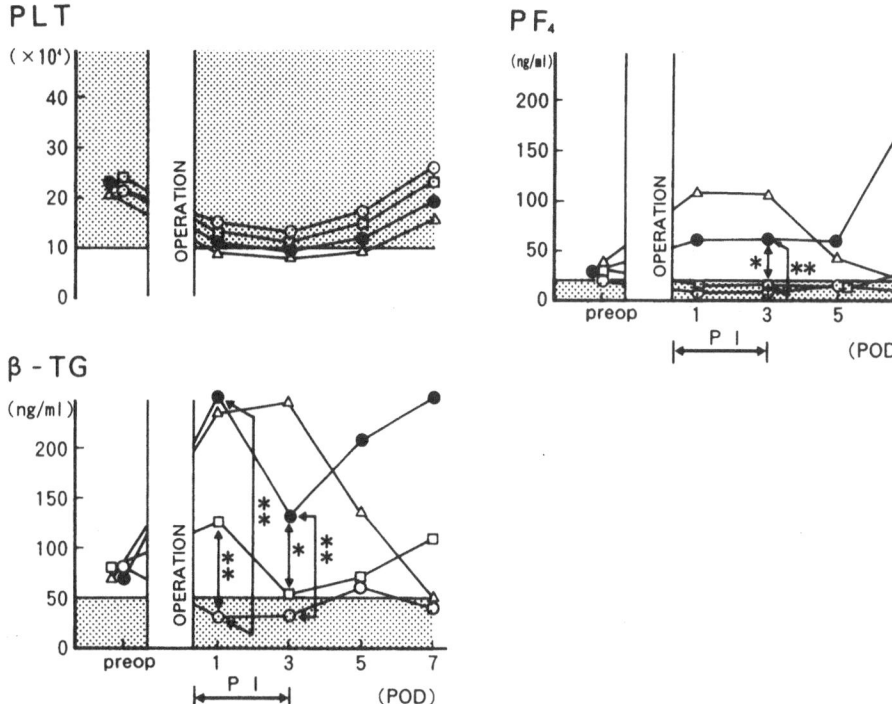

Fig. 1. The changes of three parameters of the platelet system. *POD*, postoperative day; *PLT*,
platelet count; β-*TG*, β-thromboglobulin; *PF$_4$*, platelet factor 4; *FUT* (*open circies*, $n = 4$),
nafamostat mesilate; *FOY* (*open squares*, $n = 8$), gabexate mesilate; *MRC* (*open triangles*, $n =
3$), urinastatin; *CONT* (*closed circles*, $n = 23$), control; *$P < 0.05$; **$P < 0.01$

Measured values were expressed in terms of mean ± standard deviation (mean ± SD). The student's *t*-test was used for statistical analysis with *P* values of less than 0.05 considered significant. Intergroup comparison was carried out on postoperative days 1 and 3 when PI were administered.

Results

In all test patients, preoperaive coagulability was within the normal range. Immediately after surgery, the platelet count (PLT) decreased to approx. 1/2 of the preoperative level at the 3rd POD, and recovered to the preoperative level by the 7th POD. There were no significant differences among the four groups. Both β-TG and PF4 showed a constantly high tendency in MRC and control groups compared with those in FUT and FOY groups (Fig. 1).

PT decreased and APTT and FBG increased rapidly in the four groups immediately after operation. There were no significant differences among the groups. AT III also decreased immediately after surgery, and recovered to the normal range by the 7th POD. FPA increased remarkably at the 1st and 3rd POD in MRC and control groups . On the other hand, in both the FUT and FOY groups, the FPA did not increase and significant differences between first two groups (MRC and control groups) and the second two groups (FUT and FOY groups) were noted on the 1st and 3rd POD. The TAT was stable in the FUT group at the 1st POD compared with this control group (Fig. 2).

In the fibrinopeptide B β_{15-42} (B β), plasminogen (PLG), antiplasmin (α_2PI) and t-PA, there were significant differences between the control group and FUT and/or FOY groups at the 1st POD. In ELT and DD, there were significant differences between the control group and FUT and/or FOY groups at the 1st POD (Fig. 3).

Discussion

Immediately after surgery, both the control and MRC groups were in a hypercoagulable state, showing a marked decrease in PLT, PT, AT III, and PLG, and an increase in APTT, FPA, and B β.

FUT, FOY, and MRC, PI inhibiting trypsin activity, were developed for the treatment of acute pancreatitis. FUT and FOY inhibit serine proteinases, such as thrombin and plasmin, and are thus termed serine PI. We clinically compared the effects of PI on the hypercoagulability following resection of esophageal cancer.

In the platelet system, FUT and FOY controlled increases in β-TG and PF_4, and the effect of the former was more marked. Since there are no reports on the effect of these drugs to control platelet aggregation or release, our findings were thought to be indirect results. In the coagulation system, there were no significant intergroup differences for PT, APTT, or FBG, but the AT III levels recovered rapidly in the FUT and FOY groups. FUT and FOY inhibited thrombin of FPA, the former showing a marked effect. As for the fibrinolytic system, FUT and FOY showed considerable antifibrinolytic effects. In particular, FUT had a marked effect on ELT, but the FUT group showed a DD

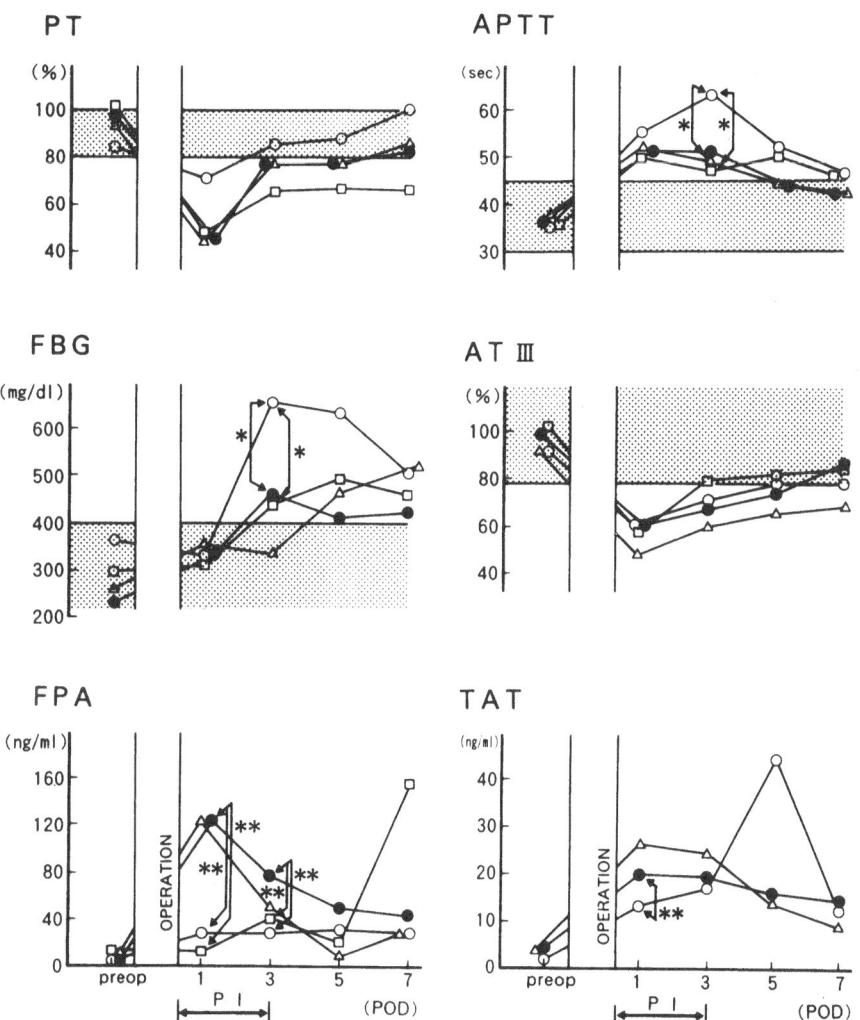

Fig. 2. The changes of six parameters of the coagulation system. *PT*, prothrombin time activity; *FBG*, fibrinogen; *FPA*, fibrinopeptide A; *APTT*, activated partial thromboplastin time; *AT III*, antithrombin III; *TAT*, thrombin-AT III complex; *Symbols* and *n* as for Fig. 1 legend; *P < 0.05; **P < 0.01

level similar to that of the control group. The anti-secondary fibrinolytic action of FUT was negligible. MRC had no effect on the coagulation or fibrinolytic systems.

Conclusion

Hypercoagulability developed after surgery for esophageal carcinoma. FUT and FOY completely checked the abnormal increase in thrombin activty which might

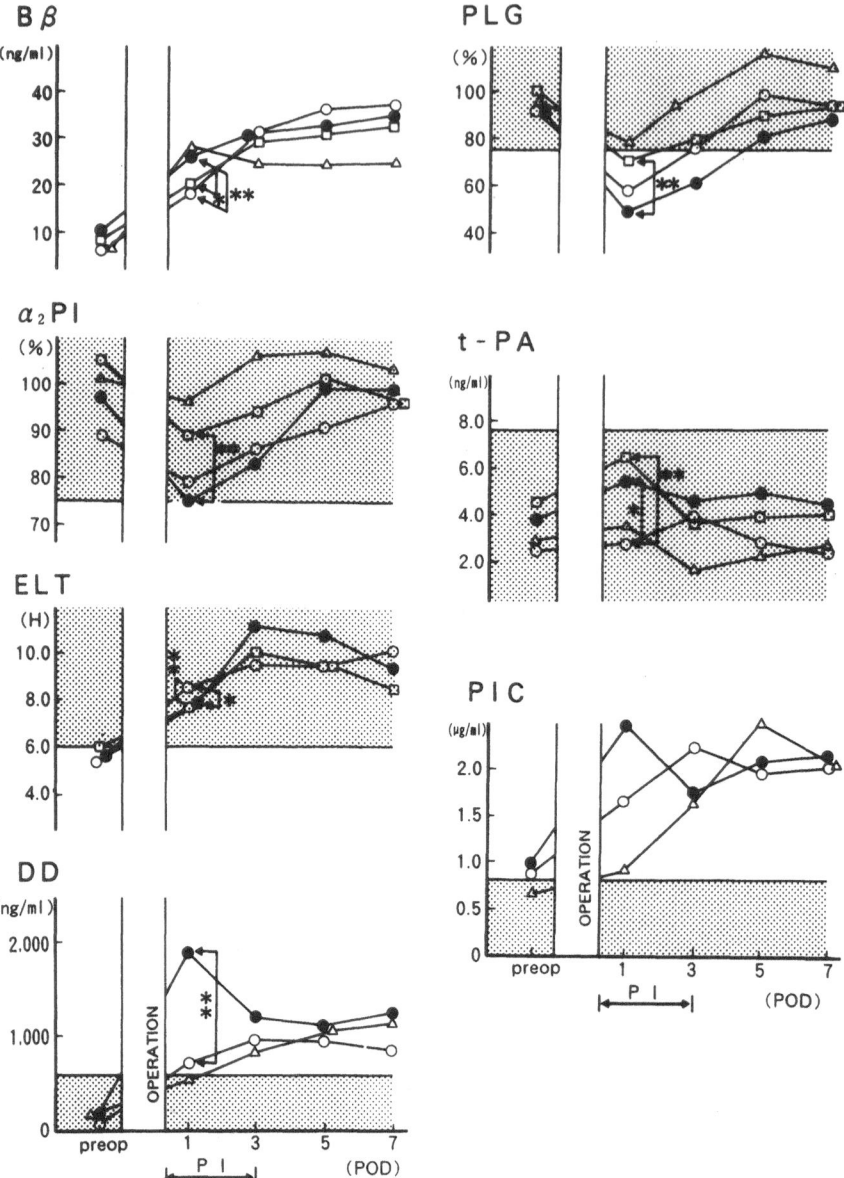

Fig. 3. The changes of seven parameters of the fibrinolytic system. *B* β, fibrinopeptide B
β_{15-42}; $\alpha_2 PI$, antiplasmin; *ELT*, euglobulin lysis time; *DD*, D-dimer; *PLG*, plasminogen; *t-PA*,
tissue plasminogen activator; *PIC*, $\alpha_2 PI$ complex; *Symbols* and *n* as for Fig. 1 lenged; *P <
0.05; **P < 0.01

trigger the hypercoagulability, but MRC had no such effect. FUT had a more marked effect than that of FOY, posing no particular problem of anti–secondary fibrinolytic action.

References

1. McKay DG (1973) Intravenous coagulation—acute and chronic—disseminated and local. In: Schmer G, Strandjord PE (eds) Coagulation current research and clinical applications. Academic, New York, pp 45–72
2. Usuba A, Motoki R, Watanabe M, Koizumi Y, Kanno R, Matayoshi K, Ohishi A, Endoh Y, Konno O, Inoue H (1990) Hypercoagulability after surgery for esophageal carcinoma. J Jpn Assoc Thorac Surg 38:401–411
3. Miyamoto Y, Hirose H, Matsuda H, Nakano S, Ohtani N, Kaneko M, Nishigaki K, Nomura F, Kitamura H, Kawashima Y (1985) Analysis of complement activation profile drug cardiopulmonary bypass and its inhibition by FUT-175. Trans Am Soc Artif Intern Organs 31:508–561
4. Ohno H, Kosaki G, Kambayashi J, Imaoka S, Hirata F (1980) FOY [Ethyl p-(6-guanidino-hexanoyloxy) benzoate] methansulfonate as a serine proteinase inhibitor. I. Inhibition of thrombin and factor Xa in vitro. Thromb Res 19:579–588

Experimental Study on Function of the Upper Esophageal Sphincter After Radical Operation for Esophageal Cancer

Yosuke Fukunaga, Masayuki Higashino, Harushi Osugi,
Noriaki Maekawa, Taigo Tokuhara, Shinya Tanimura,
and Hiroaki Kinoshita[1]

Introduction

The upper esophageal sphincter (UES), located between the esophagus and the pharynx, provides a barrier against esophagopharyngeal reflux and subsequent aspiration of intraesophageal contents such as food or digestive juices. This consists of the cricopharyngeus muscle and the upper part of esophageal circular muscle. The UES is presented as a high pressure zone manometrically, with the pressure (UESP) higher than pharyngeal or esophageal pressure, i.e., around 39 mmHg as reported by Tokuhara et al. [1], and the length of this high pressure zone is about 2–4 cm.

The function of the cervical esophagus including the UES is hampered after radical surgery for esophageal cancer, especially when the lymph nodes in the upper mediastinal region are dissected. Tokuhara et al. [1] evaluated the function of the UES after radical surgery for esophageal cancer and showed that response of the UES to balloon inflation in the cervical esophagus was less after surgery than in healthy controls. We thought that the decreased response of the UES could be attributed to the dissection along the recurrent laryngeal nerves. Consequently, we performed experiments in dogs to find out the role of recurrent laryngeal nerves in the function of the cervical esophagus including the UES.

Materials and Methods

A 6-French silicone catheter was used for manometry. This catheter had a conventional small transducer attached 3 cm from the tip and a new type of pressure sensor attached at the tip (Gaeltec Corporation, England). The latter

[1] Second Department of Surgery, Osaka City University Medical School, 1-5-7 Asahimachi, Abeno-ku, Osaka, 545 Japan

could measure pressure all around the circumference of the sensor. This sensor is equipped with the same type of small transducer placed within a silicone rubber column 3 mm in length and filled with oil (Circumferentially sensitive Catheter tip Transducer, CCT).

Gastrostomy at the fundus of the stomach was made under anesthesia at least 2 days before manometry in the controls to be able to measure UESP without anesthesia. We inserted a catheter for manometry through the gastrostomy towards the esophagus.

We used ten mongrel dogs weighing between 8–15 kg, of either sex. The catheter for manometry was inserted through the gastrostomy and moved up the esophagus so that the sensor at the tip of the catheter reached the pharynx, and the intrapharyngeal pressure was taken as the zero point. After measurement of the UESP at rest following the stationary pull-through method, another silicone tube with a balloon at the tip was inserted through the stoma so that the balloon could be placed at 5–10 cm below the UES. Then, the balloon was inflated to the diameter of 1.5, 2.0, and 2.5 cm at 5 cm and 10 cm below the UES, and the UESP was measured according to the same method. Next, another silicone tube for perfusion was inserted through the stoma and the tip was placed 10 cm below the UES. When HCl 0.1 N or NaOH 0.1 N was perfused into the esophagus at a rate of 0.5 ml/min, the UESP was measured at 5 min intervals for 35 min, as mentioned above.

The dogs were fasted for 1 day and manometry was done without anesthesia. They were divided into three groups: controls, ten dogs with both recurrent laryngeal nerves intact; L group, the same ten dogs with their left recurrent laryngeal nerve severed; and B group, the same ten dogs with both recurrent laryngeal nerves severed. The left recurrent laryngeal nerve was cut at the level of the cranial point of the aortic arch, and the right one was cut at the level of the cranial point of the aortic arch, and the right one was cut at the level of the cranial point of the right subclavian artery under intravenous anesthesia.

Results

The UESP at rest which was 32.9 mmHg, 30.0 mmHg, and 30.2 mmHg, in controls, L group, and B group, respectively, and the difference was not significant. When the balloon was inflated 5 cm below the UES, the UESP at each diameter of the balloon was significantly higher than that at rest in all groups, but the UESP in the L and B groups was significantly lower than that in the controls at each diameter of the balloon (Fig. 1).

When the balloon was inflated 10 cm below the UES, the UESP at each diameter of the balloon was significantly higher than that at rest in controls and in the L group. When the balloon was inflated to the diameter of 2.0 cm and 2.5 cm, the UESP was significantly higher than that at rest in the B group, but in the L group the UESP was significantly lower than that in the controls when the balloon diameter was 2.0 and 2.5 cm. The UESP in the B group was significantly lower than that in the controls only when the balloon diameter was 2.5 cm (Fig. 1).

When the acid was perfused into the esophagus, the UESP increased gradually, and became significantly higher than that at rest 15 min after the start of perfusion

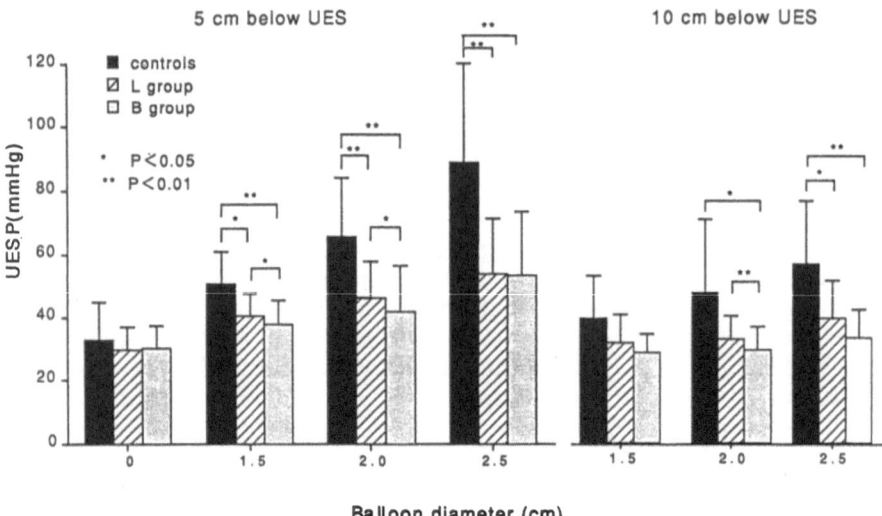

Fig. 1. Upper esophageal sphincter pressure (*UESP*) at balloon distension

in the controls. In the L and B groups, the UESP did not increase with the perfusion of acid. There were significant differences between the UESP in the controls and those in the L and B groups 15 min after the start of perfusion (Fig. 2).

When alkaline was perfused into the esophagus, the UESP increased gradually, and became significantly higher than that at rest 5 min after the start of perfusion in the controls and after 15 min in the L group. There was no significant increase of the UESP in the B group. There were significant differences between the UESP in the controls and those in the L and B groups 5 min after the start of perfusion (Fig. 2).

Discussion

The UES is a high pressure zone found by manometry and the pressure is reported to be between 30–120 mmHg in humans, measured according to the perfused open tip method. Its value varies greatly among the studies published in the literature, and this is probably due to the difficulties encountered when measuring the UESP because it changes according to the direction of the sensor. Several studies in which the UESP was measured by the perfused open tip method showed that the UESP in sagittal direction is higher than that in frontal direction. In this study, we used a new sensor to measure UES pressure which was 32.9 mmHg in dogs without anesthesia.

Recently, surgical procedures for esophageal cancer have become safer and have tended to involve extended lymph node dissection to attain a better prognosis, but this kind of extended surgery is sometimes accompanied by complications such as respiratory dysfunction and palsy of the recurrent laryngeal

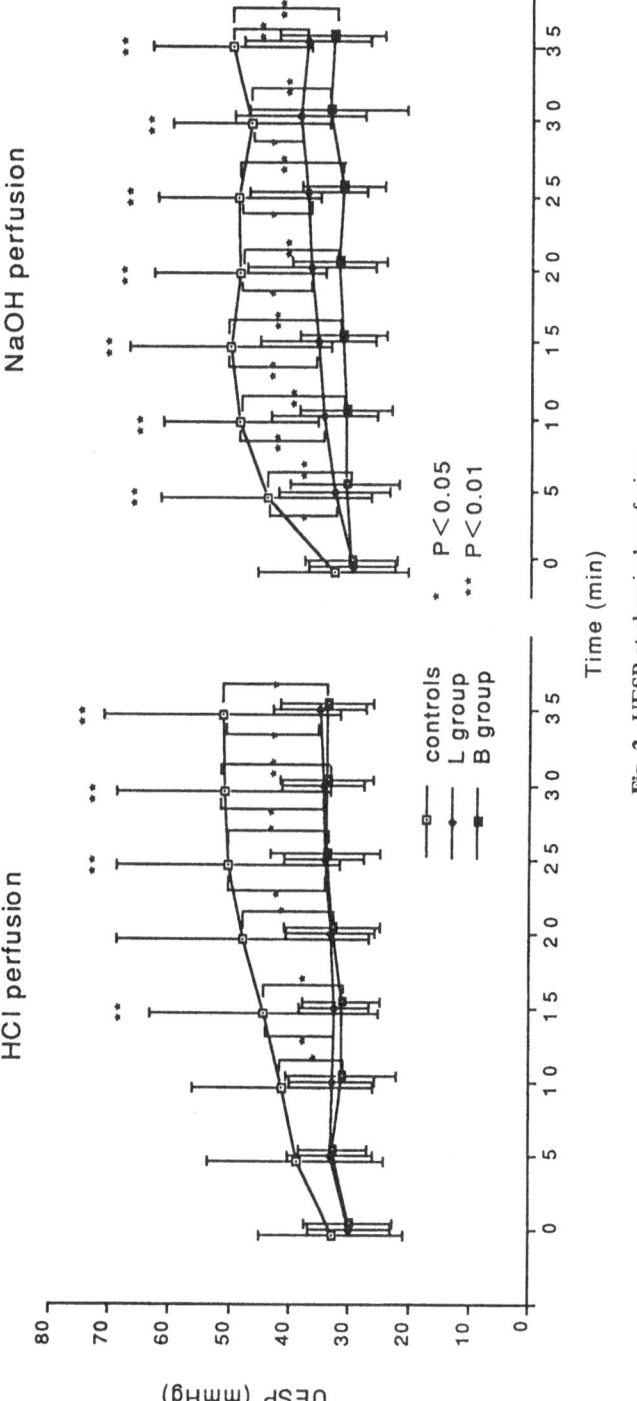

Fig. 2. UESP at chemical perfusion

nerves. There is a high incidence of dissection of the lymph nodes in the upper mediastinum, mainly those nodes found along bilateral recurrent laryngeal nerves in patients with thoracic esophageal cancer. Tokuhara et al. [1] demonstrated in a clinical study that UES dysfunction and palsy of these nerves are related. In this experimental study, we have confirmed that UES dysfunction is related to damage of recurrent laryngeal nerves because dysfunction increased as more laryngeal nerves were severed.

Moreover, we have demonstrated that the UES contracted on the response to balloon inflation, and these results are in agreement with those reported by Freiman et al. [2]. After severing the left recurrent laryngeal nerve, the responses decreased in intensity but did not disappear. And when both recurrent laryngeal nerves were severed, the responses were weaker than those observed after left denervation alone. These results agree with our own and suggest that the recurrent laryngeal nerves are one of the pathways of the UES reflex in response to stretching of the esophageal wall by balloon inflation, and that intramural innervation of the cervical esophagus might be another pathway.

The UES also contracted in response to chemical perfusion in the cervical esophagus. The response to perfusion of acid disappeared after severing the left recurrent laryngeal nerve, whereas the response to perfusion of alkaline fluid decreased after severing the left recurrent laryngeal nerve and disappeared after bilateral denervation. These results suggest that the pathway of the UES reflex induced by perfusion of acid or alkaline is mainly through recurrent laryngeal nerves. The responses of the UES to perfusion of acid or alkaline were weaker than those to wall stretching by balloon inflation.

We conclude that the response of the upper esophageal sphincter, which is an important barrier against aspiration pneumonia, is mainly controlled by recurrent laryngeal nerves. These nerves are a direct sensory pathway for reflex of the UES to various stimuli in the cervical esophagus, but there might be other pathways involved in this reflex as well such as intramural innervation.

References

1. Tokuhara T, Higashino M, Osugi H, Maekawa N, Tanimura S, Fukunaga Y, Kinoshita H (1992) Clinical study on responses of the upper esophageal sphincter after subtotal esophagectomy for esophageal cancer. Jpn J Surg 93:578–588
2. Freiman JM, El-Sharkawy TY, Diamant NE (1981) Effect of bilateral vagosympathetic nerve blockade on response of the dog upper esophageal sphincter (UES) to intraesophgeal inflation and acid. Gastroenterology 81:78–84

The Immunological Changes After Operation for Esophageal Cancer and the Effect of Lentinan

Satoru Hayashi, Masayuki Matsumori, Tetsuya Hattori,
Yoshihisa Watanabe, Takashi Koyama, Hisao Yoshihara,
Katsuhiro Sawada, and Masayoshi Okada[1]

Introduction

It has generally accepted that surgical intervention produces immunodeficiency [1, 2]. Malnutrition is also immunosuppressive [3]. So, in the patient with esophageal cancer, with the presence of preoperative starvation, the host defense mechanism is markedly suppressed by operations which involve intra-abdominal and intrathoracic procedures.

We have investigated immunological changes, mainly cell mediated immunity, before and after surgery for esophageal cancer and have assessed the effect of the administration of the polysaccharide lentinan on the host immunity following surgery in the patients with esophageal cancers.

Patients and Methods

Thirty-three patients who underwent operation for esophageal cancer were studied. The patients were divided into two groups. One group of 18 patients was administrated 2 mg of lentinan per week intravenously from 2 weeks before operation. The other group, 15 patients, who did not receive lentinan, acted as controls. Between the two groups, there were no statistical differences in the distribution of age, sex, stage of the disease, preoperative serum albumin level, and blood lymphocyte count (Table 1). Blood samples were collected 2 weeks and 1 week preoperatively, and 1 day and 1, 2, 4, and 8 weeks postoperatively. Immunological parameters, such as leukocyte count, lymphocyte count, immunoglobulins, subsets of lymphocytes, antibody-dependent cell mediated cytotoxicity (ADCC) and natural killer (NK) activity, were measured

[1] Department of Surgery, Division II, Kobe University School of Medicine, Kusuroku-cho, Chuo-ku, Kobe, 650 Japan

Table 1. Background factors in groups with and without lentinan administration

	Group with lentinan administration ($n = 18$)	Group with lentinan administration ($n = 15$)	Significance
Age (years)	64 ± 7.0	65 ± 8.0	n.s.
Sex	male 15	male 13	n.s.
	female 3	female 2	
Preoperative serum albumin levels (g/dl)	3.48 ± 0.29	3.46 ± 0.35	n.s.
Preoperative blood lymphocytes counts per mm³	2326 ± 855	2362 ± 874	n.s.
P.N.I.[a]	47.0 ± 5.8	46.2 ± 5.5	n.s.
Pathological stage	st.0 2	st.0 0	n.s.
	st.1 1	st.1 2	
	st.2 2	st.2 0	
	st.3 4	st.3 5	
	st.4 9	st.4 8	

[a] P.N.I. (serum albumin level) × (10 + blood lymphocytes count × 0.005)

for immunological assessment. Subsets of lymphocytes (LEU 4, LEU 3A, LEU 2A, LEU 7, LEU 11) were tested by the direct antibody method with laser flow cytometry. ADCC was tested for cytotoxicity against ^{51}Cr-labeled CRBC target cells. NK activity was tested for cytotoxicity against ^{51}Cr-labeled K-562 target cells.

Results have been expressed as mean ±SE. Pre- and postoperative results were compared with using paired t-test, and comparisons between two groups were made using unpaired t-test.

Results

Operation was followed by a significant rise in blood leukocyte counts. This reached significance ($P < 0.0001-0.05$) over 4 weeks in both groups.

There was a slight fall in blood lymphocyte count at 1 week following surgery in the control group. This fall returned to preoperative levels within 2 weeks. In the control group, the ratio of postoperative lymphocyte count to preoperative value (1 week before operation) was reduced by 66% at 1 week, while there was no fall shown in lentinan-administrated group. In control groups, immunoglobulins (IgG and IgA) and CH 50 fell on the first postoperative day ($P < 0.05$) but recovered to preoperative levels within 1 week.

LEU 4 was depressed ($P < 0.0005$) following surgery in both groups, and had not recovered by 4 weeks.

LEU 3A was depressed ($P < 0.0005-0.05$) following surgery in the control group, and the depression lasted over 8 weeks. There was no fall shown in postoperative changes of LEU 2A in both groups. Consequently, LEU 3A/LEU 2A declined from 1.7 preoperatively to 1.1–1.4 after surgery in the control group ($P < 0.05$), and had not recovered by 4 weeks. There was a significant difference between the two groups at 2 weeks after surgery ($P < 0.05$). The results were detailed in Fig. 1.

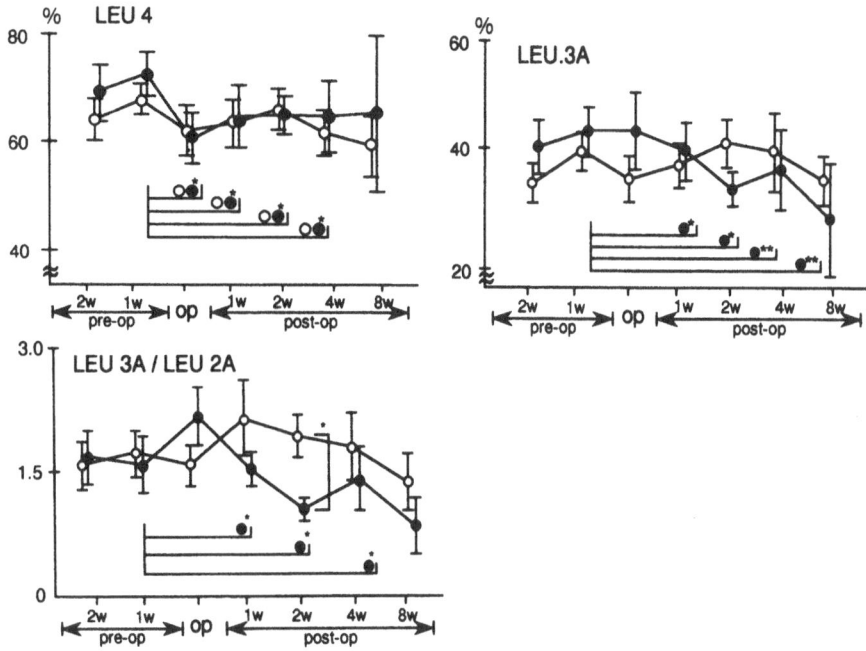

Fig. 1. Changes of LEU 4, LEU 3A and LEU 3A/LEU 2A in lentinan-administrated group (*open circles*) and control group (*closed circles*). *Significant differences from preoperative values and significant differences between two groups, $P < 0.05$; ** significant differences from preoperative values, $P < 0.0005$

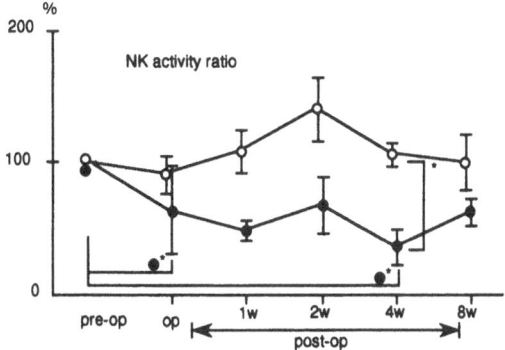

Fig. 2. Changes of % ratio of postoperative natural Killer (*NK*) activity to preoperative value (1 week before operation) in lentinan-administered group (*open circles*) and control group (*closed circles*). *Significant differences between two groups, $P < 0.05$

No remarkable postoperative change was found in LEU 7 and LEU 11. No statistical difference was found between two groups.

NK activity was depressed following surgery in the control group. In the control group, % ratio of postoperative NK activity to preoperative value

Table 2. Comparison of frequency in postoperative leukocytosis between two groups (WBC > 10000/mm^3 at 14 days after operation)

	Group with lentinan administration ($n = 18$)	Group without lentinan administration ($n = 15$)
Frequency of postoperative leukocytosis	6/18 (33%)	11/15 (73%)

* Significant difference between two groups by χ^2 test and Fisher's test ($P < 0.05$)

(1 week before operation) declined to 35% at the end of 4 weeks postoperatively, while the ratio increased to 140% at 2 weeks postoperatively in the lentinan-administered group. The difference is statistically significant at 4 weeks between the two groups ($P < 0.05$). The results are shown in Fig. 2.

In the control group, the ADCC level declined slightly postoperatively, but no statistical difference was found between the two groups.

In 17 patients, blood leukocyte counts were more than 10,000/mm^3 at 2 weeks after surgery. We considered these cases as postoperative leukocytosis. There were 6 patients in the lentinan-administrated group, and 11 patients in control group. All cases diagnosed as having lung complications were included this category. The frequency in postoperative leukocytosis was much fewer the lentinan administered group ($P < 0.05$). The results are shown in Table 2.

Discussion

Major surgery for malignant tumors have been shown to cause immunodeficiency, and the depression of immunity correlates to the degree of surgical intervention [1, 2]. With few exceptions, many investigators have observed that cellular immunity was more likely to be affected than not [1, 4]. The reason for this depression is not clear but Gupta has reported that lymphopenia and probably the number of T4+ cells had an inverse relationship with plasma cortisol [5].

In this study, parameters related to cellular immunity (LEU 4, LEU 3A, NK activity) were further suppressed. The depression of helper T cells (LEU 3A) was larger than those of suppressor T cells (LEU 2A), and cytotoxic cells (LEU 7 and LEU 11). NK cells have an important role in the first line of defense against the dissemination of tumor cells [6, 7]. Surgical procedures increase the possibility of disseminating cancer cells so the depression of NK activity may hasten the development metastasic foci. On the other hand, helper T cells not only activate cytotoxicic cells but regulate B cell function, so depression of helper T cells may suppress B cells' immune response. The disadvantage of B cells deficiency is that the risk of acquiring postoperative infection is increased. The depression of NK cells and helper T cells affect the patients' prognosis, and the correction of postoperative immunosuppression may help to prevent these problems [8].

We attempted to support host immunity following surgery by using lentinan which reduced the degree of postoperative depression on lymphocyte count, LEU 3A, and NK activity. Our results agree to the hypothesis that lentinan activates helper T cells through potentiation of IL-2 production from PMN and macropharges [9]. Lentinan did not activate LEU 2A, LEU 7, or LEU 11. Lentinan also did not increase suppressor T cells and cytotoxic T cells activity. It seemed that NK activity was potentiated increasing the sensitivity of the cells, not the number of cells.

The frequency in postoperative leukocytosis was lower in the lentinan-administrated group. There are some observations that lentinan has a protective effect against some bacterias, fungis, and viruses [10]. Potential clinical usefulness of lentinan against postoperative infection was indicated.

References

1. Lennard TWJ, Shenton BK, Borzotta A, Donelly PK, White M, Gerrie LM, Proud G, Taylor RMR (1985) The influence of surgical operation of the human immune system. Br J Surg 72:771–776
2. Meakins JL (1988) Host defence mechanisms in surgical patients: Effect of surgery and trauma. Acta Chir Scand [Suppl] 550:43–53
3. Saito T (1986) Evaluation, analysis and treatments of host-defense impairment in esophageal cancer patients under surgery. J Jpn Surg Soc 19:1856–1864
4. Singh G, Khanna NN (1985) Nutritional status in advanced upper gastrointestinal cancers. J Surg Oncol 29:269–272
5. Gupta S (1987) Immune response following surgical trauma. Crit Care Clin 3:405–415
6. Herberman RB (1984) Natural killer cells and their positive roles in host resistance against tumors. Transplant Proc 16:476–478
7. Hanna N, Fidler I (1981) Relationship between metastatic potential and resistance to natural killer cell-mediated cytotoxity in three murine tumor system. JNCI 66:1183–1190
8. Cole WH, Humphrey L (1985) Need of immunologic stimurators during immunosuppression produced by major cancer surgery. Ann Surg 202:9–20
9. Suzuki M, Hamuro J (1990) Anti-tumor polysaccharide, lentinan its biological function leading to anti-tumor activity. Biotherapy 4:1114–1126
10. Chen HY, Kaneda S, Mikami Y, Arai T, Igarashi K (1987) Protective effect of various BRMs against *Candida albicans* infection in mice. Jpn J Med Mycol 28:306–308

Study of Postoperative Arrhythmias After Operation for Esophageal Cancer

Osamu Konno, Yoshiharu Haga, Tomohiro Ogawa, Hitoshi Inoue, and Ryoichi Motoki[1]

Introduction

Postoperative complications, such as respiratory failure and circulatory insufficiency, occasionally occur in patients who have undergone surgery for esophageal cancer because they are aged, undernourished, and the reserve function of their vital organs is low.

Especially, postoperative cardiac arrhythmias are frequently observed in these cases, but the incidence and causes of the arrhythmias are not generally recognized. Little or no reference to these problems are found in textbooks or articles on esophageal surgery.

This study was undertaken to investigate the incidence and factors leading to postoperative cardiac arrhythmias.

Materials and Methods

Seventy-seven patients (69 male, 8 female, mean age 63.9 ± 8.7 years) who underwent esophagectomy and esophageal reconstruction for esophageal cancer were studied with respect to the incidence of cardiac arrhythmias (excluding sinus tachycardia), type of arrhythmia and time of onset, duration, and response to treatment.

The cases were also studied to see whether any correlation could be found between the occurrence of arrhythmias and the age of the patients, their preoperative electrocardiogram (ECG) findings, operative procedures, and various factors in the postoperative period.

[1] First Department of Surgery, Fukushima Medical College, 1 Hikarigaoka, Fukushima, 960-12 Japan

Table 1. Findings of preoperative ECG

Findings	Cases (%)	Mean age and distribution	
Normal	32 (41.6)	63.3 ± 9.3	
Abnormal	45 (58.4)	64.3 ± 8.3	
SVPC or/and VPC	13	age years	Incidence (%)
Chronic af	6[a]	$-\leqq 55$	7/13 (53.8)
First degree A-V block	2	$56\leqq-\leqq 65$	21/33 (63.3)
Bundle branch block	2	$66\leqq-\leqq 75$	13/24 (54.2)
Bradycardia	1	$76\leqq-$	4/7 (57.1)
ST segment changes	16		
Complete A-V block	1[a]		45/77 (58.4)
Other	4		

[a] Excluded from postoperative arrhythmia

ECG, electrocardiogram; *SVPC*, supraventricular premature contraction; *VPC*, ventricular premature contraction; *af*, atrial fibrillation; *A-V*, atrioventricular

Investigation of the postoperative ECG findings was based on continuous ECG monitoring and regular ECG performed when necessary.

Statistical analysis was performed by the Student's *t*-test and data were expressed as mean ± standard deviation. Values for *P* of less than 0.05 were considered significant.

Results

Preoperative ECG findings were normal in 32 cases (41.6%) and abnormal in 45 cases (58.4%). There was no significant difference between the two groups with regard to the mean age of the patients (63.3 ± 9.3 years in the former group vs 64.3 ± 8.3 years in the latter). The abnormal findings most frequently observed in preoperative ECG were ST segment changes ($n = 16$), supraventricular premature beat (SVPC) and/or ventricular premature beat (VPC) ($n = 13$), and chronic atrial fibrillation (af) ($n = 6$) (Table 1). The incidence of preoperative abnormal ECG findings in each age bracket is also shown in Table 1.

The incidence of postoperative arrhythmias in all but seven patients who had preoperative chronic af or pacemaker rhythm was 47.1% (33/70). Postoperative arrhythmias occurred in patients with abnormal preoperative ECG findings more often than in those without abnormal findings (53% vs 41%). The incidence of postoperative arrhythmias in aged patients ($\geqq 66$ years) was significantly higher than in younger patients ($\leqq 65$ years) (64% vs 35%, $P < 0.05$). Other risk factors for postoperative arrhythmias were sex and history of hypertension (Table 2).

The types of postoperative arrhythmias observed were SVPC (24.2%), VPC (18.2%), SVPC and VPC (12.1%), and af with SVPC and/or VPC (45.5%) (Table 2).

Postoperative arrhythmias occurred more often in patients who underwent blunt dissection of the thoracic esophagus and reconstruction using the whole

Table 2. Clinical features and incidence of postoperative arrhythmias

Arrhythmia	−		37 cases (52.8%)
	+		33 cases (47.1%)

Features		Incidence (%)
Sex	male	32/62 (51.6) ⎱ N.S
	female	1/8 (12.5) ⎰
Findings of	nomal	13/32 (40.6) ⎱ N.S
preoperative ECG	abnormal	20/38 (52.7) ⎰
Hypertension	+	9/17 (52.9) ⎱ N.S
	−	24/53 (45.3) ⎰
Age	~55	4/13 (30.8) ⎱ 15/42 (35.7)
	56~65	11/29 (37.9) ⎰ ↑
		$P < 0.05$
	66~75	14/22 (63.6) ⎱ 18/28 (64.3)
	76~	4/6 (66.7) ⎰ ↓

N.S., not significant

Types of postoperative arrhythmias

Type of arrhythmia	Cases (%)
SVPC	8 (24.2)
VPC	6 (18.2)
SVPC + VPC	4 (12.1)
af with SVPC or/and VPC	15 (45.5)
Total	33 (100)

stomach via the posterior mediastinal route than in those who underwent esophagectomy with right thoracotomy and reconstruction using a gastric tube via the poststernal route (60.0% vs 45.0%). The incidence of postoperative arrhythmias in cases who had preoperative arrhythmia was higher than in cases who did not have preoperative arrhythmia (Table 3).

Most SVPC and VPC occurred immediately after surgery or on the 1st postoperative day, and af often occurred either during the 1st postoperative night or on the 2nd postoperative day (Table 4).

For treatment, various antiarrhythmic agents were administered according to the patient's condition. Glucose-insulin-kalium (GIK) therapy was administered 27 times in 20 cases (some cases more than once), and clinical efficacy of this therapy was 63% (Table 5).

Discussion

The reported incidence of cardiac arrhythmias after surgery for esophageal cancer or esophagogastrectomy has ranged from 4% [1] to as high as 41.2% [2]. These differences were probably due to differences in the methods employed to investigate postoperative arrhythmias. In this study, we continuously monitored the patients using ECG in the intensive care unit, thus the overall incidence of postoperative arrhythmias (47.1%) was higher than that reported in the literature.

Table 3. Types of operation and incidence of arrhythmias

Thoracotomy	Reconstruction route	Organs for substitution	Incidence of arrhythmia (%)				
			Over-all	preoperative arrhythmia		findings of preoperative ECG	
				(−)	(+)	abnormal	normal
(+)			18/44 (40.9)	14/37 (37.8)	4/7 (57.1)	12/24 (50.0)	6/20 (30.0)
	Retrosternal		18/40 (45.0)	14/34 (41.2)	4/6 (66.7)	12/21 (57.1)	6/19 (31.6)
		Gastric tube	16/37 (43.2)	12/31 (38.7)	4/6 (66.7)	10/18 (55.6)	6/19 (31.6)
		Partial stomach	2/2 (100.0)	2/2 (100.0)	0/0 (0)	2/2 (100.0)	0/0 (0)
		Whole stomach	0/1 (0)	0/1 (0)	0/0 (0)	0/1 (0)	0/0 (0)
	Antesternal	Right hemicolon	0/4 (0)	0/3 (100.0)	0/1 (0)	0/3 (0)	0/1 (0)
	Posterior mediastinal		15/26 (57.7)	10/20 (50.0)	5/6 (83.3)	8/14 (57.1)	7/12 (58.3)
(−)	Posterior mediastinal		12/20 (60.0)	8/16 (50.0)	4/4 (100.0)	7/11 (63.6)	5/9 (55.6)
		Partial stomach	0/1 (0)	0/1 (0)	0/0 (0)	0/1 (0)	0/0 (0)
		Whole stomach	12/19 (63.2)	8/15 (53.3)	4/4 (100.0)	7/10 (70.0)	5/9 (55.6)
	Antesternal	Right hemicolon	3/ 4 (75.0)	2/2 (100.0)	1/2 (50.0)	1/2 (50.0)	2/2 (100.0)
	Other		0/2 (0)	0/2 (0)	0/0 (0)	0/1 (0)	0/1 (0)

Table 4. Day of onset of postoperative arrhythmias and incidence

POD	SVPC	VPC	SVPC + VPC	Total (%)	af with			Total (%)
					SVPC	VPC	SVPC + VPC	
0	0	2	2	4 (22.2)	2 [0]	2 [1]	1 [0]	5 (33.3) [1] (6.7)
1	3	0	1	4 (22.2)	1 [2]	1 [1]	4 [4]	6 (40.0) [7] (46.7)
2	2	2	1	5 (27.8)	2 [2]	1 [1]	0 [1]	3 (20.0) [4] (26.7)
3	1	0	1	2 (11.1)	0 [0]	1 [1]	0 [0]	1 (6.7) [1] (6.7)
4	2	0	0	2 (11.1)	0 [0]	0 [0]	0 [0]	0 (0) [0] (0)
5	0	0	0	0 (0)	0 [1]	0 [0]	0 [0]	0 (0) [1] (6.7)
6	0	1	0	1 (5.6)	0 [0]	0 [1]	0 [0]	0 (0) [1] (6.7)
7–	0	0	0	0 (0)	0 [0]	0 [0]	0 [0]	0 (0) [0] (0)
Total	8	5	5	18 (100.0)	5	5	5	15 (100.0)

POD, postoperative day; [ ], number of cases which had atrial fibrillation at the time of onset

Table 5. Effect of GIK therapy

Type of arrhythmia	Cases	Times
SVPC	3	3
SVPC + VPC	2	3
af	15	21
Total	20	27

Treatment	Effective rate
GIK therapy	66.7% (8/12)
GIK therapy + other agents	60% (9/15)
Total	62.9% (17/27)

GIK solution: 50% glucose, 80 ml; KCl, 20 ml
(20 mEq); regular insulin 10–20 IU

Risk factors for developing postoperative arrhythmias were advanced age, history of hypertension, and abnormal findings in preoperative ECG. On the other hand, postoperative arrhythmias also occurred in 40% of the patients who had normal preoperative ECG findings, therefore it seems very difficult to predict the occurrence of postoperative arrhythmias from preoperative ECG findings alone [3].

As for the types of postoperative arrhythmias, af was the most frequently observed, which is in agreement with data reported by other authors [4], and in 90% of the cases it occurred within the first 3 postoperative days when surgical stress was most influential on circulatory kinetics [5]. Regarding the relation between type of surgical procedure and incidence, the patients who had undergone blunt dissection showed a higher incidence of arrhythmia than others. This is probably due to the physical pressure caused by the whole stomach on cardiac function when pulled up to the narrow posterior mediastinal space for reconstruction. These results support the findings of Kitamura et al. [2]; that is the incidence of postoperative arrhythmias after reconstruction can be as much as twice that observed after esophagectomy in patients who had undergone second-staged operation.

Generally, we must always consider the imbalance of serum electrolytes and hypoxia as causes of arrhythmias, therefore it is important to measure these biochemical parameters. However, all the patients in this study were within normal limits, so hypoxia or/and imbalance of serum electrolytes are not always the cause of arrhythmia. On the other hand, reports in the relevant literature have mentioned vagal reflex, insomnia, mental or physical stress, and pain as causes of paroxysmal af in patients who had other underlying illnesses, thus these causes must also be taken into consideration after esophagectomy.

Cardiac output and left ventricular stroke index as measured by Swan-Ganz catheter were decreased, and circulatory kinetics were transiently unstable during af; however, none of the patients died, thus, in our study population, postoperative arrhythmias were not a serious complication. Nonetheless, severe arrhythmias can (induce by myocardial infarction, and) cause changes in circulatory kinetics as cardiac failure [6] occasionally. Consequently, it is very important to define the causes of arrhythmia and to restore the regular sinus rhythm as soon as possible.

Various antiarrhythmic agents were administered according to the type of arrhythmia, but we employed mainly the Glucose-insulin-kalium therapy to correct the intracellular potassium of the myocardium because we think that the myocardium is deficient in intracellular potassium, in spite of the normal levels of serum potassium [7]. Patients were infused with GIK solution (50% glucose 80 ml, KCl 20 mEq, regular insulin 10–20 IU) using a catheter for intravenous hyperalimentation, for 90–120 min.

Because its precise mechanism of action is unknown and other antiarrhythmic agents were also administered to half the cases at the same time, it is difficult to assess the efficacy of GIK therapy. However, healing or transient disappearance of arrhythmias were observed in 66.7% of the patients who were treated by GIK therapy only, and in 60% of the patients administered GIK concomitantly with other antiarrhythmic agents.

Therefore, it is our belief that GIK therapy should be attempted in patients who have postoperative cardiac arrhythmias.

References

1. Ellis FH, Gibb SP (1979) Esophagogastrectomy for carcinoma. Ann Surg 190:699–705
2. Kitamura M, Nishihira T, Hirayama K, Kawachi S, Kano T, Akaishi T, Shineha R, Sekine Y, Sanekata K, Mori S (1989) Cardiocirculatory disturbances after surgery for carcinoma of the thoracic esophagus. JJATS 37:17–24
3. Nabeya K, Motojima T (1980) Analysis on the resection and reconstruction for the cancer of the thoracic esophagus. Gastroenterological Surgery 3:645–651
4. Ohno H, Kawasaki S, Yoshida Y (1989) Atrial fibrillation following non-cardiac thoracic surgery: A retrospective study. JJSCA 9:69–74
5. Tsuboi M (1977) Studies on the postoperative pulmonary complications of the esophageal cancer. J Jpn Surg Soc 78:223–232
6. Motoki R (1987) Circulatory failure. In: Jinnai D, Nabeya K, Kakegawa T (eds) Surgery of the esophagus, 1st edn. Kanehara, Tokyo, pp 332–344
7. Okano M (1980) Studies on red cell kalium in surgical disease, especially on significance of G.I.K. therapy. J Jpn Surg Soc 81:1–14